Thieme

MRI in Orthopaedics and Sports Medicine

The Essentials

Uma Srikumaran, MD, MBA, MPH
Associate Professor and Vice Chair of Quality, Safety and Service;
Director, Shoulder Fellowship;
Core Faculty, Hopkins Business of Health Initiative (HBHI)
Department of Orthopaedic Surgery
Johns Hopkins University
Baltimore, Maryland, USA

Amit Jain, MD, MBA
Associate Professor of Orthopaedic Surgery and Neurosurgery;
Chief, Minimally-Invasive Spine Surgery
Department of Orthopaedic Surgery;
Director
Value-Based Care, Johns Hopkins Health System;
Co-Director
Johns Hopkins Spine Surgery Fellowship
Johns Hopkins University
Baltimore, Maryland, USA

A. Jay Khanna, MD, MBA
D'Aniello Department Chair and Professor
Department of Orthopaedic Surgery
Georgetown University School of Medicine and MedStar Georgetown University Hospital;
Physician Executive Director
MedStar Orthopaedic Institute
Washington, DC, USA

1077 illustrations

Thieme
New York • Stuttgart • Delhi • Rio de Janeiro

Library of Congress Cataloging-in-Publication Data is available with the publisher.

Important note: Medicine is an ever-changing science undergoing continual development. Research and clinical experience are continually expanding our knowledge, in particular our knowledge of proper treatment and drug therapy. Insofar as this book mentions any dosage or application, readers may rest assured that the authors, editors, and publishers have made every effort to ensure that such references are in accordance with **the state of knowledge at the time of production of the book**.

Nevertheless, this does not involve, imply, or express any guarantee or responsibility on the part of the publishers in respect to any dosage instructions and forms of applications stated in the book. **Every user is requested to examine carefully** the manufacturers' leaflets accompanying each drug and to check, if necessary, in consultation with a physician or specialist, whether the dosage schedules mentioned therein or the contraindications stated by the manufacturers differ from the statements made in the present book. Such examination is particularly important with drugs that are either rarely used or have been newly released on the market. Every dosage schedule or every form of application used is entirely at the user's own risk and responsibility. The authors and publishers request every user to report to the publishers any discrepancies or inaccuracies noticed. If errors in this work are found after publication, errata will be posted at www.thieme.com on the product description page.

Some of the product names, patents, and registered designs referred to in this book are in fact registered trademarks or proprietary names even though specific reference to this fact is not always made in the text. Therefore, the appearance of a name without designation as proprietary is not to be construed as a representation by the publisher that it is in the public domain.

Thieme addresses people of all gender identities equally.We encourage our authors to use gender-neutral or gender-equal expressions wherever the context allows.

Thieme Publishers New York
333 Seventh Avenue, 18th Floor
New York, NY 10001, USA
www.thieme.com
+1 800 782 3488, customerservice@thieme.com

Cover design: © Thieme
Cover image source: Cover illustration created by Brenda L. Bunch, MAMS / © Thieme
Typesetting by TNQ Technologies, India

Printed in India by Replika Press Pvt. Ltd. 5 4 3 2 1

MIX
Paper | Supporting responsible forestry
FSC™ C016779

DOI: 10.1055/b000000315

ISBN: 978-1-62623-394-2

Also available as an e-book:
eISBN (PDF): 978-1-62623-395-9
eISBN (epub): 978-1-63853-422-8

We dedicate this book to the person who inspired all three of us to pursue careers in orthopaedic surgery and then mentored and guided us from being medical students to colleagues. We strive to emulate his passionate care of patients, dedication to the training of future orthopaedic surgeons, and commitment to the advancement of our field: Paul D. Sponseller, MD, MBA

Contents

Preface

Although the ability to evaluate magnetic resonance imaging (MRI) studies is critical to the practice of orthopaedic surgery, most orthopaedic surgeons, sports specialists, spine specialists, and other clinicians learn this skill in an informal fashion during their training and independent clinical practice. As a result, we may not have (or need) a thorough understanding of the science and physics of MRI and the various pulse sequences that are available for obtaining the images. Additional sequences also become available with technological advancement. Many of us—those in general orthopaedic surgery practice as well as those in subspecialties such as sports medicine, spine surgery, hand and upper extremity, foot and ankle, and orthopaedic oncology—prefer to read our patients' MRI studies in addition to reviewing the "official" radiologist's report. We learn to make preoperative, intraoperative, and postoperative decisions based on those readings and benefit from correlating the imaging findings with our clinical examination. However, unlike radiologists who are trained to evaluate MRI studies in a systematic fashion, we may be more likely to evaluate the images in a less organized manner and to rely on our anatomic expertise and experience, which may not be the most effective method.

This text, *MRI in Orthopaedics and Sports Medicine: The Essentials*, is the third in a series of three textbooks, with the prior two entitled *MRI for Orthopaedic Surgeons* and *MRI Essentials for the Spine Specialist*. Given the success of the two prior books and our personal interest in continuing to work, teach, and develop new technologies at the intersection of clinical care and imaging, Thieme Publishers has graciously allowed us to use some of the relevant text, images, and drawings from our prior two texts. We have built upon that content with current theories and practices, contributions authored by acknowledged experts, and additional illustrative material for the creation of this third and most comprehensive text.

Our goal remains to help teach orthopaedic surgeons, sports specialists, and spine specialists how to systematically evaluate and interpret MRI studies of the musculoskeletal system in order to directly improve clinical practice. This text is unique in that it is written by orthopaedic surgeons, spine surgeons, spine specialists, and radiologists specifically for those who treat and operate on patients with conditions of the musculoskeletal system on a daily basis. As such, this text is clinically oriented and presents the information from the perspective of a clinician. This text is also an excellent reference for radiologists and others—such as physical medicine and rehabilitation clinicians, rheumatologists, interventional and noninterventional pain specialists, neurologist, sports medicine specialists, and nonoperative musculoskeletal care specialists—who evaluate musculoskeletal MRI studies and who would like to gain a better appreciation of the associated clinical aspects.

Our desire to create this book stems from our interest and background in musculoskeletal imaging, experience in working with musculoskeletal radiologists, and recognition that the ability to accurately evaluate MRI studies is critical to the practice of orthopaedic surgery. In performing our research for each chapter of this book and the prior two, we realized that many of the textbooks and other resources on the topic of musculoskeletal MRI are written by radiologists and directed toward radiologists and radiologists in training. This perceived void of imaging resources for orthopaedic surgeons, sports specialists, and spine specialists led us to compile and edit this textbook.

The chapters of this textbook are organized into five parts: (1) MRI Essentials, (2) Upper Extremity, (3) Lower Extremity, (4) Neurological Imaging, and (5) Tumors. Each of these five parts, or each chapter, can be read independently, but the chapters of the textbook are best read in sequential order. In particular, before reading the chapters on individual anatomic areas, the clinician should review Chapter 2 on Normal MRI Anatomy of the Musculoskeletal System and Chapter 13 on Normal Spine MRI Anatomy. These chapters provide a moderately comprehensive evaluation of the key anatomic structures and concepts with which one should be familiar when reviewing an MRI study of a particular region. They also serve as a reference point when evaluating the pathologic images in a region-specific chapter.

The book features two different types of chapters: region-specific and concept-specific. The region-specific chapters (for example, The Shoulder and The Cervical Spine) share a common organization, with sections on specialized pulse sequences and protocols, traumatic pathology, degenerative pathology, infectious conditions, and postoperative findings. The concept-specific chapters (for example, Articular Cartilage and MRI of the Peripheral Nervous System) are organized in a fashion that best suits the individual chapter's content and the goal of providing clinicians and radiologists with the information they need to maximize their proficiency in evaluating and interpreting MRI studies. In addition, this book contains a new feature in the form of a set of Common Clinical Questions (with answers and explanations) for each chapter. These questions will allow the reader to review the material efficiently and test his or her comprehension of many of the key concepts in each chapter.

MRI in Orthopaedics and Sports Medicine: The Essentials contains more than 820 MR images and 250 illustrations that have been carefully selected and created to help illustrate and teach the essential anatomy and pathology that an orthopaedic surgeon, sports specialist, spine specialist, other clinician, or radiologist should be able to recognize and define when evaluating an MRI study of the musculoskeletal system. As such, much of the material can be learned effectively by reviewing the images and illustrations along with the associated figure legends.

Most of the chapters have been authored by both clinicians and radiologists. Some, such as the region-specific chapters, have orthopaedic surgeons as the primary authors, with radiologists as co-authors for accuracy and clarity from their standpoint. Others (for example, Essentials of MRI Physics and Pulse Sequences) were written solely by radiologists, but the presentation of the material was specifically designed with a clinician audience in mind. The collaboration between clinicians and radiologists that we have used for producing this textbook emulates the optimal relationship between these subspecialties in clinical practice.

This book was envisioned to be a practical aid to develop and/or refine the skills needed to effectively and systematically evaluate MRI studies of the musculoskeletal system to enhance clinical practice. We hope that it accomplishes this goal for you.

Uma Srikumaran, MD, MBA, MPH
Amit Jain, MD, MBA
A. Jay Khanna, MD, MBA

Contributors

Shivani Ahlawat, MD
Associate Professor
Department of Radiology and Radiological Sciences
Johns Hopkins University School of Medicine
Baltimore, Maryland, USA

Raj M. Amin, MD
Orthopaedic Surgeon
Department of Orthopaedic Surgery
Community Health Partners
Fresno, California, USA

Mark W. Anderson, MD
Professor of Radiology
Department of Radiology and Medical Imaging
Charlottesville, Virginia, USA

Keith T. Aziz, MD
Assistant Professor
Department of Orthopaedic Surgery
Mayo Clinic
Jacksonville, Florida, USA

Douglas P. Beall, MD, FSIR, ABIPM, FIPP
Chief of Services
Interventional Radiology
Comprehensive Specialty Care
Edmond, Oklahoma, USA

Lance M. Brunton, MD
Chief
Musculoskeletal Service Line
Orthopaedics and Sports Medicine
Independence Health
Latrobe, Pennsylvania, USA

Jacob M. Buchowski, MS, MD
Professor of Orthopaedic Surgery
Orthopaedic Surgery
Washington University
St. Louis, Missouri, USA

John A. Carrino, MD, MHA, FACR
Vice Chairman
Radiology and Imaging
Hospital for Special Surgery
New York, New York, USA

Rebecca Cerrato, MD
Orthopaedic Surgeon
Institute for Foot and Ankle Reconstruction at Mercy Medical Center
Baltimore, Maryland, USA

A. Bobby Chhabra, MD
Lillian T. Pratt Distinguished Professor and Chair
Department of Orthopaedic Surgery
University of Virginia Health
Charlottesville, Virginia, USA

Andrew J. Cosgarea, MD
Professor
Department of Orthopaedic Surgery
Johns Hopkins University
Baltimore, Maryland, USA

Aditya R. Daftary, MBBS
Director
Department of Imaging
InnoVision Imaging
Mumbai, Maharashtra, India

Shadpour Demehri, MD
Professor of Radiology and Radiological Science
Department of Radiology and Orthopaedic Surgery
Johns Hopkins School of Medicine Faculty
Baltimore, Maryland, USA

Swati Deshmukh, MD
Assistant Professor
Department of Radiology
New York University
New York, New York, USA

Jason D. Dunleavy, MD
Director
Interventional and Vascular Services
Windsong
Buffalo, New York, USA

Laura M. Fayad, MD
Professor of Radiology, Orthopaedic Surgery & Oncology;
Chief of Musculoskeletal Imaging;
Director of Translational Research for Advanced Imaging
The Russell H. Morgan Department of Radiology and Radiological Science
Johns Hopkins University School of Medicine
Baltimore, Maryland, USA

James R. Ficke, MD, FACS, FAAOS
Professor and Chair
Department of Orthopaedic Surgery
Johns Hopkins University School of Medicine
Baltimore, Maryland, USA

Li Foong Foo, MBBCH, MRCP, FRCR, MD
Attending Radiologist
Department of Radiology & Imaging
Hospital for Special Surgery
New York, New York, USA

Jonathan A. Forsberg, MD, PhD
Attending Surgeon
Department of Surgery, Orthopaedic Service
Memorial Sloan Kettering Cancer Center
New York, New York, USA

Ziya L. Gokaslan, MD, FAANS, FACS
Julius Stoll, MD Professor and Chair
Department of Neurosurgery
The Warren Alpert Medical School of Brown University
Providence, Rhode Island, USA;
Neurosurgeon-in-Chief
Rhode Island Hospital and The Miriam Hospital
Providence, Rhode Island, USA;
Clinical Director
Norman Prince Neurosciences Institute;
President
Neurosurgery Foundation

Marc Greenberg, MD
Orthopaedic Surgery Resident, PGY-4
Johns Hopkins University School of Medicine
Baltimore, Maryland, USA

Colin Haines, MD
Director of Research
Department of Spine Surgery
Virginia Spine Institute
Reston, Virginia, USA

Andrew B. Harris, BS, MD
Resident Physician
Department of Orthopaedic Surgery
Johns Hopkins Hospital
Baltimore, Maryland, USA

Casey Jo Humbyrd, MD, MBE
Associate Professor
Department of Orthopaedic Surgery
University of Pennsylvania
Philadelphia, Pennsylvania, USA

Amit Jain, MD, MBA
Associate Professor of Orthopaedics Surgery and Neurosurgery;
Chief, Minimally-Invasive Spine Surgery
Department of Orthopaedic Surgery;
Director
Value-Based Care, Johns Hopkins Health System;
Co-Director
Johns Hopkins Spine Surgery Fellowship
Johns Hopkins University
Baltimore, Maryland, USA

Bryan T. Kelly, MD, MBA
President & CEO, Surgeon-in-Chief Emeritus
Hospital for Special Surgery, HSS - The Pavilion
New York, New York, USA

A. Jay Khanna, MD, MBA
D'Aniello Family Department Chair and Professor
Department of Orthopaedic Surgery
Georgetown University School of Medicine and MedStar Georgetown University Hospital;
Physician Executive Director
Medstar Orthopaedic Institute
Washington, DC, USA

Kelly G. Kilcoyne, MD, LTC, MC, USA
Professor of Surgery
USU;
Vice Chairman
Department of Orthopaedics
Walter Reed National Military Medical Center
Bethesda, Maryland, USA

Adam S. Levin, MD
Associate Professor
Department of Orthopaedic Surgery
Johns Hopkins University
Baltimore, Maryland, USA

Shih-Chun Lin, MD, PhD, MBA, FAANS, FACS
Chair
Department of Surgery
Suburban Hospital
Johns Hopkins University School of Medicine
Bethesda, Maryland, USA;
Assistant Professor
Department of Neurosurgery (Primary)
Department of Neuroscience (Secondary)
Department of Otolaryngology, Head and Neck Surgery (Secondary)
Johns Hopkins University School of Medicine
Baltimore, Maryland, USA

Majd Marrache, MD
Orthopaedic Resident
Department of Orthopaedics Surgery
Johns Hopkins Hospital
Baltimore, Maryland, USA

Edward F. McCarthy, MD
Pathologist
Department of Pathology
Johns Hopkins Hospital
Baltimore, Maryland, USA

Emmanuel L. McNeely, MD, MS, MHA
Surgery Resident Physician
Department of Surgery
Florida Atlantic University
Boca Raton, Florida, USA

Douglas N. Mintz, AB, MD
Attending Radiologist;
Professor
Department of Radiology & Imaging
Hospital for Special Surgery;
Professor of Clinical Radiology
Department of Radiology
Weill Cornell Medicine
Cornell University
New York, New York, USA

Carol D. Morris, MD, MS
Chief
Department of Orthopaedic Surgery
Memorial Sloan Kettering Cancer Center
New York, New York, USA

Luis E. Moya, MD
Chief Medical Officer
Agreements Unit
Adult Traumatology and Orthopaedics
Vitacura German Clinic
Vitacura, Región Metropolitana, Chile

Rick W. Obray, MD
Pain Management Specialist
Southwest Spine & Pain Center
St. George, Utah, USA

Joseph R. O'Brien, MD
Specialist in Minimally Invasive Spine Surgery
Orthopaedic Surgery
Spine & Scoliosis Institute at OrthoBethesda
Bethesda, Maryland, USA

Gbolahan O. Okubadejo, MD, FAAOS
Orthopaedic Spine Surgeon
Institute of Comprehensive Spine Care
Englewood, New Jersey, USA

Marc J. Philippon, MD
Doctor
Department of Orthopaedics
Steadman Philippon Research Institute
Vail, Colorado, USA

Hollis G. Potter, MD
Radiologist
Radiology and Imaging
Hospital for Special Surgery
New York, New York, USA

John D. Reeder, MD
Musculoskeletal Division
Lenox Hill Radiology
New York, New York, USA

Daniel M. Sciubba, BS, MD, MBA
Professor & Chair
Department of Neurosurgery
Hofstra University/Northwell Health
Great Neck, New York, USA

Delaram Shakoor, MD
Resident
Department of Radiology
Yale New Haven Hospital
New Haven, Connecticut, USA

Michael K. Shindle, MD
Orthopaedic Surgeon
New Jersey Orthopaedics Institute
Wayne, New Jersey, USA

Andrea M. Spiker, MD
Assistant Professor
Department of Orthopaedics & Rehabilitation
University of Wisconsin-Madison
Madison, Wisconsin, USA

Paul D. Sponseller, MD, MBA
Professor and Head, Pediatric Orthopaedics
Orthopaedic Surgery
Johns Hopkins Medical Institutions
Baltimore, Maryland, USA

Uma Srikumaran, MD, MBA, MPH
Associate Professor and Vice Chair of Quality, Safety and Service;
Director, Shoulder Fellowship;
Core Faculty, Hopkins Business of Health Initiative (HBHI)
Department of Orthopaedic Surgery
Johns Hopkins University
Baltimore, Maryland, USA

Miho J. Tanaka, MD, PhD
Associate Professor
Orthopaedic Surgery
Massachusetts General Hospital
Harvard Medical School
Boston, Massachusetts, USA

Bruce A. Wasserman, MD
Vice Chair of Research;
Professor of Radiology, Neurosurgery, and Surgery;
Director of Neurovascular Imaging
Department of Diagnostic Radiology & Nuclear Medicine
University of Maryland School of Medicine;
Adjunct Professor
Department of Radiology and Radiological Sciences
Johns Hopkins University School of Medicine
Baltimore, Maryland, USA

Monica D. Watkins, MD
Neuroradiology
Johns Hopkins University School of Medicine
Baltimore, Maryland, USA

Ariel A. Williams, MD
Associate Professor
Department of Orthopaedics and Rehabilitation
Yale University School of Medicine
New Haven, Connecticut, USA

Patricia L. Zadnik, MD
Director
Center for Spine Tumor and Chordoma Research
Norman Prince Neurosciences Institute;
Director
Spinal Surgery Oncology;
Member
Legoretta Cancer Center
Providence, Rhode Island, USA

Lukas P. Zebala, MD
Orthopaedic Surgeon
Department of Orthopaedic Surgery
Northshore - Endeavor Health Medical Group
Skokie, Illinois, USA

Bashir Zikria, MD, MSc
Chief of Sports Medicine Division
Department of Orthopaedics
Johns Hopkins University School of Medicine
Baltimore, Maryland, USA

Part I

MRI Essentials

I

1 Essentials of MRI Physics and Pulse Sequences

Marc Greenberg, A. Jay Khanna, Rick W. Obray, Douglas P. Beall, John D. Reeder, John A. Carrino, and Laura M. Fayad

Abstract

The goal of this chapter is to introduce some of the main topics which will be covered later in this book. In order to properly understand, read, and interpret magnetic resonance imaging (MRI), one must have a solid foundation of certain specific concepts related to how MRIs work and how MRIs can be altered to produce the various different types of imaging available to physicians. This introductory chapter will include information regarding the basic physics behind how MRI functions, the various ways in which MRI images are produced, the different characteristics of MRIs which can be altered, and the reasons why different MRI imaging modalities are necessary depending upon what is being imaged. The following chapters will then expand upon these essential concepts and explain the various concepts in greater detail.

Keywords: MRI, spine, T1, STIR, contrast-enhanced, artifacts

1.1 Introduction

Magnetic resonance imaging (MRI) is an essential tool for physicians in the accurate diagnosis and treatment of musculoskeletal diseases. The number of MRI applications has increased dramatically over the past three decades and will continue to increase as new techniques are developed. While a detailed understanding of the fundamentals of MRI physics is not required for surgeons to review images, a basic working knowledge of certain key principles is important for the accurate utilization of the increasingly diverse options available. This chapter provides the reader with a basic understanding of the physics behind MRI. It does this by both addressing specific applications of MRI within musculoskeletal radiology and describing how an MR image is generated and what basic sequences are important for optimally showing musculoskeletal anatomy. The goal of this chapter is to provide the reader with sufficient working knowledge of the technology to determine the correct type of high-quality images in a reasonable amount of time. This chapter is only a brief introduction to what most would consider a complex technology, and the reader is referred to additional sources for more detailed explanations.[1,2,3,4,5,6,7,8]

1.2 Fundamentals of MRI

1.2.1 Magnetization of Nuclei and Tissues and the Larmor Equation

In order to understand how an MR image is generated, one must have the requisite knowledge of the basic physical properties of the nucleus of an atom and its components: neutrons and protons. All neutrons and protons within the nucleus spin about their axes and generate a magnetic field called a magnetic dipole (▶ Fig. 1.1). The magnetic dipoles of protons and neutrons of even-numbered nuclei cancel each other out. However, odd-numbered nuclei generate a magnetic moment, which can be represented as a vector. When placed in a magnetic field, odd-

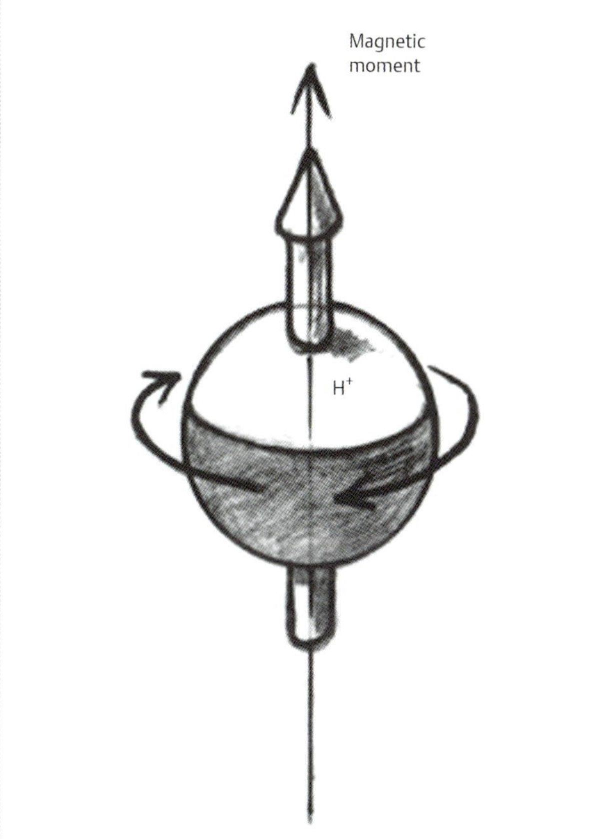

Fig. 1.1 Neutrons and protons within the nucleus spin about their axes and generate a directional magnetic field called a magnetic dipole. In this illustration, the dipole is pointing upward. (Reproduced with permission from Obray RW, Beall DP, Reeder JD, Carrino JA, Fayad LM. Essentials of MRI Physics and Pulse Sequences. In: Khanna AJ, ed. MRI for orthopaedic surgeons. New York: Thieme; 2010:3–16.)

numbered nuclei, because of their magnetic moments, align parallel to the external magnetic field in one of two orientations: spin-up or spin-down (▶ Fig. 1.2).[9] The individual particles have a preference to remain in their lowest energy state possible. A small excess of nuclei align in a spin-up orientation (slightly greater stability) and generate an overall small net magnetization vector (▶ Fig. 1.3). Conveniently, the human body is replete with hydrogen, a ubiquitous atom with odd-numbered nuclei (hydrogen has one proton and no neutrons) and, to a lesser extent, with fluorine. For almost all MR images, the neutrons and protons utilized come from these abundantly distributed hydrogen atoms.[9] It is the manipulation within an external magnetic field of this small number of excess spin-up, odd-numbered nuclei that is the basis for the signal that ultimately generates an MR image.[1,2,9]

When spinning nuclei are exposed to an external magnetic field, the magnetic fields of the spinning nuclei and the external magnetic field interact and cause the nuclei to precess, or "wobble" (▶ Fig. 1.4). For a physical analogy, one can think of

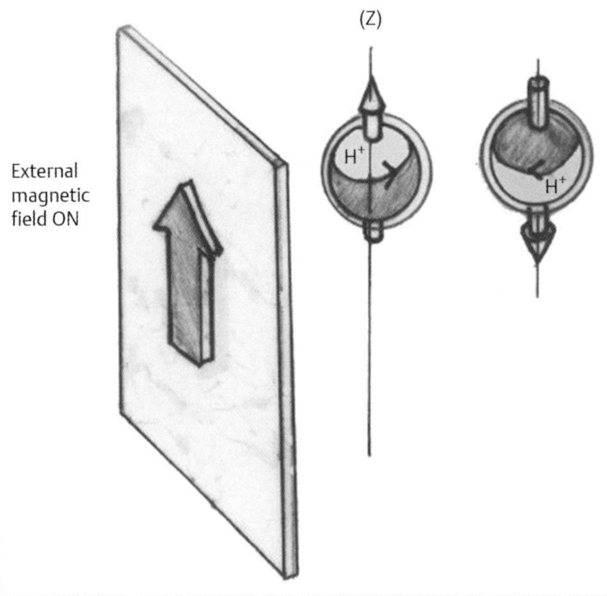

Fig. 1.2 Odd-numbered nuclei are able to exist in one of two energy states when placed in an external magnetic field: spin-up or spin-down orientation, that is, parallel to and aligned with the external magnetic field (*large arrow*) or parallel to and in an opposite direction to the external magnetic field. The spin-up orientation (*z*) is a slightly more stable, preferred energy state. (Reproduced with permission from Obray RW, Beall DP, Reeder JD, Carrino JA, Fayad LM. Essentials of MRI Physics and Pulse Sequences. In: Khanna AJ, ed. MRI for orthopaedic surgeons. New York: Thieme; 2010:3–16.)

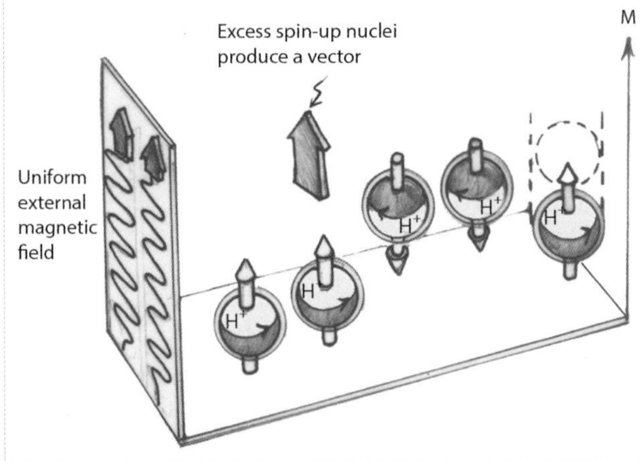

Fig. 1.3 The slight excess nuclei in the spin-up orientation is the result of the increased stability of the spin-up orientation relative to the spin-down orientation. It produces a net magnetization vector (*large arrow*) that can be manipulated to create a radiofrequency (RF) signal, which in turn can be used to create a magnetic resonance (MR) image. The two *smaller arrows* depict the direction of the external magnetic field (*M*). (Reproduced with permission from Obray RW, Beall DP, Reeder JD, Carrino JA, Fayad LM. Essentials of MRI Physics and Pulse Sequences. In: Khanna AJ, ed. MRI for orthopaedic surgeons. New York: Thieme; 2010:3–16.)

precession as similar to a "spinning top." The frequency of precession can be described by the Larmor equation:

$$\omega_0 = B_0 \times \gamma$$

where ω_0 is the precessional frequency, B_0 is the external magnetic field strength measured in tesla (T) units, and γ is the gyromagnetic ratio measured in megahertz per tesla unit. In summary, the Larmor frequency states that precessional frequency is in direct proportion to the magnetic field strength.[9] Conveniently, the ω_0 is constant for every atom at a particular magnetic field strength, and it is key for the localization of the MRI signal within space (see details below).

When the patient is within the MRI machine, a radiofrequency (RF) pulse (at the Larmor frequency for hydrogen at a given field strength) is applied and the net magnetization vector flips from its longitudinal direction by a certain angle (flip angle). This flipping process produces a transverse magnetization vector (perpendicular to the external magnetic field) and a longitudinal magnetization vector (parallel to the external magnetic field) (▶ Fig. 1.5). The magnitude of the flip angle is determined by the strength and duration of the RF pulse applied. In order for this to occur and for an image to ultimately be generated, the RF pulse must occupy the same frequency as the hydrogen protons. In addition, it must also remain in correct alignment. A 90-degree RF pulse, for instance, aligns the magnetization vector in a plane perpendicular to the external magnetic field, whereas a 180-degree RF pulse aligns the magnetization vector in a plane parallel to but in a direction opposite to that of the external magnetic field. After the RF pulse, the precessing nuclei are initially "in phase" with one another; that is, they are precessing in synch

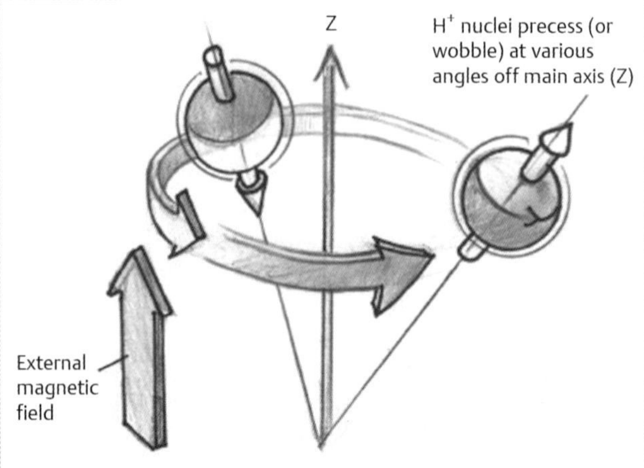

Fig. 1.4 All nuclei, including hydrogen nuclei precess about their axes when placed in an external magnetic field, which is similar to a "spinning top" as discussed above. The frequency of precession is related to the strength of the external magnetic field as determined by the Larmor equation ($\omega_0 = B_0 \times \gamma$). (Reproduced with permission from Obray RW, Beall DP, Reeder JD, Carrino JA, Fayad LM. Essentials of MRI Physics and Pulse Sequences. In: Khanna AJ, ed. MRI for orthopaedic surgeons. New York: Thieme; 2010:3–16.)

with one another. This synchronized precession maximizes the transverse magnetization vector (additive effect). Once the RF pulse is turned off, the precessing nuclei relax, the longitudinal vector returns, and the transverse vector dissipates (▶ Fig. 1.6). This relaxation occurs in two distinct ways which will be discussed later in this chapter, T2 or transverse relaxation and T1 or longitudinal relaxation.[9] The transverse magnetization vector produces a signal as it precesses around a receiver coil; this signal can be optimized, recorded, and ultimately transformed into MRI images by Fourier analysis.[1,9]

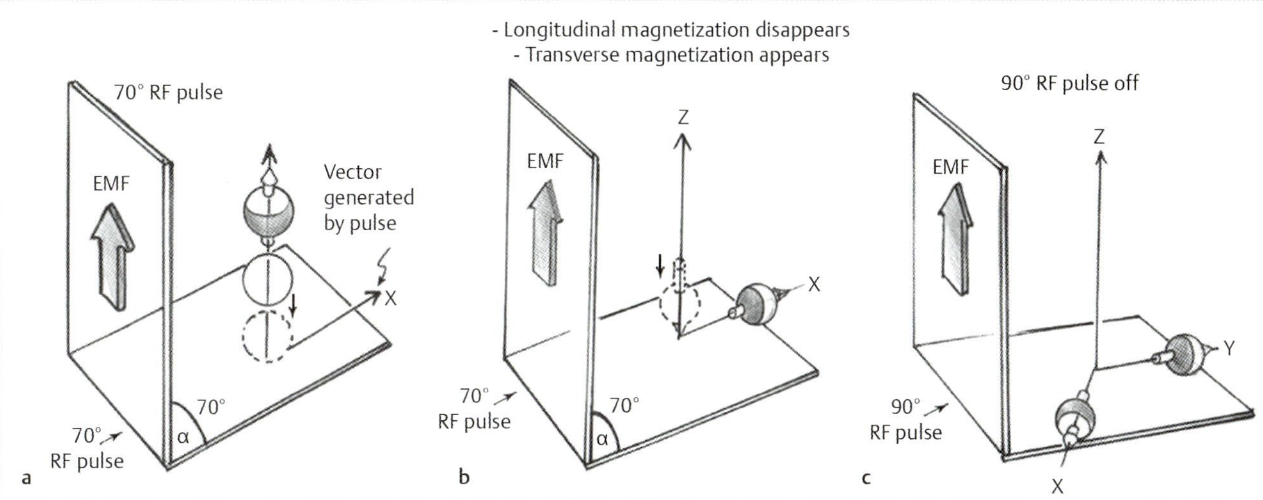

Fig. 1.5 The manipulation of the magnetization vector (*EMF*, external magnetic field) is demonstrated. **(a)** An external radiofrequency (RF) pulse administered at the Larmor frequency can flip the direction of the magnetization vector from the longitudinal to the transverse direction. **(b)** The longitudinal component of the magnetization vector decreases and the transverse component of the magnetization vector increases. This process is based upon the strength and duration of the applied RF pulse. The angle the net magnetization vector makes with the longitudinal axis, in essence, the external magnetic field, is called the flip angle. **(c)** For example, a 90-degree RF pulse will flip the direction of the net magnetization vector 90 degrees relative to the external magnetic field. (Reproduced with permission from Obray RW, Beall DP, Reeder JD, Carrino JA, Fayad LM. Essentials of MRI Physics and Pulse Sequences. In: Khanna AJ, ed. MRI for orthopaedic surgeons. New York: Thieme; 2010:3–16.)

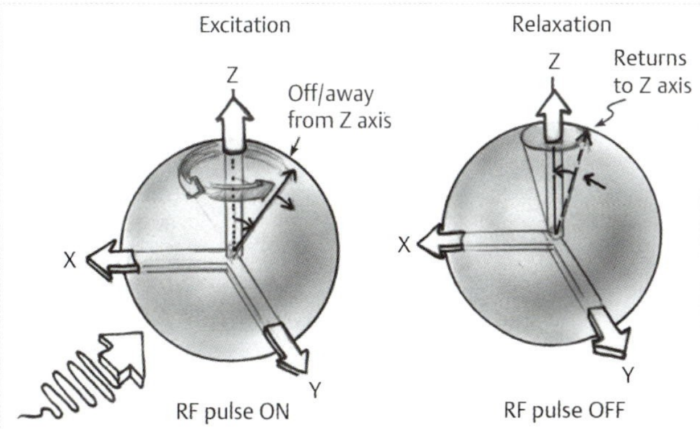

Fig. 1.6 After the discontinuation of a radiofrequency (RF) pulse, the net magnetization vector will relax, or return, to a more stable energy state, via the recovery of the longitudinal component and loss of the transverse component of the magnetization vector. The strength of the transverse component of the magnetization vector is what is ultimately used to generate the MR image. (Reproduced with permission from Obray RW, Beall DP, Reeder JD, Carrino JA, Fayad LM. Essentials of MRI Physics and Pulse Sequences. In: Khanna AJ, ed. MRI for orthopaedic surgeons. New York: Thieme; 2010:3–16.)

By using an RF pulse to flip the excess spin-up hydrogen nuclei and ultimately transform the longitudinal magnetization vector within a sample or tissue into a transverse magnetization vector, a signal is generated and subsequently used to create an image via the phenomenon of resonance. This term of resonance is indicated in the name: Magnetic Resonance Imaging.[9]

1.2.2 T1, T2, and T2*

The transverse and longitudinal magnetization vectors and the generation of the MRI signal should be addressed in relation to T1, T2, and T2*. When an RF pulse that is interacting with nuclei in an external magnetic field is turned off, the precessing nuclei return to their original equilibrium state and realign with the external magnetic field. This desire to return to their original state is related to the nuclei preference to exist in their lowest energy state. Each molecule has a specific rate by which it relaxes, determined by the molecules' "tumbling rate." Tumbling refers to the rate of motion for each molecule.[9] It is this variety of tumbling that creates fluctuation in the magnetic field surrounding the individual protons. During this tumbling process, the longitudinal magnetization vector returns to its equilibrium value before the RF pulse does. The return or recovery of the longitudinal magnetization is known as *T1 recovery*, with T1 being defined as the time constant representing 63% recovery of the equilibrium longitudinal magnetization vector.[2,9] Conversely, after the RF pulse is turned off, the transverse magnetization vector decays exponentially, with a decay rate constant, or T2. The T2 decay relates to spin dephasing secondary to the interaction of the local magnetic fields of the individual nuclei. The time necessary for T2 decay quantitatively represents the time in which the transverse magnetization vector has decayed by 63% of its maximum. The T1 relaxation time is also known as the longitudinal or spin-lattice relaxation, and T2 is also known as the transverse or spin-spin relaxation. The T2* relaxation time represents the loss of the transverse magnetization vector secondary to T2 effects and the spin dephasing secondary to local magnetic field inhomogeneities. Therefore, the T2* relaxation time is inherently shorter than T2. An important distinction between T2 and T1 is that T2 relaxation does not require the overall loss of energy. As such, T2 relaxation is almost always equal to or less than T1 values.[9] T1, T2, and T2* also differ for individual tissues. Tissues with a long T1 include water and large protein molecules, and tissues with a short T1 include fats and intermediate-size molecules. Tissues with a long T2 include liquids, whereas large molecules and solids generally have short T2 times. The T2* relaxation time is typically short for fat and water.[2,3,9,10] Fats, as an example, demonstrate short T1 times because of the carbon bonds at the end of fatty tails which have frequencies close to the Larmor frequency. The closer the frequency between the two, the more efficiently energy is able to transfer.[9]

In summary, individual tissues, such as fat and water, have reasonably well-defined T1, T2, and T2* time constants related to the recovery of the longitudinal magnetization signal (T1) and the decay of the transverse magnetization signal (T2, T2*) after an RF pulse. These differences in T1, T2, and T2* directly impact the strength of the RF signal emitted from a particular type of tissue (e.g., fat or water) at a given time and ultimately can be converted to visual differences in tissue contrast on the final image.[2,3,10] It is the MRI's ability to resolve subtle differences in the T1, T2, and T2* characteristics of various tissues and assign the differences to a discrete location (pixel/voxel, see below) within the patient that allows for the production of images of such high spatial resolution. These high-resolution images are able to provide the information about the anatomy and pathology within the musculoskeletal system that we as physicians rely upon for fast and precise diagnosis.

1.2.3 Gradient Coils and Signal Localization

The transverse magnetization signal is localized within tissue via the use of gradient coils. Nuclei in an external magnetic field precess at a particular frequency when subjected to an RF pulse, as described by the Larmor equation. By altering the external magnetic field and creating gradients in the x, y, and z planes, it is possible to identify the location of the signal within tissue based on its emitted RF and phase. Gradient coils superimpose small field gradients in the x, y, and z directions on the main magnetic field and include section-selection gradients, phase-encoding gradients, and frequency-encoding gradients.[1] Section-selective gradients select the section to be imaged.[1] The phase-encoding gradient causes a phase shift that allows for localization of the signal by its phase. Protons within a given field will have differing Larmor frequencies because of this gradient field. A frequency-encoding gradient causes a frequency shift, allowing for localization by frequency.[1] Frequency-encoding gradient leads to protons rotating differently based upon their relative position within the gradient itself.[9] The determination of which plane (i.e., x, y, z) each gradient is applied depends on the orientation of the image (i.e., axial, sagittal, coronal).[1,4] Data within the MR image are divided into pixels and voxels, which localize the signal in two or three dimensions, respectively. A pixel is a 2D unit in the x-y, x-z, or y-z planes, whereas a voxel is a 3D unit, representing a unit of volume within the data set/image. The data representing spatial frequency is stored as a data matrix termed the "k-space."[9]

1.2.4 MRI Pulse Sequence and TE, TR, and Inversion Time

An MRI pulse sequence is the sequence of RF pulses and magnetic field gradients used to generate an image. Several other concepts in addition to those discussed above are important when interpreting an MRI pulse sequence: echo time (TE), repetition time (TR), and inversion time.

In conventional spin-echo (SE) and gradient-echo (GRE) sequences, the TE is the time from the initial RF pulse (used to flip the longitudinal magnetization vector into the transverse plane/transverse magnetization vector) to the center of the echo signal (the time when the signal is at its maximum) (▶ Fig. 1.7). In conventional SE sequences, a phase-encoding gradient is applied at TE/2 to allow for spin rephasing at TE. This technique maximizes the recorded signal at readout (▶ Fig. 1.7). In GRE sequences, gradients are used to "recall the echo" at TE and use a negative gradient followed by a positive gradient (GRE) to refocus the signal at readout (▶ Fig. 1.8). GRE sequences themselves are therefore

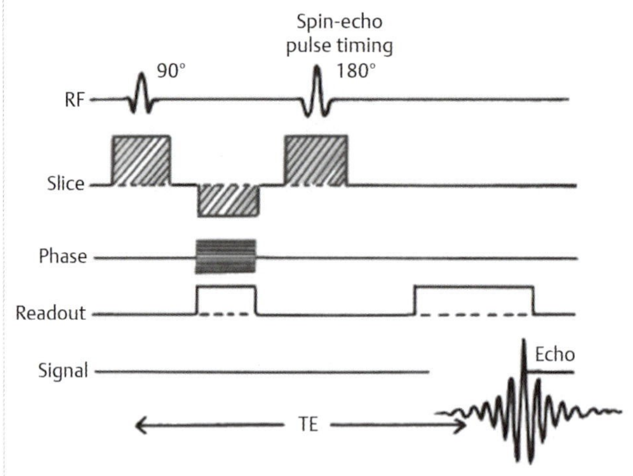

Fig. 1.7 In this example of a conventional spin-echo (SE) pulse sequence, the *top line* shows a radiofrequency (RF) pulse sequence which is a 90-degree pulse followed by a 180-degree refocusing pulse. Section-selection gradients, a phase-encoding gradient, and a readout or frequency-encoding gradients are also shown in this example. The *bottom line* depicts the RF signal or "echo" recorded at echo time (TE). The 180-degree pulse is responsible for the echo at a specific time, that is, TE. (Reproduced with permission from Obray RW, Beall DP, Reeder JD, Carrino JA, Fayad LM. Essentials of MRI Physics and Pulse Sequences. In: Khanna AJ, ed. MRI for orthopaedic surgeons. New York: Thieme; 2010:3–16.)

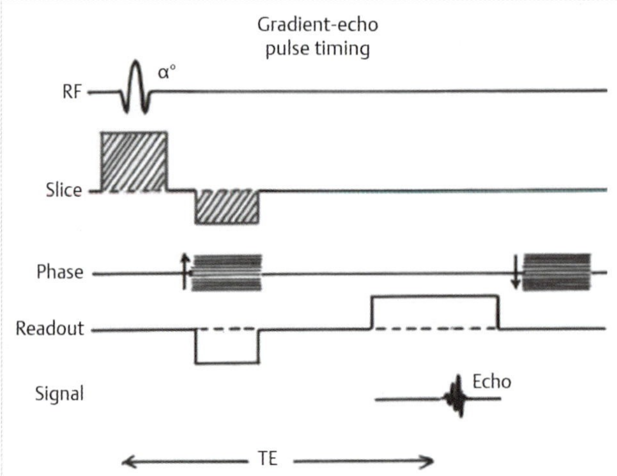

Fig. 1.8 In this example of a standard gradient-echo pulse sequence, the *top line* shows the radiofrequency (RF) pulse resulting in a predetermined flip angle. Section-selection gradients, a phase-encoding gradient, and readout or frequency-encoding gradients also are shown. A refocusing gradient (readout or frequency selection gradient sequence), which refocuses signal, produces an echo at echo time (TE), hence the name gradient echo. (Reproduced with permission from Obray RW, Beall DP, Reeder JD, Carrino JA, Fayad LM. Essentials of MRI Physics and Pulse Sequences. In: Khanna AJ, ed. MRI for orthopaedic surgeons. New York: Thieme; 2010:3–16.)

relatively short in duration.[9] There are several distinct differences between SE and GRE: GRE only uses one pulse and utilizes low flip angle excitations (5–40 degrees) as opposed to the 90-degree angle excitation of SE.[9] As a consequence of the speed of GRE, there is the risk of potential signal loss.[9] One might question why it is necessary to refocus at all. The transverse magnetization degrades secondary to dephasing effects, as described above, and is represented quantitatively by T2 and T2*. Dephasing weakens the transverse magnetization vector/signal, and rephasing (using a perfectly timed GRE) rephases, or resynchronizes, the precessing nuclei. When all the nuclei are in phase, or precessing in synch (i.e., vectors pointing in the same direction), the recorded signal is at a maximum. TE primarily affects T2 in conventional SE sequences and T2* in GRE sequences.[1,2]

TR is the time interval between the initial RF pulse of the basic pulse sequence and the subsequent repetition of the initial RF pulse.[1] In conventional SE sequences, TR primarily affects T1 or the recovery of the longitudinal magnetization vector. TR is a variable that can be specifically altered within the MRI machine. The purpose of this is to magnify differences in intensities between different tissues.[9] Both TE and TR can be manipulated to visualize the inherent differences in T1 and T2 among tissues on MRI sequences. In conventional SE sequences, a short TE (< 30 ms) and a relatively short TR (< 1,000 ms) result in T1-weighted images (T1 effects maximized and T2 effects minimized). A relatively long TE (> 60 ms) and a relatively long TR (> 2,000 ms) result in T2-weighted images on the T2 SE sequences (i.e., T2 effects maximized and T1 effects minimized). An intermediate TR (> 1,000 ms but < 2,000 ms) and a short TE (< 30 ms) minimize differences in T1 and T2 within tissues. This results in an image based primarily on the density of the protons within that tissue on conventional SE sequences. This minimization of the differences in T1 and T2 effects within tissue when creating an MR image is known as proton-density weighting. In GRE sequences, TR varies and is related to the flip angle and the TE. A larger flip angle (70–110 degrees) and a short TE favor T1 weighting, whereas a smaller flip angle (5–20 degrees) and a larger TE favor T2* weighting. A low flip angle and a short TE result in a proton-density-weighted image.[1,2,3]

Inversion time is the time to inversion used in inversion recovery MRI pulse sequences, such as STIR (short tau inversion recovery) and FLAIR (fluid-attenuated inversion recovery). More specifically, it represents the time interval between the initial 180-degree pulse used to invert the longitudinal magnetization vector and the subsequent 90-degree pulse used to convert the longitudinal magnetization vector into the transverse plane.[9] A second 180-degree pulse is used at TE/2 that generates an echo at TE, at which time the signal is recorded. Why use a 180-degree pulse followed by a 90-degree pulse? By applying a 90-degree pulse as the longitudinal vector of a certain tissue (e.g., water) crosses from a negative to a positive value (near zero), the transverse magnetization vector generated by the RF pulse from that type of tissue is very small or zero,[1,2,4] which essentially nulls the signal from that tissue. It is the knowledge of these null points that allow for the suppression of various tissue signals.[9] As an example, FLAIR sequences (fluid-attenuated inversion recovery) are used commonly in neurological fields to suppress CSF fluid signal.[9] The most common tissue that is suppressed is fat, and STIR sequences are commonly used in musculoskeletal radiology for this purpose.[1,2,3]

In summary, it is important to note that occasionally there is confusion regarding the terms T1, T2, TR, and TE. T1 and T2 are characteristics of a given tissue and are intrinsic to that tissue. As a result, they cannot be altered without altering the nature of the tissue itself. Conversely, TR and TE are parameters of the pulse sequence and, as such, are extrinsic to the tissue and may be modified by the radiologist. By altering the TE and TR in a pulse sequence, it is possible to manipulate the visually perceived differences within tissue and the MRI generated from that tissue. It is this manipulation of TE and TR that allows for differentiation, not the alteration of the tissue itself. MR pulse sequences are, in fact, designed to take advantage of the intrinsic differences within the tissue, that is, differences in T1, T2, and T2*, to create an image that allows these differences to be perceptible visually. The fact that disease processes often alter the intrinsic properties of the affected tissue and subsequently alter the T1, T2, and T2* effects is the reason that MRI is helpful in the detection of disease.

1.3 MRI Applications

1.3.1 Standard Sequences

Standard MRI pulse sequences used in musculoskeletal radiology include T1-weighted, T2-weighted, and proton-density-weighted SE (and fast spin echo [FSE]) sequences, STIR-weighted sequences, T2* GRE sequences, 3D imaging techniques, and contrast-enhanced imaging techniques. Standard MRI pulse sequences typically use a two coil system in which current runs opposite to each other. This creates the magnetic gradient utilized to generate the image.[9] For the purposes of this text, the authors have simplified the nomenclature as it relates to the "standard" pulse sequences used for most musculoskeletal MRI by using the following terms:

- T1-weighted image.
- T2-weighted image.
- Intermediate-weighted or proton-density-weighted image.
- Fluid-sensitive sequence, such as STIR or fat-suppressed T2-weighted image.
- GRE image.
- Postgadolinium T1-weighted image.

Various other proprietary terms and acronyms (e.g., fast low-angle shot [FLASH], gradient recalled acquisition in the steady state [GRASS], FLAIR, etc.) commonly used primarily in the radiologic literature have been avoided for brevity.

Unlike imaging techniques based on electron absorption, such as conventional radiography and CT, the appearance of biologic tissue with MRI, that is, its relative brightness or darkness, is determined to a great extent by the operator-chosen parameters of the MR pulse sequence used to acquire the images. Thus, a joint effusion may appear bright, dark, or intermediate in signal intensity, depending on the MR pulse sequence and the selective parameters in that sequence. Each MR pulse sequence has its own specific strengths and weaknesses, and typically a combination of pulse sequences is used in a standard examination.

Conventional SE (and FSE) sequences make up the bulk of sequences in the MRI assessment of musculoskeletal anatomy. They take a relatively significant amount of time to generate an

Table 1.1 Basic Pulse Sequences for MRI

Sequence	Fat Intensity	Water Intensity	Advantage	Disadvantage
T1-weighted	Bright	Dark	Excellent anatomic details	Poor visualization of pathology and edema
T2-weighted	Intermediate	Bright	Excellent for visualizing edema and pathology	Poor spatial resolution
Fluid sensitive: Fat-suppressed T2-weighted or STIR	Very dark	Very Bright	Most sensitive for edema and pathology	Poor spatial resolution
Gradient echo	Intermediate	Intermediate	Excellent for articular cartilage	Susceptible to metal artifacts

Source: Reproduced with permission from Khanna AJ, Cosgarea AJ, Mont MA, Andres BM, Domb BG, Evans PJ, Bluemke DA, Frassica FJ. Magnetic resonance imaging of the knee: current techniques and spectrum of disease. J Bone Joint Surg Am 2001;83(suppl 2, part 2):128–141.

image.[9] Proton-density-weighted sequences are useful because they produce images with the highest signal-to-noise ratio and, therefore, provide better resolution than do T2-weighted FSE images. T1-weighted images, which provide nearly as high a signal-to-noise ratio, are also useful in showing musculoskeletal anatomy. T2-weighted sequences tend to have the poorest signal-to-noise ratio, and therefore the poorest resolution, but they are used primarily for their fluid sensitivity and their ability to detect pathology that has a high fluid content (e.g., tendon or ligament tears, tumors). T2 sequences can also give a rough depiction of anatomy, although it is inferior to that of proton-density-weighted and T1-weighted sequences.

Fluid-sensitive sequences include T2, fat-suppressed T2-weighted, and STIR sequences. Depending on the clinical situation, each specific MRI sequence has some optimal and some less than optimal characteristics (▶ Table 1.1).

1.3.2 T1-Weighted SE

Standard T1-weighted SE sequences use a short TR (250–700 ms) and a short TE (10–25 ms) to maximize T1 differences of the tissues being imaged.[1] The ability to depict anatomic detail, bone marrow abnormalities (including marrow infiltrating processes and fractures), meniscal pathology, blood products, melanin, and enhancement after the administration of gadolinium are the strengths of T1-weighted SE sequences.[3] Generally speaking, these gadolinium agents are well tolerated and have a low adverse reaction rate according to recent studies.[9] Proton-poor substances, such as air, and substances that do not have mobile protons, such as cortical bone or other calcified structures (e.g., calcific tendinitis), produce no detectable signal and produce a relative signal void. Fast-flowing blood may generate a flow void and appear dark on T1-weighted sequences, mostly because of a lack of refocusing of the blood, which is excited by the 90-degree pulse but not by the 180-degree pulse. Other tissues, such as fat, melanin, fatty bone marrow, and certain blood products (intracellular and extracellular methemoglobin), appear bright on T1-weighted images (▶ Fig. 1.9). Fat signaling can be suppressed through the use of short T1 inversion recovery.[9] Collagenous tissue, such as ligaments, tendons, hyaline cartilage, and fluids (urine, simple cysts, edema), show low signal on standard T1-weighted sequences (▶ Fig. 1.10). Tissue with mixed characteristics (with some fluid and some collagenous tissue), such as abscesses, synovium, and complex cysts, tend to show intermediate signal intensity that is somewhere between that of collagenous tissue and fat. Usually, the higher the protein content of the fluid, the brighter the fluid appears on T1-weighted images. For the assessment of tumors or musculoskeletal infection, fat-suppressed T1-weighted imaging after gadolinium contrast administration represents the sequence of choice because the high signal from fat is suppressed, making enhancement of abnormal tissue more conspicuous (▶ Fig. 1.11). Short scan times (because of the relatively short TRs) and excellent spatial resolution and depiction of

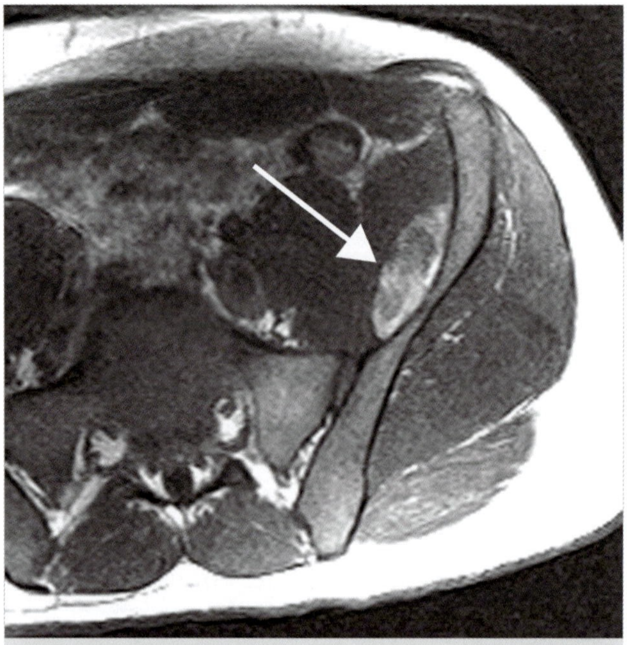

Fig. 1.9 An axial T1-weighted conventional spin-echo (SE) image through the left pelvis shows a lesion in the iliac fossa with areas of increased signal (*arrow*). This demonstrates a hematoma in a patient with hemophilia. The differential diagnosis for T1 hyperintense material includes fat, hemorrhage in the form of methemoglobin, gadolinium-based contrast material, proteinaceous material, some forms of calcium (when in solution), and melanin (as may be seen in melanoma). (Reproduced with permission from Obray RW, Beall DP, Reeder JD, Carrino JA, Fayad LM. Essentials of MRI Physics and Pulse Sequences. In: Khanna AJ, ed. MRI for orthopaedic surgeons. New York: Thieme; 2010:3–16.)

anatomic detail are the major advantages of a T1-weighted pulse sequence. Its major weakness is the relatively lower sensitivity for detecting soft-tissue edema compared with fluid-sensitive sequences such as fat-suppressed T2-weighted and STIR sequences.[3,9]

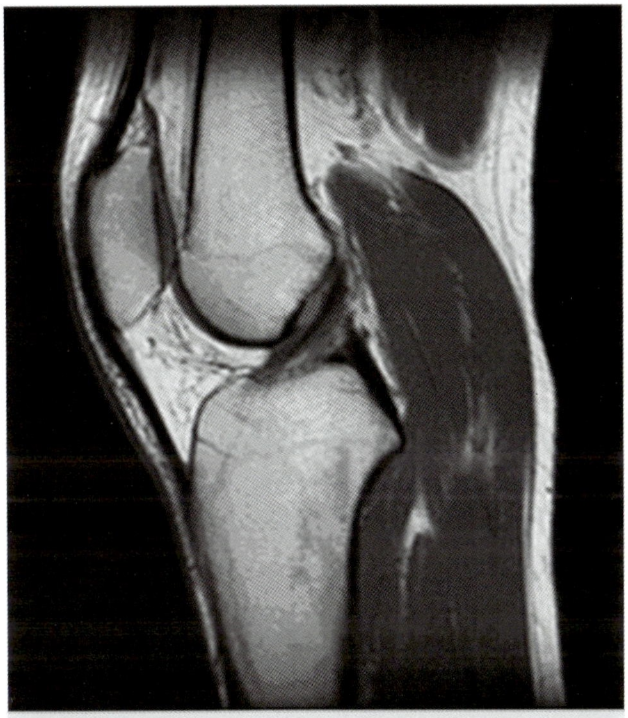

Fig. 1.10 A sagittal T1-weighted spin-echo (SE) image of the knee. The tendons and ligaments appear dark, fat appears predominantly bright, and the muscle has an intermediate signal. (Reproduced with permission from Obray RW, Beall DP, Reeder JD, Carrino JA, Fayad LM. Essentials of MRI Physics and Pulse Sequences. In: Khanna AJ, ed. MRI for orthopaedic surgeons. New York: Thieme; 2010:3–16.)

1.3.3 T2-Weighted SE and T2-Weighted FSE

T2-weighted SE and FSE sequences use a relatively long TE and long TR to maximize the T2 differences in the tissues. Both sequences, when combined with fat suppression, are excellent for detecting edema/fluid, which appears bright and is often associated with pathologic processes such as tumors, infection, fractures, tenosynovitis, and bone contusions (▶ Fig. 1.12). The T2-weighted SE and FSE sequences also are good for evaluating ligaments and tendons, cartilage, and fluid-filled structures such as cysts. As on T1-weighted SE sequences, air, cortical bone, calcified structures, and fast-flowing blood appear darker on T2-weighted sequences. Hyperacute blood (oxyhemoglobin) and subacute blood (extracellular methemoglobin) are bright on T2-weighted SE and FSE sequences. These sequences are useful for differentiating between fluid and tissue with a high fluid content, such as articular cartilage. The T2-weighted sequences (especially the FSE sequences) may also be used in the evaluation of articular cartilage defects. T2-weighted sequencing has been demonstrated to be both accurate and fast for the detection of articular cartilage defects in the knee for example.[11]

One of the major limitations of standard T2-weighted SE sequences is the relatively long image acquisition times. FSE imaging represents a technical innovation that permits much more rapid imaging with T2 contrast[12] through the use of multiple 180-degree RF pulses to create multiple echoes during a single TR period.[14] The series of echoes is called the echo train, and the number of echoes produced in a single TR period is known as the echo train length. Because of their fast acquisition times, T2-weighted FSE sequences largely have replaced standard T2-weighted SE sequences.[1,13,14]

The major weakness of T2-weighted SE and T2-weighted FSE sequences is their inability to detect marrow pathology when not combined with fat-suppression techniques (▶ Fig. 1.13). This limitation is made more apparent because both fat and water are bright on non–fat-suppressed T2-weighted FSE and SE sequences.[3]

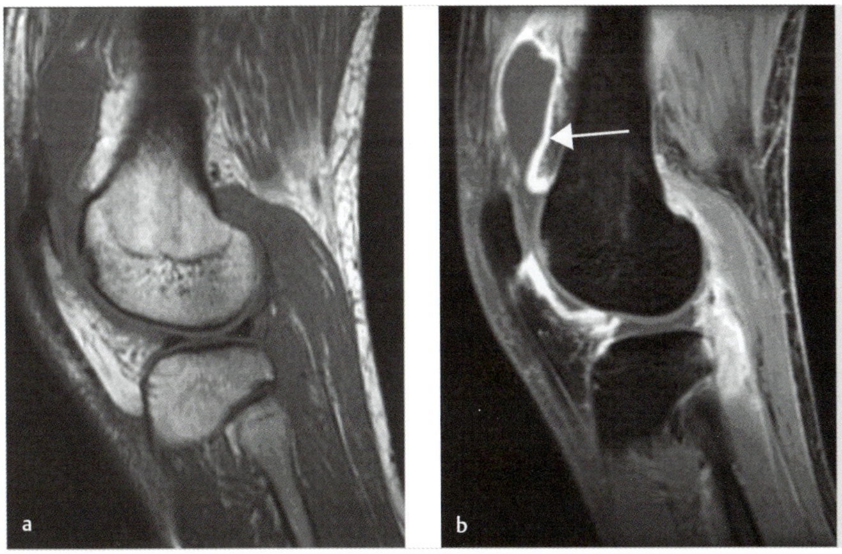

Fig. 1.11 Sagittal T1-weighted spin-echo (SE) images after the intravenous administration of a gadolinium-based contrast material without **(a)** and with **(b)** fat suppression. The diffuse enhancement of the synovium (*arrow on* **b**) is much more apparent with fat suppression in this patient with septic arthritis. The improved conspicuity is a major benefit of using fat suppression. (Reproduced with permission from Obray RW, Beall DP, Reeder JD, Carrino JA, Fayad LM. Essentials of MRI Physics and Pulse Sequences. In: Khanna AJ, ed. MRI for orthopaedic surgeons. New York: Thieme; 2010:3–16.)

1.3.4 Proton-Density SE and Proton-Density FSE

Proton-density SE sequences and proton-density FSE sequences are excellent for depicting anatomic detail[3] because of the high signal-to-noise ratio of proton-density-weighted images. Proton-density SE sequences also are used to evaluate regions obscured by the high signal on T2-weighted images. Fat-suppressed proton-density imaging is often used for the MRI evaluation of meniscal and articular cartilage (▶ Fig. 1.14).[15]

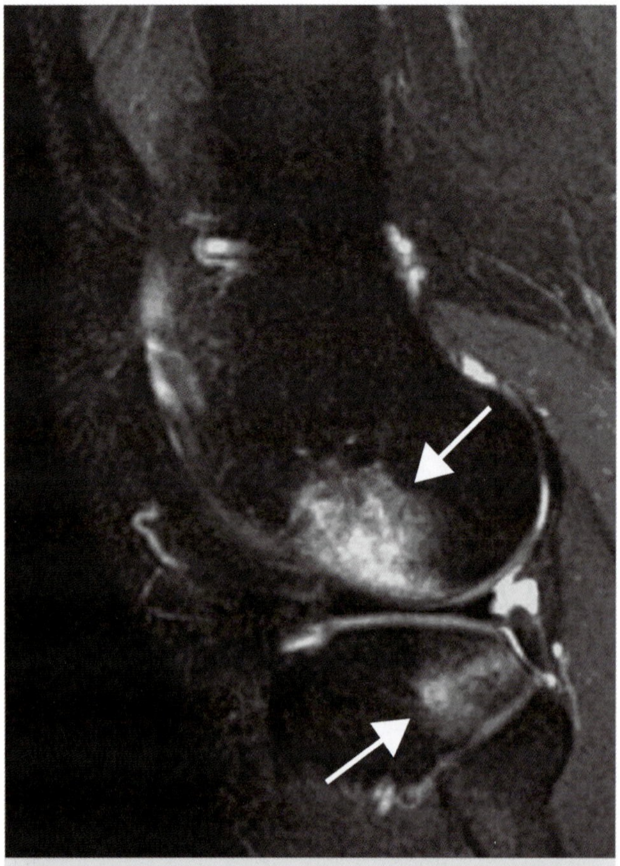

Fig. 1.12 A sagittal T2-weighted fast spin-echo (FSE) image with fat suppression through the lateral compartment of the knee demonstrates high signal within the distal femur and proximal tibia related to bone contusions (*arrows*). (Reproduced with permission from Obray RW, Beall DP, Reeder JD, Carrino JA, Fayad LM. Essentials of MRI Physics and Pulse Sequences. In: Khanna AJ, ed. MRI for orthopaedic surgeons. New York: Thieme; 2010:3–16.)

The major weakness of proton-density-weighted images is that tissue contrast is not as pronounced in comparison to either T1-weighted or T2-weighted images. This is the result of proton-density-weighted images functioning as a combination of T1 and T2 weighting.[3] Therefore, proton-density-weighted SE sequences are not as sensitive for the detection of both fluid and marrow pathology.[3]

1.3.5 Fat Suppression with T1-Weighted, T2-Weighted, and Proton-Density SE and FSE

Fat suppression commonly is achieved by spectral fat suppression or a STIR technique.[16,17] Spectral fat-suppression imaging is restricted to MRI systems with mid-level and high magnetic field strength because of the necessity for identifying distinct fat and water resonance peaks and selectively suppressing the signal arising from adipose tissue, a process dependent on the presence of a relatively strong magnetic field. When combined with T2-weighted or proton-density-weighted imaging, this technique is particularly useful in detecting bone bruises and osseous stress injury[17]; the hyperintense intraosseous fluid that accumulates secondary to osseous contusion and microtrabecular fractures appears particularly conspicuous in contrast to the adjacent suppressed normal marrow fat signal.[17,18]

On T1-weighted images, fat suppression can allow for the differentiation of fat-containing masses, for example, lipoma/liposarcoma, from other tissue that may contain elements of increased signal (e.g., hemorrhage within tissue).[17] In addition, it can be used to verify the presence of fat within a lesion and to increase the conspicuity of enhancing masses on contrast-enhanced T1-weighted images.

One of the disadvantages of T2, T1, and proton-density fat-suppression sequences is incomplete suppression of the signal from fat secondary to local magnetic field inhomogeneities and susceptibility effects (▶ Fig. 1.15).[3,17] This effect is most prominent with images of curved surfaces, such as in the shoulder and ankle,

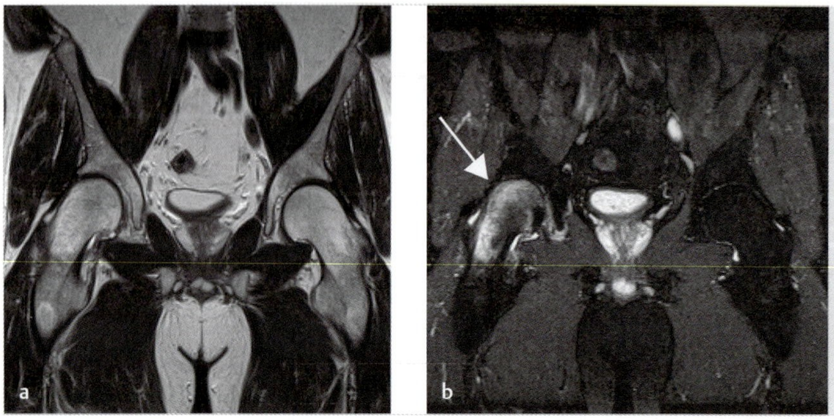

Fig. 1.13 Coronal T2-weighted fast spin-echo (FSE) images of the pelvis and hips without (**a**) and with (**b**) fat suppression. The increased signal within the right proximal femur related to transient osteoporosis (transient bone marrow edema syndrome) is seen much more easily with fat suppression (*arrow on* **b**). It is inconspicuous on the FSE image that is not fat suppressed. (Reproduced with permission from Obray RW, Beall DP, Reeder JD, Carrino JA, Fayad LM. Essentials of MRI Physics and Pulse Sequences. In: Khanna AJ, ed. MRI for orthopaedic surgeons. New York: Thieme; 2010:3–16.)

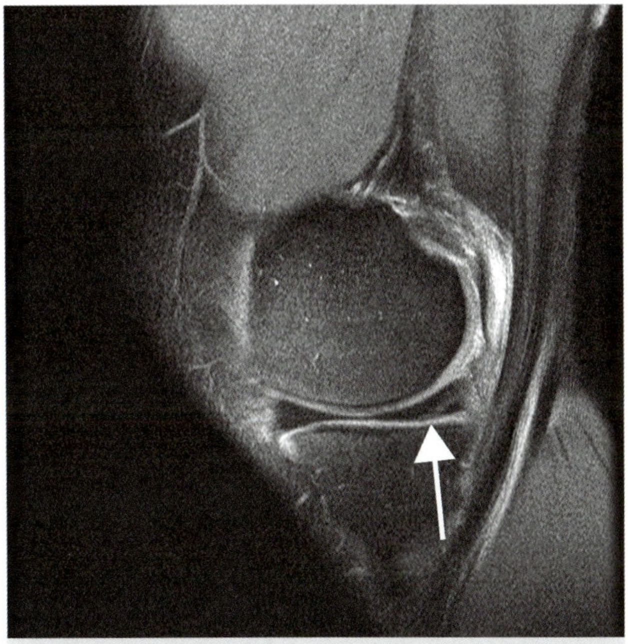

Fig. 1.14 A sagittal proton-density (intermediate)-weighted fast spin-echo (FSE) image with fat suppression through the medial compartment of the knee that demonstrates an arthroscopically proven meniscal tear. Linear signal is present in the posterior horn of the medial meniscus extending obliquely to the undersurface (*arrow*). This type of sequence is very useful for evaluating the internal derangement of joints. (Reproduced with permission from Obray RW, Beall DP, Reeder JD, Carrino JA, Fayad LM. Essentials of MRI Physics and Pulse Sequences. In: Khanna AJ, ed. MRI for orthopaedic surgeons. New York: Thieme; 2010:3–16.)

or of any body part in the presence of metal or air. As mentioned previously, fat suppression requires higher strength magnets (> 1 T) in order to ensure proper fat suppression than what is generally required for non–fat-suppression MRI. STIR sequences often are used to overcome the effects of magnetic field inhomogeneities seen with fat-suppression techniques (see the section below).[17]

1.3.6 STIR

STIR is another MRI pulse sequence commonly used in musculoskeletal imaging and, like T2-weighted sequences with fat suppression, is excellent for detecting fluid and edema when administered with a long TE. STIR can be used as an alternative to T2-weighted imaging. On fluid-sensitive images such as STIR, fluid appears bright which helps to make the edema and fluid associated with certain types of pathology more conspicuous (▶ Fig. 1.16) in comparison to non-fluid-sensitive sequences. Such pathology includes osteomyelitis, fasciitis, abscesses, metastases, primary bone tumors, fractures, tenosynovitis, tendon tears, and bone contusions.[19] Unlike T1-weighted and T2-weighted fat-suppression sequences, STIR uses a 180-degree RF inversion pulse, followed by a 90-degree RF pulse after inversion time to nullify the signal from fat.[19] Because of this phase-refocusing inversion pulse, STIR sequences are less susceptible to magnetic field inhomogeneities and subsequent susceptibility effects that often occur in inhomogeneous fat suppression on SE and FSE sequences. One of the major weaknesses of the STIR sequence, however, is that it suppresses the signal from all tissue

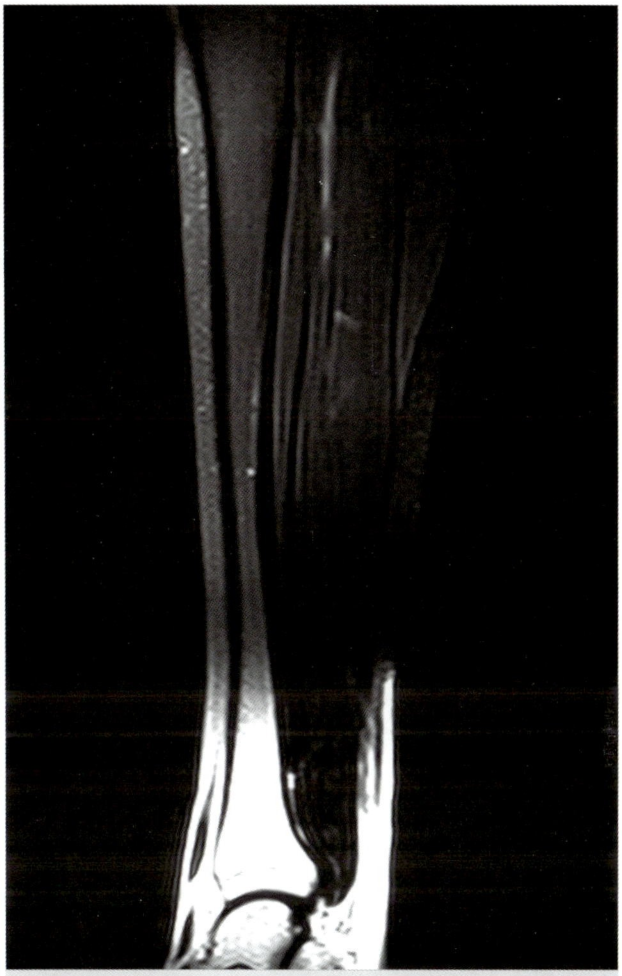

Fig. 1.15 A sagittal T1-weighted spin-echo (SE) image of the leg shows suppression of the signal from fat; the distal leg shows bright signal in the marrow and subcutaneous regions. One of the weaknesses of chemically selective fat-suppression techniques is this incomplete fat suppression, which results from local field heterogeneity. This incomplete fat suppression may arise if the imaging is off isocenter (outside of the "sweet spot" of the magnet), such as in the wrist or elbow, when there are noncylindrical structures with materials of substantially different magnetic susceptibilities next to each other (soft tissue and air), such as the foot, or with large field of views. (Reproduced with permission from Obray RW, Beall DP, Reeder JD, Carrino JA, Fayad LM. Essentials of MRI Physics and Pulse Sequences. In: Khanna AJ, ed. MRI for orthopaedic surgeons. New York: Thieme; 2010:3–16.)

with T1 signal characteristics similar to those of fat. Therefore, STIR pulse sequences should not be used with gadolinium contrast because gadolinium has relaxation properties similar to those of fat tissue, and thus all tissue with the same inversion time as fat (e.g., certain types of hemorrhage, melanin, and proteinaceous fluid) also will have its signal suppressed.[3] As an example, a study in 2006 demonstrated that STIR was less effective at visualizing a normal appendix with gadolinium.[20]

1.3.7 Gradient Echo, 3D Gradient Echo

GRE MRI pulse sequences use gradients to recall the echo at TE.[9] Specifically, a negative gradient is followed by a positive gradient to refocus the signal at the readout. In GRE sequences,

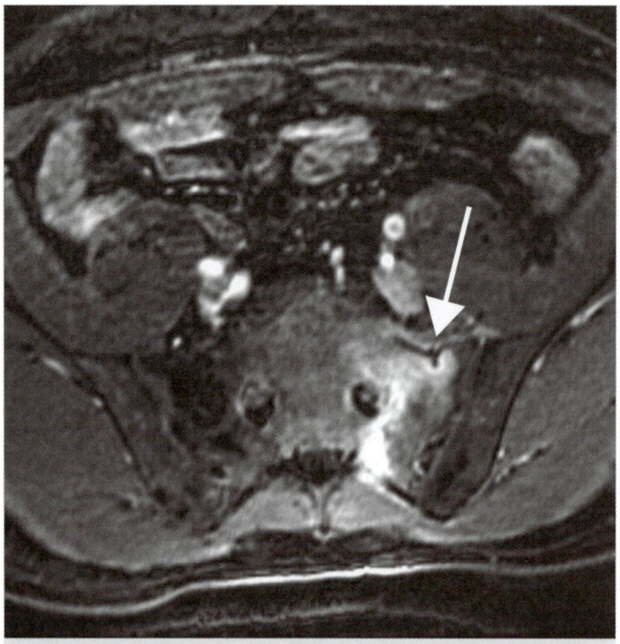

Fig. 1.16 An axial short tau inversion recovery (STIR) image of the pelvis shows increased signal within the left side of the sacrum. A small, incomplete fracture line is present within the anterior cortex (*arrow*). These findings represent an insufficiency-type stress fracture. Note that the signal from fat is very uniformly suppressed with the use of this pulse sequence. (Reproduced with permission from Obray RW, Beall DP, Reeder JD, Carrino JA, Fayad LM. Essentials of MRI Physics and Pulse Sequences. In: Khanna AJ, ed. MRI for orthopaedic surgeons. New York: Thieme; 2010:3–16.)

the TR varies and is related to the flip angle and the TE. A large flip angle (70–110 degrees) and a short TE favor T1 weighting, whereas a small flip angle (5–20 degrees) and a large TE favor T2* weighting. A low flip angle and a short TE result in a proton-density-weighted image.

GRE sequences are more sensitive than SE sequences to local magnetic field inhomogeneities.[9] These inhomogeneities can be created by blood, air, or calcium within a tissue or can be intrinsic to the MRI unit itself.[21] As a result, GRE sequences are very sensitive for the detection of certain types of tissue, such as calcification, focal air collections, and blood products, that produce magnetic field inhomogeneity.[22] Similarly, GRE sequences of tissue that contains surgical instrumentation (metal) tend to produce substantial artifact secondary to the disturbance in the local magnetic field created by that instrumentation. Because of the susceptibility effects of the trabecular bone, GRE images also tend to overestimate the size or prominence of osteophytes within the spine and marrow pathology when the trabecular bone is not destroyed.[3]

Susceptibility artifacts seen on GRE sequences can be helpful in identifying diseases such as pigmented vilonodular synovitis (PVNS) because the hemosiderin deposits that are characteristic of the disease produce local magnetic field inhomogeneities that result in focal susceptibility artifacts. GRE sequences also can be used to detect abnormalities involving the glenoid labrum and menisci of the knee.[23] Despite these utilities, the contrast between other soft tissues (such as muscle and fat) is relatively poor compared with that of other pulse sequences. GRE sequences may be T2* weighted, T1 weighted, or proton-density weighted, depending on what tissue is being evaluated which makes the technique adaptable to a variety of imaging needs.

In 3D GRE sequences, the signal from an entire volume of tissue (i.e., in the x, y, and z planes) is acquired at the same time. This volume of tissue then may be partitioned into sections in any plane.[9] These sections obtained from the 3D volume data set may be isotropic, or nearly so, and can be oriented in any way that is helpful for interpreting the data set. In general, 3D sequences (also known as volume acquisitions) have a higher signal-to-noise ratio because an entire volume of tissue is sampled rather than a single thin section. This optimal signal-to-noise ratio makes the 3D acquisition pulse sequences especially useful at low field strengths.[4] In addition, relatively high resolution and the high signal-to-noise ratio make the 3D GRE sequences good for detecting abnormalities within small structures, such as the ligaments in the wrist[3] and the articular cartilage.[3,4,24] The major disadvantages of 3D GRE pulse sequences are the relatively long acquisition times and the tendency toward susceptibility and motion artifacts.[9]

1.3.8 Contrast-Enhanced Imaging

Gadolinium is commonly used as an intravenous and intra-articular contrast agent in musculoskeletal imaging.[25] Its function in intravenous imaging is analogous to that of the iodinated contrast agent used in CT, and tissues that show increased vascularity generally show enhancement on postcontrast T1-weighted images. Fat-suppression techniques are commonly used with gadolinium because of their sensitivity to detecting gadolinium.[24,26] Areas in which there is breakdown of the blood–brain barrier also show enhancement. Specific uses for intravenous contrast include the evaluation of spinal lesions and differentiation of the following[3,24,27]:

- Solid from cystic lesions.
- Soft-tissue phlegmon from inflammation from an abscess.
- Surgical scars from disk fragments.

Intravenous administration also can be used in indirect MR arthrography.

MR arthrography and the intra-articular administration of gadolinium involve the direct injection of a gadolinium contrast solution into the joint. MR arthrography has the advantage of being able to provide joint distention and is especially helpful in delineating labral tears in the hip and shoulder, ligamentous injuries, and TFCC tears in the wrist (▸ Fig. 1.17). In the knee, MR arthrography has also been proposed as a technique that may improve sensitivity and specificity in detecting articular cartilage pathology, loose bodies, and meniscal tears, particularly in the postoperative knee.[28,29,30] Disadvantages include the relatively invasive nature of the procedure, the potential for introducing air bubbles that could simulate loose bodies, and leakage of paramagnetic contrast material into the periarticular tissues that could obscure or mimic pathology.[31]

Indirect arthrography involves the intravenous injection of gadolinium contrast material and imaging the joint approximately 5 to 10 minutes after injection, followed by movement of the joint through its range of motion. An alternative technique images the joint immediately after injection, focusing upon the enhancement of abnormal periarticular tissue or hyperemia rather than utilizing the arthrographic effect

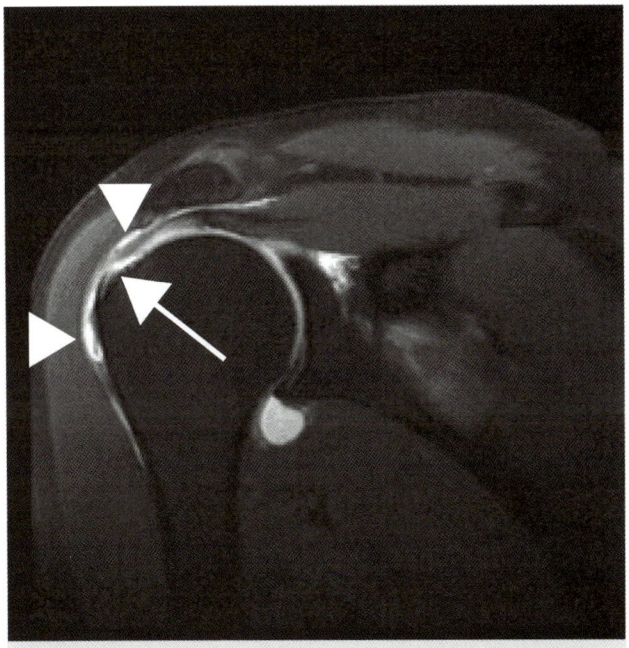

Fig. 1.17 This coronal T1-weighted spin-echo (SE) image through the right shoulder with fat suppression after the intra-articular administration of dilute gadolinium-based contrast material demonstrates a full-thickness rotator cuff tear as a defect involving the supraspinatus tendon (*arrow*). Note that the hyperintense contrast material extends from the full-thickness defect and is present within the subacromial/subdeltoid bursa (*arrowheads*). (Reproduced with permission from Obray RW, Beall DP, Reeder JD, Carrino JA, Fayad LM. Essentials of MRI Physics and Pulse Sequences. In: Khanna AJ, ed. MRI for orthopaedic surgeons. New York: Thieme; 2010:3–16.)

provided by direct and indirect MR arthrography. Facilitated by joint movement, the technique allows contrast material to rapidly diffuse into the synovial fluid. This provides the arthrographic appearance without directly violating the joint.[32,33] In patients with inflammatory arthritis, this technique proves particularly useful in evaluating synovial thickening and in the detection of full- and partial-thickness tears of the supraspinatus tendon.[34]

1.4 Artifacts

Common artifacts seen in MRI include motion artifacts, truncation artifacts, the *magic angle effect*, and susceptibility effects.[35] Motion artifacts in MRI are common and are directly related to patient motion within the scanner. Patient motion results in misregistration of the MR signal and subsequent blurring of the MR image. Motion from the pulsation of arteries results in a particular type of motion artifact or pulsation artifact. This type of artifact produces partial reproductions of the pulsating vessel in the phase-encoding direction.

Truncation artifacts occur in MRI and are related to the way the MR signal is processed during image creation and, in particular, to the Fourier transformation method used to process the MR signal data.[36,37] Truncation artifacts that can be seen include ring artifacts, artificial edge widening at parallel high-contrast interfaces, interface edge enhancement, and distortion of adjacent tissues at parallel high contrast interfaces.[36]

Susceptibility artifacts seen in MRI, briefly discussed above, are the result of local field inhomogeneities within the scan field, which create areas of focal signal loss. These magnetic field inhomogeneities can be related to the magnet or to metal, air, calcium, or blood products within the tissues being imaged.[3,4,9]

The magic angle effect is the result of the prolongation of T2 within tissues with highly ordered structures that are at a 55-degree angle relative to the main magnetic field.[24] This effect can simulate pathology by producing an increased signal, such as that seen within a normal supraspinatus tendon. To avoid overtreating a normal patient or structure, care should be taken when evaluating highly structured tissues such as tendons and cartilage when they are oriented at or near 55 degrees to the main magnetic field.

1.5 Summary

A fundamental knowledge base of MRI physics is important for the optimal use of MRI technology. This imaging modality is well suited and frequently utilized for evaluating musculoskeletal diseases. This is because MRI is capable of providing an accurate anatomic assessment, which is of paramount importance. RF pulses, appropriately applied within a graded magnetic field, can localize the tissue of interest, and the signal produced can be Fourier-transformed into an image. This image is defined not only by the T1, T2, and T2* relaxation time constants of the specific tissue but also by the variety of parameters that are used and manipulated to assess the region of interest.

The primary pulse sequence parameters in MRI are TE, TR, and inversion time, and these values determine the weighting of the image (e.g., T1, T2, or proton-density), the strength of the signal, and whether a certain type of tissue (e.g., fat) is suppressed. Each of the standard pulse sequences used in musculoskeletal imaging (SE, FSE, STIR, and GRE) has its own strengths and weaknesses, and a combination of various sequences is typical for evaluation of the joints and spine. T1-weighted images are optimal for showing anatomic detail, bone/bone marrow abnormalities, and cartilage tears. Subsequently, they are excellent when combined with fat suppression for showing abnormal contrast enhancement. As a result, T1-weighted images are not optimal for showing soft-tissue edema. T2-weighted images are excellent for detecting edema/fluid and processes associated with increased fluid content, such as trauma and tumors. They also may be useful for articular cartilage evaluation but are relatively insensitive to marrow fluid unless combined with a fat-suppression technique. Proton-density images provide the highest signal-to-noise ratio and are excellent for the evaluation of anatomic detail. The primary limitation of proton-density sequences is the lack of pure contrast compared with that of T1-weighted and T2-weighted images. GRE sequences are useful for the detection of fibrocartilage tears and identification of tissue such as blood or metal that causes magnetic inhomogeneity. 3D GRE sequences can be obtained in one sequence and then be examined in any plane as a volume of tissue. The primary disadvantage of 3D GRE imaging is the long acquisition time; this same susceptibility to magnetic field inhomogeneity that may be useful is also a disadvantage when it obscures the tissue of interest. Fat suppression may be accomplished by frequency-specific suppression or by inversion recovery techniques. Frequency-specific suppression is a useful technique but may be limited by magnetic field heterogeneity. Inversion recovery fat suppression is homogeneous but also suppresses tissue with the same inversion time as fat. Gadolinium is used as a contrast agent, most often with frequency-specific fat suppression (because inversion recovery techniques may suppress the signal from the gadolinium). Intravenous injections also may be used for indirect arthrography, although direct injection of gadolinium may often be necessary to achieve optimal joint distention and visualization of the appropriate anatomy.

MRI can be an incredibly useful tool that often requires some degree of compromise; no gain in image quality is obtained without sacrificing some other portion of the sequence or the examination. A clear understanding of the basic elements of MRI, along with how these elements interact, allows the imager to adjust the scanning techniques and image protocols to obtain the highest quality images possible. This optimization is important in all subspecialty imaging but is especially so in musculoskeletal imaging, where elucidating the anatomy is fundamental to analyzing the structure for the presence or absence of pathology.

1.6 Common Clinical Questions

1. Which MRI sequence is best for detecting pathology and edema?
   a) T1 weighted.
   b) T2 weighted.
   c) Gradient echo.
   d) Proton weighted.

2. MRI leverages what physical property of tissue?
   a) Electron spin.
   b) Proton magnetization.
   c) Neutrino emission.
   d) Electrical charge.

3. In a T1 and T2 sequence, fat and water appear as follows:
   a) Fat and water both appear bright on T1.
   b) Fat appears bright on T1 and water appears bright on T2.
   c) Fat appears bright on T2 and water appears bright on T1.
   d) Fat and water both appear bright on T2.

4. Which MRI techniques is best for visualizing abscess?
   a) T1 weighted with gadolinium contrast.
   b) T2 weighted.
   c) Gradient echo.
   d) Proton weighted.

5. What is the magic angle effect on MRI?
   a) Appearance of pathology within normal ordered tissues such as tendons and cartilage due to prolongation of T2.
   b) MRI sequences performed with patient laying at a certain angle with respect to the machine.
   c) Motion artifact from patient movement within MRI machine.
   d) Motion from pulsation of arteries.

References

[1] Bitar R, Leung G, Perng R, et al. MR pulse sequences: what every radiologist wants to know but is afraid to ask. Radiographics. 2006; 26(2):513–537

[2] Huda W, Slone RM. Review of radiologic physics. 2nd ed. Philadelphia, PA: Lippincott William & Wilkins; 2003

[3] Kaplan PA, Helms CA, Dussault R, Anderson MW, Major NM. Basic principles of musculoskeletal MRI. In: Kaplan PA, et al., eds. Musculoskeletal MRI. Philadelphia, PA: WB Saunders; 2001:1–21

[4] Runge VM, Nitz WR, Schmeets SH, Faulkner WH Jr, Desai NK. The physics of clinical MR taught through images. New York: Thieme; 2005

[5] Lejay H, Holland BA. Technical advances in musculoskeletal imaging. In: Stoller DW, ed. Magnetic resonance imaging in orthopaedics and sports medicine. 3rd ed. Baltimore, MD: Lippincott Williams & Wilkins; 2007:1–28

[6] Wehrli FW, Shaw D, Kneeland JB. Biomedical magnetic resonance imaging: principles, methodology, and applications. New York: VCH Publishers; 1988

[7] Martin AR, Aleksanderek I, Cohen-Adad J, et al. Translating state-of-the-art spinal cord MRI techniques to clinical use: A systematic review of clinical studies utilizing DTI, MT, MWF, MRS, and fMRI. Neuroimage Clin. 2015; 10: 192–238

[8] Nouri A, Martin AR, Mikulis D, Fehlings MG. Magnetic resonance imaging assessment of degenerative cervical myelopathy: a review of structural changes and measurement techniques. Neurosurg Focus. 2016; 40(6):E5

[9] Currie S, Hoggard N, Craven IJ, Hadjivassiliou M, Wilkinson ID. Understanding MRI: basic MR physics for physicians. Postgrad Med J. 2013; 89(1050):209–223

[10] Chavhan GB, Babyn PS, Thomas B, Shroff MM, Haacke EM. Principles, techniques, and applications of T2*-based MR imaging and its special applications. Radiographics. 2009; 29(5):1433–1449

[11] Bredella MA, Tirman PF, Peterfy CG, et al. Accuracy of T2-weighted fast spin-echo MR imaging with fat saturation in detecting cartilage defects in the knee: comparison with arthroscopy in 130 patients. AJR Am J Roentgenol. 1999; 172(4):1073–1080

[12] Mirowitz SA. Fast scanning and fat-suppression MR imaging of musculoskeletal disorders. AJR Am J Roentgenol. 1993; 161(6):1147–1157

[13] Escobedo EM, Hunter JC, Zink-Brody GC, Wilson AJ, Harrison SD, Fisher DJ. Usefulness of turbo spin-echo MR imaging in the evaluation of meniscal tears: comparison with a conventional spin-echo sequence. AJR Am J Roentgenol. 1996; 167(5):1223–1227

[14] Loening AM, Saranathan M, Ruangwattanapaisarn N, Litwiller DV, Shimakawa A, Vasanawala SS. Increased speed and image quality in single-shot fast spin echo imaging via variable refocusing flip angles. J Magn Reson Imaging. 2015; 42(6):1747–1758

[15] Potter HG, Linklater JM, Allen AA, Hannafin JA, Haas SB. Magnetic resonance imaging of articular cartilage in the knee. An evaluation with use of fast-spin-echo imaging. J Bone Joint Surg Am. 1998; 80(9):1276–1284

[16] Delfaut EM, Beltran J, Johnson G, Rousseau J, Marchandise X, Cotten A. Fat suppression in MR imaging: techniques and pitfalls. Radiographics. 1999; 19 (2):373–382

[17] Del Grande F, Santini F, Herzka DA, et al. Fat-suppression techniques for 3-T MR imaging of the musculoskeletal system. Radiographics. 2014; 34(1):217–233

[18] Kapelov SR, Teresi LM, Bradley WG, et al. Bone contusions of the knee: increased lesion detection with fast spin-echo MR imaging with spectroscopic fat saturation. Radiology. 1993; 189(3):901–904

[19] Morikawa M, Demura Y, Ishizaki T, et al. The effectiveness of 18F-FDG PET/CT combined with STIR MRI for diagnosing nodal involvement in the thorax. J Nucl Med. 2009; 50(1):81–87

[20] Nikolaidis P, Hammond N, Marko J, Miller FH, Papanicolaou N, Yaghmai V. Incidence of visualization of the normal appendix on different MRI sequences. Emerg Radiol. 2006; 12(5):223–226

[21] Atlas SW, Grossman RI, Hackney DB, et al. Calcified intracranial lesions: detection with gradient-echo-acquisition rapid MR imaging. AJR Am J Roentgenol. 1988; 150(6):1383–1389

[22] Thamburaj K, Radhakrishnan VV, Thomas B, Nair S, Menon G. Intratumoral microhemorrhages on T2*-weighted gradient-echo imaging helps differentiate vestibular schwannoma from meningioma. AJNR Am J Neuroradiol. 2008; 29(3): 552–557

[23] Lee MJ, Motamedi K, Chow K, Seeger LL. Gradient-recalled echo sequences in direct shoulder MR arthrography for evaluating the labrum. Skeletal Radiol. 2008; 37(1):19–25

[24] Stoller DW. Magnetic resonance imaging in orthopaedics and sports medicine. 3rd ed. Philadelphia, PA: Lippincott Williams & Wilkins; 2007

[25] Hopkins KL, Li KC, Bergman G. Gadolinium-DTPA-enhanced magnetic resonance imaging of musculoskeletal infectious processes. Skeletal Radiol. 1995; 24(5):325–330
[26] Gabata T, Matsui O, Kadoya M, et al. Small pancreatic adenocarcinomas: efficacy of MR imaging with fat suppression and gadolinium enhancement. Radiology. 1994; 193(3):683–688
[27] Longo M, Granata F, Ricciardi K, Gaeta M, Blandino A. Contrast-enhanced MR imaging with fat suppression in adult-onset septic spondylodiscitis. Eur Radiol. 2003; 13(3):626–637
[28] Brossmann J, Preidler KW, Daenen B, et al. Imaging of osseous and cartilaginous intraarticular bodies in the knee: comparison of MR imaging and MR arthrography with CT and CT arthrography in cadavers. Radiology. 1996; 200(2):509–517
[29] Magee T, Shapiro M, Rodriguez J, Williams D. MR arthrography of postoperative knee: for which patients is it useful? Radiology. 2003; 229(1):159–163
[30] White LM, Schweitzer ME, Weishaupt D, Kramer J, Davis A, Marks PH. Diagnosis of recurrent meniscal tears: prospective evaluation of conventional MR imaging, indirect MR arthrography, and direct MR arthrography. Radiology. 2002; 222(2):421–429
[31] Hodler J. Technical errors in MR arthrography. Skeletal Radiol. 2008; 37 (1):9–18
[32] Drapé JL, Thelen P, Gay-Depassier P, Silbermann O, Benacerraf R. Intraarticular diffusion of Gd-DOTA after intravenous injection in the knee: MR imaging evaluation. Radiology. 1993; 188(1):227–234
[33] Winalski CS, Aliabadi P, Wright RJ, Shortkroff S, Sledge CB, Weissman BN. Enhancement of joint fluid with intravenously administered gadopentetate dimeglumine: technique, rationale, and implications. Radiology. 1993; 187 (1):179–185
[34] Herold T, Bachthaler M, Hamer OW, et al. Indirect MR arthrography of the shoulder: use of abduction and external rotation to detect full- and partial-thickness tears of the supraspinatus tendon. Radiology. 2006; 240 (1):152–160
[35] Zaitsev M, Maclaren J, Herbst M. Motion artifacts in MRI: A complex problem with many partial solutions. J Magn Reson Imaging. 2015; 42(4):887–901
[36] Czervionke LF, Czervionke JM, Daniels DL, Haughton VM. Characteristic features of MR truncation artifacts. AJR Am J Roentgenol. 1988; 151(6): 1219–1228
[37] Block KT, Uecker M, Frahm J. Suppression of MRI truncation artifacts using total variation constrained data extrapolation. Int J Biomed Imaging. 2008; 2008:184123

Answers to Common Clinical Questions

1. Answer: b. T2 weighted.
2. Answer: b. Proton magnetization.
3. Answer: b. Fat appears bright on T1 and water appears bright on T2.
4. Answer: a. T1 weighted with gadolinium contrast.
5. Answer: a. Appearance of pathology within normal ordered tissues such as tendons and cartilage due to prolongation of T2.

2 Normal MRI Anatomy of the Musculoskeletal System

Emmanuel L. McNeely, A. Jay Khanna, Jason D. Dunleavy, and John A. Carrino

Abstract

The purpose of this chapter is to provide a basic outline of normal musculoskeletal anatomy shown on magnetic resonance imaging (MRI). A fundamental overview of normal MRI anatomy is required to successfully evaluate changes in the musculoskeletal system. This chapter will review key anatomical regions and structures to equip clinicians and radiologists to effectively recognize and interpret musculoskeletal anatomy on MRI.

Keywords: MRI, MSK, musculoskeletal system, imaging, radiology, joints

2.1 Introduction

To evaluate effectively an MRI examination of a particular joint or region in the musculoskeletal system, it is essential to have at least a basic understanding of the normal MRI anatomy of that region. Many excellent texts and atlases have been written to serve this need for clinicians and radiologists.[1,2] This chapter provides a brief overview of the most clinically important anatomy for each major region of the musculoskeletal system. The figures and line drawings in this chapter serve to highlight the structures with which the musculoskeletal medicine provider should be familiar before interpreting an imaging examination of the region. Reviewing the normal anatomy images pertinent to a specific anatomic region before reading the corresponding region-specific chapter will enhance the clinician's understanding of the relevant pathologic conditions and facilitate recognition and differentiation of the subtle regional anatomic alternations that represent various pathologic conditions.

2.2 Shoulder

2.2.1 Axial Images

Axial images are obtained from the superior aspect of the acromioclavicular (AC) joint through the inferior glenoid margin.

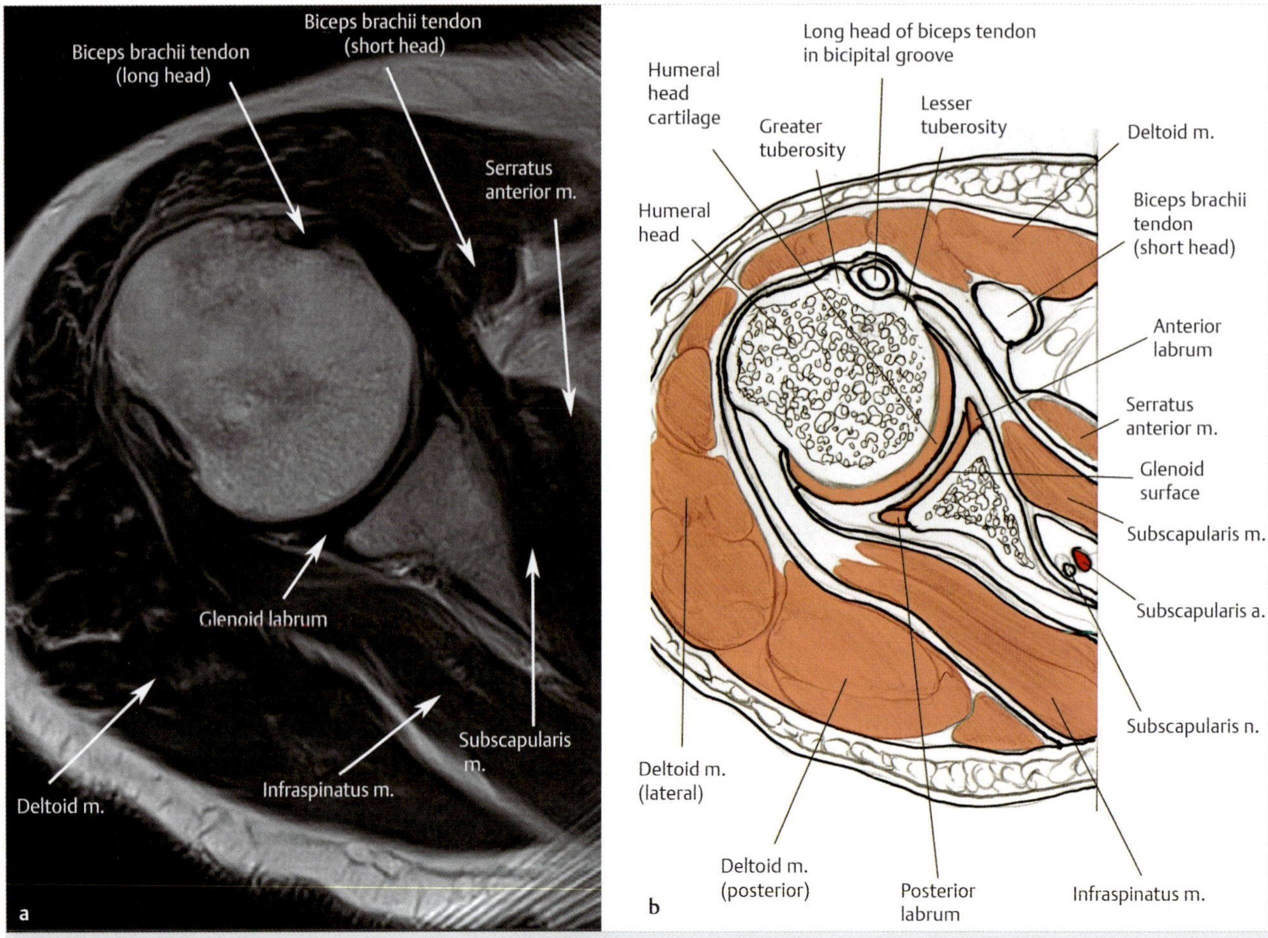

Fig. 2.1 An axial T2-weighted image **(a)** and artist's sketch **(b)** of the right shoulder at the level of the glenoid labrum showing the long head of the biceps tendon as it courses along the bicipital groove. (Reproduced with permission from Dunleavy JD, Khanna AJ, Carrino JA. Normal MRI Anatomy of the Musculoskeletal System. In: Khanna AJ, ed. MRI for orthopaedic surgeons. New York: Thieme; 2010:17–76.)

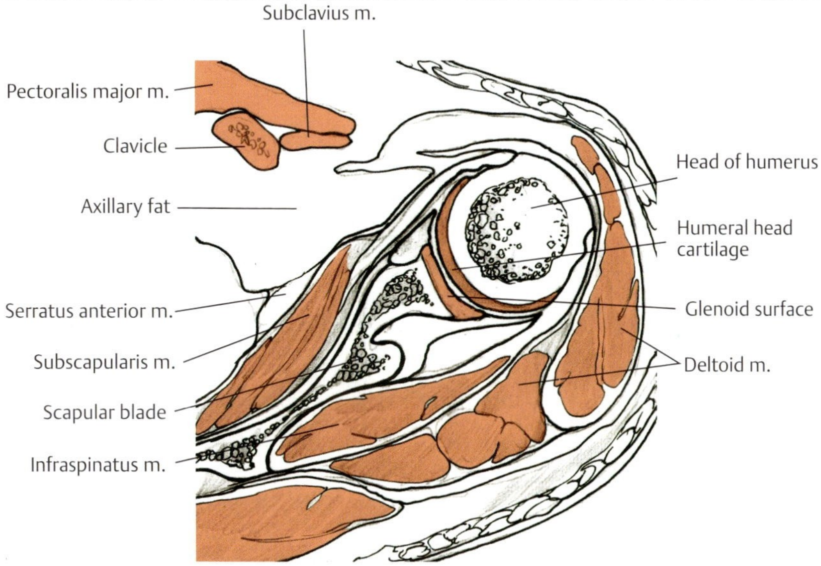

Fig. 2.2 An axial illustration of the left shoulder showing the anterior position of the subscapularis muscle and the articular cartilage of the glenoid and humeral head. (Reproduced with permission from Dunleavy JD, Khanna AJ, Carrino JA. Normal MRI Anatomy of the Musculoskeletal System. In: Khanna AJ, ed. MRI for orthopaedic surgeons. New York: Thieme; 2010:17–76.)

Axial plane images are best used for evaluating the glenoid labrum (anterior and posterior portions) (▶ Fig. 2.1) and capsular structures as well as the long head of the biceps tendon in the bicipital groove.[3] In addition, these images provide good visualization of the subscapularis muscle and tendon, the humeral head, and the glenoid (▶ Fig. 2.2). On superior axial images, the normal oblique course of the supraspinatus muscle is displayed with intermediate signal intensity, and the supraspinatus tendon is low in signal intensity. In cross-section, the tendon of the long head of the biceps is seen as a low-signal-intensity structure within the bicipital groove. Glenoid articular cartilage follows the concave shape of the glenoid cavity and shows intermediate signal intensity on T1-weighted and T2-weighted images. Articular cartilage is best evaluated on gradient-echo or fat-suppressed T2-weighted sequences.[4,5,6,7,8] The glenohumeral ligaments, best visualized on axial images, have low signal intensity on all pulse sequences. The superior glenohumeral ligament is identified at the level of the coracoid and the biceps tendon. The middle glenohumeral ligament (MGHL) is highly variable and may be identified as a thin band or a cord between the anterior labrum and subscapularis or may not be visualized at all without capsular distention. The anterior band of the inferior glenohumeral ligament (IGHL) is visualized more inferiorly between the anterior-inferior labrum and the subscapularis tendon.

2.2.2 Coronal Oblique Images

Coronal oblique images are obtained in a plane that is parallel to the course of the supraspinatus tendon; they tend to show shoulder anatomy and pathology in a plane that is familiar to most. The osseous structures of the shoulder are easily recognized (▶ Fig. 2.3a) as they would be seen on an anteroposterior (AP) shoulder radiograph. Similarly, the sagittal oblique images show the osseous structures as they would be seen from a lateral view (▶ Fig. 2.3b). The coronal oblique images should include the subscapularis muscle anteriorly and the infraspinatus and teres minor muscles posteriorly. Coronal oblique images are best used to evaluate the supraspinatus muscle and tendon (▶ Fig. 2.4), the subacromial and subdeltoid bursa, and the AC joint. The long head of the biceps tendon and biceps attachment, the infraspinatus muscle and tendon, the glenoid labrum (superior and inferior portions), and the glenohumeral joint space can also be visualized in the coronal oblique plane. Each coronal oblique image should be evaluated systematically from anterior to posterior. On anterior coronal oblique images, the subscapularis muscle and tendon can be identified as the tendon courses from its origin in the subscapularis fossa to its insertion on the lesser tuberosity. However, the subscapularis muscle and tendon can be seen more clearly on axial images (▶ Fig. 2.2). The long head of the biceps tendon is best seen in its intra-articular location on coronal oblique images. On anterior and midcoronal oblique images, the supraspinatus muscle and tendon are seen in continuity (▶ Fig. 2.5). The supraspinatus originates in the supraspinatus fossa of the scapula and inserts on the superior facet of the greater tuberosity of the humerus. On coronal oblique images, the anatomy of the AC joint is best displayed at the level of the supraspinatus tendon. The AC joint should be evaluated for the shape of the acromion (▶ Fig. 2.4) and the various ligaments around the shoulder (▶ Fig. 2.6). The superior and inferior portions of the glenoid labrum, as well as the axillary pouch, are also clearly shown on coronal oblique images. The superior and inferior glenoid labrums are seen as low-signal-intensity structures, in contrast to high-signal-intensity fluid on T2-weighted images. The axillary pouch usually is collapsed or has a small amount of fluid in the recess (▶ Fig. 2.5). Humeral head articular cartilage, intermediate in signal intensity on T1-weighted and T2-weighted images, is interposed between the low-signal-intensity supraspinatus tendon superiorly and the cortex inferiorly.

The subclavian artery courses laterally between the anterior scalene and middle scalene muscles. The axillary artery continues

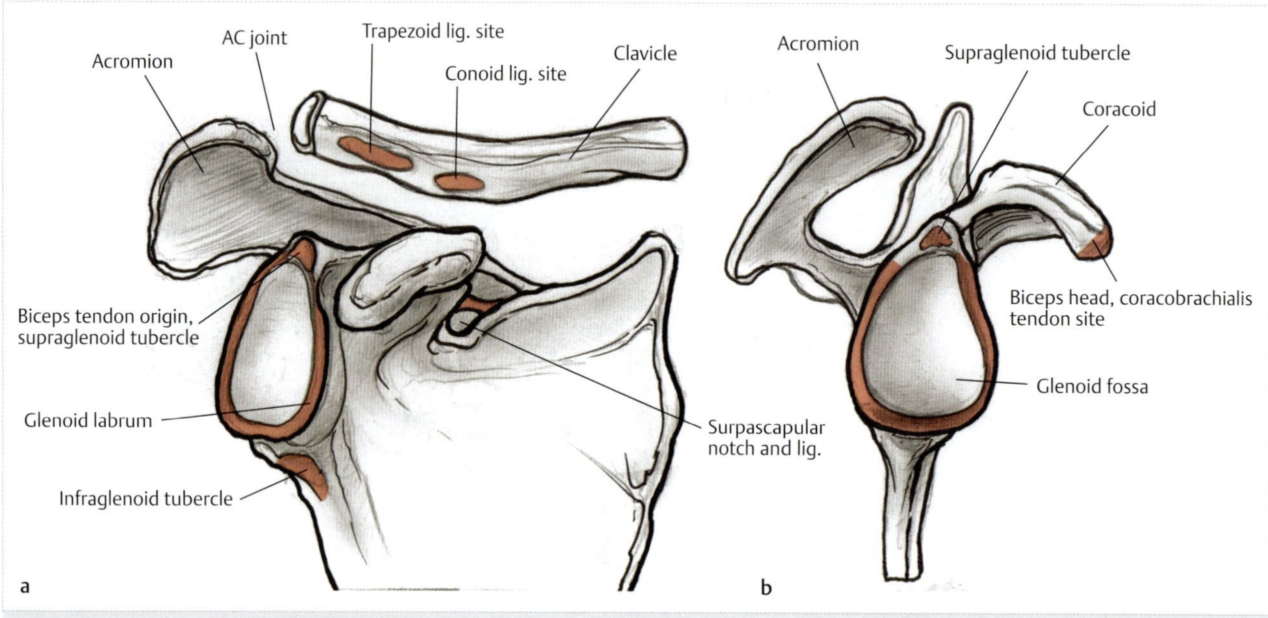

Fig. 2.3 Anterior **(a)** and lateral **(b)** 3D illustrations of the osseous structures of the right shoulder. Abbreviations: AC, acromioclavicular. (Reproduced with permission from Dunleavy JD, Khanna AJ, Carrino JA. Normal MRI Anatomy of the Musculoskeletal System. In: Khanna AJ, ed. MRI for orthopaedic surgeons. New York: Thieme; 2010:17–76.)

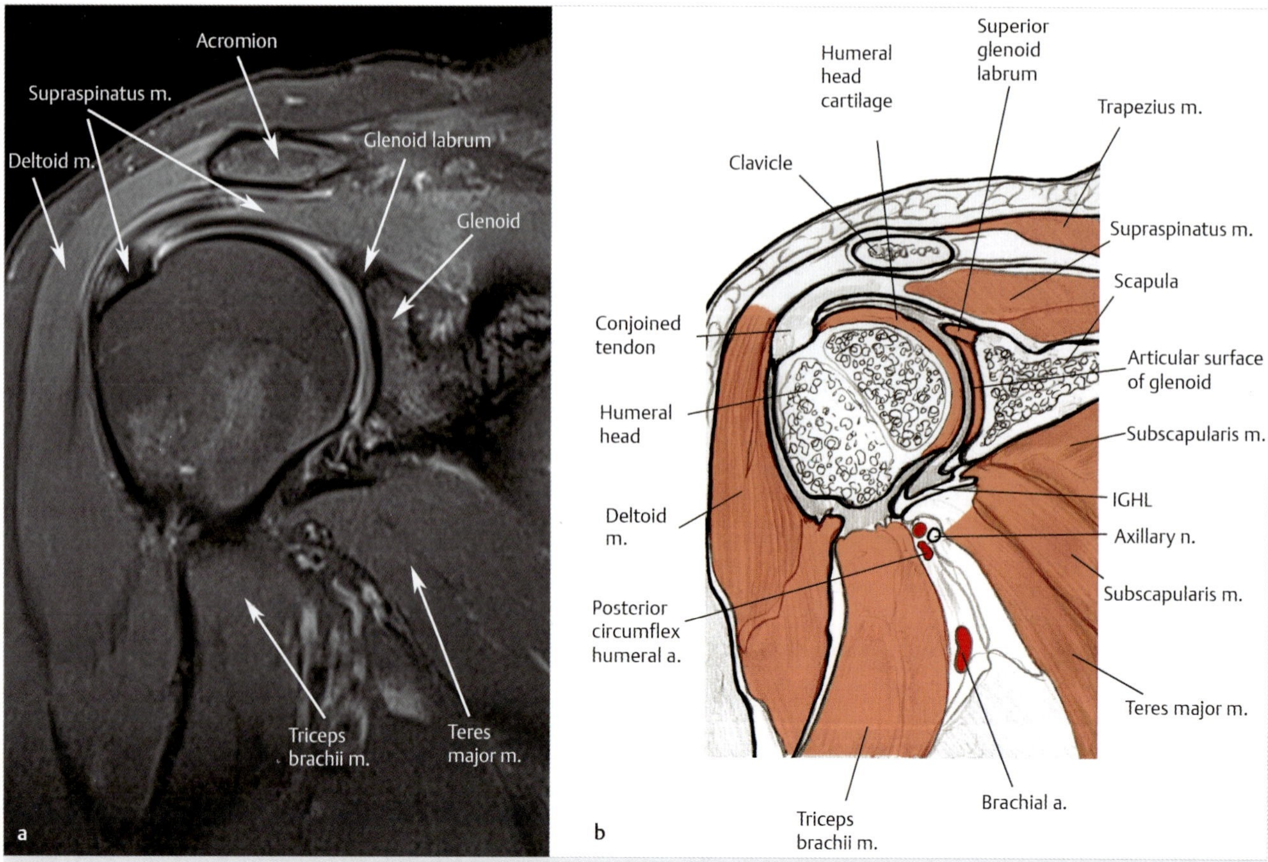

Fig. 2.4 A coronal proton-density fat-suppressed image **(a)** and artist's sketch **(b)** of the right shoulder at the level of the supraspinatus muscle and the insertion of the conjoined tendon, a site that is very prone to rotator cuff injury. The normal, flat acromion is also seen at this level, without evidence of supraspinatus impingement. Abbreviations: IGHL, inferior glenohumeral ligament. (Reproduced with permission from Dunleavy JD, Khanna AJ, Carrino JA. Normal MRI Anatomy of the Musculoskeletal System. In: Khanna AJ, ed. MRI for orthopaedic surgeons. New York: Thieme; 2010:17–76.)

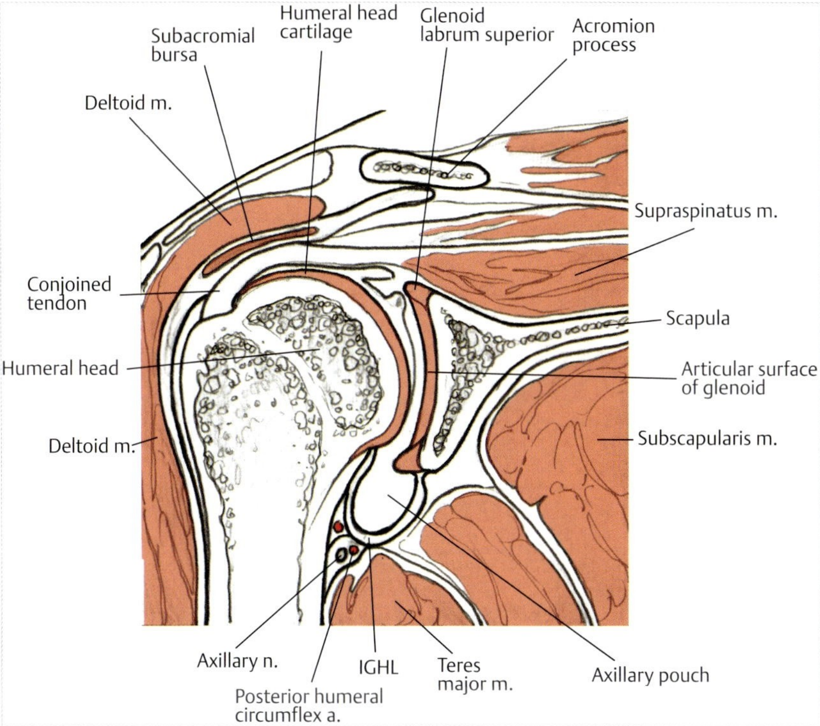

Fig. 2.5 A coronal illustration of the right shoulder at the level of the supraspinatus muscle and tendon showing the glenoid and humeral head cartilage and the superior and inferior glenoid labrum. Abbreviations: IGHL, inferior glenohumeral ligament. (Reproduced with permission from Dunleavy JD, Khanna AJ, Carrino JA. Normal MRI Anatomy of the Musculoskeletal System. In: Khanna AJ, ed. MRI for orthopaedic surgeons. New York: Thieme; 2010:17–76.)

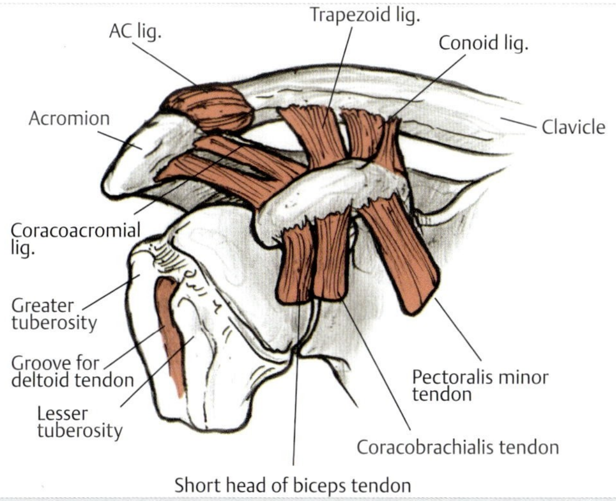

Fig. 2.6 A 3D coronal illustration of the right shoulder, identifying the insertion locations of the rotator cuff tendons at the greater and lesser tuberosities of the humerus. Also shown are the coracoclavicular and coracoacromial ligaments and other ligaments that stabilize the shoulder. Abbreviations: AC lig., acromioclavicular ligament. (Reproduced with permission from Dunleavy JD, Khanna AJ, Carrino JA. Normal MRI Anatomy of the Musculoskeletal System. In: Khanna AJ, ed. MRI for orthopaedic surgeons. New York: Thieme; 2010:17–76.)

from the subclavian artery at the lateral border of the first rib. Branches of the axillary artery are the supreme thoracic artery, thoracoacromial artery, lateral thoracic artery, subscapular artery, and anterior and posterior humeral circumflex arteries. The brachial artery continues from the axillary artery at the lateral border of the teres major muscle (▶ Fig. 2.7). The brachial artery passes posterior to the bicipital aponeurosis, and its branches provide arterial flow to the forearm and hand.

2.2.3 Sagittal Oblique Images

Sagittal oblique images, obtained in a plane that is perpendicular to the supraspinatus tendon, should extend from the most lateral aspect of the humeral head to the midscapula (to evaluate rotator cuff muscle atrophy). The osseous structures (▶ Fig. 2.3b) can be used to orient oneself to the location of the rotator cuff muscles, tendons, and other nonosseous structures (▶ Fig. 2.8). These oblique images are well suited for evaluating the rotator cuff muscles and tendons (▶ Fig. 2.9), coracoacromial arch, rotator interval, and acromial morphology.[3,4] The glenoid labrum and the long head of the biceps can also be evaluated on the sagittal oblique images. However, both structures are better visualized on axial and coronal oblique images. Sagittal oblique images should be reviewed systematically from medial to lateral. Medial sagittal sections display the clavicle and AC joint in profile. On midsagittal and lateral sagittal images, the supraspinatus, the infraspinatus, and the confluence of the cuff tendons are visualized between the acromion and the superior articular surface of the humeral head. The supraspinatus originates from the supraspinatus fossa of the scapula, and the infraspinatus originates from the infraspinatus fossa of the scapula. The teres minor originates from the posterolateral aspect of the scapula. All three of these rotator cuff structures (the supraspinatus, infraspinatus, and teres minor) insert at the greater tuberosity of the humerus: the supraspinatus, along the most superior aspect of the greater tuberosity; the infraspinatus, along the middle facet of the greater tuberosity; and the teres minor, along the inferior facet of the greater tuberosity. The subscapularis is the most anterior rotator cuff muscle, and it originates from the subscapularis fossa of the scapula. It is unique in that it is the only rotator cuff structure to insert along the lesser tuberosity of the humerus rather than the greater tuberosity (▶ Fig. 2.6). The biceps tendon can be followed from

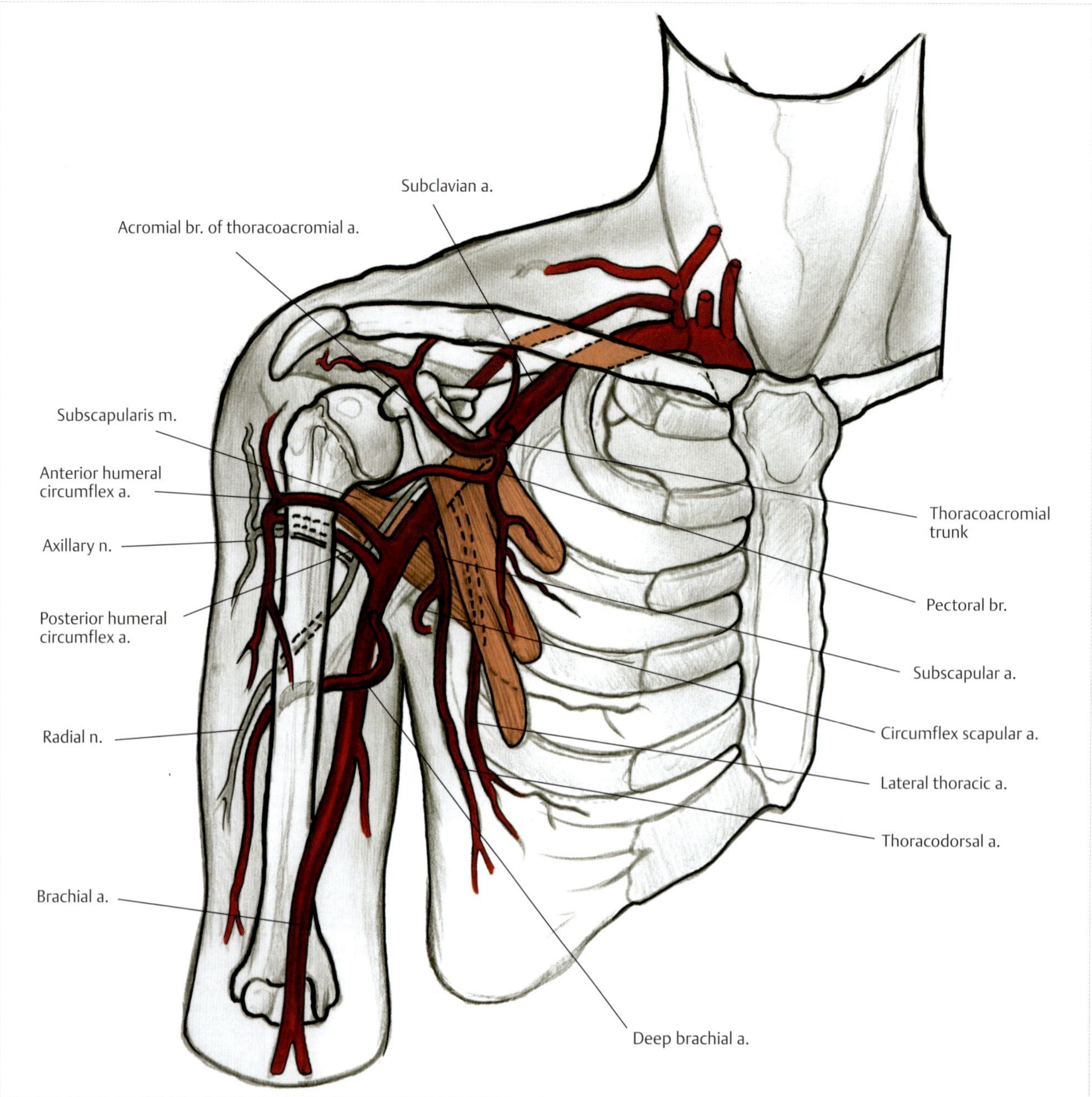

Fig. 2.7 A 3D coronal illustration of the neurovascular structures of the right shoulder and arm showing the subclavian, axillary, and brachial arteries, as well as smaller branch vessels such as the anterior humeral circumflex artery, a tributary of the axillary artery, which is seen coursing anterior to the surgical neck of the humerus. (Reproduced with permission from Dunleavy JD, Khanna AJ, Carrino JA. Normal MRI Anatomy of the Musculoskeletal System. In: Khanna AJ, ed. MRI for orthopaedic surgeons. New York: Thieme; 2010:17–76.)

medial to lateral as it courses from its intra-articular origin within the synovial sheath to its more lateral extracapsular location in the bicipital groove. The long head of the biceps originates from the supraglenoid tubercle, and the short head of the biceps originates from the coracoid (▶ Fig. 2.3).

2.3 Elbow

2.3.1 Axial Images

Axial images of the elbow should extend from above the humeral epicondyles (▶ Fig. 2.10) to a level distal to the radial tuberosity. The tendons related to the elbow are best evaluated in the axial plane. The major muscles in the anterior compartment of the arm are the biceps brachii and the brachialis; the major muscle in the posterior compartment is the triceps brachii. Ventrally, the biceps tendon is seen as a low-signal-intensity structure, which courses from its musculotendinous junction, beneath the lacertus fibrosis, to its insertion on the radial tuberosity (▶ Fig. 2.11). Some fibers of the distal biceps brachii also contribute to the bicipital aponeurosis. The aponeurosis extends from the myotendinous junction of the biceps to the fascia overlying the anteromedial muscles (flexors and pronators) and is identified as a thin, black, low-signal-intensity line on an axial image. The biceps brachii spans the

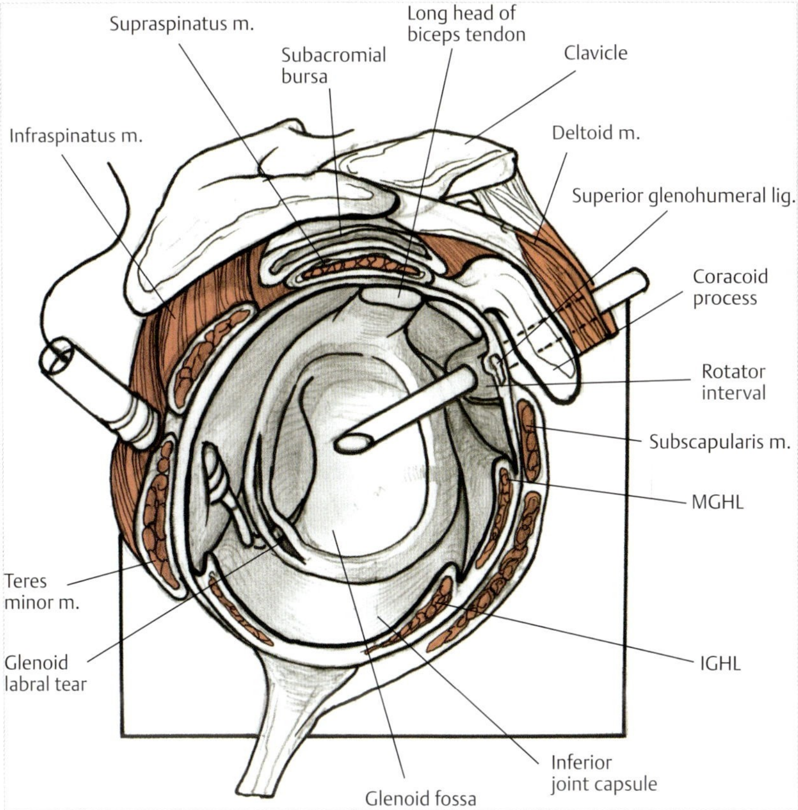

Fig. 2.8 A 3D sagittal illustration of the right glenoid showing a labral tear. Abbreviations: IGHL, inferior glenohumeral ligament; MGHL, middle glenohumeral ligament. (Reproduced with permission from Dunleavy JD, Khanna AJ, Carrino JA. Normal MRI Anatomy of the Musculoskeletal System. In: Khanna AJ, ed. MRI for orthopaedic surgeons. New York: Thieme; 2010:17–76.)

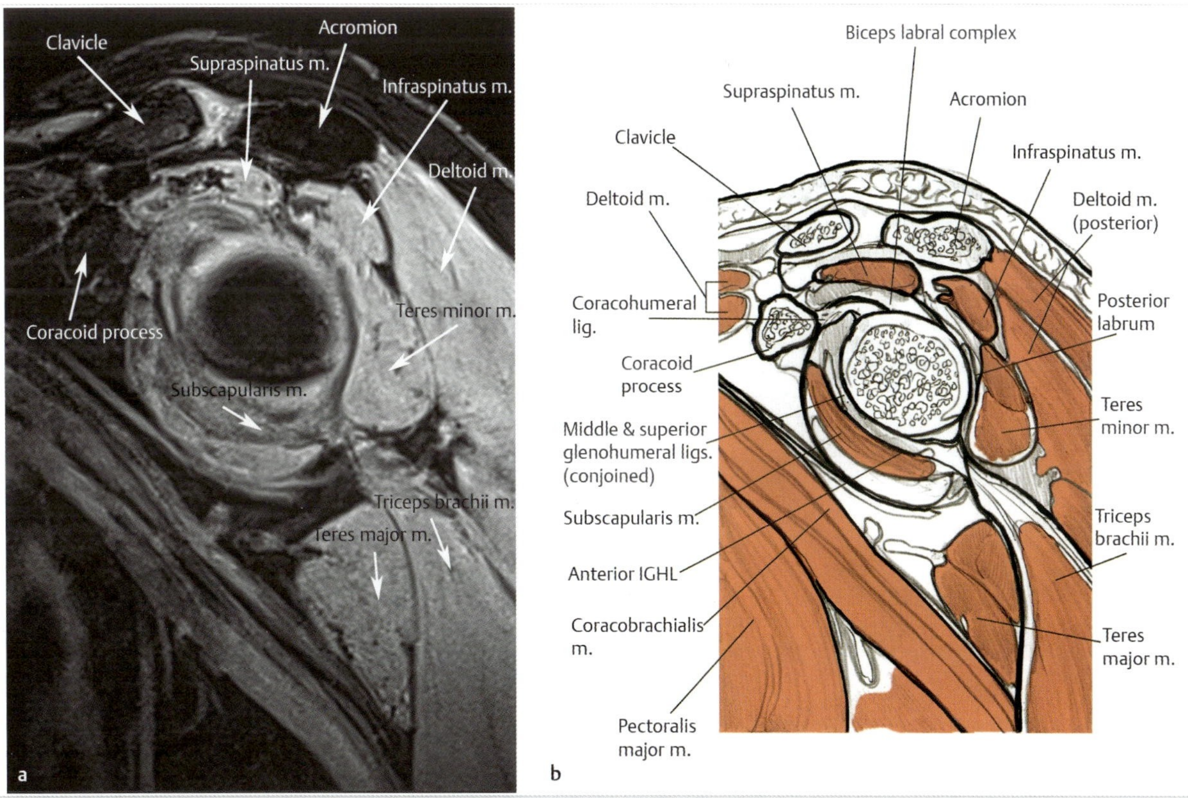

Fig. 2.9 A sagittal proton-density image with fat suppression **(a)** and artist's sketch **(b)** of the left shoulder at the level of the rotator cuff muscles. Although it takes some practice to evaluate the shoulder in the sagittal plane, the rotator cuff muscles are often best visualized on this view. (Reproduced with permission from Dunleavy JD, Khanna AJ, Carrino JA. Normal MRI Anatomy of the Musculoskeletal System. In: Khanna AJ, ed. MRI for orthopaedic surgeons. New York: Thieme; 2010:17–76.)

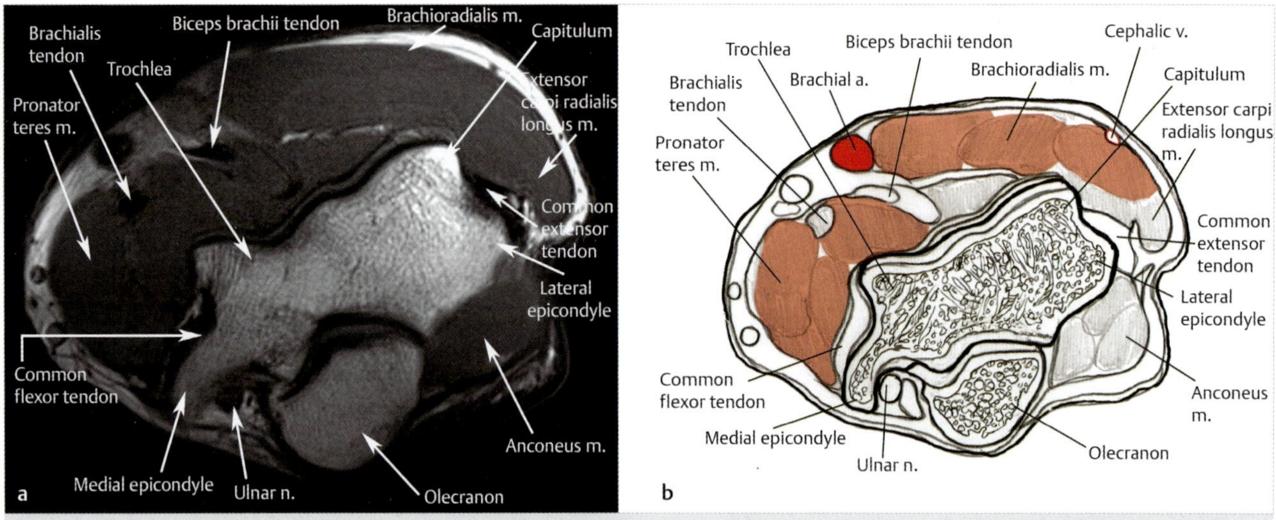

Fig. 2.10 An axial proton-density image **(a)** and artist's sketch **(b)** of the left elbow at the level of the humeral epicondyles illustrating the muscle architecture of the distal arm. The biceps brachii tendon, the common flexor tendon, and the common extensor tendon show normal thickness and low signal intensity. (Reproduced with permission from Dunleavy JD, Khanna AJ, Carrino JA. Normal MRI Anatomy of the Musculoskeletal System. In: Khanna AJ, ed. MRI for orthopaedic surgeons. New York: Thieme; 2010:17–76.)

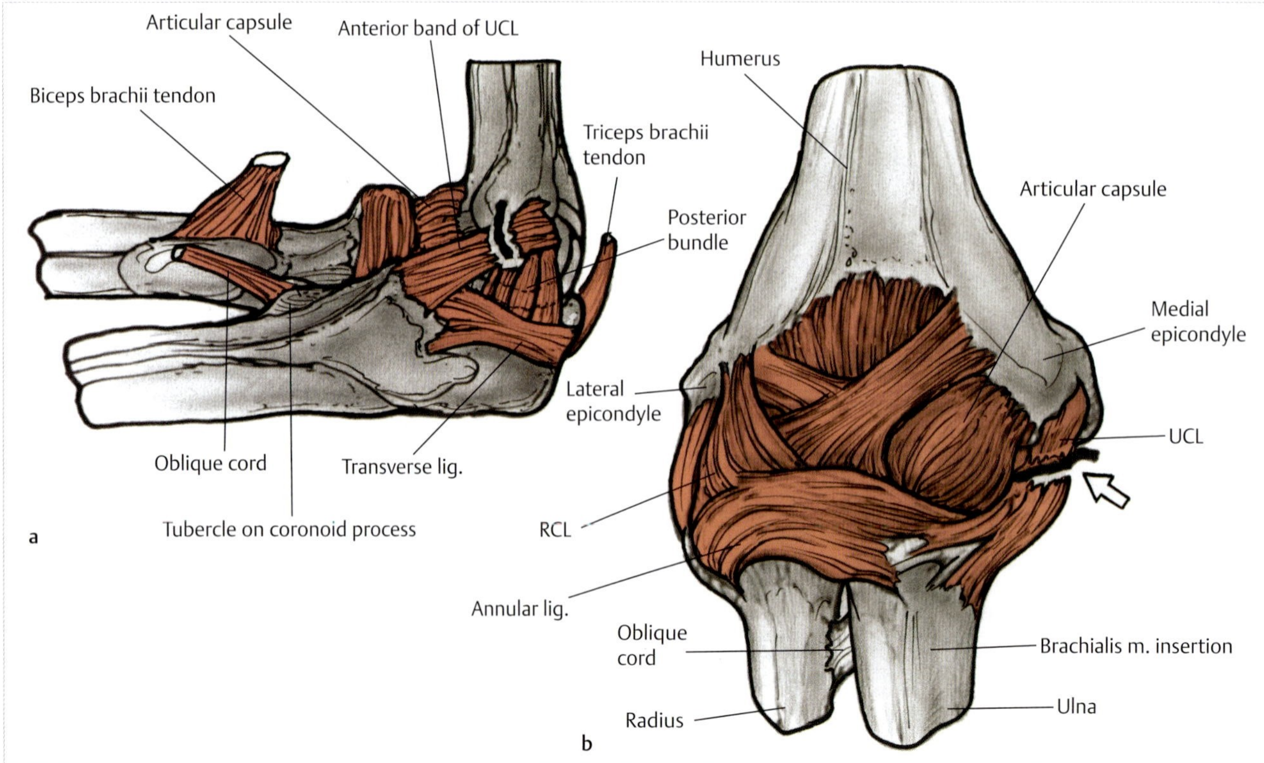

Fig. 2.11 Lateral (ulnar side) **(a)** and posterior **(b)** 3D illustrations of the left elbow showing the ligamentous structures that stabilize the elbow joint and a tear of the ulnar collateral ligament (UCL) (*arrow* on **b**). Abbreviations: RCL, radial collateral ligament. (Reproduced with permission from Dunleavy JD, Khanna AJ, Carrino JA. Normal MRI Anatomy of the Musculoskeletal System. In: Khanna AJ, ed. MRI for orthopaedic surgeons. New York: Thieme; 2010:17–76.)

shoulder and elbow joints and has a short and long head. The brachialis originates from the anterior aspect of the distal humerus, and its tendon courses immediately deep and slightly medial to the biceps and inserts on the ventral surface of the coronoid process of the ulna. The brachialis muscle is intermediate in signal intensity. Posteriorly, the triceps brachii has three heads with three separate origins; the distal triceps tendon attaches to the olecranon process of the ulna (▶ Fig. 2.12, ▶ Fig. 2.13).

Axial images also show the muscle architecture well. Because of the relative complexity of the forearm musculature compared with the arm musculature, forearm muscles are often grouped by location (superficial or deep) or by compartment (anterior,

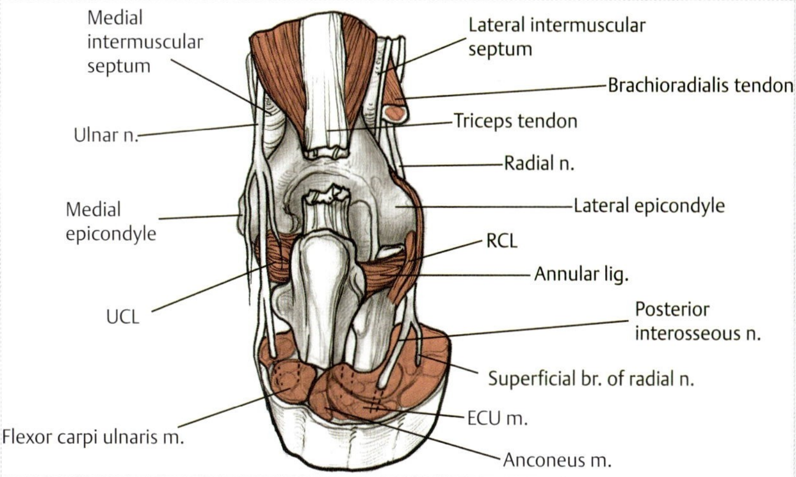

Fig. 2.12 A posterior 3D illustration of the right elbow showing the insertion of the triceps tendon (cut) onto the olecranon process of the ulna. Also seen are other neural and ligamentous structures. Abbreviations: RCL, radial collateral ligament; UCL, ulnar collateral ligament; ECU, extensor carpi ulnaris. (Reproduced with permission from Dunleavy JD, Khanna AJ, Carrino JA. Normal MRI Anatomy of the Musculoskeletal System. In: Khanna AJ, ed. MRI for orthopaedic surgeons. New York: Thieme; 2010:17–76.)

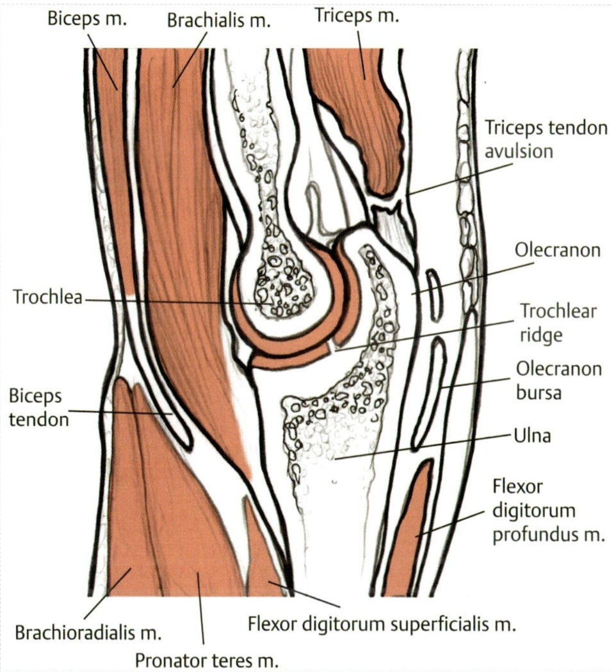

Fig. 2.13 A sagittal illustration of the elbow at the ulnotrochlear articulation showing an avulsion of the distal triceps tendon near its insertion. (Reproduced with permission from Dunleavy JD, Khanna AJ, Carrino JA. Normal MRI Anatomy of the Musculoskeletal System. In: Khanna AJ, ed. MRI for orthopaedic surgeons. New York: Thieme; 2010:17–76.)

lateral, or posterior). Both classification schemes are acceptable, although individual radiologists or clinicians may have a preference; it may be helpful to review both classification schemes.

2.3.2 Muscle Classification by Location

There are seven superficial muscles within the dorsal aspect of the proximal forearm:

- Extensor carpi radialis brevis.
- Extensor carpi radialis longus.
- Brachioradialis.
- Extensor digitorum.
- Extensor digiti minimi.
- Extensor carpi ulnaris (ECU).
- Anconeus (not always present).

Five superficial muscles are found within the volar aspect of the proximal forearm:

- Pronator teres.
- Flexor carpi radialis.
- Flexor carpi ulnaris.
- Flexor digitorum superficialis.
- Palmaris longus (absent in approximately 15% of the population[9]).

In the proximal forearm, there is only one superficial muscle within the dorsal aspect, the supinator, and one deep muscle within the volar aspect, the flexor digitorum profundus (for the superficial and deep muscles within the distal forearm, see section "Wrist/Hand").

2.3.3 Muscle Classification by Compartment

The anterior compartment of the forearm contains the following five muscles:

- Pronator teres.
- Flexor carpi radialis.
- Flexor digitorum superficialis.
- Flexor carpi ulnaris.
- Flexor digitorum profundus.

There are four muscles in the lateral compartment of the forearm:

- Brachioradialis.
- Extensor carpi radialis longus.
- Extensor carpi radialis brevis.
- Extensor digitorum.

Two muscles are found in the posterior compartment of the forearm:

- Anconeus.
- ECU.

Tendons, Ligaments, and Neurovascular Structures

It is helpful to identify the origin and insertion sites of forearm tendons that involve the elbow because these locations are often the sites of tears and avulsions. Medially, the common flexor tendon is seen on axial images in cross-section as an ovoid, low-signal-intensity structure originating from the medial epicondyle of the humerus (▶ Fig. 2.14). It is shared by several superficial flexor muscles in the forearm:

- Pronator teres.
- Flexor carpi radialis.
- Palmaris longus.
- Flexor digitorum superficialis.
- Flexor carpi ulnaris.

Not surprisingly, given their shared origin at the medial epicondyle via the common flexor tendon, the pronator teres and flexor carpi radialis are both involved in medial epicondylitis.

The medial epicondyle is not only the origin of the common flexor tendon, but also the origin of the medial collateral ligament (MCL) (or ulnar collateral ligament [UCL]). The common flexor tendon is superficial to the MCL, which also attaches to the sublime tubercle, the most proximal and medial portion of the ulna. The sublime tubercle is a helpful landmark, which can be used to easily identify the MCL, especially given that the common flexor tendon and the MCL are similarly low in signal intensity.

The lateral ulnar collateral ligament (LUCL) and radial collateral ligament (RCL) are low-signal-intensity structures originating along the lateral epicondyle in the lateral compartment of the elbow (▶ Fig. 2.11). The common extensor tendon is not only located more posteriorly but also attaches to the lateral epicondyle (▶ Fig. 2.14). It is seen in cross-section on axial images and is low in signal intensity. The common extensor tendon is shared by several extensor muscles in the forearm, including the following:

- Extensor digitorum.
- Extensor carpi radialis brevis.
- ECU.
- Extensor digiti minimi.

The anconeus is fairly isolated from other musculature, located posterolateral to the elbow. Normal muscles are usually intermediate in signal intensity, so the isolation of the anconeus from other structures with similar signal intensity makes it more easily identifiable. The anconeus is a short muscle, spanning only the elbow joint, with its origin at the lateral epicondyle and its insertion along the proximal ulna. The anconeus is a weak extensor, but it also functions to tighten the joint capsule. The supinator is also seen in this general region, although it originates directly from the lateral epicondyle and the olecranon, rather than attaching to the lateral epicondyle via the common extensor tendon. The supinator runs along the radius laterally and inserts along the lateral aspect of the proximal radius.

The axial plane allows for evaluation of the neurovascular structures (▶ Fig. 2.15). The median nerve, which lies in close association with the pronator teres and flexor carpi radialis, can often be identified as a thin, intermediate signal structure located between the ulnar and humeral heads of the pronator teres. The brachial artery, seen in close association with the origin of the pronator teres, lies lateral to the median nerve.

The ulnar nerve is well visualized posterior to the medial epicondyle within the cubital tunnel (▶ Fig. 2.14), just deep to the cubital tunnel retinaculum, where it is surrounded by high-signal fat on non–fat-suppressed images. The ulnar nerve is normally intermediate in signal intensity. Although not present in most individuals, the anconeus epitrochlearis muscle is a normal variant structure that may overlie the cubital tunnel

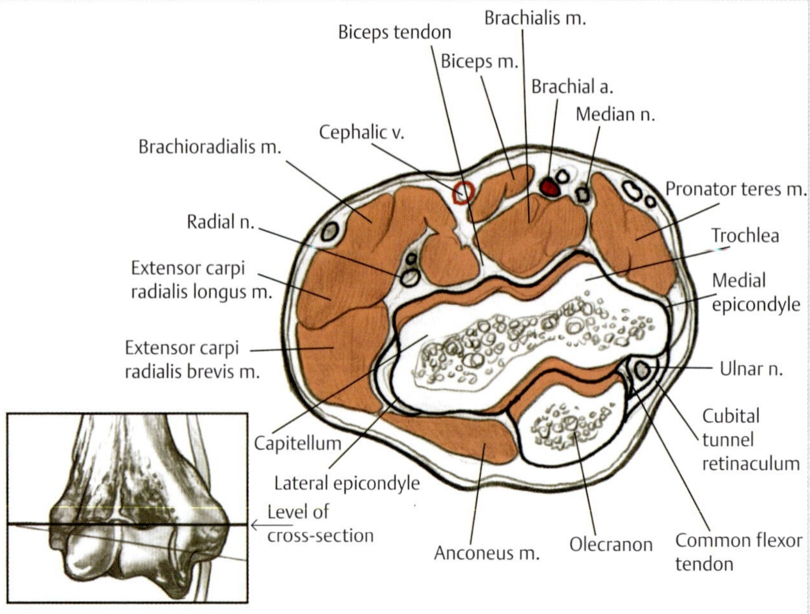

Fig. 2.14 An axial illustration of the elbow at the level of the medial and lateral epicondyles (see inset) showing the radial and ulnar nerves and the common flexor and common extensor tendons. (Reproduced with permission from Dunleavy JD, Khanna AJ, Carrino JA. Normal MRI Anatomy of the Musculoskeletal System. In: Khanna AJ, ed. MRI for orthopaedic surgeons. New York: Thieme; 2010:17–76.)

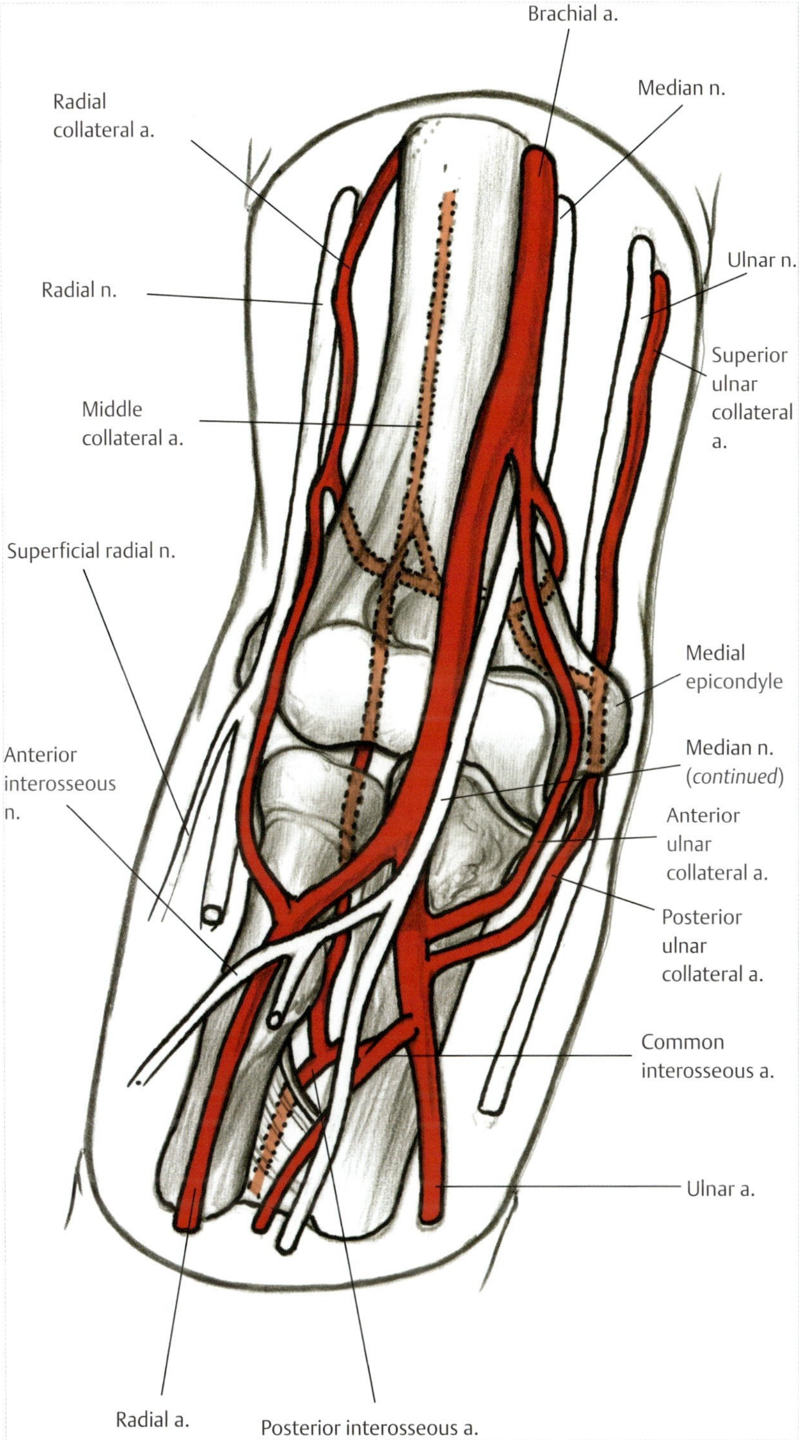

Fig. 2.15 An anterior 3D illustration of the neurovascular structures about the right elbow. (Reproduced with permission from Dunleavy JD, Khanna AJ, Carrino JA. Normal MRI Anatomy of the Musculoskeletal System. In: Khanna AJ, ed. MRI for orthopaedic surgeons. New York: Thieme; 2010:17–76.)

and ulnar nerve, extending from the posterior aspect of the medial epicondyle to the medial aspect of the ulna. Proximal to the elbow, the ulnar nerve is located along the medial border of the triceps muscle. Distal to the elbow, the ulnar nerve is seen between the two heads of the flexor carpi ulnaris muscle.

The radial nerve runs between the brachioradialis and brachialis muscles. At the level of the biceps myotendinous junction, the radial nerve can be seen dividing into its superficial and deep branches within the radial tunnel (▶ Fig. 2.12). The posterior interosseous nerve (deep branch of the radial nerve) is located between the two origins of the supinator. The median nerve lies centrally but is difficult to distinguish from the adjacent brachial vessels.

2.3.4 Coronal Images

Coronal images of the elbow are obtained in a plane parallel to the interepicondylar line. Although the common flexor and

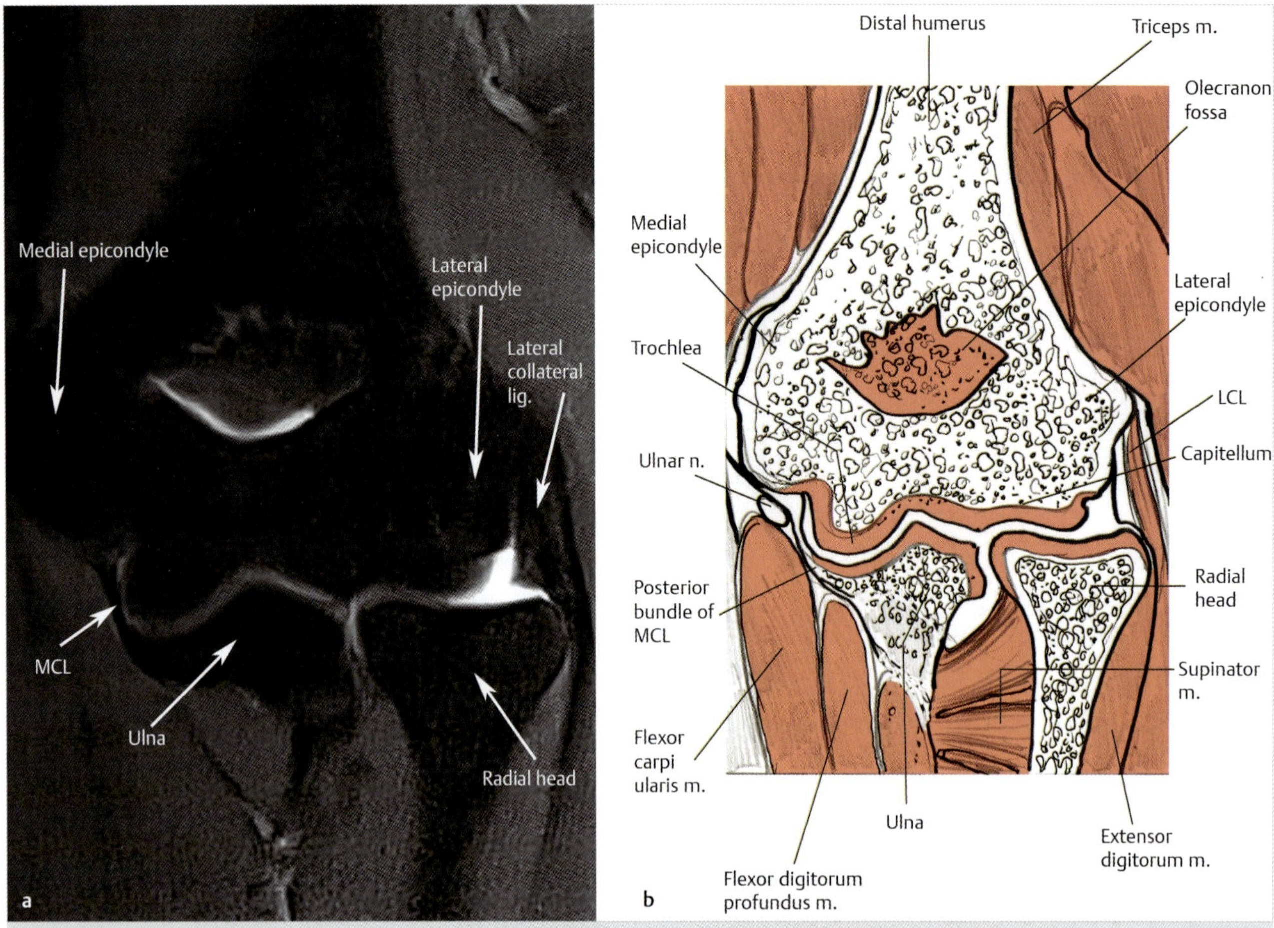

Fig. 2.16 A coronal proton-density fat-suppressed image **(a)** and artist's sketch **(b)** of the left elbow showing the medial collateral ligament (MCL) and lateral collateral ligament (LCL) in the long axis at the level of the radiocapitellar and ulnotrochlear articulations. (Reproduced with permission from Dunleavy JD, Khanna AJ, Carrino JA. Normal MRI Anatomy of the Musculoskeletal System. In: Khanna AJ, ed. MRI for orthopaedic surgeons. New York: Thieme; 2010:17–76.)

common extensor tendons are seen on axial images, these structures are also well visualized in the coronal plane. The collateral ligament complexes (▶ Fig. 2.16) are best evaluated on coronal images. Starting with the medial aspect of the elbow, the common flexor tendon is seen as it arises from the medial epicondyle. Just deep to this tendon, the anterior band of the UCL courses from the distal margin of the medial epicondyle to its attachment on the sublime tubercle of the proximal ulna. The posterior and oblique bands of the UCL are generally not evaluated well on MRI examinations.

The ulnar nerve can be identified posterior to the medial epicondyle and is shown in long axis on the coronal images, allowing for large segments of the ulnar nerve to be visualized on a single image. When evaluating the lateral aspect of the elbow, the common extensor tendon can be identified arising from the lateral epicondyle of the humerus. The RCL lies deep to the common extensor tendon and extends from the anterior aspect of the lateral epicondyle to the radial head, where it inserts onto the annular ligament. The LUCL is also deep to the common flexor tendon but is more posteriorly located relative to the RCL; the LUCL extends from the tubercle of the supinator crest of the ulna to the posterolateral aspect of the radius. The lateral collateral ligament (LCL) complex comprises the following:

- RCL.
- LUCL.
- Annular ligament.

The articular cartilage of the radiocapitellar and ulnotrochlear joints is well visualized in the coronal plane, but a "pseudodefect" is often identified on the capitellum on more posterior coronal images. This appearance in the coronal plane relates to the fact that the surface of the posterior capitellum is not covered with articular cartilage, often resulting in the appearance of a dark, thin line at the junction of the distal humerus and the capitellum; fluid accumulation in this region may accentuate the appearance of a defect because of its high signal intensity. Awareness of the normal appearance of this pseudodefect is critical: the dark line at the junction of the distal humerus and capitellum could otherwise be misinterpreted as an impacted fracture, and the accumulation of fluid in this region could be confused with an OCD. Another area that may mimic a cartilage defect is along the lateral aspect of the radial head, where the articular cartilage is generally thinner than the cartilage in other areas of the elbow.

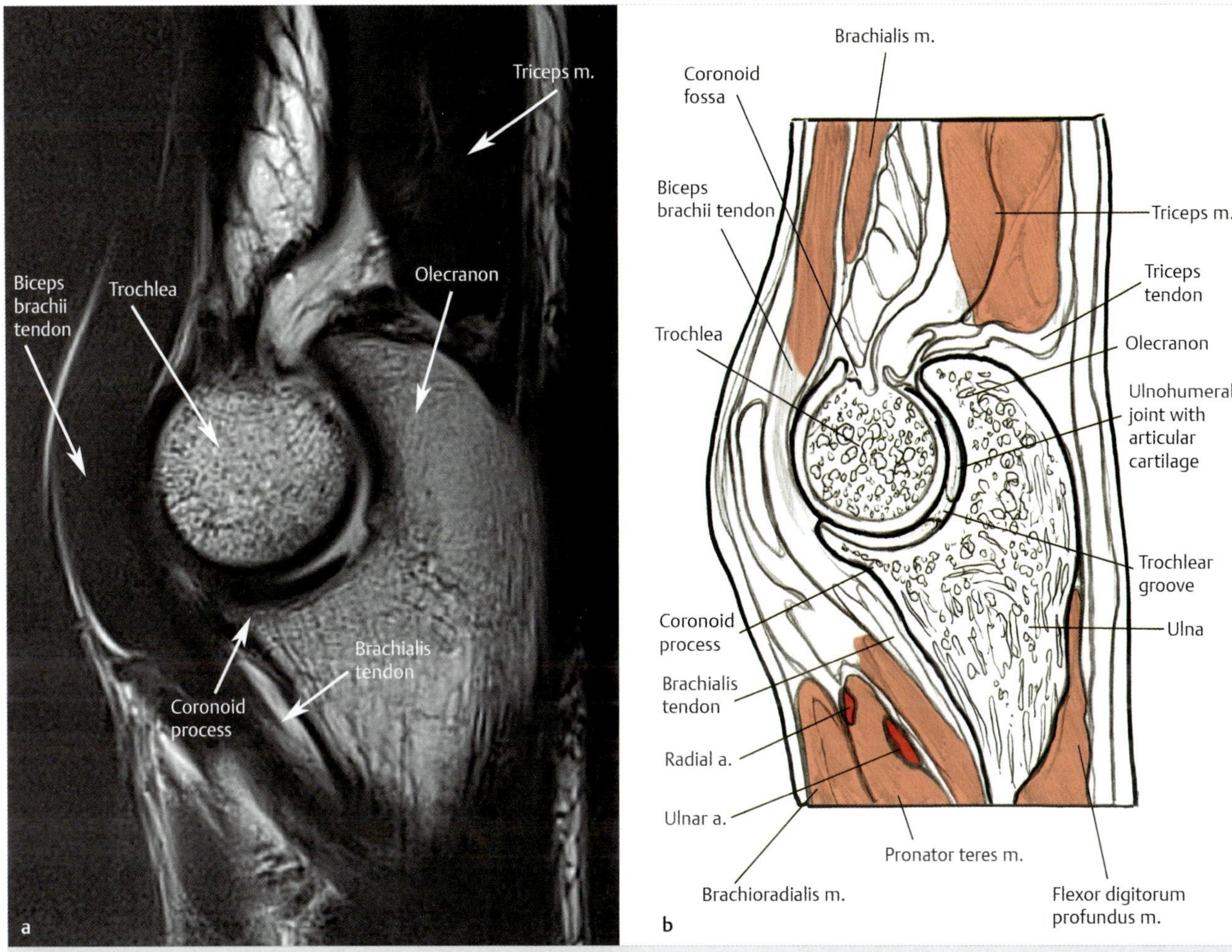

Fig. 2.17 A sagittal T2-weighted image **(a)** and artist's sketch **(b)** of the elbow showing the ulnotrochlear joint and articular cartilage, and the normal appearance of the biceps and triceps muscles in long. (Reproduced with permission from Dunleavy JD, Khanna AJ, Carrino JA. Normal MRI Anatomy of the Musculoskeletal System. In: Khanna AJ, ed. MRI for orthopaedic surgeons. New York: Thieme; 2010:17–76.)

2.3.5 Sagittal Images

The sagittal plane is useful for evaluating osseous architecture and relationships, especially the humerotrochlear and radiocapitellar articulations (▶ Fig. 2.17). Intra-articular bodies are occasionally difficult to identify because they may have signal characteristics similar to those of joint fluid. The brachialis muscle can be followed to its insertion on the ulnar tuberosity and is seen just anterior to the joint capsule. The biceps muscle can be followed distally to its tendinous insertion on the radial tuberosity. The triceps is best seen on the midline image as it inserts onto the olecranon. Each of these structures can usually be visualized on several images in the sagittal plane. The lateral images show the components of the common axis. The normal appearance of the trochlear groove as shown should not be misinterpreted as a cartilaginous defect. Extensor tendon originating from the lateral epicondyle and the medial images show the components of the common flexor tendon originating from the medial epicondyle. In the sagittal plane, the ulnar nerve is often well visualized running posterior to the medial epicondyle. The common flexor tendon lies in close association with the ulnar nerve, and both structures can often be visualized on the same sagittal image.

2.4 Wrist/Hand

2.4.1 Axial Images

The best use of axial images is for evaluating the median and ulnar nerves (▶ Fig. 2.18) and the contents of the carpal tunnel and Guyon canal. In addition, the flexor and extensor tendons crossing the wrist joint are best visualized in this plane (▶ Fig. 2.19). Many of the muscles in the forearm exert force not only on the elbow but also on the wrist and hand. Muscles in the distal forearm can be classified by location (superficial or deep).

There are five superficial muscles in the dorsal aspect of the distal forearm:

- Extensor carpi radialis brevis.
- Extensor carpi radialis longus.
- Extensor digitorum.
- Extensor digiti minimi.
- ECU.

Four superficial muscles are found in the distal forearm:

- Flexor carpi radialis.
- Flexor carpi ulnaris.

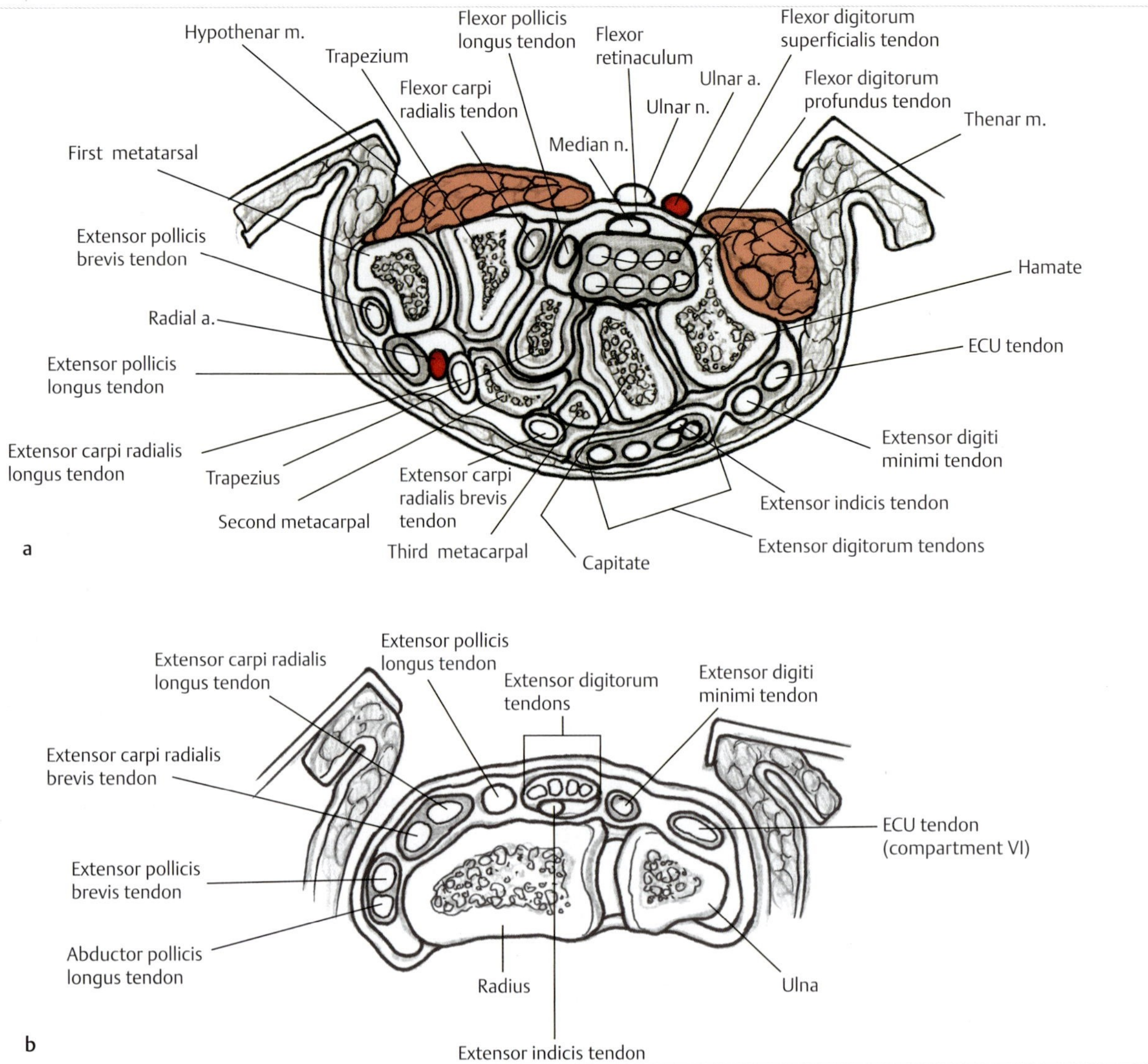

Fig. 2.18 Axial illustrations of the musculotendinous units and neurovascular structures of the wrist with retraction of the skin and subcutaneous tissues along the volar **(a)** and dorsal **(b)** aspect of the wrist. Abbreviations: ECU, extensor carpi ulnari. (Reproduced with permission from Dunleavy JD, Khanna AJ, Carrino JA. Normal MRI Anatomy of the Musculoskeletal System. In: Khanna AJ, ed. MRI for orthopaedic surgeons. New York: Thieme; 2010:17–76.)

- Flexor digitorum superficialis.
- Palmaris longus (not always present).

There are four deep muscles in the dorsal aspect of the distal forearm:

- Abductor pollicis longus.
- Extensor pollicis brevis.
- Extensor pollicis longus.
- Extensor indicis.

Three deep muscles are found in the volar aspect of the distal forearm:

- Flexor digitorum profundus.
- Flexor pollicis longus..
- Pronator quadratus.

The flexor carpi radialis originates from the common flexor tendon at the medial epicondyle and inserts on the base of the second and third metacarpals. The muscle belly of the flexor carpi radialis is intermediate in signal intensity, and its tendon should be low in signal intensity. The palmaris longus lies medial to the flexor carpi radialis, originating from the common flexor tendon at the medial epicondyle and inserting along the flexor retinaculum and palmar aponeurosis. Both the flexor retinaculum and palmar aponeurosis are seen as dark bands within the superficial palmar aspect of the wrist. The flexor carpi ulnaris originates from the common flexor tendon and the olecranon; inserts on the fifth metacarpal, hamate, and pisiform; and lies in close association with the ulnar nerve, which is seen as a thin, intermediate signal intensity structure running just deep and lateral to the flexor carpi ulnaris (► Fig. 2.20).

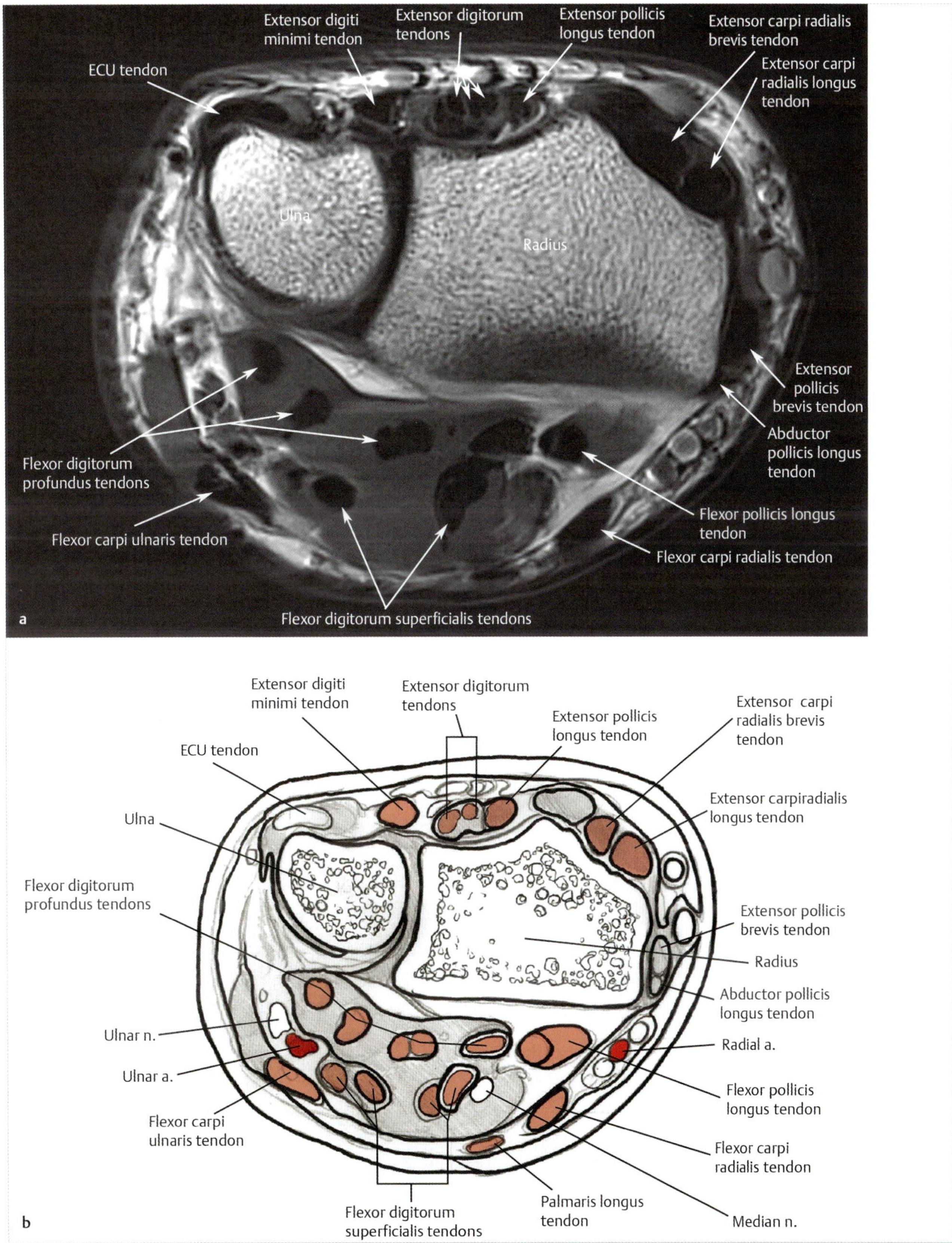

Fig. 2.19 An axial proton-density image **(a)** and artist's sketch **(b)** of the wrist, proximal to the carpal tunnel, showing the large, low-signal-intensity musculotendinous units along the volar and dorsal aspects of the left distal forearm. Abbreviations: ECU, extensor carpi ulnari. (Reproduced with permission from Dunleavy JD, Khanna AJ, Carrino JA. Normal MRI Anatomy of the Musculoskeletal System. In: Khanna AJ, ed. MRI for orthopaedic surgeons. New York: Thieme; 2010:17–76.)

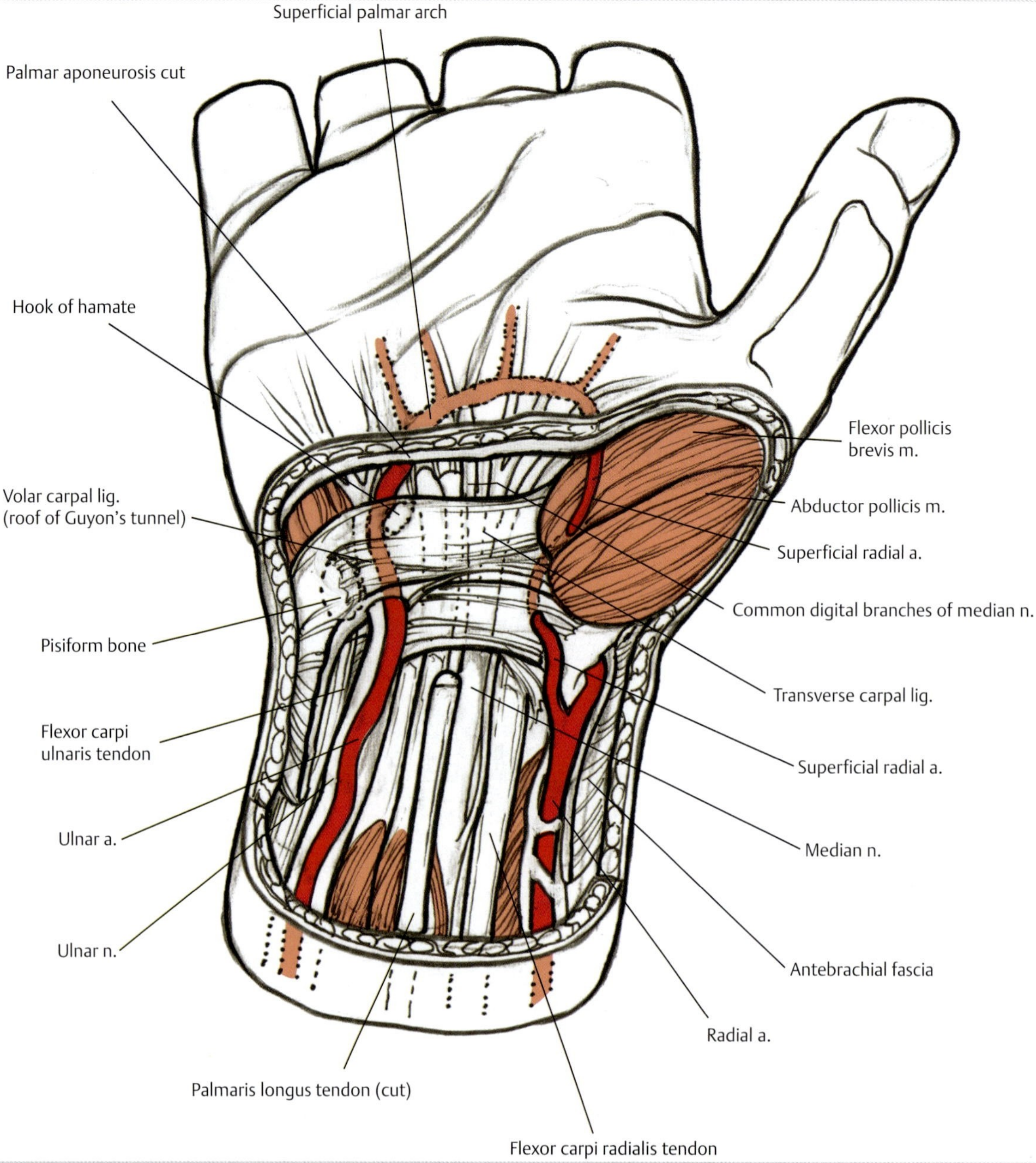

Fig. 2.20 A 3D illustration of the volar aspect of the dissected right wrist and hand, revealing the neurovascular structures, including the ulnar and median nerves and ulnar and radial arteries. (Reproduced with permission from Dunleavy JD, Khanna AJ, Carrino JA. Normal MRI Anatomy of the Musculoskeletal System. In: Khanna AJ, ed. MRI for orthopaedic surgeons. New York: Thieme; 2010:17–76.)

The flexor digitorum superficialis originates at the medial epicondyle, coronoid process, and radial head. It inserts along the volar aspect of the middle phalanx of each finger (▶ Fig. 2.21). Proximal to its insertions, the flexor digitorum superficialis divides into four musculotendinous units within the distal forearm, before entering the carpal tunnel. Within the carpal tunnel, the median nerve most often lies immediately superficial to the flexor digitorum superficialis tendons (▶ Fig. 2.18, ▶ Fig. 2.19, ▶ Fig. 2.20), although it may have an intertendinous position. However, within the forearm, the median nerve lies immediately deep to the flexor digitorum superficialis muscle. The large, dark musculotendinous units of the flexor digitorum superficialis are easily identified as they converge within the forearm to enter the carpal tunnel. In contrast to the large, low-signal-intensity musculotendinous units of the flexor digitorum superficialis, the median nerve is a thinner structure with intermediate signal intensity, which can be more challenging to identify. Thus, the musculotendinous units of the flexor digitorum superficialis may be used as a landmark for the adjacent median nerve. The flexor digitorum profundus (▶ Fig. 2.22) originates from the anteromedial aspect of the ulnar and interosseous membrane and inserts along the distal phalanges of each finger (▶ Fig. 2.21). As does the flexor digitorum

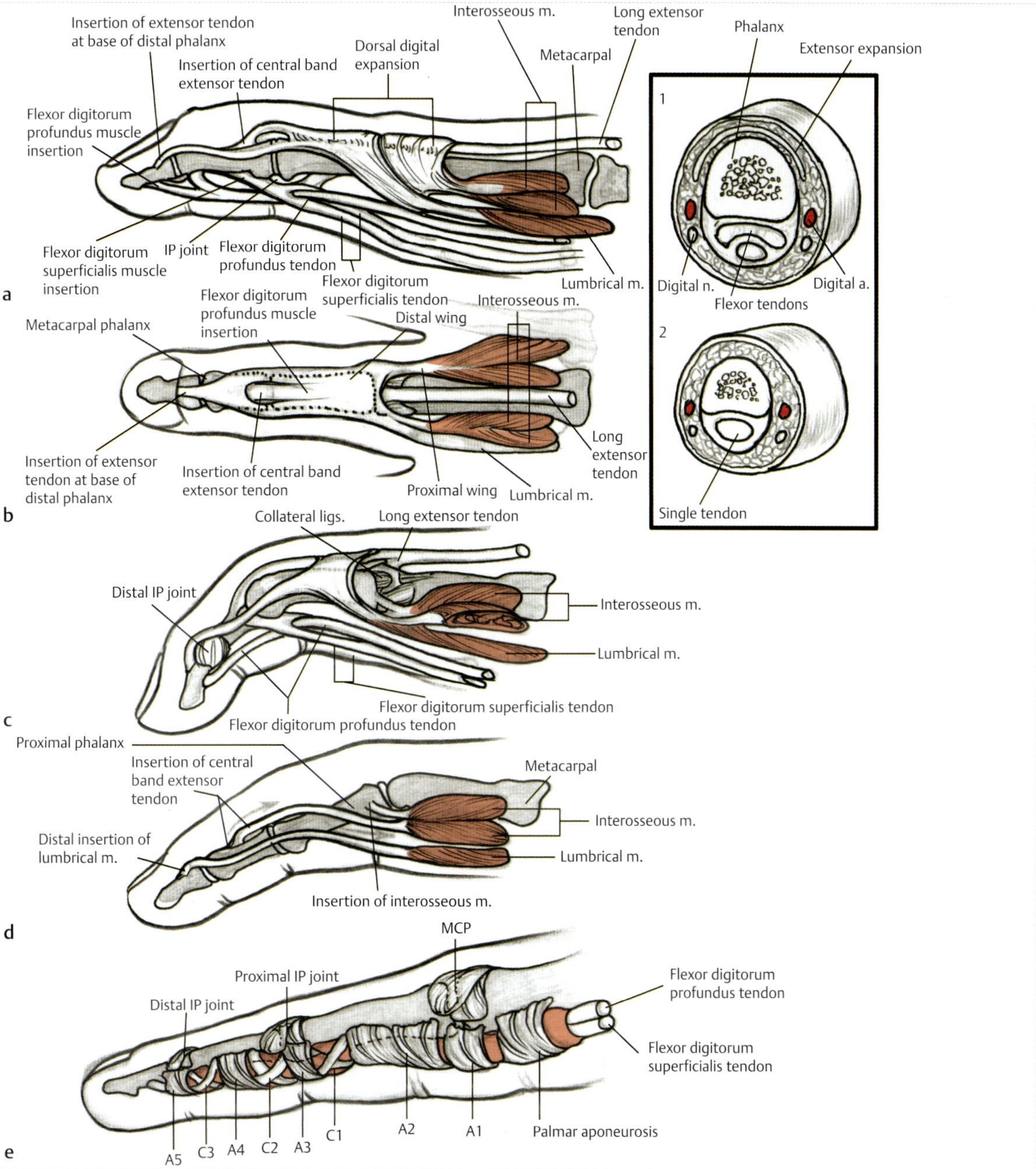

Fig. 2.21 Multiview illustrations of the muscles and ligaments in the fingers: **(a)** lateral superficial, **(b)** dorsal superficial, **(c)** lateral superficial in flexion, **(d)** lateral deep, and **(e)** pulley system (numbers and letters designate specific pulleys). *Inset*: axial cross-section through the middle (*1*) and distal (*2*) phalanxes. Abbreviations: IP, Interphalangeal; MCP, metacarpophalangeal. (Reproduced with permission from Dunleavy JD, Khanna AJ, Carrino JA. Normal MRI Anatomy of the Musculoskeletal System. In: Khanna AJ, ed. MRI for orthopaedic surgeons. New York: Thieme; 2010:17–76.)

superficialis, the flexor digitorum profundus divides into four musculotendinous units within the forearm before entering the carpal tunnel. Within the carpal tunnel, the tendons of the flexor digitorum profundus lie immediately deep to the tendons of the flexor digitorum superficialis and are easy to identify based on this predictable relationship. The flexor pollicis longus originates from the coronoid process of the ulna, the midradius, and the interosseous membrane. It inserts along the volar aspect of the base of the distal phalanx of the thumb. The pronator quadratus originates from the volar aspect of the distal ulna and inserts along the volar aspect of the distal radius.

The extensor carpi radialis longus originates along the supracondylar ridge of the humerus and the lateral intermuscular septum. It inserts along the dorsal aspect of the second (index finger) metacarpal base. The extensor carpi radialis brevis originates from the common extensor tendon at the lateral epicondyle and inserts at the dorsal aspect of the third metacarpal base. The extensor digitorum (▶ Fig. 2.18) originates from the common extensor tendon

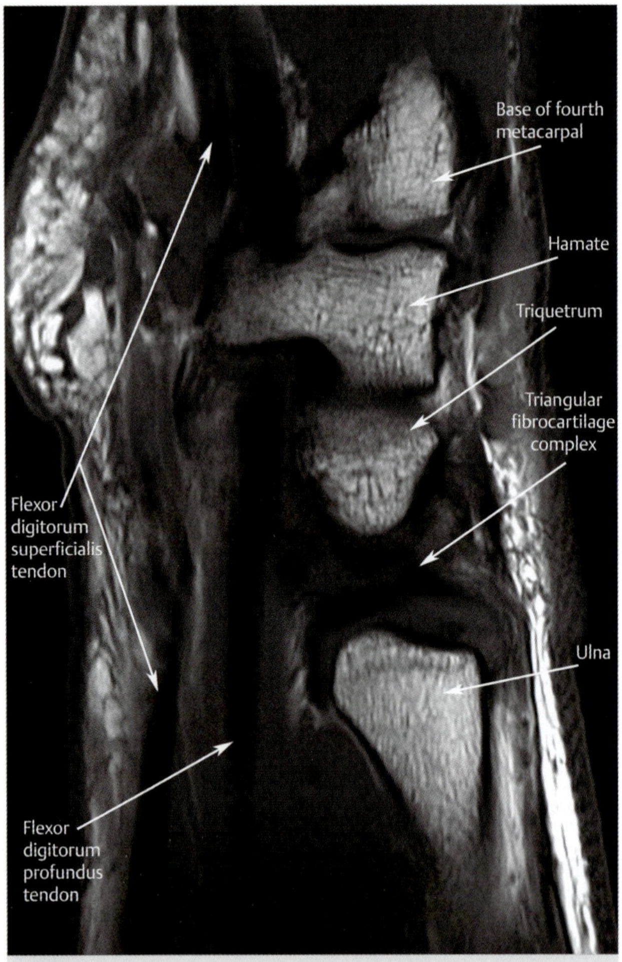

Fig. 2.22 A sagittal T1-weighted image of the wrist showing the normal appearance of the flexor digitorum profundus and flexor digitorum superficialis tendons, as well as the triangular fibrocartilage. (Reproduced with permission from Dunleavy JD, Khanna AJ, Carrino JA. Normal MRI Anatomy of the Musculoskeletal System. In: Khanna AJ, ed. MRI for orthopaedic surgeons. New York: Thieme; 2010:17–76.)

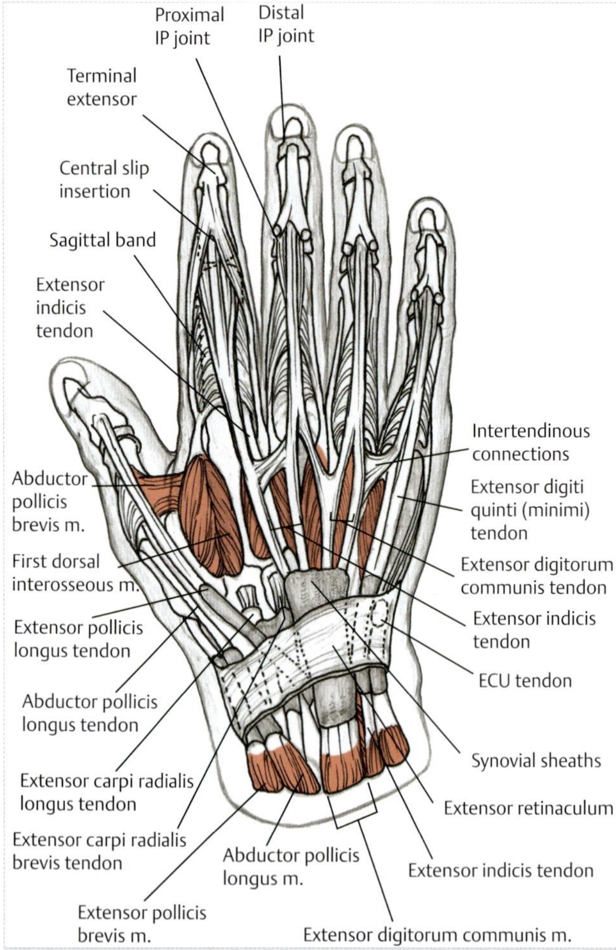

Fig. 2.23 Illustration of the dorsal aspect of the right hand showing the muscles and tendons. Abbreviations: IP, Interphalangeal; ECU, extensor carpi ulnaris. (Reproduced with permission from Dunleavy JD, Khanna AJ, Carrino JA. Normal MRI Anatomy of the Musculoskeletal System. In: Khanna AJ, ed. MRI for orthopaedic surgeons. New York: Thieme; 2010:17–76.)

at the lateral epicondyle and inserts along the dorsal aspect of each finger (digits 2 through 5) (▶ Fig. 2.21). The extensor digiti minimi (▶ Fig. 2.23) originates from the common extensor tendon at the lateral epicondyle and inserts along the dorsal aspect of the fifth digit. The extensor digiti minimi runs immediately superficial to the radioulnar joint. The ECU originates from the dorsal aspect of the mid-ulna and from the lateral epicondyle. It inserts at the base of the fifth metacarpal. Proximal to its insertion, it can be seen coursing along the groove of the distal ulna. The pisiform is actually a sesamoid bone within the ECU. The triangular fibrocartilage complex (TFCC) is composed of the following:

- Fibrocartilaginous articular disk.
- Dorsal and volar radioulnar ligaments.
- Ulnolunate ligament.
- Ulnotriquetral ligament.
- UCL.
- ECU subsheath.
- A variable meniscus homologue.

The abductor pollicis longus originates from the dorsal aspect of the proximal third of the radius and ulna and from the interosseous membrane. It inserts at the dorsal aspect of the first metacarpal base. The extensor pollicis brevis originates at the posterior aspect of the distal third of the radius and the interosseous membrane. It inserts at the dorsal aspect of the base of the proximal phalanx of the thumb, forms the lateral margin of the anatomic snuff box, and runs in close association with the abductor pollicis longus. These tendons run deep to the extensor retinaculum at the level of the distal radial groove (▶ Fig. 2.23). The extensor retinaculum is seen in the dorsal aspect of the wrist as a thin, dark band immediately deep to the subcutaneous tissues, which are very bright on non–fat-suppressed images. The extensor pollicis longus originates from the posterior aspect of the mid-ulna and the interosseous membrane, and it inserts at the dorsal aspect of the base of the distal phalanx of the thumb. The extensor indicis originates from the posterior aspect of the distal ulna and the interosseous membrane, and it inserts at the dorsal aspect of the second digit

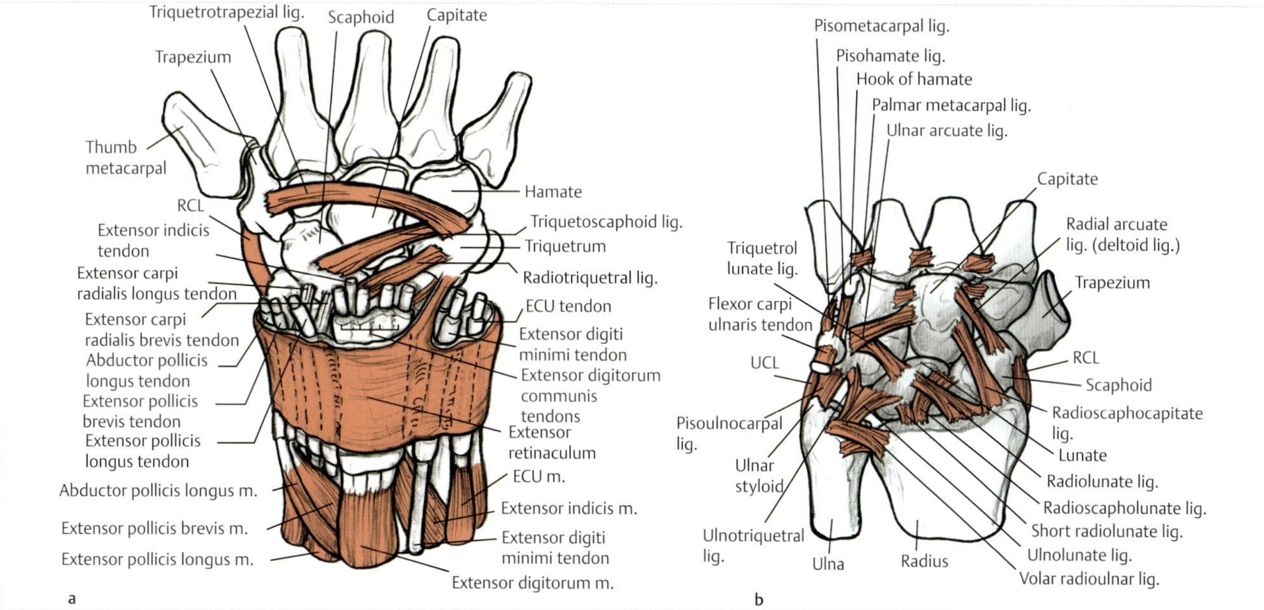

Fig. 2.24 Illustrations of the wrist showing the dorsal **(a)** and volar **(b)** aspects of the left distal radius and ulna, carpal bones, musculotendinous units, and intercarpal ligaments. Abbreviations: RCL, radial collateral ligament; UCL, ulnar collateral ligament; ECU, extensor carpi ulnaris. (Reproduced with permission from Dunleavy JD, Khanna AJ, Carrino JA. Normal MRI Anatomy of the Musculoskeletal System. In: Khanna AJ, ed. MRI for orthopaedic surgeons. New York: Thieme; 2010:17–76.)

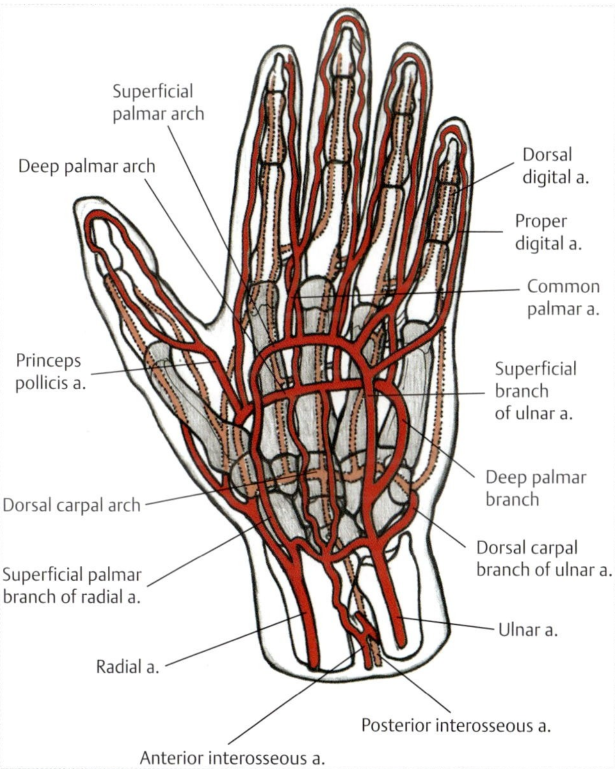

Fig. 2.25 A 3D illustration of the volar (*red*) and dorsal (*pink*) vasculature in the left wrist and hand. (Reproduced with permission from Dunleavy JD, Khanna AJ, Carrino JA. Normal MRI Anatomy of the Musculoskeletal System. In: Khanna AJ, ed. MRI for orthopaedic surgeons. New York: Thieme; 2010:17–76.)

(index finger). The abductor pollicis brevis originates at the scaphoid, trapezius, and flexor retinaculum. It inserts at the base of the proximal phalanx of the thumb. Unlike the other muscles described in this section, the abductor pollicis brevis has no function at the wrist joint, and thus is considered a hand muscle.

In the axial plane, the distal radioulnar joint is examined at the sigmoid notch of the radius. Particular osseous structures, such as the hook of the hamate, and the articulations between carpal bones can be assessed on axial images. The extrinsic carpal ligaments (▶ Fig. 2.24), seen as uniformly low-signal-intensity structures in close relationship with the wrist capsule, may be accentuated with intra-articular contrast. Axial images of the digits provide cross-sectional visualization of small anatomic structures such as the flexor tendons, extensor mechanism, volar plates, and neurovascular bundles (▶ Fig. 2.21, ▶ Fig. 2.25).

2.4.2 Coronal Images

Coronal plane images provide useful anatomic information about the wrist and hand, and show well the osseous structures and their respective relationships (▶ Fig. 2.26). Small structures such as the scapholunate and lunotriquetral ligaments are usually best seen on coronal images, and with thin sections; these structures are routinely well delineated. The radiocarpal compartment is separated from the radioulnar joint by the triangular fibrocartilage. Most information about the triangular fibrocartilage is also gained from coronal images. The triangular fibrocartilage looks like a curvilinear bowtie, and it extends horizontally from the ulnar surface of the distal radius to the base of the ulnar styloid process. It is

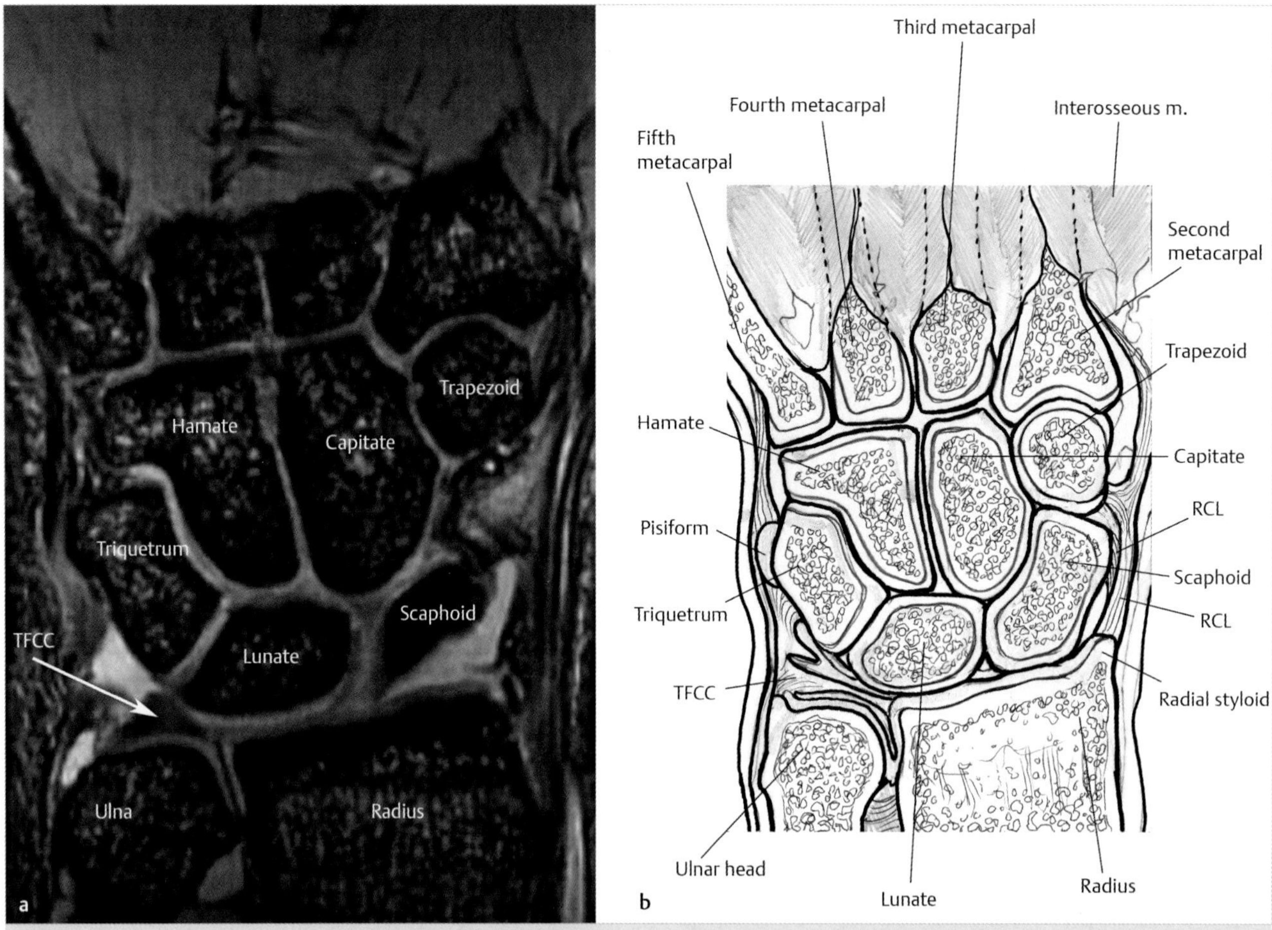

Fig. 2.26 A coronal T2*-weighted image **(a)** and artist's sketch **(b)** of the wrist at the level of the triangular fibrocartilage complex (TFCC). The carpal bone architecture is well delineated on this image, which was acquired on a high field strength magnet with an eight-channel surface coil. Abbreviations: RCL, radial collateral ligament. (Reproduced with permission from Dunleavy JD, Khanna AJ, Carrino JA. Normal MRI Anatomy of the Musculoskeletal System. In: Khanna AJ, ed. MRI for orthopaedic surgeons. New York: Thieme; 2010:17–76.)

low in signal intensity. In the coronal plane, the triangular fibrocartilage and interosseous ligaments are often seen on the same sections as the ECU tendon. Within the hand, the ligaments of the interphalangeal (IP) and metacarpophalangeal (MCP) joints (in particular, the UCL of the thumb) are most readily assessed in this plane. However, thumb imaging should be performed separately with specialized planes. The abductor pollicis longus and extensor pollicis brevis tendons are seen within the medial/volar aspect of the wrist at the level of the volar aspect of the scaphoid and lunate. Also within the volar aspect of the wrist are the radioscaphocapitate ligament and the radiolunotriquetral ligament, which extend in the ulnar direction from the radial styloid. Located slightly ulnar to these ligaments is the radioscapholunate ligament (▸ Fig. 2.24). These three carpal ligaments are low in signal intensity and are often seen on the same image in the coronal plane.

Despite the advantages of coronal images for evaluation of the TFCC and intercarpal ligaments, the variable courses of the tendons and neurovascular structures crossing the wrist and hand joints make evaluation of these structures difficult in the coronal plane, and therefore these structures are primarily assessed on axial images. On the dorsal coronal images, the extensor digiti minimi tendon is seen as it courses obliquely along the ulnar side of the triquetrum. The extensor pollicis longus and the extensor carpi radialis brevis are separated by Lister tubercle, which shows fatty marrow signal intensity. On the volar coronal images, the flexor tendons are seen coursing deep to the flexor retinaculum, which appears as a dark, transverse band. The flexor tendons appear as hypointense bands and can be followed as they pass through the carpal tunnel between the trapezium and the hook of the hamate. The median nerve is intermediate in signal, slightly brighter than that of the adjacent tendons.

The radial and ulnar styloid may be evaluated for fractures on coronal images. The joints, including the distal radioulnar, radiocarpal, intercarpal, and carpometacarpal joints, can also be evaluated for degenerative or traumatic changes. The articular surfaces of the carpal bones show intermediate signal intensity.

2.4.3 Sagittal Images

The sagittal plane is useful for depicting the longitudinal course of structures and providing an orthogonal section for bones in the wrist and hand. Information from sagittal images can be used to evaluate the TFCC (▶ Fig. 2.22) and overall carpal alignment, especially with regard to the scapholunate and capitolunate articulations (▶ Fig. 2.27, ▶ Fig. 2.28). Deformity of the scaphoid and abnormalities of the pisotriquetral joint are also examined in this plane. Fractures of the other carpal bones, including the hook of the hamate and the lunate, are also well visualized. The course of the flexor and extensor tendons is well shown on sagittal images of the digits, as is the course of the median nerve in the wrist.

2.5 Hip

2.5.1 Axial Images

The hip (femoroacetabulum), a diarthrodial joint, is an articulation between the acetabulum and the head of the femur (▶ Fig. 2.29). The acetabulum is formed by the union of the ilium, ischium, and pubis; is normally oriented approximately 45 degrees caudally; and has between 14 and 26.5 degrees of anteversion (averages: men, 18.5 ± 4.5 degrees; women, 21.5 ± 5.0 degrees).[10] The normal femoral neck–shaft angle ranges between 125 and 140 degrees.[10,11] Given the complex 3D geometry of the hip joint, MRI of the hip should use all three standard planes of imaging and a specialized plane along (parallel to) the femoral neck. The muscles of the hip can be grouped according to function or anatomic location (medial, anterior, lateral, and posterior). There is no single accepted grouping technique, but some form of a systematic review should be performed. Functional muscle grouping is a logical technique:

- Abductors: gluteus medius, gluteus minimus, and tensor fascia lata.
- Adductors: pectineus, gracilis, adductor longus, adductor brevis, and adductor magnus.
- Flexors: iliopsoas, rectus femoris, sartorius.
- Extensors: gluteus maximus, hamstrings.
- External rotators: piriformis, obturator externus, obturator internus, superior gemelli, inferior gemelli, and quadratus femoris.

Although most of the musculature in the region of the hip is best evaluated on axial images (▶ Fig. 2.30, ▶ Fig. 2.31), the hamstrings and gluteus medius and minimus are more easily evaluated in the coronal plane (▶ Fig. 2.32).

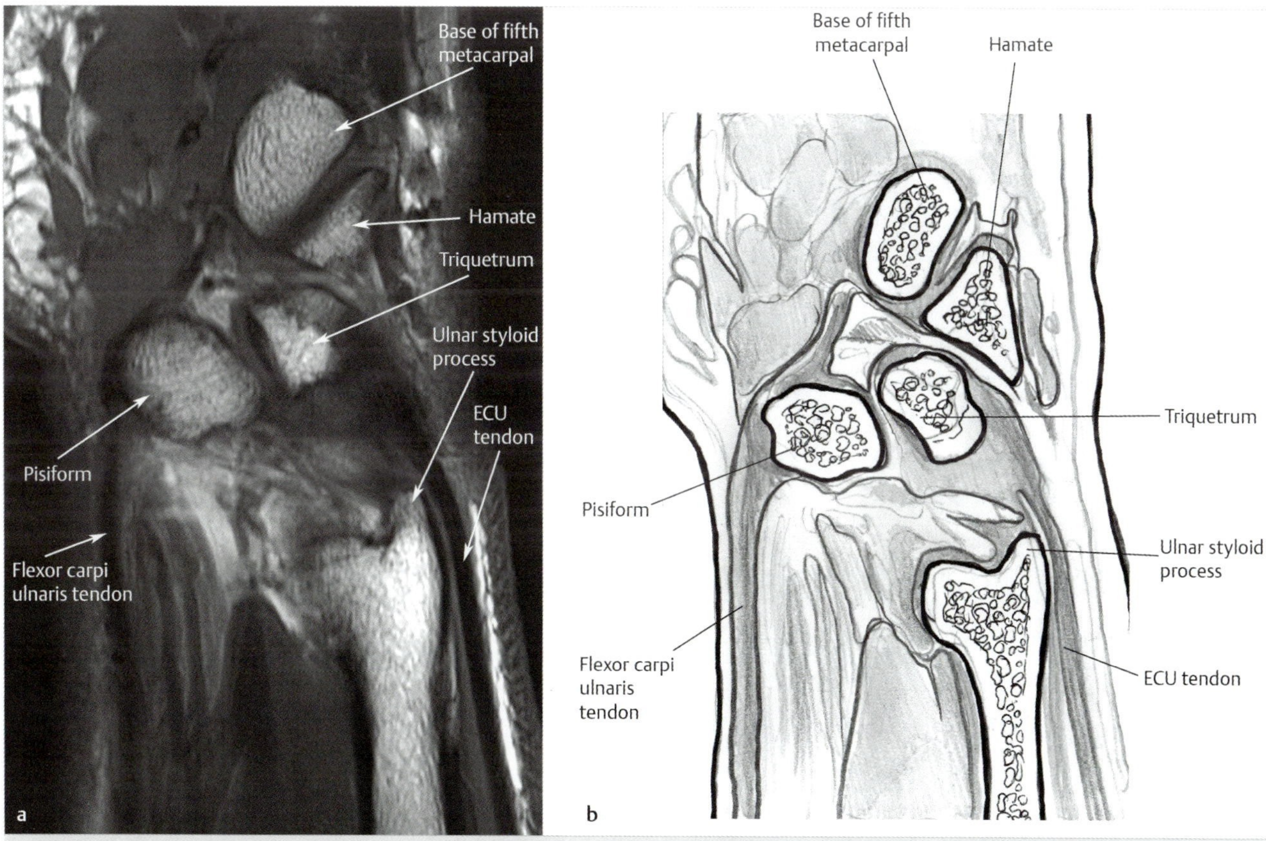

Fig. 2.27 A sagittal T1-weighted image **(a)** and artist's sketch **(b)** of the wrist at the level of the pisiform, showing the flexor and extensor carpi ulnaris (ECU) tendons within the forearm and wrist. (Reproduced with permission from Dunleavy JD, Khanna AJ, Carrino JA. Normal MRI Anatomy of the Musculoskeletal System. In: Khanna AJ, ed. MRI for orthopaedic surgeons. New York: Thieme; 2010:17–76.)

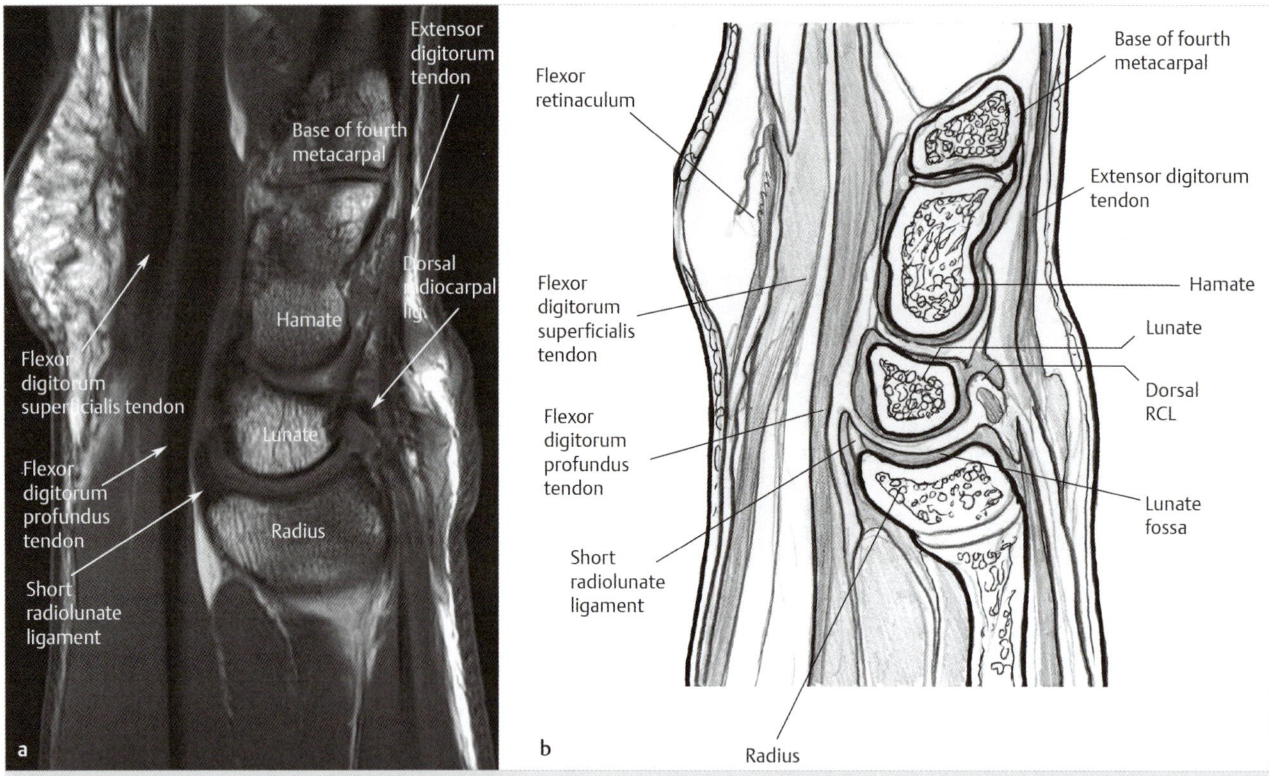

Fig. 2.28 A sagittal T1-weighted image **(a)** and artist's sketch **(b)** of the wrist at the radiolunate articulation showing the normal relationship of the radius, lunate, hamate, and fourth (ring finger) metacarpal. Long segments of the flexor digitorum superficialis and profundus tendons are seen as they pass through the carpal tunnel. (Reproduced with permission from Dunleavy JD, Khanna AJ, Carrino JA. Normal MRI Anatomy of the Musculoskeletal System. In: Khanna AJ, ed. MRI for orthopaedic surgeons. New York: Thieme; 2010:17–76.)

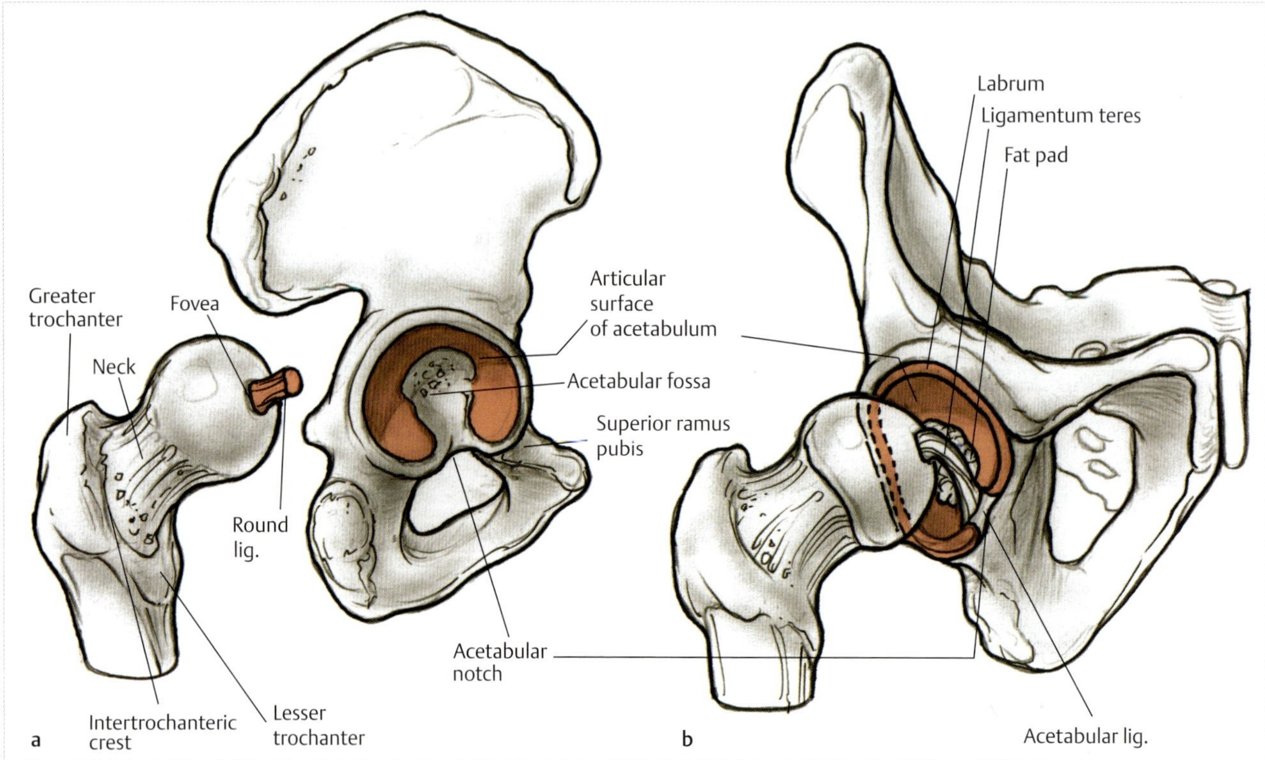

Fig. 2.29 Disarticulated lateral **(a)** and partially disarticulated anterior oblique **(b)** 3D illustrations of the femoroacetabular articular surfaces. (Reproduced with permission from Dunleavy JD, Khanna AJ, Carrino JA. Normal MRI Anatomy of the Musculoskeletal System. In: Khanna AJ, ed. MRI for orthopaedic surgeons. New York: Thieme; 2010:17–76.)

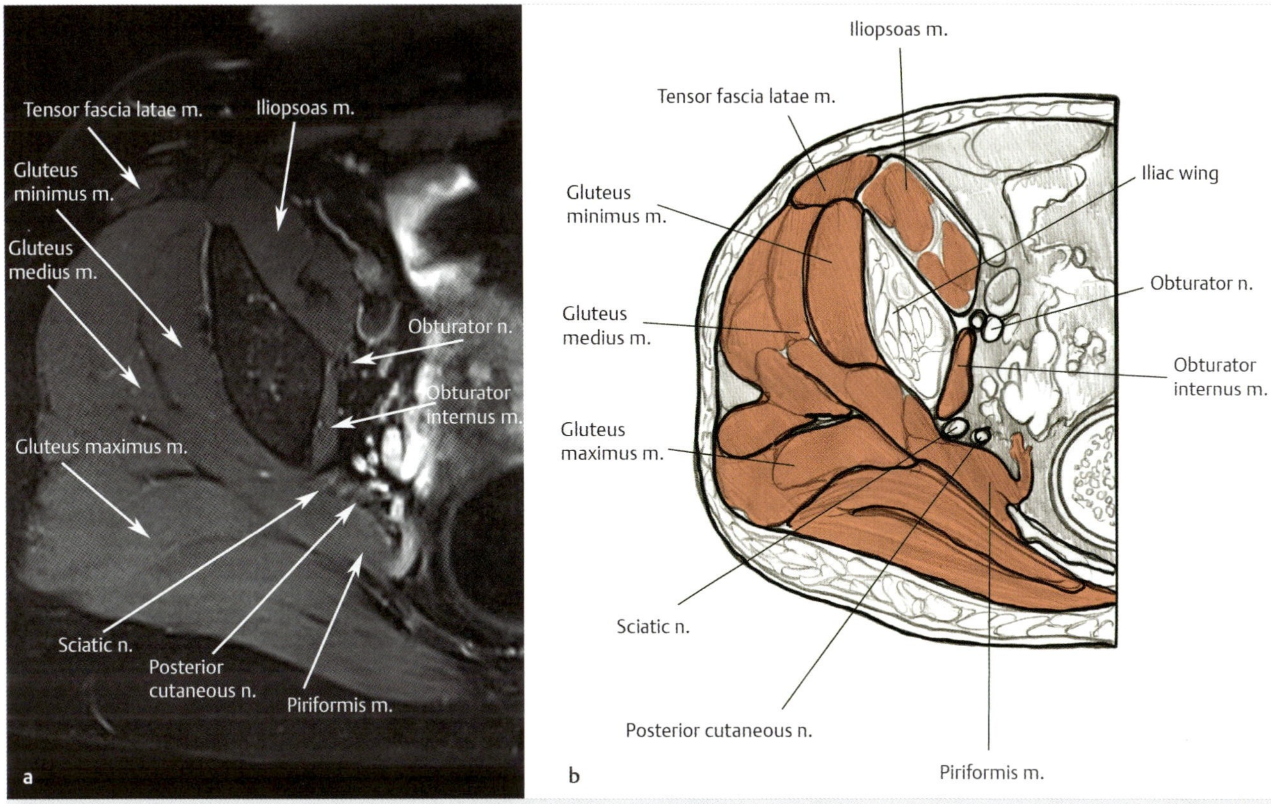

Fig. 2.30 An axial proton-density fat-suppressed image **(a)** and artist's sketch **(b)** of the right hip at the level of the iliac wing, showing the fascial layers separating the gluteus maximus, gluteus medius, and gluteus minimus musculature. The sciatic nerve is also seen. (Reproduced with permission from Dunleavy JD, Khanna AJ, Carrino JA. Normal MRI Anatomy of the Musculoskeletal System. In: Khanna AJ, ed. MRI for orthopaedic surgeons. New York: Thieme; 2010:17–76.)

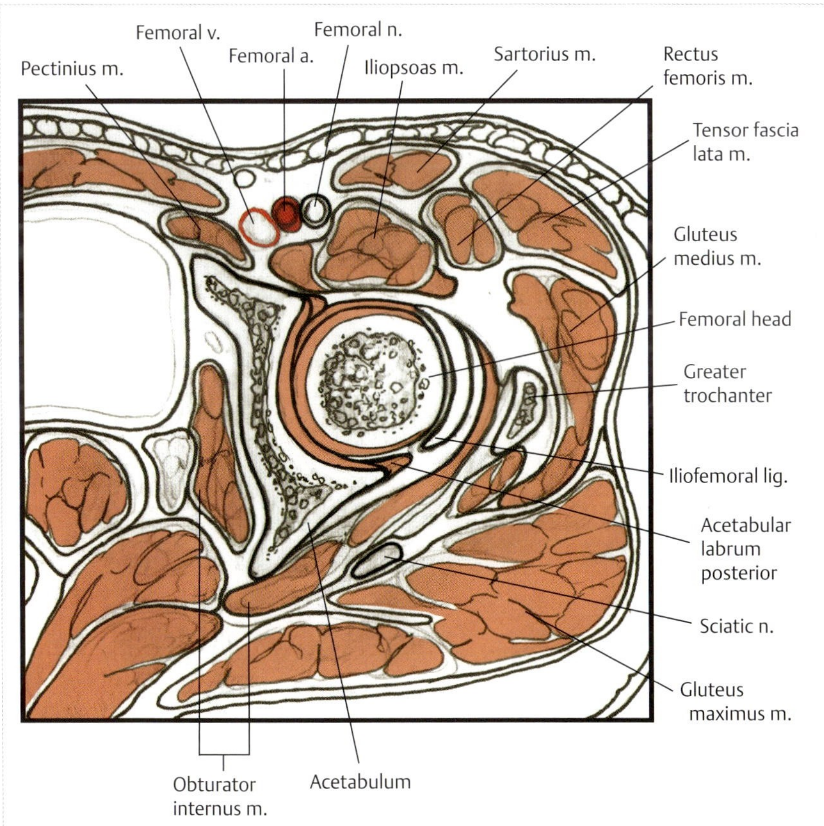

Fig. 2.31 An axial illustration of the left hip at the level of the femoroacetabular joint showing the anterior and posterior labrum, articular cartilage, and surrounding musculature. (Reproduced with permission from Dunleavy JD, Khanna AJ, Carrino JA. Normal MRI Anatomy of the Musculoskeletal System. In: Khanna AJ, ed. MRI for orthopaedic surgeons. New York: Thieme; 2010:17–76.)

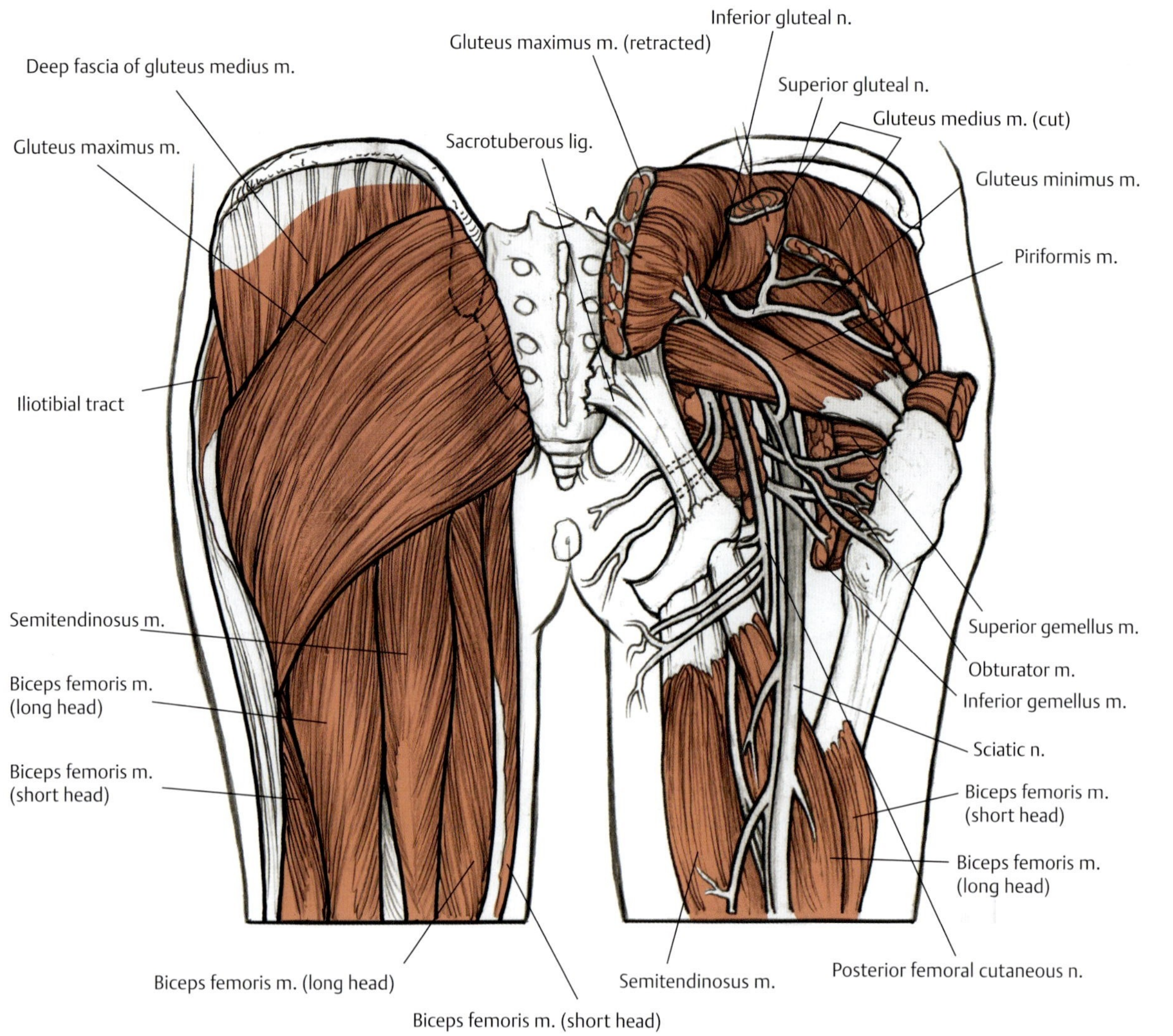

Fig. 2.32 A 3D posteroanterior illustration of the intact and removed musculature of the posterior thigh overlying the sciatic nerve and other neural structures. (Reproduced with permission from Dunleavy JD, Khanna AJ, Carrino JA. Normal MRI Anatomy of the Musculoskeletal System. In: Khanna AJ, ed. MRI for orthopaedic surgeons. New York: Thieme; 2010:17–76.)

Generally, in addition to the conventional axial images, oblique axial images oriented along the axis of the femoral neck are also obtained. These oblique images allow visualization of the head–neck junction and can aid in evaluating anatomy associated with femoroacetabular impingement. Axial images allow for good visualization of the anterior and posterior portions of the labrum (▶ Fig. 2.31), which are seen as low-signal-intensity structures. Axial images are also useful for identifying the regional neurovascular bundles, specifically the sciatic nerve, obturator, and femoral neurovascular bundles; in these bundles, the nerves are seen in cross-section as intermediate signal structures, and often discrete fascicles can be discerned.

The gluteus maximus, gluteus medius, and gluteus minimus can be identified and differentiated by fascial divisions. The tensor fascia latae is located anterior to the gluteus medius (▶ Fig. 2.31). At the level of the inferior pubic ramus, the iliopsoas inserts along the lesser trochanter. The iliotibial band (ITB) is identified laterally. The external iliac vessels are seen anterior to the anterior column of the acetabulum and medial to the iliopsoas muscle.

2.5.2 Coronal Images

The coronal plane is helpful for evaluating the weight-bearing, suprafoveal aspect of the femoral head and acetabular dome (▶ Fig. 2.33), the trochanteric bursa, and the superior labrum (▶ Fig. 2.34). The normal labrum appears as a triangular structure of low signal at the lateral (peripheral) margin of the acetabulum (▶ Fig. 2.35). To view the anterior superior, superior, and posterior superior labrum, images should be examined

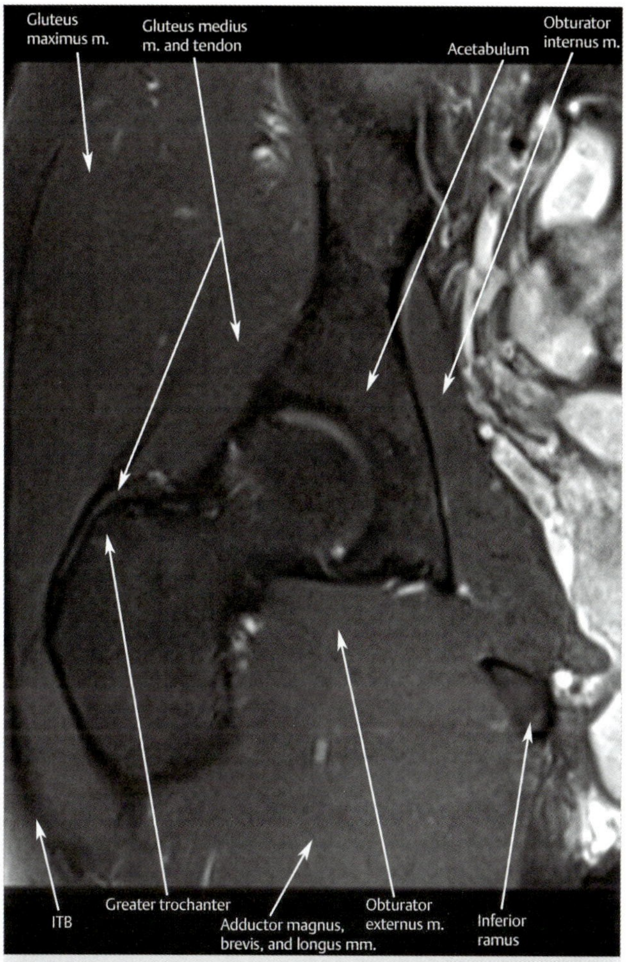

Fig. 2.33 A coronal proton-density image of the right hip showing the suprafoveal aspect of the femoral head and acetabular dome. (Reproduced with permission from Dunleavy JD, Khanna AJ, Carrino JA. Normal MRI Anatomy of the Musculoskeletal System. In: Khanna AJ, ed. MRI for orthopaedic surgeons. New York: Thieme; 2010:17–76.)

successively from anterior to posterior. The inferior portion of the acetabulum is not covered by the labrum and contains the transverse ligament. The joint capsule and capsular ligaments surround the femoral neck and appear as a low-signal-intensity structure.

The trochanteric bursa, the iliopsoas tendon, and the distal insertions of the gluteus medius and minimus tendons onto the greater trochanter are well visualized in the coronal plane. The articular cartilage appears as an intermediate signal overlying the low-signal cortical bone.

2.5.3 Sagittal Images

The sagittal images are helpful for evaluating the weight-bearing portion of the femoral head and acetabular dome, as well as the anterior superior labrum (▶ Fig. 2.36). Articular cartilage is also well evaluated in the sagittal plane. The entire course of the labrum should be evaluated from medial to lateral. The hip adductors are visualized in cross-section in the sagittal plane, which is helpful in localizing pathologic changes to specific muscles in this group. The origin of the reflected tendon of the rectus femoris muscle can be visualized at the anterior inferior iliac spine.

Sagittal images also visualize the following:

- Iliopsoas muscle (which runs anterior to the hip joint as it courses toward its insertion on the lesser trochanter).
- Iliofemoral ligament (at its insertion on the anterior labrum).
- Ischiofemoral ligament (located posterior to the iliofemoral ligament).

2.6 Knee

2.6.1 Axial Images

Axial images are useful for examining the patellofemoral joint and the medial and lateral retinaculum, and for assessing tilt and subluxation (▶ Fig. 2.37). The patellar cartilage surfaces also are well visualized in this plane, and plicae can be seen (▶ Fig. 2.38). The suprapatellar bursa can be evaluated for knee effusions. The axial images can also be used to correlate quadriceps or patellar tendon anatomy seen on sagittal images, as well as collateral ligament anatomy seen on coronal images.

The anterior cruciate ligament (ACL) can be followed as it courses in an anteromedial direction through the intercondylar notch (▶ Fig. 2.37a) to the surface of the tibia just lateral and slightly posterior to the anterior horn of the medial meniscus. The tibial insertion of the posterior cruciate ligament (PCL) is just medial to midline. This position can be verified on sagittal images because the PCL is in the same plane as the anterior and posterior horns of the medial meniscus.

The menisci can be visualized on axial images, although meniscal pathology is better evaluated in the sagittal and coronal planes. The transverse ligament usually can be seen running from the anterior horn of the medial meniscus to the lateral meniscus.

The MCL and LCL complex components are seen as low-signal-intensity structures. The popliteal neurovascular structures can be seen just posterior to the joint capsule and are surrounded by fat. The popliteus tendon and posterolateral complex structures can also be seen in this plane.

2.6.2 Coronal Images

The coronal images are best for evaluating the collateral ligaments and the posterolateral and posteromedial corner complexes (▶ Fig. 2.39), but they should be viewed in conjunction with the axial and sagittal sequences to better understand the location in all three dimensions.

Posterolateral and Posteromedial Corners

This complex layer of tissues lies deep to the popliteal neurovascular structures (▶ Fig. 2.40). The posterolateral corner is

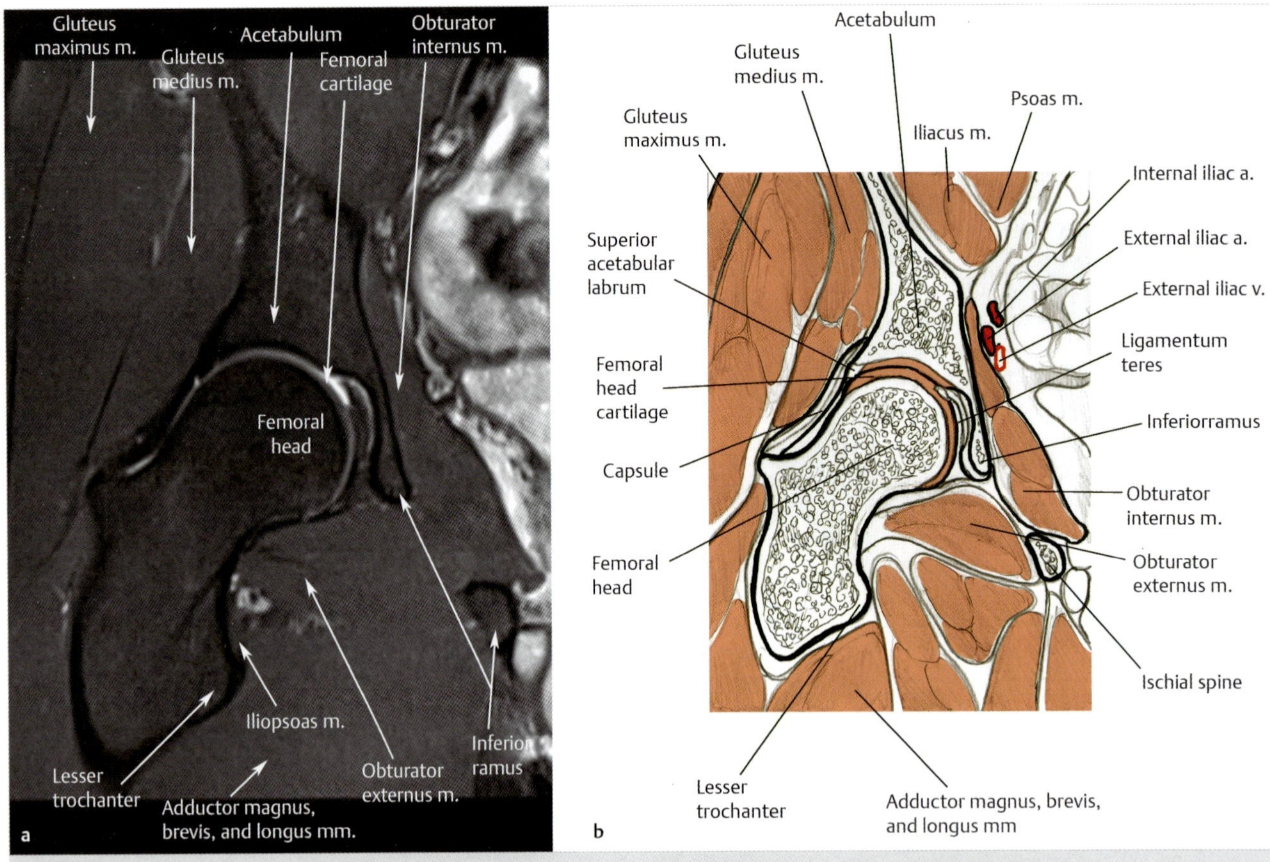

Fig. 2.34 A coronal proton-density image **(a)** and artist's sketch **(b)** of the right hip at the level of the lesser trochanter showing the articular cartilage of the femoral head and acetabulum. (Reproduced with permission from Dunleavy JD, Khanna AJ, Carrino JA. Normal MRI Anatomy of the Musculoskeletal System. In: Khanna AJ, ed. MRI for orthopaedic surgeons. New York: Thieme; 2010:17–76.)

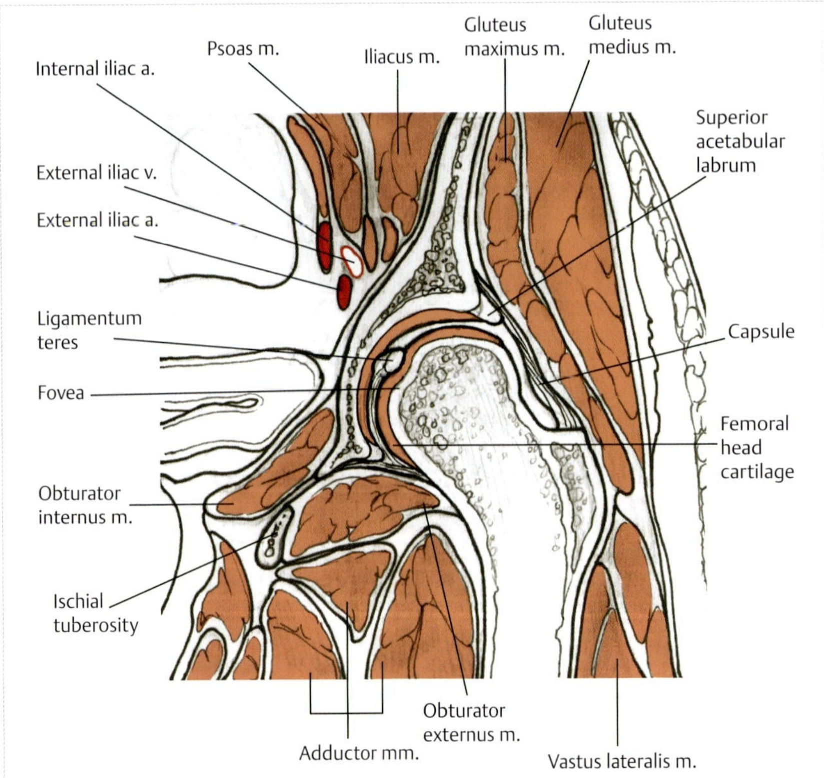

Fig. 2.35 A coronal illustration of the left hip showing the articular cartilage of the femoral head and acetabulum, the labrum, and the surrounding musculature. (Reproduced with permission from Dunleavy JD, Khanna AJ, Carrino JA. Normal MRI Anatomy of the Musculoskeletal System. In: Khanna AJ, ed. MRI for orthopaedic surgeons. New York: Thieme; 2010:17–76.)

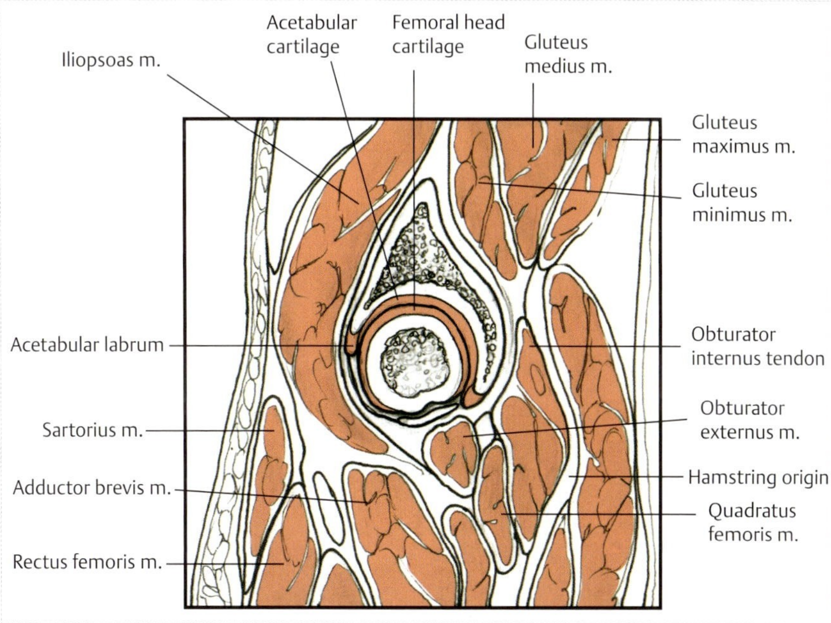

Fig. 2.36 A sagittal illustration of the left hip showing the articular cartilage, labrum, and surrounding musculature. (Reproduced with permission from Dunleavy JD, Khanna AJ, Carrino JA. Normal MRI Anatomy of the Musculoskeletal System. In: Khanna AJ, ed. MRI for orthopaedic surgeons. New York: Thieme; 2010:17–76.)

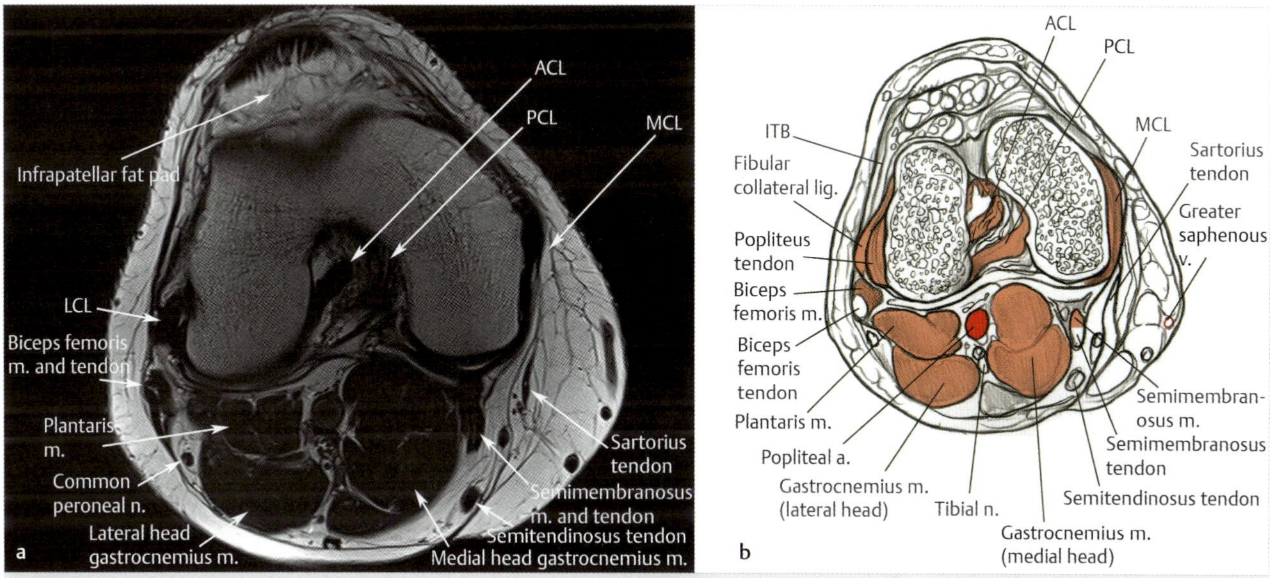

Fig. 2.37 An axial T2-weighted image **(a)** and artist's sketch **(b)** of the right knee at the level of the intercondylar notch showing the anterior cruciate ligament (ACL) and posterior cruciate ligament (PCL). (Reproduced with permission from Dunleavy JD, Khanna AJ, Carrino JA. Normal MRI Anatomy of the Musculoskeletal System. In: Khanna AJ, ed. MRI for orthopaedic surgeons. New York: Thieme; 2010:17–76.)

composed of the arcuate ligament, fabellofibular ligament, popliteofibular ligament, popliteal tendon, fibular collateral ligament, and biceps femoris tendon.[12] The posteromedial ligament corner is composed of the posterior oblique ligament and the insertion of the semimembranosus tendon with its five extensions, including the oblique popliteal ligament.[13] The fabella (variably present) can be seen as a circular structure superior to the most proximal aspect of the fibular head. The fabella frequently contains marrow and can be bright on T1-weighted sequences. Differentiating the individual components of these two complexes is difficult because they vary in consistency and are relatively thin. MR images acquired with thick sections may capture only a small portion of the complexes. The intricacy of the posterolateral complex structures makes evaluation especially sensitive to artifact in this region, particularly from patient motion or limited technical quality of the scan.

Collateral Ligaments

The MCL, which runs from the medial femoral epicondyle to the proximal tibia, deep to the pes anserinus tendon, has

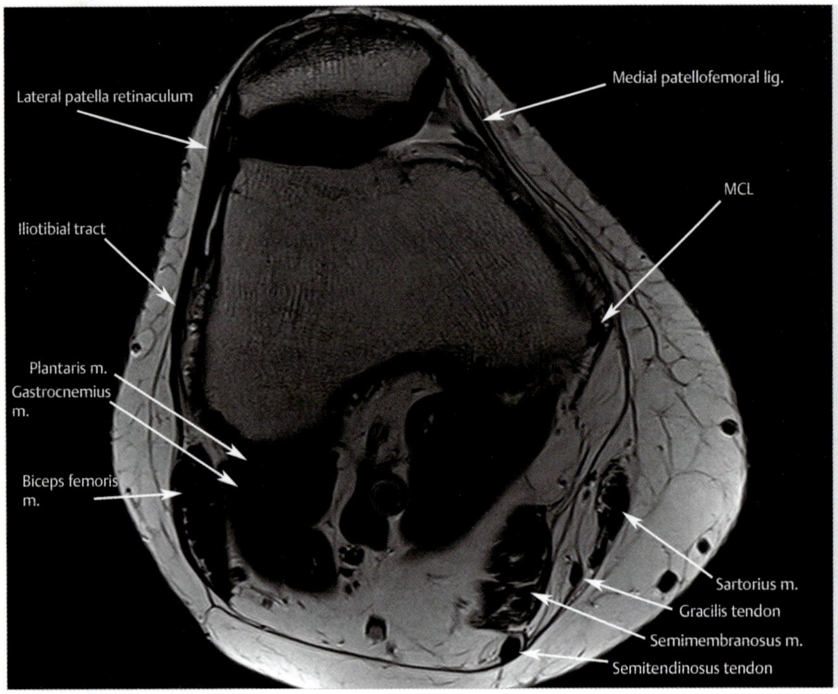

Fig. 2.38 An axial T2-weighted image of the right knee showing the patellofemoral joint, including the articular cartilage. (Reproduced with permission from Dunleavy JD, Khanna AJ, Carrino JA. Normal MRI Anatomy of the Musculoskeletal System. In: Khanna AJ, ed. MRI for orthopaedic surgeons. New York: Thieme; 2010:17–76.)

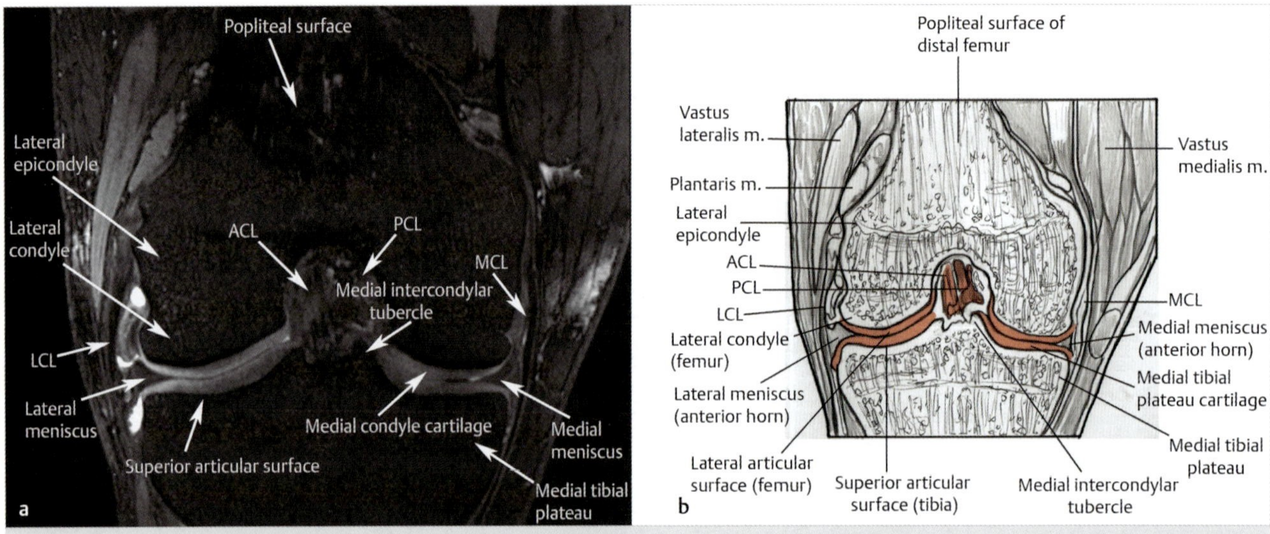

Fig. 2.39 A coronal T2-weighted image **(a)** and artist's sketch **(b)** of the right knee at the level of the intercondylar notch showing the medial collateral ligament (MCL) and lateral collateral ligament (LCL). The femoral and tibial articular cartilage is well shown. Abbreviations: ACL, anterior cruciate ligament; PCL, posterior cruciate ligament. (Reproduced with permission from Dunleavy JD, Khanna AJ, Carrino JA. Normal MRI Anatomy of the Musculoskeletal System. In: Khanna AJ, ed. MRI for orthopaedic surgeons. New York: Thieme; 2010:17–76.)

deep and superficial components. The lateral side is composed of a multistructure tendon and ligament unit known as the lateral collateral ligament (LCL) complex. It comprises the ITB, the fibular collateral ligament, and the biceps femoris tendon. The fibular collateral ligament (▶ Fig. 2.40) extends from the lateral femoral epicondyle to the fibular head, anterior to the insertion of the biceps femoris tendon. The MCL and LCL are low-signal-intensity structures (▶ Fig. 2.41). The ITB is seen on anterior coronal sections and inserts into Gerdy tubercle on the anterolateral proximal tibia.

ACL and PCL

The ACL, which can be visualized running just anterior to the PCL, fills up the lateral aspect of the intercondylar notch, whereas the PCL is located in the medial aspect of the notch. The ACL can be seen almost in its entirety, whereas the PCL is captured by successive sections through its substance as it courses posteriorly and inferiorly. It should be noted that although the ACL and PCL are more easily evaluated on sagittal images, these structures are also well visualized in the coronal plane (▶ Fig. 2.41).

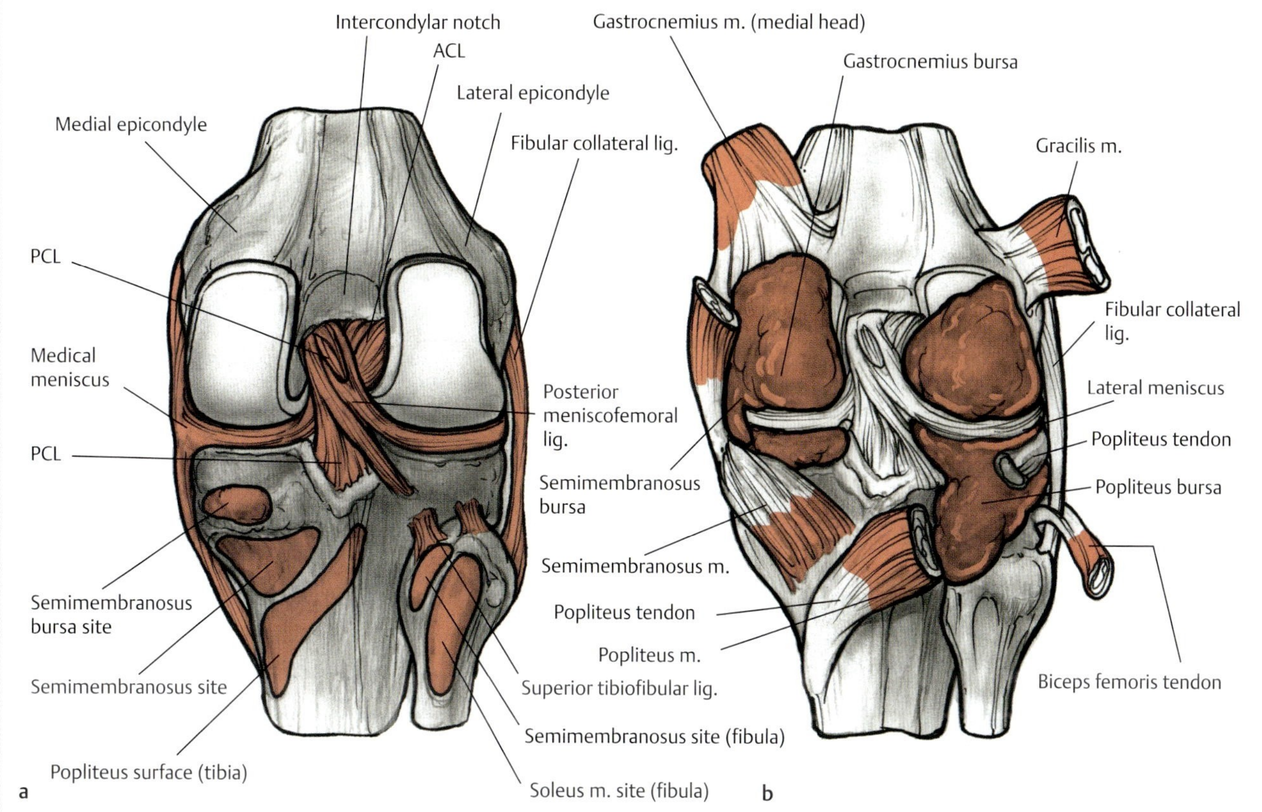

Fig. 2.40 Posteroanterior 3D illustrations of the ligamentous structures **(a)** and bursa **(b)** at the posterior aspect of the right knee. Abbreviations: ACL, anterior cruciate ligament; PCL, posterior cruciate ligament. (Reproduced with permission from Dunleavy JD, Khanna AJ, Carrino JA. Normal MRI Anatomy of the Musculoskeletal System. In: Khanna AJ, ed. MRI for orthopaedic surgeons. New York: Thieme; 2010:17–76.)

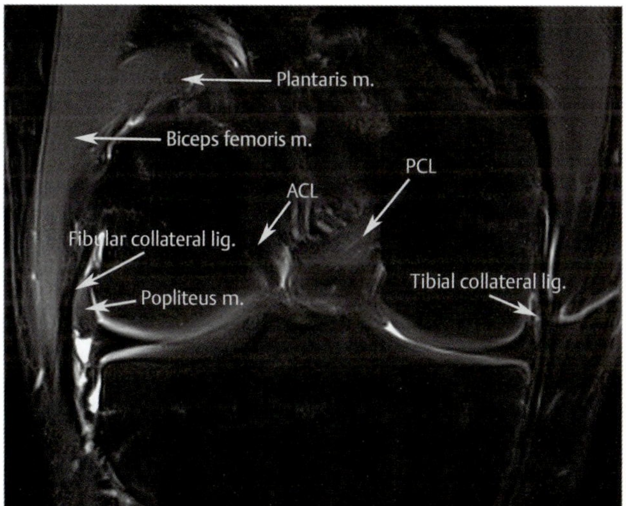

Fig. 2.41 A coronal T2-weighted image of the right knee showing the normal appearance of the collateral ligaments. The cruciate ligaments are shown coursing through the intercondylar notch. Abbreviations: ACL, anterior cruciate ligament; PCL, posterior cruciate ligament. (Reproduced with permission from Dunleavy JD, Khanna AJ, Carrino JA. Normal MRI Anatomy of the Musculoskeletal System. In: Khanna AJ, ed. MRI for orthopaedic surgeons. New York: Thieme; 2010:17–76.)

2.6.3 Sagittal Images

Structures that are well visualized on sagittal images include the cruciate ligaments, menisci, articular cartilage, and extensor mechanism (▶ Fig. 2.42, ▶ Fig. 2.43). It is important to localize the images to the lateral or medial compartment. Medial or lateral compartment localization on sagittal images is guided by the presence of the fibular head and the convex lateral tibial condyle. Another clue to medial or lateral location is that the ACL is seen before the PCL when progressing from lateral to medial images. It may also be helpful to have a coronal image with localizer lines available as a reference guide while scrolling through the sagittal plane images.

ACL

The ACL is best evaluated on sagittal images but should be identified in all planes. The ligament runs obliquely from its origin on the posteromedial aspect of the lateral femoral condyle to its insertion site just lateral to the anterior horn of the medial meniscus. The ACL is composed of the anteromedial and posterolateral bundles. The ligament is intra-articular but extrasynovial. Because of this anatomic feature, the ACL may have fatty as well as fluid signal interspersed between the fibers.

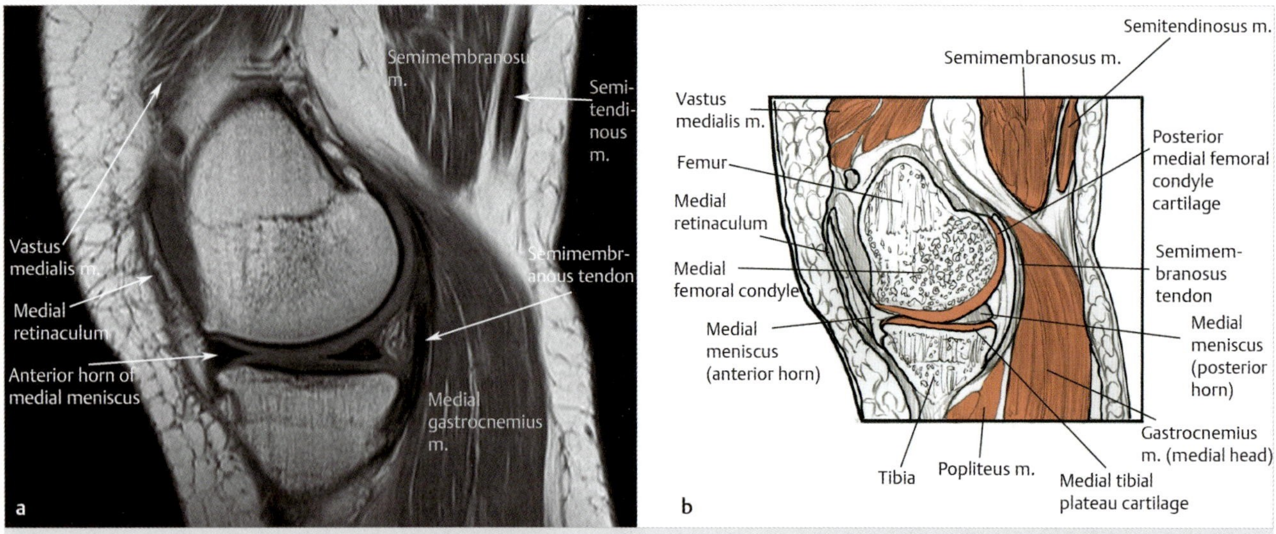

Fig. 2.42 A sagittal proton-density image **(a)** and artist's sketch **(b)** of the knee showing the articular cartilage and the anterior and posterior horns of the medial meniscus. (Reproduced with permission from Dunleavy JD, Khanna AJ, Carrino JA. Normal MRI Anatomy of the Musculoskeletal System. In: Khanna AJ, ed. MRI for orthopaedic surgeons. New York: Thieme; 2010:17–76.)

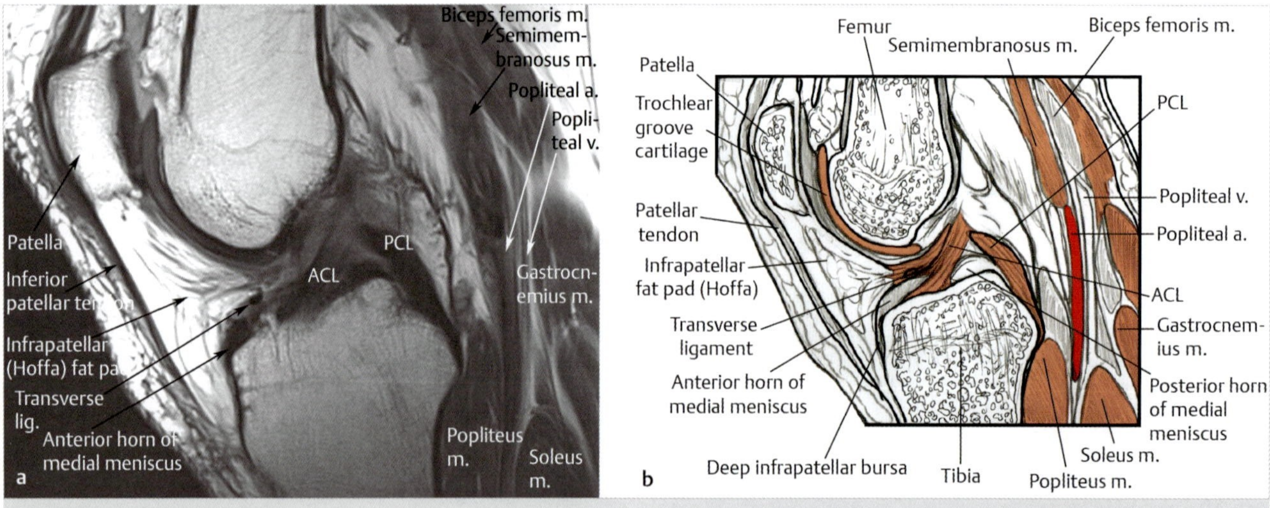

Fig. 2.43 A sagittal proton-density image **(a)** and artist's sketch **(b)** of the knee at the level of the intercondylar notch showing the anterior cruciate ligament (ACL) and posterior cruciate ligament (PCL). The transverse ligament is seen in close association with the anterior horn of the medial meniscus. Also shown are the patellofemoral cartilage and the patellar and quadriceps tendons. (Reproduced with permission from Dunleavy JD, Khanna AJ, Carrino JA. Normal MRI Anatomy of the Musculoskeletal System. In: Khanna AJ, ed. MRI for orthopaedic surgeons. New York: Thieme; 2010:17–76.)

On 5-mm sagittal sections, the ACL is usually visualized on at least one section. However, 3-mm sections for spin-echo (SE) imaging and 1- to 2-mm sections for gradient-echo imaging are preferable because they allow for better visualization of the ACL. Normally, the ligament takes a straight course and has low signal intensity. However, the normal ACL does have some variation in its signal pattern, and subtle regions of increased T2-weighted signal may be seen in the uninjured ACL. Compared with the PCL, the ACL is less well defined and has higher signal intensity. Appreciating this normal appearance will help prevent inappropriate interpretations of a normal ACL as an ACL strain or partial tear. In a normal ACL, there should be at least one identifiable dark fiber bundle, and the ACL often appears as one thick dark band. There should be a clear anterior edge to the ligament. The ACL should not show marked increased signal on T2-weighted imaging, but it may have minimally increased signal on T1-weighted images because of the presence of fatty tissue. The normal ACL should follow the contour of the

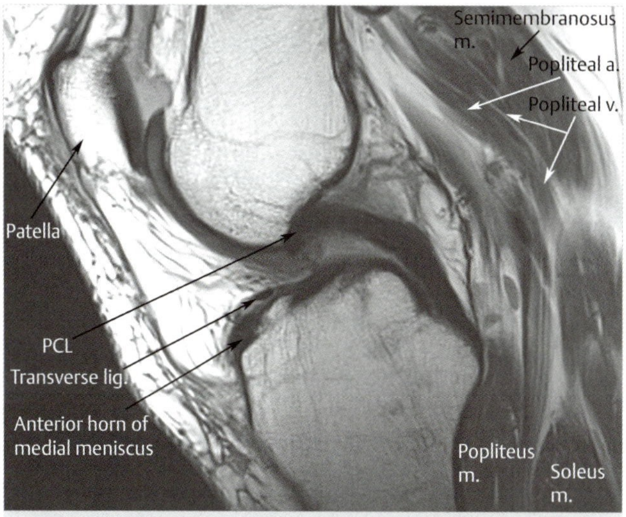

Fig. 2.44 A sagittal proton-density image of the knee showing the entire course of the posterior cruciate ligament (PCL). (Reproduced with permission from Dunleavy JD, Khanna AJ, Carrino JA. Normal MRI Anatomy of the Musculoskeletal System. In: Khanna AJ, ed. MRI for orthopaedic surgeons. New York: Thieme; 2010:17–76.)

intercondylar roof, and attachments should be well delineated. Again, clinicians should be aware of these characteristics to avoid misdiagnosing ACL injuries.[14]

PCL

The PCL attaches on the posterior proximal tibia, inferior to the tibial joint surface. In contrast to the straight course of the ACL, the PCL curves anteriorly to insert on the anterolateral aspect of the medial femoral condyle (▶ Fig. 2.44) because the knee is always imaged in extension. The PCL is usually seen on at least two images, even on examinations acquired with thick sections. The PCL usually appears as a thicker, darker, curved band compared with the ACL. When present, the ligaments of Humphry and Wrisberg (anterior and posterior meniscofemoral ligaments, which occur concurrently in 70% of knees[15]) can be seen adjacent to the PCL.

Menisci

The medial and lateral menisci are uniformly low-signal-intensity, triangle-shaped structures (when imaged in cross-section) under the femoral condyles. The menisci increase in thickness toward the periphery of the joint. At the edge of the joint, near the capsule, the menisci can be seen as thick, dark bands running parallel to the articular surface.

The transverse ligament can be seen as a tiny dark circle or triangle just superior to the anterior aspect of the tibial surface in midsagittal images. The transverse ligament also can be seen just superior to the anterior horns of the menisci, separated from the menisci in some images by a thin line of high signal intensity (▶ Fig. 2.44). Clinicians unaware of this normal appearance may interpret the hyperintense line between the menisci and the transverse ligament as pathologic, leading to a mistaken diagnosis of a meniscal tear.

The so-called *magic-angle phenomenon* can cause the false diagnosis of a lateral meniscus tear. Specifically, the upsloping portion of the posterior horn of the lateral meniscus may have increased signal on short-TE images secondary to this phenomenon.[16]

Extensor Mechanism

The structures of the extensor mechanism of the knee (the patella, patella tendon, quadriceps tendon, and medial and lateral retinaculum) are well seen on midsagittal images (▶ Fig. 2.43). The fat pad is just posterior to the patellar tendon. The patellar and femoral bone marrow signal should be uniform without edema. The signal of the patellar tendon should be uniformly dark. The quadriceps tendon may have a laminated appearance reflecting its multiple tendon composition. There should be no areas of focal thickening of the tendons. The cartilage surfaces of the patella are particularly thick (up to 1 cm). There should be no areas of signal change, fibrillation, or thinning; the presence of these findings is indicative of chondromalacia.

Neurovascular Structures

The popliteal artery courses several millimeters posterior to the knee joint. The popliteal vein is just posterior and lateral to the artery (▶ Fig. 2.43) and has a large cross-section. The tibial nerve runs just posterior and lateral to the vein. The common peroneal nerve arises from the tibial nerve above the joint line and may be seen coursing inferiorly and laterally toward the fibular head. The relationships between these structures are easily identified on coronal images.

2.7 Foot/Ankle

2.7.1 Axial Images

Axial images are extremely helpful in identifying normal and abnormal anatomy of the ankle (▶ Fig. 2.45, ▶ Fig. 2.46) and are usually evaluated from superior to inferior (proximal to distal). These images are acquired perpendicular to the plane of the tibia and fibula. The tibia and fibula expand distally to form the tibial plafond, medial malleolus, and lateral malleolus. Axial images also show the distal tibiofibular joint and ankle syndesmosis, with the fibula located laterally and posteriorly in the syndesmotic notch. More inferiorly, the talar dome is visualized, followed sequentially by the calcaneus and the midfoot osseous structures (▶ Fig. 2.47). The navicular bone can be seen on axial images and can be evaluated in this plane. More distally, the tarsometatarsal joints and metatarsals are seen. These structures are not all in the same axial plane because of the transverse arch of the foot. Therefore, they must be examined on sequential images, which is facilitated by correlation with the coronal and sagittal images. The forefoot structures (▶ Fig. 2.48) are usually best evaluated with specialized planes for the hallux and separate planes for the lesser metatarsals.

On axial images, most tendon structures in the ankle are seen in cross-section. Therefore, it is important to identify and follow each tendon from image to image along its course.

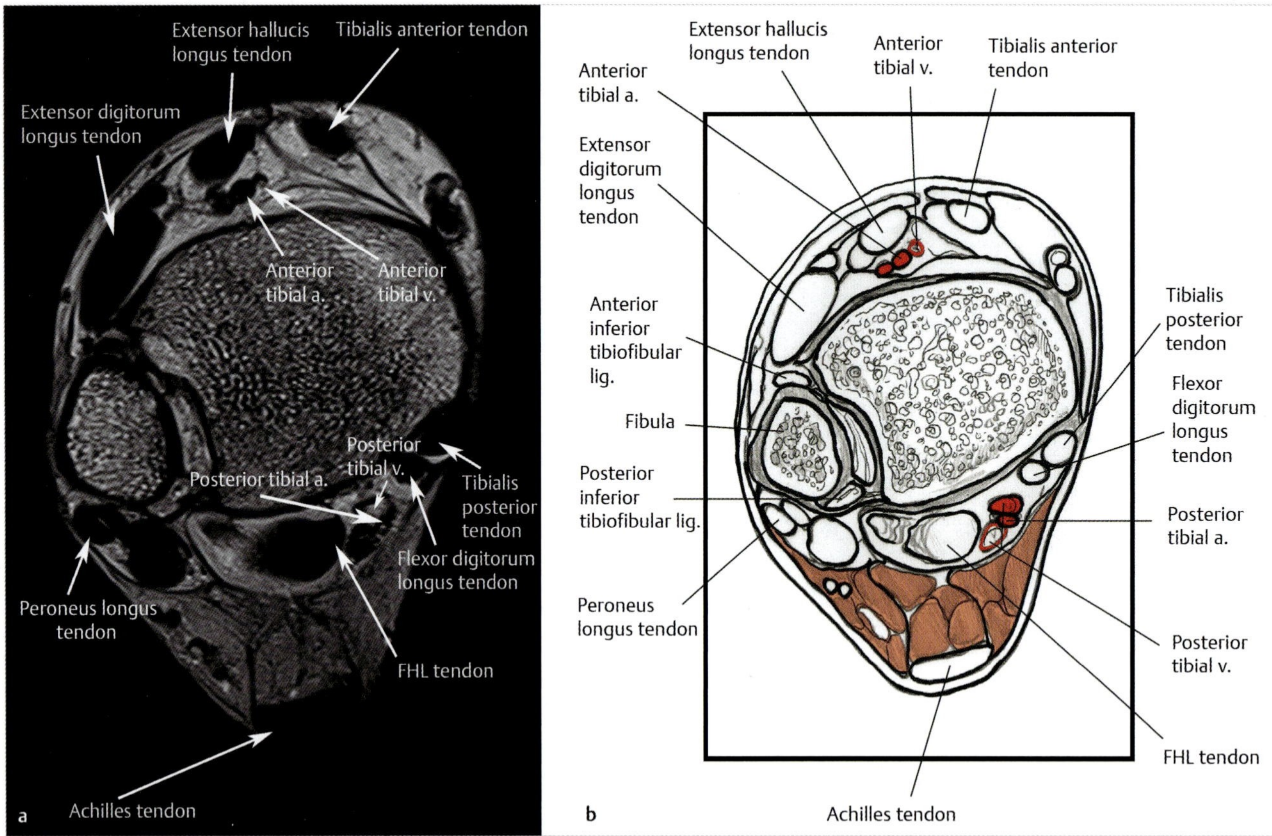

Fig. 2.45 An axial T2-weighted image **(a)** and artist's sketch **(b)** of the right ankle at the level of the tibial plafond. The tibialis posterior, flexor digitorum longus, and flexor hallucis longus (FHL) tendons are seen posterior to the medial malleolus. The normal concave appearance of the Achilles tendon is seen in the midline posteriorly. The peroneus longus and brevis tendons are shown posterior to the lateral malleolus. (Reproduced with permission from Dunleavy JD, Khanna AJ, Carrino JA. Normal MRI Anatomy of the Musculoskeletal System. In: Khanna AJ, ed. MRI for orthopaedic surgeons. New York: Thieme; 2010:17–76.)

These tendons should be dark on all sequences. At the level of the ankle joint, the tibialis anterior and extensor hallucis longus tendons are the most anteromedial structures, anterior to the neurovascular bundle. The extensor digitorum longus tendon (▶ Fig. 2.49) has a more muscular, broad appearance at the level of the ankle joint and lies more laterally than does the extensor hallucis longus. The most anterolateral structure is the peroneus tertius tendon (variably present), which can sometimes be difficult to visualize because of its small size.

The posterior tibialis tendon is the most obvious tendon structure just posterior to the medial malleolus. The flexor digitorum longus tendon is just posterior to the posterior tibialis tendon and medial to the posterior neurovascular bundle. It is approximately one-third the diameter of the posterior tibialis tendon. Lateral and deep to the posterior neurovascular bundle is the flexor hallucis longus (FHL), which has a broad muscular cross-section at the level of the ankle joint. This tendon can be followed further distally in its sheath between the posteromedial and posterolateral processes of the talus. These three tendons can be identified not only by their appearance and insertions but also by their predictable relationships to each other as they pass posterior to the medial malleolus.

The peroneus brevis and longus (▶ Fig. 2.50, ▶ Fig. 2.51) are easily identified posterior to the fibula. The peroneus brevis lies directly against the fibula, and the longus is more superficial at the level of the ankle joint. The overlying superior peroneal retinaculum should be assessed for integrity.

The Achilles tendon is the most posterior tendinous structure in the ankle. At its insertion on the calcaneus, it has an oblong appearance on axial images and should appear concave more proximally on the anterior surface.

The anterior and posterior tibiofibular ligaments, along with the dense interosseous tibiofibular ligament, constitute the syndesmotic complex between the tibia and fibula. The anterior and posterior tibiofibular ligaments are identified easily as low-signal-intensity ligamentous connections between the distal tibia and fibula at the level of the ankle joint.

Of the lateral ligamentous complex structures, the anterior and posterior talofibular ligaments are best seen on axial images. They appear as dark, thin, ligamentous bands extending distally from the fibula anteriorly and posteriorly to insert on the talus. The anterior band attaches to the neck of the talus, and the posterior band attaches to the posterior lateral process of the talus. However, the structures of the lateral ligamentous complex do not all run in the same plane, and thus, the calcaneofibular

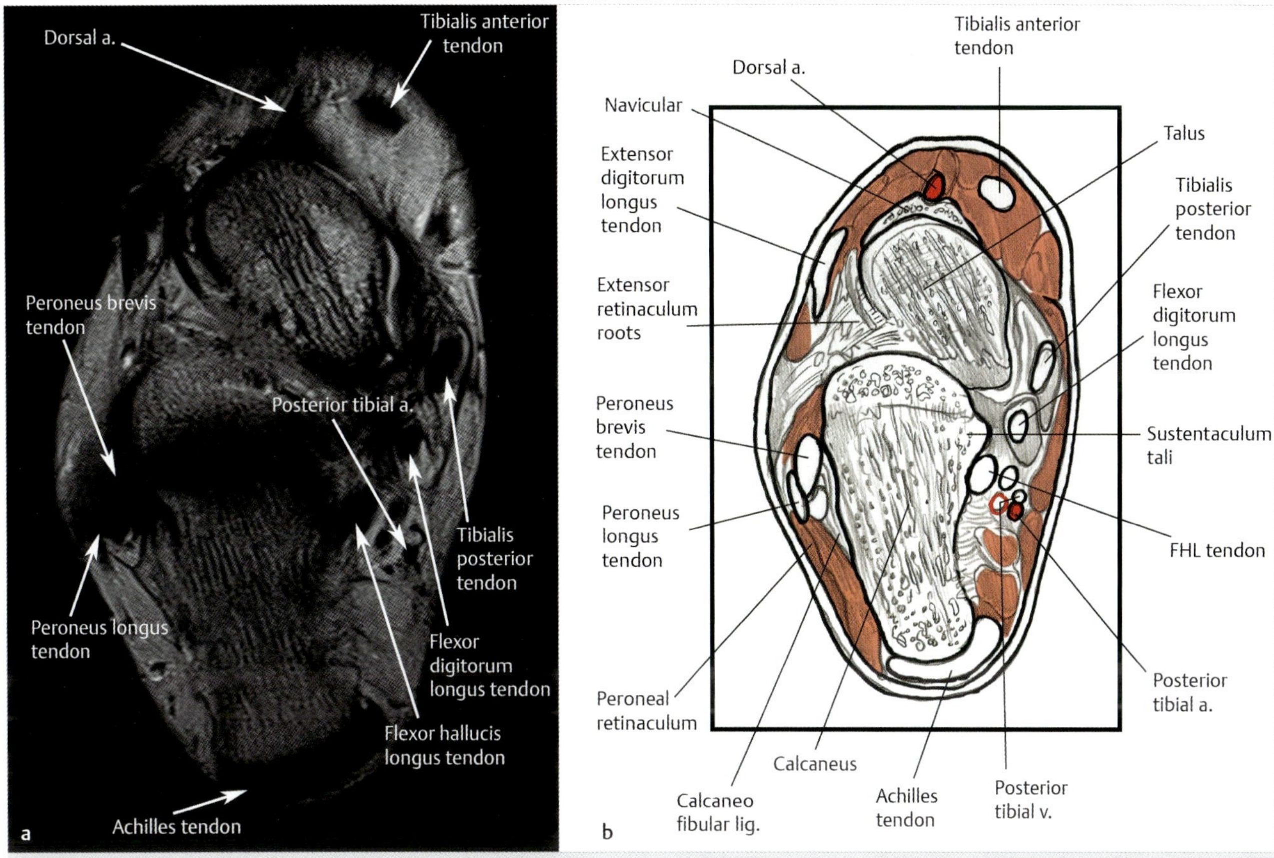

Fig. 2.46 An axial T2-weighted image **(a)** and artist's sketch **(b)** of the right ankle at the level of the calcaneus, showing the posterior tibialis, flexor digitorum longus, and flexor hallucis longus (FHL) tendons in their expected locations from anteromedial to posterolateral, respectively. The peroneus longus and brevis tendons are seen coursing along the lateral aspect of the calcaneus. (Reproduced with permission from Dunleavy JD, Khanna AJ, Carrino JA. Normal MRI Anatomy of the Musculoskeletal System. In: Khanna AJ, ed. MRI for orthopaedic surgeons. New York: Thieme; 2010:17–76.)

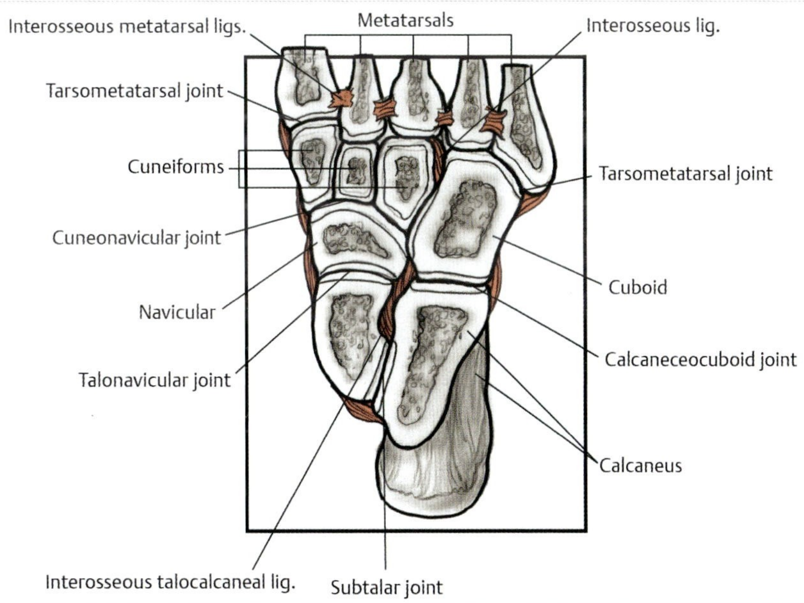

Fig. 2.47 Illustration of an axial section through the osseous structures of the right foot showing the tarsometatarsal and intertarsal joints and the interosseous ligaments. (Reproduced with permission from Dunleavy JD, Khanna AJ, Carrino JA. Normal MRI Anatomy of the Musculoskeletal System. In: Khanna AJ, ed. MRI for orthopaedic surgeons. New York: Thieme; 2010:17–76.)

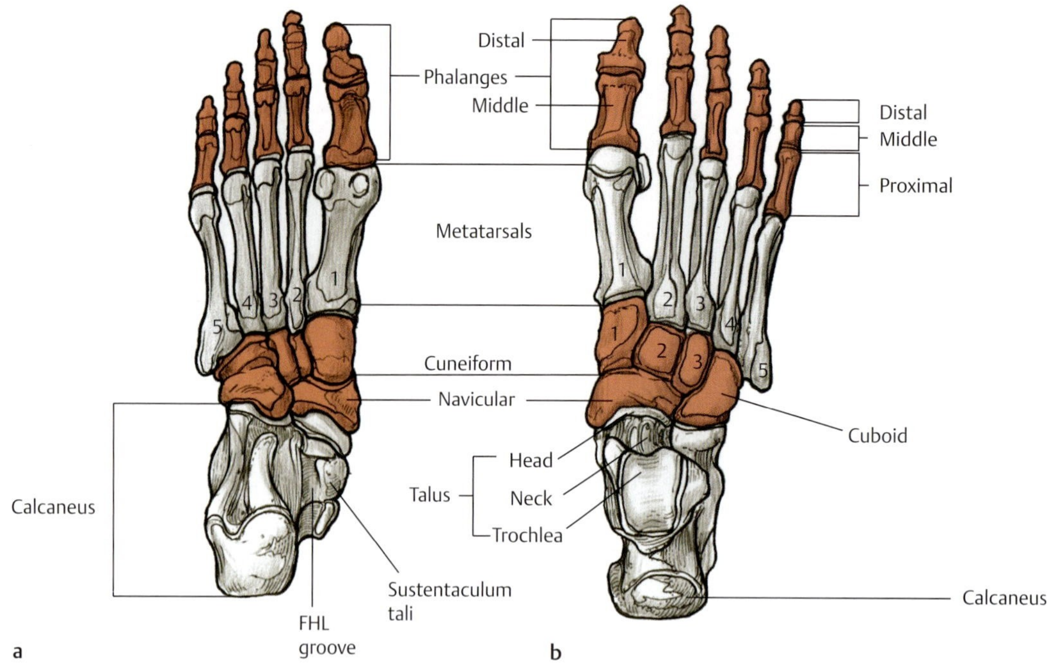

Fig. 2.48 Illustrations of the osseous structures of the plantar **(a)** and dorsal **(b)** surface views of the right foot. Abbreviations: FHL, flexor hallucis longus. (Reproduced with permission from Dunleavy JD, Khanna AJ, Carrino JA. Normal MRI Anatomy of the Musculoskeletal System. In: Khanna AJ, ed. MRI for orthopaedic surgeons. New York: Thieme; 2010:17–76.)

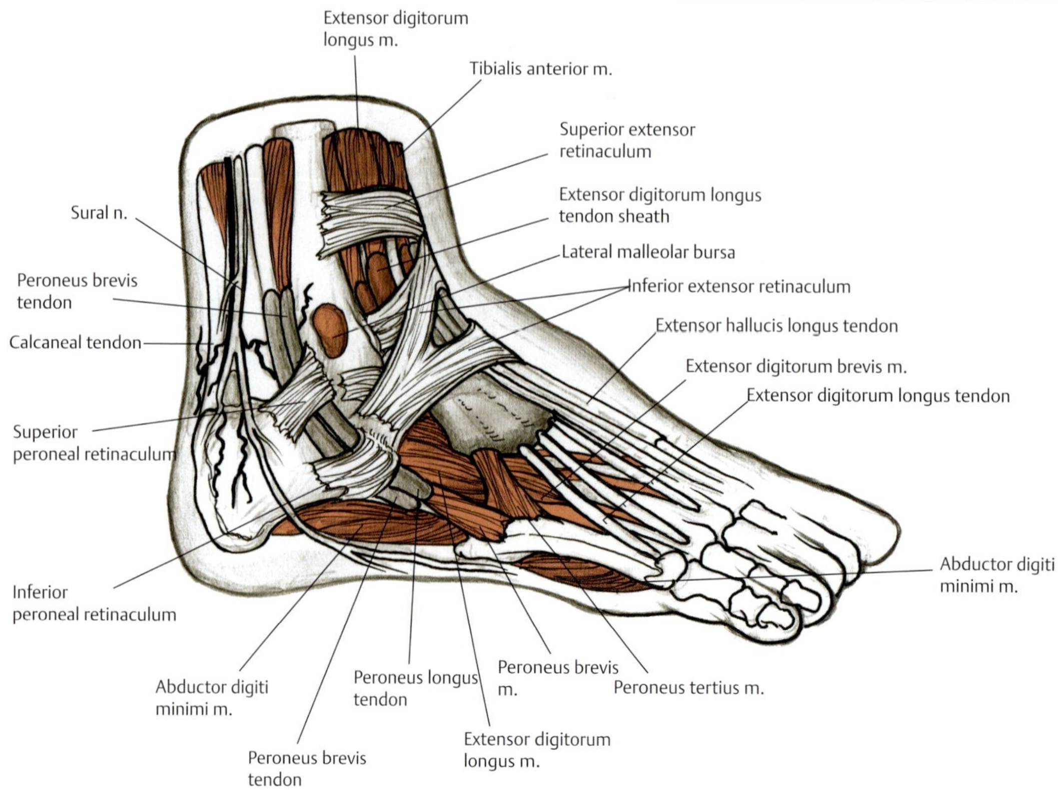

Fig. 2.49 A 3D illustration of the ankle and foot from the lateral aspect showing the musculotendinous units passing deep to the superior and inferior extensor retinacula. (Reproduced with permission from Dunleavy JD, Khanna AJ, Carrino JA. Normal MRI Anatomy of the Musculoskeletal System. In: Khanna AJ, ed. MRI for orthopaedic surgeons. New York: Thieme; 2010:17–76.)

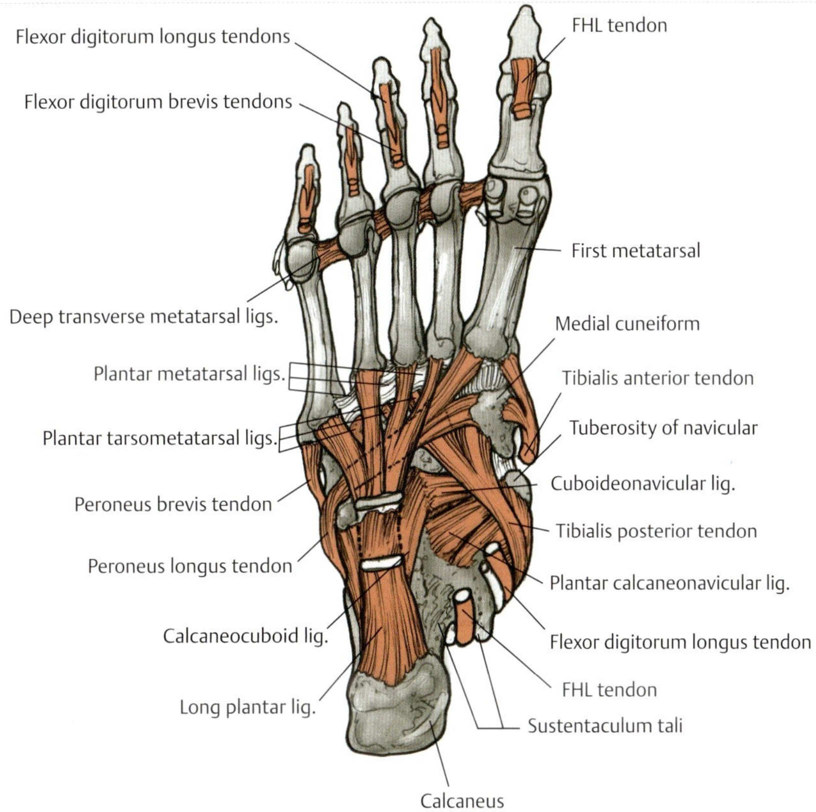

Fig. 2.50 An axial 3D illustration of the plantar aspect of the right foot showing the tarsometatarsal and intertarsal ligaments, as well as the tendons crossing the ankle into the foot. Abbreviations: FHL, flexor hallucis longus. (Reproduced with permission from Dunleavy JD, Khanna AJ, Carrino JA. Normal MRI Anatomy of the Musculoskeletal System. In: Khanna AJ, ed. MRI for orthopaedic surgeons. New York: Thieme; 2010:17–76.)

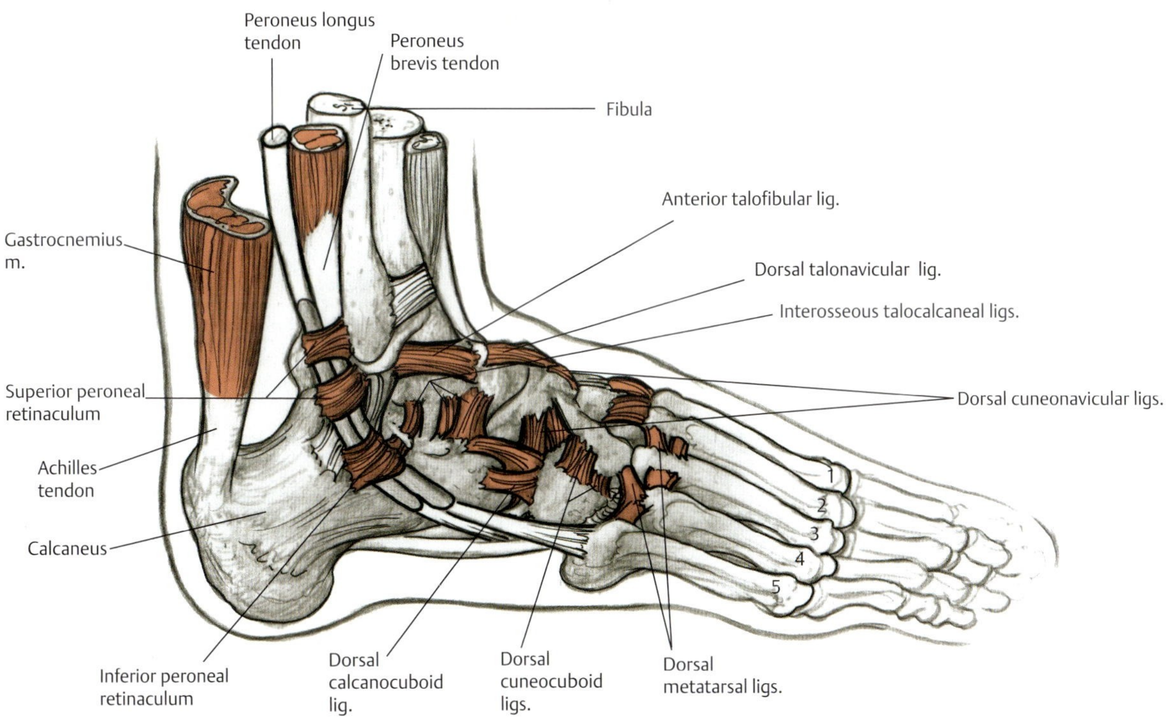

Fig. 2.51 A 3D illustration of the ankle and foot from the lateral aspect showing the deep ligaments and the peroneus longus and brevis tendons passing posterior to the lateral malleolus, deep to the peroneal retinaculum. (Reproduced with permission from Dunleavy JD, Khanna AJ, Carrino JA. Normal MRI Anatomy of the Musculoskeletal System. In: Khanna AJ, ed. MRI for orthopaedic surgeons. New York: Thieme; 2010:17–76.)

ligament component of the lateral ligamentous complex is best seen on the coronal images, whereas the anterior and posterior talofibular ligaments are best seen on axial images.

The anterior neurovascular bundle (anterior tibial artery, anterior tibial vein, and deep peroneal nerve) is slightly lateral and deep to the extensor hallucis longus (▶ Fig. 2.52). The posterior neurovascular bundle (posterior tibial artery, vein, and nerve) lies between the flexor digitorum longus and FHL and deep to the flexor retinaculum.

2.7.2 Coronal Images

Coronal images of the ankle are obtained in the plane of the tibia (▶ Fig. 2.53, ▶ Fig. 2.54). The tibial plafond, medial and lateral malleoli, and talar dome are well visualized on proton-density and T2-weighted coronal images. Such images are useful in diagnosing osseous pathology such as occult fractures, stress fractures, OCDs, degenerative arthritis, osseous infections, and neoplastic processes.

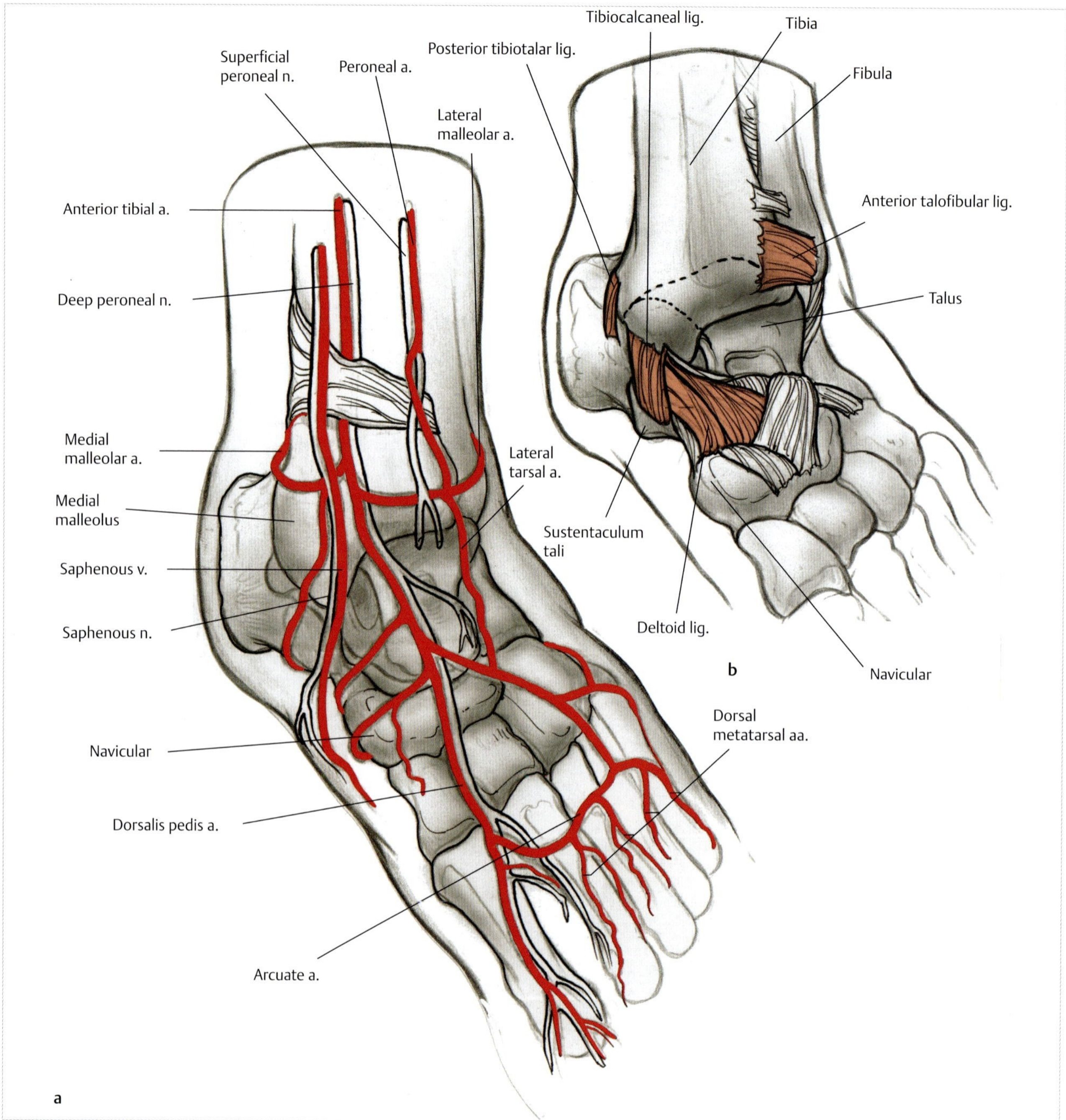

Fig. 2.52 Anterior oblique illustrations of the left foot and ankle showing the neurovascular **(a)** and ligamentous **(b)** structures. (Reproduced with permission from Dunleavy JD, Khanna AJ, Carrino JA. Normal MRI Anatomy of the Musculoskeletal System. In: Khanna AJ, ed. MRI for orthopaedic surgeons. New York: Thieme; 2010:17–76.)

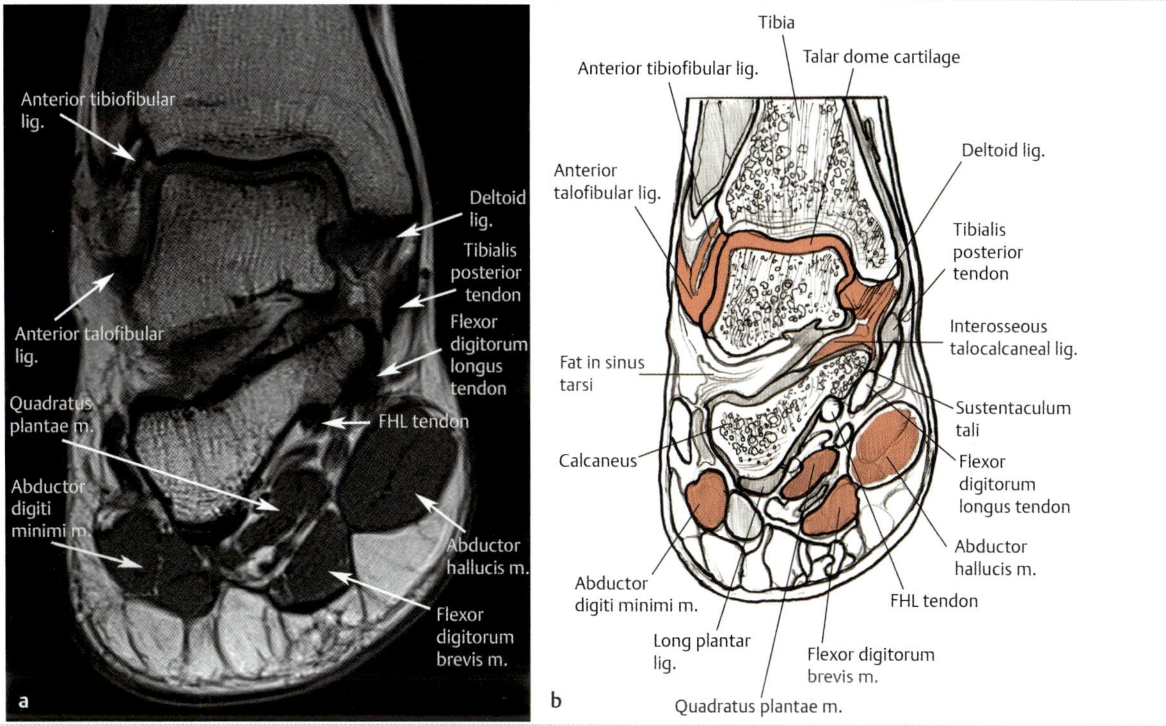

Fig. 2.53 A coronal T1-weighted image **(a)** and artist's sketch **(b)** of the right ankle at the level of the tibial plafond and talus. Abbreviations: FHL, flexor hallucis longus. (Reproduced with permission from Dunleavy JD, Khanna AJ, Carrino JA. Normal MRI Anatomy of the Musculoskeletal System. In: Khanna AJ, ed. MRI for orthopaedic surgeons. New York: Thieme; 2010:17–76.)

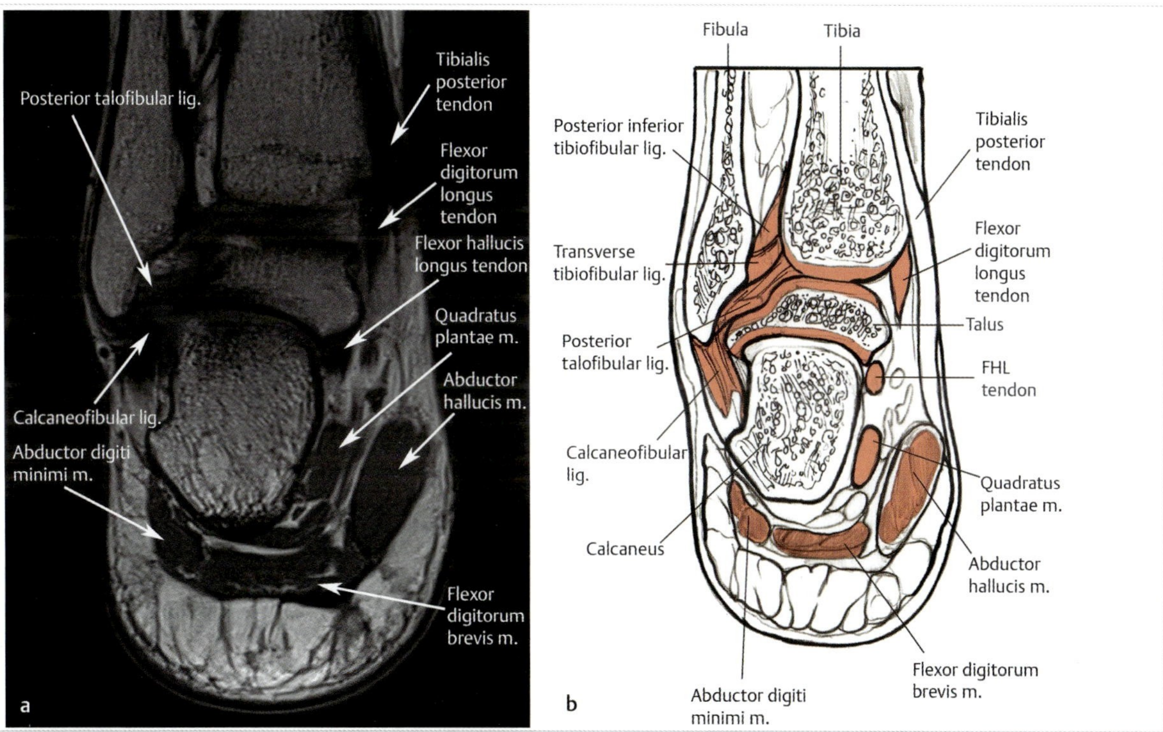

Fig. 2.54 A coronal T1-weighted image **(a)** and artist's sketch **(b)** of the right ankle through the posterior aspect of the joint showing the posterior tibialis, flexor digitorum longus, and flexor hallucis longus (FHL) tendons coursing posterior to the medial malleolus in their expected locations from anteromedial to posterolateral, respectively. (Reproduced with permission from Dunleavy JD, Khanna AJ, Carrino JA. Normal MRI Anatomy of the Musculoskeletal System. In: Khanna AJ, ed. MRI for orthopaedic surgeons. New York: Thieme; 2010:17–76.)

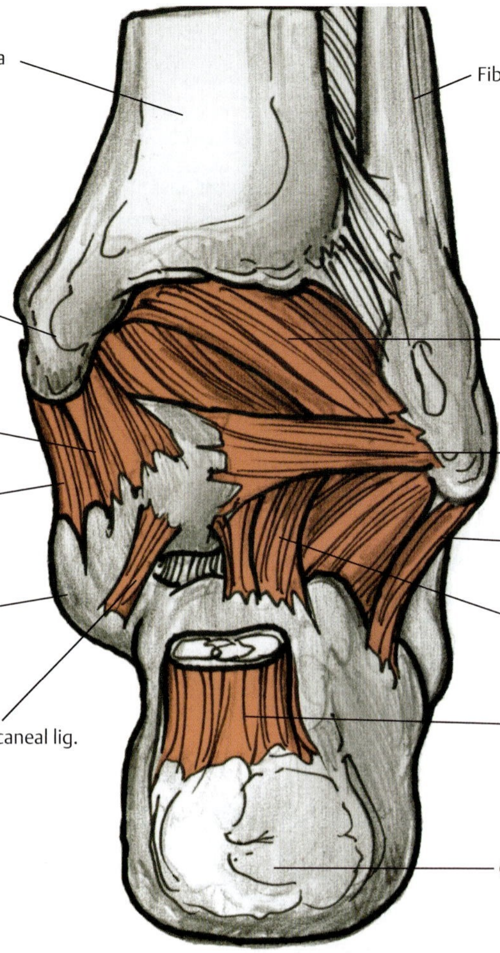

Fig. 2.55 A posteroanterior 3D illustration of the right ankle showing the posterior ligamentous structures, including the tibiocalcaneal and posterior tibiotalar parts of the deltoid ligament. (Reproduced with permission from Dunleavy JD, Khanna AJ, Carrino JA. Normal MRI Anatomy of the Musculoskeletal System. In: Khanna AJ, ed. MRI for orthopaedic surgeons. New York: Thieme; 2010:17–76.)

The ankle structures identified on coronal images are the medial and lateral ligament complexes. The deltoid ligament forms the MCL complex of the ankle and consists of superficial and deep layers. The tibionavicular and tibiocalcaneal ligaments constitute the superficial layer, and the tibiotalar ligament constitutes the deep layer (▶ Fig. 2.55). The tibionavicular ligament originates from the medial malleolus and attaches to the tuberosity of the navicular. The tibiocalcaneal ligament is seen as a thick, dark band extending from the medial malleolus inferiorly to the sustentaculum tali of the calcaneus. The tibiotalar ligament extends from the medial malleolus to the entire nonarticular medial aspect of the talus.

The lateral ligamentous complex of the ankle consists of the calcaneofibular, anterior talofibular, and posterior talofibular ligaments. Of these three structures, the calcaneofibular ligament is best seen on coronal images, extending from the tip of the lateral malleolus to the lateral wall of the calcaneus. Despite the fact that many tendinous structures can be difficult to identify in the coronal plane, the posterior tibial tendon and the peroneus longus and brevis tendons can be identified inferior to the medial and lateral malleoli, respectively. The posterior tibial tendon should be seen as a longitudinal dark signal structure just posterior to the medial malleolus. The FHL can be identified at its broad origin from the posterior two-thirds of the fibula. The peroneus longus and brevis tendons are seen as longitudinal dark signal structures on most coronal images, passing just posterior to the lateral malleolus.

The osseous structures of the foot can also be evaluated on the coronal images. The hindfoot, including the talar body, calcaneus, and subtalar joint, can be examined for occult talocalcaneal coalitions or arthritic processes. The talocalcaneal ligaments and soft-tissue contents of the sinus tarsi can be examined on T2-weighted images or fat-suppressed proton-density images for evidence of increased signal secondary to ligament injury or soft-tissue impingement that supports a diagnosis of sinus tarsi syndrome. Coronal imaging of the midfoot also shows the talonavicular and calcaneocuboid joints, the navicular body and cuboid, and the tarsometatarsal joints. Coronal images through the midfoot are useful for diagnosing navicular or cuboid stress fractures, arthritis of the midfoot joints, or soft-tissue injuries of the tarsometatarsal (Lisfranc) complex. These images can show the plantar tarsometatarsal ligament complex and facilitate evaluation of tendinitis or tearing of the extensor and flexor tendons. Coronal imaging of the forefoot osseous structures includes the following:

- Metatarsals.
- Phalanges.
- Metatarsophalangeal (MTP) and IP joints.
- Sesamoids.

The flexor and extensor tendons can be visualized at the forefoot, particularly the extensor hallucis longus tendon and prominent flexor tendons at the first MTP level. The capsuloligamentous structures (plantar plate) of the MTP joints are also visualized in the coronal plane, allowing for diagnosis of MTP sprain injuries, such as the common turf-toe injury at the first MTP joint.

2.7.3 Sagittal Images

Like coronal images, sagittal images allow most structures to be visualized longitudinally along their courses (▶ Fig. 2.56). The osseous structures of the ankle and foot can be visualized in sequence from medial to lateral (▶ Fig. 2.57). The tibial plafond, talar dome, and lateral malleolus can be inspected for arthritic, degenerative, neoplastic, infectious, or traumatic conditions. Sagittal imaging shows the midfoot bones (particularly the talar head, navicular, and cuboid) and can permit sequential examination of the cuneiforms and metatarsals. Precise identification of the central osseous structures is facilitated by concurrent correlation with the axial and coronal images. The first MTP joint structures are visualized particularly well in the sagittal plane. Although coronal and axial images are better suited for identification of the ligamentous complexes of the ankle, the plantar plate and ligament structures of the MTP joints can be identified in the sagittal plane.

The Achilles tendon, easily identified as the most posterior tendon inserting onto the posterior calcaneal tuberosity, can be inspected for thickening, intratendinous signal heterogeneity, partial tearing, or complete rupture with retraction (▶ Fig. 2.58). Immediately deep to this structure is the retrocalcaneal bursa, which can show increased signal intensity on T2-weighted images, suggestive of retrocalcaneal bursitis. The posterior tibial tendon is the first structure posterior to the medial malleolus. The course of this tendon can be appreciated as it curves around the medial malleolus to insert onto the tuberosity of the navicular bone. The next two medial tendons are the flexor digitorum longus and FHL (▶ Fig. 2.59). The flexor digitorum longus tendon is located just posterior

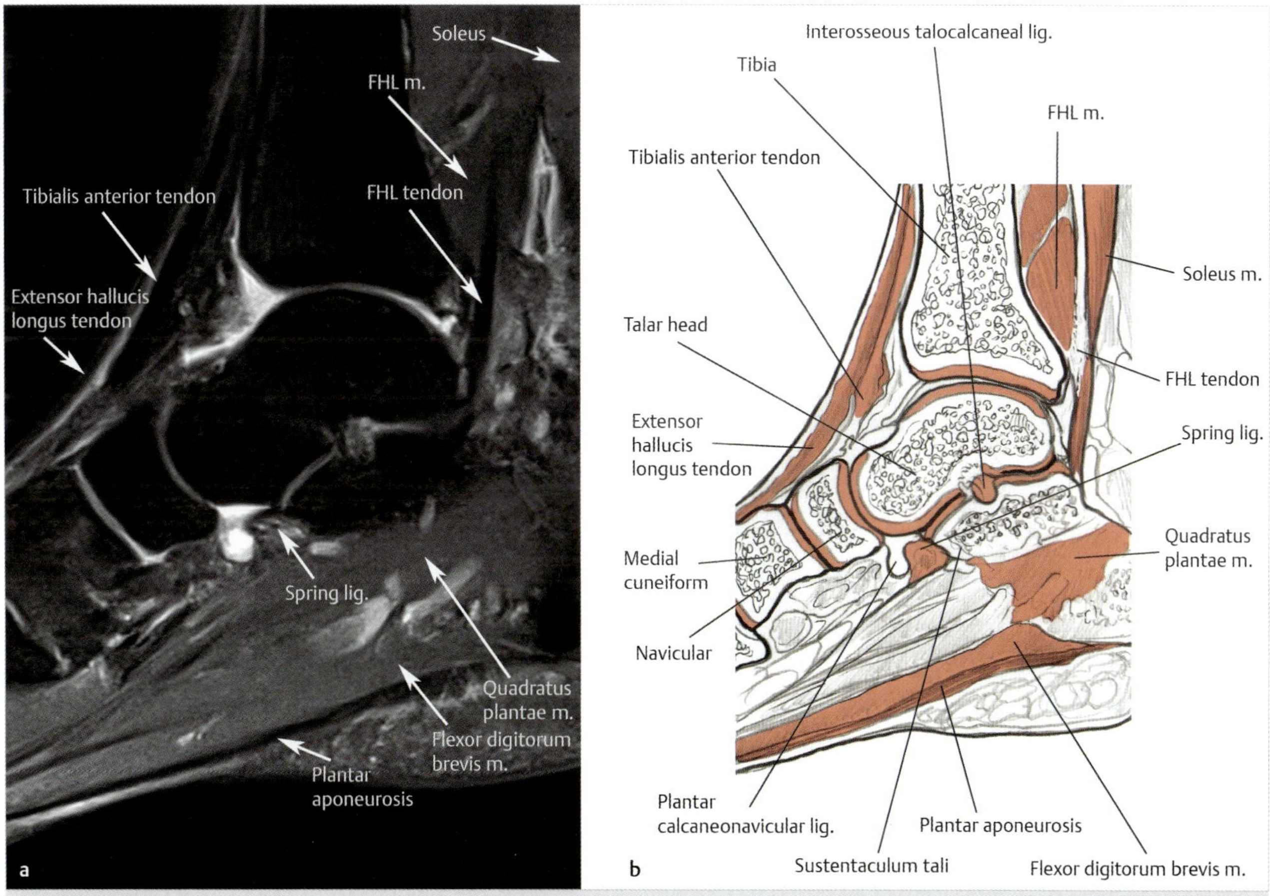

Fig. 2.56 A sagittal proton-density fat-suppressed image **(a)** and artist's sketch **(b)** of the medial aspect of the ankle at the level of the navicular. Abbreviations: FHL, flexor hallucis longus. (Reproduced with permission from Dunleavy JD, Khanna AJ, Carrino JA. Normal MRI Anatomy of the Musculoskeletal System. In: Khanna AJ, ed. MRI for orthopaedic surgeons. New York: Thieme; 2010:17–76.)

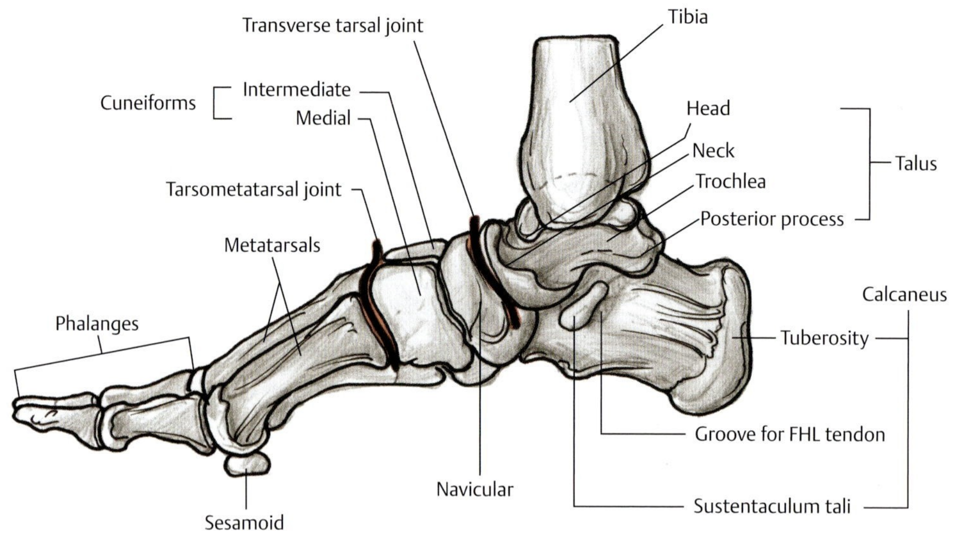

Fig. 2.57 An illustration of the osseous structures of the right foot from a medial view. Abbreviations: FHL, flexor hallucis longus. (Reproduced with permission from Dunleavy JD, Khanna AJ, Carrino JA. Normal MRI Anatomy of the Musculoskeletal System. In: Khanna AJ, ed. MRI for orthopaedic surgeons. New York: Thieme; 2010:17–76.)

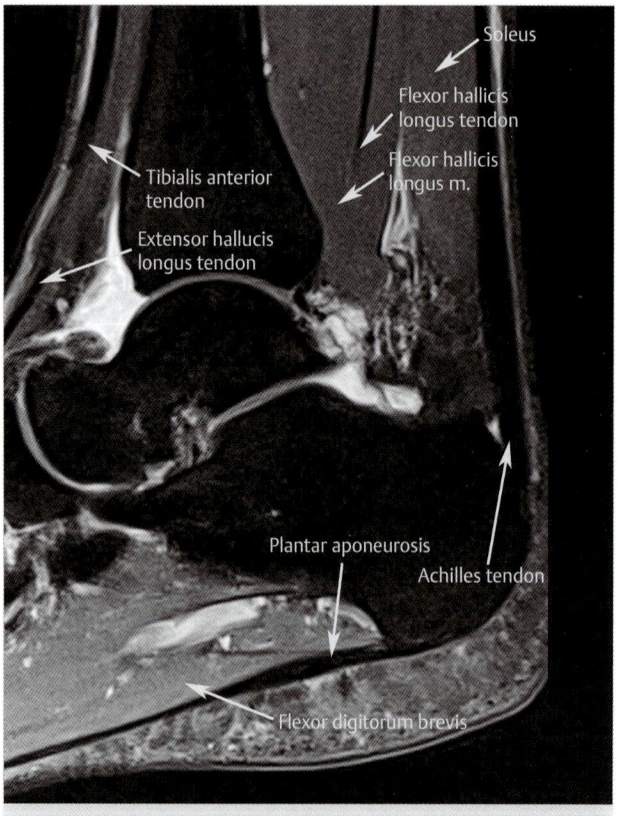

Fig. 2.58 A sagittal proton-density fat-suppressed image of the ankle showing the Achilles tendon and plantar aponeurosis. Flexor and extensor tendons crossing the ankle are also seen. (Reproduced with permission from Dunleavy JD, Khanna AJ, Carrino JA. Normal MRI Anatomy of the Musculoskeletal System. In: Khanna AJ, ed. MRI for orthopaedic surgeons. New York: Thieme; 2010:17–76.)

to the posterior tibialis tendon and medial to the posterior neurovascular bundle. The FHL, the deepest muscle in the posterior compartment, lies against the tibia. Lateral to the FHL are the peroneal tendons, which course posterior to the lateral malleolus and then toward the plantar midfoot. The anterior tibialis, extensor hallucis longus, and extensor digitorum longus tendons can be visualized anteriorly. In particular, the anterior tibialis tendon can be identified on sagittal imaging and should be evaluated for tenosynovitis, partial tear, or rupture.

2.8 General Spine Anatomy

2.8.1 Intervertebral Disks

The normal discovertebral complex has three components:

- Cartilaginous end plate.
- Annulus fibrosus.
- Nucleus pulposus.

Overall, the intervertebral disks show intermediate signal intensity on T1-weighted images and high signal intensity on T2-weighted images. The outer annulus appears hypointense on T2-weighted images, whereas the inner annulus, which is composed of fibrocartilage and a high proportion of type II collagen, is indistinguishable from the hyperintense nucleus pulposus. Compared with normal vertebral marrow, the nucleus pulposus, which is composed of a proteoglycan matrix and type II collagen, appears hyperintense on T2-weighted images and hypointense on T1-weighted images.[17] As the disk degenerates and as patients age, the signal intensity of the nucleus pulposus decreases on T2-weighted images and becomes dark on all pulse sequences with advanced degenerative changes. Additional

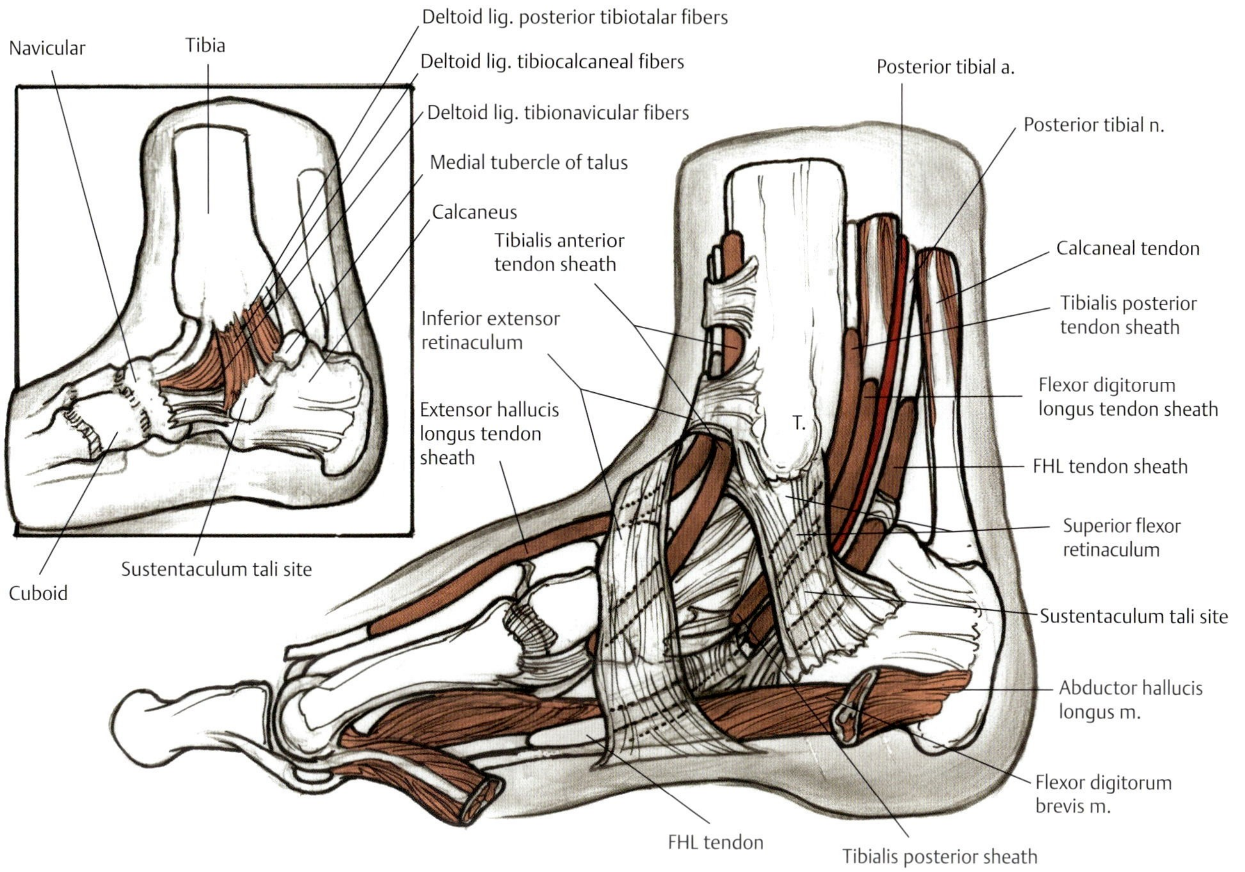

Fig. 2.59 Medial 3D illustrations of the right ankle showing the tibialis posterior tendon, flexor digitorum longus tendon, and the flexor hallucis longus (FHL) tendon coursing posterior to the medial malleolus, deep to the flexor retinaculum. The inset shows the various components of the deltoid ligament. (Reproduced with permission from Dunleavy JD, Khanna AJ, Carrino JA. Normal MRI Anatomy of the Musculoskeletal System. In: Khanna AJ, ed. MRI for orthopaedic surgeons. New York: Thieme; 2010:17–76.)

pulse sequences, such as fat-suppressed T2-weighted images, are useful for accentuating fluid and edema, which may help in delineating spine pathology. Special attention should be given to the posterior aspect of the disk on both sagittal and axial T2-weighted images to evaluate for disk protrusion, extrusion, sequestration, or other pathology that may be contributing to central canal or neural foraminal stenosis.

The end plate is a flat, osseous disk with a slightly elevated rim secondary to the attached ring apophysis, which produces a central depression in the end plate that is occupied by hyaline cartilage.[17] The annulus is composed of type I collagen fibers (Sharpey fibers) that are attached to the ring apophysis periosteum. The annulus also blends with the anterior and posterior longitudinal ligaments. T1-weighted images provide optimal evaluation of anatomy, fracture lines, and other osseous detail. T1-weighted images also clearly delineate the relationships of the vertebral bodies, intervertebral disks, central canal, and posterior elements.

2.8.2 Vertebral Bodies

Normal lordosis should be seen in the cervical and lumbar spine, and normal kyphosis should be present in the thoracic spine. The superior and inferior end plates should be intact and parallel to one another in the absence of vertebral compression fractures, other fractures, or infection. The subaxial cervical vertebral bodies all have a similar appearance (▶ Fig. 2.60), whereas the atlas (C1) has no vertebral body and the axis (C2) has an odontoid process. Each of the lumbar vertebral bodies also has a similar appearance (▶ Fig. 2.61), as do the thoracic vertebral bodies (▶ Fig. 2.62). The anterior and posterior longitudinal ligaments, seen along the vertebral bodies, have low signal

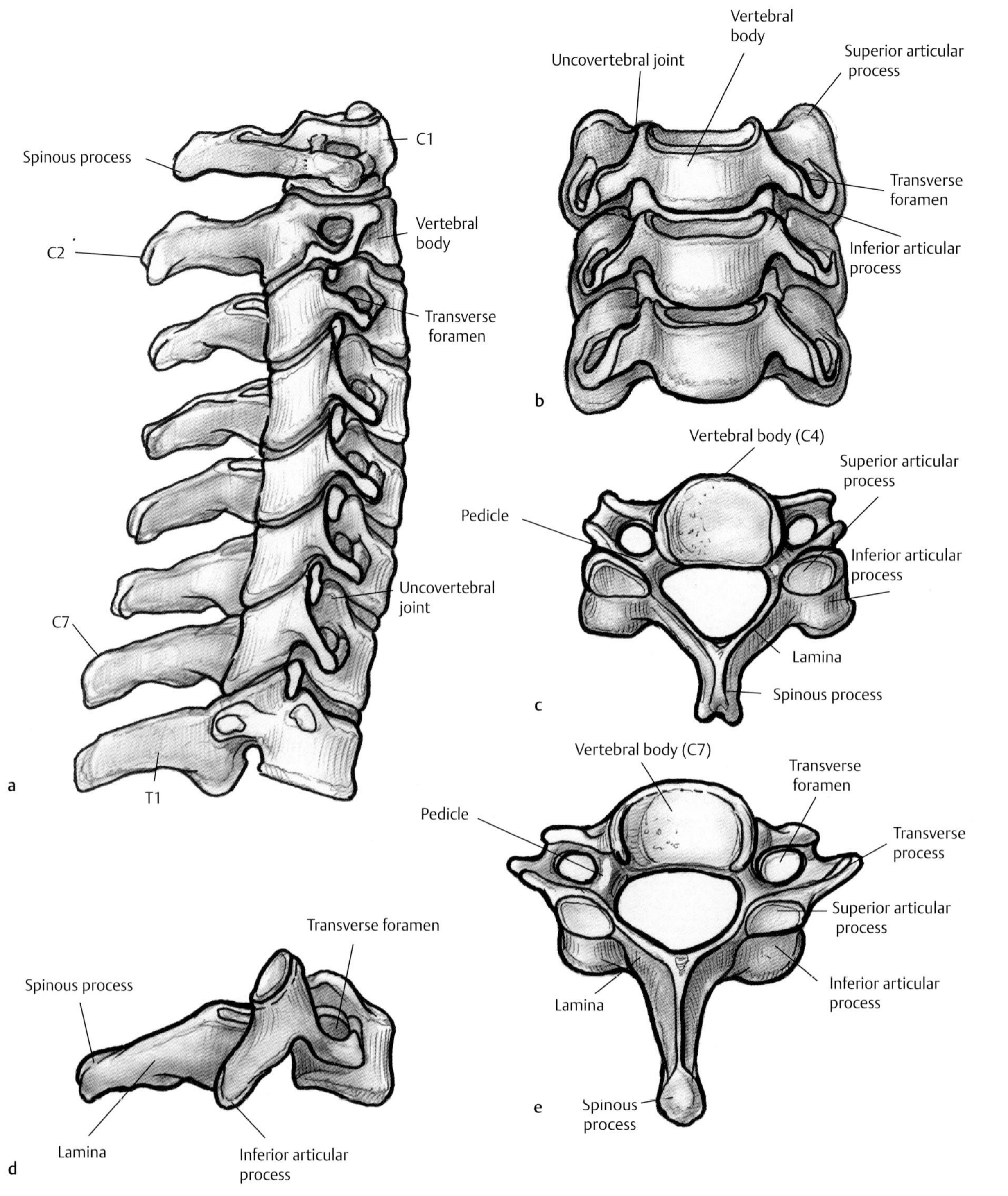

Fig. 2.60 Various views of the cervical vertebral bodies: **(a)** lateral vertebral body at C1–T1, **(b)** lateral anteroposterior (AP) vertebral body at C4–C7, **(c)** axial vertebral body at C4, **(d)** lateral vertebral body at C7, and **(e)** axial vertebral body at C7. (Reproduced with permission from Dunleavy JD, Khanna AJ, Carrino JA. Normal MRI Anatomy of the Musculoskeletal System. In: Khanna AJ, ed. MRI for orthopaedic surgeons. New York: Thieme; 2010:17–76.)

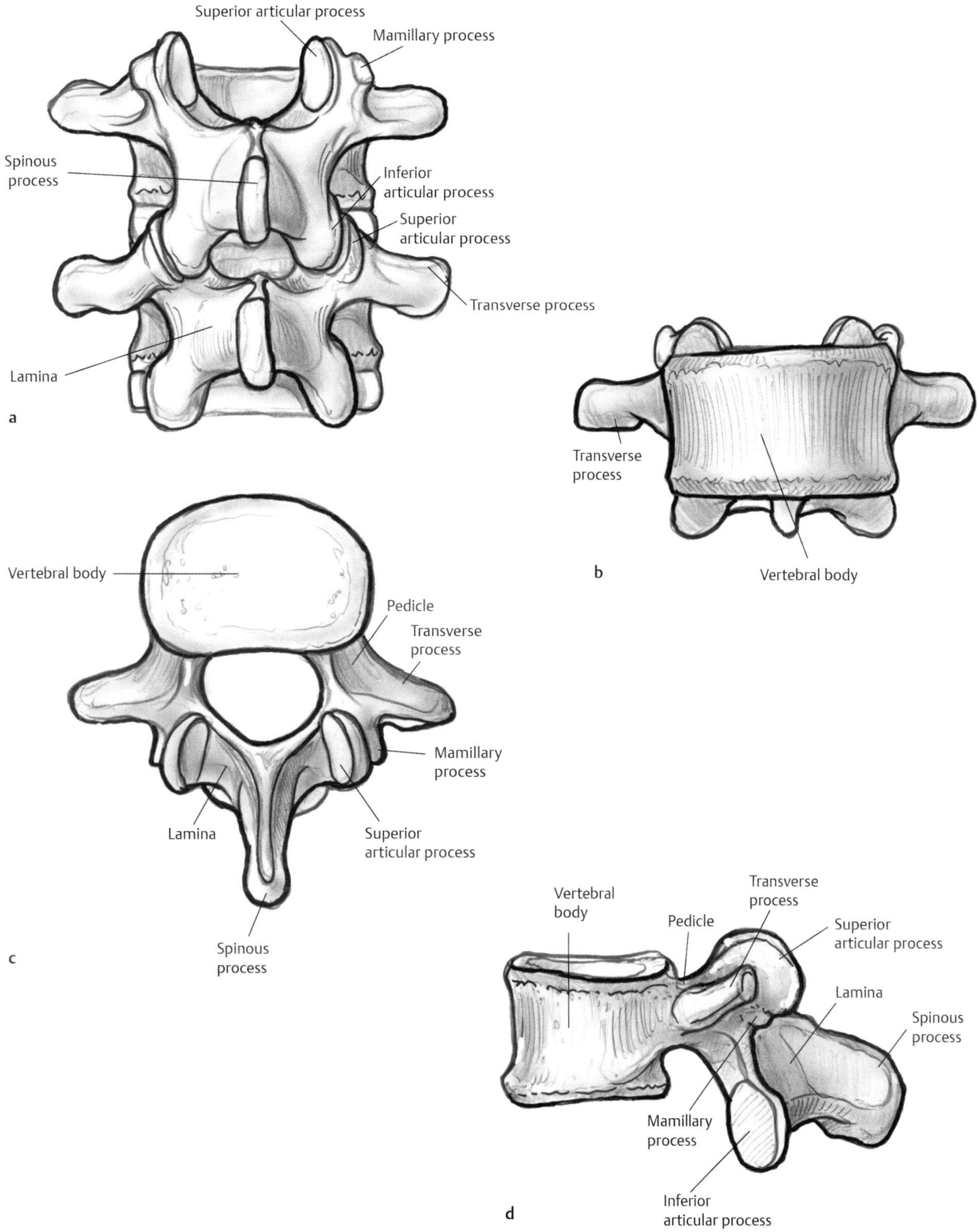

Fig. 2.61 Various views of the L3 and L4 lumbar vertebral bodies: **(a)** posterior, **(b)** anterior, **(c)** axial, and **(d)** lateral. (Reproduced with permission from Dunleavy JD, Khanna AJ, Carrino JA. Normal MRI Anatomy of the Musculoskeletal System. In: Khanna AJ, ed. MRI for orthopaedic surgeons. New York: Thieme; 2010:17–76.)

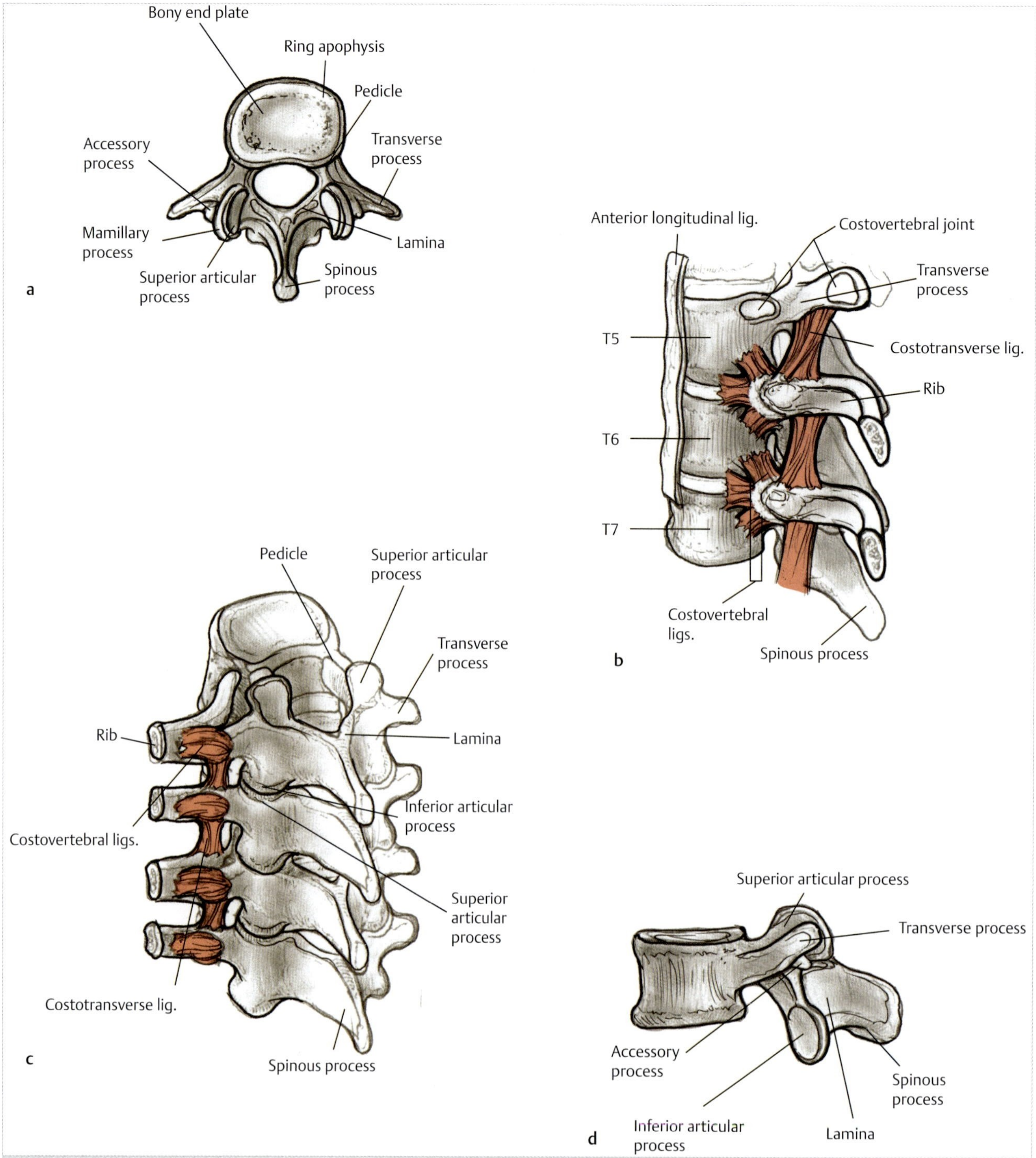

Fig. 2.62 Axial **(a)**, lateral **(b)**, posterior oblique **(c)**, and lateral **(d)** illustrations of the osseous structures of the thoracic spine, the costovertebral joints, and the costotransverse and costovertebral ligaments. (Reproduced with permission from Dunleavy JD, Khanna AJ, Carrino JA. Normal MRI Anatomy of the Musculoskeletal System. In: Khanna AJ, ed. MRI for orthopaedic surgeons. New York: Thieme; 2010:17–76.)

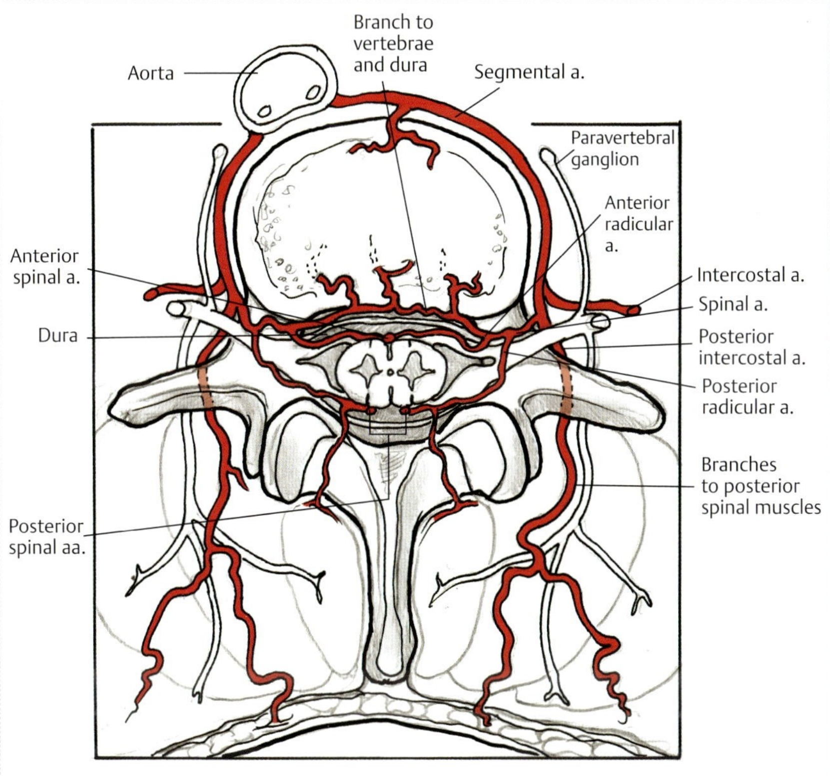

Fig. 2.63 A 3D illustration (axial view) of the spinal, intercostal, and other arteries that supply the thoracic spine. (Reproduced with permission from Dunleavy JD, Khanna AJ, Carrino JA. Normal MRI Anatomy of the Musculoskeletal System. In: Khanna AJ, ed. MRI for orthopaedic surgeons. New York: Thieme; 2010:17–76.)

intensity. The entry site of the basivertebral veins is seen at the midportion of the posterior vertebral bodies. The spinal and radicular arteries course around the cord's anterior, posterior, and lateral aspects within the vertebral canal (▶ Fig. 2.63). Fat-suppression techniques can be used to nullify marrow signal and increase the sensitivity in the evaluation of neoplastic and infiltrative processes.

2.8.3 CSF

Like other fluids, cerebrospinal fluid (CSF) has low signal intensity on T1-weighted images and high signal intensity on T2-weighted images. On sagittal and axial images, CSF is seen surrounding the spinal cord in the cervical, thoracic, and lumbar spine and around the cauda equina in the lower lumbar spine. Thus, T2-weighted images provide a myelographic appearance that allows for the detection of spinal stenosis.

2.8.4 Spinal Cord

Sagittal T2-weighted images provide a myelographic effect that allows for the evaluation of spinal cord morphology and the presence of extrinsic compression. The cord should have homogeneous signal intensity in the absence of intrinsic pathology. On axial T2-weighted images, the central gray matter can be faintly identified. Specialized sequences obtained with high magnetic field magnets allow for detailed evaluation of central gray matter (▶ Fig. 2.64). The spinal cord should terminate at or above the L1–L2 level in adults.

2.8.5 Ligaments

Normal ligaments should have low signal intensity on all pulse sequences. The transverse ligament can be seen posterior to the odontoid process (▶ Fig. 2.65) and is best visualized on axial images. The ligamentum flavum connects the lamina of adjacent vertebrae and is seen as a hypointense band posterior to the dura. The anterior longitudinal ligament is broad, thick, and adherent to the anterior vertebral bodies. The posterior longitudinal ligament is thin, attached to the posterior vertebral cortex via the midline septum, and defines the posterior margin of the anterior epidural space at the midline (▶ Fig. 2.66). The anterior epidural space is not apparent at the disk level because the posterior longitudinal ligament fuses to the disks. Visualization of these structures may be limited with MRI because of partial volume averaging with the adjacent vertebral body.[18]

2.8.6 Roots and Foramina

The dorsal and ventral nerve roots can be identified within the neural foramina on the parasagittal images and the axial images, and the exiting nerve root is located just posterior to the vertebral artery in the cervical spine (▶ Fig. 2.67). Additional neural structures, including the sympathetic chain, are

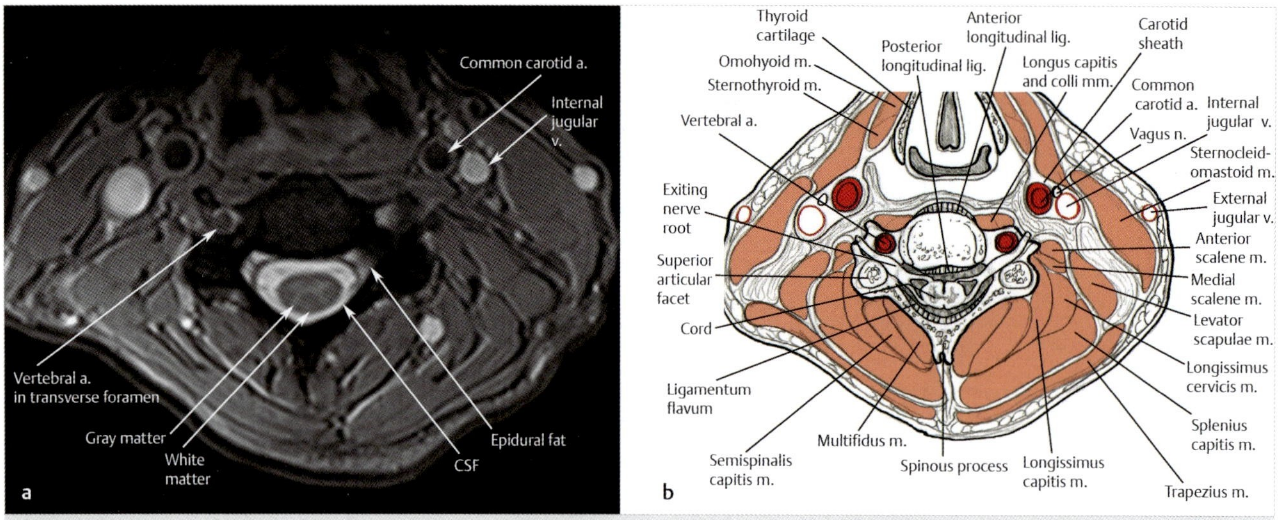

Fig. 2.64 An axial T2-weighted image **(a)** and artist's sketch **(b)** clearly defining the gray and white matter of the cervical spinal cord, the cerebrospinal fluid (CSF) within the subarachnoid space, and epidural fat. Normal flow voids are seen within the carotid and vertebral arteries. (Reproduced with permission from Dunleavy JD, Khanna AJ, Carrino JA. Normal MRI Anatomy of the Musculoskeletal System. In: Khanna AJ, ed. MRI for orthopaedic surgeons. New York: Thieme; 2010:17–76.)

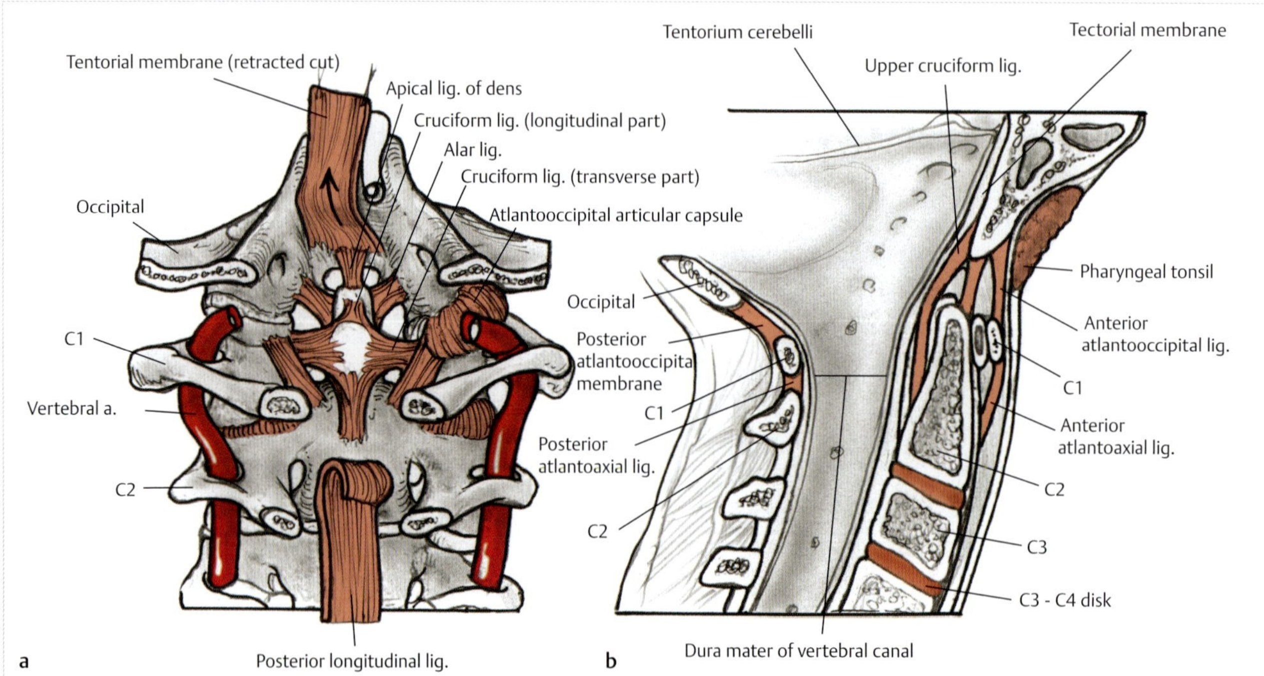

Fig. 2.65 Posteroanterior **(a)** and sagittal **(b)** illustrations showing the ligamentous structures of the skull base and cervical spine, including the alar ligament, cruciform ligament, and atlantooccipital ligaments. (Reproduced with permission from Dunleavy JD, Khanna AJ, Carrino JA. Normal MRI Anatomy of the Musculoskeletal System. In: Khanna AJ, ed. MRI for orthopaedic surgeons. New York: Thieme; 2010:17–76.)

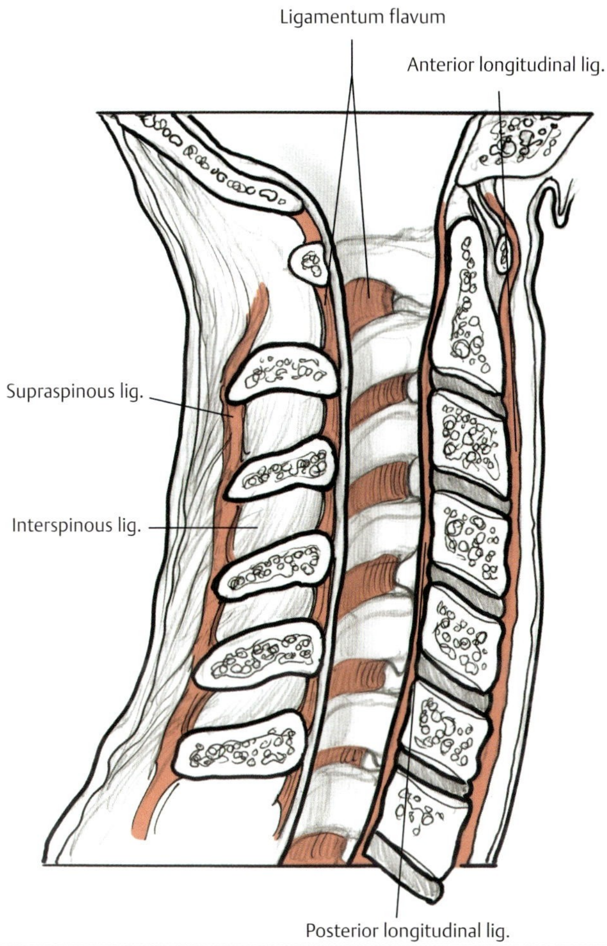

Fig. 2.66 An illustration (lateral view) of the cervical spine showing the midsagittal ligaments. (Reproduced with permission from Dunleavy JD, Khanna AJ, Carrino JA. Normal MRI Anatomy of the Musculoskeletal System. In: Khanna AJ, ed. MRI for orthopaedic surgeons. New York: Thieme; 2010:17–76.)

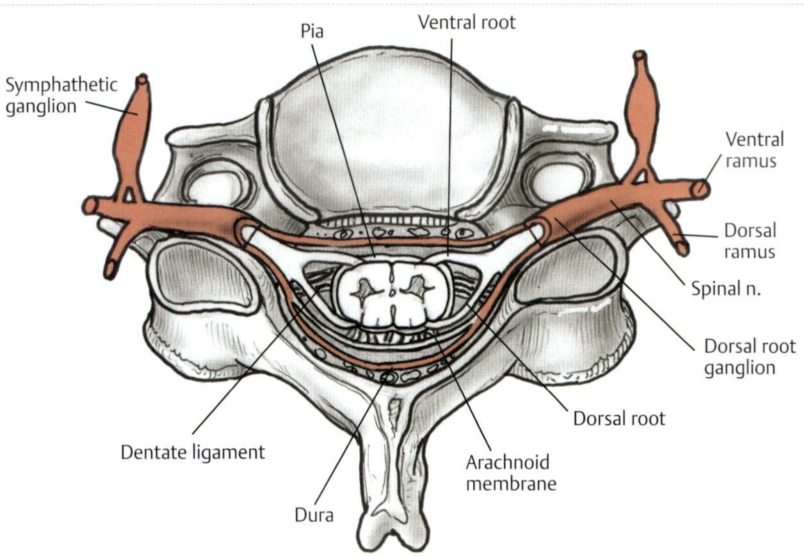

Fig. 2.67 An illustration (axial view) of the neural structures originating from the cervical spinal cord. (Reproduced with permission from Dunleavy JD, Khanna AJ, Carrino JA. Normal MRI Anatomy of the Musculoskeletal System. In: Khanna AJ, ed. MRI for orthopaedic surgeons. New York: Thieme; 2010:17–76.)

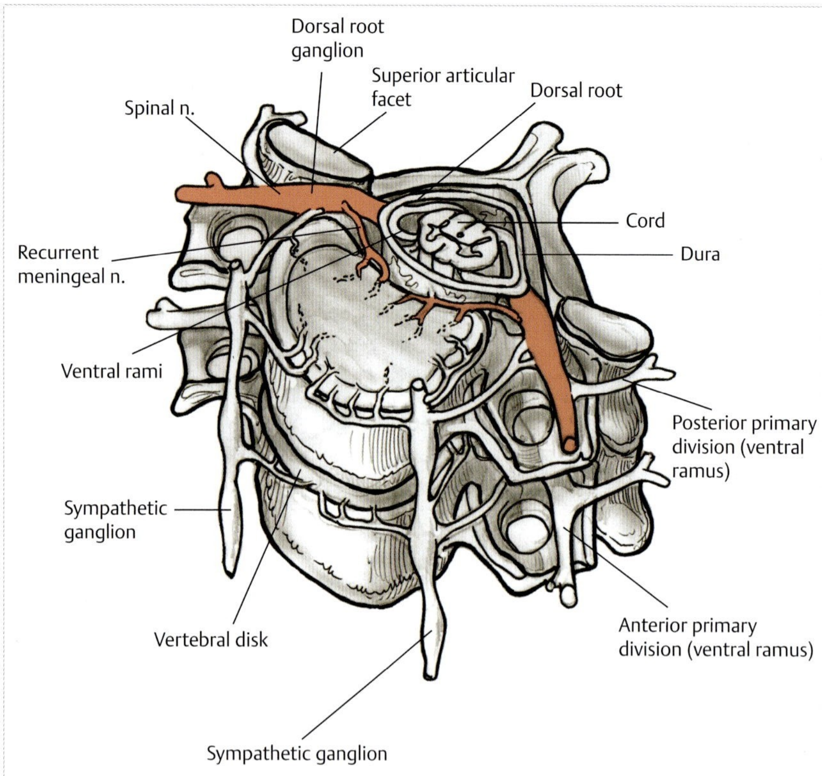

Fig. 2.68 A 3D illustration (anterosuperior view) of the neural structures in and around the cervical spine. (Reproduced with permission from Dunleavy JD, Khanna AJ, Carrino JA. Normal MRI Anatomy of the Musculoskeletal System. In: Khanna AJ, ed. MRI for orthopaedic surgeons. New York: Thieme; 2010:17–76.)

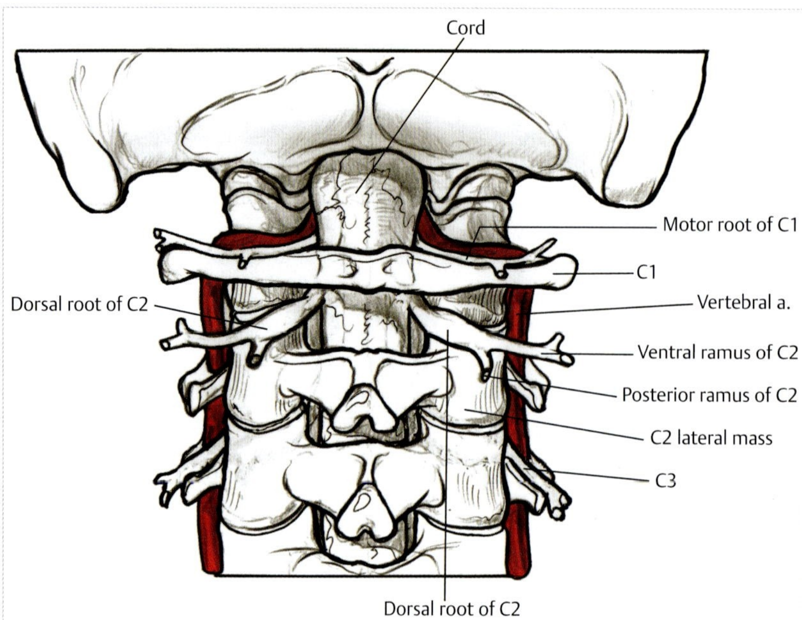

Fig. 2.69 A posterior 3D illustration of the upper cervical spine showing the location of the vertebral artery relative to the posterior arch of C1 and the exit of the C2 nerve root above the pedicle of C2. (Reproduced with permission from Dunleavy JD, Khanna AJ, Carrino JA. Normal MRI Anatomy of the Musculoskeletal System. In: Khanna AJ, ed. MRI for orthopaedic surgeons. New York: Thieme; 2010:17–76.)

located in and around the cervical vertebral bodies (▶ Fig. 2.68). Note that the C2 nerve root exits the spine above the C2 pedicle and runs parallel to the C1–C2 facet joint (▶ Fig. 2.69). The nerve roots have intermediate signal intensity and are surrounded by high-signal-intensity fat on T1-weighted images and by high-signal-intensity CSF on T2-weighted images.

2.9 Cervical Spine

2.9.1 Sagittal Images

The T1-weighted and T2-weighted sagittal images should be reviewed first to evaluate the spinal anatomy (▶ Fig. 2.70). The midsagittal image from the cervicomedullary to cervicothoracic

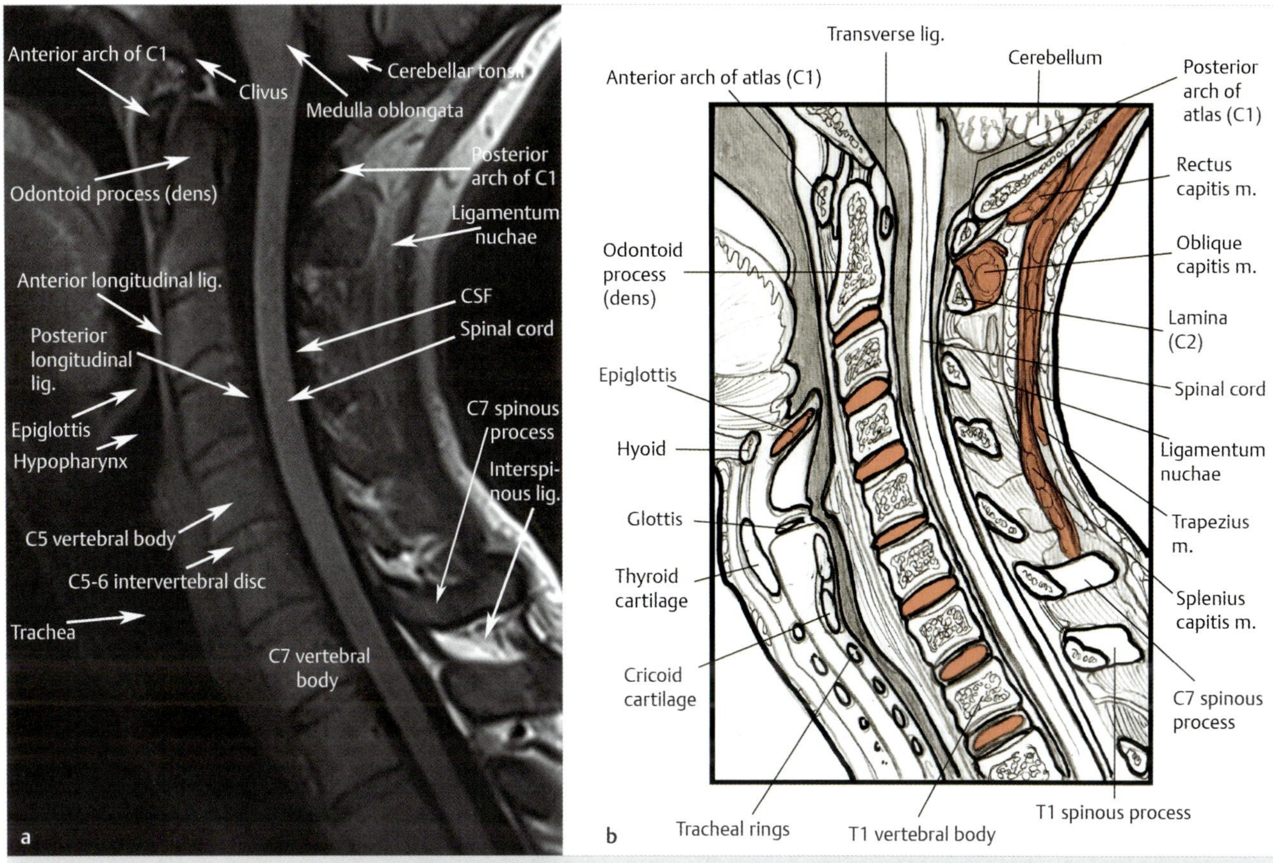

Fig. 2.70 A sagittal T1-weighted midline image **(a)** and artist's sketch **(b)** of the cervical spine depicting the cervical cord, cerebrospinal fluid (CSF), and the anterior and posterior longitudinal ligaments, as well as the anterior and posterior elements of the cervical spine and the intervertebral disks. (Reproduced with permission from Dunleavy JD, Khanna AJ, Carrino JA. Normal MRI Anatomy of the Musculoskeletal System. In: Khanna AJ, ed. MRI for orthopaedic surgeons. New York: Thieme; 2010:17–76.)

junctions is a good anatomic screen of the cervical vertebral bodies, intervertebral disks, spinal cord, thecal sac, and posterior elements. To find the midsagittal image, the sagittal series should be reviewed for the image that best shows the entire cervical spinal cord and the odontoid process, basion, opisthion, midbrain, and fourth ventricle.

Sequential evaluation of the sagittal series away from the midsagittal image allows for assessment of facet joints and neural foramina (▶ Fig. 2.71). The foramina have an oblique orientation to the sagittal plane, which can cause distortion and lead to artifactual narrowing. T1-weighted images are somewhat limited because they afford poor differentiation of the vertebral body, the annular-posterior longitudinal ligament complex, and the CSF in the adjacent thecal sac[19]; the posterior longitudinal ligament, a disk herniation, an osseous spur, and CSF all appear as a low-intensity signal on T1-weighted sagittal images.[19] The CSF–extradural interface is well defined on T2-weighted images, and a myelographic appearance is produced on T2-weighted sagittal images because of the CSF's high signal. The intervertebral disks show intermediate signal intensity on T1-weighted images and high signal intensity on T2-weighted and gradient-echo images.

The cervical vertebral body has bright signal intensity on T1-weighted images because of the presence of normal fatty bone marrow. Normal cervical spine lordosis should be observed. The AP diameter of the canal tapers from the first to third cervical levels and then is relatively constant. Parasagittal images show the short cervical pedicles. The anterior and posterior longitudinal ligaments are depicted as low-signal-intensity linear structures along the vertebral bodies.[18,20,21] Often, a small cortical defect is seen in the midportion of the posterior vertebral body; this defect represents a vascular channel and is a normal finding.

2.9.2 Axial Images

Evaluation of the cervical spine on axial MRI initially requires the correct identification of the spinal level, which can be accomplished by using the localizing sagittal images or by evaluating signal intensity differences between the intervertebral disks and vertebral bodies and sequentially numbering the levels caudal to the odontoid process. Given the potential risk of wrong-level surgery, special care should be taken to identify the correct spinal level by using a combination of sagittal and axial labeling techniques. In addition, most imaging

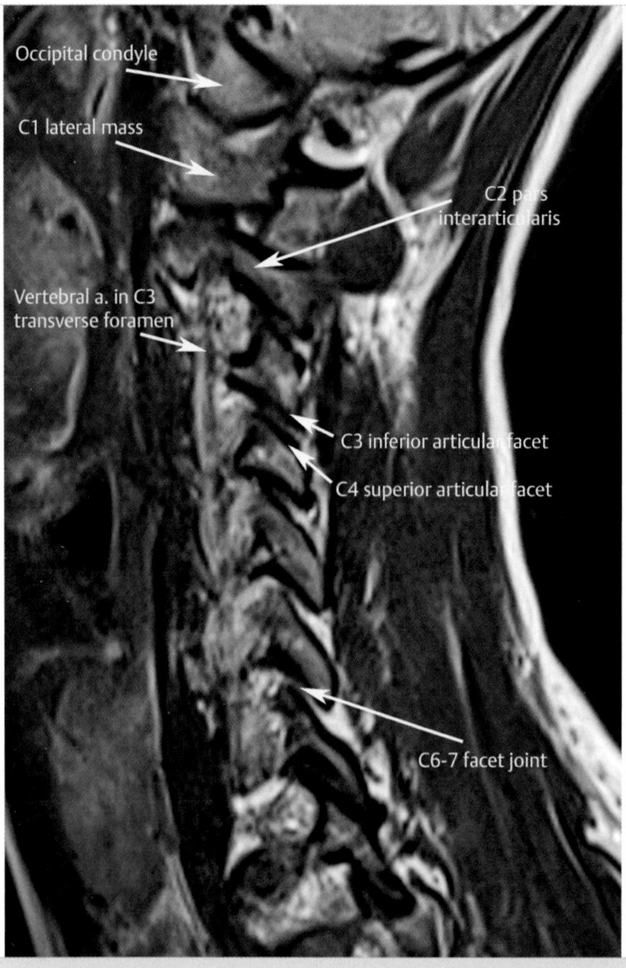

Fig. 2.71 A sagittal T2-weighted paramidline image of the cervical spine showing the vertebral artery in long axis coursing through the transverse foramina of the cervical spine. The facet joints are most easily evaluated in the parasagittal plane, as shown here. (Reproduced with permission from Dunleavy JD, Khanna AJ, Carrino JA. Normal MRI Anatomy of the Musculoskeletal System. In: Khanna AJ, ed. MRI for orthopaedic surgeons. New York: Thieme; 2010:17–76.)

workstations have a tool that allows the vertebral bodies to be identified using the numbering techniques outlined above, which facilitates rapid localization on the midsagittal images while evaluating the associated axial images.

Cervical spine anatomy and anatomic pathology are well visualized on axial T1-weighted images; T2-weighted images have good CSF-to-cord contrast (▶ Fig. 2.64), which allows evaluation of spinal cord or nerve root compression.[18,20,21] Knowledge of the location of the various spinal tracts can allow a clinician to correlate the clinical and radiographic findings in a patient with known or suspected spinal cord injury (▶ Fig. 2.72). Compared with sagittal images, axial T2-weighted images can provide a higher resolution depiction of the cord (because of the smaller field of view), enabling a more sensitive assessment of its signal intensity. Sagittal images are also helpful in evaluating signal abnormalities in the spinal cord because one image can show a long segment of the spinal cord. Neural foramina are best depicted with gradient-echo and T2-weighted images and should be evaluated on axial and parasagittal images. Evaluation of the neural foramina in the axial and sagittal planes takes experience and training, especially with patients who have scoliosis or poor positioning in the scanner, which can cause each neural foramen to be visualized on individual parasagittal images. Care should be taken to evaluate the axial T2-weighted images and to recognize the normal shape and size of the central canal and the neural foramina. Specifically, the degree of contribution of the three primary contributors to cervical spinal stenosis (disk pathology, facet arthropathy, and ligamentum flavum hypertrophy) should be noted, and their combined contribution to the degree of central and foraminal stenosis should be assessed. The anterior border of the neural foramen is the disk, and the posterior border is the facet joint (▶ Fig. 2.73). It is important to note the location and course of the vertebral arteries on the axial images. Aberrant vertebral arteries should be identified preoperatively, especially if a cervical corpectomy is being considered. Furthermore, the vertebral arteries should show normal hypointense pulsation signal. Incidentally imaged structures should also be evaluated. For instance, lymph nodes in the neck should be evaluated for size and the presence of a normal fatty hilum. The thyroid should also be evaluated for size and to exclude large nodules.

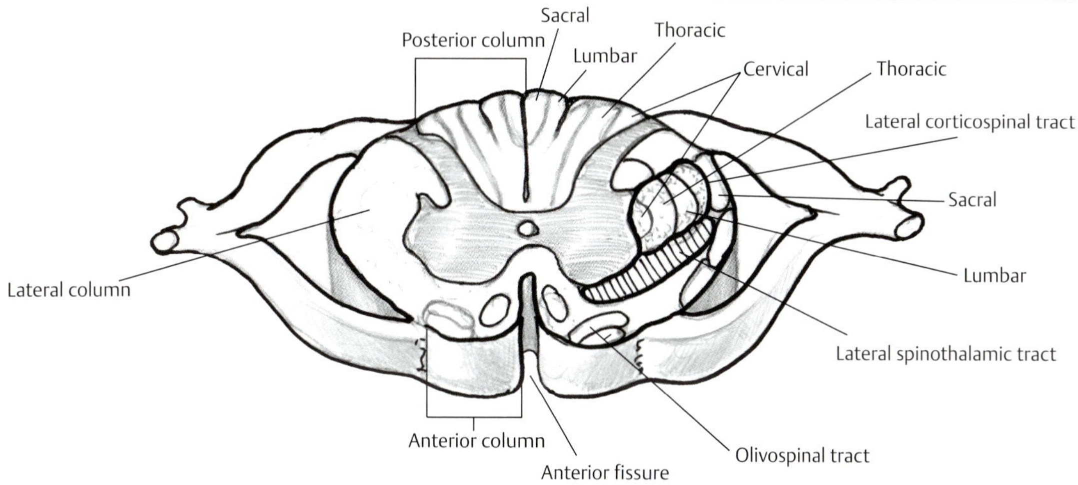

Fig. 2.72 An axial 3D illustration of cervical spinal cord anatomy with location of various spinal tracts. (Reproduced with permission from Dunleavy JD, Khanna AJ, Carrino JA. Normal MRI Anatomy of the Musculoskeletal System. In: Khanna AJ, ed. MRI for orthopaedic surgeons. New York: Thieme; 2010:17–76.)

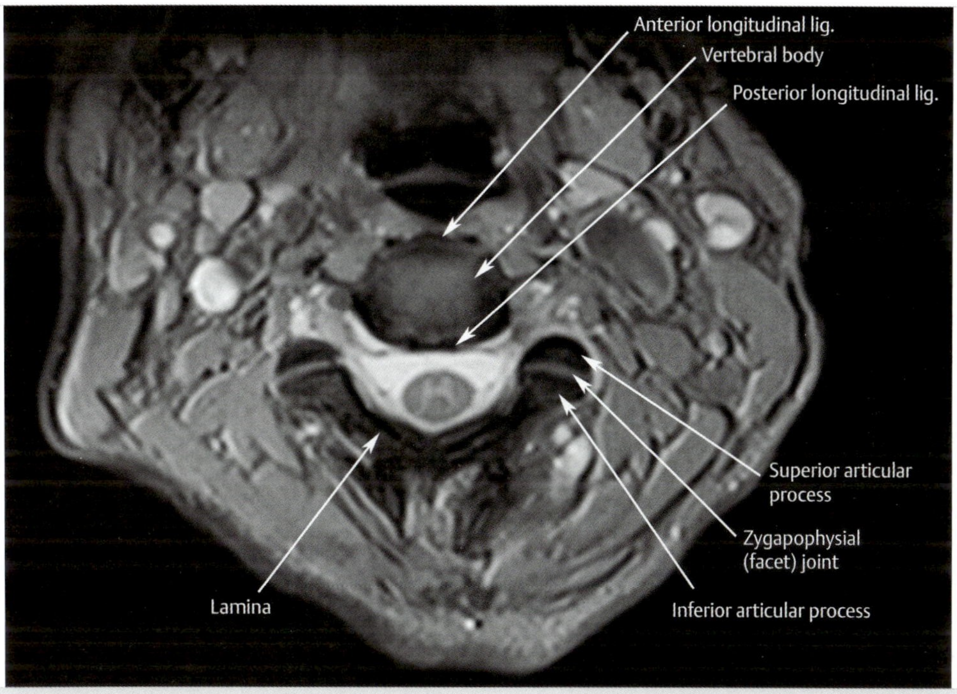

Fig. 2.73 An axial T2-weighted image of the cervical spine showing the anterior and posterior longitudinal ligaments and the superior and inferior articular processes of the facet joints. (Reproduced with permission from Dunleavy JD, Khanna AJ, Carrino JA. Normal MRI Anatomy of the Musculoskeletal System. In: Khanna AJ, ed. MRI for orthopaedic surgeons. New York: Thieme; 2010:17–76.)

2.9.3 Coronal Images

Coronal images show the craniocervical spine articulations, intervertebral disks, uncinate processes, atlantooccipital joints, and lateral atlantoaxial joints.[18] Although the sagittal and axial images provide enough information for diagnosis in most cases, coronal images may be especially valuable for evaluating the craniocervical junction or assessing for spinal tumors. Coronal plane MR images, along with conventional radiographs, also facilitate evaluation of the rarely occurring cervical scoliosis because the entire scoliotic spine can be included within a single imaging plane.

2.10 Thoracic Spine

MRI of the thoracic spine is obtained relatively less frequently than that of the lumbar and cervical spine. The anatomic structures in the thoracic spine are unique, in that the ribs form two additional articulations with the vertebrae: the costocentral joint (between the vertebral body and the rib head) and the costotransverse joint (between the transverse process and proximal rib). The thoracic intervertebral disks are fairly uniform and monotonous. The facet joints are coronally oriented.

2.11 Lumbar Spine

2.11.1 Sagittal Images

Sagittal imaging of the lumbar spine is usually obtained with T1-weighted and T2-weighted pulse sequences (▶ Fig. 2.74, ▶ Fig. 2.75). The T1-weighted images are best used for evaluating the anatomic detail of the lumbar spine. The midsagittal image should be evaluated first. This image shows the full profile of the sacrum and most of the lumbar vertebral bodies, spinal cord, and cauda equina in patients without substantial scoliosis. After evaluating the midsagittal image, the sagittal images are sequentially evaluated toward each side to assess the facet joints and neural foramina. The sagittal images can be concurrently evaluated with the axial sequence to confirm laterality. The bright signal from CSF on T2-weighted images provides a myelographic effect. T1-weighted gradient-echo images assist by providing improved evaluation of end plate and osteophyte anatomy and differentiation of the anterior and posterior longitudinal ligaments from the cortical bone.

2.11.2 Axial Images

When evaluating axial MR images, it is important to accurately identify the level at which the pathology exists, which can be achieved by using the localizing sagittal image. In addition, each level can be identified by starting at the sacrum and numbering each vertebral body from L5 to L1. In complex cases where severe pathology is present at multiple levels, it may also be helpful to use the spine labeling tool (see section "Cervical Spine"). On axial images, the difference in signal intensity between the intervertebral disks and vertebral bodies allows for the distinction between vertebral levels. Evaluation of the axial images requires more experience and training than does the evaluation of the sagittal images. Care should be taken to evaluate the axial T2-weighted images and recognize the normal shape and size of the central canal and the neural foramina (▶ Fig. 2.76). Specifically, the degree of contribution of the three primary contributors to spinal stenosis (disk pathology, facet arthropathy, and ligamentum flavum hypertrophy) should be noted, and their combined contribution to the

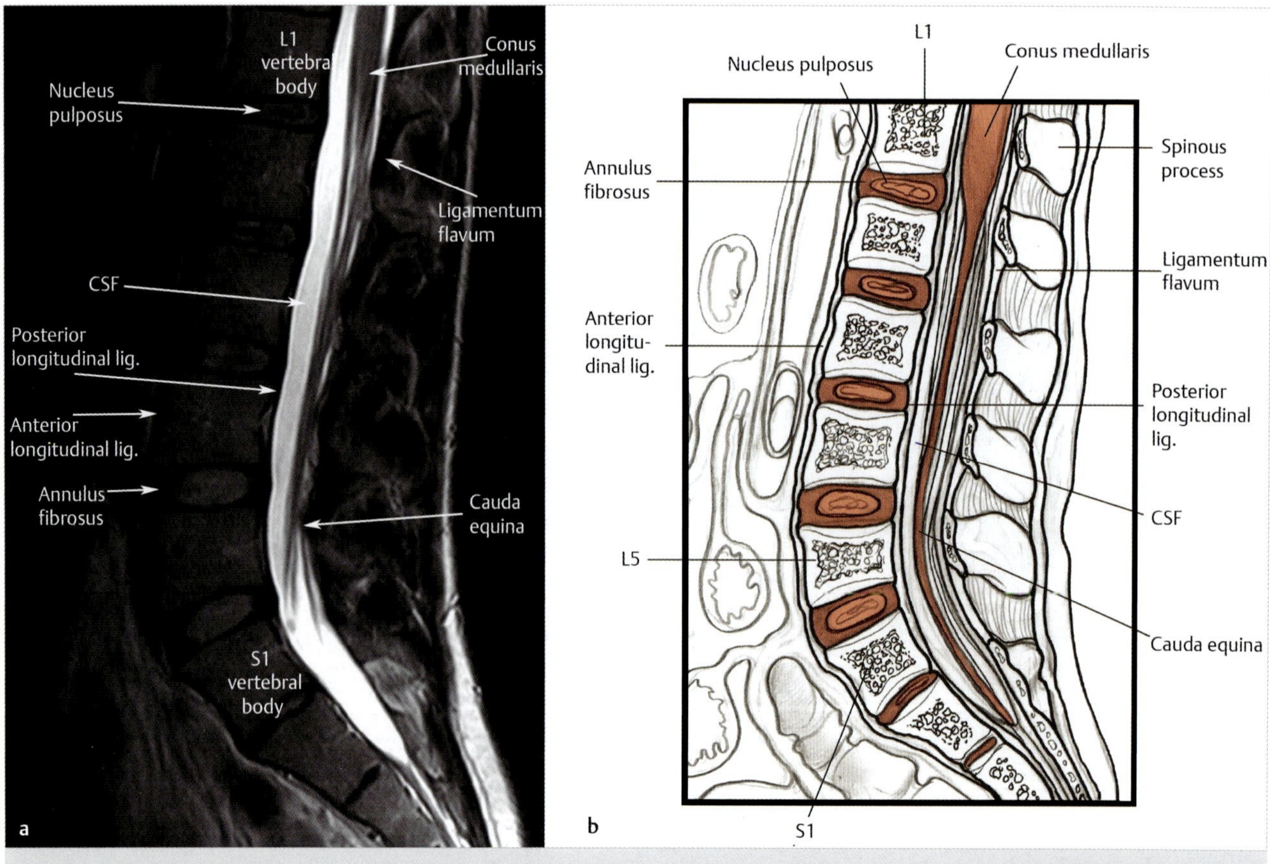

Fig. 2.74 A sagittal T2-weighted midline image (a) and artist's sketch (b) of the lumbar spine showing the conus medullaris. The posterior longitudinal ligament, intervertebral disks, and vertebral bodies are better differentiated on the T2-weighted images than on T1-weighted images (see ▶ Fig. 2.70). Abbreviations: CSF, cerebrospinal fluid. (Reproduced with permission from Dunleavy JD, Khanna AJ, Carrino JA. Normal MRI Anatomy of the Musculoskeletal System. In: Khanna AJ, ed. MRI for orthopaedic surgeons. New York: Thieme; 2010:17–76.)

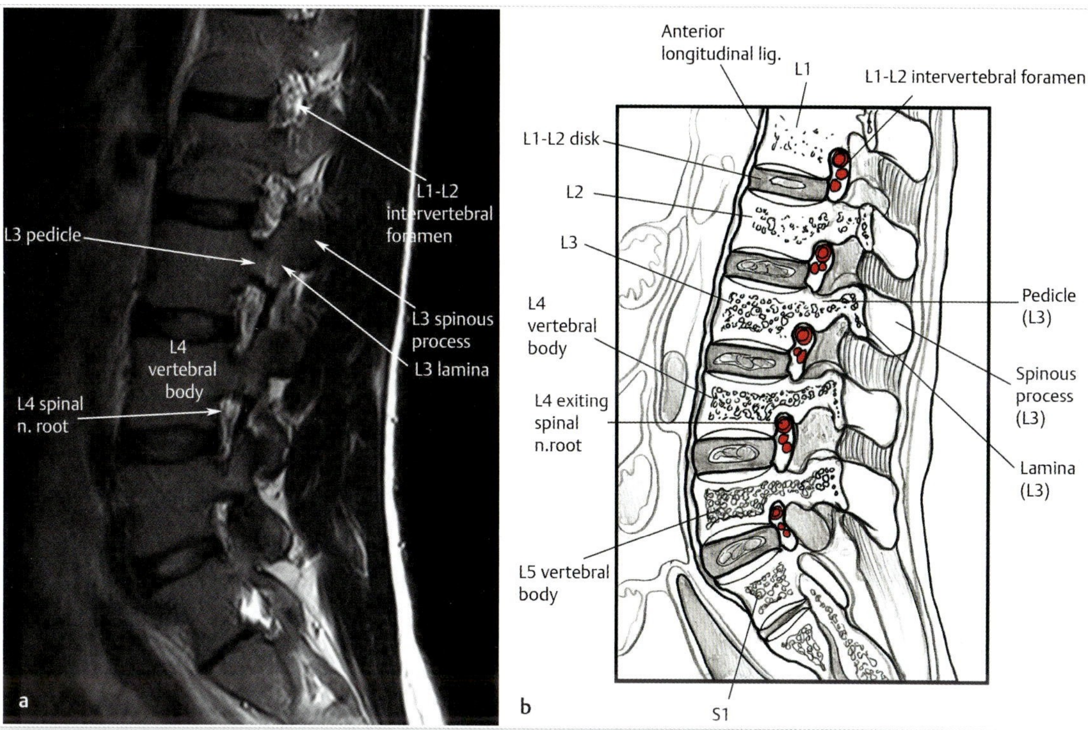

Fig. 2.75 A parasagittal T2-weighted image **(a)** and artist's sketch **(b)** of the lumbar spine showing the neural foramina and exiting nerve roots at multiple levels. (Reproduced with permission from Dunleavy JD, Khanna AJ, Carrino JA. Normal MRI Anatomy of the Musculoskeletal System. In: Khanna AJ, ed. MRI for orthopaedic surgeons. New York: Thieme; 2010:17–76.)

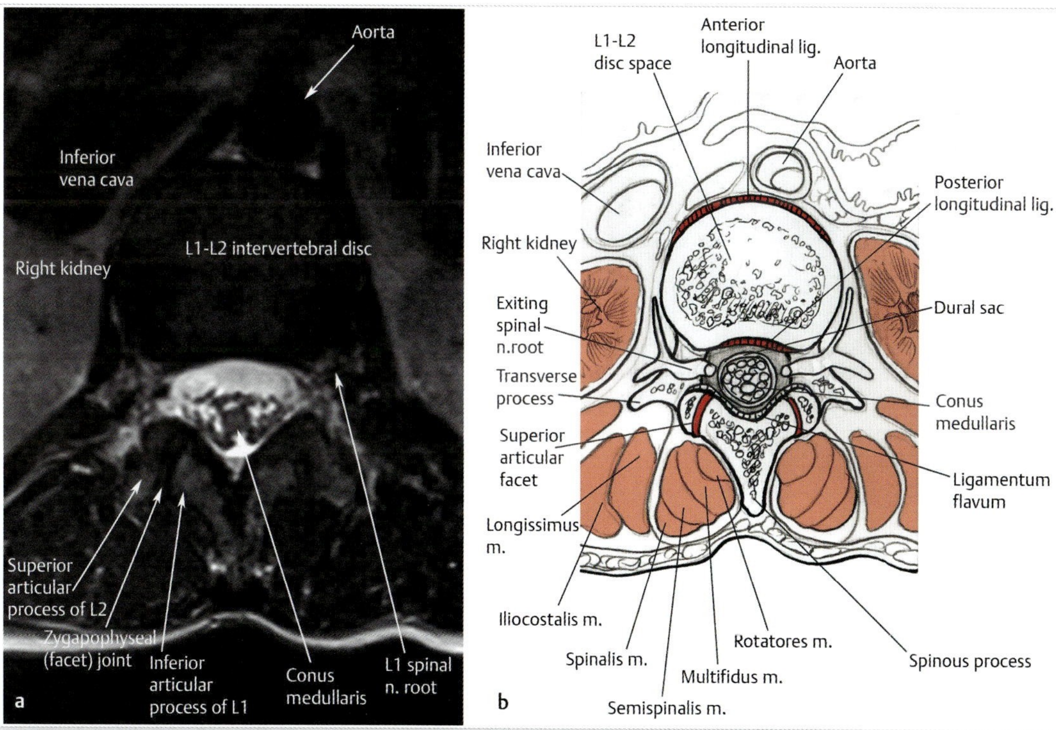

Fig. 2.76 An axial T2-weighted image **(a)** and artist's sketch **(b)** of the spine at the level of the L1–L2 intervertebral disk showing the conus medullaris and the L1 spinal nerve root, as well as the superior and inferior articular processes of the L1–L2 facet joint. (Reproduced with permission from Dunleavy JD, Khanna AJ, Carrino JA. Normal MRI Anatomy of the Musculoskeletal System. In: Khanna AJ, ed. MRI for orthopaedic surgeons. New York: Thieme; 2010:17–76.)

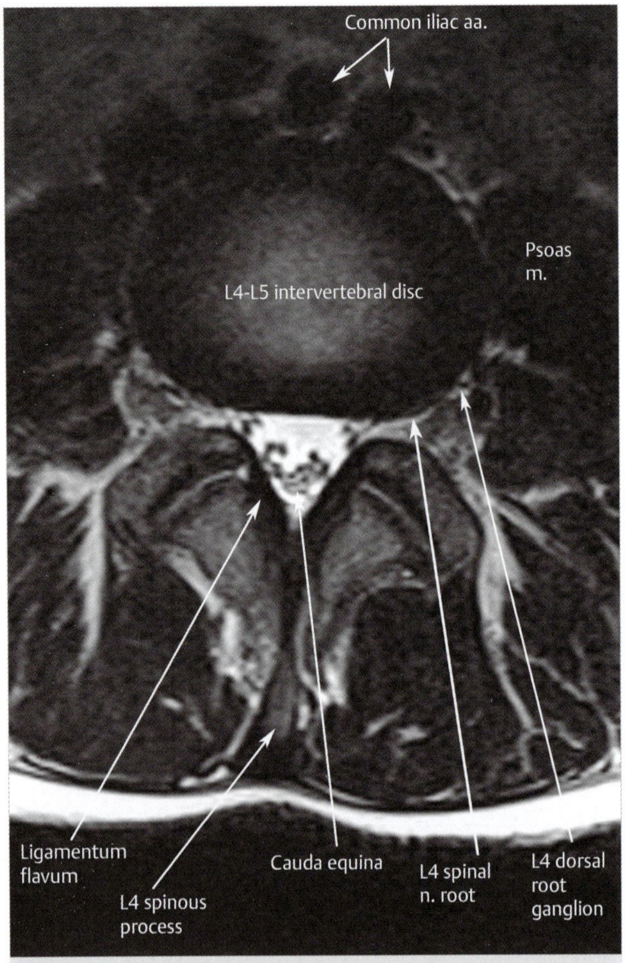

Fig. 2.77 An axial T2-weighted image at the level of the L4–L5 intervertebral disk showing the cauda equina, L4 spinal nerve root, and L4 dorsal root ganglion. Normal flow voids are seen within the common iliac arteries, just below the aortic bifurcation. (Reproduced with permission from Dunleavy JD, Khanna AJ, Carrino JA. Normal MRI Anatomy of the Musculoskeletal System. In: Khanna AJ, ed. MRI for orthopaedic surgeons. New York: Thieme; 2010:17–76.)

degree of central and foraminal stenosis should be carefully assessed (▶ Fig. 2.77). The relationship between the superior articular process from the caudal level and the exiting nerve root should be evaluated because hypertrophy of this structure leads to lateral recess and foraminal stenosis. The extraforaminal zone should also be studied at each level to rule out far lateral disk pathology. The psoas muscles are seen adjacent to the vertebral bodies in the lumbar spine (▶ Fig. 2.77), and the major vessels (including the aorta and vena cava) are seen anterior to the vertebral bodies. Along with the spine, these structures should also be evaluated for pathologic processes such as aneurysm, thrombosis, and infection.

2.11.3 Coronal Images

Coronal images provide a clear evaluation of the general alignment and anatomy of the lumbar spine, allowing for the identification of the vertebrae and intervertebral disks. Because lordosis increases toward the caudal aspect of the lumbar spine, it is impossible to obtain one image that visualizes the entire spinal canal and its contents. The coronal plane images can be used to evaluate spinal alignment and transitional anatomy at the lumbosacral junction.

2.12 Common Clinical Questions

1. Which MRI sequence is best for evaluating articular cartilage?
   a) T1 weighted.
   b) T2 weighted.
   c) Gradient echo.
   d) Proton weighted.

2. Which MRI sequence is best for assessment of ACL injury?
   a) Axial T1 weighted.
   b) Sagittal proton density.
   c) Coronal T2 weighted.
   d) Axial STIR.

3. Which MRI sequence is best for assessment of retrocalcaneal bursitis?
   a) Axial T1 weighted.
   b) Sagittal T2 weighted.
   c) Coronal Gradient echo.
   d) Axial Proton density.

4. Which MRI image is best for assessment of glenoid labrum and long head of biceps?
   a) Sagittal oblique images.
   b) Axial and coronal oblique images.
   c) True sagittal images.
   d) True coronal images.

5. Which MRI image is best for assessment of knee collateral ligaments?
   a) Sagittal oblique images.
   b) Axial images.
   c) Coronal images.
   d) Coronal oblique images.

References

[1] Stoller DW, ed. Stoller's atlas of orthopaedics and sports medicine. Baltimore, MD: Lippincott Williams & Wilkins; 2008

[2] Anderson MW, Fox MG, El-Khoury GY. Sectional anatomy by MRI and CT. 4th ed. Philadelphia, PA: Elsevier; 2016

[3] Uri DS. MR imaging of shoulder impingement and rotator cuff disease. Radiol Clin North Am. 1997; 35(1):77–96

[4] Fritz RC. Magnetic resonance imaging of sports-related injuries to the shoulder: impingement and rotator cuff. Radiol Clin North Am. 2002; 40(2): 217–234, vi

[5] Bredella MA, Tirman PFJ, Peterfy CG, et al. Accuracy of T2-weighted fast spin-echo MR imaging with fat saturation in detecting cartilage defects in the knee: comparison with arthroscopy in 130 patients. AJR Am J Roentgenol. 1999; 172(4):1073–1080

[6] Disler DG, Recht MP, McCauley TR. MR imaging of articular cartilage. Skeletal Radiol. 2000; 29(7):367–377

[7] Potter HG, Linklater JM, Allen AA, Hannafin JA, Haas SB. Magnetic resonance imaging of articular cartilage in the knee. An evaluation with use of fast-spin-echo imaging. J Bone Joint Surg Am. 1998; 80(9):1276–1284
[8] Crema MD, Roemer FW, Marra MD, et al. Articular cartilage in the knee: current MR imaging techniques and applications in clinical practice and research. Radiographics. 2011; 31(1):37–61
[9] Blease S, Stoller DW, Safran MR, Li AE, Fritz RC. The elbow. In: Stoller DW, ed. Magnetic resonance imaging in orthopaedics and sports medicine. Philadelphia, PA: Lippincott Williams & Wilkins; 2007:1463–1625
[10] Werlen S, Leunig M, Ganz R. Magnetic resonance arthrography of the hip in femoracetabular impingement: technique and findings. Oper Tech Orthop. 2005; 15:191–203
[11] Fitzgerald RH, Jr. Acetabular labrum tears. Diagnosis and treatment. Clin Orthop Relat Res. 1995(311):60–68
[12] Munshi M, Pretterklieber ML, Kwak S, Antonio GE, Trudell DJ, Resnick D. MR imaging, MR arthrography, and specimen correlation of the posterolateral corner of the knee: an anatomic study. AJR Am J Roentgenol. 2003; 180(4): 1095–1101
[13] Loredo R, Hodler J, Pedowitz R, Yeh LR, Trudell D, Resnick D. Posteromedial corner of the knee: MR imaging with gross anatomic correlation. Skeletal Radiol. 1999; 28(6):305–311
[14] Cone RO III. Knee. Section B. Imaging sports-related injuries of the knee. In: DeLee JC, Drez D Jr, Miller MD, eds. DeLee and Drez's orthopaedic sports medicine: principles and practice. Philadelphia, PA: WB Saunders; 2003:1595–1652
[15] Stanitski CL. Knee. Section D. Meniscal injuries. Part 2. Meniscal injuries in the skeletally immature patient. In: DeLee JC, Drez D Jr, Miller MD, eds. DeLee and Drez's orthopaedic sports medicine: principles and practice. Philadelphia, PA: WB Saunders; 2003:1686–1696
[16] Peterfy CG, Janzen DL, Tirman PFJ, van Dijke CF, Pollack M, Genant HK. "Magic-angle" phenomenon: a cause of increased signal in the normal lateral meniscus on short-TE MR images of the knee. AJR Am J Roentgenol. 1994; 163(1):149–154
[17] Morgan S, Saifuddin A. MRI of the lumbar intervertebral disc. Clin Radiol. 1999; 54(11):703–723
[18] White ML. Cervical spine: MR imaging techniques and anatomy. Magn Reson Imaging Clin N Am. 2000; 8(3):453–470
[19] Kaiser JA, Holland BA. Imaging of the cervical spine. Spine. 1998; 23(24): 2701–2712
[20] Khanna AJ, Carbone JJ, Kebaish KM, et al. Magnetic resonance imaging of the cervical spine. Current techniques and spectrum of disease. J Bone Joint Surg Am. 2002; 84-A Suppl 2:70–80
[21] Boden SD, Lee RR, Herzog RJ. Magnetic resonance imaging of the spine. In: Frymoyer JW, ed. The adult spine: principles and practice. Philadelphia: Lippincott-Raven; 1997:563–629

Answers to Common Clinical Questions

1. Answer: c. Gradient echo.
2. Answer: b. Sagittal proton density.
3. Answer: b. Sagittal T2 weighted.
4. Answer: b. Axial and coronal oblique images.
5. Answer: c. Coronal images.

3 A Systematic Approach to the Review of Spine MRI Studies

Andrew B. Harris, Amit Jain, and A. Jay Khanna

Abstract

The purpose of this chapter is to provide the clinician or radiologist with a method for evaluating magnetic resonance imaging (MRI) studies in an organized and systematic fashion, given that a systematic approach to reviewing spinal MRI studies has the potential to reduce errors in interpretation and diagnosis. To simplify and standardize the approach to review and interpret spinal MRI studies, we break the process down into five steps: (1) determination of MRI pulse sequences available for review; (2) evaluation of T2-weighted images; (3) evaluation of T1-weighted images; (4) evaluation of specialized MRI pulse sequences; (5) correlation of the imaging information from Steps 1–4 with the patient's history, physical examination, and laboratory study results. Subsequent chapters will build upon the general process of systematically reviewing MRI studies outlined in this chapter.

Keywords: MRI, spine, systematic approach, structured reporting, checklist

3.1 Introduction

As with any new skill, learning the technique of evaluating a magnetic resonance imaging (MRI) study begins with a systematic approach. Given that a checklist approach has been well demonstrated to reduce errors in medicine, a systematic approach to reviewing MRI studies has the potential to reduce errors in interpretation and diagnosis.[1,2,3] Less experienced clinicians may have a tendency to review imaging studies without paying special attention to the type of pulse sequences that are being evaluated or to the plane in which they are being evaluated. When reviewing MRI studies on a computer workstation, they may also tend to review only one pulse sequence or one or two imaging planes. These shortcuts, especially early in a clinician's experience in evaluating MRI studies, may lead to less accurate and less reliable MR study interpretation compared with a structured reporting methodology.[4]

Chapter 1 (Essentials of MRI Physics and Pulse Sequences) provided a summary of the technical foundation that radiologists often use to select the appropriate pulse sequences and imaging techniques for the study of a given region or pathologic process. The purpose of this more clinically oriented chapter is to provide the clinician or radiologist with a method for evaluating MRI studies in an organized and systematic fashion. The adoption of such a system early in a clinician's experience is believed to lead to improved accuracy and reliability in the interpretation of MRI studies. Over time, clinicians may be able to incorporate a more informal method of evaluating MRI studies and rely more on their own experience and personalized method of study evaluation.

The evaluation of an MRI study of the spine can be divided into the following five steps:

1. Determination of which conventional and specialized MRI pulse sequences are available for review.
2. Evaluation of T2-weighted images for recognition of areas of increased T2-weighted signal that are not expected or physiologic.
3. Evaluation of T1-weighted images for improved detection of anatomic detail and correlation of the alteration in local and regional anatomy on the T1-weighted images with areas of increased signal intensity on the T2-weighted images.
4. Evaluation of specialized MRI pulse sequences that may be specific to the region or disease process that is being evaluated.
5. Correlation of the imaging information from Steps 1–4 with the patient's history, physical examination, and laboratory study results to identify the most likely differential diagnostic considerations.

The use of a general technique of MRI study evaluation described in this chapter, in conjunction with the more region- and concept-specific information provided in subsequent chapters, will help improve a clinician's ability to interpret MRI studies of the spine accurately.

3.2 Step 1: Determination of Pulse Sequences Available for Review

The first step in the evaluation of an MRI study is to determine which pulse sequences are available for review. For most cases, such sequences include at least T1-weighted and conventional T2-weighted images, acquired in the sagittal and axial planes. For patients with spinal deformities such as scoliosis, images may also be obtained in the coronal plane.

In addition to conventional T1-weighted and T2-weighted pulse sequences, there are other pulse sequences that are often acquired and that should be recognizable, including the following:

- Fat-suppressed T2-weighted images or short tau inversion recovery (STIR) images.
- Postgadolinium T1-weighted images.
- MR angiography images.

3.2.1 T1-Weighted and T2-Weighted Images

One should be able to determine whether an image is T1-weighted or T2-weighted using the following techniques:

- Recognition of an area within an image that is known to contain fluid, such as cerebrospinal fluid (CSF) (▶ Fig. 3.1). If this fluid is noted to be bright or of high signal intensity, then the image is likely T2-weighted. If the region of the fluid is noted to be dark, then the image is likely T1 weighted.

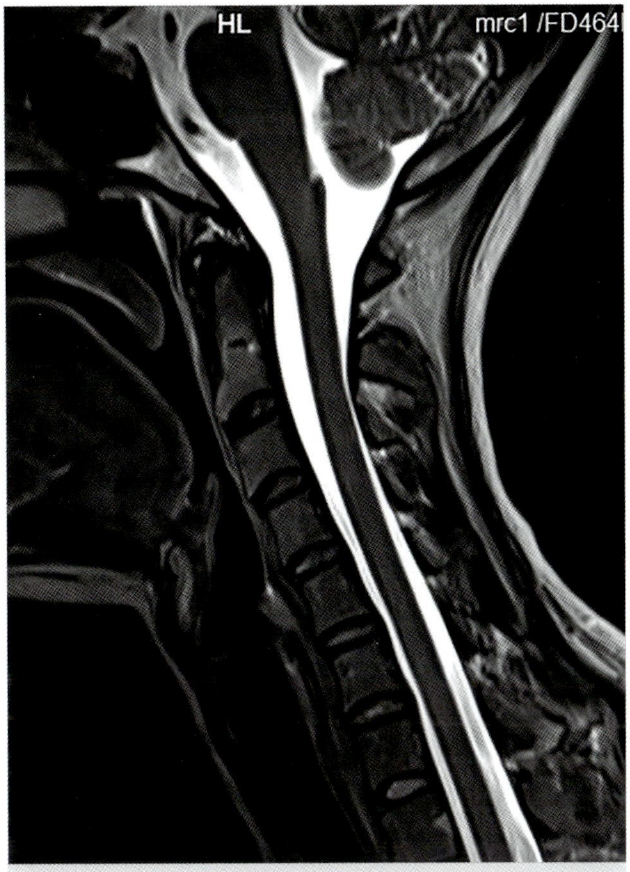

Fig. 3.1 A sagittal T2-weighted image of the cervical spine. Note that the cerebrospinal fluid (CSF) is of high signal intensity. (Reproduced with permission from, A Systematic Approach to the Review of Spine MRI Studies. In: Khanna A, ed. MRI Essentials for the Spine Specialist. 1st Edition. New York: Thieme; 2014.)

- Recognition of the repetition time (TR) and time to echo (TE) values, which are often printed on the film or are visible on the workstation screen. Recognizing these values may enable the clinician to determine whether an image is T1-weighted or T2-weighted. In most institutions and in most cases, images are acquired using a spin-echo (SE) technique (for additional details, see Chapter 1, Essentials of MRI Physics and Pulse Sequences). When this technique or similar techniques are used, the TR value is usually 300 to 800 ms for T1-weighted images and 2,000 to 5,000 ms for T2-weighted images. If the clinician evaluates the image and is unable to use the technique in which fluid recognition allows the differentiation of T1-weighted and T2-weighted images, this technique is a good second option. If the TR number is noted to be in the hundreds range, the image likely is T1-weighted. If the TR number is found to be in the thousands range, the image likely is T2-weighted. With newer and more variable pulse sequences, this method may be less reliable.

3.2.2 Fat-Suppressed T2-Weighted Images or STIR Images

Fat-suppressed T2-weighted images are acquired using techniques similar to those for conventional T2-weighted images, and then various computer algorithms and processes are used to "suppress" the signal that is coming from fat. A more "pure" way of achieving

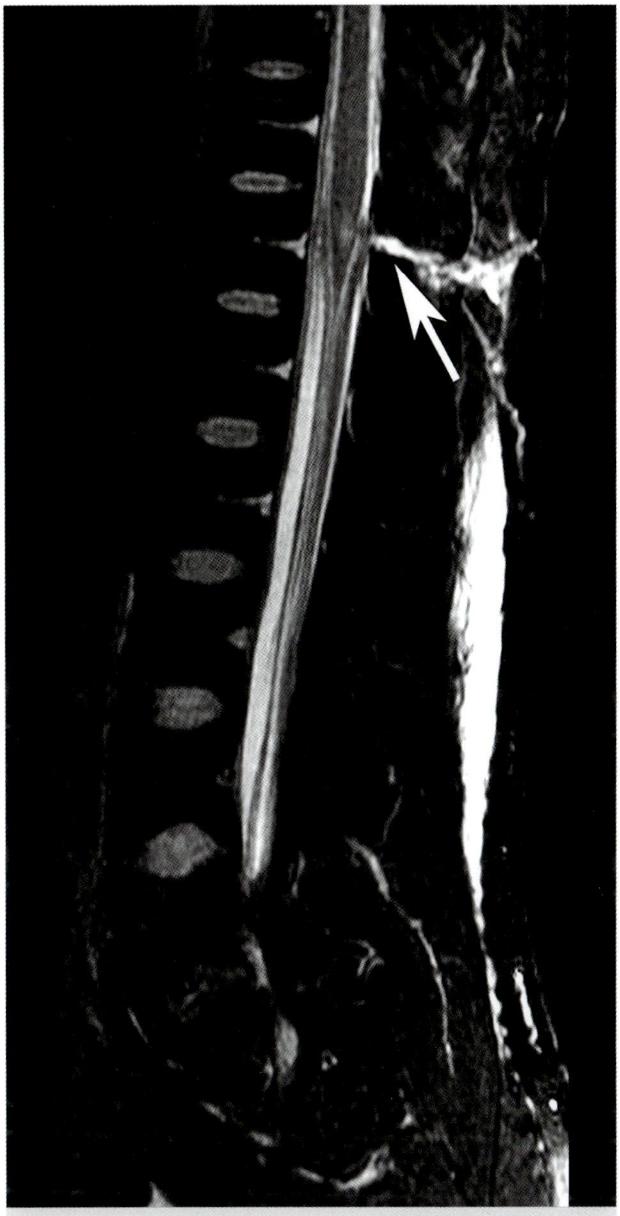

Fig. 3.2 A sagittal short tau inversion recovery (STIR) image of the thoracolumbar spine accentuates the edema along the track (*arrow*) of a stab injury to the conus medullaris. Note that, aside from the pathologic fluid, the hydrated disks in this young patient, and the CSF within the spinal canal, this image is quite "dark." (Reproduced with permission from, A Systematic Approach to the Review of Spine MRI Studies. In: Khanna A, ed. MRI Essentials for the Spine Specialist. 1st Edition. New York: Thieme; 2014.)

this goal is to acquire a STIR image, in which case the signal from fat is not acquired. Because of the suppression of signal from fat in either of these techniques, the images tend to appear quite a bit "darker" than images obtained via other techniques (such as conventional T2-weighted images) and thus help accentuate the increase in T2-weighted signal (relative to the adjacent tissues), which may otherwise be missed (▶ Fig. 3.2). Specifically, this technique facilitates the evaluation of bone-marrow edema and edema secondary to other pathologic processes. Fat-suppressed T2-weighted images or STIR images show areas of edema with markedly greater conspicuity than that seen on conventional T2-weighted images (see individual chapters for applications of these techniques for region-specific pathology).

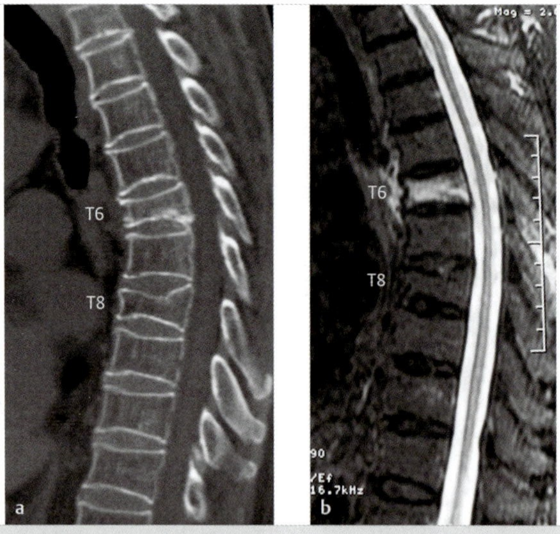

Fig. 3.3 Vertebral compression fracture. **(a)** A sagittal reconstructed computed tomography (CT) image shows vertebral compression fractures at the T6 and T8 levels. **(b)** A sagittal short tau inversion recovery (STIR) image shows that the T6 vertebral compression fracture has increased signal compatible with edema within it, which is representative of an acute or subacute fracture. The T8 vertebral compression fracture shows no increase in signal within it, which is compatible with a chronic vertebral compression fracture. (Reproduced with permission from, A Systematic Approach to the Review of Spine MRI Studies. In: Khanna A, ed. MRI Essentials for the Spine Specialist. 1st Edition. New York: Thieme; 2014.)

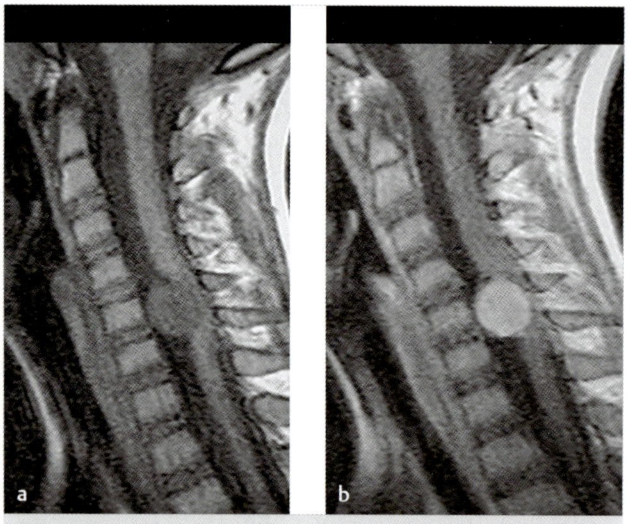

Fig. 3.4 Postgadolinium contrast enhancement. **(a)** A pregadolinium sagittal T1-weighted image shows an intradural-extramedullary mass at the C5–C6 level. **(b)** The associated postgadolinium T1-weighted image shows that the mass has uniform contrast enhancement. This mass was found to be a schwannoma. (Reproduced from Khanna AJ, Carbone JJ, Kebaish KM, Cohen DB, Riley LH, III, Wasserman BA, Kostuik JP. Magnetic resonance imaging of the cervical spine: current techniques and spectrum of disease. J Bone Joint Surg Am. 2002;84(suppl 2, pt 2):70–80 with permission from Wolters Kluwer Health, Inc.)

As an example, in the evaluation of a patient with back pain secondary to vertebral compression fractures, sagittal T1-weighted or T2-weighted images may not show edema in an acute or subacute vertebral compression fracture, whereas a fat-suppressed T2-weighted image or a STIR image would make such a finding quite obvious (▶ Fig. 3.3). These latter images are also useful for determining whether a vertebral compression fracture represents a chronic fracture or an acute or subacute fracture (▶ Fig. 3.3).

3.2.3 Postgadolinium T1-Weighted Images

Postgadolinium T1-weighted images and fat-suppressed postgadolinium T1-weighted images are typically obtained for the evaluation of infection, tumor, postsurgical changes, or scar. These images can sometimes be confused with T2-weighted images because they may show areas of increased signal in the presence of pathology (▶ Fig. 3.4); the distinction can be made using the techniques just outlined. Specifically, the clinician should evaluate the areas in which one may expect to find physiologic fluid, such as CSF in the spine. If this fluid is bright, then the images are T2 weighted. If this fluid seems to be dark, and the pathology seems to be bright, then the image is likely a postgadolinium T1-weighted image. In addition, the technique of TR evaluation described previously can also be used to differentiate a postgadolinium T1-weighted image (TR is in the hundreds range) from a T2-weighted image (TR is in the thousands range).

3.2.4 MR Angiography Images

MR angiography images highlight the blood vessels and enable evaluation of the arterial and venous vascular structures (▶ Fig. 3.5). These images are obviously different in appearance from the images

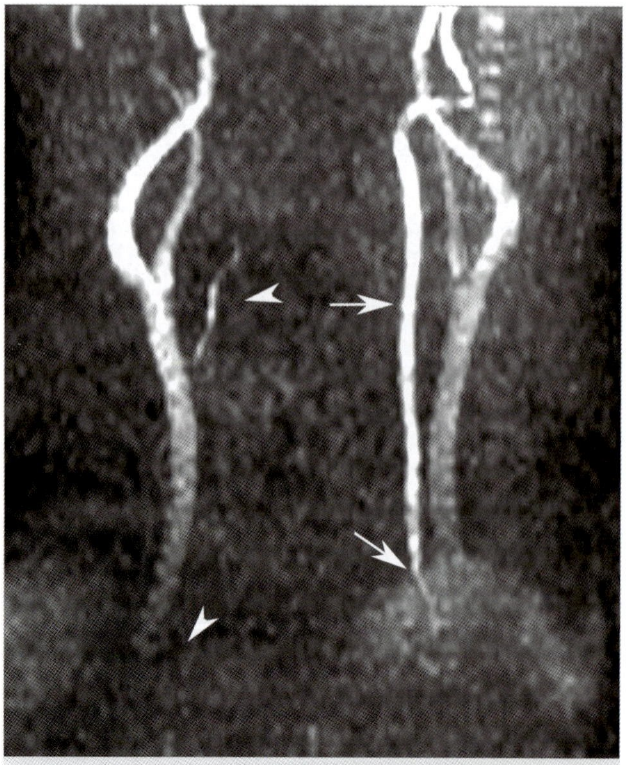

Fig. 3.5 A magnetic resonance (MR) angiogram (anterior view) from a 2D time-of-flight acquisition shows absence of signal intensity in the expected course of the right vertebral artery (*arrowheads*). Note the normal course of the left vertebral artery (*arrows*). (Reproduced with permission from, A Systematic Approach to the Review of Spine MRI Studies. In: Khanna A, ed. MRI Essentials for the Spine Specialist. 1st Edition. New York: Thieme; 2014.)

acquired using the more conventional pulse sequences and MRI techniques.

3.3 Step 2: Evaluation of T2-Weighted Images

After the clinician has identified all of the T2-weighted images, they should be systematically evaluated, plane by plane. In almost all instances, the clinician should begin with sagittal T2-weighted images of the cervical or lumbar spine. In rare instances, such as for the patient with a spinal deformity (e.g., degenerative or congenital scoliosis), it may be best to begin with the coronal T2-weighted images.

If the images are being evaluated as films on a light box, they should be viewed in sequential order, starting with all sagittal images, then all axial images, and then all coronal images. The same process should be used when evaluating an imaging study on a computer workstation.

3.3.1 Cervical Spine Example

A description of the evaluation of the cervical spine serves as an illustrative example.

- First, evaluate the sagittal T2-weighted images. Ensure that all of the sagittal T2-weighted images are being visualized in order from one side to the other (in this case, from left to right) (▶ Fig. 3.6).

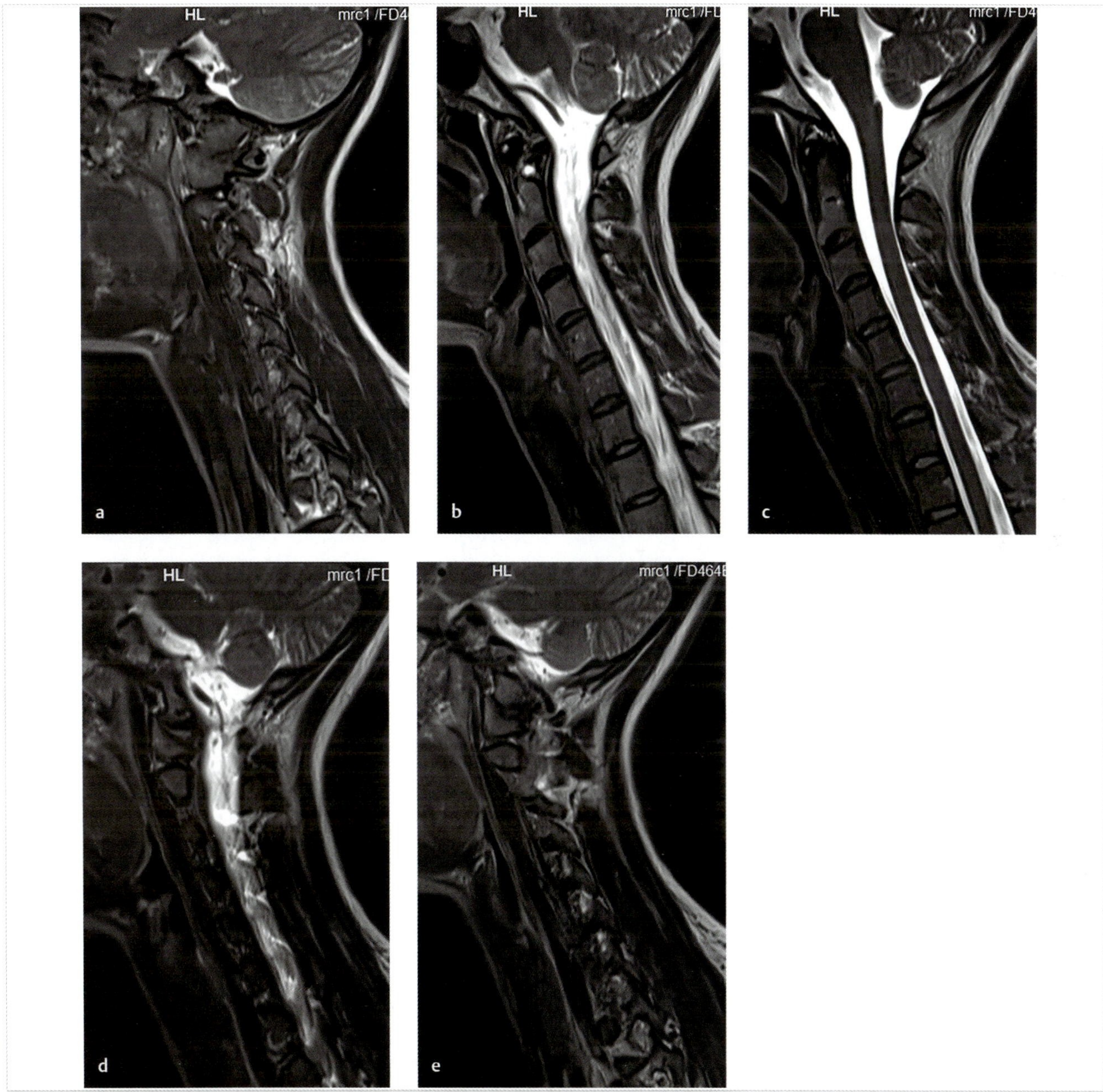

Fig. 3.6 Sequential sagittal imaging of the cervical spine. These T2-weighted images should be viewed in order from **(a)** left to **(e)** right. The midline image **(c)** should be identified. (Reproduced with permission from, A Systematic Approach to the Review of Spine MRI Studies. In: Khanna A, ed. MRI Essentials for the Spine Specialist. 1st Edition. New York: Thieme; 2014.)

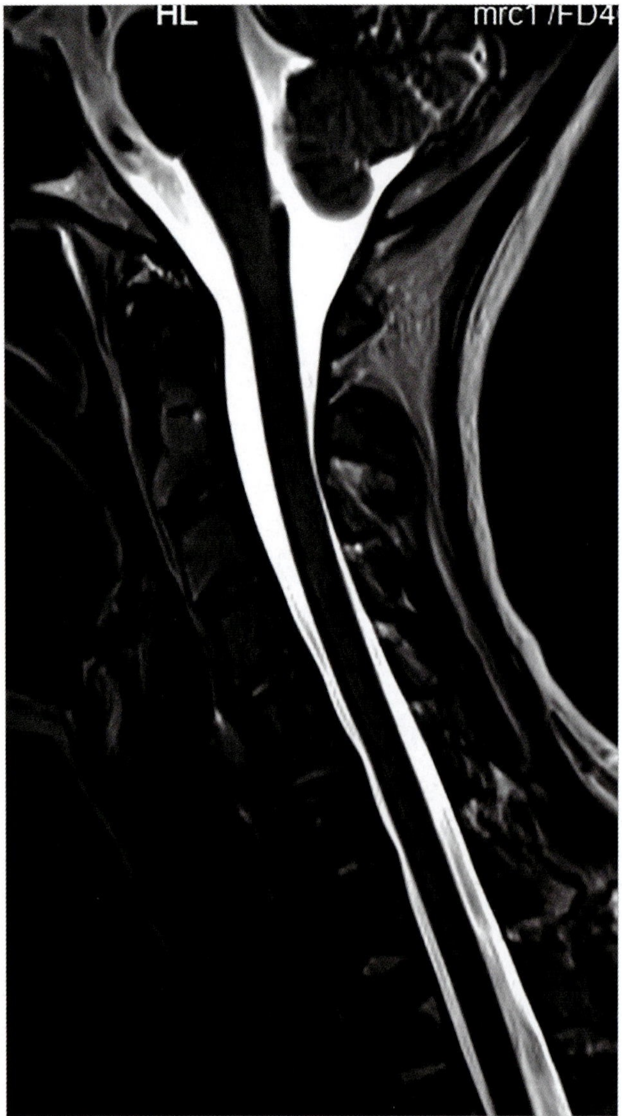

Fig. 3.7 A midline sagittal T2-weighted image of the cervical spine. Note that the spinal cord is seen in its entirety; cerebrospinal fluid (CSF) is seen anterior and posterior to the spinal cord; and the vertebral bodies, odontoid process, and fourth ventricle are seen in profile. (Reproduced with permission from, A Systematic Approach to the Review of Spine MRI Studies. In: Khanna A, ed. MRI Essentials for the Spine Specialist. 1st Edition. New York: Thieme; 2014.)

- Next, look for the midline image (▶ Fig. 3.7, ▶ Fig. 3.8).
  - For the cervical spine, recognize the midline image by noting that the spinal cord is seen in its entirety (in the patient without scoliosis), extending from the midbrain to the upper thoracic spine.
  - Visualize the CSF anterior and posterior to the cervical spinal cord.
  - Confirm that the midline image is being evaluated by noting the basion and opisthion at the foramen magnum. In addition, the fourth ventricle is visualized, the vertebral bodies are seen as rectangular or square structures, and the odontoid process is seen in profile with its domed tip.
- After evaluating all of the structures in the midline, continue the review to the left or right side to evaluate for foraminal or lateral recess stenosis.
  - Each institution has its own convention as to whether the images for sagittal images are acquired from left to right or right to left.
  - The only way to be 100% positive about which side of the cervical spine is being visualized is to evaluate the coronal localizing pulse sequence, which often displays numbers that correspond to the numbers seen on the sagittal images. The other way to determine whether a specific pathologic finding (for example, a disk herniation) is right or left or paracentral is to correlate the sagittal images with the findings seen on the axial images.
- Next, evaluate all of the axial T2-weighted images from the OCJ to the lower cervical spine (▶ Fig. 3.9).
  - The only way to ensure that all of the images are seen in sequence and that none is missed is to look at the image numbers on the printed film or on the workstation screen and to confirm that the image number at the beginning of one sheet of film is, indeed, the next sequential number after that on the previous sheet.
  - Confirm the location at the OCJ by noting that the odontoid process appears different from the remaining cervical vertebral bodies in the subaxial cervical spine.
  - Finally, evaluate all of the images in sequence to view the cervical spinal cord and note that there is CSF (bright signal) around it and adequate space available for the nerve roots at the neural foramina; correlating the axial image number with the sagittal localizing image, which contains lines corresponding with numbers that indicate the level of the axial image, will ensure accurate identification of the spinal level being evaluated. Another option is to "link" the sagittal and axial images with the available image-viewing software so that a line on the sagittal midline image shows the level of the axial image.

3.3.2 Lumbar Spine Example

The same technique just described for the cervical spine can also be used for the lumbar spine.

- First, evaluate the sagittal T2-weighted images. Ensure that all of the sagittal T2-weighted images are being visualized in order from one side to the other.
- Next, look for the midline image (▶ Fig. 3.10). For the lumbar spine, recognize the midline image by noting that the spinal cord is seen in its entirety (in the patient without scoliosis), descending from the thoracolumbar spine to the level of L1–L2 (which is the typical location of the conus medullaris).
  - Visualize the CSF anterior and posterior to the spinal cord and around the nerve roots of the cauda equina in the lumbar spine below the conus medullaris.

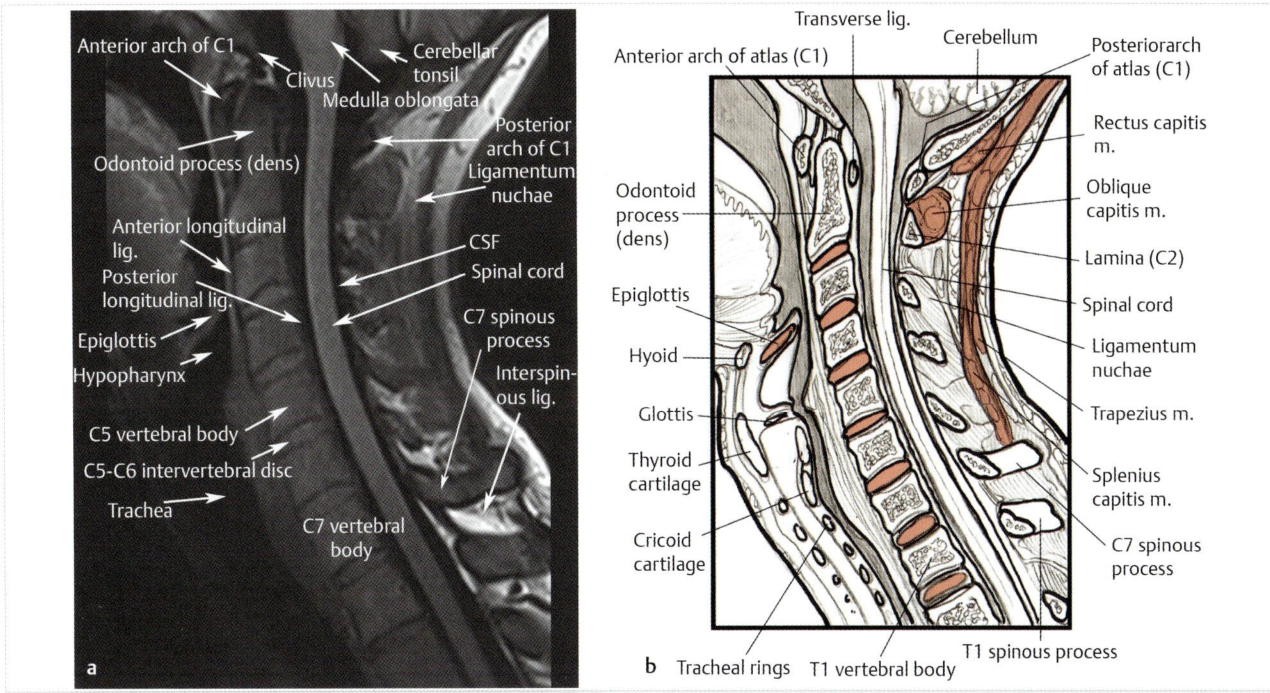

Fig. 3.8 This **(a)** sagittal T1-weighted midline image and **(b)** artist's sketch of the cervical spine depict the cervical spinal cord, cerebrospinal fluid (CSF), and anterior and posterior longitudinal ligaments, as well as the anterior and posterior elements of the cervical spine and the intervertebral disks. (Reproduced with permission from, A Systematic Approach to the Review of Spine MRI Studies. In: Khanna A, ed. MRI Essentials for the Spine Specialist. 1st Edition. New York: Thieme; 2014.)

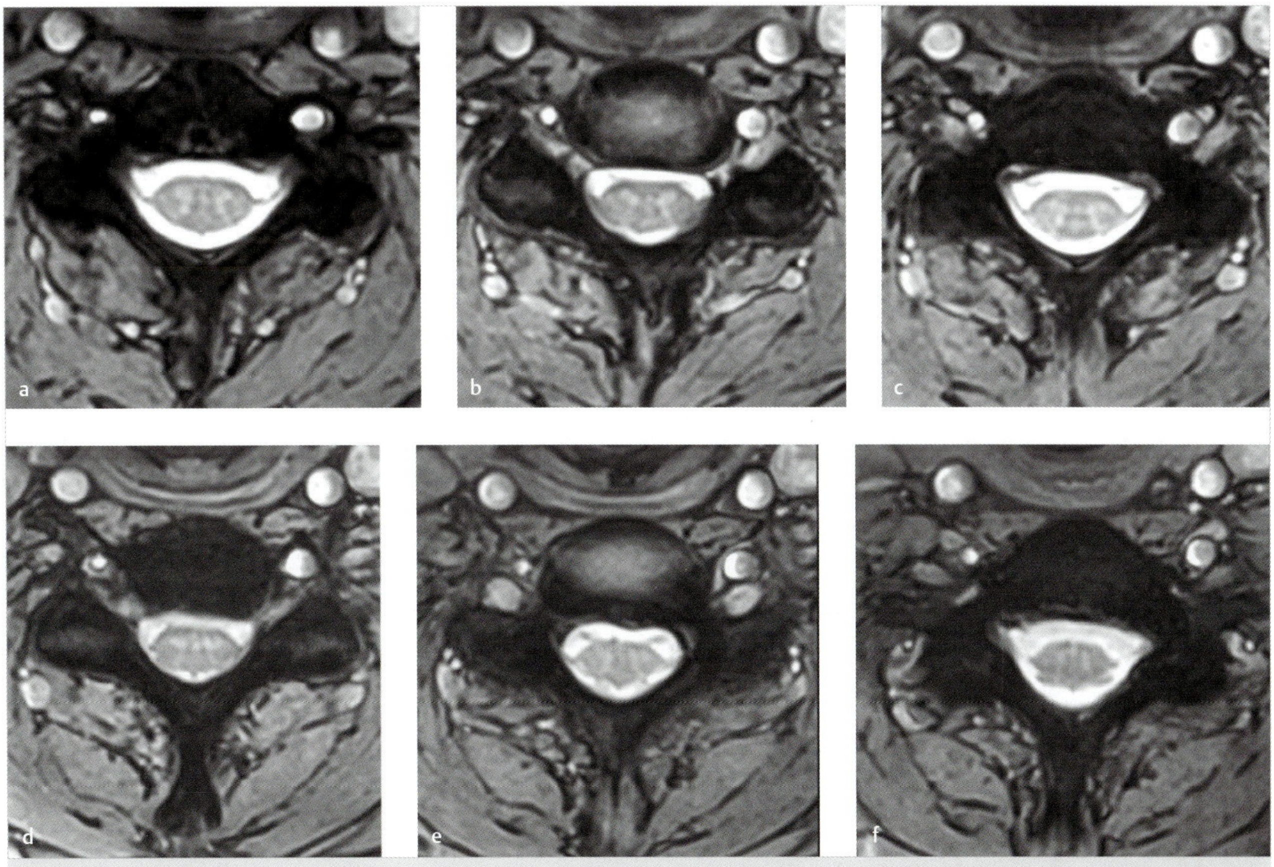

Fig. 3.9 Sequential axial imaging of the cervical spine. These T2-weighted images should be viewed in order from **(a)** C6 to **(f)** T1. (Reproduced with permission from, A Systematic Approach to the Review of Spine MRI Studies. In: Khanna A, ed. MRI Essentials for the Spine Specialist. 1st Edition. New York: Thieme; 2014.)

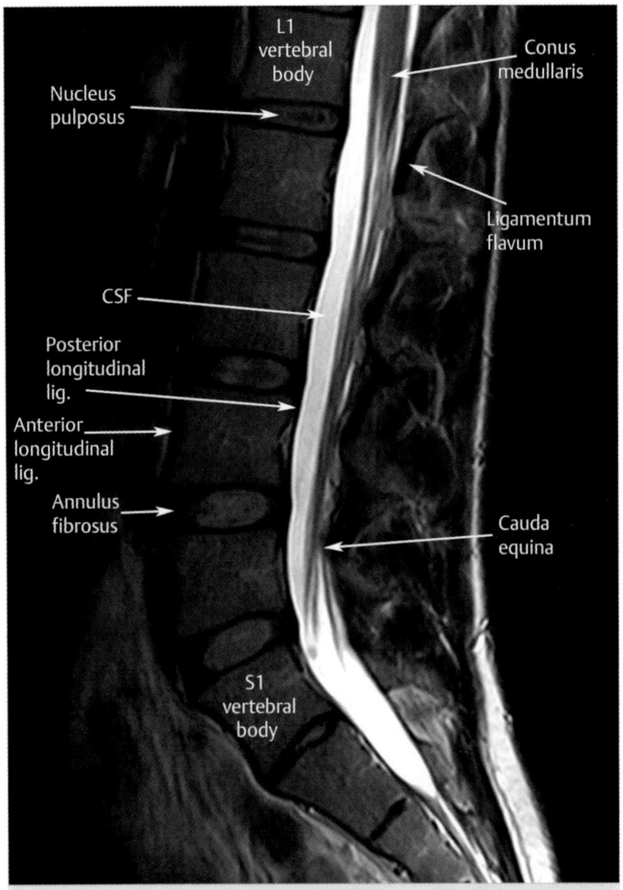

Fig. 3.10 A midline sagittal T2-weighted image of the lumbar spine. Note that the spinal cord is seen in its entirety; cerebrospinal fluid (CSF) is seen anterior and posterior to the spinal cord; and the vertebral bodies and sacrum are seen in profile. (Reproduced with permission from, A Systematic Approach to the Review of Spine MRI Studies. In: Khanna A, ed. MRI Essentials for the Spine Specialist. 1st Edition. New York: Thieme; 2014.)

  - Confirm that the midline image is being evaluated by noting the spinal cord and conus medullaris. In addition, the sacrum should be seen in sagittal cross-section with a normal AP length equal to that of the L5–S1 disk and the other intervertebral disks of the lumbar spine. Lastly, the lumbar vertebral bodies should be seen as square or rectangular structures.
- After evaluating all of the structures in the midline, continue the review to the left or right side to evaluate for foraminal or lateral recess stenosis (▶ Fig. 3.11).
  - Each institution has its own convention as to whether the images for sagittal images are acquired from left to right or from right to left.
  - As with the cervical spine example just discussed, the only way to be 100% positive about which side of the lumbar spine is being visualized is to evaluate the coronal localizing pulse sequence, which often displays numbers that correspond to the numbers seen on the sagittal images. The other way to see whether a specific pathologic finding (e.g., a disk herniation) is right or left or paracentral is to correlate the sagittal images with the findings seen on the axial images.
- Next, evaluate all of the axial T2-weighted images from the lumbosacral junction to L4–L5 (▶ Fig. 3.12), to the upper lumbar spine (▶ Fig. 3.13).
  - As with the cervical spine example discussed previously, the only way to ensure that all of the images are seen in sequence and that none is missed is to look at the image numbers on the printed film or on the screen and to confirm that the image number at the beginning of one sheet is the next sequential number after that on the previous sheet.
  - Confirm the location at the lumbosacral junction by noting that the sacrum appears different (similar to Napoleon's hat; see ▶ Fig. 3.14) from the remaining lumbar vertebral bodies in the lumbar spine.

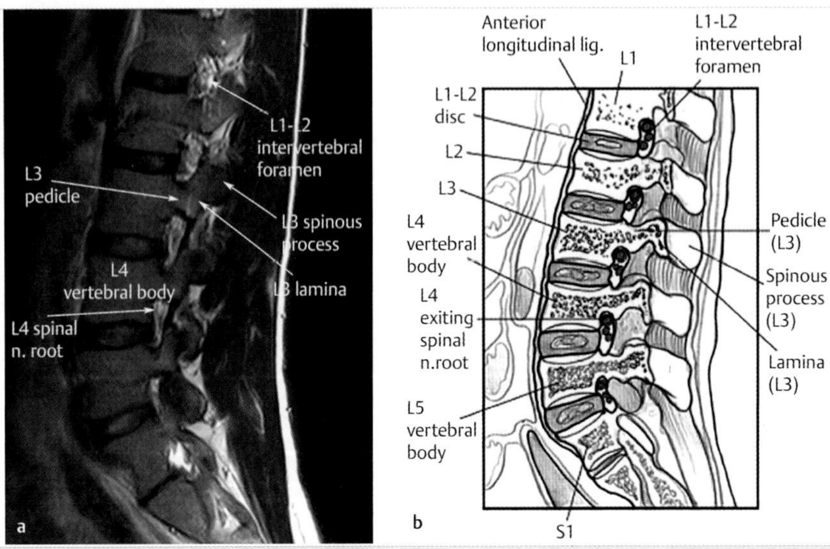

Fig. 3.11 This **(a)** parasagittal T2-weighted image and **(b)** artist's sketch of the lumbar spine show the neural foramina and exiting nerve roots at multiple levels. (Reproduced with permission from, A Systematic Approach to the Review of Spine MRI Studies. In: Khanna A, ed. MRI Essentials for the Spine Specialist. 1st Edition. New York: Thieme; 2014.)

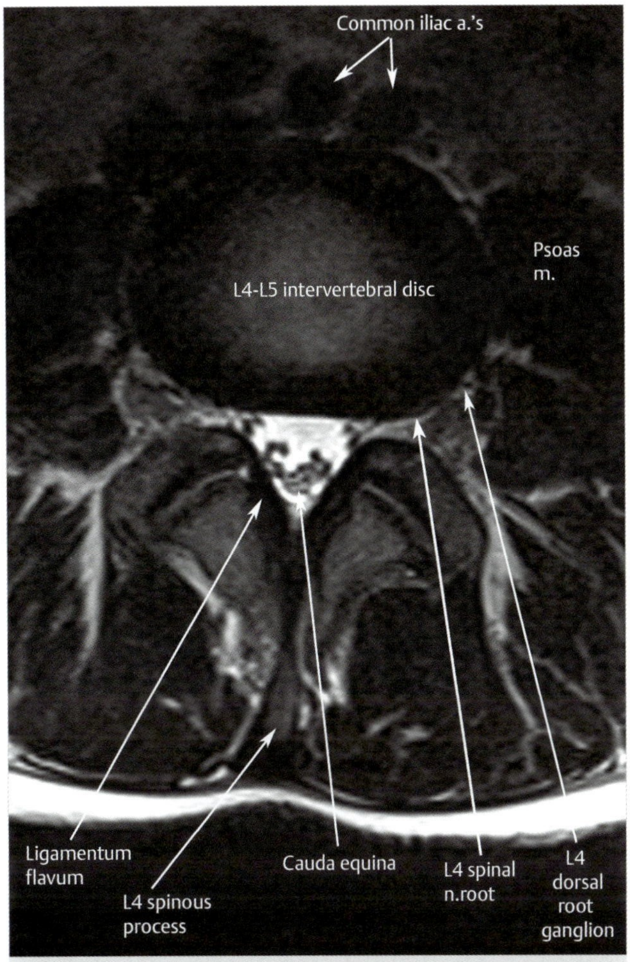

Fig. 3.12 An axial T2-weighted magnetic resonance (MR) image at the level of the L4–L5 intervertebral disk shows the cauda equina, L4 spinal nerve root, and L4 dorsal root ganglion. Normal flow voids are seen within the common iliac arteries, just below the aortic bifurcation. (Reproduced with permission from, A Systematic Approach to the Review of Spine MRI Studies. In: Khanna A, ed. MRI Essentials for the Spine Specialist. 1st Edition. New York: Thieme; 2014.)

  - Finally, evaluate all of the images in sequence to view the neural structures in the lumbar spine (spinal cord, conus medullaris, and cauda equina) and note whether there is CSF (bright signal) around them and adequate space available for the nerve roots at the neural foramina. Correlating the axial image number with the sagittal localizing image, which contains lines corresponding with numbers that indicate the level of the axial image, will ensure accurate identification of the level being evaluated. Another option is to "link" the sagittal and axial images with the available image-viewing software so that a line on the sagittal midline image shows the level of the axial image.

3.3.3 Pattern Recognition

The next step is to evaluate for any areas of increased T2-weighted signal that should not have increased T2-weighted signal. This evaluation may be relatively easy for a clinician with extensive experience in evaluating MRI studies of a particular region. Most clinicians would agree that in determining these areas of increased T2-weighted signal, they tend to use a gestalt method. However, for the less experienced clinician or the clinician in training, several techniques can be used to determine whether or not an area should show increased T2-weighted signal. These techniques rely on the concepts of pattern recognition and experience:

- Recall the evaluations of the last 20 to 50 MRI studies of the region of interest and attempt to remember exactly where the increase in T2-weighted signal was seen.
  - Increased T2-weighted signal outside of that pattern on the current study may represent an area of pathology.
  - This technique of pattern recognition is commonly used by experienced radiologists to read imaging studies. Although clinicians tend to use this technique for in-office patient evaluation, it may or may not be a safe-and-effective technique.[5]

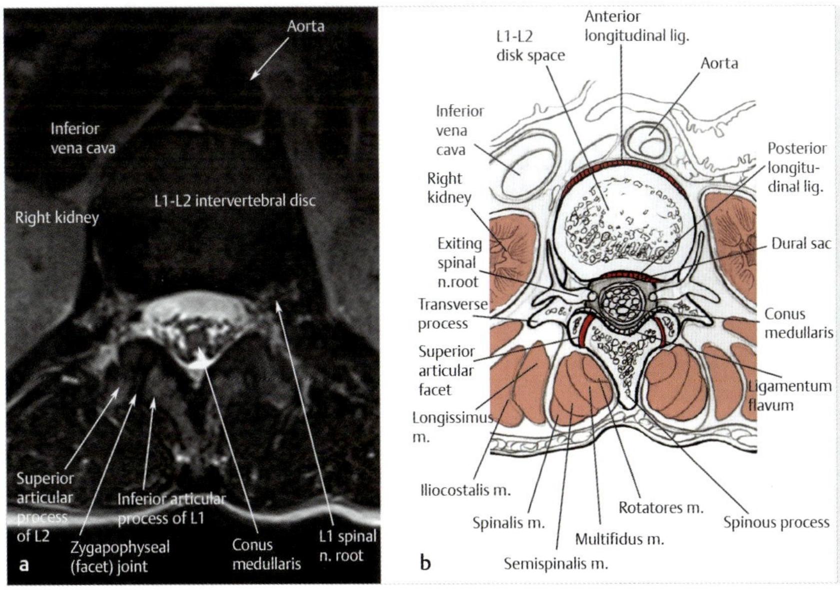

Fig. 3.13 This **(a)** axial T2-weighted image and **(b)** artist's sketch of the spine at the level of the L1–L2 intervertebral disk show the conus medullaris and the L1 spinal nerve root, as well as the superior and inferior articular processes of the L1–L2 facet joint. (Reproduced with permission from, A Systematic Approach to the Review of Spine MRI Studies. In: Khanna A, ed. MRI Essentials for the Spine Specialist. 1st Edition. New York: Thieme; 2014.)

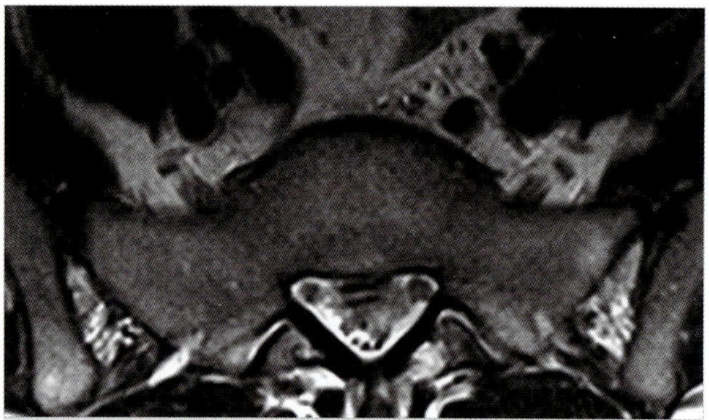

Fig. 3.14 An axial T2-weighted image of the sacrum at the S1 level shows the "Napoleon's hat" configuration of this level. (Reproduced with permission from, A Systematic Approach to the Review of Spine MRI Studies. In: Khanna A, ed. MRI Essentials for the Spine Specialist. 1st Edition. New York: Thieme; 2014.)

- The other method that one can use to evaluate for areas of abnormal increased T2-weighted signal is to note all areas of increased T2-weighted signal within a given image and then ask oneself whether water does, indeed, "belong" in that area. For example, if the sagittal T2-weighted images of a cervical spine MRI study are being evaluated and a small region of high signal is seen within the spinal cord (an anatomic structure that is obvious to even the least experienced clinician), then one may assume that it represents fluid (or edema) within the spinal cord (▶ Fig. 3.15). The question, then, is whether it is a normal (physiologic) or an excessive (pathologic) amount of fluid. The ability to make this determination comes from experience (i.e., the recognition of lack of such a region of increased T2-weighted signal within the spinal cord on many previous studies of other patients) or from a developed fund of knowledge (such as the review of Chapter 6, The Cervical Spine) that would enable the clinician to develop a focused differential diagnosis for this finding.

3.4 Step 3: Evaluation of T1-Weighted Images

T1-weighted images enable optimal evaluation of anatomic detail. However, with current improvements in MRI techniques and equipment, including dedicated surface and other coils, T2-weighted images also often show excellent anatomic detail. This improvement may be the reason that the author believes the routine use of T1-weighted images by clinicians and radiologists is declining. Nevertheless, the most appropriate way to evaluate an MRI study fully and most effectively is to review all of the images and pulse sequences.

Therefore, after identification of the pulse sequences obtained (Step 1) and evaluation of the T2-weighted images (Step 2), the next step is to review the T1-weighted images for improved evaluation of anatomic detail. This author's routine is to correlate the areas of increased T2-weighted signal seen during the very detailed and systematic evaluation of the T2-weighted images just described with the same region on the T1-weighted images. The improved spatial resolution of the T1-weighted images facilitates the evaluation of regional and local disturbances in anatomic detail. For example, if a sagittal fat-suppressed T2-weighted image of a vertebral compression fracture shows a somewhat indistinct area of increased T2-weighted signal within a vertebral body, the clinician may decide that it represents a vertebral compression fracture, but the clinician may also consider the possibility of other diagnoses such as tumor or infection. However, a relatively sharp and discrete fracture line seen within the sagittal T1-weighted image would likely leave no doubt in the clinician's mind that it represents a fracture and not some other process.

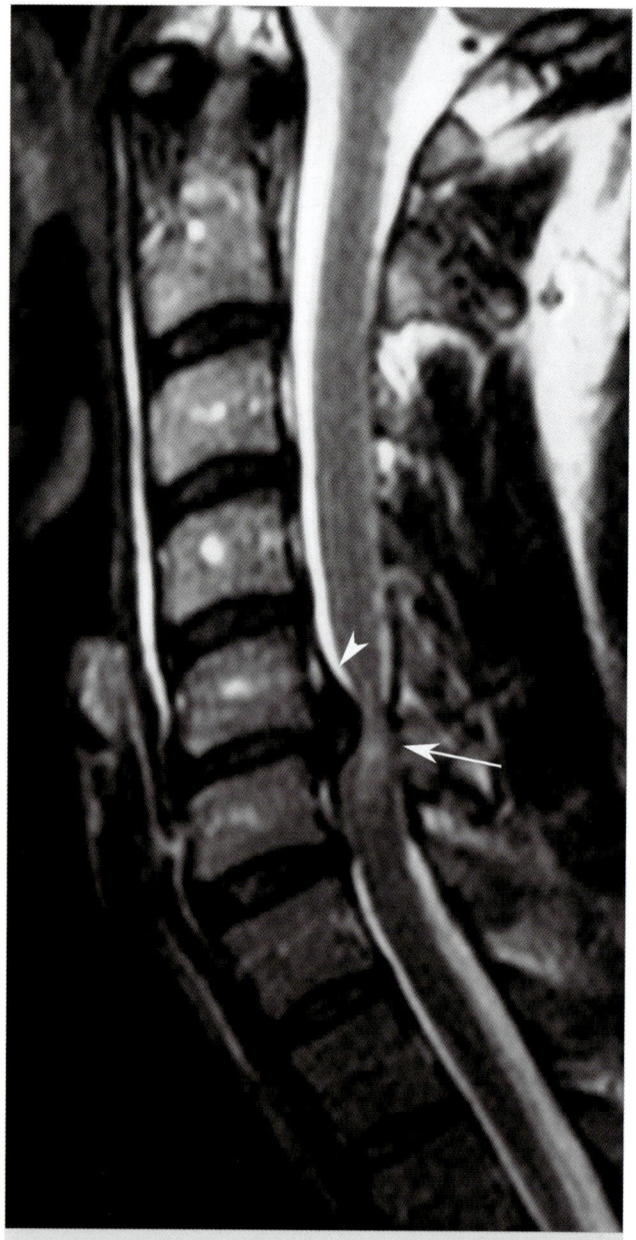

Fig. 3.15 A sagittal T2-weighted image shows a large central disk extrusion at the C5–C6 level with associated increased cord signal intensity (*arrow*) compatible with myelomalacia. Note the elevation of the posterior longitudinal ligament (*arrowhead*). (Reproduced with permission from, A Systematic Approach to the Review of Spine MRI Studies. In: Khanna A, ed. MRI Essentials for the Spine Specialist. 1st Edition. New York: Thieme; 2014.)

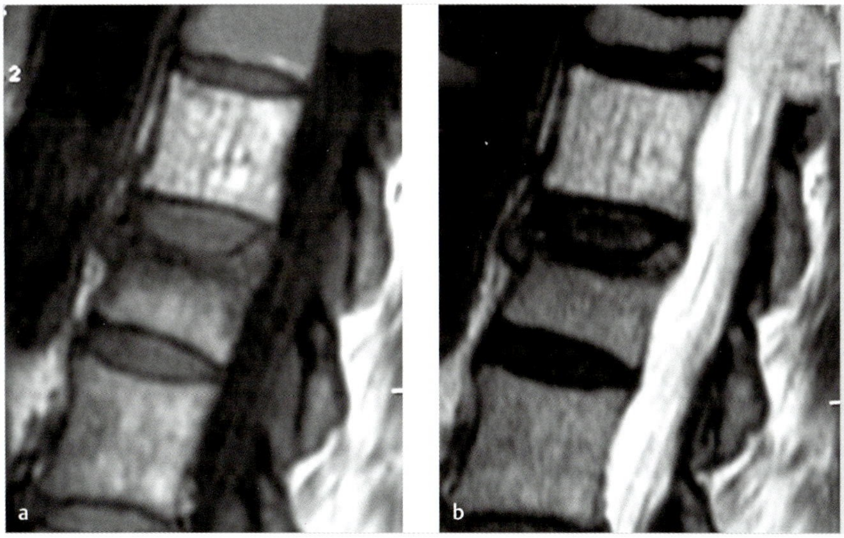

Fig. 3.16 These sagittal **(a)** T1 -weighted and **(b)** T2-weighted images show a lesion at the T12 level with high signal intensity on both images and with the typical striations compatible with a vertebral body hemangioma. An incidentally noted vertebral compression fracture is seen at the L1 level. (Reproduced with permission from, A Systematic Approach to the Review of Spine MRI Studies. In: Khanna A, ed. MRI Essentials for the Spine Specialist. 1st Edition. New York: Thieme; 2014.)

In addition, the T1-weighted images may help the clinician determine the type of tissue that is present in a lesion. Central to this concept is the fact that T1-weighted images tend to show fat as bright signal and fluid as dark signal. Therefore, lesions such as a lipoma are noted to be bright on T1-weighted images and, in fact, follow the signal of subcutaneous fat on all pulse sequences, including fat-suppressed or STIR pulse sequences. As another example, one of the few lesions that is bright on both T2-weighted and T1-weighted images is a hemangioma, which is often seen in the vertebral body (▶ Fig. 3.16). Thus, if the lesion is seen to be bright on both of these images and displays the typical pattern of serpentine vascular channels, the diagnosis of vertebral body hemangioma can be made with relative certainty.[6]

Like T2-weighted images, T1-weighted images should be evaluated in all planes and in the same sequence as described in Step 2.

3.5 Step 4: Evaluation of Specialized Pulse Sequences

3.5.1 Fat-Suppressed T2-Weighted or STIR Images

The fat-suppressed T2-weighted or STIR pulse sequences are used to accentuate the increase in signal and edema seen in pathologic processes such as fracture, infection, and tumor. On conventional T2-weighted images, the signal from bone-marrow fat is maintained, and one attempts to recognize edema by noting the presence or absence of a very bright region (marrow pathology or edema) within a bright background (fatty marrow) (▶ Fig. 3.17a). On fat-suppressed T2-weighted images, all of the subcutaneous, bone-marrow, and other fat is suppressed, and one can more easily recognize an area of edema as a bright region within a dark background (▶ Fig. 3.17b). This author considers fat-suppressed T2-weighted and STIR images to be somewhat like a three-phase nuclear scintigraphy (bone scan) study (see Chapter 4, Correlation of MRI with Other Imaging Modalities), which is relatively sensitive to increased bone turnover but not very specific. Similarly, if a region is evaluated with fat-suppressed T2-weighted imaging or STIR imaging and there is no area of increased signal, one can be somewhat reassured that a pathologic process is not present in that region. Conversely, if an area of increased signal is noted, it may represent pathologic change or a normal region of increased signal such as physiologic fluid within a facet joint or CSF. Other pulse sequences, such as T2-weighted and T1-weighted images, provide better anatomic detail for evaluation and help the clinician identify a more specific diagnosis. As discussed previously and in the subsequent region-specific chapters, fat-suppressed T2-weighted images can be used to evaluate nondisplaced fractures and to determine the approximate age or chronicity of fractures, including vertebral compression fractures.

3.5.2 Postgadolinium T1-Weighted Images

Postgadolinium T1-weighted images are often acquired to evaluate for the presence or absence of infection and tumor and to assess the postoperative spine. For example, postgadolinium T1-weighted images can help differentiate recurrent disk herniation from epidural fibrosis and scar (▶ Fig. 3.18). The recommended method for evaluating these images is to place the postgadolinium T1-weighted images side by side with the pregadolinium T1-weighted images. The region of interest is then compared in the same planes and on matching images. Higher signal intensity in the region or structure of interest on the postgadolinium T1-weighted images is termed *postgadolinium* (or contrast) enhancement. An evaluation can then be made with regard to the degree and pattern of enhancement. For example, peripheral rim enhancement with a central region of nonenhancement in a relatively well-circumscribed lesion is considered, in the appropriate clinical setting, to be a finding suggestive of an abscess.[7]

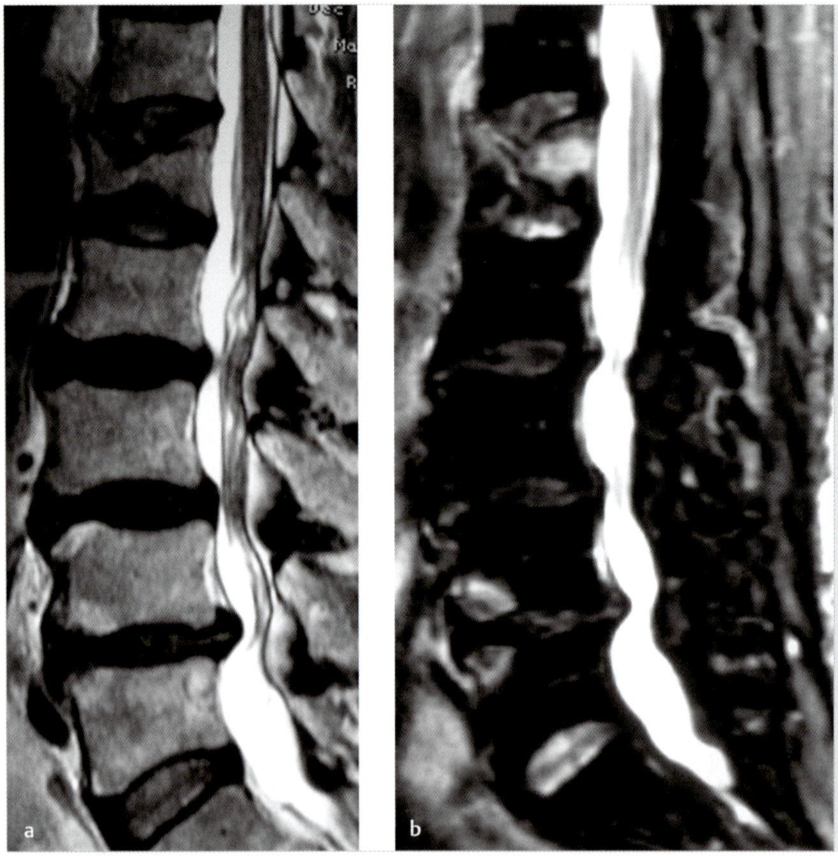

Fig. 3.17 Vertebral compression fracture. **(a)** A sagittal T2-weighted image of the lumbar spine shows an L1 vertebral body compression fracture of an indeterminate age, given that edema is not definitely seen. **(b)** A sagittal short tau inversion recovery (STIR) image of the same patient shows edema within the L1 vertebral body, which is compatible with an acute or subacute vertebral compression fracture. (Reproduced with permission from, A Systematic Approach to the Review of Spine MRI Studies. In: Khanna A, ed. MRI Essentials for the Spine Specialist. 1st Edition. New York: Thieme; 2014.)

3.6 Step 5: Correlation of Imaging Findings with Patient History and Examination Findings to Determine the Most Likely Diagnosis

Clinicians and radiologists have distinct advantages and disadvantages relative to one another in terms of evaluating MRI studies of the spine. Radiologists have the advantage of often being trained with a process similar to the one just described and frequently have, and take, the time to evaluate the images in a systematic fashion. However, clinicians have the advantage of knowing the patient's history and physical examination findings, laboratory results, and other parameters. It is essential that clinicians use this advantage to help maximize the accuracy and reliability of their MRI interpretations. This point is especially true for the evaluation of patients with spinal pathologies because it is well known that many patients with pathology seen on their spine MRI studies are asymptomatic,[8,9,10,11] and it is imperative that the clinician treat the patient and not just the MRI findings.

The authors believe that an accurate diagnosis, or differential diagnosis, occurs at the "intersection" of a patient's history, physical examination results, radiographic findings, and laboratory study results (▶ Fig. 3.19). With an understanding of the clinical scenario, clinicians can arrive at an accurate diagnosis, especially when they are armed with the appropriate techniques for evaluating the MRI studies. One way to leverage the strengths of clinicians and radiologists is to use a collaborative and team approach to the evaluation of patients with complex spinal pathologies.

For example, if a patient presents with low back pain after trauma and is point-tender at the thoracolumbar junction, and the MR image shows a region of increased STIR signal within the T12 vertebral body, the diagnosis of a vertebral compression fracture can be suggested, especially if the region of edema has a linear appearance on the T2-weighted and T1-weighted images. However, if a patient with similar imaging findings presents with no history of trauma, is elderly, has a history of insidious onset of low back pain (particularly at night), and has a history of a primary malignancy, another diagnosis (e.g., metastatic disease) might be higher on the differential diagnosis. To help determine the correct diagnosis, the clinician would likely obtain a CT scan to evaluate further the osseous anatomy in both patients. The second patient might also benefit from a primary malignancy survey, a three-phase bone scan, and a CT-guided biopsy.

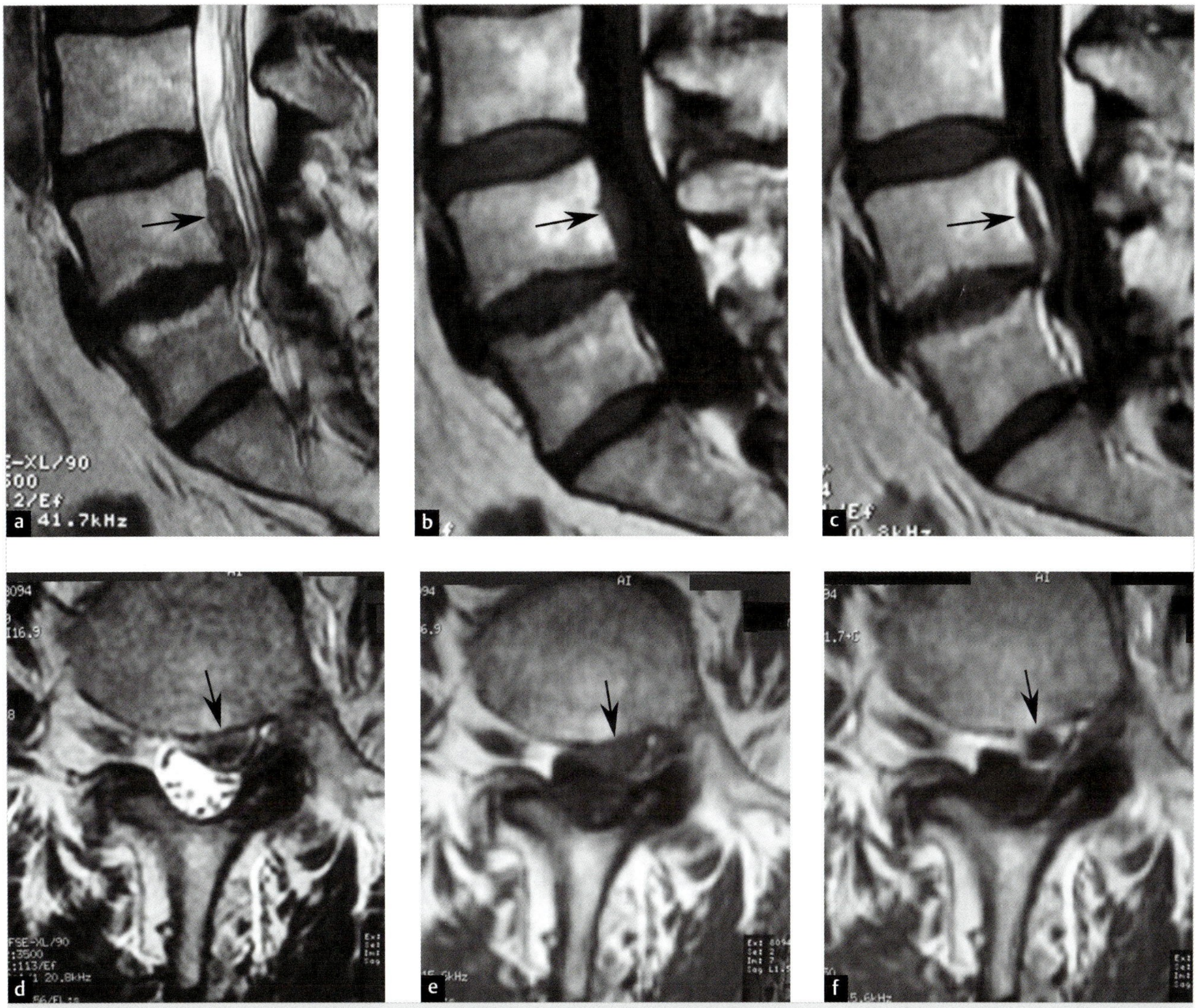

Fig. 3.18 Recurrent lumbar disk extrusion. **(a)** Sagittal T2-weighted, **(b)** T1-weighted, and **(c)** postgadolinium T1-weighted images in a patient with a history of previous L4–L5 diskectomy show a large disk extrusion (*arrow* on each) that has migrated proximally and is located behind the L4 vertebral body. Note that the disk is difficult to see on **(b)** the T1-weighted image and shows peripheral enhancement on **(c)** the postgadolinium T1-weighted image. **(d)** Axial T2-weighted, **(e)** T1-weighted, and **(f)** postgadolinium T1-weighted images at the L4–L5 level show the left paracentral extradural lesion (*arrows* on each) that appears to be disk material on **(d)** the T2-weighted image and shows peripheral enhancement on **(f)** the postgadolinium T1-weighted image compared with **(e)** the pregadolinium T1-weighted image. (Reproduced with permission from, A Systematic Approach to the Review of Spine MRI Studies. In: Khanna A, ed. MRI Essentials for the Spine Specialist. 1st Edition. New York: Thieme; 2014.)

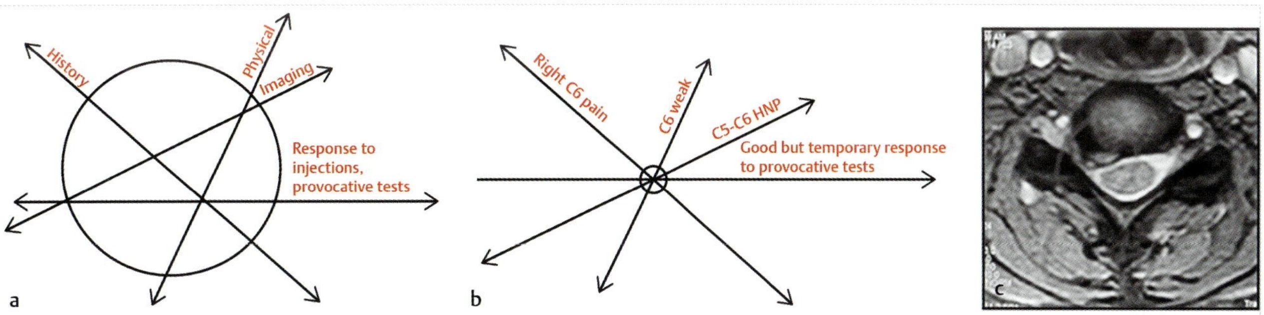

Fig. 3.19 The concept of intersecting lines for diagnosis and surgical decision making. **(a)** In a patient for whom the history, physical examination, imaging findings, and response to provocative tests do not "intersect" within a small circle, it is difficult to identify a diagnosis or to narrow a differential diagnosis. Conversely, for a patient with a smaller region of intersection, such as one with a right C6 radiculopathy **(b)**, one may expect to see a C5–C6 disk protrusion on magnetic resonance imaging (MRI) **(c)**. HNP, herniated nucleus pulposus. (Reproduced with permission from, A Systematic Approach to the Review of Spine MRI Studies. In: Khanna A, ed. MRI Essentials for the Spine Specialist. 1st Edition. New York: Thieme; 2014.)

3.7 Summary

In summary, the five-step technique described in this chapter will help guide the clinician in systematically evaluating MRI studies of the spine. This author strongly believes that such a systematic technique should be used for the evaluation of all MRI studies and that the tendency to become less meticulous and systematic over time should be avoided. One additional suggestion is to always attempt to read the MRI study using this technique and then to evaluate the "official" radiologist's reading to determine the degree of correlation between the two readings. Occasionally, the clinician notes findings that were not reported by the radiologist, and vice versa.[12] Over time, this method of checking one's own evaluation against that of another trained specialist will serve as a method of quality control and assurance and will likely result in a continuously improving ability to evaluate MRI studies accurately.

3.8 Common Clinical Questions

1. One should begin the interpretation of an MRI study of the cervical or lumbar spine with which imaging plane and pulse sequence?
   a) Sagittal, T1-weighted images.
   b) Axial, T1-weighted images.
   c) Sagittal, T2-weighted images.
   d) Axial, T2-weighted images.
   e) Coronal, T2-weighted images.

2. Evaluation of what structure or region will enable one to differentiate T1-weighted and T2-weighted images?
   a) Muscle.
   b) Bone.
   c) Tendon.
   d) CSF.
   e) It is not possible to differentiate these two pulse sequences by viewing an image.

3. What is the most common MRI manifestation of almost all pathology such as tumor, fracture, or infection in the spine?
   a) Loss of signal on all pulse sequences.
   b) Increased T2-weighted signal.
   c) Decreased T2-weighted signal.
   d) Increased T1-weighted signal.
   e) Increased signal on all pulse sequences.

4. What is the primary advantage that clinicians have relative to radiologists when evaluating MRI studies of the spine?
   a) Better understanding of spinal anatomy.
   b) Greater likelihood of having formal training in the evaluation of MRI studies.
   c) Greater knowledge of the range of the various disease processes that can affect the spine.
   d) Greater likelihood of being able to correlate the imaging findings with patient's history and physical examination findings to determine the most likely diagnosis.
   e) B and D.

5. Aside from "counting" levels up from the sacrum, what is the best way to confirm the spinal level of an axial image in the lumbar spine?
   a) Determine the level based on the shape of the vertebral body.
   b) Determine the level based on the size of the spinal canal.
   c) Utilize the sagittal localizing pulse sequence and correlate the image number on the axial image with those on the localizing pulse sequence/image.
   d) "Link" the sagittal and axial images with the available image-viewing software so that a line on the sagittal midline image demonstrates the level of the axial image.
   e) C and D.

References

[1] Pronovost P, Needham D, Berenholtz S, et al. An intervention to decrease catheter-related bloodstream infections in the ICU. N Engl J Med. 2006; 355 (26):2725–2732

[2] Alessandrino F, Cristiano L, Cinnante CM, et al. Value of structured reporting in neuromuscular disorders. Radiol Med (Torino). 2019; 124(7):628–635

[3] Marcovici P, Blume-Marcovici A. Intuition versus rational thinking: psychological challenges in radiology and a potential solution. J Am Coll Radiol. 2013; 10(1):25–29

[4] Lin E, Powell DK, Kagetsu NJ. Efficacy of a checklist-style structured radiology reporting template in reducing resident misses on cervical spine computed tomography examinations. J Digit Imaging. 2014; 27(5):588–593

[5] Groopman J. How doctors think. Houghton Mifflin; 2007

[6] Gaudino S, Martucci M, Colantonio R, et al. A systematic approach to vertebral hemangioma. Skeletal Radiol. 2015; 44(1):25–36

[7] Chima-Melton C, Pearl M, Scheiner M. Diagnosis of spinal epidural abscess: a case report and literature review. Spinal Cord Ser Cases. 2017; 3:17013

[8] Boden SD, Davis DO, Dina TS, Patronas NJ, Wiesel SW. Abnormal magnetic-resonance scans of the lumbar spine in asymptomatic subjects. A prospective investigation. J Bone Joint Surg Am. 1990; 72(3):403–408

[9] Bogduk N. Degenerative joint disease of the spine. Radiol Clin North Am. 2012; 50(4):613–628

[10] Borenstein DG, O'Mara JW, Jr, Boden SD, et al. The value of magnetic resonance imaging of the lumbar spine to predict low-back pain in asymptomatic subjects: a seven-year follow-up study. J Bone Joint Surg Am. 2001; 83(9):1306–1311

[11] Teresi LM, Lufkin RB, Reicher MA, et al. Asymptomatic degenerative disk disease and spondylosis of the cervical spine: MR imaging. Radiology. 1987; 164(1):83–88

[12] Rihn JA, Yang N, Fisher C, et al. Using magnetic resonance imaging to accurately assess injury to the posterior ligamentous complex of the spine: a prospective comparison of the surgeon and radiologist. J Neurosurg Spine. 2010; 12(4):391–396

Answers to Common Clinical Questions

1. Answer: c. In almost all instances, the clinician should begin with the midline sagittal T2-weighted images of the cervical or lumbar spine because the high contrast between the CSF and the neural elements provides a myelographic view of the spine, which provides a good "overview" of the condition of the spine. In rare instances, such as for the patient with a spinal deformity (e.g., degenerative or congenital scoliosis), it may be best to begin with the coronal T2-weighted images.
2. Answer: d. Recognition of an area within an image that is known to contain fluid, such as CSF, will allow one to differentiate T1-weighted and T2-weighted images. If this fluid is noted to be bright or of high signal intensity, then the image is likely T2-weighted. If the region of the

fluid is noted to be dark, then the image is likely T1-weighted.

3. Answer: b. The most common MRI manifestation of almost all pathology such as tumor, fracture, or infection in the spine (or any other structure in the musculoskeletal system) is increased T2-weighted signal because it represents the edema (free extracellular fluid) that is common to most pathologic processes.
4. Answer: d. Clinicians and radiologists have distinct advantages and disadvantages relative to one another in terms of evaluating MRI studies of the spine. Radiologists have the advantage of often being trained, and frequently have, and take, the time to evaluate the images in a systematic fashion. However, clinicians have the advantage of knowing the patient's history and physical examination findings, laboratory results, and other parameters. It is essential that clinicians use this advantage to help maximize the accuracy and reliability of their MRI interpretations.
5. Answer: e. Aside from "counting" levels up from the sacrum, the best way to confirm the spinal level of an axial image in the lumbar (or cervical) spine is to use the localizing sagittal pulse sequence. One can correlate the image number on the axial image with that on the localizing pulse sequence/image or "link" the sagittal and axial images with the available image-viewing software so that a line on the sagittal midline image shows the level of the axial image. The size, shape, and configuration of the vertebral body or spinal canal are not reliable methods of determining a spinal level.

4 Correlation of MRI with Other Imaging Modalities

Laura M. Fayad, Shivani Ahlawat, Uma Srikumaran, and A. Jay Khanna

Abstract

For the appropriate evaluation of patients with musculoskeletal diseases, clinicians should use all of the available imaging tools and techniques, as necessary. Efficacy, cost, availability, and patient limitations influence imaging modality selection. Often, most of the clinically important information can be obtained with conventional radiography and a cross-sectional study (typically magnetic resonance imaging [MRI]). However, for some patients, the clinician must request other or alternative imaging studies such as ultrasonography, computed tomography (CT), nuclear scintigraphy, or positron emission tomography (PET). As technology improves and new imaging modalities are developed, the role of each modality will evolve for diagnosis and integration into treatment algorithms.

Keywords: conventional radiography, CT, imaging modality, magnetic resonance imaging, nuclear scintigraphy, PET, ultrasonography

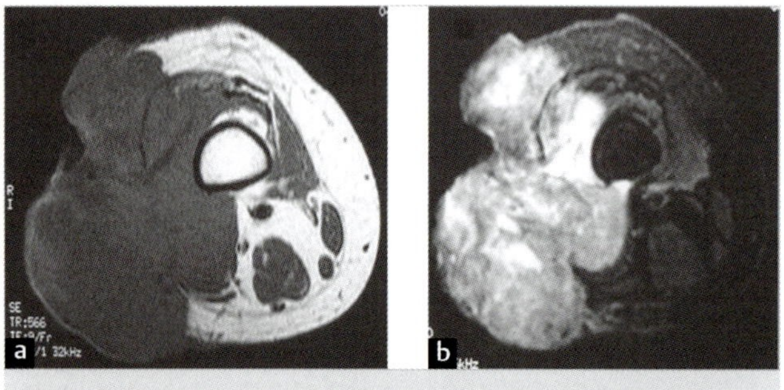

Fig. 4.1 Magnetic resonance imaging (MRI): excellent contrast resolution for evaluation of the soft tissues and bone marrow. **(a)** Axial T1-weighted and **(b)** fat-suppressed T2-weighted images of the left distal femur show a large mass involving the soft tissues around the femur. Note the excellent contrast between the different soft-tissue layers provided by MRI that allows for an accurate and detailed assessment of the compartmental involvement. (Reproduced with permission from Srikumaran U, Fayad LM, Khanna AJ. Correlation of MRI with other imaging studies. In: Khanna AJ, ed. MRI for orthopaedic surgeons. New York: Thieme; 2010:414–424.)

4.1 Introduction

Although magnetic resonance imaging (MRI) plays a central role in musculoskeletal imaging, it is important for the clinician to recognize that other imaging modalities also contribute to the evaluation of patients with musculoskeletal disorders. These other commonly used imaging modalities include conventional radiography, computed tomography (CT), nuclear scintigraphy, positron emission tomography (PET), and ultrasonography. When evaluating the patient for a particular disease process, a basic understanding of the strengths and weaknesses of these modalities is important in deciding which imaging study to use. For many patients, one or more imaging modalities will be superior to MRI alone. After the patient has been evaluated with MRI, the other modalities may provide additional anatomic, functional, or metabolic information that can help narrow the differential diagnosis and guide treatment.

4.2 MRI

MRI provides excellent visualization of the tissues in the musculoskeletal system in multiple planes because of its high-contrast resolution compared with other modalities. One of its major advantages is that its multiple pulse sequences enable the detection of soft-tissue and bone-marrow pathology with great sensitivity (▶ Fig. 4.1). In general terms, an MRI study is often obtained to evaluate the water content of tissues because most acute and subacute pathology results in free extracellular fluid. MRI pulse sequences use the magnetization and relaxation properties of protons to assess and differentiate various tissue types. Tissues that contain larger amounts of water (e.g., CSF or joint fluid) are bright on fluid-sensitive sequences, and tissues that contain lesser amount of water (e.g., cortical bone or physeal scar) are dark on all routine pulse sequences. Structures that contain little or no water are not well assessed by MRI with usual clinical sequences, and tissue types associated with susceptibility are also not well assessed by MRI. For example, the lungs contain primarily air; therefore, MRI is not used to evaluate pathology of the lung parenchyma. Cortical bone also contains little water; therefore, MRI is limited (compared with CT, for example) in its ability to evaluate cortical osseous abnormalities.

4.3 Conventional Radiography

As most clinicians learn during their training, conventional radiography is often the initial step in evaluating a patient who has (or is suspected of having) a musculoskeletal disorder. Conventional radiographs are obtained by using ionizing irradiation. The radiation beam is attenuated by structures between the image intensifier and the cassette. Structures with high density (e.g., cortical bone, metallic implants) block a larger amount of the radiation and thus leave a white region on the film. Structures with lower density (e.g., air, subcutaneous tissues) block less radiation and thus leave a dark or gray region on the film.

Conventional radiography is widely available and is good for evaluating osseous detail. It is also time- and cost-effective, and the large field of view it affords allows for the study of "global" deformities (e.g., spine deformities such as scoliosis) or deformity or malalignment of the lower extremities. For these reasons, conventional radiography is frequently used in musculoskeletal imaging to evaluate the joints and spine (▶ Fig. 4.2). Conventional radiography is the study of choice for the initial evaluation of patients with traumatic injury to joints, long bones, or

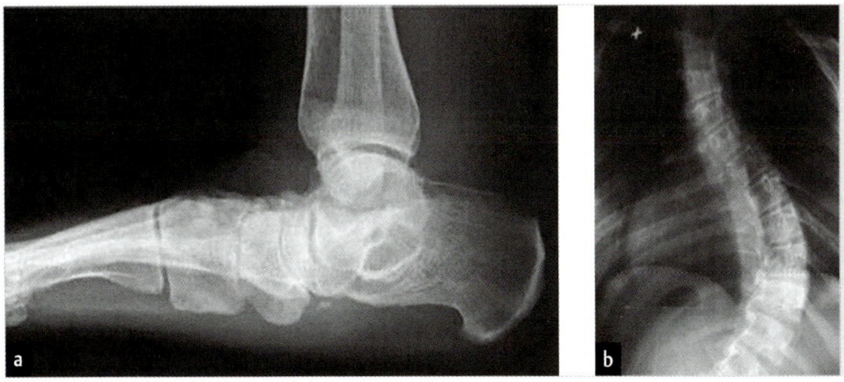

Fig. 4.2 Conventional radiographs: visualization of local and global deformity. **(a)** A lateral view of the foot shows a pes planus deformity and midfoot fault in an elderly woman. This deformity may indicate posterior tibial dysfunction, although assessment of the posterior tibial tendon is not possible by conventional radiography alone. **(b)** A posteroanterior (PA) radiograph of the spine shows a large right thoracic scoliosis. (Reproduced with permission from Srikumaran U, Fayad LM, Khanna AJ. Correlation of MRI with other imaging studies. In: Khanna AJ, ed. MRI for orthopaedic surgeons. New York: Thieme; 2010:414–424.)

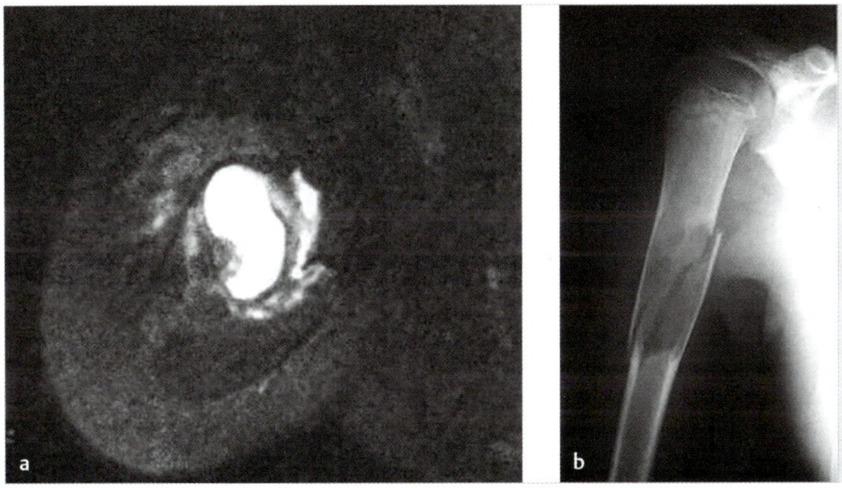

Fig. 4.3 Pathologic fracture through a unicameral bone cyst. **(a)** An axial fat-suppressed T2-weighted MR image of the right mid-humerus of a young woman shows a nodule at the periphery of a lesion occupying the humerus. The lesion is indeterminate by magnetic resonance imaging (MRI). The diagnosis of a unicameral bone cyst with a pathologic fracture would be impossible with MRI alone; that diagnosis requires **(b)** a radiograph showing the specific features. (Reproduced with permission from Srikumaran U, Fayad LM, Khanna AJ. Correlation of MRI with other imaging studies. In: Khanna AJ, ed. MRI for orthopaedic surgeons. New York: Thieme; 2010:414–424.)

the spine. Radiography is also required as an adjunct to MRI when evaluating skeletal lesions (▶ Fig. 4.3) or arthritis.

However, conventional radiographs are less valuable when evaluating patients with low back pain, neck pain, or spinal stenosis. Radiography does not provide optimal visualization of soft-tissue structures such as ligaments, menisci, and the spinal cord. In addition, radiography is less sensitive than CT or MRI for evaluating osseous destruction, and particularly less sensitive than MRI for detecting abnormalities of the bone marrow. For example, a 30% decrease in bone mass is often required before osteoporosis can be appreciated on radiographs.[1,2] Similarly, early osteomyelitis is best evaluated by MRI rather than radiography because bone changes related to osteomyelitis are not apparent on radiographs until 2 to 3 weeks.[3]

As a first-line imaging modality, conventional radiography helps the clinician determine the need for radiographic studies in other anatomic locations or for more advanced imaging studies of the local region. For example, a patient reporting arm pain after trauma may be initially evaluated with humerus and elbow radiographs. Findings of an elbow fracture would then necessitate imaging of the forearm with conventional radiography to rule out associated injuries. If the fracture appeared to be intra-articular and comminuted, CT imaging may be used to study the elbow further, to delineate the fracture pattern, and to provide information for preoperative planning. In another example, a patient presenting with a history of thigh pain may undergo conventional radiography to evaluate the hip, femur, and knee. If a lytic lesion were found in the proximal femur, MRI would then be required to determine, more precisely, the extent of disease and to aid in characterizing the lesion.

Conventional radiographs are also extremely useful for the preoperative evaluation of patients undergoing orthopaedic surgery. For example, in spine surgery, preoperative radiographs facilitate the evaluation of spinal alignment and localization of the level of pathology. This information can then be used intraoperatively and correlated with intraoperative radiographs or fluoroscopy to confirm the operative level.

4.4 CT

CT images, which are acquired using principles similar to those for conventional radiography, can be considered multiplanar high-resolution conventional radiographic images because the radiation is transmitted through the patient in multiple planes, which permits the acquisition of a large-volume dataset. Unlike conventional radiography, in which the images are acquired in one plane, this dataset can be manipulated using computer software algorithms to provide images in any plane. Current-generation multidetector CT scanning devices allow for the

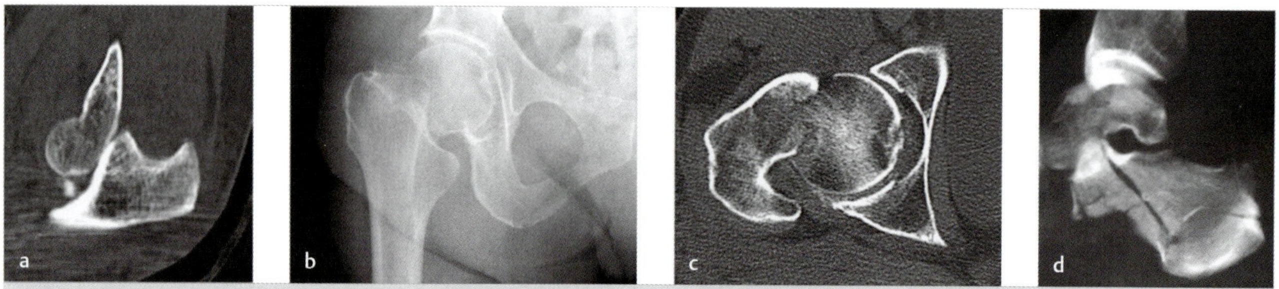

Fig. 4.4 Computed tomography (CT): excellent osseous detail. **(a)** A sagittal CT image of the elbow shows a posterior elbow dislocation and fracture fragment in the joint. **(b)** An anteroposterior (AP) radiograph of the right femur shows a varus deformity at the femoral neck that was noted on all views. **(c)** Given this deformity, CT was requested and more clearly showed a femoral neck fracture. **(d)** A 3D sagittal reconstructed CT image of the foot and ankle shows a complex calcaneal fracture. (Reproduced with permission from Srikumaran U, Fayad LM, Khanna AJ. Correlation of MRI with other imaging studies. In: Khanna AJ, ed. MRI for orthopaedic surgeons. New York: Thieme; 2010:414–424.)

acquisition of very large volumes of data in exceptionally small amounts of time. For example, studies of the entire body can be completed in < 10 seconds, which is particularly useful in pediatric and trauma patients, and for those who cannot lie still.[4]

With regard to its use in orthopaedic surgery, CT is most valuable for assessing anatomic detail for which radiography is limited, such as determining the location of bone fragments or the inter-relationship of structures (▶ Fig. 4.4). CT is also used secondarily to help characterize disease processes in areas where conventional radiography is generally suboptimal, such as the sacrum and pelvic structures. Although CT does not provide physiologic information about the status of the various tissues (except for cases in which intravenous contrast is used), it does provide excellent spatial resolution. Hence, CT is particularly useful for imaging the axial skeleton and for evaluating the extent of cortical destruction.[5,6,7] With the development of multiplanar 3D reconstructions, CT imaging provides additional guidance in preoperative planning, fracture assessment and classification, and evaluation of complex deformities.[8,9] Although CT images provide excellent osseous detail and can precisely localize fracture extent and fragmentation (information that can guide operative intervention), as a general rule, in current clinical practice, CT imaging does not provide resolution of high enough contrast for optimal evaluation of soft tissues such as the menisci and ligaments.[10] With the recent introduction of 16- and 64-multidetector CT and the advent of isotropic datasets, volume-rendered 3D CT evaluation of the tendons has emerged as a new indication for CT imaging (for patients in whom MRI is not possible).[11] With the introduction of dual-energy CT, the potential for defining the soft tissues with resolution of greater contrast is now being investigated. Dual-energy CT offers imaging with two X-ray generation sources that operate at different energies. Tissues will appear with different attenuation values on such images, favoring the differentiation of the soft tissues by CT.[11]

CT can also be used for preoperative planning of orthopaedic surgical procedures. For example, a patient who presented with knee pain after direct trauma had normal-appearing conventional radiographs (▶ Fig. 4.5a, b). Because the patient had a large knee effusion associated with severe pain, suspicion was high for a ligamentous injury or an occult fracture. Coronal and sagittal CT images confirmed a lateral anterior femoral condyle comminuted fracture and an avulsion fracture of the inferior pole of the patella (▶ Fig. 4.5c–e). MR images showed osseous edema of the lateral anterior femoral condyle and the inferior pole of the patella, as well as the disruption of the medial retinaculum (▶ Fig. 4.5f, g).

4.5 Nuclear Scintigraphy

Although the imaging studies described above provide excellent anatomic information, they are limited in their abilities to provide high-quality physiologic information, specifically information related to bone turnover. In this regard, the imaging modality of choice is three-phase bone scintigraphy. For a bone scan, the patient is injected with technetium-99 m phosphate or another radiopharmaceutical agent that emits gamma rays. Subsequently, the patient is placed under a scintillation camera to detect the presence and distribution of the radiotracer activity. The typical three-phase bone scan acquires the radiotracer activity information in the following phases (although for the identification of metastatic disease, only the delayed phase is acquired):

- Blood-flow phase.
- Soft-tissue phase.
- Delayed or bone phase.

Each of these phases provides different information. In the blood-flow phase, increased uptake is found in areas of mature blood vessels. The soft-tissue phase shows areas of neovascularity such as with acute inflammation or vascular neoplasms. In the delayed or bone phase, the radiotracer has had time to adsorb newly formed crystals at the site of bone turnover.[12,13]

The advantages of bone scans are that they provide physiologic information regarding bone (more specifically, mineral turnover) and can survey the entire body and detect lesions early in their course. Their disadvantages are that the images are nonspecific and provide poor spatial and anatomic resolution. Thus, when using bone scans, one trades the anatomic detail provided by other imaging techniques for physiologic information regarding metabolic activity in the bone. Fortunately, systems have been developed that, in combination with CT scanning, allow scintigraphy and anatomic localization to occur simultaneously. The indications for scintigraphy include the evaluation of osseous lesions, metastatic disease, benign and malignant primary

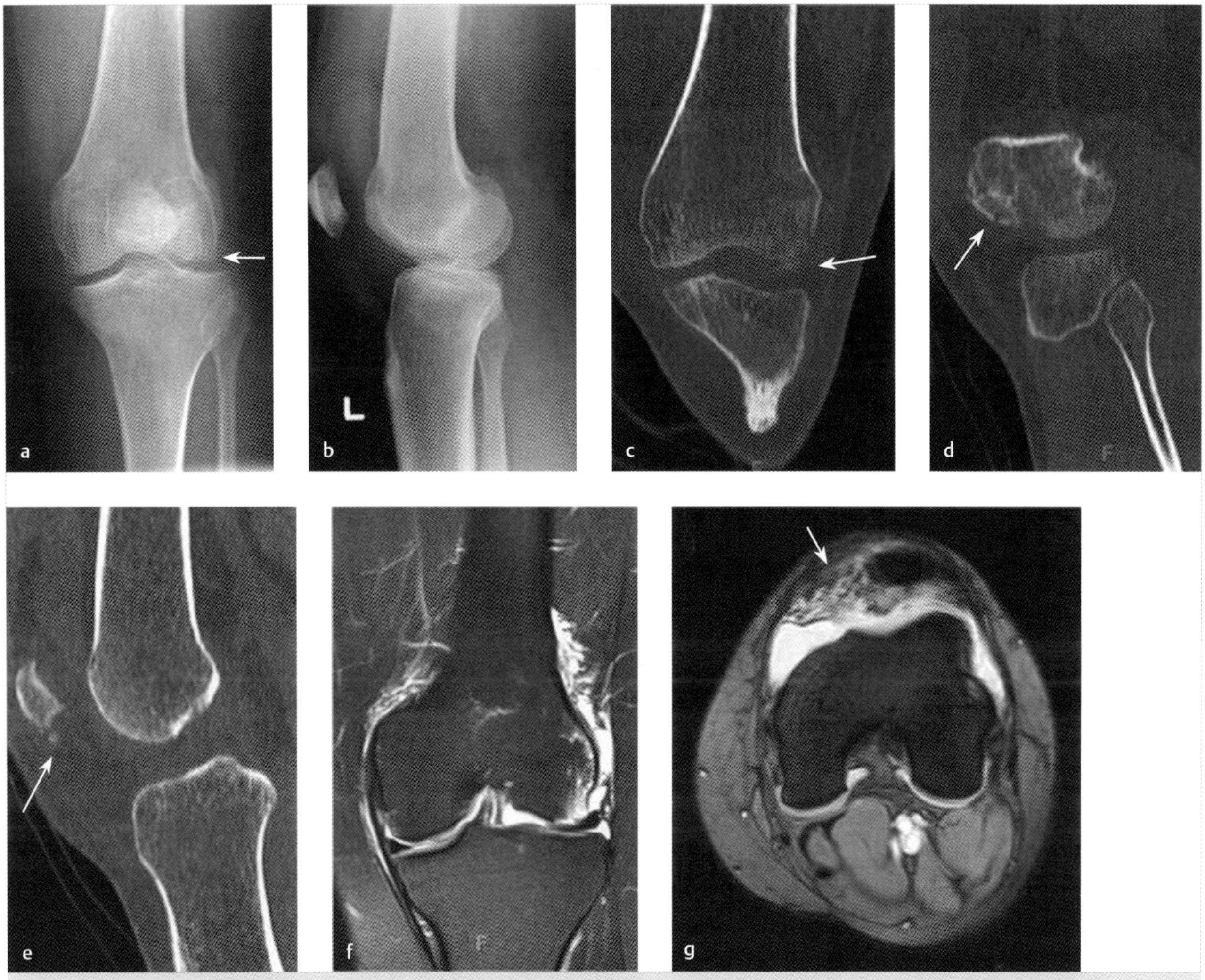

Fig. 4.5 Value of multimodal imaging. **(a)** Posteroanterior (PA) and **(b)** lateral radiographs of a young woman involved in a motor vehicle accident show a mild cortical irregularity at the left lateral femoral condyle (*arrow on* **a**). **(c)** A coronal reconstructed computed tomography (CT) image toward the anterior aspect of the knee better shows a small fracture fragment adjacent to the anterolateral femoral condyle (*arrow*). **(d)** A sagittal reconstructed CT image also shows the fracture (*arrow*) at the anterior aspect of the lateral femoral condyle. **(e)** A midline sagittal CT reconstructed image shows a small avulsion fracture at the inferior pole of the patella (*arrow*). **(f)** A coronal short tau inversion recovery (STIR) image shows the bone marrow edema at the anterolateral aspect of the lateral femoral condyle associated with the fracture, in addition to disruption of medial ligamentous structures. **(g)** An axial T2-weighted image better depicts disruption of the medial retinaculum (*arrow*). (Reproduced with permission from Srikumaran U, Fayad LM, Khanna AJ. Correlation of MRI with other imaging studies. In: Khanna AJ, ed. MRI for orthopaedic surgeons. New York: Thieme; 2010:414–424.)

tumors, metabolic disorders, infection, and sometimes, stress fractures.[12,1415,16] Different findings in the phases of a three-phase bone scan can help differentiate osteomyelitis from soft-tissue infection without osseous involvement.[17,18]

In the setting of osteomyelitis, conventional radiographs are the initial study of choice, but additional imaging modalities are often required for a definitive diagnosis because osteomyelitis is not detectable by radiography until ~40% of the bone has been destroyed. MRI and nuclear scintigraphy provide greater diagnostic sensitivity and specificity. MRI is extraordinarily sensitive to the presence of bone marrow abnormalities and can show associated soft-tissue involvement. Hence, MRI is considered the modality of choice for the early detection of osteomyelitis. Nuclear scintigraphy has an advantage, in that it can quickly show other areas of involvement, which is particularly important for pediatric patients who may have multiple sites of infection.[19] It is important to note that when bone turnover is exceptionally high, such as in a patient with multiple myeloma and other lytic processes, conventional bone scan techniques may produce false-negative findings, and other whole-body modalities (e.g., PET or whole-body MRI) should be considered.[20,21]

Nuclear scintigraphy can also be used to help determine the age or physiologic activity of vertebral compression and other fractures (▸ Fig. 4.6).[22,23,24] In such cases, nuclear scintigraphy may be indicated in patients for whom MRI is contraindicated

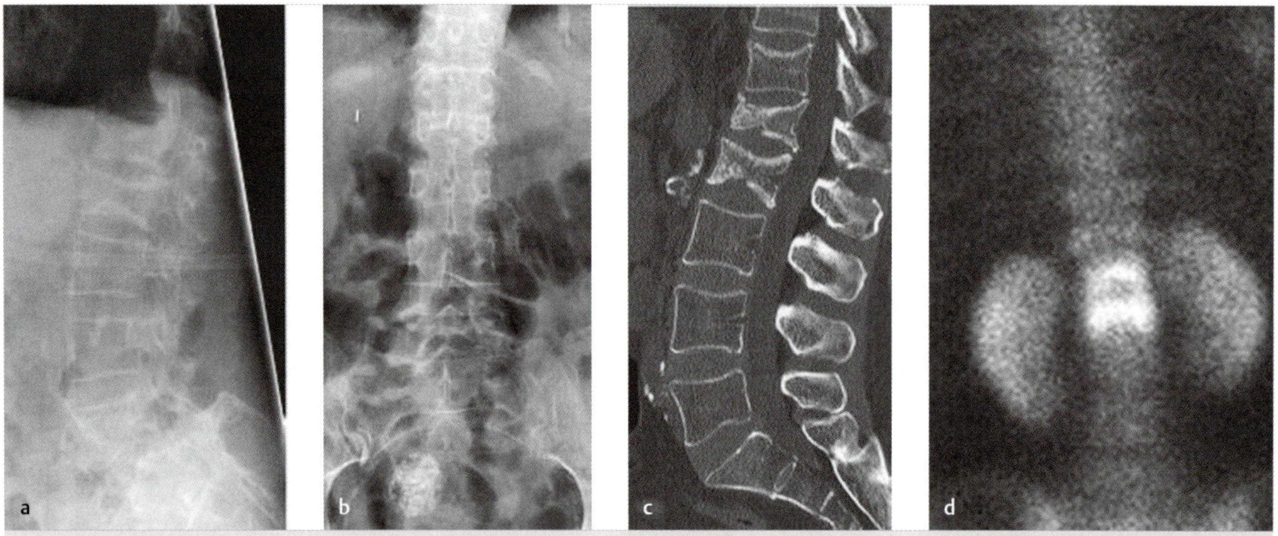

Fig. 4.6 Three-phase bone scan: to evaluate age and activity of vertebral compression fractures. **(a)** Lateral and **(b)** posteroanterior (PA) radiographs of an elderly woman with osteoporosis showing L2 and L3 vertebral compression fractures. **(c)** A sagittal reconstructed computed tomography (CT) image better shows the osseous detail and configuration of the fractures but it does not allow for accurate assessment of the relative age or physiologic activity of the fracture. **(d)** A PA delayed bone-phase image from a three-phase bone scan shows intense radiotracer uptake within the L2 and L3 vertebral bodies, suggestive of an acute or subacute fracture that is physiologically active. (Reproduced with permission from Srikumaran U, Fayad LM, Khanna AJ. Correlation of MRI with other imaging studies. In: Khanna AJ (ed). MRI for orthopaedic surgeons. New York: Thieme; 2010:414–424.)

such as those with claustrophobia or non–MRI-compatible pacemakers or defibrillators.

4.6 PET

As does nuclear scintigraphy, PET facilitates evaluation of the physiologic activity in the tissues, most typically that of glucose metabolism. Although other agents can be used, current common clinical practice is to inject a patient with 18F-labeled 2-fluoro-2-deoxyglucose, which emits gamma rays according to the rate of glucose metabolism. Whereas in the past, the availability of PET was limited to a few centers in North America, access is now more widely available.

The most common indication for PET scanning is for the evaluation of malignant metastases, tumor recurrence, or treatment response; PET has shown limited promise in differentiating benign and malignant lesions.[25,26,27,28] In one study of 45 heterogeneous lesions,[26] PET scanning provided high sensitivity (91%) and specificity (100%) for the differentiation of malignant and benign lesions but false-positive results have been shown with PET,[29,30,31] including in insufficiency fractures that are common in patients with cancer, inflammatory conditions such as sarcoidosis, and benign soft-tissue tumors.

Applications of PET continue to be developed. Preliminary studies have shown that PET can effectively determine whether vertebral compression fractures are pathologic or secondary to osteoporosis alone,[32,33] although MRI is usually the test of choice for assessing whether a fracture is associated with an underlying bone lesion.[34] Recent work has shown a potential role for PET in patients with arthroplasty in terms of evaluating osteolysis and determining whether prosthetic loosening is aseptic or infectious.[35,36,37] The combined technique of PET and CT has recently been advocated for use in diagnostically difficult cases of adolescent back pain.[38] The strength of this technique is in the combination and correlation of functional data with the detailed anatomic findings of CT. Of note, imaging of metallic implants is evolving to include MRI with metal reduction techniques rather than CT, such that optimal evaluation of the soft tissues can occur.[39]

4.7 Ultrasonography

Musculoskeletal applications for ultrasonography have been expanding, and in some centers ultrasonography is offered as a first-line study of the joints because it is more readily available than MRI, is relatively inexpensive, and is not associated with the radiation exposure of CT imaging.[40] The main advantage of ultrasonography in musculoskeletal imaging is that it provides a focused examination that can be tailored to the patient's point of pain. Dynamic ultrasound imaging can detect abnormalities in tendons or nerve subluxation.[40,41] Ultrasonography is also useful in the setting of metal because it is not susceptible to artifacts, unlike CT and MRI. Increasingly, ultrasonography is used for interventions, particularly for common joint injections and aspirations, as well as for more complex procedures.[40,42]

The disadvantages of ultrasonography, however, include the need for expertise in performing the ultrasound examination. Another disadvantage is that ultrasound images provide only a limited view and not a global assessment of a body part or allow comprehensive evaluation for internal derangement. For example, when assessing the postoperative shoulder, detection of a recurrent rotator cuff tendon tear is possible with ultrasonography (▶ Fig. 4.7) but detection of recurrent subacromial spurs and evaluation of the labrum are not.

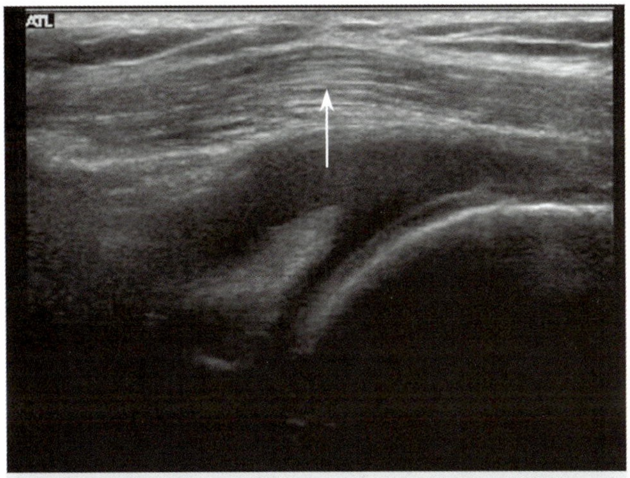

Fig. 4.7 Ultrasound image of the shoulder showing a full-thickness tear of the supraspinatus tendon with retraction (*arrow*), and fluid in the bursa.

4.8 Common Clinical Questions

1. Which of the following is the modality of choice for detecting early osteomyelitis?
   a) Radiography.
   b) CT.
   c) Nuclear scintigraphy.
   d) MRI.

2. Which modality is most appropriate for imaging of an obtunded trauma patient's body?
   a) Radiography.
   b) CT.
   c) MRI.
   d) Bone scan.

3. Which of the following indications would be appropriate for a bone scan?
   a) Evaluation of a sclerotic bone lesion.
   b) Whole body evaluation for soft-tissue and bone metastasis.
   c) Evaluation of multiple myeloma.
   d) Three-phase bone scan for a calcified soft-tissue mass.

4. When imaging with ultrasound, the following is true:
   a) A focused examination of the site of pain is more possible with ultrasonography than MRI.
   b) Although ultrasonography can be used for assessing shoulder tendons, labral and osseous abnormalities are not well-assessed.
   c) Ultrasonography is an ideal modality for joint aspiration because fluid in the joint can be targeted.
   d) All of the above.

5. Which modality should be used for first detecting a bone tumor?
   a) Radiography.
   b) Bone scintigraphy.
   c) CT.
   d) MRI.

References

[1] Kamholtz R, Sze G. Current imaging in spinal metastatic disease. Semin Oncol. 1991; 18(2):158–169

[2] Steinbach HL. The roentgen appearance of osteoporosis. Radiol Clin North Am. 1964; 2:191–207

[3] Fayad LM, Carrino JA, Fishman EK. Musculoskeletal infection: role of CT in the emergency department. Radiographics. 2007; 27(6):1723–1736

[4] Fayad LM, Johnson P, Fishman EK. Multidetector CT of musculoskeletal disease in the pediatric patient: principles, techniques, and clinical applications. Radiographics. 2005; 25(3):603–618

[5] Fayad LM, Bluemke DA, Fishman EK. Musculoskeletal imaging with computed tomography and magnetic resonance imaging: when is computed tomography the study of choice? Curr Probl Diagn Radiol. 2005; 34(6):220–237

[6] Genant HK, Wilson JS, Bovill EG, Brunelle FO, Murray WR, Rodrigo JJ. Computed tomography of the musculoskeletal system. J Bone Joint Surg Am. 1980; 62(7):1088–1101

[7] Wilson JS, Korobkin M, Genant HK, Bovill EG, Jr. Computed tomography of musculoskeletal disorders. AJR Am J Roentgenol. 1978; 131(1):55–61

[8] Geijer M, El-Khoury GY. MDCT in the evaluation of skeletal trauma: principles, protocols, and clinical applications. Emerg Radiol. 2006; 13(1): 7–18

[9] Newton PO, Hahn GW, Fricka KB, Wenger DR. Utility of three-dimensional and multiplanar reformatted computed tomography for evaluation of pediatric congenital spine abnormalities. Spine. 2002; 27(8):844–850

[10] Mui LW, Engelsohn E, Umans H. Comparison of CT and MRI in patients with tibial plateau fracture: can CT findings predict ligament tear or meniscal injury? Skeletal Radiol. 2007; 36(2):145–151

[11] Demehri S, Chalian M, Farahani SJ, Fishman EK, Fayad LM. Detection and characterization of tendon abnormalities with multidetector computed tomography. J Comput Assist Tomogr. 2014; 38(2):299–307

[12] Lee E, Worsley DF. Role of radionuclide imaging in the orthopedic patient. Orthop Clin North Am. 2006; 37(3):485–501, viii

[13] McCarthy EF, Frassica FJ. Diagnosing bone disease. In: Pathology of bone and joint disorders: with clinical and radiographic correlation. Philadelphia, PA: WB Saunders; 1998:1–24

[14] Abdel-Dayem HM. The role of nuclear medicine in primary bone and soft tissue tumors. Semin Nucl Med. 1997; 27(4):355–363

[15] Deutsch AL, Coel MN, Mink JH. Imaging of stress injuries to bone. Radiography, scintigraphy, and MR imaging. Clin Sports Med. 1997; 16(2): 275–290

[16] Greenspan A, Stadalnik RC. A musculoskeletal radiologist's view of nuclear medicine. Semin Nucl Med. 1997; 27(4):372–385

[17] Alazraki NP. Radionuclide imaging in the evaluation of infections and inflammatory disease. Radiol Clin North Am. 1993; 31(4):783–794

[18] El-Maghraby TAF, Moustafa HM, Pauwels EKJ. Nuclear medicine methods for evaluation of skeletal infection among other diagnostic modalities. Q J Nucl Med Mol Imaging. 2006; 50(3):167–192

[19] Santiago Restrepo C, Giménez CR, McCarthy K. Imaging of osteomyelitis and musculoskeletal soft tissue infections: current concepts. Rheum Dis Clin North Am. 2003; 29(1):89–109

[20] Ghanem N, Lohrmann C, Engelhardt M, et al. Whole-body MRI in the detection of bone marrow infiltration in patients with plasma cell neoplasms in comparison to the radiological skeletal survey. Eur Radiol. 2006; 16(5): 1005–1014

[21] Mulligan ME. Myeloma update. Semin Musculoskelet Radiol. 2007; 11(3): 231–239

[22] Fernandez-Ulloa M, Klostermeier TT, Lancaster KT. Orthopaedic nuclear medicine: the pelvis and hip. Semin Nucl Med. 1998; 28(1):25–40
[23] Masala S, Schillaci O, Massari F, et al. MRI and bone scan imaging in the preoperative evaluation of painful vertebral fractures treated with vertebroplasty and kyphoplasty. In Vivo. 2005; 19(6):1055–1060
[24] Maynard AS, Jensen ME, Schweickert PA, Marx WF, Short JG, Kallmes DF. Value of bone scan imaging in predicting pain relief from percutaneous vertebroplasty in osteoporotic vertebral fractures. AJNR Am J Neuroradiol. 2000; 21(10):1807–1812
[25] Bastiaannet E, Groen H, Jager PL, et al. The value of FDG-PET in the detection, grading and response to therapy of soft tissue and bone sarcomas; a systematic review and meta-analysis. Cancer Treat Rev. 2004; 30(1):83–101
[26] Feldman F, van Heertum R, Manos C. 18FDG PET scanning of benign and malignant musculoskeletal lesions. Skeletal Radiol. 2003; 32(4):201–208
[27] Lodge MA, Lucas JD, Marsden PK, Cronin BF, O'Doherty MJ, Smith MA. A PET study of 18FDG uptake in soft tissue masses. Eur J Nucl Med. 1999; 26 (1):22–30
[28] Schwarzbach MH, Dimitrakopoulou-Strauss A, Willeke F, et al. Clinical value of [18-F]] fluorodeoxyglucose positron emission tomography imaging in soft tissue sarcomas. Ann Surg. 2000; 231(3):380–386
[29] Ahlawat S, Baig A, Blakeley JO, Jacobs MA, Fayad LM. Multiparametric whole-body anatomic, functional, and metabolic imaging characteristics of peripheral lesions in patients with schwannomatosis. J Magn Reson Imaging. 2016; 44(4):794–803
[30] Fayad LM, Cohade C, Wahl RL, Fishman EK. Sacral fractures: a potential pitfall of FDG positron emission tomography. AJR Am J Roentgenol. 2003; 181(5): 1239–1243
[31] Liepe K. False-positive finding in FDG-PET in a patient with seminoma and sarcoidosis. Acta Clin Belg. 2015; 70(2):138–140
[32] Schmitz A, Risse JH, Textor J, et al. FDG-PET findings of vertebral compression fractures in osteoporosis: preliminary results. Osteoporos Int. 2002; 13(9): 755–761
[33] Shin DS, Shon OJ, Byun SJ, Choi JH, Chun KA, Cho IH. Differentiation between malignant and benign pathologic fractures with F-18-fluoro-2-deoxy-D-glucose positron emission tomography/computed tomography. Skeletal Radiol. 2008; 37(5):415–421
[34] Fayad LM, Kawamoto S, Kamel IR, et al. Distinction of long bone stress fractures from pathologic fractures on cross-sectional imaging: how successful are we? AJR Am J Roentgenol. 2005; 185(4):915–924
[35] Delank KS, Schmidt M, Michael JWP, Dietlein M, Schicha H, Eysel P. The implications of 18F-FDG PET for the diagnosis of endoprosthetic loosening and infection in hip and knee arthroplasty: results from a prospective, blinded study. BMC Musculoskelet Disord. 2006; 7:20–28
[36] Manthey N, Reinhard P, Moog F, Knesewitsch P, Hahn K, Tatsch K. The use of [18 F]fluorodeoxyglucose positron emission tomography to differentiate between synovitis, loosening and infection of hip and knee prostheses. Nucl Med Commun. 2002; 23(7):645–653
[37] Mumme T, Reinartz P, Alfer J, Müller-Rath R, Buell U, Wirtz DC. Diagnostic values of positron emission tomography versus triple-phase bone scan in hip arthroplasty loosening. Arch Orthop Trauma Surg. 2005; 125(5):322–329
[38] Ovadia D, Metser U, Lievshitz G, Yaniv M, Wientroub S, Even-Sapir E. Back pain in adolescents: assessment with integrated 18F-fluoride positron-emission tomography-computed tomography. J Pediatr Orthop. 2007; 27(1):90–93
[39] Fritz J, Lurie B, Miller TT, Potter HG. MR imaging of hip arthroplasty implants. Radiographics. 2014; 34(4):E106–E132
[40] Patil P, Dasgupta B. Role of diagnostic ultrasound in the assessment of musculoskeletal diseases. Ther Adv Musculoskelet Dis. 2012; 4(5):341–355
[41] Corazza A, Orlandi D, Fabbro E, et al. Dynamic high-resolution ultrasound of the shoulder: how we do it. Eur J Radiol. 2015; 84(2):266–277
[42] Finnoff JT. The evolution of diagnostic and interventional ultrasound in sports medicine. PM R. 2016; 8(3) Suppl:S133–S138

Answers to Common Clinical Questions

1. Answer: d. In the setting of osteomyelitis, conventional radiography is often the first-line test but additional imaging modalities are often required for a definitive diagnosis because osteomyelitis is not detectable by radiography until ~40% of the bone has been destroyed. MRI is extraordinarily sensitive to the presence of bone marrow abnormalities and can show associated soft-tissue involvement. Hence, MRI is considered the modality of choice for the early detection of osteomyelitis.
2. Answer: b. CT offers high spatial resolution and speed of acquisition. Hence, a whole-body CT scan can be performed in less than 10 seconds, which is particularly beneficial to trauma patients or patients who cannot hold their breath.
3. Answer: a. Bone scanning is appropriately used to detect activity within an indeterminate sclerotic lesion, typically to differentiate metastatic disease from a bone island. Bone scanning is not sensitive to the detection of processes that present as lytic lesions (such as myeloma). In the latter, PET scanning is used instead.
4. Answer: d. Ultrasonography in musculoskeletal imaging provides a focused examination that can be tailored to the patient's point of pain. Ultrasonography is also advantageous for assessing superficial tendons and is increasingly used for interventions, particularly for common joint injections and aspirations, because fluid visualized by ultrasound can be targeted for aspiration. However, ultrasound images provide only a limited view of a joint and do not provide a comprehensive evaluation of the joint for internal derangement.
5. Answer: a. Radiography is the first-line modality for detecting a bone tumor. However, 40% of osseous destruction is needed before a pathologic process is identifiable by radiography. If radiography is negative and a cause of bone pain is unknown, then MRI is the best test for ruling out a bone marrow lesion because of the high-contrast resolution offered by this technique.

5 Articular Cartilage

Andrea M. Spiker, Michael K. Shindle, Li Foong Foo, Bryan T. Kelly, and Hollis G. Potter

Abstract
Articular cartilage imaging is used to determine the cause of joint pain, to evaluate the success of cartilage restorative procedures, and to perform thorough preoperative planning. Recent advances in magnetic resonance imaging (MRI) technology have allowed better visualization of articular cartilage. These include delayed gadolinium-enhanced MRI of cartilage, T2 mapping, T1ρ, and glycosaminoglycan (GAG) chemical exchange saturation transfer. Our preferred sequences for evaluating articular cartilage include an intermediate echo time, 2-dimensional (2D) non-fat-suppressed fast-spin-echo (FSE) sequence without the use of intra-articular or intravenous contrast. The Modified International Cartilage Repair Society Classification is helpful for applying the classic arthroscopic Outerbridge classification to MRI. In the knee, MRI can identify chondral shear and delamination and can differentiate between a stable and unstable osteochondral defect. In the hip, MRI can be used to evaluate articular and labral cartilage, as well as capsular integrity and status of periarticular structures, which clarify abnormalities and is very important when referring patients for surgical treatment of femoroacetabular impingement. MRI can also be used to diagnose and monitor infection and inflammatory arthritis and as part of follow-up after cartilage restoration procedures.

Keywords: articular cartilage, fat-suppression sequence, high signal intensity, magnetic resonance imaging, pulse sequence

5.1 Introduction

Our ability to image articular cartilage has improved recently with advances in magnetic resonance imaging (MRI). This has provided greater insight into the structure and health of articular cartilage in the setting of injury and/or pain, which has improved clinical diagnosis, helped determine the most appropriate surgical candidates, and allowed surgeons to better counsel patients regarding expected outcomes.

Cartilage-sensitive pulse sequences should be included in all joint imaging MRI protocols. Cartilage-sensitive sequences can detect traumatic cartilage injury, evaluate the presence and/or extent of osteoarthritic changes, and monitor disease progression in inflammatory and degenerative arthritis. Cartilage repair techniques such as autologous chondrocyte implantation, juvenile allogeneic implantation, microfracture, and allogeneic or autologous osteochondral grafting are being performed with increased frequency, and MRI offers a noninvasive and objective method for evaluating postoperative integration after cartilage restorative procedures. Preoperatively, MRI helps determine cartilage quality and lesion size, which can influence the extent and appropriateness of surgery and indicate successful integration with the host tissue.

To differentiate the MR appearance between normal and abnormal cartilage morphology, it is necessary to understand the structure of articular cartilage. Articular cartilage, a metabolically active tissue, has viscoelastic properties and consists of chondrocytes (approximately 1%) and an extracellular matrix that consists of water (65–80%), proteoglycan, and collagen.[1] Type II collagen is the most common type (95%), but other types have been identified (types IV, VI, IX, X, and XI).[1] Collagen provides the tensile strength of articular cartilage. The hydrophilic proteoglycans are mainly chondroitin and keratin sulfates, which provide compressive strength to the cartilage.

Articular cartilage ranges in thickness from 2 to 5 mm, reflecting the contact pressures that occur across a given joint. The patellofemoral joint has the thickest articular cartilage in the body and is the site of very high peak pressures. Articular cartilage can be categorized structurally and functionally into the following four zones (▶ Fig. 5.1):

- Superficial.
- Transitional or middle.
- Deep or radial.
- Calcified.

The superficial zone accounts for 10 to 20% of the total thickness of cartilage, has the highest collagen content of any zone, and has highly organized collagen fibers that are oriented parallel to the articular surface.[2] This zone has a low proteoglycan content and functions to resist shear stress. Depending on the spatial resolution of the MR acquisition at clinically relevant field strengths, this zone may be distinguishable from the transitional zone (▶ Fig. 5.2). The middle or transitional zone accounts for 40 to 60% of the cartilage thickness, has collagen fibers that are oriented randomly, and has a higher compressive modulus than the superficial zone because the inhomogeneity of fiber orientation distributes the stress more uniformly across the loaded tissue.[3] The deep or radial zone accounts for 30% of cartilage thickness and has highly organized collagen fibers that are oriented perpendicular to the cartilage surface. This zone also has the lowest water content and highest proteoglycan content. The collagen fibers have a radial orientation that

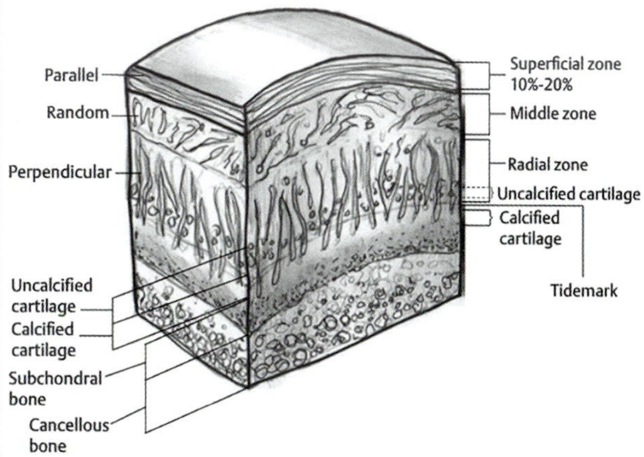

Fig. 5.1 Artist's depiction of cartilage zonal histology.

crosses the tidemark (the interface between the articular cartilage and the calcified cartilage beneath it), which anchors the cartilage to the underlying bone.[4] The calcified cartilage layer is the deepest zone. This zone is separated from the radial zone by the tidemark, which can be a potential shear plane for articular cartilage defects.[5] At clinically relevant field strengths using traditional pulse sequences, the tidemark cannot be differentiated from the subchondral plate.

The distribution of water, proteoglycan, and collagen content all account for MR signal characteristics of articular cartilage. However, the bulk of MR signal comes from the free water present and not from the water that is electrostatically bound to proteoglycan or the water that is associated with collagen. Depending on the pulse sequence used, cartilage will have a bilaminar or trilaminar appearance secondary to the highly ordered structure of the collagen of the deeper radial zone, which yields a shorter T2 relaxation time and corresponding lower signal intensity. Understanding the normal signal characteristics and anatomy of articular cartilage is imperative for detecting abnormal cartilage morphology.

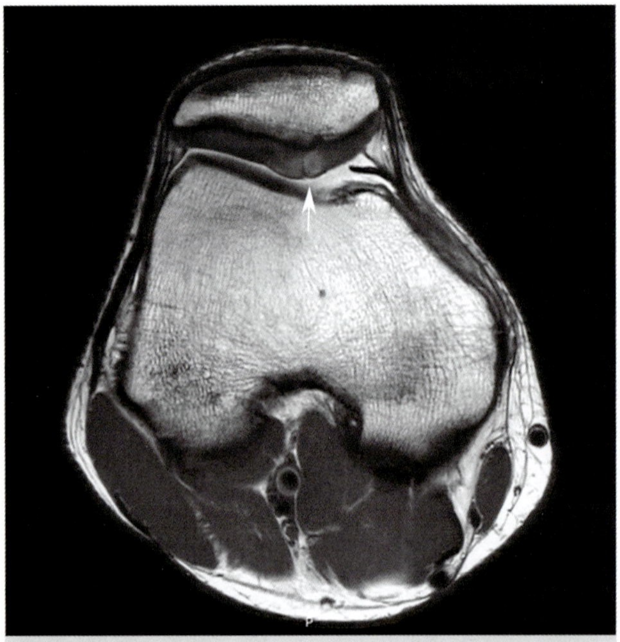

Fig. 5.2 Axial magnetic resonance imaging (MRI) of a 27-year-old athlete with anterior knee pain. The *arrow* shows cartilage with loss of grayscale stratification, deformity of the tidemark, and a fissure at the patellar apex as a focal defect in the lamina splendens. An incidental medial plica is noted.

5.2 Systematic Approach to Reviewing Cartilage on MRI

When evaluating articular cartilage on MRI, it is our preference to begin with fat-suppression sequences. These provide information regarding subchondral bone marrow edema patterns, which may herald basilar delamination, traumatic chondral shear, or stress reaction in the setting of osteoarthritis (OA) (▶ Fig. 5.3, ▶ Fig. 5.4). Use of a consistent approach ensures that the entire joint surface is evaluated, and we typically begin with the sagittal images followed by the coronal and then the axial series.

First, the structural integrity of the cartilage can be evaluated by following the superficial edge of the cartilage from lateral to medial and anterior to posterior, in which large defects can be seen as a break in the line representing the cartilage edge. Second, the signal intensity can be evaluated for homogeneity. Also evaluate for fluid imbibition within the cartilage, among the cartilage zones, or in the subchondral bone, which will indicate areas of abnormal cartilage.

Articular cartilage on sagittal and coronal imaging in the shoulder, knee, and hip can be followed from lateral to medial (sagittal) and anterior to posterior (coronal) in the glenohumeral, femorotibial, and acetabular-femoral joints, respectively. At the knee, axial imaging is helpful to evaluate the patellar and trochlear cartilage.

5.3 Specialized Pulse Sequences and Imaging Protocols

MRI provides soft-tissue contrast superior to that of traditional imaging techniques. However, standardized conventional radiographs are still a valuable part of cartilage assessment. When planning for cartilage repair, standing hip-to-ankle

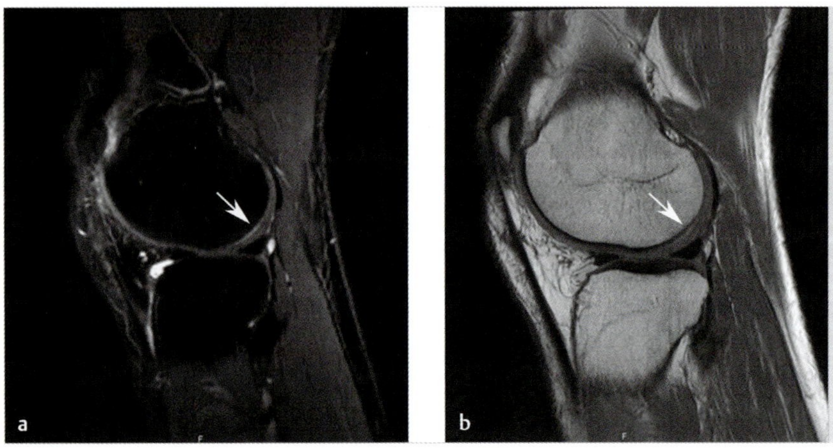

Fig. 5.3 (a) Sagittal inversion recovery and (b) moderate echo time magnetic resonance imaging (MRI) of a 49-year-old man's knee showing (*arrow*) signal intensity and reversal of grayscale intensity with basilar separation at the tidemark. This is in contrast to the lateral tibial plateau, where a normal lower signal intensity in the basilar layer of the cartilage is noted.

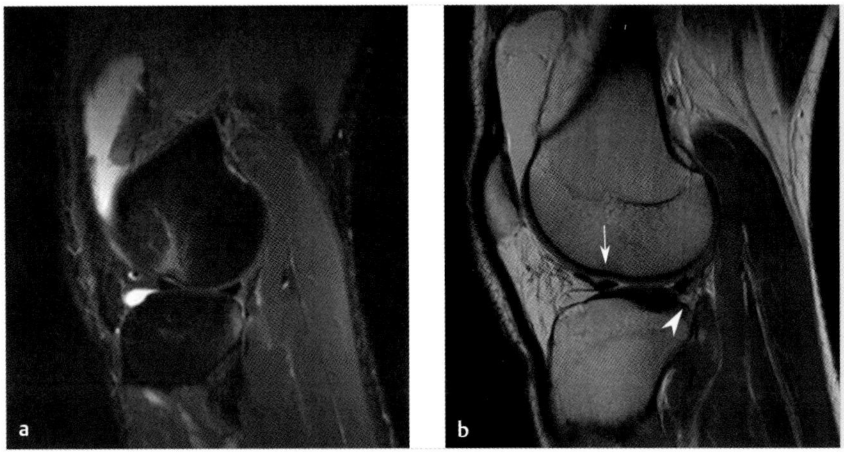

Fig. 5.4 Magnetic resonance imaging (MRI) showing traumatic chondral injury after an acute anterior cruciate ligament tear. This 29-year-old man has compression in the cartilage over the anterior aspect of the lateral femoral condyle on the **(a)** sagittal inversion recovery and **(b)** sagittal moderate echo-time image. Note full-thickness shear with debris in the meniscosynovial recess (*arrow*) over the tibial plateau (*arrow head*).

radiographs are useful for preoperative planning to determine the following:

- The mechanical axis of the limb, to identify any pre-existing deformity that may limit the clinical success of cartilage repair.
- Whether concomitant procedures (i.e., high tibial osteotomy) should be performed.

The orthopaedic surgeon should be aware that different pulse sequences are available for evaluating articular cartilage and should be included in all joint imaging protocols. Traditional sequences include a T1-weighted 3-dimensional (3D) fat-suppressed gradient-echo sequence, which renders high contrast between the low signal intensity of the fat-suppressed bone and the high signal intensity of articular cartilage (▶ Fig. 5.5). This sequence has several drawbacks: it requires a long scan time (although this has been mitigated recently by faster scanning techniques); it is not ideal for meniscal or ligamentous evaluation; it is less sensitive to partial-thickness cartilage defects; and the image signal degrades in the presence of metal.[6,7,8]

For these reasons, we prefer an intermediate echo time, 2D non–fat-suppressed FSE sequence that provides good differential contrast among the intermediate signal intensity of articular cartilage, the high signal intensity of synovial fluid, and the low signal intensity of fibrocartilage (▶ Fig. 5.6).[7,8] With proper technique, this sequence offers several advantages, including the following:

- Short scan time.
- Effectiveness in the presence of instrumentation.
- Detection of partial-thickness chondral lesions.
- Very good differential contrast among the underlying bone, cartilage, ligaments, joint fluid, and menisci.

This pulse sequence shows cartilage as a laminar grayscale appearance that corresponds to the different orientations of collagen within the cartilage zones: a hypointense radial zone and a higher-signal-intensity transitional zone (▶ Fig. 5.7).[7]

The three most commonly used pulse sequences in cartilage imaging include 2D fat-suppressed moderate echo FSE, 2D non–fat-suppressed moderate echo time FSE, and 3D fat-suppressed T1-weighted gradient echo. The 2D FSE sequences demonstrate high joint fluid signal intensity and intermediate cartilage

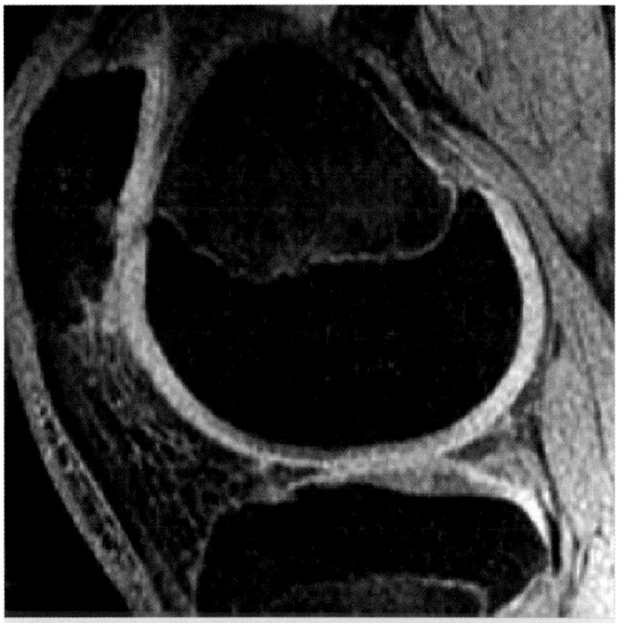

Fig. 5.5 Sagittal 3-dimensional fat-suppressed T1-weighted gradient-echo image of the knee showing high contrast between hyperintense articular cartilage and hypointense bone. (Reproduced with permission from, Shindle MK, Foo LF, Kelly BT, et al. Magnetic resonance imaging of cartilage in the athlete: current techniques and spectrum of disease. J Bone Joint Surg Am. 2006; 88 Suppl 4:27–46.)

signal intensity, whereas the 3D fat-suppressed T1-weighted echo has low joint fluid and high cartilage signal intensity. The ability to see meniscus and ligamentous tissue in 3D fat-suppressed T1-weighted gradient echo is poor, whereas it is good in both 2D sequences. Fat in subchondral bone marrow shows up as very low signal, low signal, and high signal in 3D fat-suppressed T1, 2D fat-suppressed, and 2D non–fat-suppressed sequences, respectively. The image quality in the presence of instrumentation is poor in 3D fat-suppressed T1-weighted gradient echo, fair in 2D fat-suppressed moderate echo time FSE, and good in 2D non–fat-suppressed moderate echo time FSE.[7]

Intra-articular or intravenous contrast agents were advocated for evaluating articular cartilage.[9,10,11,12] However, use of such agents with MRI can be invasive and may be associated with long imaging time and higher costs. With new MR capabilities,

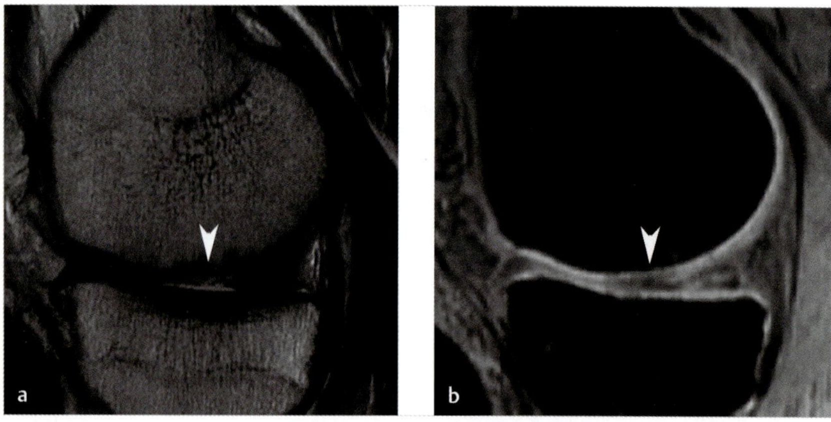

Fig. 5.6 **(a)** Sagittal fast-spin-echo sequence showing a focal partial-thickness cartilage defect overlying the medial femoral condyle (*arrowhead*). **(b)** Sagittal fat-suppressed T1-weighted gradient-echo sequence, in which the lesion is less clear. Image acquisition took twice as long as the fast-spin-echo image. (Reproduced with permission from, Potter HG, Foo LF. Magnetic resonance imaging of articular cartilage: trauma, degeneration, and repair. Am J Sports Med 2006;34(4)661–677.)

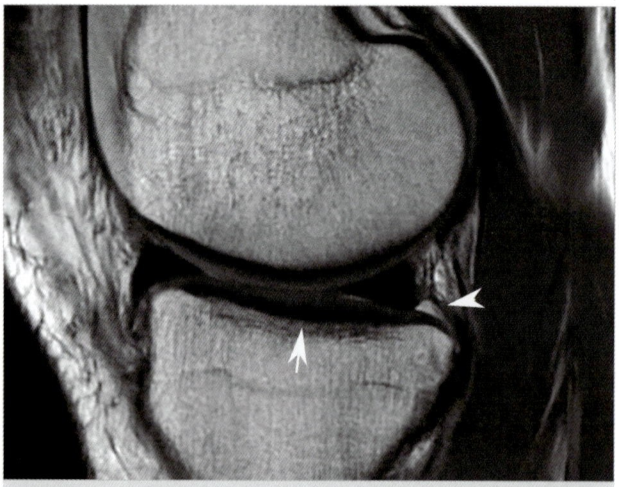

Fig. 5.7 Sagittal fast-spin-echo image of the knee of a 32-year-old patient showing grayscale stratification of the tibial plateau articular cartilage (*arrow*). Note the differential contrast for the high-signal-intensity joint fluid within the meniscosynovial recess (*arrowhead*), the intermediate signal intensity of hyaline cartilage, and the low signal intensity of meniscal fibrocartilage.

higher quality and clear visualization of the cartilage does not require contrast agents. Delayed gadolinium-enhanced MRI of cartilage (dGEMRIC) uses the contrast agent gadopentetate,[2] which moves through the cartilage and measures proteoglycan content within hyaline cartilage indirectly via its inverse relationship with glycosaminoglycan (GAG).[13] These techniques require injecting intravenous gadolinium followed by a brief period of joint exercise and then a 90-minute delay for assessment, which limits their use in multi-institutional trials.

Most MR signal derives from the free water content of the cartilage. Approaches have been developed to supplement traditional MRI techniques by targeting additional "bound" components of the extracellular matrix, specifically collagen or proteoglycan. For example, with OA and after traumatic cartilage injuries, there is a loss of negatively charged glycosaminoglycan, and thus MRI techniques such as positively charged sodium (^{23}Na) MRI,[14] T1ρ, and dGEMRIC were developed to detect these changes.[14,15,16,17,18] T2 mapping is an imaging technique that reflects the collagen component of the extracellular matrix. T2 relaxation time is a function of the internuclear reactions among the excited hydrogen dipoles and is influenced partially by the water content of the tissue, varying depending on the zone of articular cartilage.[19] For example, in the middle zone, collagen orientation is random and water is more mobile, corresponding to longer T2 values. In contrast, the deep zone has highly ordered collagen, and therefore T2 values are short because water is immobilized with shorter relaxation times (▶ Fig. 5.8). Clinically, T2 mapping is useful because of its ability to detect changes in cartilage structure before substantial loss of cartilage thickness or the development of gross signal alterations in the cartilage grayscale. This early detection can help surgical decision-making by optimizing the timing of surgery such as meniscal transplantation or patellofemoral realignment.

T1ρ is another means of visualizing cartilage composition, which uses spin locking in the rotating frame. However, this sequence is less readily available among MRI vendors. T1ρ and T2 have been shown to predict progressive cartilage loss in the knee and the hip.[20,21] T1ρ and T2 mapping have been shown to be reproducible across sites and scanners.[22]

Chemical exchange saturation transfer is a new method of imaging that functions as a biomarker for GAG within cartilage. Frequencies of off-resonance saturation pulses are used to isolate the protons located on cartilage GAG hydroxyl groups.[23] Although initially GAG chemical exchange saturation transfer was described using an ultra-high-field MR system, it has now shown noninferiority to dGEMRIC and T2 mapping in detecting articular cartilage defects.[24]

The aforementioned techniques are useful in quantifying and characterizing the articular cartilage.[13] Three-dimensional turbo spin-echo and gradient echo–based pulse sequences have also been described as useful for identifying cartilage defects[25] and can provide isotropic datasets that can be reformatted and serve as a template for tissue engineering.[26]

5.4 Clinical Cartilage Imaging

Cartilage imaging can be clinically important for diagnosing joint articular cartilage injury or abnormality; preoperative planning according to type and extent of cartilage disease; monitoring degenerative processes such as hip dysplasia, femoroacetabular impingement (FAI), OA, or rheumatic disease; and assessing success of cartilage reconstructive surgery.

5.5 Classification

Multiple scoring systems are used to classify articular cartilage lesions.[27,28,29,30] The most commonly used is the Outerbridge system,[30] an arthroscopic system that categorizes lesions into the following five grades:

- Grade 0: normal cartilage.
- Grade I: cartilage with softening and swelling.
- Grade II: a partial-thickness defect with fissures on the surface that do not reach subchondral bone or that are < 1.5 cm in diameter.
- Grade III: fissuring to the level of subchondral bone in an area with a diameter > 1.5 cm.
- Grade IV: exposed subchondral bone.

This classification system was originally used to describe chondromalacia patellae but is now commonly used to classify chondral lesions throughout the body[31]; however, it is limited because it does not describe the lesion depth for grade-II and grade-III lesions. The International Cartilage Repair Society has validated a standardized system for evaluating cartilage injury and repair, which can be applied to MRI (▶ Table 5.1).[27,32]

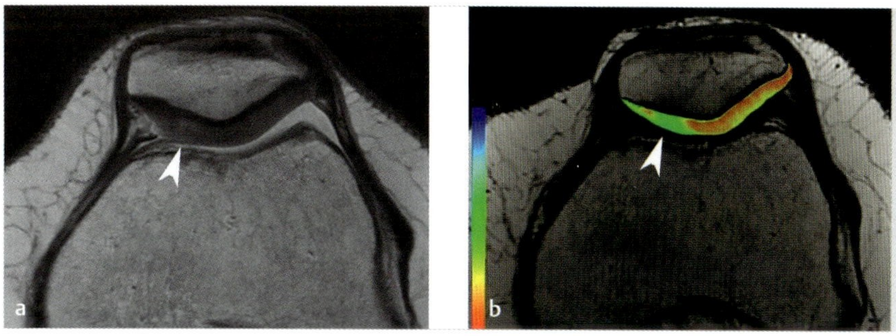

Fig. 5.8 Images of the knee of a patient with anterior knee pain. **(a)** Axial fast-spin-echo image showing focal increased signal (*arrowhead*) affecting normal-thickness cartilage in the medial patella facet. **(b)** Corresponding quantitative T2 relaxation time map showing geographic loss of stratification and prolongation in T2 values (*arrowhead*) throughout the thickness of the cartilage at this site.

Table 5.1 Modified International Cartilage Repair Society classification: MRI, arthroscopic, and anatomy correlations

Grade[a]	Pathologic change	Arthroscopic findings	MRI findings	MR images	Anatomic illustration
0	Normal articular cartilage	None	Normal cartilage with grayscale stratification		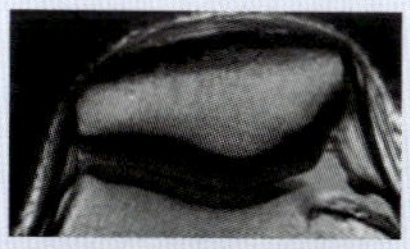
1	Superficial lesions: chondral softening	Softening to probe	Increased signal in articular cartilage		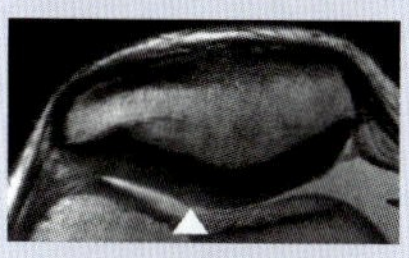
2	Superficial lesions extending down to ≤ 50% of cartilage depth	Fissures/ fibrillation involving ≤ 50% thickness	Linear to ovoid foci of increased signal involving ≤ 50% thickness	Fibrillation ≤ 50%	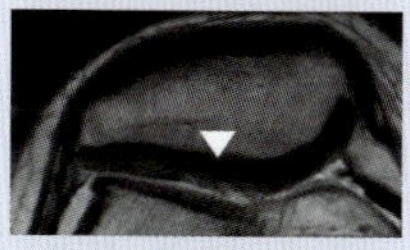
				Fissure ≤ 50%	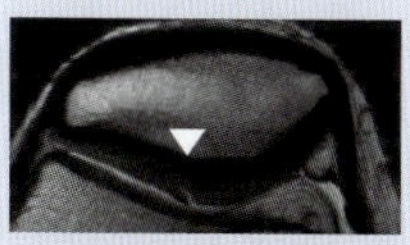
3	Cartilage defects extending down to > 50% of depth but not through subchondral bone	Blisters/fissures/ fibrillation involving > 50% thickness	Linear to ovoid foci of increased signal involving > 50% of cartilage thickness but not extending down to bone		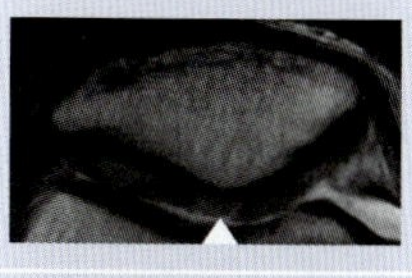
4	Ulceration to subchondral bone	Exposed subchondral bone	Complete loss of articular cartilage or surface flap		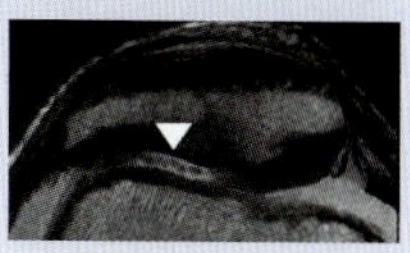

Abbreviations: MR, magnetic resonance; MRI, magnetic resonance imaging.
[a]Modified Outerbridge classification.[27,32]
Source: Reproduced with permission from, Shindle MK, Foo LF, Kelly BT, et al. Magnetic resonance imaging of cartilage in the athlete: current techniques and spectrum of disease. J Bone Joint Surg Am. 2006; 88 Suppl 4:27-46.

5.6 Traumatic Conditions

MRI after injury allows for noninvasive evaluation of cartilage and can detect clinically relevant lesions such as a cartilage shear injury or a displaced cartilage flap, which can mimic other injuries such as a displaced meniscal tear (▶ Fig. 5.9).[33]

5.6.1 Knee

In the knee, articular cartilage injuries have been associated with poor clinical outcomes.[34,35,36] Thus, MRI before surgery can aid in diagnosis, help predict prognosis, and identify patients who may benefit from cartilage repair techniques.[35]

Sheer stresses across the articular cartilage can result in chondral delamination from the underlying subchondral bone at the tidemark (▶ Fig. 5.10).[37,38] Isolated cartilage shearing injury is a different entity than osteochondral fracture, and carefully scrutinizing traumatic cartilage injury is necessary to distinguish the two. Osteochondral injuries are recognized by the presence of a hyperintense fatty marrow signal attached to the cartilage fragment and/or by the absence of the subchondral plate (thin, low-signal-intensity line) and tidemark between the bone and cartilage (▶ Fig. 5.11).[6]

Osteochondral defect is associated with separation of the subchondral bone adjacent to the articular surface secondary to an ischemic insult to the bone. It most commonly occurs at the lateral aspect of the medial femoral condyle. In this setting, MRI is useful for assessing lesion stability (▶ Fig. 5.12). Signs of an unstable fragment include the following[39]:

- High signal intensity surrounding the fragment on water-sensitive pulse sequences (e.g., proton density) and T2-weighted images.
- Size > 5 mm.
- Subchondral sclerosis on the deep side of the lesion, depicting a "mature bed."
- Defect in the overlying cartilage.
- Prominent cystic changes of ≥ 5 mm between the fragment and host bone.

5.6.2 Hip

Articular cartilage injuries of the hip are difficult to evaluate because of the deep ball-and-socket configuration. Focal chondral injuries on the femoral side are uncommon but they may result from axial loading or a shear injury of the head within the socket during a subluxation event. Cartilage injuries on the acetabular side are more common and typically present as localized cartilage delamination in the anterosuperior weight-bearing zone of the acetabular rim. One common mechanism for cartilage injury in this area is FAI (see section "Degenerative Conditions").

Although some research advocates using MR arthrography to improve contrast between the articular cartilage and synovial fluid, this addition converts MRI to an invasive procedure.[40,41,42] Mintz et al[43] evaluated 92 patients with noncontrast imaging before hip arthroscopy and concluded that an optimized protocol can identify labral and chondral abnormalities. Our protocol includes a screening examination of the whole pelvis, acquired using coronal inversion recovery and axial proton-density sequences. This procedure is followed by use of a surface coil over the hip joint with high-resolution cartilage-sensitive images acquired in three planes (sagittal, coronal, and oblique axial) using an FSE pulse sequence and proton density–weighted contrast.

Acute isolated traumatic articular surface injuries most commonly occur from impact loading across the hip joint. The type

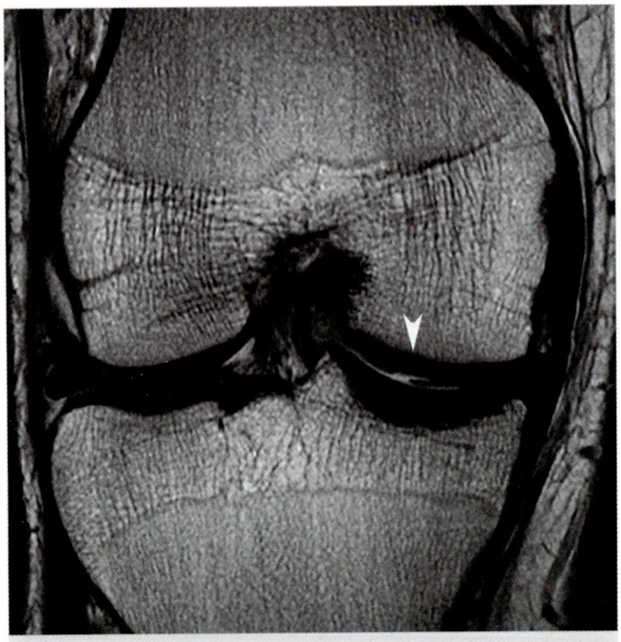

Fig. 5.9 Coronal cartilage-sensitive image of the knee of a 31-year-old man with a clinically suspected meniscal tear showing a focal chondral flap *(arrowhead)* over the right medial femoral condyle. (Reproduced with permission from, Potter HG, Foo LF. Magnetic resonance imaging of articular cartilage: trauma, degeneration, and repair. Am J Sports Med 2006;34(4)661–677.)

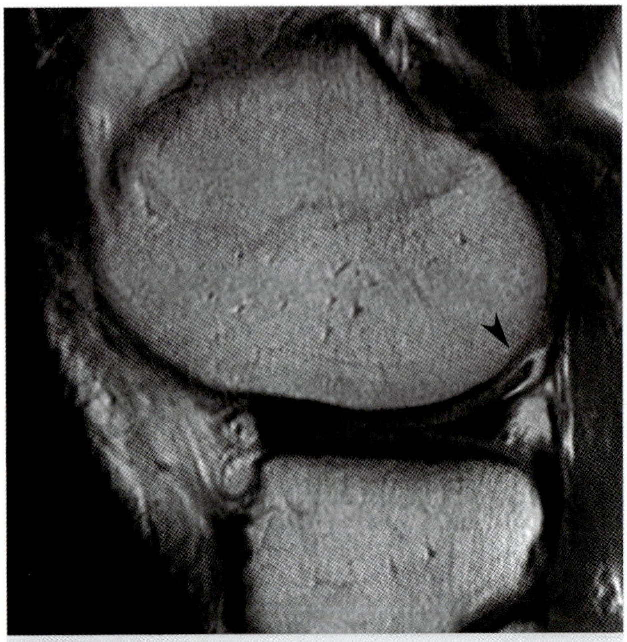

Fig. 5.10 Sagittal fast-spin-echo image of the knee showing articular cartilage delaminating *(arrowhead)* with fluid signal intensity between the cartilage flap and the underlying subchondral bone. (Reproduced with permission from, Shindle MK, Foo LF, Kelly BT, et al. Magnetic resonance imaging of cartilage in the athlete: current techniques and spectrum of disease. J Bone Joint Surg Am. 2006; 88 Suppl 4:27–46.)

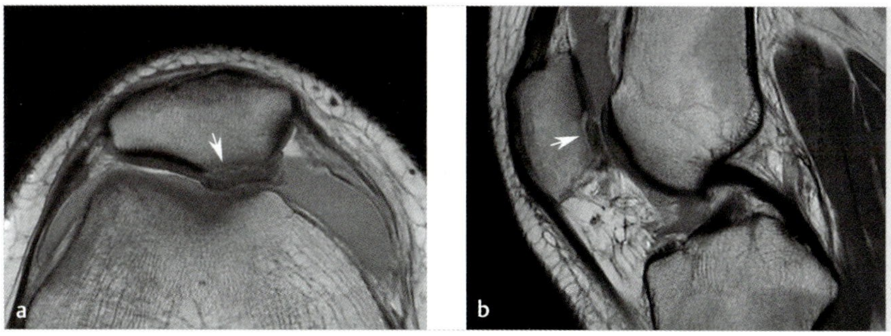

Fig. 5.11 **(a)** Axial and **(b)** sagittal fast-spin-echo images after a right patellar dislocation in a 15-year-old girl showing an osteochondral fracture of the patella apex (*arrow*). This injury can be distinguished from an isolated chondral shear injury because there is absence of the subchondral plate and tidemark at the site of injury.

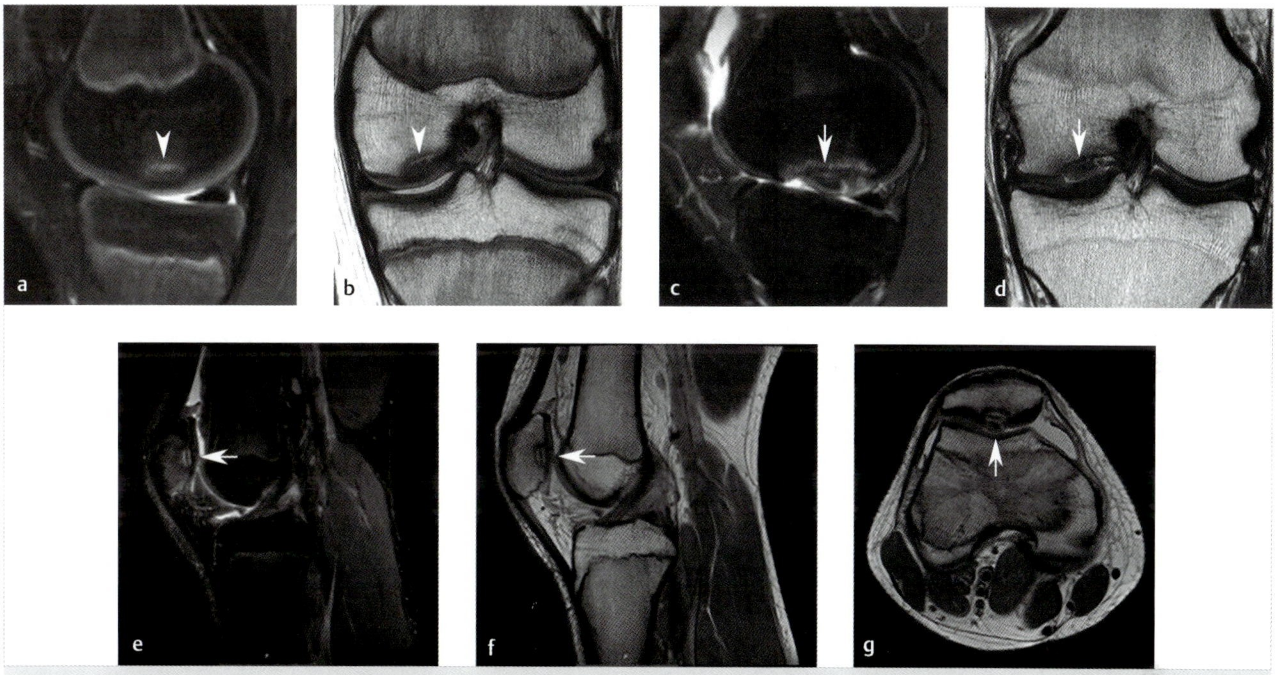

Fig. 5.12 **(a)** Sagittal fat-suppressed and **(b)** coronal non–fat-suppressed fast-spin-echo images of the knee showing a small stable osteochondral defect lesion (*arrowhead on each*). In comparison, **(c)** sagittal fat-suppressed and **(d)** coronal non–fat-suppressed fast-spin-echo images showing a large unstable lesion (*arrow on each*) with low-signal-intensity sclerosis at the margins of the underlying bone, indicating the presence of a "mature" bed. Sagittal **(e)** inversion recovery and **(f)** non–fat-suppressed and **(g)** axial non–fat-suppressed images of the knee showing an unstable osteochondral defect lesion of the patella (*arrow*) with sclerosis at the deep margin of the lesion. (Figure parts a, b, c, and d: Reproduced with permission from, Shindle MK, Foo LF, Kelly BT, et al. Magnetic resonance imaging of cartilage in the athlete: current techniques and spectrum of disease. J Bone Joint Surg Am. 2006; 88 Suppl 4:27–46.)

and degree of injury vary depending on the amount and direction of the impact load. A posteriorly directed force can lead to hip subluxation, in which the femoral head is forced against the labrum and rim of the posterior wall. This subluxation can lead to shear injuries at the level of the articular cartilage and associated fractures of the subchondral bone (▶ Fig. 5.13). Moorman et al[44] described the characteristic MRI triad of posterior acetabular lip fracture, hemarthrosis, and iliofemoral ligament disruption. In addition, MRI is useful to detect and monitor subsequent osteonecrosis and to help determine whether an athlete may return to play.

5.6.3 Shoulder

Cartilage injuries are noted in 5 to 17% of all routine shoulder arthroscopies.[45] Acute and chronic shoulder instability can lead to cartilage lesions in the glenohumeral joint. In first-time shoulder dislocations, chondral shear injuries or osteochondral compression fractures have been reported in 47 to 100% of cases.[46]

5.7 Degenerative Conditions

MRI can offer much more detailed information on the status of articular cartilage compared with plain radiographs. With information on the presence or extent of cartilage degeneration, the surgeon can indicate patients appropriately for surgery. MRI also allows the surgeon to monitor the development or progression of articular cartilage degeneration.

5.7.1 Hip

The previous standard of evaluating hip OA was the Tönnis Classification on conventional anteroposterior pelvis radiographs, in

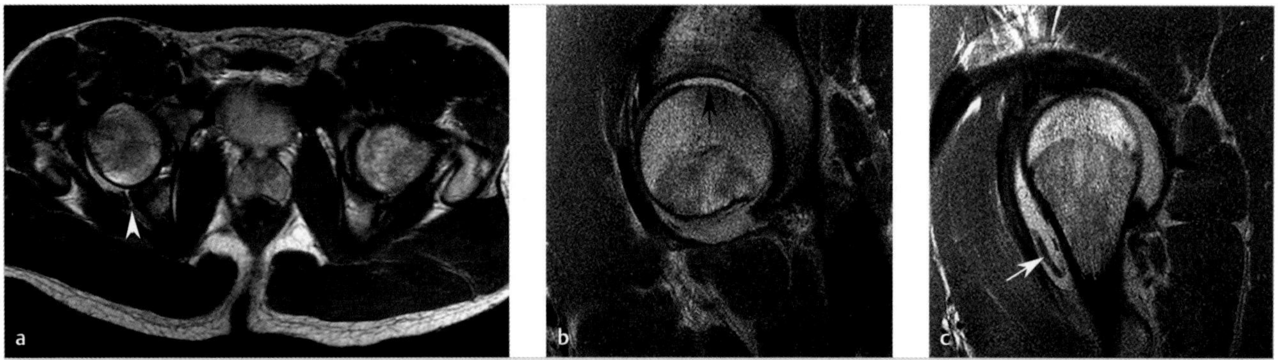

Fig. 5.13 Posterior hip subluxation sequelae in an 18-year-old patient. **(a)** Axial body coil fast-spin-echo image shows an intact right posterior hip capsule (*arrowhead*) attached to a posterior wall fracture. **(b)** Sagittal surface coil fast-spin-echo image shows a large full-thickness chondral shear injury (*black arrow*) of the femoral head. **(c)** Sagittal surface coil fast-spin-echo image shows cartilaginous debris (*white arrow*) within the anteroinferior dependent recess of the joint. (Reproduced with permission from, Shindle MK, Foo LF, Kelly BT, et al. Magnetic resonance imaging of cartilage in the athlete: current techniques and spectrum of disease. J Bone Joint Surg Am. 2006; 88 Suppl 4:27–46.)

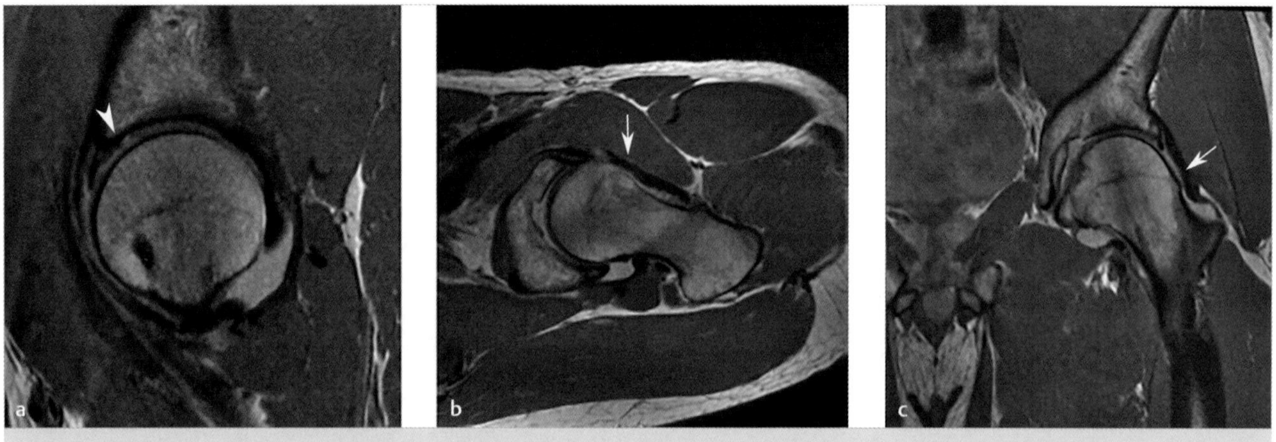

Fig. 5.14 **(a)** Sagittal, **(b)** axial, and **(c)** coronal moderate-echo-time MRI images of a 38-year-old man with left hip femoroacetabular impingement. All three planes of imaging are needed to identify full-thickness defect (*arrowhead*) in the articular cartilage and insufficient offset of the anterior neck-head junction (*arrows*). Note the associated mild synovitis in all three planes.

which the joint space was classified as 0, no signs of OA; 1, slight narrowing of the joint space, slight lipping at the joint margin, and slight sclerosis of the femoral head or acetabulum; 2, small cysts in the femoral head or acetabulum, increasing narrowing of the joint space, and moderate loss of sphericity of the femoral head; or 3, large cysts, severe narrowing or obliteration of the joint space, severe deformity of the femoral head, and osteonecrosis.[13] MRI of the hip gives us much more detailed information about the structure and state of the articular cartilage, although it cannot yet provide prognostic information about the cartilage.

Traditionally, chondral damage to the hip has been associated with progressive generalized joint deterioration from conditions like OA or inflammatory arthritis. However, several other mechanisms result in more focal chondral lesions and articular cartilage degeneration such as the sequelae of trauma, osteonecrosis, FAI, and developmental dysplasia. FAI is the most common underlying condition resulting in cartilage defects of the acetabulum and the anterosuperior weight-bearing zone. The articular surfaces of the acetabulum and femoral head should be evaluated using all three imaging planes.

The concept of FAI as a source of anterosuperior chondral and labral damage was introduced by Ganz et al.[47] Abnormal contact between the femoral head-neck junction and the anterior acetabulum during terminal hip flexion leads to a reproducible pattern of anterosuperior labral and chondral injury. According to anatomic features, they classified FAI into two distinct entities: cam and pincer. Cam impingement is associated with abnormal contact between an abnormal femoral head and neck with a morphologically normal acetabulum. During hip flexion, this abnormal region engages the anterior acetabulum and is associated with the characteristic chondrolabral junction chondral injury with potential detachment of the labrum (▶ Fig. 5.14).[48] Pincer impingement is the result of contact between a typically normal femoral head-neck junction and an abnormal acetabular rim. This abnormal anterior acetabular "over-coverage" can be the consequence of anatomic variants, including the following:

- Acetabular retroversion.
- Coxa profunda (protrusio).
- Deformity after trauma or periacetabular osteotomies.

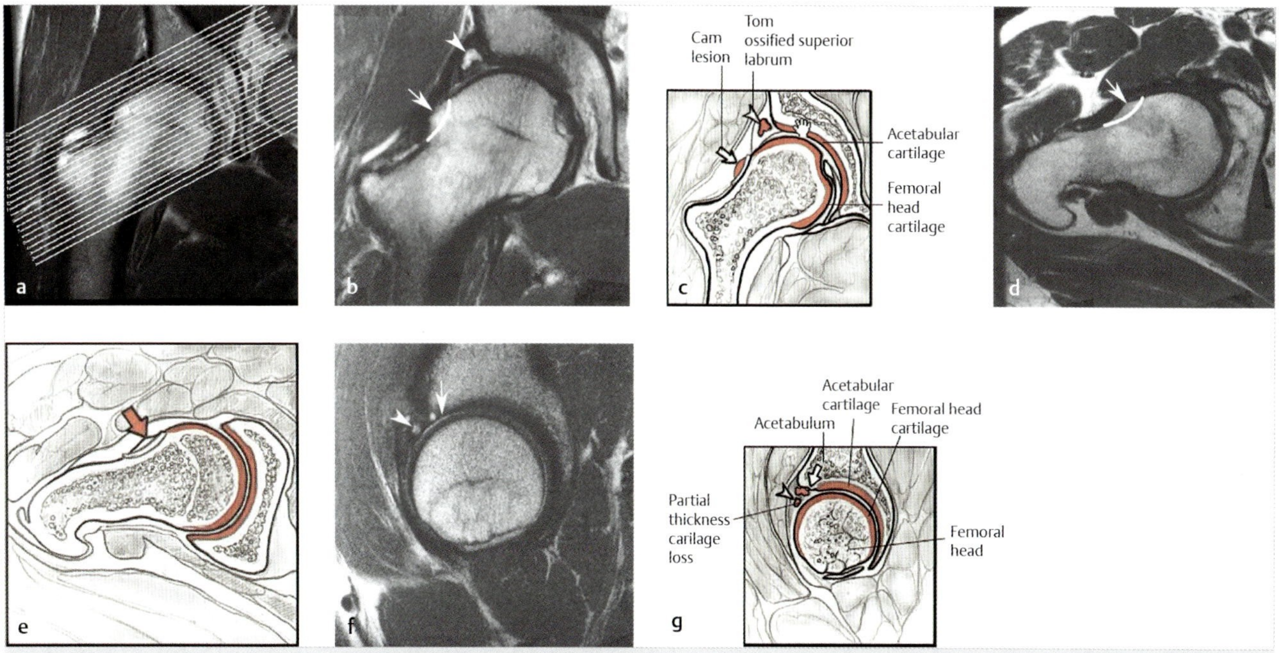

Fig. 5.15 Fast-spin-echo images and illustrations of a 41-year-old patient with combined femoroacetabular impingement of the right hip. **(a)** Segment prescription, **(b)** coronal image, and **(c)** illustration showing a torn ossified superior labrum (*arrowhead on each*) and a cam lesion at the neck-shaft junction (*arrow on each*). **(d)** Oblique axial view and **(e)** illustration (*arrow on each*) accentuate the osseous defect (cam lesion). **(f)** Sagittal image and **(g)** illustration shows full-thickness cartilage loss over the anterior acetabular dome (*arrow on each*) and an ossified labral tear (*arrowhead on each*). (Figure parts a, b, c, d: Reproduced with permission from, Shindle MK, Foo LF, Kelly BT, et al. Magnetic resonance imaging of cartilage in the athlete: current techniques and spectrum of disease. J Bone Joint Surg Am. 2006; 88 Suppl 4:27–46.).

This type of impingement can lead to degeneration, ossification, and tears of the anterosuperior labrum, as well as a characteristic posteroinferior contrecoup pattern of cartilage loss over the femoral head and corresponding acetabulum. Despite the two types of distinct anatomic variants of FAI, most cases involve a combination of femoral-side and acetabular-side lesions (see Chapter 10, The Hip) (▶ Fig. 5.15).[48,49,50]

5.7.2 Shoulder

A 13% incidence of articular cartilage lesions has been reported in the setting of rotator cuff abnormality, with a chondral wear pattern that is different than that seen in typical shoulder arthritis. When the rotator cuff is intact, glenohumeral articular cartilage degenerates at the posterior glenoid and superior/central humeral head (best visualized on axial MRI). With chronic rotator cuff insufficiency, the humeral head chondral wear occurs inferiorly, correlating with anterior and superior subluxation of the humeral head. In this setting, glenoid wear occurs more anterosuperior.[46]

5.7.3 Smaller Joints

Cartilage imaging in the elbow and smaller joints such as those in the hands and feet is also possible but superior surface coil design and meticulous attention to pulse sequence parameters are necessary to allow detection of partial-thickness defects in the thinner cartilage lining these joints (▶ Fig. 5.16).[6,7,8]

5.7.4 OA and Inflammatory Arthritis

With progression of OA, articular cartilage changes include thinning and degeneration, with fissuring, ulceration, and eventually full-thickness loss of the articular surface. Factors associated with OA may include the following:

- Subchondral sclerosis.
- Osteophyte formation.
- Subchondral cysts.
- Bone marrow changes.

In longstanding OA, a bone marrow edema pattern may develop secondary to subchondral osseous remodeling in the presence of substantial cartilage loss. This bone marrow edema pattern is a nonspecific MRI finding; it does not necessarily indicate a traumatic cartilage injury but it may indicate increased risk for additional cartilage degeneration.[6,7,51] This pattern should not be misinterpreted as tumor infiltration of bone or osteonecrosis, especially in the absence of a segmental subchondral fracture or demarcation of a necrosis-viable bone interface.

In contrast to OA, cartilage thinning associated with inflammatory arthritis is uniform and diffuse and does not typically involve focal chondral defects, except where the pannus erodes the cartilage and subchondral bone.[51] In a rheumatoid joint, conventional radiographs may remain normal for at least 6 to 12 months after the onset of symptoms.[52] MRI may show thickened and hyperintense synovium and debris, as well as periarticular marrow edema.[53] In the hands and wrists of patients with rheumatoid arthritis, osseous erosions can be seen much earlier on MRI than on conventional radiographs.[54] MRI has clinical applications for diagnosing inflammatory arthritis and for predicting prognosis, which has the potential to influence treatment of early disease.[55]

5.8 Infection

Septic arthritis can be associated with MRI findings of synovial enhancement, perisynovial edema, joint effusion, and synovial thickening.[56] MRI has been shown to have a 100% sensitivity for showing changes as early as 24 hours after presentation of septic arthritis; however, it lacks specificity to distinguish between inflammatory arthritis and viral or immunogenic synovitis.[57]

5.9 Cartilage Imaging after Repair

Articular cartilage injuries are common but there is little to no inherent capacity for spontaneous repair because of the avascular nature of hyaline cartilage. Several techniques have been described for repairing articular injuries but the clinical outcomes and results have varied widely. To evaluate these techniques, researchers relied on second-look surgery combined with biopsies.[58] However, with advances in imaging techniques, MRI has become a noninvasive alternative for evaluating the results of articular cartilage repair procedures.[6] After a cartilage repair procedure, the following variables can be assessed on MRI[59]:

- Degree of defect filling.
- Signal intensity of the regenerated cartilage compared with the surrounding native tissue.
- Absence or presence of displacement.
- Degree of peripheral integration to adjacent cartilage or underlying bone.
- Surface geometry and morphology of the repaired tissue.
- Presence of proud subchondral bone formation.
- Presence of any reactive synovitis.

Microfracture was a commonly used technique, in which perforations in the underlying subchondral bone were created using a drill or pick.[60,61] This procedure releases multipotent stem cells from the bone marrow that create a covering of reparative fibrocartilage (type I collagen). At short-term follow-up, this reparative tissue after microfracture appears hyperintense compared with native hyaline cartilage (type II collagen) because it is less organized and has a higher water content.[6,62] The signal intensity of reparative cartilage decreases as it matures (▶ Fig. 5.17). Osseous overgrowth of the underlying subchondral bone has been reported after microfracture, and it may result in a thinner layer of reparative tissue.[63] Microfracture has fallen out of favor recently because it has not been shown to improve outcomes over other cartilage reparative techniques,[64,65] and the indications for its use have not been clearly defined across various joints.

Another cartilage repair technique is the use of autologous or allograft osteochondral plugs.[66] Cartilage plugs are advantageous

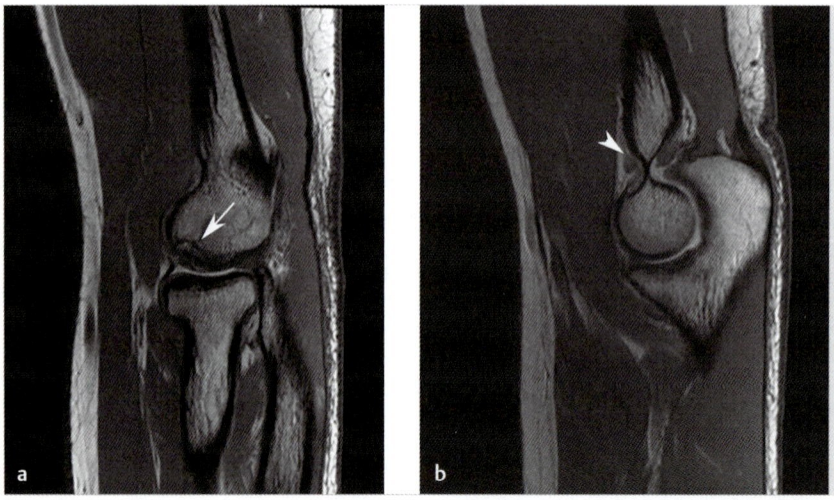

Fig. 5.16 (a) Sagittal non–fat-suppressed image of the left elbow of a 13-year-old gymnast showing an osteochondral lesion of the capitellum *(arrow)*. **(b)** This unstable osteochondral defect is collapsed and separated from the host bone with a visible region of devitalized subchondral bone. The *arrowhead* shows an anterior loose body, representing a cartilaginous fragment.

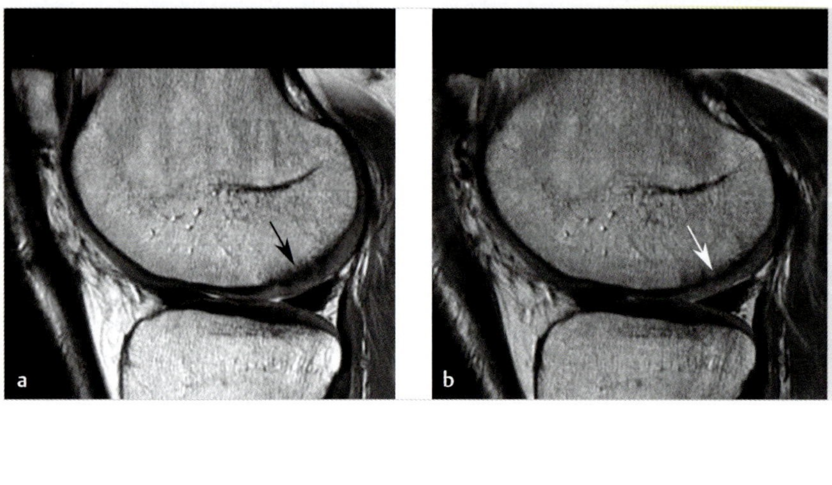

Fig. 5.17 Sagittal fast-spin-echo images of the knee in a 32-year-old patient after microfracture. **(a)** At 5 months after surgery, there is irregularity of the subchondral plate (*black arrow*) adjacent to the repair cartilage, which is hyperintense. **(b)** At 13 months after surgery, the mature reparative fibrocartilage is partially hypointense (*white arrow*) compared with the adjacent hyaline cartilage. Note the presence of subtle osseous overgrowth of the subchondral bone. (Reproduced with permission from, Shindle MK, Foo LF, Kelly BT, et al. Magnetic resonance imaging of cartilage in the athlete: current techniques and spectrum of disease. J Bone Joint Surg Am 2006;88:27–46.)

because they can be used for large defects and they contain hyaline cartilage rather than a reparative fibrocartilage. Autologous osteochondral plugs are harvested from a non-weight-bearing portion of the knee, usually the side of the intercondylar notch or anterior margin of the femoral condyle. Allograft plugs are harvested from a cadaver and are usually inserted using a press-fit technique in which the plug and the recipient site are prepared to matching sizes. Evaluation of these procedures on MRI should include assessment of the integration of the osseous portion of the plug and the accuracy of the restoration of the surface morphology and radius of curvature (▶ Fig. 5.18). Because of the press-fit technique, there is usually a hypointense signal at the osseous interface. A hyperintense signal at the native bone–graft interface may indicate failure of integration (▶ Fig. 5.19).[6] Although the osseous portion of the plug typically shows excellent incorporation, persistent gaps at the cartilaginous level have been reported between the graft and the native cartilage tissue.[67]

Autologous chondrocyte implantation is another cartilage restoration technique in which the patient's native chondrocytes are harvested arthroscopically, grown in tissue culture for 3 to 5 weeks, and then, via an open arthrotomy, injected into a periosteum cover harvested from the patient.[27,68] Similar to microfracture, the reparative tissue remains disorganized with increased water content and hyperintense signal on MRI. The overlying periosteum appears hypointense and allows differentiation from the reparative tissue.[51] One potential problem with autologous chondrocyte implantation is hypertrophy of the periosteum (▶ Fig. 5.20). Matrix-induced autologous chondrocyte implantation is similar to autologous chondrocyte implantation

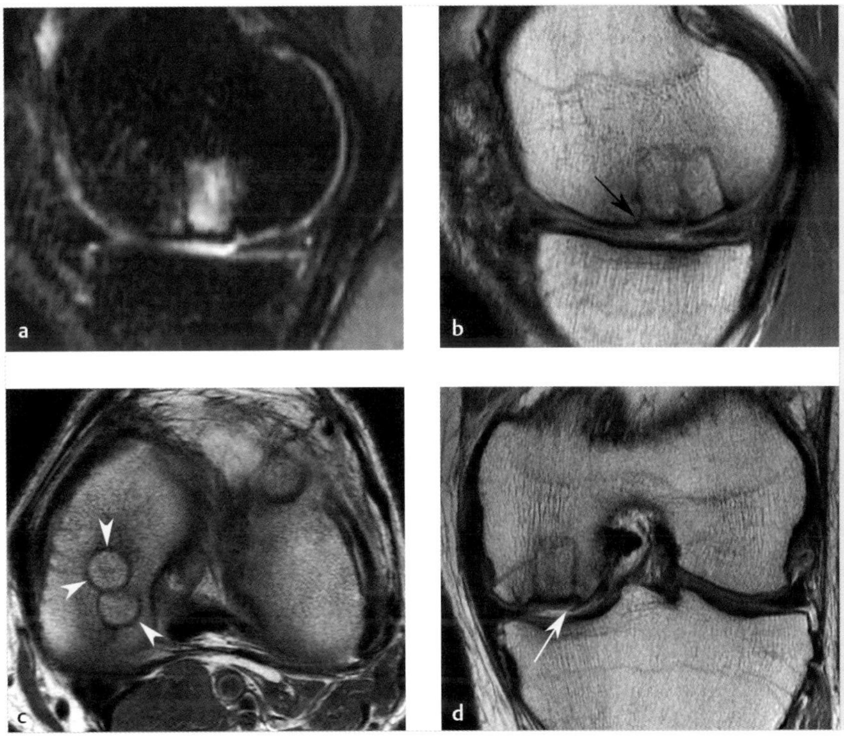

Fig. 5.18 Images of the knee in a 52-year-old patient after the transfer of two autologous osteochondral plugs. **(a)** Sagittal fat-suppressed and **(b)** non–fat-suppressed fast-spin-echo images showing osseous incorporation of the plugs. Although the cartilage surface remains flush over the anterior plug, there is slight depression of the subchondral bone (*black arrow* in **b**). **(c)** There is slight sclerosis in the side walls of the plugs in the axial plane (*white arrowheads*) reflecting the "press-fit" technique. **(d)** A fissure at the medial interface with the native cartilage (*white arrow*) is shown on the coronal image. The medial tibial plateau has a degenerative pattern of partial-thickness cartilage loss. (Reproduced with permission from, Shindle MK, Foo LF, Kelly BT, et al. Magnetic resonance imaging of cartilage in the athlete: current techniques and spectrum of disease. J Bone Joint Surg Am 2006;88:27–46.)

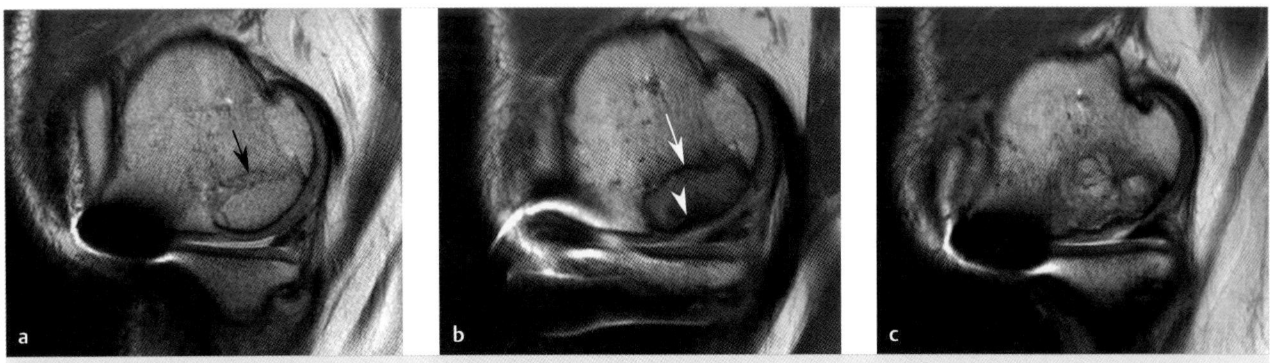

Fig. 5.19 Postoperative sagittal fast-spin-echo images of the knee of a 46-year-old patient with progressive collapse of an allograft osteochondral transfer. **(a)** Incomplete osseous incorporation of the graft (*black arrow*) is seen at early follow-up. **(b)** Nine months after surgery, there is sclerosis of the bone at the graft–host bone interface (*white arrow*). The low-signal-intensity subchondral bone (*white arrowhead*) indicates devitalized bone with partial collapse. **(c)** This scenario subsequently led to graft failure. (Reproduced with permission from, Shindle MK, Foo LF, Kelly BT, et al. Magnetic resonance imaging of cartilage in the athlete: current techniques and spectrum of disease. J Bone Joint Surg Am. 2006; 88 Suppl 4:27–46.)

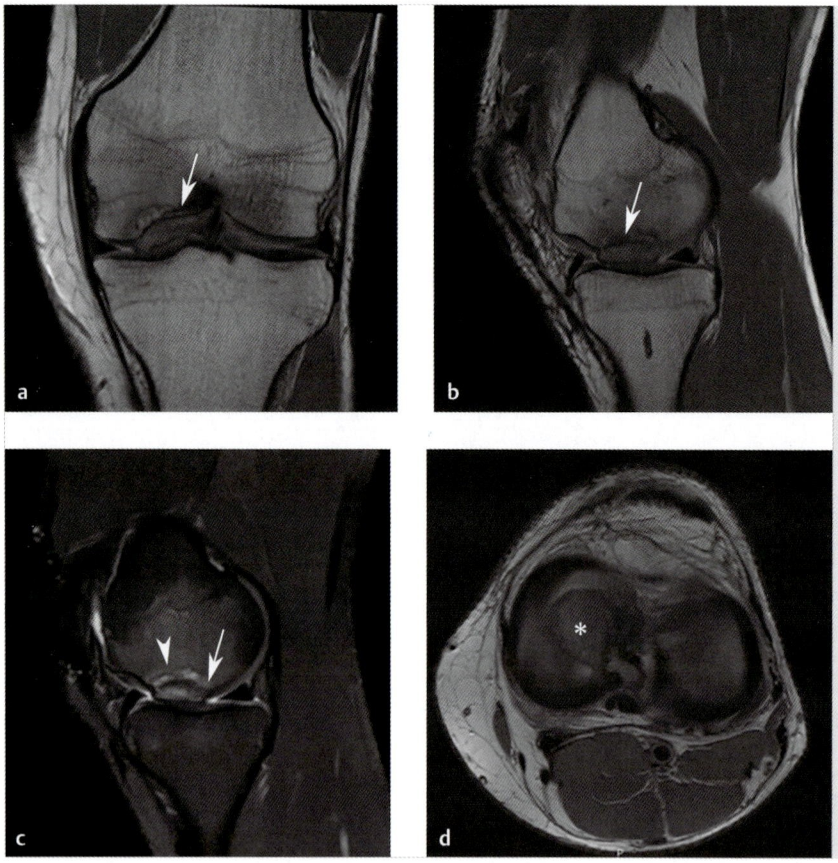

Fig. 5.20 These images show hypertrophy 4 years after autologous chondrocyte implantation. This patient had symptoms of locking in his right knee. In the **(a)** coronal and **(b)** sagittal fast-spin-echo images, there is graft hypertrophy at the site of the autologous chondrocyte implantation (*arrow*). On the **(c)** sagittal inversion recovery image, there is cystic resorption (*arrowhead*) at the interface between the repair site and host bone. On the **(d)** axial fast-spin-echo image, the proud repair extends to the level of the menisci (*asterisk*).

but the chondrocytes are cultured in a membrane that acts as a scaffold, and this membrane is then implanted directly into the joint over the cartilage defect.[69] Complete integration of cartilage may take up to 2 years, during which time a decline in the signal intensity of the reparative tissue occurs as it becomes increasingly organized and incorporated. A hyperintense fluid signal between the reparative tissue and the underlying bone may indicate delamination of the reparative tissue because of incomplete integration.[51,70] Yet another cartilage procedure that has been described is matrix-induced autologous chondroplasty, which involves performing a microfracture and then securing a resorbable collagen membrane over the defect.[69]

In addition to allowing visualization of cartilage after restorative procedures, MRI can offer useful information after arthroscopic surgery. For example, after hip arthroscopy, MRI can be used to evaluate malpositioned suture anchors (if they are placed too close to or violating the acetabular articular cartilage) or iatrogenic cartilage injury caused by instrument placement or manipulation.[71] In shoulder labral repair, erosion of the glenoid cartilage can occur from misplaced suture anchors used in labral repair, and chondrolysis has been described after thermal capsulorrhaphy.[71,72]

5.10 Common Clinical Questions

1. What are the best sequences and series to evaluate articular cartilage integrity when examining for cartilage injury or osteoarthritis?
2. How long after cartilage procedures (osteochondral autograft or autograft, autologous chondrocyte implantation, or microfracture) is it reasonable to obtain MRI to evaluate successful intervention?
3. What factors can affect the image quality of articular cartilage on MRI?

References

[1] West RV, Fu FH. Soft tissue physiology and repair. In: Vaccaro AR, ed. Orthopaedic knowledge update home study syllabus. Rosemont, IL: Journal of the American Academy of Orthopaedic Surgeons; 2005:15–28
[2] Mow V, Proctor C, Kelly M. Biomechanics of articular cartilage. In: Nordin M, Frankel VH, eds. Basic biomechanics of the musculoskeletal system. Philadelphia, PA: Lea & Febiger; 1989:60–101
[3] Askew MJ, Mow VC. The biomechanical function of the collagen fibril ultrastructure of articular cartilage. J Biomech Eng. 1978; 100(3):105–115
[4] Bullough PG, Jagannath A. The morphology of the calcification front in articular cartilage. Its significance in joint function. J Bone Joint Surg Br. 1983; 65(1):72–78
[5] Bullough P, Goodfellow J. The significance of the fine structure of articular cartilage. J Bone Joint Surg Br. 1968; 50(4):852–857
[6] Potter HG, Foo LF. Magnetic resonance imaging of articular cartilage: trauma, degeneration, and repair. Am J Sports Med. 2006; 34(4):661–677
[7] Potter HG, Foo LF. Articular cartilage. In: Stoller DW, ed. Magnetic resonance imaging in orthopaedics and sports medicine. Philadelphia, PA: Lippincott Williams & Wilkins; 2006:1099–1130
[8] Shindle MK, Foo LF, Kelly BT, et al. Magnetic resonance imaging of cartilage in the athlete: current techniques and spectrum of disease. J Bone Joint Surg Am. 2006; 88 Suppl 4:27–46

[9] Kassarjian A, Yoon LS, Belzile E, Connolly SA, Millis MB, Palmer WE. Triad of MR arthrographic findings in patients with cam-type femoroacetabular impingement. Radiology. 2005; 236(2):588–592

[10] Kramer J, Recht MP. MR arthrography of the lower extremity. Radiol Clin North Am. 2002; 40(5):1121–1132

[11] Schmid MR, Nötzli HP, Zanetti M, Wyss TF, Hodler J. Cartilage lesions in the hip: diagnostic effectiveness of MR arthrography. Radiology. 2003; 226(2): 382–386

[12] Vahlensieck M, Peterfy CG, Wischer T, et al. Indirect MR arthrography: optimization and clinical applications. Radiology. 1996; 200(1):249–254

[13] Beaulé PE, Kim YJ, Rakhra KS, Stelzeneder D, Brown TD. New frontiers in cartilage imaging of the hip. Instr Course Lect. 2012; 61:253–262

[14] Reddy R, Insko EK, Noyszewski EA, Dandora R, Kneeland JB, Leigh JS. Sodium MRI of human articular cartilage in vivo. Magn Reson Med. 1998; 39(5):697–701

[15] Bashir A, Gray ML, Boutin RD, Burstein D. Glycosaminoglycan in articular cartilage: in vivo assessment with delayed Gd(DTPA)(2-)-enhanced MR imaging. Radiology. 1997; 205(2):551–558

[16] Duvvuri U, Charagundla SR, Kudchodkar SB, et al. Human knee: in vivo T1(rho)-weighted MR imaging at 1.5 T—preliminary experience. Radiology. 2001; 220(3):822–826

[17] Wheaton AJ, Dodge GR, Elliott DM, Nicoll SB, Reddy R. Quantification of cartilage biomechanical and biochemical properties via T1rho magnetic resonance imaging. Magn Reson Med. 2005; 54(5):1087–1093

[18] Williams A, Gillis A, McKenzie C, et al. Glycosaminoglycan distribution in cartilage as determined by delayed gadolinium-enhanced MRI of cartilage (dGEMRIC): potential clinical applications. AJR Am J Roentgenol. 2004; 182 (1):167–172

[19] David-Vaudey E, Ghosh S, Ries M, Majumdar S. T2 relaxation time measurements in osteoarthritis. Magn Reson Imaging. 2004; 22(5):673–682

[20] Gallo MC, Wyatt C, Pedoia V, et al. T1ρ and T2 relaxation times are associated with progression of hip osteoarthritis. Osteoarthritis Cartilage. 2016; 24(8): 1399–1407

[21] Prasad AP, Nardo L, Schooler J, Joseph GB, Link TMT. $T_1\rho$ and T_2 relaxation times predict progression of knee osteoarthritis. Osteoarthritis Cartilage. 2013; 21(1):69–76

[22] Li X, Pedoia V, Kumar D, et al. Cartilage T1ρ and T2 relaxation times: longitudinal reproducibility and variations using different coils, MR systems and sites. Osteoarthritis Cartilage. 2015; 23(12):2214–2223

[23] Guermazi A, Alizai H, Crema MD, Trattnig S, Regatte RR, Roemer FW. Compositional MRI techniques for evaluation of cartilage degeneration in osteoarthritis. Osteoarthritis Cartilage. 2015; 23(10):1639–1653

[24] Rehnitz C, Kupfer J, Streich NA, et al. Comparison of biochemical cartilage imaging techniques at 3 T MRI. Osteoarthritis Cartilage. 2014; 22(10):1732–1742

[25] Abdulaal OM, Rainford L, MacMahon P, et al. 3 T MRI of the knee with optimised isotropic 3D sequences: accurate delineation of intra-articular pathology without prolonged acquisition times. Eur Radiol. 2017; 27(11): 4563–4570

[26] Ballyns JJ, Gleghorn JP, Niebrzydowski V, et al. Image-guided tissue engineering of anatomically shaped implants via MRI and micro-CT using injection molding. Tissue Eng Part A. 2008; 14(7):1195–1202

[27] Brittberg M, Winalski CS. Evaluation of cartilage injuries and repair. J Bone Joint Surg Am. 2003; 85-A Suppl 2:58–69

[28] Dougados M, Ayral X, Listrat V, et al. The SFA system for assessing articular cartilage lesions at arthroscopy of the knee. Arthroscopy. 1994; 10(1):69–77

[29] Noyes FR, Stabler CL. A system for grading articular cartilage lesions at arthroscopy. Am J Sports Med. 1989; 17(4):505–513

[30] Outerbridge RE. The etiology of chondromalacia patellae. 1961. Clin Orthop Relat Res. 2001(389):5–8

[31] Cameron ML, Briggs KK, Steadman JR. Reproducibility and reliability of the outerbridge classification for grading chondral lesions of the knee arthroscopically. Am J Sports Med. 2003; 31(1):83–86

[32] Smith GD, Taylor J, Almqvist KF, et al. Arthroscopic assessment of cartilage repair: a validation study of 2 scoring systems. Arthroscopy. 2005; 21(12): 1462–1467

[33] Curl WW, Krome J, Gordon ES, Rushing J, Smith BP, Poehling GG. Cartilage injuries: a review of 31,516 knee arthroscopies. Arthroscopy. 1997; 13(4): 456–460

[34] McCauley TR, Disler DG. MR imaging of articular cartilage. Radiology. 1998; 209(3):629–640

[35] McCauley TR, Disler DG. Magnetic resonance imaging of articular cartilage of the knee. J Am Acad Orthop Surg. 2001; 9(1):2–8

[36] Northmore-Ball MD, Dandy DJ. Long-term results of arthroscopic partial meniscectomy. Clin Orthop Relat Res. 1982(167):34–42

[37] Kendell SD, Helms CA, Rampton JW, Garrett WE, Higgins LD. MRI appearance of chondral delamination injuries of the knee. AJR Am J Roentgenol. 2005; 184(5):1486–1489

[38] Levy AS, Lohnes J, Sculley S, LeCroy M, Garrett W. Chondral delamination of the knee in soccer players. Am J Sports Med. 1996; 24(5):634–639

[39] De Smet AA, Ilahi OA, Graf BK. Reassessment of the MR criteria for stability of osteochondritis dissecans in the knee and ankle. Skeletal Radiol. 1996; 25(2): 159–163

[40] Chan YS, Lien LC, Hsu HL, et al. Evaluating hip labral tears using magnetic resonance arthrography: a prospective study comparing hip arthroscopy and magnetic resonance arthrography diagnosis. Arthroscopy. 2005; 21 (10):1250

[41] Leunig M, Podeszwa D, Beck M, Werlen S, Ganz R. Magnetic resonance arthrography of labral disorders in hips with dysplasia and impingement. Clin Orthop Relat Res. 2004(418):74–80

[42] Werlen S, Leunig M, Ganz R. Magnetic resonance arthrography of the hip in femoroacetabular impingement: technique and findings. Oper Tech Orthop. 2005; 15(3):191–203

[43] Mintz DN, Hooper T, Connell D, Buly R, Padgett DE, Potter HG. Magnetic resonance imaging of the hip: detection of labral and chondral abnormalities using noncontrast imaging. Arthroscopy. 2005; 21(4):385–393

[44] Moorman CT, III, Warren RF, Hershman EB, et al. Traumatic posterior hip subluxation in American football. J Bone Joint Surg Am. 2003; 85(7):1190–1196

[45] Cole BJ, Yanke A, Provencher MT. Nonarthroplasty alternatives for the treatment of glenohumeral arthritis. J Shoulder Elbow Surg. 2007; 16(5) Suppl:S231–S240

[46] Coris EE, Zwygart K, Fletcher M, Pescasio M. Imaging in sports medicine: an overview. Sports Med Arthrosc Rev. 2009; 17(1):2–12

[47] Ganz R, Parvizi J, Beck M, Leunig M, Nötzli H, Siebenrock KA. Femoroacetabular impingement: a cause for osteoarthritis of the hip. Clin Orthop Relat Res. 2003(417):112–120

[48] Beck M, Kalhor M, Leunig M, Ganz R. Hip morphology influences the pattern of damage to the acetabular cartilage: femoroacetabular impingement as a cause of early osteoarthritis of the hip. J Bone Joint Surg Br. 2005; 87(7): 1012–1018

[49] Bredella MA, Stoller DW. MR imaging of femoroacetabular impingement. Magn Reson Imaging Clin N Am. 2005; 13(4):653–664

[50] Meislin R, Abeles A. Role of hip MR imaging in the management of sports-related injuries. Magn Reson Imaging Clin N Am. 2005; 13(4):635–640

[51] Verstraete KL, Almqvist F, Verdonk P, et al. Magnetic resonance imaging of cartilage and cartilage repair. Clin Radiol. 2004; 59(8):674–689

[52] van der Heijde DM, van Leeuwen MA, van Riel PL, et al. Biannual radiographic assessments of hands and feet in a three-year prospective followup of patients with early rheumatoid arthritis. Arthritis Rheum. 1992; 35(1):26–34

[53] Burge AJ, Nwawka OK, Berkowitz JL, Potter HG. Imaging of inflammatory arthritis in adults: Status and perspectives on the use of radiographs, ultrasound, and MRI. Rheum Dis Clin North Am. 2016; 42(4):561–585

[54] Foley-Nolan D, Stack JP, Ryan M, et al. Magnetic resonance imaging in the assessment of rheumatoid arthritis; a comparison with plain film radiographs. Br J Rheumatol. 1991; 30(2):101–106

[55] McQueen FM. Magnetic resonance imaging in early inflammatory arthritis: what is its role? Rheumatology (Oxford). 2000; 39(7):700–706

[56] Karchevsky M, Schweitzer ME, Morrison WB, Parellada JA. MRI findings of septic arthritis and associated osteomyelitis in adults. AJR Am J Roentgenol. 2004; 182(1):119–122

[57] Simpfendorfer CS. Radiologic approach to musculoskeletal infections. Infect Dis Clin North Am. 2017; 31(2):299–324

[58] Mainil-Varlet P, Aigner T, Brittberg M, et al. International Cartilage Repair Society. Histological assessment of cartilage repair: a report by the Histology Endpoint Committee of the International Cartilage Repair Society (ICRS). J Bone Joint Surg Am. 2003; 85-A Suppl 2:45–57

[59] Brown WE, Potter HG, Marx RG, Wickiewicz TL, Warren RF. Magnetic resonance imaging appearance of cartilage repair in the knee. Clin Orthop Relat Res. 2004(422):214–223

[60] Steadman JR, Rodkey WG, Briggs KK, Rodrigo JJ. [The microfracture technic in the management of complete cartilage defects in the knee joint]. Orthopade. 1999; 28(1):26–32

[61] Steadman JR, Rodkey WG, Rodrigo JJ. Microfracture: surgical technique and rehabilitation to treat chondral defects. Clin Orthop Relat Res. 2001(391) Suppl:S362–S369
[62] Knutsen G, Engebretsen L, Ludvigsen TC, et al. Autologous chondrocyte implantation compared with microfracture in the knee. A randomized trial. J Bone Joint Surg Am. 2004; 86(3):455–464
[63] Mithoefer K, Williams RJ, III, Warren RF, et al. The microfracture technique for the treatment of articular cartilage lesions in the knee. A prospective cohort study. J Bone Joint Surg Am. 2005; 87(9):1911–1920
[64] Frehner F, Benthien JP. Microfracture: State of the Art in Cartilage Surgery? Cartilage. 2018; 9(4):339–345
[65] Kraeutler MJ, Belk JW, Purcell JM, McCarty EC. Microfracture versus autologous chondrocyte implantation for articular cartilage lesions in the knee: a systematic review of 5-year outcomes. Am J Sports Med. 2017; •••: 363546517701912
[66] Hangody L, Feczkó P, Bartha L, Bodó G, Kish G. Mosaicplasty for the treatment of articular defects of the knee and ankle. Clin Orthop Relat Res. 2001(391) Suppl:S328–S336
[67] Glenn RE, Jr, McCarty EC, Potter HG, Juliao SF, Gordon JD, Spindler KP. Comparison of fresh osteochondral autografts and allografts: a canine model. Am J Sports Med. 2006; 34(7):1084–1093
[68] Brittberg M, Lindahl A, Nilsson A, Ohlsson C, Isaksson O, Peterson L. Treatment of deep cartilage defects in the knee with autologous chondrocyte transplantation. N Engl J Med. 1994; 331(14):889–895
[69] Jannelli E, Fontana A. Arthroscopic treatment of chondral defects in the hip: AMIC, MACI, microfragmented adipose tissue transplantation (MATT) and other options. SICOT J. 2017; 3:43
[70] Alparslan L, Winalski CS, Boutin RD, Minas T. Postoperative magnetic resonance imaging of articular cartilage repair. Semin Musculoskelet Radiol. 2001; 5(4):345–363
[71] Black BR, Chong R, Potter HG. Cartilage imaging in sports medicine. Sports Med Arthrosc Rev. 2009; 17(1):68–80
[72] Good CR, Shindle MK, Kelly BT, Wanich T, Warren RF. Glenohumeral chondrolysis after shoulder arthroscopy with thermal capsulorrhaphy. Arthroscopy. 2007; 23(7):797.e1–797.e5
[73] Neri JP, Koff MF, Koch KM, Tan ET. Validating the accuracy of multispectral metal artifact suppressed diffusion-weighted imaging. Med Phys. 2022 Oct;49(10):6538–6546

Answers to Common Clinical Questions

1. Answer: Begin with fat-suppression sequences, which highlight bone marrow edema and can alert the MRI reader to areas of potential cartilage damage. Then use a consistent approach to evaluate the entire joint surface on moderate echo time non–fat-suppressed images, typically with sagittal images followed by coronal and then axial series.
2. Answer: Imaging after cartilage restorative procedures is most useful when activity level will be advanced or modified. MRI at 6 months after microfracture and at 12 months after other restorative procedures will offer clinically applicable information on cartilage integration and healing.
3. Answer: The presence of nearby metal alters the magnetic field and lowers the precision of cartilage imaging. Metal-suppressing protocols can be used to improve visualization around a metal artifact, and use of a field strength of 1.5 T instead of 3 T is recommended, though a tradeoff occurs because of a lower signal-to-noise ratio. Multispectral imaging techniques include multiacquisition variable-resonance imaging combination and slice encoding for metal artifact correction and have been useful in reducing distortion near metal artifact.[73]

6 MRI Safety Considerations for the Referring Clinician

Monica D. Watkins and Bruce A. Wasserman

Abstract
Although magnetic resonance imaging (MRI) facilities are mandated to present patients with a prescreening checklist, the referring physician can prevent the need to reschedule or cancel the procedure by beginning the screening process and alleviating some of the concerns the patient may have regarding the examination. It is imperative that physicians be familiar with the few absolute contraindications to MRI and that they identify patients for whom additional information is needed. Furthermore, brief questions to screen for claustrophobia, pregnancy, and known gadolinium contrast allergy, combined with identification of potential safety hazards via knowledge of the patient's history, can facilitate obtaining the most informative and safest study possible.

Keywords: claustrophobia, gadolinium-based contrast, magnetic fields, magnetic resonance imaging, nephrogenic systemic fibrosis, pregnancy, safety

6.1 Introduction

The year 2017 marked the 40th anniversary of the first magnetic resonance imaging (MRI) scan for medical use.[1] Since those first examinations, the use of diagnostic imaging, particularly MRI and computed tomography (CT), has had exponential growth. The total number of MRI scans increased twofold from 2000 to 2013, estimated at 107 per 1,000 people in the United States in 2015.[2] Increased use of medical imaging has brought renewed scrutiny of the ordering practices of clinicians, focusing on factors ranging from value of the examination for the suspected diagnosis to cost. Recent public health initiatives urge clinicians to "choose wisely" by selecting the examination most appropriate for the clinical question. Clinicians are also encouraged to "image wisely" for adults and "image gently" for children, making an effort to be judicious in the use of radiation.[3,4,5] These initiatives will continue to modify the diagnostic decisions of ordering physicians. For example, an increasing focus on reducing radiation doses may shift more patients from CT scanning toward MRI. However, this will be balanced with increasing concern for repeated use of MRI contrast agents. Patient safety remains paramount, and although the MRI center is typically responsible for safety screening, the referring physician can minimize the chance of adverse effects by being aware of important contraindications to MRI and of safety concerns that might put a patient at risk. This chapter reviews these issues and provides guidelines for maximizing safety.

6.2 Physiologic Effects of the Magnetic Field

In the MRI scanner, a patient is exposed to magnetic fields from two sources. The first is the baseline static magnetic field that aligns hydrogen atoms in the body. The second source comes from far weaker time-varying magnetic fields created by a radiofrequency (RF) field generator with receiver coils that rapidly switch on and off to identify the location of the hydrogen nuclei for generating images. The strength of these magnetic fields is measured in gauss or tesla (T) units; 1 T equals 10,000 gauss. For comparison, the strength of the earth's magnetic field is 0.6 gauss.[6] The static magnetic field of a clinical MRI scanner typically ranges from 0.5 to 3.0 T, although there are magnets up to 11.7 T for use in human research. The FDA has guidelines, last updated in 2014,[7] for the exposure of patients to static and time-varying magnetic fields.

6.2.1 Static Magnetic Fields

Currently, the FDA approves clinical imaging using a static magnetic field strength of up to 4.0 T for patients < 1-month-old and up to 8.0 T for older patients.[7] Many studies have evaluated the potential biologic effects of a static magnetic field, and there has been no clear evidence of deleterious effects.[8] Although there have been concerns about an elevation of skin and core body temperatures induced by the magnetic field, investigators have concluded that harmful heating does not occur in humans.[9,10] Reversible electrocardiographic changes (e.g., an increase in the amplitude of the T-wave or a nonspecific wave form) secondary to the conductive nature of blood have been noted with field strength up to 8 T.[11] However, this "magnetohydrodynamic effect" has not been associated with a clinically adverse effect. Transient increase in systolic blood pressure by 3.6 mm Hg has been noted at 8 T in some patients.[12]

At strengths of 4 T, patients may experience transient reversible biologic effects such as nausea (which may be caused by stimulation of the vestibulolabryrinthine complex) or a flashing light sensation (magnetophosphenes, thought to be caused by direct excitation of the optic nerves or retina, by changing magnetic fields, or by rapid eye movements).[13]

6.2.2 Time-Varying Magnetic Fields

Time-varying magnetic fields or gradient magnetic fields can induce current in the body, which can have two biologic effects: heating and neuromuscular stimulation. With substantial exposure, tingling or tapping sensations and minor temperature changes (i.e., < 0.6 °C) have been described.[14] The FDA has suggested guidelines to limit the risk of these effects and ensure heat dissipation by restricting the strength of time-varying magnetic fields.[7] The intensity of the RF energy absorbed by tissue is termed the *specific absorption rate* and is measured in watts per kilogram. The FDA reports that specific absorption rates of ≤ 3.2 W/kg for the head and ≤ 4 W/kg (averaged) for the rest of the body pose no substantial risk.[7] Usually, higher specific absorption rate exposures are a concern with faster pulse sequences.

6.3 Metallic Substances

6.3.1 Field Distortion

Image quality depends on the ability to maintain homogeneity of the magnetic field surrounding the patient. Metallic artifacts can result in misregistered spatial information or signal loss, leading to image distortion. Three types of magnetic materials may cause artifacts because of their inherent ability to disturb the uniformity of magnetic fields used for imaging: ferromagnetic, paramagnetic, and diamagnetic materials. Of these, ferromagnetic materials (e.g., iron, nickel, and martensitic stainless steel) concentrate and retain magnetism the most, resulting in severe distortion of the images. Paramagnetic or weakly ferromagnetic materials (e.g., platinum) have a minimal effect on magnetic field homogeneity and result in less image distortion. Diamagnetic materials (e.g., zinc, gold, and copper) do not affect or affect only minimally the static or local magnetic field homogeneity.

6.3.2 Metallic Objects in Magnetic Fields

The clinical value of an MRI examination in a patient with a metallic implant typically depends on the proximity of the implant to the site of interest. For example, one can anticipate a limited evaluation of neural foramina adjacent to an instrumented anterior cervical fusion or an inability to detect an epidural abscess adjacent to pedicle screw instrumentation. However, multiple techniques can be applied to limit artifact during scanning. Myelography remains a viable alternative for the postoperative spine. CT also is a valuable alternative in patients after surgery, particularly in conjunction with myelography.

In addition to distorting images, some metallic foreign bodies or surgical implants move or generate heat in the presence of a magnetic field, possibly leading to injury or death.[15,16] There is a baseline risk from the metallic device entering the static field with secondary risks caused by currents created from time-varying gradient fields. Research using metallic rods to model heating during the use of time-varying gradient fields shows that the orientation relative to the magnetic field is also important in predicting heating. For example, an implant perpendicular to the magnetic field can double heating as opposed to parallel positioning.[17]

For these reasons, each patient must be screened for metallic objects in the body, usually with a verbal interview and a written checklist. Of particular concern are metallic foreign bodies in the orbit that may dislodge and rupture the ocular globe or damage the optic nerve. To the authors' knowledge, there is only one reported case of a patient who experienced a vitreous hemorrhage, caused by a dislodged metal fragment (measuring 2.0 × 3.5 mm), leading to blindness.[18]

Although it is standard for MRI facilities to prescreen for metallic orbital foreign bodies, methods of accomplishing this screening vary. Conventional radiographs of the orbits are said to detect metallic fragments as small as 0.1 × 0.1 × 0.1 mm. However, there is debate over which patients should be referred for conventional radiography. Many MRI centers obtain orbital radiographs of patients with an occupational history of welding, but some experts advocate obtaining radiographs only if the patient is aware of a previous orbital exposure to metal without removal of the fragment by an ophthalmologist.[19] At the authors' institutions, patients with a history of working with metal undergo screening with orbital radiographs. Alternatively, review of a previous CT scan, including the entirety of the orbits, is often considered sufficient.

In addition to assessing for orbital foreign bodies and surgical implants, the clinician should question the patient regarding history of metallic foreign bodies such as bullet fragments, pellets, and shrapnel that could move and cause local damage. Although most tested ammunition is made of nonferrous material, it may have traces of ferromagnetic components; most shrapnel is ferromagnetic.[20] It is important to learn whether these foreign bodies are near other vital structures such as the lungs or spinal cord. For example, bullet fragments in the spinal canal in a patient without complete cord injury contraindicate MRI because they may be ferromagnetic.

6.3.3 Implant Safety Profiles

The FDA requires testing of all medical implants to evaluate their safety profiles for MRI scanning. Certain implants are contraindicated because of the possibility of dislodgement, induction of electrical current, and heating. Other implants can be imaged but only under certain conditions to reduce the risk of focal heating with gradient switching sequences.[21]

The FDA classifies implants as MRI unsafe, conditionally safe, or safe. The list of these devices is extensive and constantly changing, especially as more objects are tested at 3 T and higher, precluding a complete review of these devices in this chapter. A regularly updated list of reviewed implants and devices is available online at www.MRIsafety.com.

Unsafe

It is important to be aware of the devices that most commonly contraindicate MRI scanning, including the following:

- Implantable medication infusion pumps.
- Ferromagnetic aneurysm clips (e.g., stainless steel).
- Pacemakers/implantable defibrillators.
- Neurostimulation systems.
- Brain stimulators.
- Cochlear implants.
- Spine/bone fusion stimulators.
- Swan-Ganz thermodilution catheters.
- Poppen-Blaylock carotid artery clamps.
- Tissue expanders.

Certain models of some of the above devices such as implantable cardiac defibrillators, cardiac pacemakers, neurostimulation systems, deep brain stimulators, spinal/bone fusion stimulators, and cochlear implants have been developed specifically for MRI scanning or may be scanned under strict criteria on a case-by-case basis, taking into consideration the manufacturers' restrictions and the relative risk versus benefit of the study.[22,23,24,25,26,27,28] A collaborative effort between the referring specialist and radiologist might be needed, along with informed consent of the patient.

Of note, the Starr-Edwards Model Pre-6000 heart valve prosthesis (Baxter Healthcare, Santa Ana, CA) is now designated as conditionally MRI safe, although previously it was thought to be an absolute contraindication to an MRI examination.[29]

In the past, residual epicardial pacing wires were also considered a contraindication to MRI. However, the current consensus is that patients with such wires may undergo MRI if the wires are cut short (flush with skin) and there are no loops of wire outside the patient. Again, consultation with the patient's cardiologist may be necessary.[30] Retained intracardiac pacing leads remain a contraindication.[31]

Programmable cerebral spinal shunt valves may need to be reset after MRI scanning. In most cases, external and implantable insulin pumps should be removed before entering the scanner.

Conditionally Safe

Devices that are conditionally safe for MRI are implants that may be scanned if certain guidelines are satisfied. These devices include weakly magnetic intravascular filters, stents, and coils. MRI of patients with such devices may require a waiting period of 6 to 8 weeks after implantation to ensure that movement of the device caused by the magnetic field does not disturb its implantation onto the vessel wall.[32,33] The evolving list of all such devices is beyond the scope of this chapter, but one should acquire additional information (e.g., brand name of the device and date of implantation) for patients who have undergone recent placement of such devices. Most MRI centers require documentation of this information before scanning is allowed.

Safe Devices

Devices that are safe for MRI are those known to produce no clinical hazard in the MRI environment. These devices have no electronically or magnetically activated component, are made from nonferromagnetic material (such as titanium or nitinol), and may undergo MRI scanning at $\leq 1.5\,T$ immediately after implantation.[34,35] Many of these devices have been tested in the 3-T environment. It is important to obtain the brand name of the device from patients (who may have the package insert) or from their records. Furthermore, it is helpful for the surgeon to provide the patient with a written record of the device name so the patient can present this information at the time of scanning to avoid delays and unnecessary cancelations if this information is otherwise inaccessible to the MRI technologists. Safe devices also include orthopaedic implants placed firmly in the bone because, although they may be weakly magnetic, they do not dislodge or generate substantial heat.

6.3.4 Superficial Metal

There are safety concerns not only with internal metallic devices but also with skin surface metal, such as medicine patches containing a metal foil, surgical staples, tattoos, or permanent cosmetics that could cause skin burns. It is standard practice to remove transdermal medicine patches containing metallic foil at the time of an MRI. Tope and Shellock[36] reviewed the results of a questionnaire given to 1,032 patients with cosmetic tattoos. Only two patients experienced any sensory consequences (i.e., "slight tingling" or a "burning" sensation). These sensations are thought to be caused by heating from iron oxide or other metal-based pigment. The FDA Center for Food Safety and Applied Nutrition, Office of Cosmetics and Colors fact sheet states, "The risks of avoiding an MRI when your doctor has recommended one are likely to be much greater than the risk of complications from the interaction between the MRI and tattoo or permanent makeup."[37] Most practices agree that an ice pack or cold compress can be applied during scanning to the site of the tattoo, permanent cosmetics, or surgical staples to reduce the chance of thermal injury.

6.3.5 External Metallic Objects

In addition to precautions about internal foreign bodies, MRI centers screen for external metallic devices that may become projectiles in the MRI suite. Injuries and death have occurred when large metallic objects, such as a ferrous oxygen tank, have been brought into the MRI suite.[38,39,40] Even small objects that may not seem dangerous to many patients, such as jewelry or hairpins, can become projectiles and cause injury. It is standard procedure to ask patients to remove such objects and to empty their pockets or change out of street clothes.

6.4 Pregnancy

Since long there have been theoretical concerns that the electromagnetic fields of MRI could disrupt cell division at any stage of pregnancy. Because cell division is most rapid during the first trimester, scanning at this time would present a greater potential risk. However, the current consensus of the American College of Radiology is that "no special consideration is recommended for the first, versus any other, trimester in pregnancy."[24] MRI during pregnancy continues to be obtained on a case-by-case basis, weighing the risk and benefit for each examination. The American College of Radiology advises radiologists to confer with referring physicians and to document that, "1. The information requested from the MR study cannot be acquired by means of nonionizing means (e.g., ultrasonography); 2. The data is needed to potentially affect the care of the patient or fetus during the pregnancy; 3. The referring physician believes that it is not prudent to wait until the patient is no longer pregnant to obtain this data."[24] In almost all institutions, written, informed consent is obtained.

6.5 Gadolinium-Based Contrast

Gadolinium-based intravenous contrast agents are used to increase the sensitivity of MRI for multiple diagnoses such as suspected infection in the postoperative patient, musculoskeletal tumors, and vascular abnormalities. Gadolinium paramagnetic properties are the result of its seven unpaired electrons, which shorten the relaxation rates of nearby water protons and accentuate differences in adjacent tissue. Currently, nine agents are approved for use in the United States.

Gadolinium itself is toxic; however, chelation with other substances renders it nontoxic for intravenous use. These chelates are characterized by whether they have a linear structure or a macrocyclic structure. Macrocyclic agents include gadobutrol (Gadavist, Bayer HealthCare Pharmaceuticals, Leverkusen, Germany), gadoteridol (ProHance, Bracco

Diagnostics, Singen, Germany), and gadoterate meglumine (Dotarem, Guerbet, Bloomington, IN). Linear agents can be classified as ionic or nonionic and include gadopentetate dimeglumine (Magnevist, Bayer HealthCare Pharmaceuticals), gadobenate dimeglumine (MultiHance, Bracco Diagnostics), gadodiamide (Omniscan, GE Healthcare, Oslo, Norway), and gadoversetamide (OptiMARK, Liebel-Flarsheim Company, Raleigh, NC). Over time, in the body, the gadolinium ion can dissociate from its chelate. Because of their structure that encases the gadolinium ion centrally, the macrocyclic chelates are more stable, releasing less free gadolinium than the linear agents. An in vitro study using human serum showed that macrocyclic agents release < 0.1% of gadolinium ion after 15 days, as opposed to linear chelates, which release between 1% for ionic and 20% for nonionic chelates.[41]

In vivo, the amount of free ion that remains in the body after injection is almost undetectable, with rapid clearance by the kidneys, except those that are partly excreted through the hepatobiliary system such as gadoxetate, which is approved for evaluation of the liver. Most agents have an elimination half-life of approximately 90 minutes, with most of the dose eliminated within a few days in healthy patients.[42,43] In patients with severe renal impairment, the elimination half-life can be 18 to 34 hours.[44,45]

6.5.1 Nephrogenic Systemic Fibrosis

The delayed clearance time in patients with renal impairment, which increases the potential for free gadolinium to disassociate from its chelate, is considered one of the main factors contributing to nephrogenic systemic fibrosis. Nephrogenic systemic fibrosis is a progressive and sometimes fatal disease seen in patients with reduced renal function resulting in fibrosis of the skin and connective tissues throughout the body, including muscles of the extremities or abdomen, the diaphragm, and pulmonary vessels. Gadolinium has been detected in the soft tissues of several patients with nephrogenic systemic fibrosis who were exposed to it as a radiographic contrast agent, supporting its association with this disease.[46] The onset of disease is typically weeks to months after the exposure to gadolinium, although a delayed onset of multiple years has been reported.[47] Currently, there are 380 confirmed cases of nephrogenic systemic fibrosis listed in an international pathology registry.[48] The exact pathogenesis of nephrogenic systemic fibrosis has not been determined; however, the fibrotic changes are a result of circulating fibrocyte cells that are incited to leave the circulation and deposit within soft tissues.[49] To date, there is no known cure, with multiple treatments used to slow progression of the fibrosis, including steroids, immunoglobulin therapy, and renal transplant.[48]

Patients at greatest risk for developing nephrogenic systemic fibrosis are those with acute kidney injury or chronic severe dysfunction with an eGFR < 30 mL/min/1.73 m^2, with the risk among these patients estimated to be between 1 and 7%.[48,50,51,52,53] Since the early health advisories regarding a link between nephrogenic systemic fibrosis and gadolinium contrast, the disease has been associated with the following FDA-approved gadolinium agents: gadobutrol, gadopentetate dimeglumine, gadobenate dimeglumine, gadodiamide, gadoversetamide, gadoterate meglumine, and gadoteridol.[53] However, the greatest number of cases have been associated with gadopentetate dimeglumine, gadodiamide, and gadoversetamide with the remaining agents associated with only a few cases.[54] In 2010, the FDA advised that the use of gadopentetate dimeglumine, gadodiamide, and gadoversetamide is contraindicated for patients with acute kidney injury or chronic, severe kidney disease (eGFR < 30 mL/min/1.73m^2).[55] The American College of Radiology also warns against using gadolinium contrast agents in patients with an eGFR of < 45 mL/min/1.73 m^2 and in patients with acute kidney injury regardless of calculated eGFR because of potential rapid fluctuations in kidney function.[53] In most institutions, the benefits of gadolinium administration are weighed against the risk for patients with eGFRs between 30 and 60 mL/min/1.73 m^2. At the authors' institutions, a creatinine/eGFR measurement is obtained for patients at risk for renal dysfunction, including those ≥ 60 years of age, those with a history of diabetes, those with renal disease or transplantation, and those with hepatorenal syndrome. The adoption of guidelines to identify patients with renal impairment and limit the use of gadolinium in those patients has led to decreased incidence of new cases of nephrogenic systemic fibrosis.[56,57,58]

6.5.2 Accumulation of Free Gadolinium Ion

Although the amount of free gadolinium that remains in the body after a single dose is small in a patient with competent renal function, there is growing concern about the possibility of toxicity to the tissues, particularly when accumulated after multiple doses. Recent research has focused on deposition of gadolinium in the brain parenchyma, particularly the basal ganglia and the dentate nuclei of the cerebellum. Retrospective studies have shown progressive increase in T1 signal intensity with cumulative doses of gadolinium contrast.[59,60] Studies have suggested that linear agents have a greater association with brain signal changes versus macrocyclic agents, which have shown no or little increased signal changes.[60,61,62,63]

Currently, there are no reported adverse effects of gadolinium deposition in the brain parenchyma, but research to establish safety remains in its early stages. There are evolving recommendations from government agencies regarding the use of gadolinium. Currently under appeal is the decision by the Pharmacovigilance Risk Assessment Committee (PRAC) of the European Medicine Agency (EMA) to recommend suspension of marketing of four linear gadolinium agents because of high retention of gadolinium in the brain.[64] In May 2017, the FDA issued an updated safety announcement to outline its commitment to further investigation, as well as to urge clinicians to be judicious in the use of contrast, making sure that contrast is required for diagnosis and to consider carefully the need for repeat gadolinium contrast imaging.[65]

6.5.3 Contrast Allergies

It is important to obtain a patient's allergy history, especially regarding whether the patient has had a reaction to gadolinium contrast previously and, if so, the nature of that reaction. A history of a mild reaction (such as hives) to gadolinium typically requires premedication with prednisone and diphenhydramine.

A history of severe reactions such as respiratory or circulatory compromise is a contraindication to the use of MRI contrast. An adverse reaction to MRI contrast is expected to occur in < 1% of patients.[66] Reactions range from headache to weakness and, very rarely, anaphylaxis.[54]

Clinicians and radiologists are often faced with the decision as to whether to administer gadolinium contrast to a patient with a history of an allergy to ionic contrast agents such as those used for CT. Studies have shown that patients with a history of allergy to an ionic contrast agent are at higher risk for a reaction to gadolinium, as are those with asthma and multiple medication allergies.[54,67] Often, MRI centers require consent from such patients before giving contrast, and some centers may require that the patient be premedicated. In addition to premedication, a gadolinium contrast agent that differs from the one that elicited the previous reaction can be used if a contrast-enhanced MRI scan is deemed clinically important.

6.5.4 Pregnancy and Contrast

In pregnant patients, contrast agents cross the placenta, enter the fetal collecting system, and are excreted into the amniotic fluid. To the authors' knowledge, no studies show the clearance rate of MRI contrast agents in the fetus, but it is possible that a chelated gadolinium agent could stay in the amniotic fluid long enough to allow toxic free ions to accumulate. Gadolinium-based intravenous MR contrast is labeled by the FDA as a category C medication; that is, there is a lack of controlled studies with which to evaluate the effects. Contrast is typically not administered to pregnant patients unless its potential benefit outweighs its risks and unless written, informed consent has been obtained.[53,68] The theoretic risk of free ion accumulation is smaller if the agent is administered in the third trimester, leaving less time for dissociation and accumulation of free ions before delivery.

When a breastfeeding mother receives contrast, it is expected that most of the contrast will have cleared by 24 hours, leaving minimal residual contrast (< 1%) to be excreted into the breast milk.[54,68] However, a breastfeeding mother should be given information about abstaining from breastfeeding for 24 hours and pumping and discarding breast milk during this period.

6.5.5 Other Special Populations and Contrast

Other patient populations have a theoretic risk of toxicity from gadolinium, although no direct clinical evidence has been established. For example, patients with elevated levels of copper (such as those with Wilson disease) or zinc may have increased free ion accumulation after contrast administration because these metals may compete with gadolinium for the chelate. Previous studies have shown that fully deoxygenated sickle erythrocytes align perpendicular to the magnetic field.[69,70] It has been speculated that this alignment could be exacerbated by the administration of gadolinium, possibly leading to the slowing of flow and vasoocclusive crisis in patients with sickle cell disease. However, to the authors' knowledge, there is no documented clinical evidence to suggest that these agents can precipitate a sickle cell crisis.[41,53]

6.6 Claustrophobia

The key to obtaining an informative MRI study is a cooperative patient who is able to remain still for the duration of the examination. Scanning an uncooperative patient often leads to poor image quality with motion artifact, and it increases the anxiety level of the patient for future examinations. It is important to identify claustrophobic patients who may be unable to tolerate the examination and to determine whether sedation is needed. For some patients, their anxieties may be alleviated by being told they can communicate with the technicians via an intercom and can stop the examination if needed. A benzodiazepine such as diazepam may be used to sedate a nervous patient, with additional monitoring provided by the nursing staff. Occasionally, a patient may be unable to tolerate imaging, even with sedation. In such cases, an open (unenclosed) or wide-bore MRI examination might be best. However, image quality may be sacrificed because of the lower field strength of some open or semiopen MRI systems.

6.7 Common Clinical Questions

1. Which is correct regarding image quality in the MRI scanner?
   a) The static magnetic field aligns oxygen atoms within the body.
   b) A homogenous magnetic field surrounding the patient is needed for the optimal image quality.
   c) Platinum causes more distortion in the magnetic field than iron.
   d) The baseline static magnetic field of the MRI scanner is weaker than the time-varying magnetic fields applied during the examination.

2. All of the following implants are absolute contraindications to MRI scanning, except:
   a) Stainless steel brain aneurysm clips.
   b) Swan-Ganz thermodilution catheters.
   c) Bilateral rod and pedicle screw spine fixation.
   d) Poppen-Blaylock carotid artery clamps.

3. Regarding pregnant/postpartum patients:
   a) A pregnant patient may be scanned only in the third trimester.
   b) Contrast agents do not enter the amniotic fluid.
   c) A patient must stop breastfeeding for one week after receiving intravenous gadolinium.
   d) Written informed consent is typically obtained before a pregnant patient enters the scanner.

4. Which of the following is true regarding gadolinium-based contrast agents?
   a) Most gadolinium-based contrast agents are processed mainly through the liver.
   b) A patient who has had hives caused by gadolinium contrast should not receive contrast again.

c) Patients with a history of reaction to ionic contrast for CT scan and multiple medicine allergies are at higher risk for a reaction to gadolinium.
d) Twenty percent of patients will have an adverse reaction to gadolinium contrast.

5. Which is true regarding nephrogenic systemic fibrosis?
a) Nephrogenic systemic fibrosis can be cured with dialysis.
b) Gadolinium has been identified in the soft tissue of patients with nephrogenic systemic fibrosis.
c) Nephrogenic systemic fibrosis is typically seen in patients with eGFR between 50 and 70 mL/min/1.73 m^2.

References

[1] Damadian R, Goldsmith M, Minkoff L. NMR in cancer: XVI. FONAR image of the live human body. Physiol Chem Phys. 1977; 9(1):97–100, 108
[2] OECD. Health at a Glance 2015: OECD Indicators. http://www.oecd-ilibrary.org/docserver/download/8115071e.pdf?expires=1493740208&id=id&accname=guest&checksum=60FD299A8DA66C8D4A453960F720EA6A. Accessed on May 2, 2017
[3] American Board of Internal Medicine. Choosing Wisely: An initiative of the ABIM Foundation. http://www.choosingwisely.org/. Accessed on May 2, 2017
[4] Brink JA, Amis ES, Jr. Image Wisely: a campaign to increase awareness about adult radiation protection. Radiology. 2010; 257(3):601–602
[5] Don S, Macdougall R, Strauss K, et al. Image gently campaign back to basics initiative: ten steps to help manage radiation dose in pediatric digital radiography. AJR Am J Roentgenol. 2013; 200(5):W431–6
[6] Westbrook C, Roth CK, Talbot J. MRI safety. In: MRI in practice. Oxford: Blackwell Publishing; 2005:329–351
[7] U. S. Food and Drug Administration. Guidance for industry and FDA staff: criteria for significant risk investigations of magnetic resonance diagnostic devices. http://www.fda.gov/MedicalDevices/DeviceRegulationandGuidance/GuidanceDocuments/ucm072686.htm. Accessed on May 1, 2016
[8] Schenck JF. Health effects and safety of static magnetic fields. In: Shellock FG, ed. Magnetic resonance procedures: health effects and safety. Boca Raton, FL: CRC Press; 2001:1–29
[9] Shellock FG, Schaefer DJ, Crues JV. Exposure to a 1.5-T static magnetic field does not alter body and skin temperatures in man. Magn Reson Med. 1989; 11(3):371–375
[10] Shellock FG, Schaefer DJ, Gordon CJ. Effect of a 1.5 T static magnetic field on body temperature of man. Magn Reson Med. 1986; 3(4):644–647
[11] Chakeres DW, Kangarlu A, Boudoulas H, Young DC. Effect of static magnetic field exposure of up to 8 Tesla on sequential human vital sign measurements. J Magn Reson Imaging. 2003; 18(3):346–352
[12] Chakeres DW, de Vocht F. Static magnetic field effects on human subjects related to magnetic resonance imaging systems. Prog Biophys Mol Biol. 2005; 87(2–3):255–265
[13] Schenck JF, Dumoulin CL, Redington RW, Kressel HY, Elliott RT, McDougall IL. Human exposure to 4.0-Tesla magnetic fields in a whole-body scanner. Med Phys. 1992; 19(4):1089–1098
[14] Shellock FG, Crues JV. MR procedures: biologic effects, safety, and patient care. Radiology. 2004; 232(3):635–652
[15] Boutin RD, Briggs JE, Williamson MR. Injuries associated with MR imaging: survey of safety records and methods used to screen patients for metallic foreign bodies before imaging. AJR Am J Roentgenol. 1994; 162(1):189–194
[16] Klucznik RP, Carrier DA, Pyka R, Haid RW. Placement of a ferromagnetic intracerebral aneurysm clip in a magnetic field with a fatal outcome. Radiology. 1993; 187(3):855–856
[17] El Bannan K, Handler W, Chronik B, Salisbury SP. Heating of metallic rods induced by time-varying gradient fields in MRI. J Magn Reson Imaging. 2013; 38(2):411–416
[18] Kelly WM, Paglen PG, Pearson JA, San Diego AG, Soloman MA. Ferromagnetism of intraocular foreign body causes unilateral blindness after MR study. AJNR Am J Neuroradiol. 1986; 7(2):243–245
[19] Seidenwurm DJ, McDonnell CH, III, Raghavan N, Breslau J. Cost utility analysis of radiographic screening for an orbital foreign body before MR imaging. AJNR Am J Neuroradiol. 2000; 21(2):426–433
[20] Teitelbaum GP, Yee CA, Van Horn DD, Kim HS, Colletti PM. Metallic ballistic fragments: MR imaging safety and artifacts. Radiology. 1990; 175(3):855–859
[21] Graf H, Steidle G, Schick F. Heating of metallic implants and instruments induced by gradient switching in a 1.5-Tesla whole-body unit. J Magn Reson Imaging. 2007; 26(5):1328–1333
[22] Dyer RK, Jr, Nakmali D, Dormer KJ. Magnetic resonance imaging compatibility and safety of the SOUNDTEC Direct System. Laryngoscope. 2006; 116(8): 1321–1333
[23] Jung W, Zvereva V, Hajredini B, Jäckle S. Safe magnetic resonance image scanning of the pacemaker patient: current technologies and future directions. Europace. 2012; 14(5):631–637
[24] Kanal E, Barkovich AJ, Bell C, et al. Expert Panel on MR Safety. ACR guidance document on MR safe practices: 2013. J Magn Reson Imaging. 2013; 37(3): 501–530
[25] Martinelli M. Magnetic resonance imaging and cardiac implantable electronic devices: safety barrier overtaken: is the image quality the current target? Heart Rhythm. 2013; 10(6):873–874
[26] Nazarian S, Hansford R, Roguin A, et al. A prospective evaluation of a protocol for magnetic resonance imaging of patients with implanted cardiac devices. Ann Intern Med. 2011; 155(7):415–424; W-121–412
[27] Santini L, Forleo GB, Santini M, World Society of Arrhythmias. Evaluating MRI-compatible pacemakers: patient data now paves the way to widespread clinical application? Pacing Clin Electrophysiol. 2013; 36(3):270–278
[28] Sommer T, Naehle CP, Yang A, et al. Strategy for safe performance of extrathoracic magnetic resonance imaging at 1.5 tesla in the presence of cardiac pacemakers in non-pacemaker-dependent patients: a prospective study with 115 examinations. Circulation. 2006; 114(12):1285–1292
[29] Shellock FG. Heart valve prostheses and annuloplasty rings. In: Reference manual for magnetic resonance safety, implants, and devices: 2014 edition. Los Angeles, CA: Biomedical Research Publishing Group; 2014:323–325
[30] Hartnell GG, Spence L, Hughes LA, Cohen MC, Saouaf R, Buff B. Safety of MR imaging in patients who have retained metallic materials after cardiac surgery. AJR Am J Roentgenol. 1997; 168(5):1157–1159
[31] Shellock FG. Epicardial pacing leads and intracardiac pacing leads. In: Reference manual for magnetic resonance safety, implants, and devices: 2013 edition. Los Angeles, CA: Biomedical Research Publishing Group; 2013:36–38
[32] Shellock FG, Shellock VJ. Metallic stents: evaluation of MR imaging safety. AJR Am J Roentgenol. 1999; 173(3):543–547
[33] Teitelbaum GP, Bradley WG, Jr, Klein BD. MR imaging artifacts, ferromagnetism, and magnetic torque of intravascular filters, stents, and coils. Radiology. 1988; 166(3):657–664
[34] Pride GL, Jr, Kowal J, Mendelsohn DB, Chason DP, Fleckenstein JL. Safety of MR scanning in patients with nonferromagnetic aneurysm clips. J Magn Reson Imaging. 2000; 12(1):198–200
[35] Shellock FG. Terminology for implant and devices. In: Reference manual for magnetic resonance safety, implants, and devices: 2014 edition. Los Angeles, CA: Biomedical Research Publishing Group; 2014:167–171
[36] Tope WD, Shellock FG. Magnetic resonance imaging and permanent cosmetics (tattoos): survey of complications and adverse events. J Magn Reson Imaging. 2002; 15(2):180–184
[37] United States Health Care Administration. Tattoos and permanent makeup. Rockville, MD: U.S. Food and Drug Administration; 2006
[38] Chaljub G, Kramer LA, Johnson RF, III, Johnson RF, Jr, Singh H, Crow WN. Projectile cylinder accidents resulting from the presence of ferromagnetic nitrous oxide or oxygen tanks in the MR suite. AJR Am J Roentgenol. 2001; 177(1):27–30
[39] Colletti PM. Size "H" oxygen cylinder: accidental MR projectile at 1.5 Tesla. J Magn Reson Imaging. 2004; 19(1):141–143
[40] Landrigan C. Preventable deaths and injuries during magnetic resonance imaging. N Engl J Med. 2001; 345(13):1000–1001
[41] Frenzel T, Lengsfeld P, Schirmer H, Hütter J, Weinmann HJ. Stability of gadolinium-based magnetic resonance imaging contrast agents in human serum at 37 degrees C. Invest Radiol. 2008; 43(12):817–828
[42] Ersoy H, Rybicki FJ. Biochemical safety profiles of gadolinium-based extracellular contrast agents and nephrogenic systemic fibrosis. J Magn Reson Imaging. 2007; 26(5):1190–1197
[43] Staks T, Schuhmann-Giampieri G, Frenzel T, Weinmann HJ, Lange L, Platzek J. Pharmacokinetics, dose proportionality, and tolerability of gadobutrol after single intravenous injection in healthy volunteers. Invest Radiol. 1994; 29(7): 709–715

[44] Aime S, Caravan P. Biodistribution of gadolinium-based contrast agents, including gadolinium deposition. J Magn Reson Imaging. 2009; 30(6):1259–1267
[45] Tombach B, Bremer C, Reimer P, et al. Pharmacokinetics of 1 M gadobutrol in patients with chronic renal failure. Invest Radiol. 2000; 35(1):35–40
[46] Abraham JL, Thakral C, Skov L, Rossen K, Marckmann P. Dermal inorganic gadolinium concentrations: evidence for in vivo transmetallation and long-term persistence in nephrogenic systemic fibrosis. Br J Dermatol. 2008; 158 (2):273–280
[47] Larson KN, Gagnon AL, Darling MD, Patterson JW, Cropley TG. Nephrogenic systemic fibrosis manifesting a decade after exposure to gadolinium. JAMA Dermatol. 2015; 151(10):1117–1120
[48] Cowper SE. Nephrogenic systemic fibrosis (The International Center for Nephrogenic Systemic Fibrosis Research [ICNSFR] Website), 2001–2013. http://www.icnsfr.org. Accessed on July 17, 2013
[49] Wagner B, Drel V, Gorin Y. Pathophysiology of gadolinium-associated systemic fibrosis. Am J Physiol Renal Physiol. 2016; 311(1):F1–F11
[50] Deo A, Fogel M, Cowper SE. Nephrogenic systemic fibrosis: a population study examining the relationship of disease development to gadolinium exposure. Clin J Am Soc Nephrol. 2007; 2(2):264–267
[51] Sadowski EA, Bennett LK, Chan MR, et al. Nephrogenic systemic fibrosis: risk factors and incidence estimation. Radiology. 2007; 243(1):148–157
[52] Shabana WM, Cohan RH, Ellis JH, et al. Nephrogenic systemic fibrosis: a report of 29 cases. AJR Am J Roentgenol. 2008; 190(3):736–741
[53] Wertman R, Altun E, Martin DR, et al. Risk of nephrogenic systemic fibrosis: evaluation of gadolinium chelate contrast agents at four American universities. Radiology. 2008; 248(3):799–806
[54] ACR Committee on Drugs and Contrast Media. ACR Manual on Contrast Media: Version 10.2. https://www.acr.org/Quality-Safety/Resources/Contrast-Manual. Accessed on May 2, 2017
[55] U.S. Food and Drug Administration. FDA Drug Safety Communication: New warnings for using gadolinium-based contrast agents in patients with kidney dysfunction. https://www.fda.gov/Drugs/DrugSafety/ucm223966.htm. Accessed on May 2, 2017
[56] Bruce R, Wentland AL, Haemel AK, et al. Incidence of nephrogenic systemic fibrosis using gadobenate dimeglumine in 1423 patients with renal insufficiency compared with gadodiamide. Invest Radiol. 2016; 51(11):701–705
[57] Wang Y, Alkasab TK, Narin O, et al. Incidence of nephrogenic systemic fibrosis after adoption of restrictive gadolinium-based contrast agent guidelines. Radiology. 2011; 260(1):105–111
[58] Becker S, Walter S, Witzke O, Kreuter A, Kribben A, Mitchell A. Application of gadolinium-based contrast agents and prevalence of nephrogenic systemic fibrosis in a cohort of end-stage renal disease patients on hemodialysis. Nephron Clin Pract. 2012; 121(1–2):c91–c94
[59] Errante Y, Cirimele V, Mallio CA, Di Lazzaro V, Zobel BB, Quattrocchi CC. Progressive increase of T1 signal intensity of the dentate nucleus on unenhanced magnetic resonance images is associated with cumulative doses of intravenously administered gadodiamide in patients with normal renal function, suggesting dechelation. Invest Radiol. 2014; 49(10):685–690
[60] Kanda T, Ishii K, Kawaguchi H, Kitajima K, Takenaka D. High signal intensity in the dentate nucleus and globus pallidus on unenhanced T1-weighted MR images: relationship with increasing cumulative dose of a gadolinium-based contrast material. Radiology. 2014; 270(3):834–841
[61] Cao Y, Huang DQ, Shih G, Prince MR. Signal change in the dentate nucleus on T1-weighted MR images after multiple administrations of gadopentetate dimeglumine versus gadobutrol. AJR Am J Roentgenol. 2016; 206(2):414–419
[62] Radbruch A, Weberling LD, Kieslich PJ, et al. Gadolinium retention in the dentate nucleus and globus pallidus is dependent on the class of contrast agent. Radiology. 2015; 275(3):783–791
[63] Stojanov DA, Aracki-Trenkic A, Vojinovic S, Benedeto-Stojanov D, Ljubisavljevic S. Increasing signal intensity within the dentate nucleus and globus pallidus on unenhanced T1 W magnetic resonance images in patients with relapsing-remitting multiple sclerosis: correlation with cumulative dose of a macrocyclic gadolinium-based contrast agent, gadobutrol. Eur Radiol. 2016; 26(3):807–815
[64] European Medicines Agency. Gadolinium-containing contrast agents. http://www.ema.europa.eu/ema/index.jsp?curl=pages/medicines/human/referrals/Gadolinium-containing_contrast_agents/human_referral_000182.jsp&mid=WC0b01ac05805c516f. Accessed on April 7, 2017
[65] U.S. Food and Drug Administration. FDA drug safety communication: FDA identifies no harmful effects to date with brain retention of gadolinium-based contrast agents for MRIs; review to continue. https://www.fda.gov/Drugs/DrugSafety/ucm559007.htm. Accessed on June 9, 2017
[66] Dillman JR, Ellis JH, Cohan RH, Strouse PJ, Jan SC. Frequency and severity of acute allergic-like reactions to gadolinium-containing i.v. contrast media in children and adults. AJR Am J Roentgenol. 2007; 189(6):1533–1538
[67] Nelson KL, Gifford LM, Lauber-Huber C, Gross CA, Lasser TA. Clinical safety of gadopentetate dimeglumine. Radiology. 1995; 196(2):439–443
[68] Kubik-Huch RA, Gottstein-Aalame NM, Frenzel T, et al. Gadopentetate dimeglumine excretion into human breast milk during lactation. Radiology. 2000; 216(2):555–558
[69] Brody AS, Embury SH, Mentzer WC, Winkler ML, Gooding CA. Preservation of sickle cell blood-flow patterns during MR imaging: an in vivo study. AJR Am J Roentgenol. 1988; 151(1):139–141
[70] Brody AS, Sorette MP, Gooding CA, et al. AUR memorial Award. Induced alignment of flowing sickle erythrocytes in a magnetic field. A preliminary report. Invest Radiol. 1985; 20(6):560–566

Answers to Common Clinical Questions

1. Answer: b. The key to image quality is homogeneity within the magnetic field. Ferromagnetic materials such as iron cause the greatest distortion of images. The patient is exposed to two magnetic fields in the scanner environment: the stronger is the baseline static field and the weaker is time-varying or gradient magnetic fields. The static magnetic field aligns hydrogen atoms within the body.
2. Answer: c. Metallic objects implanted firmly in bone are not at risk for movement during scanning, although they can distort images.
3. Answer: d. After MRI scanning is determined to be a medical necessity, it is typical that written informed consent is obtained. There are theoretical concerns that MRI could disrupt cell division at any stage in pregnancy and that, because cell division is most rapid during the first trimester, there would be a greater potential risk during that period. However, on a case-by-case basis, weighing the risk and benefits, patient in all trimesters can be scanned. Contrast agents enter the amniotic fluid but are administered to pregnant patients in rare circumstances. Typically, a breastfeeding mother is advised to abstain from breastfeeding and to discard breast milk for 24 hours after receiving intravenous gadolinium contrast.
4. Answer: c. Patients with multiple medicine allergies, including previous allergy to ionic CT contrast dye, are at a higher risk for reaction to gadolinium. Patients with a history of isolated hives (i.e., no shortness of breath or anaphylaxis) can receive gadolinium again after premedication, typically with prednisone and diphenhydramine. Less than 1% of patients who receive gadolinium will have an adverse reaction. Gadolinium contrast dyes are excreted primarily through the kidneys.
5. Answer: b. Nephrogenic systemic fibrosis causes progressive fibrosis of the skin and connective tissue throughout the body in patients who have received gadolinium contrast and who have reduced renal function. It can be fatal and is without a known cure. Gadolinium has been detected in the soft tissues of such patients. Patients typically have an eGFR of $< 30\ mL/min/1.73\ m^2$.

Part II

Upper Extremity

II

7 The Shoulder

Kelly G. Kilcoyne and Uma Srikumaran

Abstract

This chapter describing a systematic approach to magnetic resonance imaging (MRI) of the shoulder takes the reader on a step-by-step review of shoulder MRI, shoulder anatomy, and the most common shoulder pathologic conditions. Shoulder anatomy and its interpretation on MRI can be challenging. The purpose of this chapter is to outline how to perform a detailed and stepwise analysis of shoulder MRI, highlighting both normal anatomy and pathologic conditions. It also describes which sequences are best to assess each structure and pathologic condition. By the end of the chapter, the reader should be able to differentiate normal shoulder anatomy from pathologic conditions on MRI. The ability to evaluate shoulder MRIs is essential for any physician treating patients with shoulder conditions.

Keywords: arthritis, magnetic resonance imaging, shoulder abnormalities, shoulder anatomy, shoulder injuries

7.1 Normal Anatomy

The first section of this chapter describes the anatomic structures of the shoulder and their functions, focusing on how specific structures appear in the sagittal, coronal, and axial planes. This section also introduces an approach to systematically review magnetic resonance imaging (MRI) of the shoulder, assessing individual structures and their relationships to surrounding structures and correlating findings and anatomy between different planes and sequences.

7.1.1 Rotator Cuff

The rotator cuff consists of four muscle-tendon units: the subscapularis, which inserts on the lesser tuberosity and, anteriorly to posteriorly, the supraspinatus, infraspinatus, and teres minor, which all insert on the greater tuberosity. The rotator cuff compresses the humeral head into the glenoid, increasing the lever arm and efficiency of the deltoid muscle. The supraspinatus originates from the supraspinatus fossa, the infraspinatus from the infraspinatus fossa, and the teres minor from the dorsal surface of the scapula and two aponeurotic laminae. The subscapularis originates from the anterior scapular surface. The subscapularis has a tendinous insertion onto the upper two-thirds of the lesser tuberosity and a muscular insertion onto the lower one-third.[1]

It was thought that the supraspinatus footprint was larger than that of the infraspinatus but a recent study demonstrated that the supraspinatus occupies a smaller area of the tuberosity. In an anatomic study, the supraspinatus insertion was triangular with an average medial-to-lateral length of 6.9 mm and an anteroposterior width of 12.6 mm, and the infraspinatus insertion was trapezoidal with a medial-to-lateral length of 10.2 mm and an anteroposterior width of 32.7 mm.[2] Normal rotator cuff tendons are uniformly dark with low signal intensity on all imaging sequences.

Sagittal Anatomy

Starting medially, the sagittal plane shows the rotator cuff muscles at the level of the scapular spine, which is where one assesses for presence and degree of muscle atrophy (▶ Fig. 7.1a). The degree of rotator cuff muscle atrophy is typically graded according to the Goutallier classification.[3] Moving laterally, the musculotendinous junction is visualized near the level of the glenoid. The thick insertion of each rotator cuff tendon is seen laterally. The relative involvement of the rotator cuff tendons in a lateral tear can be determined by following the muscular transitions from their origins medially to their insertions laterally.

Coronal Anatomy

Anteriorly, the subscapularis can be seen inserting laterally onto the lesser tuberosity but it is difficult to assess and characterize on the coronal plane. In contrast, the other rotator muscles can be evaluated for atrophy or fatty infiltration medially, and the tendinous insertions are seen while scrolling anteroposteriorly where they insert on the greater tuberosity. The long head of the biceps tendon (LHBT) splits the greater and lesser tuberosities, with the insertion of the subscapularis seen anteriorly on the lesser tuberosity. The LHBT turns medially as it travels proximal to the transverse humeral ligament and toward its intra-articular insertion. At this level, as the upper border of the subscapularis disappears from view, the rotator interval can be seen laterally between the medially coursing biceps and the far lateral supraspinatus insertion.

Axial Anatomy

Although the insertions of the supraspinatus, infraspinatus, and teres minor can be seen on axial images, they are typically evaluated for abnormal changes on sagittal and coronal images. However, the subscapularis can be well visualized inserting on the lesser tuberosity. The location of the biceps and the bicipital groove are also readily seen in the axial plane. This relationship is associated with assessing for subscapularis tears, as discussed in section "Labrum." In addition to the location of the biceps, the morphology of the biceps tendon and bicipital groove; signal intensity, including any surrounding fluid; presence of partial or full-thickness tearing; and presence of loose bodies in the sheath or groove can be assessed.[4] A recent study evaluating the accuracy of MRI in detecting abnormality of the LHBT found that MRI is highly sensitive in the detection of full-thickness tears, as well as detecting the absence of complete tear and dislocation or subluxation of the tendon.[5] However, MRI had limited effectiveness in the detection of partial tearing of the LHBT.

7.1.2 Glenoid Labrum and Capsular Ligaments

The labrum is a thick, fibrocartilaginous ringlike structure attached to the glenoid rim. The joint capsule has superior, inferior,

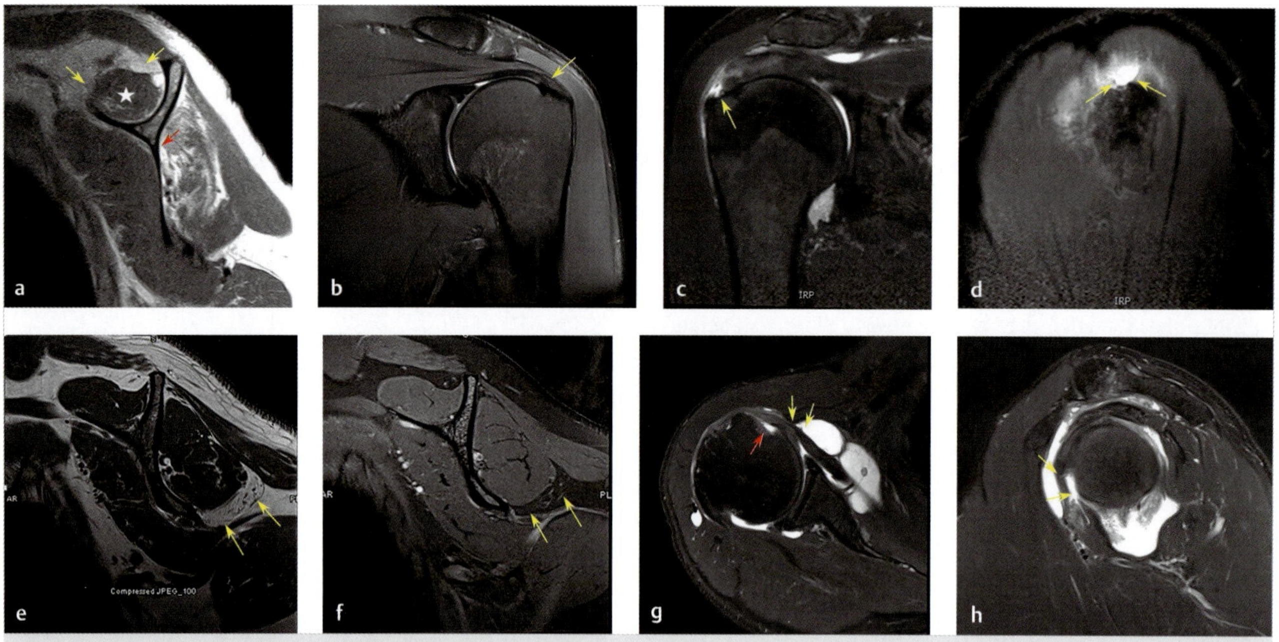

Fig. 7.1 **(a)** Sagittal T1-weighted image at the level of the scapular spine (*red arrow*), with visualization of the supraspinatus muscle belly (*white star*) and surrounding fat atrophy (*yellow arrows*). **(b)** Coronal T2-weighted image of intact supraspinatus insertion at greater tuberosity. **(c)** Coronal T2-weighted image of full-thickness supraspinatus tear with minimal retraction. **(d)** Same supraspinatus tear visualized on sagittal T2-weighted image. Note the size of the tear is more readily apparent as seen between the *yellow arrows*, which mark pathology and relevant anatomic structures. **(e)** Sagittal T1-weighted and **(f)** T2-weighted images with atrophy of the teres minor (*yellow arrows*). **(g)** Axial and **(h)** sagittal images showing subscapularis tear (*yellow arrows*) with noted absence of the biceps from the groove (*red arrow*).

and posterior attachments to the labrum. The labrum gives the otherwise shallow glenoid depth, and the anterior and posterior-inferior labrum provides a stable bumper that contributes to glenohumeral stability. The superior labrum serves as the origin of the LHBT and is a common source of shoulder abnormality (see section "Labrum"), as well as common anatomic variants (see section "Biceps"). Also notable are the superior, middle, and inferior glenohumeral ligaments (IGHLs). The superior glenohumeral ligament, which is located within the rotator interval, restricts anterior humeral head translation with the arm in adduction. The middle glenohumeral ligament, which is seen adjacent and deep to the subscapularis tendon, restricts anterior humeral head translation with the arm in 45 degrees of abduction and external rotation. An anatomic study demonstrated that the superior and middle glenohumeral ligaments attach to the labrum between the 12 o'clock and 1 o'clock positions, with little variability.[6] The IGHL has anterior and posterior bands. The anterior band restricts anteroinferior translation with the arm in 90 degrees of abduction and external rotation, whereas the posterior band restricts posteroinferior translation with the arm in internal rotation and adduction. The IGHL has greater variability in attachment, ranging from the 3 o'clock to the 5 o'clock position.[6]

Sagittal Anatomy

The articular surface of the glenoid and entirety of the glenoid labrum are best seen in the sagittal plane. This view can be helpful in visualizing glenoid bone loss that can occur in the setting of inferior labral tears and instability; however, the coronal and axial planes are more helpful in detecting signal between the glenoid and the labrum in superior labral tear from anterior to posterior (SLAP) and inferior labral tears. The glenohumeral ligaments, including their labral attachments, are typically well visualized in the sagittal plane.

Coronal Anatomy

The superior labrum is best visualized on coronal images (▶ Fig. 7.2a). The biceps tendon can be traced as it courses medially to its intra-articular attachment. Some separation between the superior aspect of the glenoid and the labrum (medial extension of signal) is often normal and correlates with the normal superior labral attachment. It is important to distinguish superior labral tears from normal labral variants, including Buford complex (cordlike middle glenohumeral ligament), sublabral foramen, and sublabral recess.[7] On coronal sequences, SLAP tears are typically posterior to the biceps complex, whereas these anatomic variants will be anterior. Abnormality is suggested when high signal extends laterally into the substance of the superior labrum or when medial signal is present with no underlying cartilage (▶ Fig. 7.2). In addition, SLAP tears will show lateral extension, whereas normal variants will show medial origin and extension.

Axial Anatomy

The anterior and posterior labrum are best visualized on axial images. Typically, T2-weighted sequences will show the labrum to be a dark, triangular-shaped structure on the rim of the glenoid cartilage. The coracoid can be used as a reference for the level (superior to inferior) on the glenoid being viewed. The glenohumeral ligaments can be visualized by scrolling through

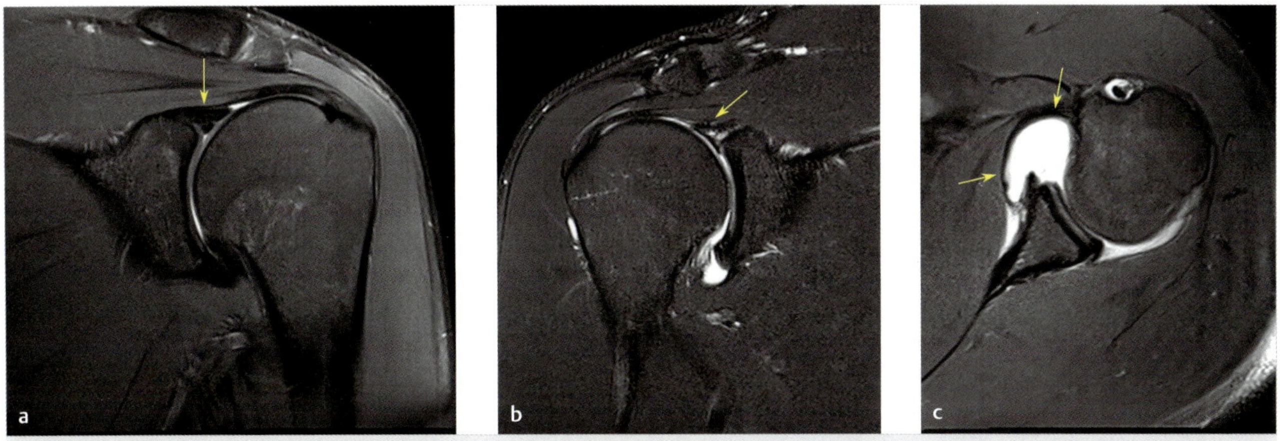

Fig. 7.2 **(a)** Coronal T2-weighted image of intact biceps/superior labral complex (*yellow arrow*). **(b)** Coronal T2-weighted image of torn superior labrum (type 2 superior labral tear from anterior to posterior) (*yellow arrow*). Note lateral extension of signal. **(c)** Superior labral tear seen on axial T2-weighted image (*yellow arrow*).

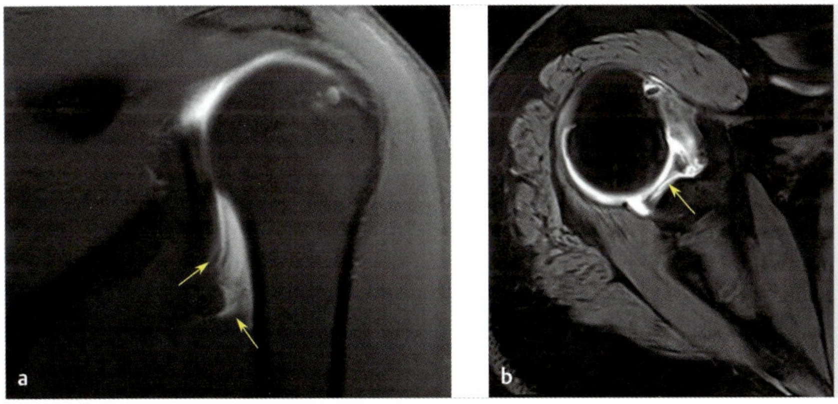

Fig. 7.3 **(a)** Normal humeral attachment of the glenohumeral ligament (*yellow arrows*) seen on axial T2-weighted image. **(b)** Humeral avulsion of the glenohumeral ligament (HAGL) lesion (*yellow arrow*) seen on coronal T2-weighted image.

the images from superior to inferior. At the inferior glenoid in the axillary pouch, the humeral attachment of the glenohumeral ligament can typically be seen attaching to the humeral head (▶ Fig. 7.3a). Superior labral tears, especially larger ones, can also be visualized on axial images.

7.1.3 Biceps

The LHBT originates in the glenohumeral joint from the supraglenoid tubercle and the superior glenoid labrum. A portion of the tendon is intra-articular. There are four variations of the origin of the LHBT. The most common is entirely posterior, followed by posterior dominant, equal, and entirely anterior.[6] As the LHBT traverses toward the bicipital groove, it is held in place by the biceps pulley, which prevents medial subluxation. The biceps pulley consists of the coracohumeral ligament and superior glenohumeral ligament with contributions from the supraspinatus and subscapularis tendons.[8] The biceps travels under the transverse humeral ligament distally.

Sagittal Anatomy

On the sagittal view, the biceps tendon is visualized laterally as it exits the groove adjacent to the lesser tuberosity. It is deep to the supraspinatus tendon and adjacent to the articular surface of the humeral head. The intra-articular portion of the LHBT is seen as it crosses the joint and inserts on the supraglenoid tubercle and the superior glenoid labrum.

Coronal Anatomy

The LHBT is found on the most anterior cuts of the coronal sequences. It appears as a distinct structure and can start to be seen when the tip of the coracoid comes into view. The tendon is seen within the groove and as it turns near the rotator interval, traversing toward its insertion.

Axial Anatomy

The LHBT is easily visualized on axial views and found within the bicipital groove unless subluxed or absent. The bicipital groove separates the greater and lesser tuberosities. The axial view best shows the extra-articular portion of the LHBT.

7.1.4 Glenoid and Scapula

The glenoid is a shallow and concave structure. It is commonly referred to as pear-shaped because of its slightly wider base.

There has been recent interest in using MRI to assess the dimensions (height, width, and depth) of the glenoid and amount of glenoid retroversion as a predictor of glenohumeral instability.[9] Normal glenoid version ranges from neutral to 5 degrees of retroversion.

The scapula is a flat, triangular-shaped bone. It is positioned on the posterior surface of the thoracic rib cage and typically spans ribs 2 to 7. The scapula comprises discrete osseous structures, including the acromion, coracoid process, glenoid, neck, scapular body, and spine. The scapula has the lateral, medial, and superior borders, and the inferior, superior, and lateral angles.

The coracoid process is a critical landmark for arthroscopic examinations and procedures and injections, as well as a critical reference in shoulder MRI review. Attached to the coracoid process are six clinically important structures: the coracoacromial ligament, the coracoclavicular ligaments (conoid and trapezoid), the conjoined tendons of the coracobrachialis and biceps brachii, and the pectoralis minor muscle.

Sagittal Anatomy

Like the glenoid labrum, the articular surface of the bony glenoid is best seen in the sagittal plane. The normal pear shape of the glenoid is seen on this plane, and presence of bone loss (see section "Labrum," shoulder instability) can be assessed. The coracoid and base of the coracoid can be seen while scrolling medially through the images. The coracoid is used as a guide to orient and help differentiate the anterior and posterior aspects of the shoulder. At the level of the scapular spine, the clear separation of the four rotator cuff muscles is seen, and on T1-weighted images at this level, rotator cuff atrophy and fatty infiltration are easily seen and characterized.

Coronal Anatomy

The tip of the coracoid is traced to the glenoid base, and this marks the anterior portion of the scapula and glenoid. Moving posteriorly, the scapular notch is seen and is a landmark for the separation and anterior-to-posterior location of the supraspinatus and infraspinatus. Like the labrum, the superior and inferior aspects of the glenoid are well visualized.

Axial Anatomy

The axial plane offers a clear delineation of the anterior and posterior rim of the glenoid. The coracoid and base of the coracoid should be used as a reference for the reader as the glenoid is assessed. This plane is also helpful to visualize bone loss seen in patients with instability and glenohumeral arthritis.

7.1.5 Humeral Head

The bony anatomy of the proximal humerus and humeral head is well visualized on MRI, and these landmarks serve as references in the review of the shoulder MRI. Important bony landmarks include the anatomic and surgical neck, articular surface, bicipital groove, greater and lesser tuberosities, and humeral shaft. T1-weighted sequences show the bony anatomy well, whereas T2-weighted sequences can further highlight changes within the bone, including cystic change (i.e., in the greater tuberosity) and bony edema. Fat-suppressed three-dimensional gradient-echo sequences are best used for evaluation of articular cartilage.[10]

The humeral head has an ellipsoidal shape with an articular surface of hyaline cartilage. The articular surface of the humeral head approximates one-third of a sphere.[11,12] The anatomic neck of the proximal humerus is the area of transition from cartilage to metaphyseal bone. The humeral head is retroverted relative to the epicondylar axis. Mean humeral head retroversion is approximately 20 degrees, with a range of 15 to 45 degrees.[11]

Sagittal Anatomy

In the sagittal plane, the greater tuberosity with the insertion of the posterior rotator cuff (supraspinatus, infraspinatus, and teres minor) is seen laterally. Cystic changes within the head, adjacent to the rotator cuff insertion, can be seen and indicate chronic rotator cuff disease. Similarly, the subscapularis is seen as it inserts on the lesser tuberosity.

Coronal Anatomy

The coronal plane offers good visualization of the superior and inferior aspects of the humeral head, in addition to visualization of the greater tuberosity and rotator cuff insertions (► Fig. 7.1b). Although the lesser tuberosity can be seen, it is better viewed on sagittal and axial images. Coronal images also give the best view of the neck of the humerus and neck-shaft angle, and they allow analysis of superior migration of the humeral head relative to the acromion (see section "Rotator Cuff").

Axial Anatomy

Axial anatomy of the humeral head gives a clear assessment of the greater and lesser tuberosities and the bicipital groove that separates them. The articular cartilage can be examined closely (see Chapter 1, Essentials of MRI Physics and Pulse Sequences) and the version of the humeral head along with any anterior or posterior translation or subluxation of the humeral head relative to the glenoid can be assessed.

7.2 Systematic Approach to Image Review

Just as the physical examination of the shoulder must include all critical structures in a systematic fashion, MRI must be reviewed in a stepwise fashion. To evaluate a shoulder MRI thoroughly, the reader must perform a systematic assessment of the critical structures in all planes and on multiple sequences. If the same steps are performed with every shoulder MRI, the interpreter ensures a full and accurate assessment of all structures and potential abnormalities. The sequence below follows the same pattern as the description of normal anatomy above.

7.2.1 Rotator Cuff

The supraspinatus and infraspinatus are readily seen on coronal and sagittal views. The subscapularis and teres minor can be seen on coronal images but are more readily seen on axial and sagittal images. A rotator cuff tear that is seen on the coronal T2-weighted image (▶ Fig. 7.1c) should be correlated with the coronal T1-weighted images. To assess the tear size, the reader can count the number of frames (i.e., 3) and multiply by the size of the cuts (3 cuts × 5 mm/cut = 1.5-cm tear). The size of the tear can also be measured directly on the sagittal sequences (▶ Fig. 7.1d). The sagittal view also aids in assessing full-thickness versus partial-thickness tears. The tendons of all four rotator cuff muscles can be followed on the sagittal sequence to their insertions on the tuberosities. In addition, at the level of the scapular spine, the presence and degree of any rotator cuff muscle atrophy can be assessed (▶ Fig. 7.1a). The more severe the grade of atrophy, the larger the tear and the more likely it is chronic.

7.2.2 Glenoid Labrum and Capsular Ligaments

The anterior and posterior labrum are best seen on axial T2-weighted images. Careful review of the axial cuts allows the reader to determine the presence of a tear and at what level on the glenoid the tear starts and ends. On axial views, the normal labrum should appear triangular and wedge-shaped with homogeneously low signal on all sequences.[13] The sagittal view also allows visualization of the entire labral complex. In addition, the sagittal view allows for assessment of any disruption of the superior, middle, or IGHLs.

The superior labrum, like the anterior and posterior labrum, not only can be seen on the axial sequences but also is well visualized on coronal T2-weighted images. The extension of signal medially under the labrum is often normal, representing the normal labral anatomy and attachment to the supraglenoid tubercle.[14] Extension of signal laterally often indicates a superior labral or SLAP tear.[15] Normal variants of labral attachment in the anterior-superior quadrant exist; therefore, potential tears in this area must be interpreted with caution and differentiated from normal anatomic variants.

7.2.3 LHBT

The biceps can be seen on coronal imaging and is a good landmark to evaluate the rotator interval (anterior) and the anterior insertion of the supraspinatus (posterior). It is visualized easily in the bicipital groove on axial sequences. Medial subluxation of the tendon can indicate a subscapularis tear or a tear of the biceps pulley, both of which should be evaluated if medial subluxation is encountered.

7.2.4 Bone and Cartilage Defects

The humeral head should be assessed in all planes. Sagittal and axial views can be used to assess for the presence and size of a Hill-Sachs lesion, which can occur with shoulder instability. The humeral head can also be assessed in the axial plane for any cartilage defects. Cystic changes, which can occur with chronic rotator cuff disease, can be seen in the coronal, sagittal, and axial planes. Changes to the articular cartilage, loss of joint space, and subchondral cystic changes of the glenoid and humeral head can be assessed on axial and coronal cuts. Subchondral bone edema that occurs with degeneration of the glenohumeral joint can best be seen on T2-weighted and gradient-echo sequences.

7.2.5 Acromioclavicular Joint

The acromioclavicular (AC) joint can be seen on axial and coronal series. Edema in the distal clavicle and/or the medial acromion can be assessed in both planes and is best seen on T2-weighted sequences. Associated osteophytes and the presence of subchondral cystic change can be seen on T1- and T2-weighted sequences.

7.3 Traumatic Conditions

Patient age is an important determiner of the most likely shoulder abnormality. In addition, the mechanism of injury is an important factor. Rotator cuff tears are common in patients older than 40 years, whereas shoulder instability and inferior labral tears are most common in patients aged 18 to 35 years. When elderly patient dislocate their shoulders, clinicians must closely evaluate not only the labrum for injury but more commonly, an injury to the rotator cuff, including possible fracture of the greater tuberosity.[16,17]

7.3.1 Labrum

Superior Labral Lesions

Tears of the labrum can occur anywhere in the 360 degrees of labrum that surrounds the glenoid. They can occur in isolation or combination (i.e., an inferior labral tear with a separate superior labral tear). Tears of the anteroinferior and posteroinferior labrum are associated with glenohumeral dislocations and instability, whereas tears of the superior labrum can be degenerative, can occur in throwers, or can result from acute injury. Magnetic resonance arthrography (MRA) has been shown to be more sensitive than noncontrast MRI for assessment of labral and capsular injury.[18]

In a retrospective review of 700 consecutive arthroscopic shoulder procedures, Snyder et al[19] described a tear of the superior labrum in 27 patients. The most common mechanism was fall onto an outstretched arm with the arm in an abducted and slightly forward flexed position. The original classification included the following types: type 1, degeneration and fraying of superior labrum with intact biceps anchor; type 2, detachment of superior labrum and biceps anchor from superior glenoid insertion; type 3, bucket handle labral tear; and type 4, bucket handle labral tear with extension into the biceps tendon (▶ Fig. 7.4h). Combined lesions that do not fit into the above groups have also been described, with types of SLAP tears expanded.[20] SLAP tears can be seen on coronal T2-weighted images (▶ Fig. 7.2b). Seen arthroscopically, the normal labrum can have some liftoff from the cartilaginous superior glenoid rim. Thus, some increased signal under the labrum medially can be normal. Signal that extends laterally on coronal imaging, however, suggests a SLAP tear. In addition, just as inferior tears are well visualized on axial imaging, superior labral tears can sometimes be seen on axial T2-weighted images depending on size and location of tear (▶ Fig. 7.2c). On MRI, SLAP tear appearance depends on the type of tear, as follows[13]: type 1, hyperintense signal with blunting/irregularity of the typically sharp labral edge; type 2, increased signal intensity and medial extent of signal under the anchor with no signal extension into the biceps tendon, which remains attached to the avulsed labrum; type 3, high signal intensity across the base of the labrum with extension beyond the equator, and if tear is displaced, this can sometimes be seen on axial images with signal interposed between the medial and lateral flap; and type 4, hyperintense signal with extension beyond the equator of the superior labrum with disruption of the superior labrum and extension of signal into the biceps tendon. In addition to acute traumatic superior labral tears, SLAP tears also occur from degeneration and are associated with chondromalacia, glenohumeral arthritis, and rotator cuff tears. In an analysis of 140 consecutive arthroscopic shoulder procedures with superior labral tears, Snyder et al[21] found that 29% of SLAP tears were associated with partial-thickness rotator cuff tears, 11% with full-thickness tears, and 22% with Bankart lesions.

Shoulder Instability

Shoulder instability includes a spectrum of conditions ranging from subluxation to complete dislocation, unidirectional instability (anterior and posterior), and multidirectional instability. MRI and MRA are essential tools in the diagnosis and treatment of shoulder instability.

The most common direction of primary shoulder instability is anterior.[22] Traumatic injuries are the most common cause of shoulder instability and account for 95% of anterior shoulder dislocations. Indirect force with the arm in an abducted and externally rotated position increases the anterior translational forces of the humerus within the glenoid. With the shoulder in this position, the anterior band of the IGHL and the anterior-inferior labrum detach from the glenoid, producing the "essential" lesion of anterior shoulder instability, known as a Bankart lesion.[23] Anteroinferior labral detachment disrupts the main anterior static restraints to the glenohumeral joint in the abducted and externally rotated position, and this must be identified and is often repaired surgically to prevent further instability events. Although a Bankart lesion can often be seen in all planes, it is typically best visualized on axial images with increased linear signal (best seen on T2-weighted imaging) between the labrum and glenoid rim (▶ Fig. 7.4a, b).[24] Tears can be nondisplaced or displaced (typically medially). An anterior labroligamentous periosteal sleeve avulsion occurs when the periosteum remains intact and the labroligamentous structures displace, and commonly scar, medially and rotate inferiorly on the scapular neck. Anterior labroligamentous periosteal sleeve avulsion lesions, like other inferior labral lesions, are best visualized on axial MRI as medial displacement and inferior rotation of a torn anterior labrum (▶ Fig. 7.4c).[24,25] A humeral avulsion of the glenohumeral ligament (HAGL) occurs in less than 10% of instability events but can easily be missed during arthroscopy if not visualized and assessed. On MRI, an HAGL lesion can be seen on axial and coronal images. On axial imaging, HAGL lesion is suggested when a wavy and irregular ligament that does not reach its normal humeral insertion is seen in the axillary pouch. On coronal sequences, the classic appearance is similar to the letter "J," which describes the characteristic wavy appearance of the avulsed ligament from its normal humeral attachment (▶ Fig. 7.3a, b).[26]

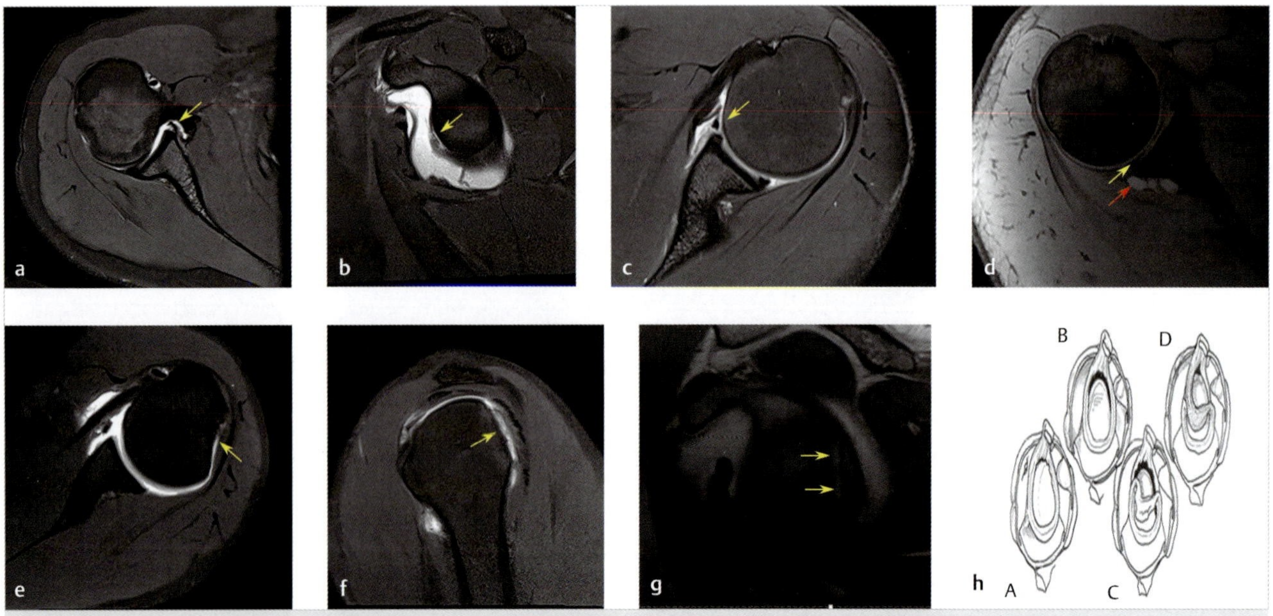

Fig. 7.4 **(a)** Anterior-inferior labral tear (Bankart lesion) (*yellow arrow*) seen on axial T2-weighted image. **(b)** Anterior-inferior labral tear (Bankart lesion) seen on sagittal T2-weighted image. **(c)** Axial T2-weighted image of anterior labral periosteal sleeve avulsion (*yellow arrow*). **(d)** Posterior-inferior labral tear (*yellow arrow*) with associated paralabral cyst (*red arrow*) seen on axial T2-weighted image. **(e)** Hill-Sachs lesion (*yellow arrow*) seen on axial T2-weighted image. **(f)** Same Hill-Sachs lesion (*yellow arrow*) seen on sagittal imaging. **(g)** Reverse bony Bankart lesion (*yellow arrows*) on T1-weighted sagittal image. **(h)** Types of SLAP lesions. A, type I, a frayed and degenerative superior labrum with a normal (stable) biceps tendon anchor. B, type II, detachment of the superior labrum and biceps anchor. C, type III, a bucket-handle tear of a meniscoid superior labrum without extension into the biceps tendon. The biceps anchor is stable and the remaining labrum is intact. D, type IV, a bucket-handle tear of a meniscoid superior labrum with extension into the biceps tendon. (Figure part h: Reprinted from Operative Techniques in Sports Medicine. Vol 12. Powell SE, Nord KD, Ryu RKN. The diagnosis, classification, and treatment of SLAP lesions. 99–110, 2004 with permission from Elsevier.)

In addition to injury to the soft-tissue structures, bony abnormality can also occur. The anteroinferior glenoid may fracture when the humeral head dislocates, creating a bony Bankart lesion. These can be seen as an avulsion or flattening of the anterior-inferior glenoid margin. Glenoid bone loss resulting from recurrent dislocation is important in treatment and predicting recurrence of instability.[27,28] Although computed tomography has historically been the modality of choice for assessment of the amount of glenoid bone loss, MRI is increasingly being used to quantify the degree of bone loss with equal accuracy.[29,30]

Sagittal views allow the best global view and assessment of glenoid bone loss. The Hill-Sachs lesion is the corresponding humeral lesion to the glenoid Bankart lesion. It occurs when the softer bone of the posterosuperior humeral head impacts against the harder anteroinferior glenoid rim. Hill-Sachs lesions are posterosuperior compression fractures on the humeral head and must be recognized because failure to address bony abnormality is associated with future instability episodes. The size of the lesion can be quantified on axial and sagittal images (▶ Fig. 7.4e, f). A glenolabral articular disruption is a defect of the articular cartilage (fibrillation, erosion, delamination) adjacent to a superficial and nondisplaced tear of the anterior-inferior labrum.[26] Best seen on axial images, high-intensity signal or contrast is seen adjacent and under but not completely between the glenoid and labrum (▶ Fig. 7.5).

Injury to the middle and inferior one-third of the subscapularis is associated with anterior shoulder dislocation and must be critically assessed. In one study of 45 consecutive patients with anterior shoulder dislocations, more than 60% (27 patients) had some degree of subscapularis injury on MRI.[31]

Posterior instability is uncommon compared with anterior instability and dislocations. The classic mechanisms include seizures or electrical shock in which the more powerful pectoralis muscles produce a posteriorly directed force on the humeral head. More commonly, however, posterior subluxation or dislocation is encountered in athletes such as football linemen. Posterior instability may produce lesions similar to those found in anterior instability and dislocations but on the posterior (or reverse) aspect of the shoulder instead of the anterior aspect. Similarly, the appearance of high-intensity signal or fluid between the posterior labrum and glenoid is characteristic of a tear: a posteroinferior glenoid lesion (reverse Bankart lesion) (▶ Fig. 7.4g) and an anterosuperior humeral head lesion (reverse Hill-Sachs lesion) Flattening and blunting of the normal, sharply contoured labrum is unique to the posterior labrum, whereas the junction between the labrum and glenoid remains intact, which is known as a Kim lesion.[32,33]

Paralabral cysts can be associated with labral tears in any quadrant. The presence of a labral cyst indicates a labral tear because the tear creates a one-way valve that allows the collection of fluid, forming the cyst. Cysts in the spinoglenoid and suprascapular notch are notable because they may cause compression of the suprascapular nerve, which can manifest as pain and/or weakness.

In older patients with shoulder dislocation, the typical mechanism of injury, as well as the pathologic findings, differs from the labral abnormality seen in younger patients.[16] In patients older than 40 years, a low-energy fall is a typical mechanism of injury, and the rotator cuff, not the labrum, is typically torn. In addition, shoulder instability can be caused by massive rotator cuff tearing. Associated bony injuries can also occur, especially in elderly patients with osteoporosis. These include impaction of the humeral head, greater tuberosity fracture, and anterior glenoid rim fracture (▶ Fig. 7.6).

7.4 Degenerative Conditions

7.4.1 Rotator Cuff: Tendinopathy, Partial- and Full-Thickness Tears

Rotator cuff disease is highly correlated with age, with 28% of patients with partial- or full-thickness tears older than 60 years and 65% of patients older than 70 years.[34] In addition, tears are bilateral in 50% of patients older than 66 years.[34]

Degeneration and inflammation of the rotator cuff can lead to rotator cuff tendinopathy. Tendinopathy can lead to partial- and full-thickness tearing. However, the tendon degeneration that occurs without actual tendon tearing is irreversible. There are different theories about the pathogenesis and cause of rotator cuff tendinosis. Neer[35] described extrinsic factors that put a critical portion of the supraspinatus at risk, including variations in acromial morphology and shape, osteophyte formation, and the acromial attachment of the coracoacromial ligament. Neer[35] hypothesized that most rotator cuff tears (95%) were the result of this rotator cuff impingement. Acromioplasty of this bone was developed in an attempt to prevent impingement and subsequent rotator cuff tearing. The shape of the undersurface of

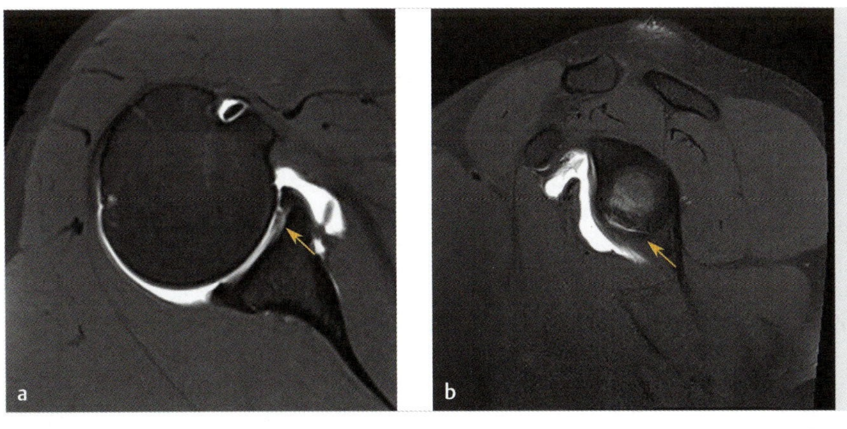

Fig. 7.5 Glenolabral articular disruption lesion (*yellow arrows*) on **(a)** axial and **(b)** sagittal T2-weighted images.

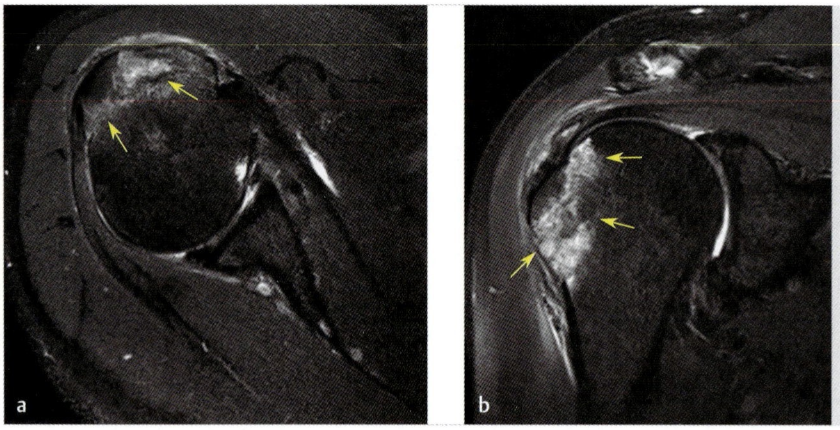

Fig. 7.6 Displaced greater tuberosity fracture (*yellow arrows*) seen on **(a)** axial and **(b)** coronal T2-weighted images.

the acromion is classified into three distinct types: type 1, flat; type 2, curved (smooth); type 3, hooked.[36] Acromial shape in the anterior-to-posterior plane is best visualized on scapular lateral radiographs and, correspondingly, sagittal MRI sequences. The shape and any associated osteophytes of the anteroinferior acromial edge can also be seen on coronal sequences with the morphology of the bone best seen on T1-weighted images and any associated edema or inflammation noted with increased signal on T2-weighted images. Most changes seen on MRI with tendinopathy or impingement are on the bursal side of the rotator cuff in the subacromial space. There is often increased signal and hypertrophy of the bursa, as well as increased signal superficial to the rotator cuff tendons. However, with chronic tendinopathy these changes can be found within the rotator cuff muscle and tendon. In addition, one should note changes to the surrounding bony structures, including the morphology of the acromion and any changes to the AC joint (see section "Acromioclavicular Arthritis").

If there is partial tearing of a rotator cuff tendon, there is a combination of hyperintense signal from the portion of the tendon that is torn and hypointense signal from the portion that remains intact. Quantifying the exact amount of tendon that remains can be difficult. MRA can be helpful in distinguishing full-thickness from partial tears, as well as partial bursal or articular tears from intrasubstance tears.[37,38,39]

After the initial evaluation of the rotator cuff and assessment for presence of a tear, it is important to assess the size and shape of the tear, the amount (if any) of tendon retraction from the greater tuberosity, and the degree of rotator cuff atrophy. The Goutallier classification that quantifies the degree of rotator cuff muscle atrophy was based on preoperative and postoperative computed tomography scans.[3] There are four stages included in the classification as follows: stage 0, absence of intramuscular fat; stage 1, presence of some fatty streaks; stage 2, presence of substantial fat that was less than the amount of muscle; stage 3, presence of a quantity of fat approximately equal to the muscle volume; and stage 4, more fat than muscle (▶ Fig. 7.1e, f). A recent study assessing the accuracy of quantifying rotator cuff atrophy showed significant intraobserver and interobserver agreement for radiologists and orthopaedic surgeons.[40]

The medial-to-lateral width of the rotator cuff tendons (depending on the tendon) ranges from 6 to 14 mm. In addition, the tendon has an articular surface (seen within the glenohumeral joint) and a bursal surface (seen within the subacromial space). Thus, the tendon can be partially or completely torn. Assessment for the degree of tearing and location of tearing is important because it often dictates treatment. If the articular side of the tendon is torn, it is described as a partial articular-sided tear. A partial articular-sided tear of the supraspinatus is described as partial sided–articular sided supraspinatus tendon avulsion lesion. Partial tears are graded as 1, 2, or 3, according to the amount of tendon torn (grade 1 [< 3 mm, < 25%], grade 2 [3–6 mm, 25–50%], grade 3 [> 6 mm, > 50%][41]). The degree of tearing typically dictates whether the tendon is repaired or debrided.

The supraspinatus and infraspinatus are the most commonly torn rotator cuff tendons. Subscapularis tears are less common, and they are more frequently missed.[1,42] A systematic assessment of tears on multiple sequences and images allows a better understanding of various aspects of the tear. Tears of the supraspinatus and infraspinatus are best seen on sagittal and coronal T2-weighted sequences. On these sequences, if increased signal at the footprint with disruption of the normal low signal intensity of an intact tendon and/or tendons is not visualized, it indicates a tear. The degree of retraction is best seen on coronal images, whereas the anterior-to-posterior size of the tear is best measured on sagittal images. The amount of medial displacement of a torn tendon often determines whether the tear can be repaired. The tendon can remain adjacent to the normal insertion, retract medially along the articular surface of the humeral head, or retract to or past the level of the glenoid.

Tears of the subscapularis, as well as of the teres minor, are best seen on sagittal images and can be correlated with axial images (▶ Fig. 7.1g, h). Sagittal images are useful in assessing the size of a subscapularis tear, as well as determining whether the tear is on the upper or lower border of the subscapularis and whether it is a full-thickness tear. Axial images can be used to assess the degree of retraction and the presence of a subluxed or medialized LHBT. Tearing of the articular upper border is most common.[42]

Glenohumeral Arthritis

Glenohumeral arthritis typically occurs in patients older than 65 years and in men more commonly than women. In addition to the common osteoarthritis findings in other joints (hip and knee) such as joint-space narrowing, periarticular osteophytes, and cystic change, glenohumeral arthritis has distinct features such as flattening and enlargement of the humeral head, and posterior glenoid erosion. Rotator cuff tears are uncommon, occurring in approximately 5 to 10% of patients with glenohumeral osteoarthritis.[43] However, because the presence of a rotator cuff tear can affect surgical treatment, it is a vital aspect of the preoperative assessment.

To assess the cartilage, gradient-echo sequences are the most helpful and accurate. The relationship of the articular surfaces of the glenoid and humeral head can be seen on coronal and axial images. Axial images are the most useful in the assessment of glenoid version (▶ Fig. 7.7a). Osteophytes of the humeral head and of the glenoid can be seen on coronal images. Although cysts within the humeral head (and more importantly, the glenoid) can be seen in all planes, the axial plane is most useful for assessing the specific location of the cyst within the glenoid. Precise cyst location is often important in preoperative planning of placement of the glenoid component (▶ Fig. 7.7b).

Evaluation of glenoid version is also an essential part of the preoperative plan and has traditionally been examined on axillary radiographs and computed tomography scans.[44] However, similar to the advantages discussed in the assessment of glenoid bone loss with instability, MRI has important advantages in the assessment of glenoid version (▶ Fig. 7.7c). A recent study demonstrated that MRI is reliable in assessment of glenoid version and wear, with the additional benefit of assessing the soft-tissue structures of the shoulder and the integrity of the rotator cuff.[45]

Acromioclavicular Arthritis

Arthritis of the AC joint can occur in isolation or in conjunction with other shoulder abnormalities, including rotator cuff tendinopathy and tears, as well as superior labral tears and biceps tendinopathy. Although radiographic and MRI evidence of degenerative changes are common, most patients are asymptomatic.[46] Changes in and around the joint include joint-space narrowing, hypertrophy of the joint capsule, cystic changes, and periarticular erosions. These changes are seen on all sequences that allow visualization of the AC joint, including axial, sagittal, and coronal sequences (▶ Fig. 7.8).

A study of MRI finding of the AC joint in asymptomatic patients reported that 82% of patients (41 of 50) had MRI findings consistent with AC joint arthritis.[46] In a subsequent study, the same authors compared 25 patients with symptomatic AC joint arthritis with 50 patients with asymptomatic AC joint arthritis.[47] The authors assessed which MRI findings predicted symptoms. They found varying degrees of arthritic changes in both groups, but a significantly higher grade of AC joint arthritis in the symptomatic group. In addition, the authors found that the presence of bone edema in the distal clavicle and/or acromion sides of the joint was not present in any asymptomatic patients. However, bone edema on one or both sides of the joint was present in 80% of symptomatic patients. They concluded that, on MRI, reactive bone edema is a more reliable predictor of a symptomatic AC joint than the commonly encountered degenerative changes.[47]

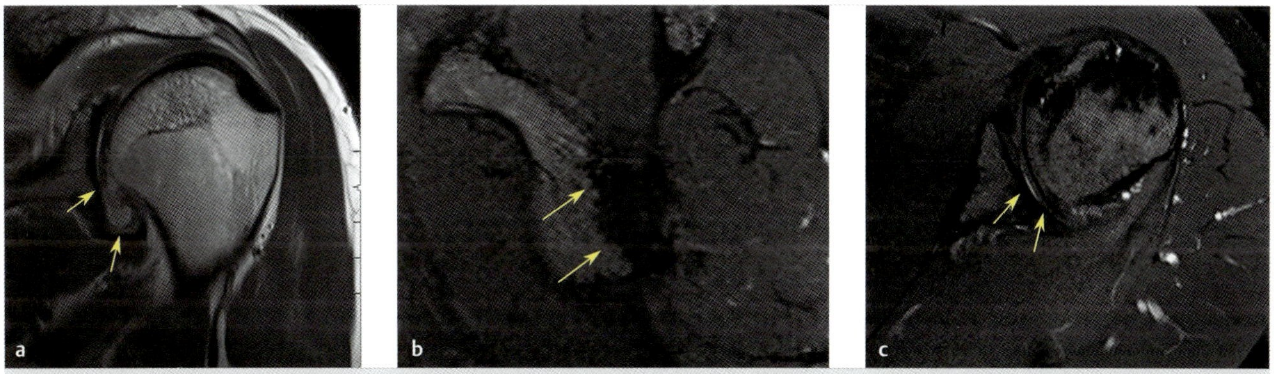

Fig. 7.7 **(a)** T1-weighted coronal image in an arthritic shoulder showing large inferior humeral head osteophyte (*yellow arrows*). **(b)** Sagittal T2-weighted image in same shoulder showing chondral wear of posterior glenoid (*yellow arrows*). **(c)** Axial T2-weighted images showing contact between humeral head and glenoid posteriorly with associated posterior glenoid wear (*yellow arrows*).

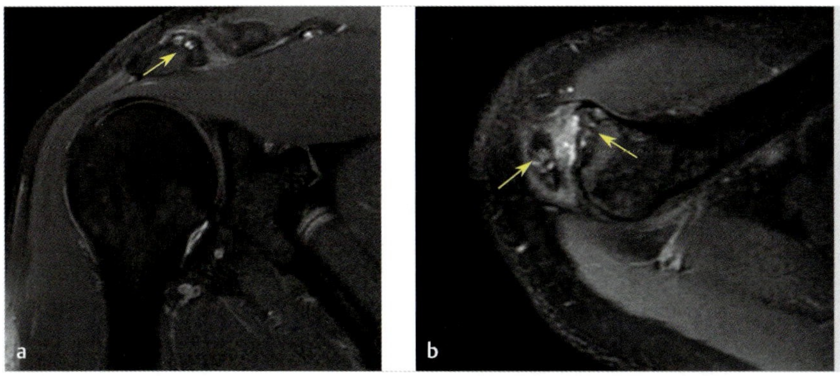

Fig. 7.8 **(a)** Coronal and **(b)** axial T2-weighted images showing acromioclavicular joint arthrosis, with joint hypertrophy and cystic change (*yellow arrows*).

7.5 Other Pathologic Conditions

7.5.1 Septic Arthritis

Septic arthritis of the shoulder is less common than septic arthritis of the hip and knee.[9,48] It can be difficult to diagnose because it often presents as vague pain that can be confused or initially misdiagnosed as a less serious subacromial bursitis, rotator cuff tendonitis, or adhesive capsulitis.[49] The confluence of symptoms can include pain (that increases with passive motion), decrease in range of motion, warmth and erythema, swelling, tenderness (typically diffuse), and fever.[49]

The work-up of a patient with possible septic arthritis of the shoulder includes radiographs, blood tests (C-reactive protein, erythrocyte sedimentation rate, and white blood cell count), laboratory analysis of joint-fluid aspirate, and a detailed history and physical examination. Patients with septic arthritis may have a history of recent shoulder surgery, injection, or illness and are typically older than 60 years. In a study of 18 patients with septic arthritis of the shoulder, 17 patients had at least 1 serious medical comorbidity, including alcoholism, cancer, diabetes, cardiac disease, cirrhosis, metabolic disease, neurologic impairment, or other infection.[49,50] Other risk factors include human immunodeficiency virus, history of intravenous drug abuse, and end-stage renal disease.[48]

Radiographs typically do not help in confirming the diagnosis of septic arthritis; however, they can aid in identifying preexisting conditions (e.g., glenohumeral arthritis, calcific tendonitis). MRI is a useful adjunct in the diagnosis and treatment of the septic shoulder. The septic shoulder typically shows a joint effusion, which can be assessed in all planes, and is best seen on T2-weighted and fat-suppressed T2-weighted MRI sequences.[51,52] Acutely, the findings that most correlate with septic arthritis are synovial enhancement, perisynovial edema, and joint effusion.[53] Postcontrast fat-suppressed T1-weighted images are helpful in evaluating for perisynovial edema and enhancement.[51] Edema within the humeral head and glenoid can also be seen in the acute stages. Chronic changes include glenoid or humeral head erosions, cartilage destruction, and with continued progression, subchondral edema and cyst formation.[51]

7.5.2 Adhesive Capsulitis

Adhesive capsulitis or "frozen shoulder" is a common condition. It classically presents in middle-aged women, diabetic patients, and patients with thyroid disorders. Patients typically present with pain that precedes progressive and global loss of glenohumeral range of motion. Unlike patients with rotator cuff tears who more typically present with decreased active range of motion and maintenance of passive range of motion, patients with adhesive capsulitis present with decreases in both active and passive range of motion, including forward elevation, abduction, and internal and external rotation.[17] Because the condition results from thickening, contracture, and inflammation of the capsule, MRI findings include thickening of the joint capsule and decreased contrast filling of the axillary pouch if MRA is obtained (▶ Fig. 7.9(a,b)).[50,54] In addition, a capsular thickness greater than 4 mm in the area of the axillary pouch, as measured on axial and coronal sequences, is often seen with this diagnosis.[55] Consistent with the physical examination finding of decreased external rotation, MRI findings can include scarring or narrowing of the rotator interval, which can be assessed on axial and coronal images.

7.5.3 Calcific Tendonitis

Similar to rotator cuff tendonitis or partial rotator cuff tears, calcific tendonitis can present as an acute or chronic painful condition of the shoulder. It can involve any of the rotator cuff tendons, most commonly the supraspinatus. Its clinical presentation is similar to that of other inflammatory conditions of the rotator cuff and includes laterally based pain that increases with overhead motion and activity, greater tuberosity tenderness, and sometimes weakness with strength testing of the rotator cuff in isolation. The intratendinous calcium deposit that characterizes the condition can be seen on conventional radiographs, typically medial to the rotator cuff footprint. MRI more clearly defines not only the specific tendon or tendons involved but also the size of the deposit (▶ Fig. 7.10). The approach to MRI review should be the same as in a patient with a rotator cuff tear, assessing the degree of involvement on coronal and sagittal images. On T1- and T2-weighted sequences, the calcium deposits are hypointense, and edema surrounding the deposits is seen as hyperintensity.

7.6 Postoperative MRI Findings

For various reasons, it is difficult to assess whether a rotator cuff tendon, labrum, or other repaired tissue has retorn after surgery. Some postoperative edema in bone and soft tissue is normal; artifact may be created by anchors or other implants; retears can be

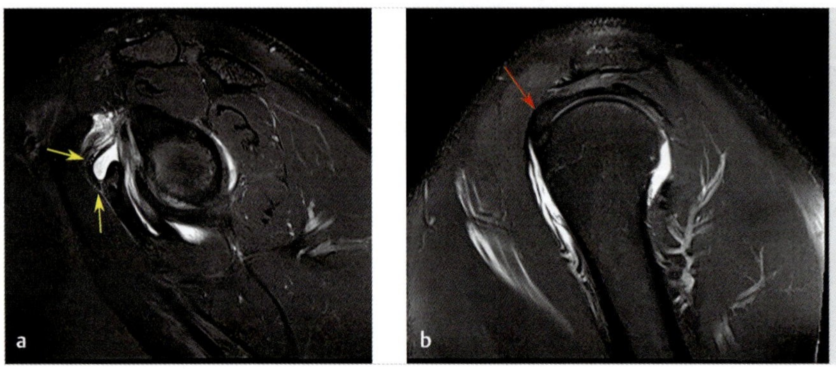

Fig. 7.9(a,b) Sagittal T1 fat saturated images post arthrography demonstrate synovial hypertrophy and synovitis seen in rotator cuff interval (*red arrow*) and subscapularis recess (*yellow arrows*).

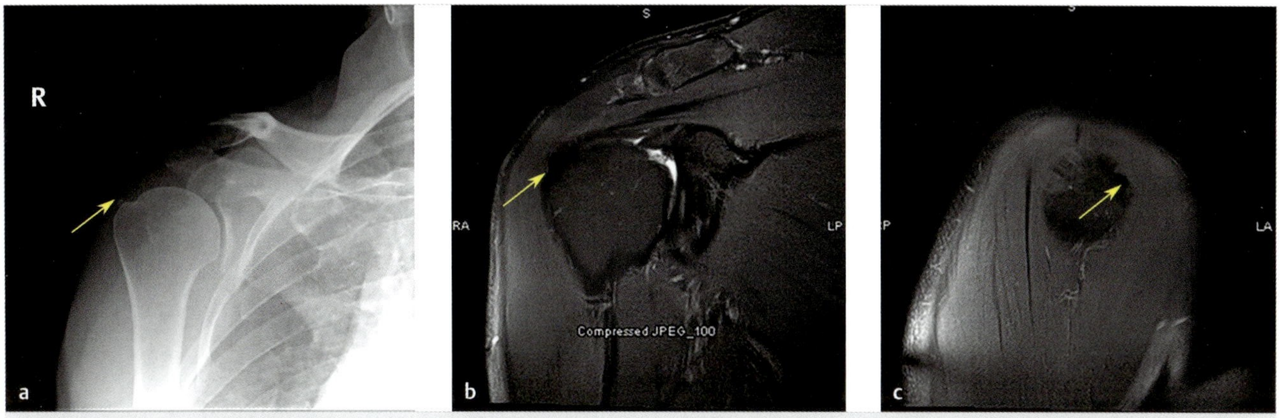

Fig. 7.10 **(a)** Plain radiograph of calcific tendonitis with typical hypointense appearance of the calcification (*yellow arrows*) on **(b)** coronal and **(c)** sagittal T2-weighted imaging.

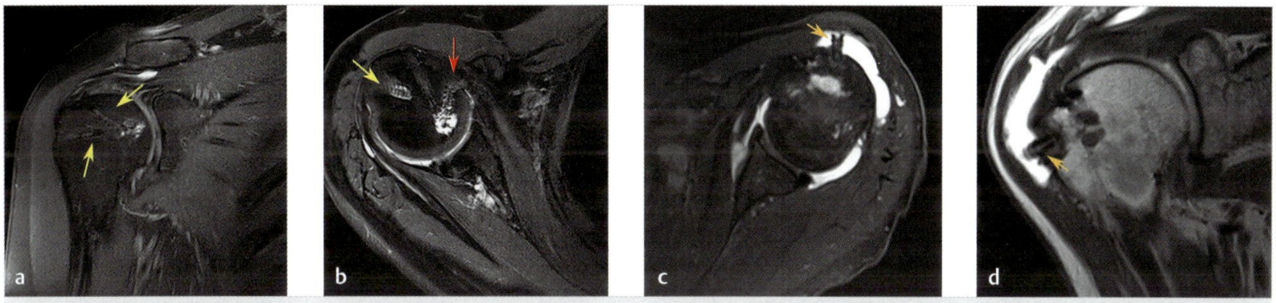

Fig. 7.11 **(a)** T2-weighted coronal image with evidence of previous double row rotator cuff repair with medial and lateral anchors in greater tuberosity (*yellow arrows*). **(b)** T2-weighted axial image showing anchors placed in greater tuberosity (*yellow anchor*) and evidence of subscapularis repair with anchors in the lesser tuberosity (*red arrow*). **(c)** Axial T2-weighted and **(d)** coronal T1-weighted images showing previous rotator cuff repair with anchor failure and pull-out (*yellow arrows*) into subacromial space.

difficult to distinguish from normal postsurgical appearance of healed tissue; and partially healed versus full-thickness rotator cuff retears can be difficult to distinguish (▶ Fig. 7.11).

There are several important tools to aid in the evaluation of the postoperative shoulder. First, one must have knowledge of the specifics of the operation performed. This allows a more accurate understanding not only of what was repaired but also where implants may have been placed and whether bone has been resected (e.g., distal clavicle excision). When available, a comparison of presurgical MRI or MRA is helpful. This allows comparison of the preoperative appearance of labral and rotator cuff tears with postoperative appearance. Challenges remain in determining the clinical relevance of an irregular appearance of a repaired tendon, including minor leakage of contrast (i.e., repair not watertight), the labrum appearing rounded but intact, as well as determining significance of fluid-like signal in the subacromial space.[56] In addition, some sequences such as spin-echo sequences tend to minimize the artifact.

Rotator cuff surgery is effective at relieving pain and, if the tendon heals, restoring function.[57,58,59] However, the retear rate after repair remains high.[58,60,61] Preoperative patient factors, tear size, number of tendons involved, amount of tendon retraction, muscle atrophy, and degree of fatty infiltration have been assessed as potential predictors of postsurgical retear. One study suggested that although MRI is sensitive for diagnosing a retear, its specificity is low. In an analysis of 37 shoulders in 33 patients with previous rotator cuff repairs who underwent revision surgery for presumed failed repair, Motamedi et al[62] found a sensitivity of 91% and a specificity of 25%. MRI correctly identified recurrent tears in 30 of 33 shoulders. However, of the four shoulders without retears, MRI was incorrectly interpreted as showing retear in three shoulders. Motamedi et al[62] concluded that, in addition to being inaccurate in diagnosing the size of retear, MRI may be associated with over diagnosis of recurrent tears in patients with symptoms consistent with retear. In this study and others, the criteria for recurrence of tear includes the absence of tendon or disruption of tendon morphology with the presence of a focal defect (tear) with high fluid signal intensity in T2-weighted imaging (coronal and sagittal views are most helpful).[16,56]

Similar to the assessment of the repaired rotator cuff tendon, the assessment of the postsurgical labrum can be challenging. Important aspects of the surgery, including repair of anterior, posterior, and superior labrum; open versus arthroscopic procedure; and use of bony augment are important to evaluate. The surgically repaired labrum loses some if its crisp, sharp edges, appearing somewhat blunted. The locations of the suture anchor tunnels, seen within the glenoid on axial, sagittal, and coronal T1-weighted images, are an obvious landmark for the site of labral repair (▶ Fig. 7.12). Thickening of the anterior or posterior capsule, depending on the site of repair, is also common.[56] However, the intact labral repair typically should not have fluid extravasation or linear high-intensity signal between the glenoid rim and labrum.

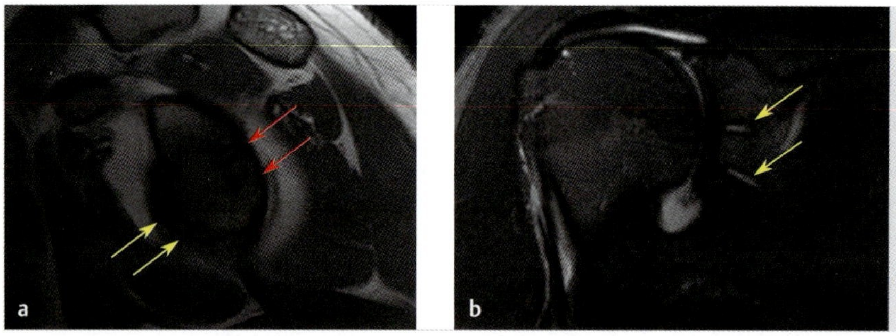

Fig. 7.12 **(a)** Sagittal T1-weighted image showing previous anterior and posterior labral repair with evidence of anchors placed anterior (*yellow arrows*) and posterior (*red arrows*). **(b)** Coronal T2-weighted image in the same patient showing anchors within the glenoid (*yellow arrows*).

Shoulder MRI after shoulder arthroplasty, including total arthroplasty and hemiarthroplasty, is substantially affected and subject to artifact. However, MRI remains helpful in the assessment of the integrity of the rotator cuff, which can play an important role in the clinical decision-making process in the setting of a failed or painful arthroplasty. In addition, in the case of hemiarthroplasty, it can allow assessment of the glenoid articular cartilage, which is important in the assessment of a patient with hemiarthroplasty who is experiencing persistent pain. Availability and implementation of metal artifact–reducing techniques and protocols also allow an accurate assessment of not only the soft-tissue structures (rotator cuff, deltoid, capsule) but also the implant itself, including loosening and osteolysis.[63]

7.7 Common Clinical Questions

1. A 22 year old male is in your office after sustaining a shoulder injury during a football game this week. What findings are evident on the T2 weighted axial MR image below?
   a) Full thickness subscapularis tear.
   b) Dislocated biceps tendon, with upper border subscapularis tear.
   c) Posterior labral tear.
   d) Anterior labral tear, with a Hill Sachs lesion of the humeral head.
   e) Pan labral tear.

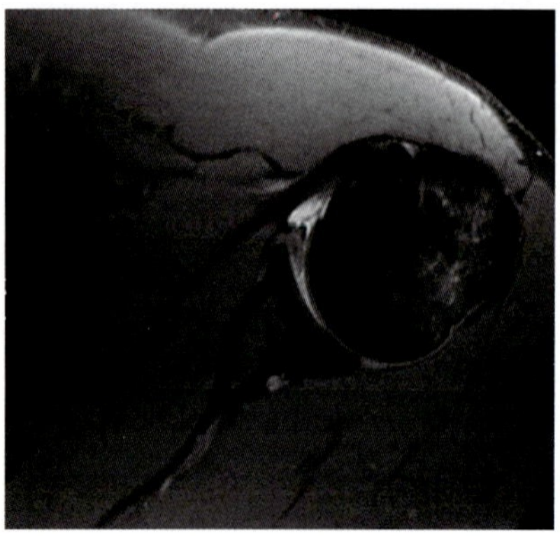

2. A 60-year-old male presents to your office with shoulder pain and overhead weakness. On examination, he has weakness in both abduction and external rotation, as well as positive provocative biceps maneuvers. Based on the T2 weight coronal and sagittal MR images below, what is his diagnosis?
   a) Full thickness supraspinatus tear.
   b) Full thickness infraspinatus tear.
   c) Full thickness subscapularis tear.
   d) Split tear of the long head of the biceps.
   e) Massive rotator cuff tear involving the teres minor

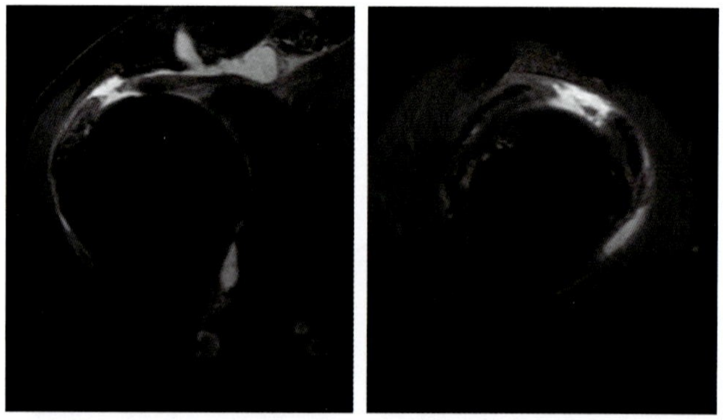

3. Based on the T1-weighted coronal MR image below, what physical examination finding would you expect based on the underlying diagnostic findings?
   a) Weakness in abduction as a result of full thickness supraspinatus tear.
   b) Pain and restricted range of motion based on glenohumeral arthritis.
   c) AC joint tenderness to palpation based on AC joint arthritis.
   d) Apprehension based on anterior labral tear.
   e) Positive liftoff based on subscapularis tear.

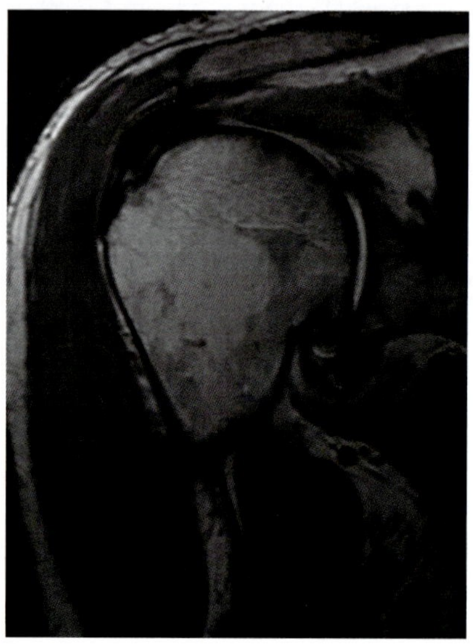

References

[1] Lyons RP, Green A. Subscapularis tendon tears. J Am Acad Orthop Surg. 2005; 13(5):353–363

[2] Mochizuki T, Sugaya H, Uomizu M, et al. Humeral insertion of the supraspinatus and infraspinatus. New anatomical findings regarding the footprint of the rotator cuff. J Bone Joint Surg Am. 2008; 90(5):962–969

[3] Goutallier D, Postel JM, Bernageau J, Lavau L, Voisin MC. Fatty muscle degeneration in cuff ruptures. Pre- and postoperative evaluation by CT scan. Clin Orthop Relat Res. 1994(304):78–83

[4] Urita A, Funakoshi T, Amano T, et al. Predictive factors of long head of the biceps tendon disorders: the bicipital groove morphology and subscapularis tendon tear. J Shoulder Elbow Surg. 2016; 25(3):384–389

[5] Razmjou H, Fournier-Gosselin S, Christakis M, Pennings A, ElMaraghy A, Holtby R. Accuracy of magnetic resonance imaging in detecting biceps pathology in patients with rotator cuff disorders: comparison with arthroscopy. J Shoulder Elbow Surg. 2016; 25(1):38–44

[6] Tuoheti Y, Itoi E, Minagawa H, et al. Attachment types of the long head of the biceps tendon to the glenoid labrum and their relationships with the glenohumeral ligaments. Arthroscopy. 2005; 21(10):1242–1249

[7] Williams MM, Snyder SJ, Buford D, Jr. The Buford complex—the "cord-like" middle glenohumeral ligament and absent anterosuperior labrum complex: a normal anatomic capsulolabral variant. Arthroscopy. 1994; 10 (3):241–247

[8] Taylor SA, O'Brien SJ. Clinically relevant anatomy and biomechanics of the proximal biceps. Clin Sports Med. 2016; 35(1):1–18

[9] Owens BD, Campbell SE, Cameron KL. Risk factors for anterior glenohumeral instability. Am J Sports Med. 2014; 42(11):2591–2596

[10] Wutke R, Fellner FA, Fellner C, Stangl R, Dobritz M, Bautz WA. Direct MR arthrography of the shoulder: 2D vs. 3D gradient-echo imaging. Magn Reson Imaging. 2001; 19(9):1183–1191

[11] Boileau P, Walch G. The three-dimensional geometry of the proximal humerus. Implications for surgical technique and prosthetic design. J Bone Joint Surg Br. 1997; 79(5):857–865

[12] Iannotti JP, Gabriel JP, Schneck SL, Evans BG, Misra S. The normal glenohumeral relationships. An anatomical study of one hundred and forty shoulders. J Bone Joint Surg Am. 1992; 74(4):491–500

[13] Connell DA, Potter HG, Wickiewicz TL, Altchek DW, Warren RF. Noncontrast magnetic resonance imaging of superior labral lesions. 102 cases confirmed at arthroscopic surgery. Am J Sports Med. 1999; 27(2):208–213

[14] Vangsness CT, Jr, Jorgenson SS, Watson T, Johnson DL. The origin of the long head of the biceps from the scapula and glenoid labrum. An anatomical study of 100 shoulders. J Bone Joint Surg Br. 1994; 76(6):951–954

[15] Jee WH, McCauley TR, Katz LD, Matheny JM, Ruwe PA, Daigneault JP. Superior labral anterior posterior (SLAP) lesions of the glenoid labrum: reliability and accuracy of MR arthrography for diagnosis. Radiology. 2001; 218(1):127–132

[16] Murthi AM, Ramirez MA. Shoulder dislocation in the older patient. J Am Acad Orthop Surg. 2012; 20(10):615–622

[17] Neviaser RJ, Neviaser TJ, Neviaser JS. Concurrent rupture of the rotator cuff and anterior dislocation of the shoulder in the older patient. J Bone Joint Surg Am. 1988; 70(9):1308–1311

[18] Amin MF, Youssef AO. The diagnostic value of magnetic resonance arthrography of the shoulder in detection and grading of SLAP lesions: comparison with arthroscopic findings. Eur J Radiol. 2012; 81(9):2343–2347

[19] Snyder SJ, Karzel RP, Del Pizzo W, Ferkel RD, Friedman MJ. SLAP lesions of the shoulder. Arthroscopy. 1990; 6(4):274–279

[20] Maffet MW, Gartsman GM, Moseley B. Superior labrum-biceps tendon complex lesions of the shoulder. Am J Sports Med. 1995; 23(1):93–98

[21] Snyder SJ, Banas MP, Karzel RP. An analysis of 140 injuries to the superior glenoid labrum. J Shoulder Elbow Surg. 1995; 4(4):243–248

[22] Krøner K, Lind T, Jensen J. The epidemiology of shoulder dislocations. Arch Orthop Trauma Surg. 1989; 108(5):288–290

[23] Bankart ASB. Recurrent or habitual dislocation of the shoulder-joint. BMJ. 1923; 2(3285):1132–1133

[24] Walz DM, Burge AJ, Steinbach L. Imaging of shoulder instability. Semin Musculoskelet Radiol. 2015; 19(3):254–268

[25] Neviaser TJ. The anterior labroligamentous periosteal sleeve avulsion lesion: a cause of anterior instability of the shoulder. Arthroscopy. 1993; 9(1):17–21

[26] Neviaser TJ. The GLAD lesion: another cause of anterior shoulder pain. Arthroscopy. 1993; 9(1):22–23

[27] Burkhart SS, De Beer JF. Traumatic glenohumeral bone defects and their relationship to failure of arthroscopic Bankart repairs: significance of the inverted-pear glenoid and the humeral engaging Hill-Sachs lesion. Arthroscopy. 2000; 16(7):677–694

[28] Lo IKY, Parten PM, Burkhart SS. The inverted pear glenoid: an indicator of significant glenoid bone loss. Arthroscopy. 2004; 20(2):169–174

[29] Gyftopoulos S, Yemin A, Mulholland T, et al. 3DMR osseous reconstructions of the shoulder using a gradient-echo based two-point Dixon reconstruction: a feasibility study. Skeletal Radiol. 2013; 42(3):347–352

[30] Markenstein JE, Jaspars KC, van der Hulst VP, Willems WJ. The quantification of glenoid bone loss in anterior shoulder instability; MR-arthro compared to 3D-CT. Skeletal Radiol. 2014; 43(4):475–483

[31] Gyftopoulos S, Carpenter E, Kazam J, Babb J, Bencardino J. MR imaging of subscapularis tendon injury in the setting of anterior shoulder dislocation. Skeletal Radiol. 2012; 41(11):1445–1452

[32] Kim SH, Ha KI, Yoo JC, Noh KC. Kim's lesion: an incomplete and concealed avulsion of the posteroinferior labrum in posterior or multidirectional posteroinferior instability of the shoulder. Arthroscopy. 2004; 20(7): 712–720

[33] Kim SH, Noh KC, Park JS, Ryu BD, Oh I. Loss of chondrolabral containment of the glenohumeral joint in atraumatic posteroinferior multidirectional instability. J Bone Joint Surg Am. 2005; 87(1):92–98

[34] Yamaguchi K, Ditsios K, Middleton WD, Hildebolt CF, Galatz LM, Teefey SA. The demographic and morphological features of rotator cuff disease. A comparison of asymptomatic and symptomatic shoulders. J Bone Joint Surg Am. 2006; 88(8):1699–1704

[35] Neer CS, II. Anterior acromioplasty for the chronic impingement syndrome in the shoulder: a preliminary report. J Bone Joint Surg Am. 1972; 54(1):41–50

[36] Bigliani LU, Ticker JB, Flatow EL, Soslowsky LJ, Mow VC. The relationship of acromial architecture to rotator cuff disease. Clin Sports Med. 1991; 10(4): 823–838

[37] Kassarjian A, Bencardino JT, Palmer WE. MR imaging of the rotator cuff. Radiol Clin North Am. 2006; 44(4):503–523, vii–viii

[38] Schaeffeler C, Mueller D, Kirchhoff C, Wolf P, Rummeny EJ, Woertler K. Tears at the rotator cuff footprint: prevalence and imaging characteristics in 305 MR arthrograms of the shoulder. Eur Radiol. 2011; 21(7):1477–1484

[39] Vinson EN, Helms CA, Higgins LD. Rim-rent tear of the rotator cuff: a common and easily overlooked partial tear. AJR Am J Roentgenol. 2007; 189(4):943–946

[40] Schiefer M, Mendonça R, Magnanini MM, et al. Intraobserver and interobserver agreement of Goutallier classification applied to magnetic resonance images. J Shoulder Elbow Surg. 2015; 24(8):1314–1321

[41] Ellman H. Diagnosis and treatment of incomplete rotator cuff tears. Clin Orthop Relat Res. 1990(254):64–74

[42] Adams CR, Brady PC, Koo SS, et al. A systematic approach for diagnosing subscapularis tendon tears with preoperative magnetic resonance imaging scans. Arthroscopy. 2012; 28(11):1592–1600

[43] Iannotti JP, Norris TR. Influence of preoperative factors on outcome of shoulder arthroplasty for glenohumeral osteoarthritis. J Bone Joint Surg Am. 2003; 85(2):251–258

[44] Nyffeler RW, Jost B, Pfirrmann CW, Gerber C. Measurement of glenoid version: conventional radiographs versus computed tomography scans. J Shoulder Elbow Surg. 2003; 12(5):493–496

[45] Raymond AC, McCann PA, Sarangi PP. Magnetic resonance scanning vs axillary radiography in the assessment of glenoid version for osteoarthritis. J Shoulder Elbow Surg. 2013; 22(8):1078–1083

[46] Stein BES, Wiater JM, Pfaff HC, Bigliani LU, Levine WN. Detection of acromioclavicular joint pathology in asymptomatic shoulders with magnetic resonance imaging. J Shoulder Elbow Surg. 2001; 10(3):204–208

[47] Shubin Stein BE, Ahmad CS, Pfaff CH, Bigliani LU, Levine WN. A comparison of magnetic resonance imaging findings of the acromioclavicular joint in symptomatic versus asymptomatic patients. J Shoulder Elbow Surg. 2006; 15 (1):56–59

[48] Cleeman E, Auerbach JD, Klingenstein GG, Flatow EL. Septic arthritis of the glenohumeral joint: a review of 23 cases. J Surg Orthop Adv. 2005; 14(2): 102–107

[49] Leslie BM, Harris JM, III, Driscoll D. Septic arthritis of the shoulder in adults. J Bone Joint Surg Am. 1989; 71(10):1516–1522

[50] Lee MH, Ahn JM, Muhle C, et al. Adhesive capsulitis of the shoulder: diagnosis using magnetic resonance arthrography, with arthroscopic findings as the standard. J Comput Assist Tomogr. 2003; 27(6):901–906
[51] Sussmann AR, Cohen J, Nomikos GC, Schweitzer ME. Magnetic resonance imaging of shoulder arthropathies. Magn Reson Imaging Clin N Am. 2012; 20 (2):349–371, xi–xii
[52] Weishaupt D, Schweitzer ME. MR imaging of septic arthritis and rheumatoid arthritis of the shoulder. Magn Reson Imaging Clin N Am. 2004; 12(1):111–124, vii
[53] Karchevsky M, Schweitzer ME, Morrison WB, Parellada JA. MRI findings of septic arthritis and associated osteomyelitis in adults. AJR Am J Roentgenol. 2004; 182(1):119–122
[54] Sofka CM, Ciavarra GA, Hannafin JA, Cordasco FA, Potter HG. Magnetic resonance imaging of adhesive capsulitis: correlation with clinical staging. HSS J. 2008; 4(2):164–169
[55] Emig EW, Schweitzer ME, Karasick D, Lubowitz J. Adhesive capsulitis of the shoulder: MR diagnosis. AJR Am J Roentgenol. 1995; 164(6): 1457–1459
[56] Zanetti M, Hodler J. MR imaging of the shoulder after surgery. Magn Reson Imaging Clin N Am. 2004; 12(1):169–183, viii
[57] Baker CL, Liu SH. Comparison of open and arthroscopically assisted rotator cuff repairs. Am J Sports Med. 1995; 23(1):99–104
[58] Bishop J, Klepps S, Lo IK, Bird J, Gladstone JN, Flatow EL. Cuff integrity after arthroscopic versus open rotator cuff repair: a prospective study. J Shoulder Elbow Surg. 2006; 15(3):290–299
[59] Wolf EM, Pennington WT, Agrawal V. Arthroscopic rotator cuff repair: 4- to 10-year results. Arthroscopy. 2004; 20(1):5–12
[60] Lindley K, Jones GL. Outcomes of arthroscopic versus open rotator cuff repair: a systematic review of the literature. Am J Orthop. 2010; 39(12): 592–600
[61] Youm T, Murray DH, Kubiak EN, Rokito AS, Zuckerman JD. Arthroscopic versus mini-open rotator cuff repair: a comparison of clinical outcomes and patient satisfaction. J Shoulder Elbow Surg. 2005; 14(5):455–459
[62] Motamedi AR, Urrea LH, Hancock RE, Hawkins RJ, Ho C. Accuracy of magnetic resonance imaging in determining the presence and size of recurrent rotator cuff tears. J Shoulder Elbow Surg. 2002; 11(1):6–10
[63] Koff MF, Shah P, Potter HG. Clinical implementation of MRI of joint arthroplasty. AJR Am J Roentgenol. 2014; 203(1):154–161

Answers to Common Clinical Questions

1. Answer: d. Anterior labral tear, with a Hill Sachs lesion of the humeral head.
2. Answer: a. Full thickness supraspinatus tear.
3. Answer: b. Pain and restricted range of motion based on glenohumeral arthritis.

8 The Elbow

Ariel A. Williams, Lance M. Brunton, Mark W. Anderson, and A. Bobby Chhabra

Abstract

The elbow is affected by a wide variety of degenerative, traumatic, inflammatory, and other Orthopaedic conditions, and magnetic resonance imaging (MRI) is often employed to guide diagnosis and treatment. This chapter presents a systematic approach to viewing and interpreting these studies. The role of MRI in evaluating common traumatic, degenerative and other elbow conditions is reviewed, and important MRI findings are described, with clinical correlation provided throughout.

Keywords: arthritis, magnetic resonance imaging, elbow abnormalities, elbow anatomy, elbow injuries

8.1 Normal Anatomy

8.1.1 Coronal Anatomy

The elbow comprises three joints: the radiocapitellar, ulnohumeral, and proximal radioulnar joints, all of which can be clearly visualized on the coronal view. Flexion and extension occur through the radiocapitellar and ulnohumeral joint whereas pronation and supination occur through the radiocapitellar and radioulnar joints.

The important ligamentous structures of the elbow are the medial and lateral collateral ligament (LCL) complexes (▶ Fig. 8.1). The medial collateral ligament (MCL) complex is seen on the coronal images as a vertically oriented, uniformly low-signal-intensity structure coursing between the medial epicondyle and the sublime tubercle. It has anterior, posterior, and transverse bundles. The anterior bundle is the most important stabilizer against valgus stress and is divided into the anterior band, the primary restraint in extension, and the posterior band, the primary restraint in flexion. The posterior bundle serves as a secondary restraint in flexion, while the transverse bundle makes minimal contribution to elbow stability. The LCL complex is a Y-shaped structure comprising the lateral ulnar collateral ligament (LUCL), the radial collateral ligament (RCL), and the annular ligament. There is some variability in normal anatomy of the LCL complex, and a fourth component, the accessory LCL, is also sometimes present.[1] The LUCLs and RCLs are seen on coronal images, both originating from the lateral epicondyle.[2] The LUCL descends obliquely from the lateral epicondyle to insert more posteriorly onto the ulna's supinator crest. The RCL comes down vertically to insert onto the annular ligament and supinator fascia. The annular ligament is best seen on axial and sagittal sections. By virtue of its Y-shape, the entire RCL complex contributes to lateral elbow stability.[3] However, the LUCL has long been felt to be the primary restraint to posterolateral rotatory instability.

The common extensor origin arises from the lateral epicondyle proximal to the LCL complex. It gives rise to the extensor carpi radialis brevis, extensor digitorum, communis, and extensor carpi ulnaris muscles. The extensor carpi radialis longus originates proximal to the common extensor origin at the distal supracondylar ridge. The common flexor origin arises from the medial epicondyle. It gives rise to the flexor carpi radialis, palmaris longus, flexor carpi ulnaris, flexor digitorum superficial humeroulnar head, and pronator teres. Distally, its fibers may appear confluent with the proximal MCL complex.

8.1.2 Sagittal Anatomy

The radiocapitellar and ulnohumeral joints are both observed on the sagittal images. The annular ligament can be appreciated as a ringlike structure encircling the radial head and stabilizing the proximal radioulnar joint.[4] On the posterior capitellum, a small depression is sometimes found. This "pseudodefect of the capitellum" is a normal variant and should not be confused for

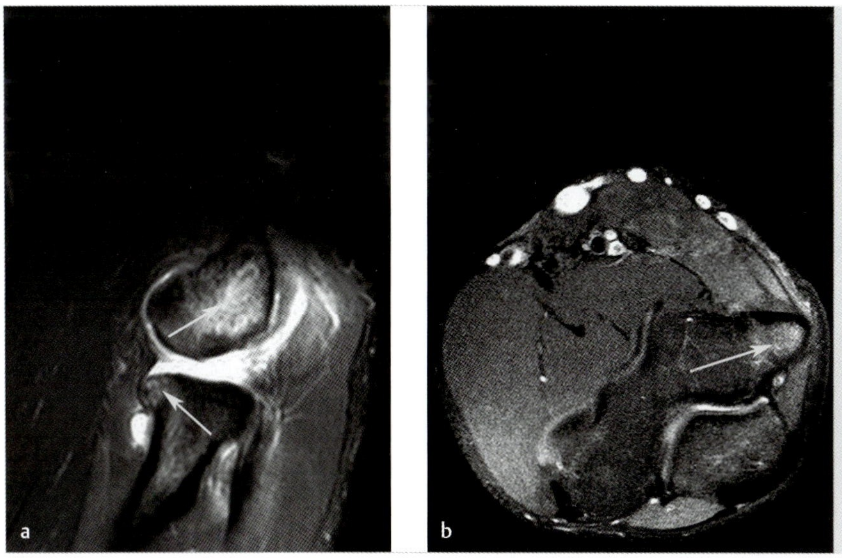

Fig. 8.1 Osseous injury. **(a)** Bone contusions. A sagittal short tau inversion recovery (STIR) image reveals high signal intensity within the capitellum and radial head, indicative of marrow edema (*arrows*). No discrete low signal fracture lines are evident. **(b)** Epiphysiolysis (Little Leaguer elbow). An axial STIR image of the right elbow showing diffuse high signal intensity within the medial epicondyle consistent with epiphysiolysis from repetitive valgus stress to the elbow (*arrow*). (Part **a**: Reproduced with permission from Brunton LM, Anderson MW, Pannunzio ME, Khanna AJ, Chhabra AB. Magnetic resonance imaging of the elbow: update on current techniques and indications. J Hand Surg Am 2006;31:1001–1011.) (Part **b**: Reproduced with permission from Brunton LM, Anderson MW, Chhabra AB. The Elbow. In: Khanna AJ, ed. MRI for orthopaedic surgeons. New York: Thieme; 2010:118–128.)

a chondral injury.[5] Although the ulnohumeral joint can also be seen on the coronal views, the articulation between the olecranon and olecranon fossa can be more clearly seen here on the sagittal as well as on the axial images.

The triceps tendon inserts onto the olecranon posterior to the elbow joint. It has three heads (medial, long, and lateral). On magnetic resonance imaging (MRI), the long and lateral head have a shared tendinous insertion that can be distinguished from the deeper and primarily muscular insertion of the medial head.[6] The biceps tendon inserts onto the radial tuberosity and onto the bicipital aponeurosis, a broad sheath of tissue that extends from the myotendinous junction to the antecubital fossa. Although the biceps tendon can usually be clearly identified on sagittal and axial images, the insertion into the bicipital aponeurosis can be difficult to visualize. The brachialis muscle can be seen deep to the biceps inserting onto the coronoid process and ulnar tuberosity.

8.1.3 Axial Anatomy

The axial sections allow excellent visualization of the radial head, the radioulnar joint, and the articulation between the olecranon and olecranon fossa. The common extensor and flexor origins are observed in cross-section as they arise from the lateral and medial epicondyles, respectively. The anconeus muscle is seen arising from the posterior aspect of the lateral epicondyle, coursing adjacent to the extensor carpi ulnaris and inserting onto the posterior ulna.[2] The triceps inserts onto the olecranon just proximal to the anconeus. Anteriorly, the biceps tendon inserts onto the radial tuberosity and the brachialis muscle lies deep to this. The brachialis's dual insertion is most clearly visualized on this view.[7]

The major nerves are best seen on the axial sections and can be traced along their lengths. The ulnar nerve lies posterior to the medial epicondyle where it courses through the cubital tunnel, the floor of which is formed by the MCL. It is the most easily visualized nerve due to its surrounding perineural fat. It then enters the forearm between the two heads of the flexor carpi ulnaris. The median nerve runs through the cubital fossa, medial to the brachial artery and biceps tendon. It then enters the forearm between the two heads of the pronator teres. The radial nerve travels adjacent to the lateral head of the triceps. It passes between the brachialis and brachioradialis, anterior to the lateral epicondyle, and after crossing the elbow joint, it gives rise to its terminal branches, the superficial sensory branch, and the posterior interosseous nerve.

8.2 Specialized Pulse Sequences and Imaging Protocols

MRI of the elbow has improved with the development of high-field systems and enhanced surface coil technology.[8] Most centers image the elbow with the patient in the supine position and the arm comfortably positioned at the patient's side, with the elbow in full extension. This position limits rotation of the proximal radioulnar joint with respect to the distal humerus and minimizes motion artifact. Alternatively, the patient can be positioned in the "Superman" position, prone with the arm over the head and the elbow extended. This position is less comfortable for the patient but places the elbow more centrally in the bore, which improves the signal-to-noise ratio and may sometimes be more feasible than supine positioning in larger patients who have difficulty fitting in the scanner.[9,10] Axial, coronal, and sagittal images are obtained routinely.

Most centers use a standard screening examination, consisting of an array of specified imaging planes and pulse sequences.[11] In addition to standard T1-weighted and T2-weighted images, fat-suppressed T2-weighted and short tau inversion recovery (STIR) sequences are extremely sensitive for detecting marrow and soft-tissue pathology by accentuating the increased signal of fluid and edema relative to the surrounding structures. These sequences are acquired with a fast spin-echo (FSE) technique that produces the desired contrast in a fraction of the time needed for conventional T2-weighted sequences. Gradient-echo sequences are often used to evaluate ligaments and articular cartilage (see Chapter 1, Essentials of MRI Physics and Pulse Sequences) and to delineate loose bodies in the elbow joint. However, these sequences should be avoided after elbow surgery (especially in the presence of metal hardware) because of the increased artifact inherent to the gradient-echo technique (see Chapter 1, Essentials of MRI Physics and Pulse Sequences). A proton-density pulse sequence is occasionally used, often with fat suppression, and combines characteristics of T1-weighted and T2-weighted images. FSE pulse sequences have substantially reduced the length of examination, a great benefit for claustrophobic patients. Imaging parameters can be refined additionally for optimal cartilage visualization when indicated (see Chapter 5, Articular Cartilage).[12]

MR arthrography is performed by injecting approximately 5 to 10 mL of diluted gadolinium contrast agent into the radiocapitellar joint from a lateral approach and acquiring fat-suppressed T1-weighted and T2-weighted images.[13] Although somewhat controversial, MR arthrography of the elbow may help evaluate undersurface collateral ligament tears, capsular disruption, osteochondritis dissecans (OCD), and intra-articular loose bodies. When investigating infectious, neoplastic, or synovial disorders involving the elbow, intravenous gadolinium is often used to evaluate for synovial hypertrophy or enhancement of pathologic tissues. Intravenous contrast is also useful for detecting soft tissue abscesses, which show a thick, enhancing wall surrounding the nonenhancing central fluid. Additional refinement of conventional MRI pulse sequences may eventually render these invasive techniques obsolete.[14]

8.3 Systematic Approach to Image Review

Coronal, sagittal, and axial views should all be examined including T1, T2, and any specialized sequences. T2-weighted images are reviewed first to look for abnormal regions of increased T2-weighted signal intensity. Findings from T2-weighted images are then correlated with T1-weighted images to allow better evaluation of anatomic detail. A systematic, structure-by-structure approach is utilized to evaluate for specific pathology. The bony structures are evaluated for the presence of stress reactions, occult fractures, evidence of infection or neoplasia, or, in the skeletally immature, apophyseal or physeal injury. Joint congruity is evaluated and osteophytes and joint space collapse are noted. The cartilage and subchondral bone are evaluated for localized or diffuse chondral injuries, OCD lesions, or erosive change. The synovium and synovial fluid should also be examined. The presence of an effusion should be noted, as well as any loose bodies or suggestion of atypical synovial proliferation. The ligamentous structures are inspected carefully. Abnormal signal intensity or frank discontinuity is strongly suggestive of partial or complete ligament injury. MR arthrogram may also show contrast extravasation. The common flexor and extensor origins are evaluated for tendinosis or tearing. Similarly, the biceps, triceps, and brachialis tendons are examined to look for abnormal signal intensity and partial or complete rupture. The adjacent soft tissues should be examined for abnormal fluid collections or masses. Finally, the major nerves should be traced down their length to evaluate for compression or signal changes.

8.4 Traumatic Conditions

Most patients with elbow trauma may be evaluated and treated adequately without the use of advanced imaging. However, for select patients, MRI may facilitate the diagnosis of suspected occult fractures, loose bodies, ligamentous injuries, and tendinous pathology.

8.4.1 Occult Fractures

Conventional radiographs often are unrevealing in a patient presenting with elbow pain after acute trauma. In this setting, a joint effusion is often detected clinically, and an elevated posterior fat pad sign may be evident on conventional radiographs. Prospective studies in adults and children have shown that the presence of a posterior fat pad sign correlates with an occult fracture in more than 75% of patients.[15,16] However, localizing the injury is a challenging endeavor, and patients often may be overtreated with immobilization in the absence of advanced imaging.

MRI may be used in the setting of elbow trauma to localize and characterize osseous injury when conventional radiographs are unrevealing or equivocal. Fat-suppressed T2-weighted (or STIR) pulse sequences are the most sensitive images for detecting radiographically occult traumatic or stress fractures. Fractures show a linear pattern of signal change on T1-weighted (decreased signal) or T2-weighted (increased signal) images, whereas an osseous contusion often has a more nonspecific appearance (▶ Fig. 8.1a). The most frequent site of occult fracture is the radial head; other sites, such as the lateral epicondyle or olecranon, are much less common.[16] The radial head fractures may be accompanied by associated injuries that are most effectively detected by MRI, such as ligament or capsular disruptions, OCD, loose bodies, or capitellar bone contusions.[17] Olecranon stress fractures can be seen in throwing athletes, possibly as a result of valgus extension overload, and may be accompanied with associated injuries such as MCL injuries and, in skeletally immature patients, medial epicondyle avulsion fractures.[18]

In children with a traumatic injury to the elbow and radiographic evidence of only a joint effusion, MRI is a sensitive and accurate modality for identifying or excluding an occult fracture.[19] MRI reveals a broad spectrum of elbow pathology in this setting, including the following[20]:

- Bone bruises.
- Ligamentous disruptions.
- Muscle injury.

MRI also may be effective in evaluating pediatric physeal injuries, especially in young children with poorly visualized ossification centers.[21] Finally, MRI has a role in the detection of Little Leaguer elbow, a valgus stress injury in skeletally immature throwing athletes in which epiphysiolysis occurs at the medial epicondylar apophysis (▶ Fig. 8.1b).[22]

8.4.2 Loose Bodies

The clinical manifestation of loose bodies within the elbow joint is typically pain with motion, often accompanied by mechanical symptoms, such as catching or locking. Loose bodies may originate from a traumatic shear injury to the osteochondral surface, synovial disorders, or OCD. The definitive treatment of symptomatic loose bodies is arthroscopic or open removal, but accurate diagnosis is imperative to prevent unnecessary surgery.

Although conventional radiographs or CT may detect the presence of osseous loose bodies in the elbow joint, MRI is especially useful for detecting intra-articular cartilaginous or osteocartilaginous loose bodies. Loose bodies are found most commonly in the olecranon or coronoid fossae on T2-weighted images (▶ Fig. 8.2). Osteophytes and synovial hypertrophy may mimic loose bodies on MRI images.[11] The use of MRI for detecting loose bodies in the elbow has been disputed, and an overall

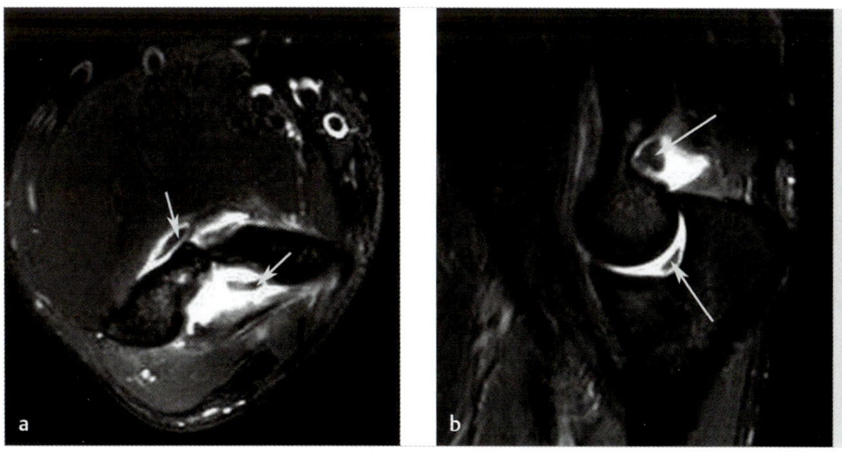

Fig. 8.2 Axial (a) and sagittal (b) T2-weighted images showing loose bodies in the coronoid and olecranon fossae and in the trochlear ulnar joint (*arrows on each*). (Reproduced with permission from Brunton LM, Anderson MW, Pannunzio ME, Khanna AJ, Chhabra AB. Magnetic resonance imaging of the elbow: update on current techniques and indications. J Hand Surg Am 2006;31:1001–1011.)

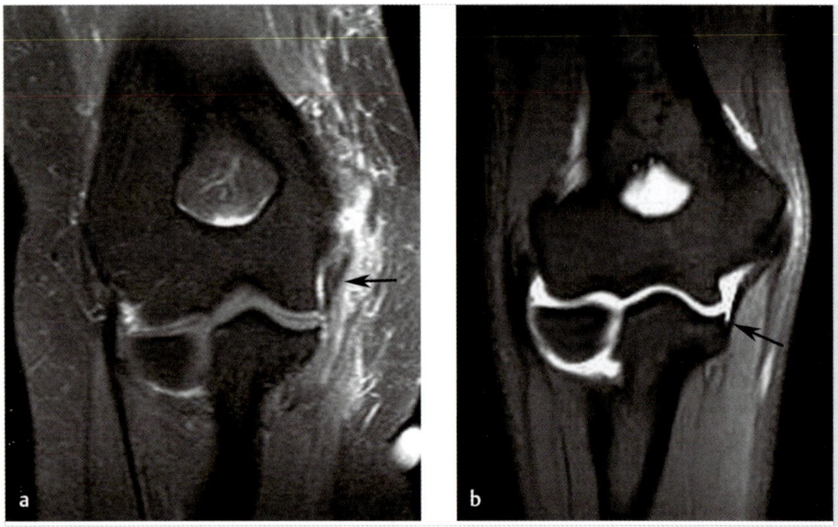

Fig. 8.3 Medial collateral ligament (MCL) injury of the right elbow. **(a)** A coronal fat-suppressed T2-weighted image showing discontinuity (complete tear) of the MCL with surrounding edema and hemorrhage (*arrow*). **(b)** A coronal fat-suppressed T1-weighted arthrogram showing a partial tear of the MCL as a "T-sign" with leakage of intra-articular contrast at the undersurface of the MCL at its distal insertion on the sublime tubercle (*arrow*). (Part **a**: Reproduced with permission from Brunton LM, Anderson MW, Pannunzio ME, Khanna AJ, Chhabra AB. Magnetic resonance imaging of the elbow: update on current techniques and indications. J Hand Surg Am 2006;31:1001–1011.) (Part **b**: Reproduced with permission from Brunton LM, Anderson MW, Chhabra AB. The Elbow. In: Khanna AJ, ed. MRI for orthopaedic surgeons. New York: Thieme; 2010:118–128.)

low specificity and sensitivity, similar to that of conventional radiography, when compared with arthroscopic findings have been reported.[23] MR arthrography may be effective in this setting, but it has not been studied adequately.

8.4.3 MCL Injury

MCL injuries have received tremendous attention because of their prevalence in throwing athletes of all ages and at all levels of competition. Accurate diagnosis of a full-thickness or partial-thickness tear of the MCL has important implications for treatment, as does the differentiation between MCL pathology and other causes of medial-side elbow pain, such as ulnar neuropathy, stress fracture, and flexor-pronator mass injury.

Full-thickness tears of the anterior bundle of the MCL can be detected accurately by MRI. The abnormalities detectable by MRI include ligament attenuation, redundancy, or discontinuity. Increased signal intensity often is found within and adjacent to the ligament on fat-suppressed T2-weighted images, indicating edema or hemorrhage (▶ Fig. 8.3a).[14] MRI is less reliable for detecting partial-thickness tears, but the addition of intra-articular contrast may improve its sensitivity (▶ Fig. 8.3b).[24,25] Other findings related to chronic MCL insufficiency are not unusual. These include adjacent muscle edema, ulnar neuritis, and chondral injuries of the radiocapitellar joint. Signs of posteromedial elbow impingement may also be present, including posterior trochlea and anterior olecranon chondrosis and marginal osteophytes of the trochlea and olecranon.[14,26]

8.4.4 LCL Complex Injury

Injury to the lateral ligamentous complex from an acute elbow dislocation may lead to chronic mechanical symptoms or recurrent instability when early treatment is inadequate. Tears of the LUCL and RCL are common in acute elbow dislocations. Chronic insufficiency of the LUCL is believed to lead to posterolateral rotatory instability, which is often difficult to diagnose clinically.[27]

The ability of MRI to visualize tears of the LCL complex has been historically less dependable, especially in patients with chronic instability.[28] One study of asymptomatic individuals revealed inconsistent MRI signal characteristics within the

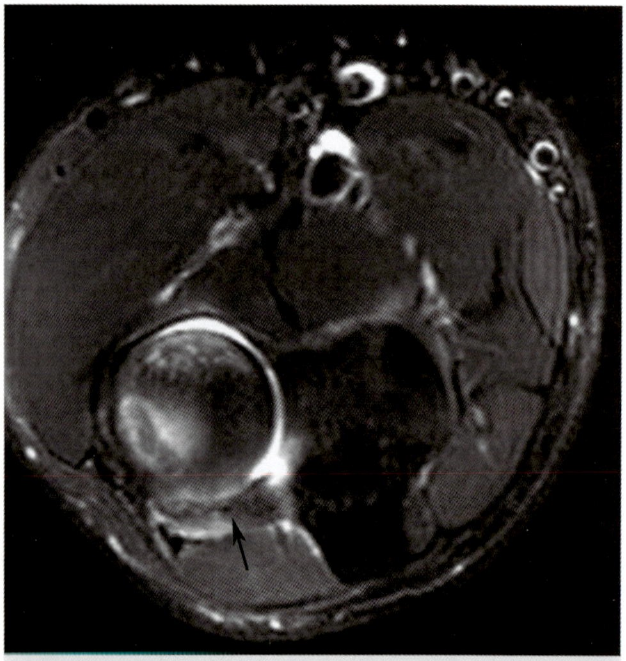

Fig. 8.4 An axial T2-weighted image of the right elbow showing thickening and abnormal signal (sprain vs. partial tear) of the lateral ulnar collateral ligament (LUCL) with adjacent high signal intensity edema posterior to the radial head (*arrow*). (Adapted with permission from Brunton LM, Anderson MW, Pannunzio ME, Khanna AJ, Chhabra AB. Magnetic resonance imaging of the elbow: update on current techniques and indications. J Hand Surg Am 2006;31:1001–1011.)

LUCL.[29] Other investigators, however, have found MRI to be effective in detecting abnormalities of the LUCL in the setting of posterolateral rotatory instability when 3D gradient-echo and FSE sequences were used.[30] Findings are similar to those seen in MCL injuries, with combinations of ligament attenuation, redundancy, and/or discontinuity evident on coronal or axial images (▶ Fig. 8.4).[21] MR arthrography may show contrast extravasation through complete LUCL tears but has not been well studied in this setting.[31] MRI also demonstrates increased radiocapitellar and ulnohumeral joint incongruity in some patients with instability.[32]

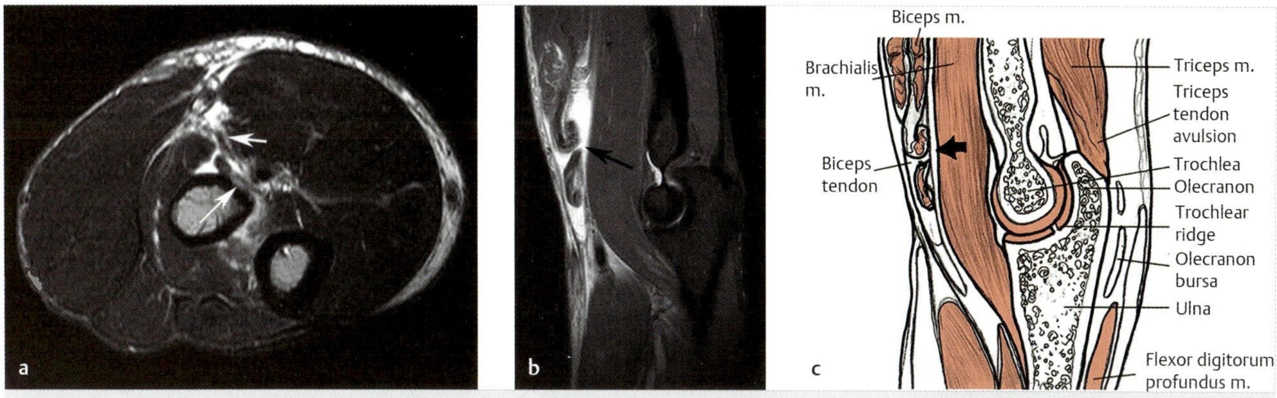

Fig. 8.5 Distal biceps tendon injury. **(a)** An axial T2-weighted image of the right elbow showing the ruptured and retracted distal biceps tendon (*arrows*) with associated surrounding edema and hematoma. **(b)** A sagittal T2-weighted image showing a complete tear of the biceps tendon with prominent edema and hemorrhage surrounding the thickened, retracted tendon (*arrow*). **(c)** Artist's sketch. (Part **a**, **c**: Reproduced with permission from Brunton LM, Anderson MW, Chhabra AB. The Elbow. In: Khanna AJ, ed. MRI for orthopaedic surgeons. New York: Thieme; 2010:118–128.) (Part **b**: Reproduced with permission from Magnetic Resonance Imaging of the Elbow: Update on Current Techniques and Indications Brunton, Lance M. et al. Journal of Hand Surgery, Volume 31, Issue 6, 1001–1011)

8.4.5 Biceps Tendon Injury

Injury to the distal biceps tendon is relatively common. Complete rupture occurs almost exclusively in men after forced extension of the flexed elbow against an eccentric load. However, symptoms arising from a partial tear may have an insidious onset, and such tears usually occur from repetitive microtrauma in an already degenerative tendon. Although MRI is not always necessary to diagnose a complete distal biceps tendon rupture, it can distinguish between tendinosis, partial tears, and complete tears. MRI may also allow for the diagnosis of concomitant injuries. A complete rupture is characterized by the absence of the low signal intensity tendon tissue at the radial tuberosity insertion on axial images. The less experienced clinician may have difficulty localizing the biceps tendon insertion on the axial images and may find it easier to make or confirm the diagnosis on the sagittal T2-weighted images. A large amount of high signal intensity fluid and/or hemorrhage in the antecubital fossa usually accompanies an acute distal biceps tendon injury. The extent of tendon retraction is assessed on sagittal images, although the course of the tendon often is oriented obliquely to this plane (▶ Fig. 8.5). An abnormally thickened or attenuated distal biceps tendon with increased signal intensity may represent tendinopathy or a partial tear. Associated bone marrow edema within the radial tuberosity is likely related to microavulsive injury. Increased fluid within the bicipitoradial bursa may accompany a partial tear in some patients.[21,33]

8.4.6 Triceps Tendon Injury

Ruptures of the triceps tendon are far less common than are injuries to the distal biceps tendon. Complete tears result from a traumatic event and are manifested clinically by the inability to extend the elbow against gravity. Extensive posterior elbow swelling, ecchymosis, and a palpable tendon defect are also common findings. The tendon typically is detached from its insertion on the olecranon process of the proximal ulna, and a small osseous avulsion may be seen on conventional radiographs.

MRI has a role in diagnosing triceps tendon injury in patients with equivocal clinical findings. A complete rupture is accompanied by extensive adjacent soft tissue edema, and the retracted tendon margin is seen on sagittal images (▶ Fig. 8.6). Partial injury or tendinopathy is more common and may result only in thickening or thinning of the tendon, sometimes without related abnormal signal intensity.[34] Findings of olecranon bursitis may accompany triceps tendon injury in some patients.

8.5 Degenerative Conditions: Lateral and Medial Epicondylitis

The term *epicondylitis* may be a misnomer because mucoid degeneration and tearing of the extensor carpi radialis brevis tendon (in the case of lateral epicondylitis), rather than inflammation, are the key histologic features of the disorder.[35]

Nevertheless, in the absence of a more accurate term, lateral epicondylitis (also known as *tennis elbow*) is the most common overuse disorder of the elbow, occurring most frequently in individuals who participate in racquet sports and in middle-aged persons who perform repetitive wrist extension in their daily activities. Patients complain of lateral elbow pain that increases with the offending activity. Examination reveals tenderness over the insertion of the common extensor tendon at the lateral epicondyle, and the pain is exacerbated by resisted wrist extension with the elbow fully extended. Although the diagnosis usually is obvious by history and physical examination, concurrent underlying pathology cannot be ruled out easily. The differential diagnosis for lateral elbow pain includes the following:

- Degenerative joint disease.
- OCD.
- Radial tunnel syndrome.
- Posterolateral rotatory instability.
- Occult fracture.
- Loose bodies.

It is important to consider these other etiologies when nonoperative treatment of lateral epicondylitis for more than 6 to 12 months has failed.

Usually, MRI is used to rule out concomitant causes of refractory elbow pain rather than to diagnose lateral epicondylitis.[36] The typical MRI finding of isolated lateral epicondylitis is

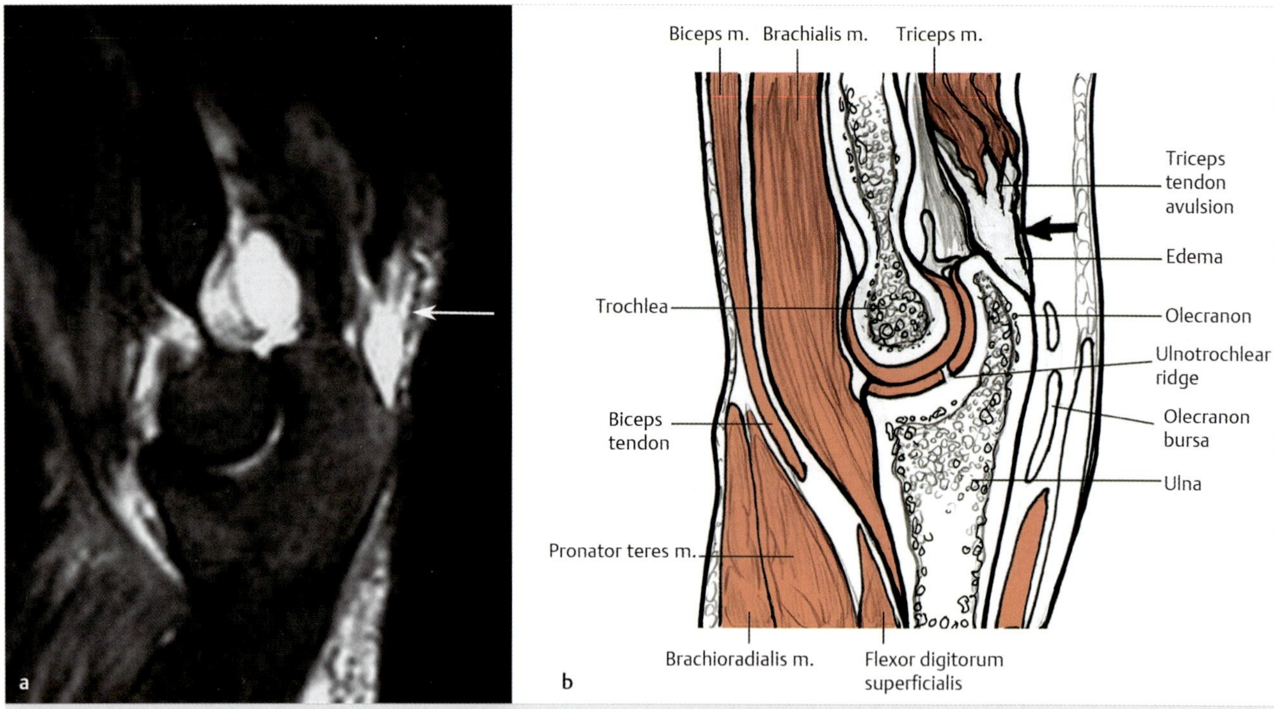

Fig. 8.6 A sagittal T2-weighted image **(a)** and artist's sketch **(b)** revealing a torn, retracted triceps tendon with a large amount of high-signal-intensity edema between the olecranon process and the tendon end (*arrows on each*). (Part **a**: Reproduced with permission from Brunton LM, Anderson MW, Pannunzio ME, Khanna AJ, Chhabra AB. Magnetic resonance imaging of the elbow: update on current techniques and indications. J Hand Surg Am 2006;31:1001–1011.) (Reproduced with permission from Brunton LM, Anderson MW, Chhabra AB. The Elbow. In: Khanna AJ, ed. MRI for orthopaedic surgeons. New York: Thieme; 2010:118–128.)

increased signal intensity and thickening of the common extensor tendon origin, in some cases with adjacent soft tissue edema (▶ Fig. 8.7).[21,37] In patients with severe lateral epicondylitis, the common extensor tendon origin may be separated off the lateral epicondyle.[36] Abnormalities of the LCL complex, especially the LUCL, are also often seen (▶ Fig. 8.8).[38] Increased signal intensity and thickening of the common extensor tendon origin can be incidental findings in some patients without symptoms of lateral epicondylitis, especially in older individuals, but in these cases soft tissue edema and other related findings are usually absent.[39]

Similar to lateral epicondylitis, the diagnosis of medial epicondylitis can usually be made clinically, and the primary role of MRI is to rule out other diagnoses, such as MCL injury or ulnar neuritis, in patients for whom nonoperative treatment fails. The MRI findings in medial and lateral epicondylitis are similar. Medial epicondylitis is characterized by a thickened common flexor tendon and local soft tissue edema.

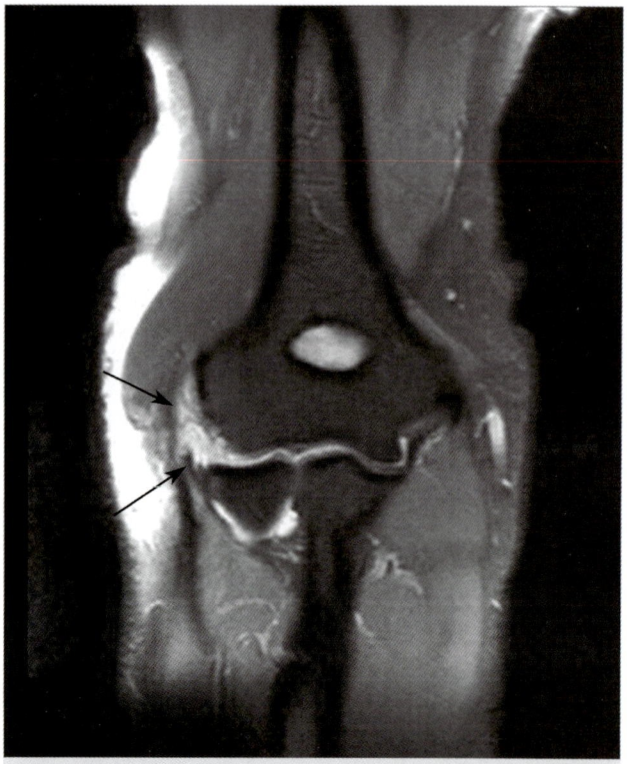

Fig. 8.7 A coronal T2-weighted image of the right elbow showing concurrent severe lateral epicondylitis (*upper arrow*) with high signal intensity within a thickened common extensor tendon and discontinuity of the underlying RCL (*lower arrow*). (Reproduced with permission from Brunton LM, Anderson MW, Chhabra AB. The Elbow. In: Khanna AJ, ed. MRI for orthopaedic surgeons. New York: Thieme; 2010:118–128.)

8.6 Other Pathologic Conditions

8.6.1 Infections

Depending on the acuity of presentation, various imaging modalities are used in the evaluation of patients with signs and symptoms of musculoskeletal infection. Conventional radiographs, computed tomography (CT), and radioisotope studies all have roles in the diagnosis of an infectious process, although MRI is the single most useful study for determining the precise anatomic location and extent of infection.

Acute osteomyelitis causes inflammation of medullary bone, which can be detected by MRI well before findings are evident on conventional radiographs. On T1-weighted images, areas of marrow involvement show a low signal intensity that contrasts with the surrounding bright normal marrow. STIR images, or other fat-suppressed T2-weighted images, are the most sensitive for infection, showing affected areas as high signal intensity. Sometimes these regions of high T2-weighted signal are accompanied by a well-defined low-intensity margin. Because these findings may be similar in patients with tumor or early osteonecrosis, correlation with the history and physical examination is critical.[40]

The role of MRI in patients with presumed septic arthritis is less clear. Although the presence of an elbow joint effusion can be well depicted by MRI, characterizing the synovial fluid as normal, bloody, or purulent is less reliable. MRI often is used to determine the extent of involvement in patients with severe cellulitis, septic bursitis, or other superficial infections that are unresponsive to nonoperative measures. MRI also is an excellent method for diagnosing a suspected deep abscess about the elbow that may require surgical incision and drainage.[41]

The MRI findings in septic and nonseptic olecranon bursitis may be markedly similar. Abnormalities may include the following:

- Marginal lobulation.
- Bursal septation.
- Heterogeneous internal signal.
- Poorly defined margins.
- Adjacent soft tissue edema.
- Thickening or edema of the triceps tendon.
- Localized bone marrow edema.

The most consistent finding in septic olecranon bursitis is rim and soft tissue enhancement on postgadolinium T1-weighted images.[42]

8.6.2 OCD

OCD of the humeral capitellum is an idiopathic disorder affecting adolescents with a history of repetitive overuse of the elbow. Affected individuals commonly present with pain and swelling of the lateral aspect of the elbow. Mechanical symptoms and/or limitations of motion may be indicative of an associated loose body. MRI can be helpful in the early detection of OCD, when conventional radiographs may show only subtle changes. Focal areas of subchondral low signal intensity on T1-weighted images are characteristic. Fat-suppressed T2-weighted images provide the most sensitive evaluation for a potential OCD lesion at the capitellar articular surface; however, these images are the least specific. With a patient in whom the clinical suspicion is relatively high, the fat-suppressed T2-weighted image can be used as a "screening" examination and then correlated with the T1-weighted image where anatomic detail may be better seen. MRI can also help to evaluate the stability and viability of the OCD fragment. Fluid surrounding the fragment on fat-suppressed T2-weighted images or surrounding contrast material on MR arthrography is a sign of an unstable fragment (▶ Fig. 8.9).[43] Enhancement of a fragment after intravenous gadolinium

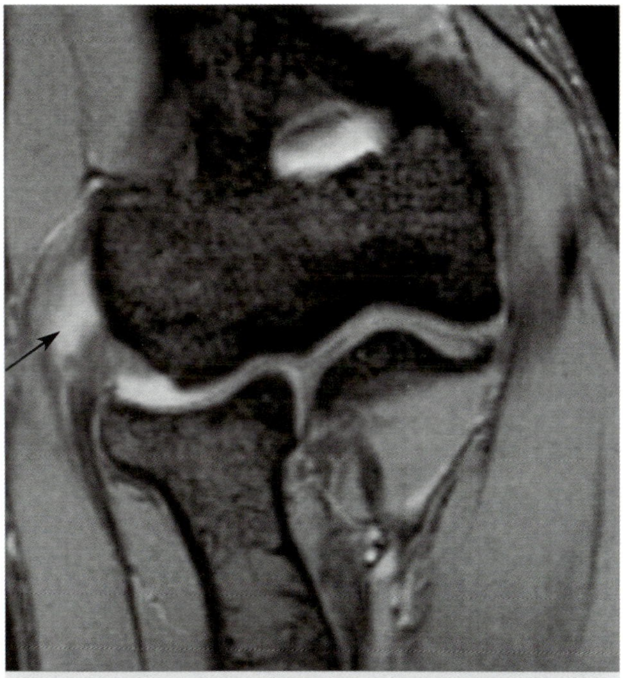

Fig. 8.8 A coronal short tau inversion recovery (STIR) image of the right elbow showing isolated lateral epicondylitis, indicated by the thickened common extensor tendon with amorphous features and high signal intensity (*arrow*). (Reproduced with permission from Brunton LM, Anderson MW, Pannunzio ME, Khanna AJ, Chhabra AB. Magnetic resonance imaging of the elbow: update on current techniques and indications. J Hand Surg Am 2006;31:1001–1011.)

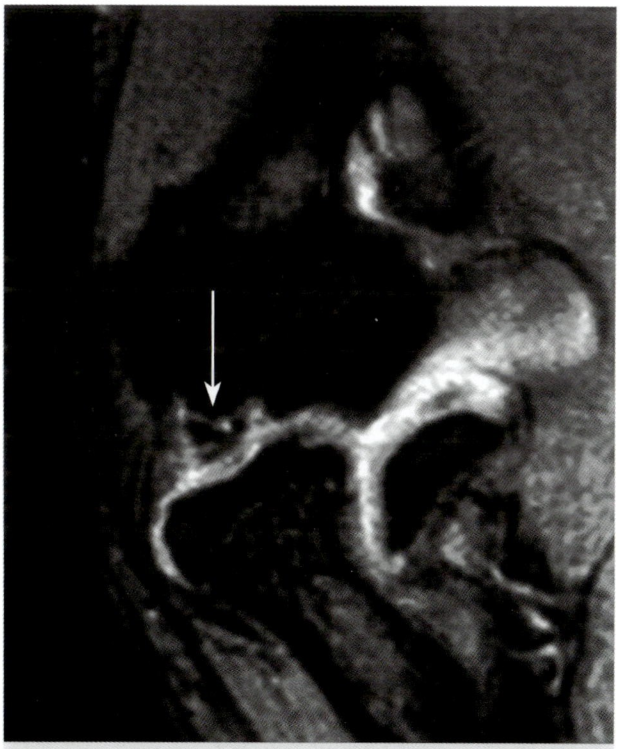

Fig. 8.9 A coronal oblique short tau inversion recovery (STIR) image of the right elbow showing an unstable osteochondritis dissecans (OCD) fragment of the capitellum with joint fluid tracking behind the fragment (*arrow*). (Reproduced with permission from Brunton LM, Anderson MW, Pannunzio ME, Khanna AJ, Chhabra AB. Magnetic resonance imaging of the elbow: update on current techniques and indications. J Hand Surg Am 2006;31:1001–1011.)

contrast has been administered suggests adequate blood supply and fragment viability.[44]

8.6.3 Compression Neuropathies

The most commonly occurring compression neuropathies about the elbow include the following:

- Cubital tunnel syndrome (ulnar nerve).
- Radial tunnel syndrome (posterior interosseous nerve—pain).
- Posterior interosseous nerve syndrome (posterior interosseous nerve—motor deficits).
- Pronator syndrome (median nerve).

Each syndrome has key historical and physical examination findings that have been addressed elsewhere.[45] Electromyography and nerve conduction studies are the most frequently used adjunctive diagnostic tests. Advanced imaging may have a role in evaluating patients for whom nonoperative treatment fails or those with recurrence after surgical intervention.

MRI is most useful for assessing cubital tunnel syndrome, especially when electrodiagnostic testing is equivocal, or for excluding accompanying pathology in patients in whom this syndrome recurs.[46,47] MRI may be more sensitive than nerve conduction studies in the diagnosis of ulnar neuropathy at the elbow.[48] Prolonged compression of peripheral nerves leads to a spectrum of MRI findings, including the following:

- Thickening of the nerve.
- Increased signal intensity within the nerve.
- A mottled appearance of the nerve.
- A surrounding fluid collection, which may represent varying degrees of inflammatory changes (▶ Fig. 8.10).

The median and radial nerves are more difficult to evaluate; however, MRI can detect adjacent space-occupying lesions that may produce compression. Patients with chronic neuropathy also may show changes within adjacent denervated muscles, such as fatty atrophy on T1-weighted images (▶ Fig. 8.11) or muscle edema on T2-weighted images.[49]

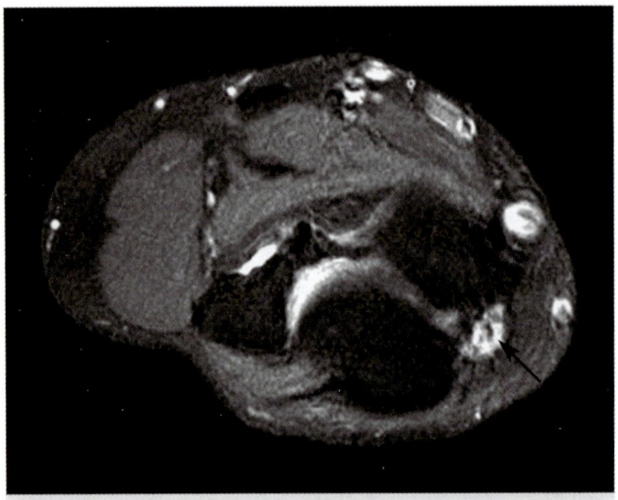

Fig. 8.10 An axial short tau inversion recovery (STIR) image of the right elbow showing a thickened ulnar nerve with a mottled appearance and surrounding increased signal intensity consistent with edema from inflammation (ulnar neuritis) (*arrow*). (Reproduced with permission from Brunton LM, Anderson MW, Pannunzio ME, Khanna AJ, Chhabra AB. Magnetic resonance imaging of the elbow: update on current techniques and indications. J Hand Surg Am 2006;31:1001–1011.)

8.6.4 Synovial Disorders

MRI can depict numerous abnormal synovial-based processes, such as rheumatoid arthritis (RA), crystal deposition disorders, pigmented villonodular synovitis (PVNS), and idiopathic synovial osteochondromatosis.[50] When synovial fluid analysis is equivocal, MRI may aid in differentiating conditions that produce a joint effusion. With the use of intravenous gadolinium, MRI has become a powerful tool for detecting the early stages of inflammatory arthritides, such as RA, because of the striking enhancement of the proliferative synovium. Although PVNS and synovial chondromatosis are commonly seen in the hip and knee and are quite rare in the elbow, these syndromes should be considered in the differential diagnosis of the patient with multiple loose bodies in the elbow. Gradient-echo imaging shows accentuated "signal dropout" in areas of PVNS, relating to the presence of hemosiderin in this disease process. Other nonspecific MRI findings of PVNS include variable synovial proliferation, bone erosion, and joint effusion.[51,52]

8.6.5 Soft Tissue Masses

Although soft tissue masses are less common around the elbow than in the lower extremity, MRI is essential for evaluating such lesions. The primary role of MRI is differentiating determinate from indeterminate lesions. Determinate lesions are those for which a well-trained musculoskeletal radiologist or clinician can provide a single diagnosis after MRI evaluation with a high degree of certainty based on the imaging appearance. Such lesions include the following[21,53,54]:

- Lipomas.
- Ganglions.
- Hemangiomas.

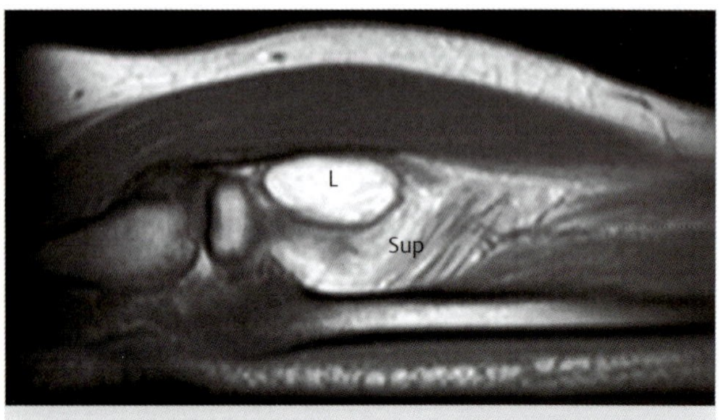

Fig. 8.11 A sagittal T1-weighted image revealing a lipoma (*L*) within the supinator muscle (*Sup*). The supinator shows diffuse high signal intensity, which matches that of the lipoma and subcutaneous fat, indicating fatty atrophy of the denervated muscle from long-standing compression of the posterior interosseous nerve by the lipoma. (Reproduced with permission from Brunton LM, Anderson MW, Pannunzio ME, Khanna AJ, Chhabra AB. Magnetic resonance imaging of the elbow: update on current techniques and indications. J Hand Surg Am 2006;31:1001–1011.)

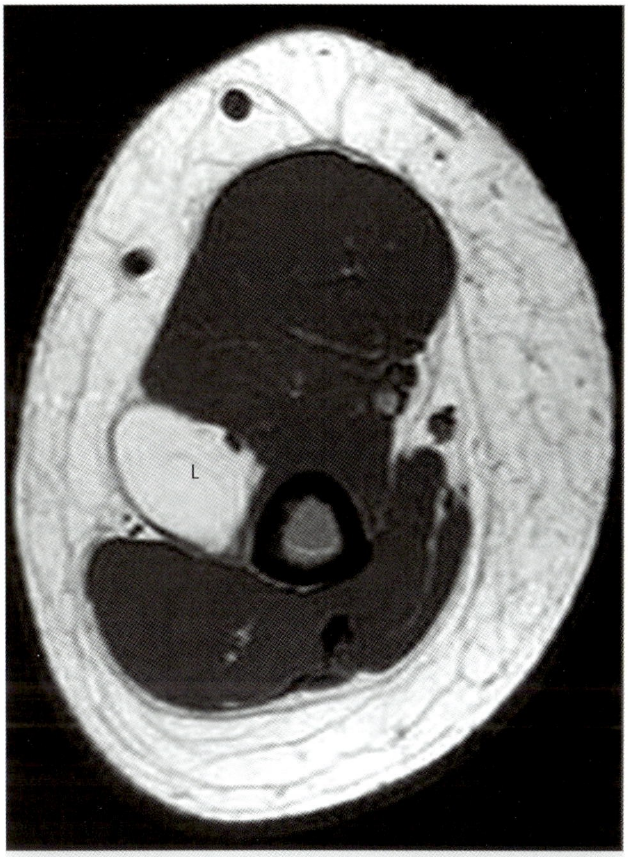

Fig. 8.12 An axial T1-weighted image showing the similarity in signal intensity between the well-circumscribed lipoma (*L*) and the adjacent subcutaneous fat. (Reproduced with permission from Brunton LM, Anderson MW, Chhabra AB. The Elbow. In: Khanna AJ, ed. MRI for orthopaedic surgeons. New York: Thieme; 2010:118–128.)

- Neurofibromas.
- Muscle tears.
- Myositis ossificans (chronic stage).
- PVNS.

Determinate lesions are those for which a well-trained musculoskeletal radiologist or clinician can provide a single diagnosis after MRI evaluation with a high degree of certainty based on the imaging appearance. Such lesions include the following: Lipomas. Ganglions, Hemangiomas. Neurofibromas. Muscle tears. Myositis ossificans (chronic stage). PVNS. Lipomas are amongst the most commonly encountered determinate lesions. A lipoma matches the signal intensity of subcutaneous fat on all pulse sequences, including fat-suppressed sequences (▶ Fig. 8.12). Indeterminate lesions are those lesions in which the radiologist or clinician is unable to provide a definitive diagnosis and therefore warrant a needle or open biopsy.[53]

8.6.6 Postoperative MRI Findings

MRI can be invaluable in evaluating patients with new or recurrent symptoms following elbow surgery. Postoperative images can sometimes be difficult to interpret due to the challenge of differentiating between normal postoperative and pathologic changes. Orthopaedic implants can also create artifact that substantially distorts the image. However, both conventional MRI with a metal artifact reduction protocols and newer techniques such as Multi-acquisition Variable-Resonance Image Combination (MAVRIC) and Slice Encoding for Metal Artifact Correction (SEMAC) imaging can produce high-quality images even when metal is present.[8,55] After successful distal biceps repair, the distal biceps tendon normally appears heterogeneous and thickened.[56,57] MRI is useful to assess for complications such as heterotopic bone formation and graft re-rupture. In patients with recurrent pain or difficulty throwing after UCL reconstruction, MR arthrography can be used to assess graft integrity and evaluate other potential issues such as posterior olecranon osteophytes, heterotopic ossification, and medial epicondyle avulsion.[58] MRI is also useful in patients with OCD of the capitellum after debridement and microfracture or with osteochondral mosaiplasty to assess the progress of healing and potentially assist with decision-making regarding return to full activity.[59,60] If the surgery is successful, the signal of the underlying bone should return to near-normal. After microfracture and debridement, the cartilage defect may or may not fill in with fibrocartilage, but some persistent thickening of the subchondral bone is common.[60] After mosaiplasty, as the graft heals, the signal intensity of the graft cartilage, which is initially hyperintense, will approach that of surrounding cartilage.[59] For patients with compressive neuropathy who have not improved after nerve release, MRI can evaluate for alternate causes of nerve compression, such as masses, and for structural or signal abnormalities within the nerve.

8.7 Common Clinical Questions

1. A 52 year-old male was water-skiing. The rope slipped. He struggled to keep his grip and felt a sudden painful pop in the elbow. He subsequently developed swelling and ecchymosis in the antecubital area. Two proton-density fat-suppressed MRI axial images are shown below. What is the diagnosis?
   a) Triceps rupture.
   b) MCL complex injury.
   c) Distal biceps rupture.
   d) Elbow hemarthrosis.

2. Which of the following is a normal variant?
   a) Pseudodefect of the radius.
   b) Pseudodefect of the olecranon.
   c) Pseudodefect of the capitellum.
   d) Pseudodefect of the trochlea.

3. A 61-year-old male has had 9 months of lateral elbow pain. He attributes his symptoms to his job as a cashier at a paint store, where he lifts dozens of heavy paint cans a day. He is now on light duty, but his symptoms have persisted. A T2 coronal MRI image is shown below. Which of the following examination findings is most likely?
   a) Pain with resisted wrist extension with the elbow extended.
   b) Pain with resisted wrist extension with the elbow flexed.
   c) Pain with supination.
   d) Varus instability.

4. A short tau inversion recovery (STIR) coronal MRI image is shown below. What is the most likely clinical scenario?
   a) A 45-year-old with overuse related medial elbow pain.
   b) A 22-year-old who dislocated his elbow playing football.
   c) A 64-year-old with rheumatoid arthritis.
   d) A 52-year-old with numbness and tingling in the small and ring finger.

5. Which of the following is most useful in ruling out septic olecranon bursitis?
   a) Well-defined margins.
   b) Bursal size.
   c) Bursal septation.
   d) Absence of rim and soft-tissue enhancement on postgadolinium T1-weighted images.

References

[1] Reichel LM, Milam GS, Sitton SE, Curry MC, Mehlhoff TL. Elbow lateral collateral ligament injuries. J Hand Surg Am. 2013; 38(1):184–201, quiz 201

[2] Zoner CS, Buck FM, Cardoso FN, et al. Detailed MRI-anatomic study of the lateral epicondyle of the elbow and its tendinous and ligamentous attachments in cadavers. AJR Am J Roentgenol. 2010; 195(3):629–636

[3] Anakwenze OA, Kancherla VK, Iyengar J, Ahmad CS, Levine WN. Posterolateral rotatory instability of the elbow. Am J Sports Med. 2014; 42 (2):485–491

[4] Mak S, Beltran LS, Bencardino J, et al. MRI of the annular ligament of the elbow: review of anatomic considerations and pathologic findings in patients with posterolateral elbow instability. AJR Am J Roentgenol. 2014; 203(6): 1272–1279

[5] Husarik DB, Saupe N, Pfirrmann CW, Jost B, Hodler J, Zanetti M. Ligaments and plicae of the elbow: normal MR imaging variability in 60 asymptomatic subjects. Radiology. 2010; 257(1):185–194

[6] Belentani C, Pastore D, Wangwinyuvirat M, et al. Triceps brachii tendon: anatomic-MR imaging study in cadavers with histologic correlation. Skeletal Radiol. 2009; 38(2):171–175

[7] Tagliafico A, Michaud J, Perez MM, Martinoli C. Ultrasound of distal brachialis tendon attachment: normal and abnormal findings. Br J Radiol. 2013; 86 (1025):20130004

[8] Johnson D, Stevens KJ, Riley G, Shapiro L, Yoshioka H, Gold GE. Approach to MR Imaging of the Elbow and Wrist: Technical Aspects and Innovation. Magn Reson Imaging Clin N Am. 2015; 23(3):355–366

[9] Wenzke DR. MR imaging of the elbow in the injured athlete. Radiol Clin North Am. 2013; 51(2):195–213

[10] Binaghi D. MR Imaging of the Elbow. Magn Reson Imaging Clin N Am. 2015; 23(3):427–440

[11] Potter HG. Imaging of posttraumatic and soft tissue dysfunction of the elbow. Clin Orthop Relat Res. 2000(370):9–18

[12] Jazrawi LM, Alaia MJ, Chang G, Fitzgerald EF, Recht MP. Advances in magnetic resonance imaging of articular cartilage. J Am Acad Orthop Surg. 2011; 19(7): 420–429

[13] Lomasney LM, Choi H, Jayanthi N. Magnetic resonance arthrography of the upper extremity. Radiol Clin North Am. 2013; 51(2):227–237

[14] Kaplan LJ, Potter HG. MR imaging of ligament injuries to the elbow. Radiol Clin North Am. 2006; 44(4):583–594, ixix.

[15] Skaggs DL, Mirzayan R. The posterior fat pad sign in association with occult fracture of the elbow in children. J Bone Joint Surg Am. 1999; 81(10):1429–1433

[16] O'Dwyer H, O'Sullivan P, Fitzgerald D, Lee MJ, McGrath F, Logan PM. The fat pad sign following elbow trauma in adults: its usefulness and reliability in suspecting occult fracture. J Comput Assist Tomogr. 2004; 28(4):562–565

[17] Kaas L, Turkenburg JL, van Riet RP, Vroemen JP, Eygendaal D. Magnetic resonance imaging findings in 46 elbows with a radial head fracture. Acta Orthop. 2010; 81(3):373–376

[18] Furushima K, Itoh Y, Iwabu S, Yamamoto Y, Koga R, Shimizu M. Classification of Olecranon Stress Fractures in Baseball Players. Am J Sports Med. 2014; 42 (6):1343–1351

[19] Pudas T, Hurme T, Mattila K, Svedström E. Magnetic resonance imaging in pediatric elbow fractures. Acta Radiol. 2005; 46(6):636–644

[20] Griffith JF, Roebuck DJ, Cheng JC, et al. Acute elbow trauma in children: spectrum of injury revealed by MR imaging not apparent on radiographs. AJR Am J Roentgenol. 2001; 176(1):53–60

[21] Melloni P, Valls R. The use of MRI scanning for investigating soft-tissue abnormalities in the elbow. Eur J Radiol. 2005; 54(2):303–313

[22] Wei AS, Khana S, Limpisvasti O, Crues J, Podesta L, Yocum LA. Clinical and magnetic resonance imaging findings associated with Little League elbow. J Pediatr Orthop. 2010; 30(7):715–719

[23] Dubberley JH, Faber KJ, Patterson SD, et al. The detection of loose bodies in the elbow: the value of MRI and CT arthrography. J Bone Joint Surg Br. 2005; 87(5):684–686

[24] Schwartz ML, al-Zahrani S, Morwessel RM, Andrews JR. Ulnar collateral ligament injury in the throwing athlete: evaluation with saline-enhanced MR arthrography. Radiology. 1995; 197(1):297–299

[25] Hill NB, Jr, Bucchieri JS, Shon F, Miller TT, Rosenwasser MP. Magnetic resonance imaging of injury to the medial collateral ligament of the elbow: a cadaver model. J Shoulder Elbow Surg. 2000; 9(5):418–422

[26] Cohen SB, Valko C, Zoga A, Dodson CC, Ciccotti MG. Posteromedial elbow impingement: magnetic resonance imaging findings in overhead throwing athletes and results of arthroscopic treatment. Arthroscopy. 2011; 27(10): 1364–1370

[27] O'Driscoll SW, Bell DF, Morrey BF. Posterolateral rotatory instability of the elbow. J Bone Joint Surg Am. 1991; 73(3):440–446

[28] Grafe MW, McAdams TR, Beaulieu CF, Ladd AL. Magnetic resonance imaging in diagnosis of chronic posterolateral rotatory instability of the elbow. Am J Orthop (Belle Mead NJ). 2003; 32(10):501–503, discussion 504

[29] Terada N, Yamada H, Toyama Y. The appearance of the lateral ulnar collateral ligament on magnetic resonance imaging. J Shoulder Elbow Surg. 2004; 13 (2):214–216

[30] Potter HG, Weiland AJ, Schatz JA, Paletta GA, Hotchkiss RN. Posterolateral rotatory instability of the elbow: usefulness of MR imaging in diagnosis. Radiology. 1997; 204(1):185–189

[31] LiMarzi GM, O'Dell MC, Scherer K, Pettis C, Wasyliw CW, Bancroft LW. Magnetic resonance arthrography of the wrist and elbow. Magn Reson Imaging Clin N Am. 2015; 23(3):441–455

[32] Hackl M, Wegmann K, Ries C, Leschinger T, Burkhart KJ, Müller LP. Reliability of magnetic resonance imaging signs of posterolateral rotatory instability of the elbow. J Hand Surg Am. 2015; 40(7):1428–1433

[33] Williams BD, Schweitzer ME, Weishaupt D, et al. Partial tears of the distal biceps tendon: MR appearance and associated clinical findings. Skeletal Radiol. 2001; 30(10):560–564

[34] Koplas MC, Schneider E, Sundaram M. Prevalence of triceps tendon tears on MRI of the elbow and clinical correlation. Skeletal Radiol. 2011; 40(5):587–594

[35] Kraushaar BS, Nirschl RP. Tendinosis of the elbow (tennis elbow). Clinical features and findings of histological, immunohistochemical, and electron microscopy studies. J Bone Joint Surg Am. 1999; 81(2):259–278

[36] Walton MJ, Mackie K, Fallon M, et al. The reliability and validity of magnetic resonance imaging in the assessment of chronic lateral epicondylitis. J Hand Surg Am. 2011; 36(3):475–479

[37] Potter HG, Hannafin JA, Morwessel RM, DiCarlo EF, O'Brien SJ, Altchek DW. Lateral epicondylitis: correlation of MR imaging, surgical, and histopathologic findings. Radiology. 1995; 196(1):43–46

[38] Qi L, Zhu ZF, Li F, Wang RF. MR imaging of patients with lateral epicondylitis of the elbow: is the common extensor tendon an isolated lesion? PLoS One. 2013; 8(11):e79498

[39] van Leeuwen WF, Janssen SJ, Ring D, Chen N. Incidental magnetic resonance imaging signal changes in the extensor carpi radialis brevis origin are more common with age. J Shoulder Elbow Surg. 2016; 25(7):1175–1181

[40] Boutin RD, Brossmann J, Sartoris DJ, Reilly D, Resnick D. Update on imaging of orthopedic infections. Orthop Clin North Am. 1998; 29(1):41–66

[41] Berquist TH. Musculoskeletal infection. In: Berquist TH, ed. MRI of the musculoskeletal system. 5th ed. Philadelphia, PA: Lippincott Williams & Wilkins; 2006

[42] Floemer F, Morrison WB, Bongartz G, Ledermann HP. MRI characteristics of olecranon bursitis. AJR Am J Roentgenol. 2004; 183(1):29–34

[43] Satake H, Takahara M, Harada M, Maruyama M. Preoperative imaging criteria for unstable osteochondritis dissecans of the capitellum. Clin Orthop Relat Res. 2013; 471(4):1137–1143

[44] Kijowski R, De Smet AA. MRI findings of osteochondritis dissecans of the capitellum with surgical correlation. AJR Am J Roentgenol. 2005; 185(6): 1453–1459

[45] Lubahn JD, Cermak MB. Uncommon nerve compression syndromes of the upper extremity. J Am Acad Orthop Surg. 1998; 6(6):378–386

[46] Keen NN, Chin CT, Engstrom JW, Saloner D, Steinbach LS. Diagnosing ulnar neuropathy at the elbow using magnetic resonance neurography. Skeletal Radiol. 2012; 41(4):401–407

[47] Bäumer P, Pham M, Ruetters M, et al. Peripheral neuropathy: detection with diffusion-tensor imaging. Radiology. 2014; 273(1):185–193

[48] Vucic S, Cordato DJ, Yiannikas C, Schwartz RS, Shnier RC. Utility of magnetic resonance imaging in diagnosing ulnar neuropathy at the elbow. Clin Neurophysiol. 2006; 117(3):590–595

[49] Kijowski R, Tuite M, Sanford M. Magnetic resonance imaging of the elbow. Part II: Abnormalities of the ligaments, tendons, and nerves. Skeletal Radiol. 2005; 34(1):1–18

[50] Chen FS, Diaz VA, Loebenberg M, Rosen JE. Shoulder and elbow injuries in the skeletally immature athlete. J Am Acad Orthop Surg. 2005; 13(3):172–185

[51] Khanna AJ, Cosgarea AJ, Mont MA, et al. Magnetic resonance imaging of the knee. Current techniques and spectrum of disease. J Bone Joint Surg Am. 2001; 83-A Suppl 2 Pt 2:128–141

[52] Cheng XG, You YH, Liu W, Zhao T, Qu H. MRI features of pigmented villonodular synovitis (PVNS). Clin Rheumatol. 2004; 23(1):31–34

[53] Frassica FJ, Khanna JA, McCarthy EF. The role of MR imaging in soft tissue tumor evaluation: perspective of the orthopedic oncologist and musculoskeletal pathologist. Magn Reson Imaging Clin N Am. 2000; 8(4):915–927

[54] Chen AL, Youm T, Ong BC, Rafii M, Rokito AS. Imaging of the elbow in the overhead throwing athlete. Am J Sports Med. 2003; 31(3):466–473

[55] Ariyanayagam T, Malcolm PN, Toms AP. Advances in metal artifact reduction techniques for periprosthetic soft tissue imaging. Semin Musculoskelet Radiol. 2015; 19(4):328–334

[56] Schmidt CC, Diaz VA, Weir DM, Latona CR, Miller MC. Repaired distal biceps magnetic resonance imaging anatomy compared with outcome. J Shoulder Elbow Surg. 2012; 21(12):1623–1631

[57] Alemann G, Dietsch E, Gallinet D, Obert L, Kastler B, Aubry S. Repair of distal biceps brachii tendon assessed with 3-T magnetic resonance imaging and correlation with functional outcome. Skeletal Radiol. 2015; 44(5):629–639

[58] Wear SA, Thornton DD, Schwartz ML, Weissmann RC, III, Cain EL, Andrews JR. MRI of the reconstructed ulnar collateral ligament. AJR Am J Roentgenol. 2011; 197(5):1198–1204

[59] Iwasaki N, Kato H, Kamishima T, Minami A. Sequential alterations in magnetic resonance imaging findings after autologous osteochondral mosaicplasty for young athletes with osteochondritis dissecans of the humeral capitellum. Am J Sports Med. 2009; 37(12):2349–2354

[60] Wulf CA, Stone RM, Giveans MR, Lervick GN. Magnetic resonance imaging after arthroscopic microfracture of capitellar osteochondritis dissecans. Am J Sports Med. 2012; 40(11):2549–2556

Answers to Common Clinical Questions

1. Answer: c. The first image shows the bicipital tuberosity, where the distal biceps tendon inserts onto the proximal radius. Normally, the distal biceps is visible here as low signal intensity tendon tissue. In this image, the bicipital tuberosity is bare as the distal biceps has ruptured and retracted proximally. The second image is a more proximal section showing the ruptured and retracted distal biceps tendon surrounded by high signal intensity fluid.
2. Answer: c. On sagittal MRI sequences of the elbow, a small depression of the posterior capitellum is sometimes seen. This can be a normal variant but is easily confused with an osteochondral fracture. Injuries of the posterior capitellum do occur, but they are uncommon. Marrow edema and other concomittant bony and/or ligamentus injuries can help distinguish between a traumatic defect and a pseudodefect.
3. Answer: a. The MRI shows interstitial tearing of the common extensor tendon, consistent with lateral epicondylitis. Lateral epicondylitis is caused by degenerative tearing of the extensor carpi radialis brevis tendon (ECRB). It is characterized by pain with wrist extension against resistance with the elbow extended, which stresses the ECRB.
4. Answer: b. The MRI shows a full-thickness tear of the ulnar collateral ligament with surrounding edema. Elbow dislocations usually result in multiple ligamentous and tendinous injuries though most often heal very well without surgery.
5. Answer: d. Nonseptic and septic olecranon bursitis can appear very similar on MRI. Poorly defined margins, marginal lobulation, bursal septation, heterogeneous internal signal, adjacent sot tissue edema, thickening/ edema of the triceps tendon, and localized bone marrow edema can be seen in both nonseptic bursitis. While rim and soft-tissue enhancement can also occur in both nonseptic and septic bursitis, when it is absent, septic bursitis can be ruled out.

9 The Wrist and Hand

Ariel A. Williams, Lance M. Brunton, Mark W. Anderson, and A. Bobby Chhabra

Abstract

MRI of the hand and wrist is particularly challenging because of the size and complexity of the anatomic structures. However, technologic advances have greatly improved image quality, and with appropriate sequences and protocols, MRI can be used to visualize many of the clinically important structures in the hand and wrist with good anatomic detail. 3-T imaging has improved detection of small anatomic structures even further, but most hand and wrist examinations are still performed with 1.5-T magnets, which are adequate in most cases. MRI now has an essential role in evaluating the full spectrum of traumatic, degenerative, and other disorders of the hand and wrist. MRI is the preferred modality for many clinicians when evaluating patients with suspected scaphoid fractures and negative radiographs. MR arthrography can be used to assess the triangular fibrocartilage complex and scapholunate and lunotriquetral ligaments, all of which have been difficult to visualize with conventional imaging. MRI can identify a variety of tendon abnormalities, including acute injuries and degenerative and inflammatory conditions. It is useful in early diagnosis of both Kienböck disease and rheumatoid arthritis and may be of prognostic value in these contexts. MRI is also useful in localizing and staging malignant and infectious conditions of the hand and wrist.

Keywords: carpal tunnel, compression neuropathies, fractures, hand, ligaments, osteonecrosis, rheumatoid arthritis, tendons, triangular fibrocartilage complex, wrist

9.1 Normal Anatomy

9.1.1 Sagittal Anatomy

The wrist is made of the distal radius and ulna, proximal and distal carpal rows, and metacarpal bases. The many osseous articulations allow tremendous range of motion. Injuries to the wrist ligaments can manifest in subtle changes in overall osseous alignment. Sagittal alignment can be assessed on magnetic resonance imaging (MRI) in a number of ways. The central column of the wrist comprises the lunate and capitate. Normally, on sagittal images, a single line can be drawn through the distal radius, central column, and third metacarpal. The capitolunate, radiolunate, and scapholunate angles can also be measured and compared with standard values. Deviations in these measurements from their norms suggest carpal instability.

A number of muscles and tendons are responsible for the full range of wrist and hand motion. Sagittal images are particularly useful for evaluating the digital flexor and extensor tendons, both of which are low-signal structures on T1- and T2-weighted images. The flexor digitorum profundus, flexor digitorum superficialis, and flexor pollicis longus tendons enter and then exit the carpal tunnel as they pass over the carpal bones. Proximally, the flexor digitorum superficialis lies superficial to the flexor digitorum profundus. At the level of the proximal phalanx, the flexor digitorum superficialis splits into two slips at the Camper chiasm, allowing the flexor digitorum profundus to pass more superficially. The two flexor digitorum superficialis slips reapproximate deep to the flexor digitorum profundus and insert individually onto the middle phalanx, and the flexor digitorum profundus inserts onto the distal phalanx. From the metacarpophalangeal joints to the distal phalanges, the digital flexor tendons are contained within the flexor tendon sheaths, which consist of a synovial lining overlain by a pulley system created by segmental bands of fibrous tissue. The five annular and three cruciate pulleys prevent tendon bowstringing and provide a biomechanical advantage during finger flexion. The pulleys are small, and advances in imaging have led to improvements in their imagery.[1] They are best seen on axial sections, in which the thicker annular pulleys are easier to see than the thinner cruciate pulleys.

The extensor tendons pass under the extensor retinaculum and over the dorsum of the distal radius and ulna within six fibroosseous extensor compartments, which are described in detail in "Axial Anatomy." The anatomy of the digital extensor tendons is unique and can be appreciated on sagittal and axial imagery. Proximal to the proximal interphalangeal joint, each digital extensor tendon divides into one central and two lateral slips. The central slip inserts on the middle phalanx. The two lateral slips become confluent with the lateral bands formed by the intrinsic muscles to produce the two conjoined lateral bands. The conjoined lateral bands then converge to form the terminal extensor tendon, which inserts onto the distal phalanx.

The volar plates are fibrocartilaginous thickenings of the volar joint capsules of the metacarpophalangeal and interphalangeal joints. They are seen on sagittal imaging as low-intensity triangular structures. The sagittal bands originate at the volar plates and then extend dorsally where they stabilize the extensor tendons over the metacarpophalangeal joints. The sagittal bands, like the pulley system, are best seen on axial sections. The collateral ligaments of the digits have attachments to the volar plates and are most apparent on coronal sections. The collateral ligaments, together with the volar plates and dorsal capsule, are the primary static stabilizers of the metacarpophalangeal and interphalangeal joints.

9.1.2 Coronal Anatomy

On coronal sections, the proximal and distal carpal rows are delineated by three arcs (one over the proximal extent of the proximal carpal row, one over the distal extent of the proximal carpal row, and one over the proximal extent of the distal carpal row). These arcs, known as Gilula lines, should be smooth and parallel. Disruption of these parallel arcs indicates carpal instability. A different measure of alignment that can be assessed on coronal sections is ulnar variance. Ulnar variance describes the relative lengths of the ulna and the radius, and although it is usually measured on radiographs, it can also be estimated on coronal sections. A difference in ulnar variance of more than 2 mm in the positive or negative direction is considered abnormal. Positive ulnar variance has been associated with triangular fibrocartilage complex injuries and ulnar impaction syndrome, and negative ulnar variance has been associated with Kienböck disease.

Most of the major intrinsic and extrinsic ligaments of the wrist can be seen on coronal sections. The most clinically important intrinsic wrist ligaments are the scapholunate and lunotriquetral ligaments. These c-shaped structures vary in thickness throughout their courses. Although carpal ligaments usually have low signal intensity on MRI, the scapholunate ligament tends to be more heterogeneous. The scapholunate and lunotriquetral ligaments are made of volar, dorsal, and membranous bands. The dorsal layer has lower signal intensity than the middle or volar layer. Mechanically, the dorsal layer of the scapholunate ligament and the volar layer of the lunotriquetral ligament are most important for joint stability.

Volar and dorsal extrinsic ligaments can also be observed on coronal images.[2] These include the volar radioscaphocapitate ligament, the volar radiolunate ligament (also called the long radiolunate and radiolunotriquetral ligaments), the dorsal intercarpal ligament, and the dorsal radiotriquetral ligament. The volar radiolunate ligament is the largest ligament in the wrist and originates medial and proximal to the volar radioscaphocapitate ligament on the radial styloid. The dorsal intercarpal and dorsal radiotriquetral ligaments attach to the dorsal tubercle of the triquetrum and diverge from one another in a V-shaped configuration to insert on the distal radius and carpus.

The triangular fibrocartilage complex encompasses the major stabilizing structure of the ulnar aspect of the wrist, spanning the distal radioulnar joint and consisting of the following components[3]:

- Dorsal and volar radioulnar ligaments.
- Fibrocartilaginous articular disk.
- Meniscal homologue.
- Extensor carpi ulnaris subsheath.
- Ulnar collateral ligament.
- Ulnolunate ligament.
- Ulnotriquetral ligament.

The normal triangular fibrocartilage complex is a low-signal-intensity, biconcave disk shaped like a bowtie in the coronal plane. The articular disk is readily apparent on coronal and sagittal images. Advances in MRI techniques have enabled visualization of other individual components of the triangular fibrocartilage complex such as the radioulnar ligaments and the extensor carpi ulnaris's subsheath.

The courses of the main arterial structures of the wrist and hand can be traced on coronal images. The radial and ulnar arteries typically anastomose at the deep and superficial palmar arches, although variations exist. After passing through the snuffbox and entering the hand, the radial artery terminates in the deep palmar arch. The ulnar artery enters the hand via Guyon canals and terminates in the superficial palmar arch. The superficial and deep palmar arches provide the main blood supply to the palm and digits.

9.1.3 Axial Anatomy

The axial sections provide optimal imaging of the carpal tunnel and Guyon canal. The carpal tunnel contains the median nerve, flexor digitorum superficialis, flexor digitorum profundus, and flexor pollicis longus tendons. The flexor pollicis longus tendon lies most radially in the tunnel. The four flexor digitorum superficialis tendons lie ulnar to the flexor pollicis longus tendon and superficial to the four flexor digitorum profundus tendons. The roof of the carpal tunnel is formed by the low-signal-intensity transverse carpal ligament, which is deep to the palmar fascia and attaches proximally to the scaphoid tubercle and pisiform and distally to the trapezium and hook of the hamate. The transverse carpal ligament is split into two layers by the flexor carpi radialis tendon, which passes through it before inserting onto the second metacarpal base. The carpal bones form the floor of the tunnel.

Guyon canal lies ulnar and superficial to the carpal tunnel in a depression between the pisiform and the hook of the hamate. Its floor is formed by the transverse carpal ligament and hypothenar muscles, and its roof is formed by the volar carpal ligament. The ulnar nerve and artery traverse the tunnel; the nerve is situated ulnar to the artery. The nerve gives rise to its terminal sensory and deep motor branches within the canal, and three zones of the canal have been defined. The first zone is located proximal to the bifurcation and contains the ulnar nerve proper. The second and third zones extend from the bifurcation distally. The second zone contains the deep motor branch, and the third zone contains the superficial sensory branch. These zones represent distinct sites of nerve compression with unique clinical manifestations.

On the dorsal side of the wrist, axial sections show the six extensor compartments clearly.

- I: Extensor pollicis brevis, abductor pollicis longus.
- II: Extensor carpi radialis brevis, extensor carpi radialis longus.
- III: Extensor pollicis longus.
- IV: Extensor digitorum communis, extensor indicis.
- V: Extensor digiti minimi.
- VI: Extensor carpi ulnaris.

The extensor tendons pass through these fibroosseous canals as they course distally over the dorsal radius and ulna. The extensor retinaculum, an intermediate-signal structure on T1- and T2-weighted sequences, forms the roof of the compartments, which have fixed relationships to the underlying osseous anatomy. Lister tubercle lies between the second and third compartments, the fifth compartment overlies the distal radioulnar joint, and the sixth compartment lies in a deep groove radial to the ulnar styloid.

9.2 Systematic Approach to Image Review

T1-weighted, T2-weighted, and specialized sequences should be viewed in all three imaging planes. T2-weighted images should be examined first for areas of increased signal intensity, which can then be correlated with T1-weighted images for improved anatomic detail. Structures should be comprehensively evaluated in a stepwise fashion. Bones and joints are evaluated first to detect abnormal areas that could represent occult fractures, osteonecrosis, infection, neoplasm, osteophytes, joint space narrowing, erosions, or chondral defects. Attention must also be paid to overall osseous alignment to detect signs of carpal instability, which can be subtle. This should include inspection of Gilula lines and measurement of capitolunate, radiolunate, and scapholunate angles. Ulnar variance should also be assessed, especially in patients with suspicion for triangular fibrocartilage complex injuries, ulnar impaction, or Kienböck disease. The synovium and synovial fluid should be examined for presence of effusion, loose bodies, or synovial proliferation. The triangular fibrocartilage complex should be assessed for signs of tearing or degeneration. If the study is an arthrogram, the presence or absence of fluid leakage should be noted. The intrinsic and extrinsic ligaments should be examined to determine whether tears or attritional changes are present. The pulleys, collateral ligaments of the digits, volar plates, and sagittal bands should be evaluated if possible. The flexor and extensor tendons should be examined along their lengths for rupture, adhesions, tenosynovitis, or subluxation. Subluxation of the extensor tendons at the metacarpophalangeal joint suggests injury to the sagittal bands. The carpal tunnel should be inspected for enlargement or enhancement of the median nerve or masses within the tunnel. Similarly, Guyon canal should be assessed for the presence of masses, hook of the hamate fractures, or abnormal ulnar nerve changes. Finally, the remaining soft tissues should be checked for fluid collections, neoplasms, or other abnormalities.

9.3 Six Specialized Pulse Sequences and Imaging Protocols

The routine use of MRI for the distal upper extremity, compared with its use for larger joints, has been hindered by the technical challenges of imaging small anatomic structures. MRI of the wrist and hand typically is performed at a magnetic field strength of 0.2 to 3.0 T, using systems with dedicated surface coils. Recent advances in high-field-strength magnets and extremity surface coil design, however, have improved image quality.[1,4] Prospective studies have shown higher contrast-to-noise ratios between muscle and bone and between bone and cartilage and greater detection of anatomic structures with 3-T than with 1.5-T systems.[5,6] The 3-T systems are now becoming available for clinical use, but most hand and wrist examinations are still performed with 1.5-T magnets.

The hand and wrist are best imaged with the patient prone and the affected extremity placed above the head with the forearm pronated. Typically, the closer the body part being imaged is to the isocenter of the magnet, the better the image quality. Because this position is uncomfortable for many patients, scanning may be performed with the patient supine, the arm positioned at the patient's side, and the forearm in neutral position, with the attendant risk of some degradation of image quality. A small field of view and 1- to 3-mm thick sections are preferable.

Scanning is performed routinely in the axial, coronal, and sagittal planes. Most centers use a standard screening examination, consisting of an array of specified imaging planes and their corresponding pulse sequences. According to the indication, other pulse sequences may be added. Standard pulse sequences include the following:

- T1-weighted.
- T2-weighted fast spin-echo (FSE) with fat suppression.
- Short tau inversion recovery (STIR).
- Gradient-echo.

T1-weighted images provide good anatomic detail and are especially useful for identifying fat (given its high signal intensity on these images) in lipomatous masses or atrophied muscles. Fat-suppressed, T2-weighted sequences are the most sensitive for detecting many pathologic conditions by accentuating the presence of abnormal fluid, edema, or hemorrhage related to traumatic injury or an inflammatory process. Gradient-echo sequences, especially with a 3D, thin-section technique, are useful for evaluating the carpal ligaments and articular cartilage (see Chapter 5, Articular Cartilage).

MR arthrography of the wrist can be performed with single-, double-, or triple-compartment (radiocarpal, intercarpal, or distal radioulnar compartments) injection of contrast material. Approximately 2 to 5 mL of contrast material is administered using sterile technique and fluoroscopic guidance. A single-compartment radiocarpal technique is used most often with normal dissemination of contrast material between the proximal carpal row and the distal radius. Fat-suppressed, T1-weighted images are typically obtained in all three planes, in addition to other sequences. MR arthrography of the wrist has proven useful in evaluating the scapholunate ligament, the lunotriquetral ligament, and the triangular fibrocartilage complex.[7]

Intravenous contrast provides valuable information for evaluating a soft tissue mass or possible synovial process involving the wrist and hand, especially when combined with fat-suppressed T1-weighted images. It is useful for differentiating solid and cystic lesions, showing rim-enhancing soft tissue abscesses, and determining bone vascularity in cases of suspected osteonecrosis. Intravenous contrast may also be used to perform indirect arthrography, in which the contrast may migrate into the joint over time. This effect is most notable in an inflamed joint. The information to be gained from these procedures must always be weighed against the additional cost and risk associated with an invasive procedure.

9.4 Traumatic Conditions

Traumatic conditions affecting the wrist and hand that are commonly evaluated by MRI include occult fractures, tears of the triangular fibrocartilage complex, and injuries to the interosseous carpal ligaments and small joint ligaments and tendons.

9.4.1 Occult Fractures of the Scaphoid and Other Bones

Initial radiographs of patients with scaphoid fractures are often negative because of the scaphoid's unique morphology. Therefore, patients with negative radiographs and tenderness in the anatomic snuffbox or scaphoid tubercle after traumatic injury to an outstretched hand may be immobilized presumptively until follow-up radiographs confirm or exclude the diagnosis to avoid the potential negative consequences of a missed fracture.

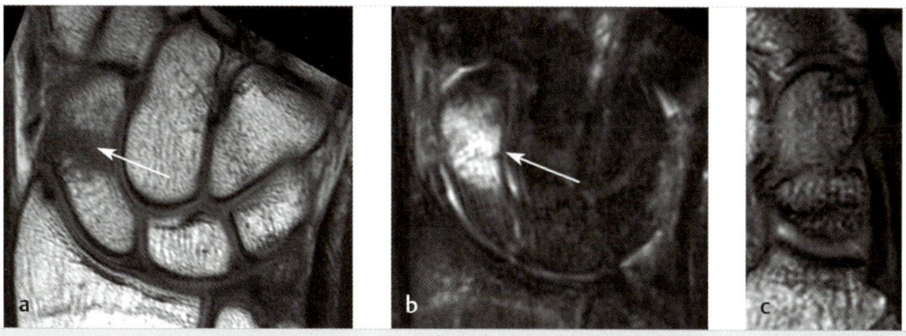

Fig. 9.1 Scaphoid fracture/deformity. **(a)** A coronal T1-weighted image of the wrist showing a fracture through the scaphoid waist (*arrow*), seen as a discrete line of low signal intensity. **(b)** A coronal fat-suppressed T2-weighted image showing the same fracture with focal marrow edema in the scaphoid waist consistent with fracture (*arrow*). **(c)** A sagittal gradient-echo image showing a humpback deformity of the scaphoid. (Reproduced with permission from Brunton LM, Anderson MW, Chhabra AB. The wrist and hand. In: Khanna AJ, ed. MRI for orthopaedic surgeons. New York: Thieme; 2010:129–143.)

Alternatively, advanced imaging modalities can be used to detect radiographically occult scaphoid fracture early to avoid unnecessary immobilization. Early advanced imaging for patients with suspected occult fractures is likely more comfortable and cost-effective than cast immobilization and repeat radiography at a later date.[8] A review of comparative studies sought to determine the superior modality for confirming the diagnosis: bone scintigraphy, CT, MRI, or ultrasonography.[9] Although there is no consensus, many surgeons favor MRI for its safety and ability to provide information about alternative diagnoses.[10,11,12]

A fracture may be identified on T1-weighted images as a distinct line of low signal intensity that contrasts with the surrounding high-signal marrow (▶ Fig. 9.1a). Fat-suppressed, T2-weighted images typically show high-signal marrow edema surrounding the fracture line (▶ Fig. 9.1b). A scaphoid humpback deformity may also be shown on sagittal images (▶ Fig. 9.1c).

MRI is sensitive in the detection of occult fractures in the distal radius, distal ulna, and other carpal bones (▶ Fig. 9.2) and can also differentiate fractures from bone bruises (contusions), which show marrow edema without a discrete fracture line.[13,14] MRI is also sensitive for diagnosing subtle physeal injuries in children (▶ Fig. 9.3) and for evaluating physeal bars and growth arrest.[15] Radiographically, occult fractures of the metacarpals and phalanges are uncommon.

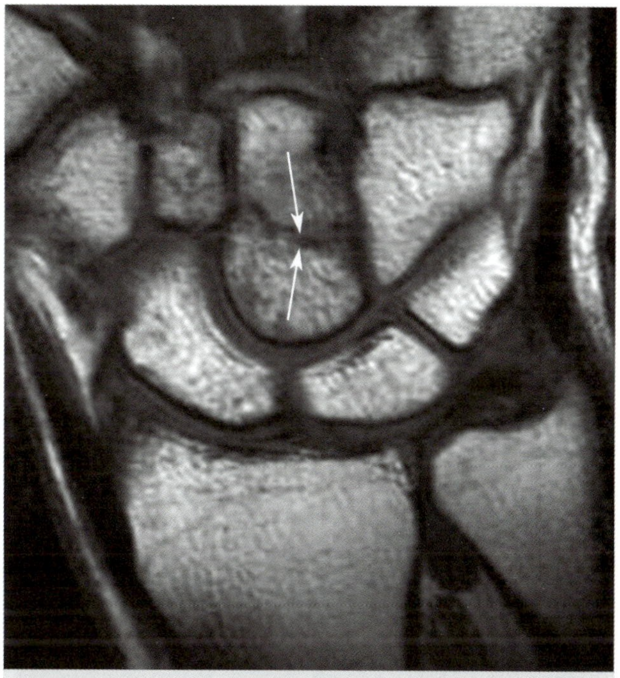

Fig. 9.2 A coronal T1-weighted image of the wrist showing a radiographically occult capitate fracture (*arrows*). (Reproduced with permission from Brunton LM, Anderson MW, Chhabra AB. The wrist and hand. In: Khanna AJ, ed. MRI for orthopaedic surgeons. New York: Thieme; 2010:129–143.)

9.4.2 Triangular Fibrocartilage Complex Injury

Tears of the triangular fibrocartilage complex may be classified as degenerative or traumatic.[16] Degenerative central perforations of the triangular fibrocartilage complex are common and often asymptomatic. Conversely, acute injuries to the triangular fibrocartilage complex frequently lead to ulnar-side wrist pain and dysfunction. It is difficult to distinguish this condition from other causes of ulnar-side wrist pain (such as occult fractures, lunotriquetral ligament injury, extensor carpi ulnaris tendinopathy or subluxation, distal radioulnar joint injury, or pisotriquetral joint injury) by history and physical examination. Historically, three-compartment wrist arthrography was the imaging test of choice for evaluation of the triangular fibrocartilage complex. However, this modality has unacceptably low sensitivity and specificity and lacks the ability to determine lesion size, location, and acuity.[17,18] Although wrist arthroscopy remains the standard for diagnosing triangular fibrocartilage complex pathology, technological advances have improved the ability to evaluate the size, location, and character of triangular fibrocartilage complex tears using MRI and MR arthrography before wrist arthroscopy. In the most specialized centers, the sensitivity and accuracy of MRI for detecting triangular fibrocartilage complex tears approaches 100%, using arthroscopy as the standard diagnostic modality.[19] Not all triangular fibrocartilage complex tears are symptomatic, hence making clinical correlation important. In one study, the prevalence of triangular fibrocartilage complex abnormalities on MRI in 103 asymptomatic volunteers was found to be 38%, with 22% of subjects having complete tears.[20] T2-weighted

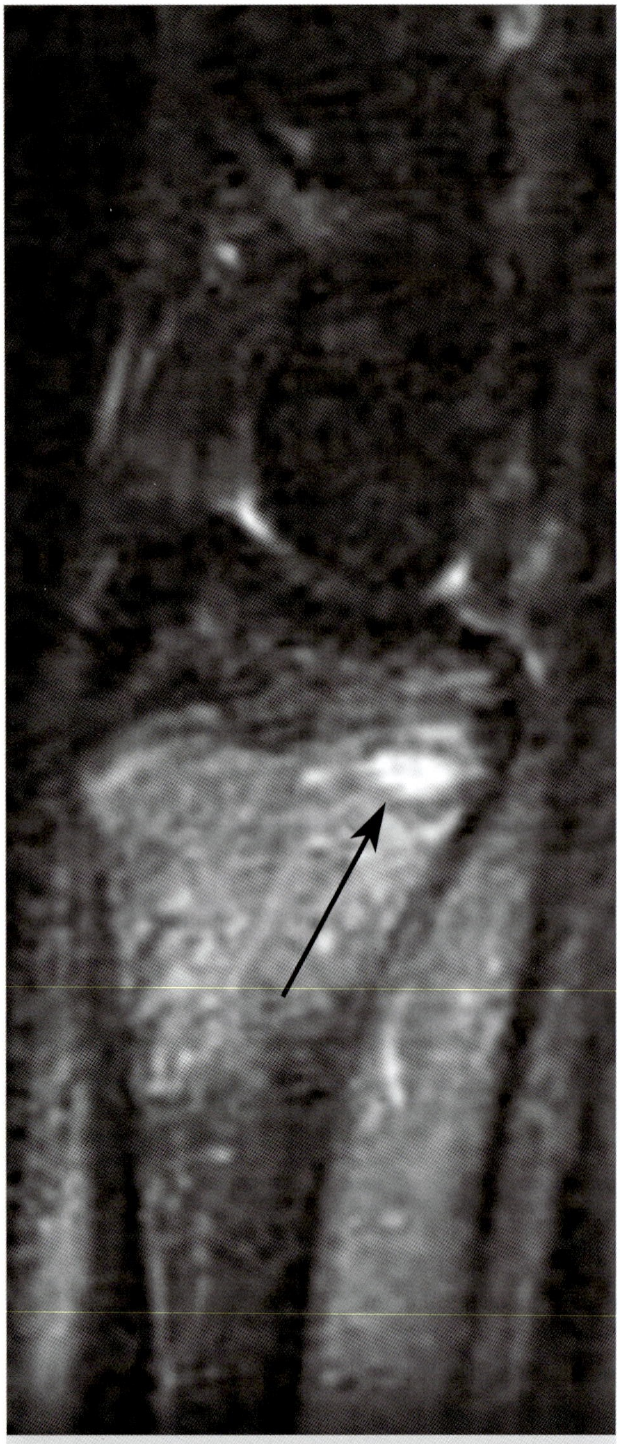

Fig. 9.3 Stress injury in the skeletally immature wrist. A sagittal short tau inversion recovery (STIR) image of the wrist showing diffuse marrow edema in the distal radius metaphysis adjacent to the growth plate, which is widened along its volar aspect (*arrow*). (Reproduced with permission from Brunton LM, Anderson MW, Chhabra AB. The wrist and hand. In: Khanna AJ, ed. MRI for orthopaedic surgeons. New York: Thieme; 2010:129–143.)

images may help to differentiate between degenerative and traumatic tears of the triangular fibrocartilage complex, with traumatic tears showing increased signal intensity in adjacent tissues. The excellent anatomic detail afforded by MRI also helps in determining the specific lesion location, with degenerative tears typically occurring in the thinner central portion and traumatic tears most often found in the periphery of the triangular fibrocartilage complex (▶ Fig. 9.4). Nonetheless, all triangular fibrocartilage complex attachments must be carefully evaluated in all three planes. Ulnar attachment tears have been consistently more difficult to diagnose.[21] Concomitant pathology of the extensor carpi ulnaris tendon, lunotriquetral ligament, and surrounding osseous structures must be pursued. MR arthrography may be superior to MRI in detecting some triangular fibrocartilage complex lesions.[22] A triangular fibrocartilage complex tear is often shown by the presence of gadolinium contrast within the tear itself and/or in the distal radioulnar joint. Strong evidence exists that observer experience is critical for the accurate detection of triangular fibrocartilage complex pathology.[23]

9.4.3 Interosseous Ligament Injury

The scapholunate and lunotriquetral ligaments are the most commonly injured wrist ligaments secondary to acute trauma. MRI has supplanted stress radiography and conventional wrist arthrography as the study of choice for suspected carpal ligament injury. Compared with arthroscopy, conventional MRI is highly specific but has an overall low sensitivity for the detection of tears of the scapholunate and lunotriquetral ligaments, although the sensitivity seems to be improving with technologic advances in imaging techniques.[24] Disruption of the interosseous ligaments is best evaluated on coronal gradient-echo (▶ Fig. 9.5) and fat-suppressed T2-weighted images. The normally heterogenous appearance of the scapholunate ligament on coronal images may lead to the misdiagnosis of a tear. Distinct linear areas of high signal intensity equal to that of fluid, especially in the thick dorsal portion of the ligament, usually indicate clinically meaningful tears, which may lead to carpal instability if not treated. Alternative findings in ligament tears include nonvisualization of the ligament or morphologic distortion.[25] MR arthrography may be more accurate than conventional MRI for the detection of interosseous ligament injuries.[4,26,27,28]

9.4.4 Extrinsic Carpal Ligament Injury

The extrinsic carpal ligaments are a complex assortment of dorsal and volar structures that lie in close relation to the wrist joint capsule.[29] The volar extrinsic ligaments are stronger and more robust than their dorsal counterparts. Isolated acute injuries to the extrinsic ligaments are rare. Typically, disruptions of these ligaments are part of a constellation of acute bone and soft tissue injuries about the wrist joint. Although MRI can distinguish the extrinsic ligament complexes with multiple image planes (▶ Fig. 9.6), the role of MRI in this clinical setting is more often to exclude occult fracture, disruption of the intrinsic carpal ligaments, or injury to the triangular fibrocartilage complex. If diagnosed, these conditions may require a change in treatment.

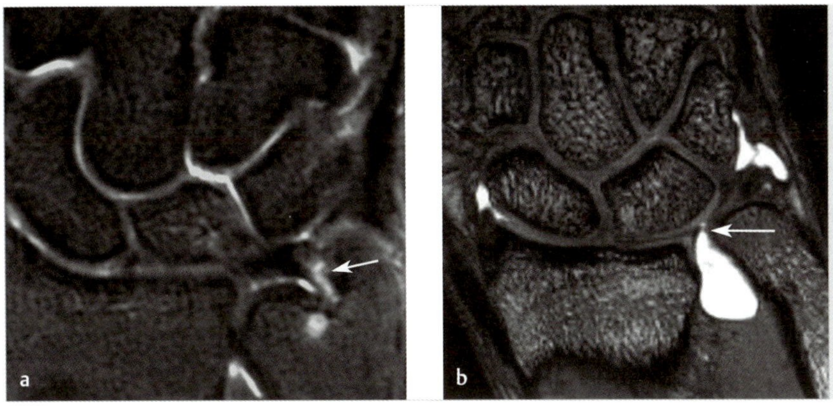

Fig. 9.4 Peripheral triangular fibrocartilage complex tear. **(a)** A coronal fat-suppressed T2-weighted image showing a tear of the peripheral portion of the triangular fibrocartilage complex near its ulnar attachment (*arrow*). **(b)** A coronal gradient-echo image showing a perforation of the central portion of the triangular fibrocartilage complex near its radial attachment (*arrow*). (Reproduced with permission from Brunton LM, Anderson MW, Chhabra AB. The wrist and hand. In: Khanna AJ, ed. MRI for orthopaedic surgeons. New York: Thieme; 2010:129–143.)

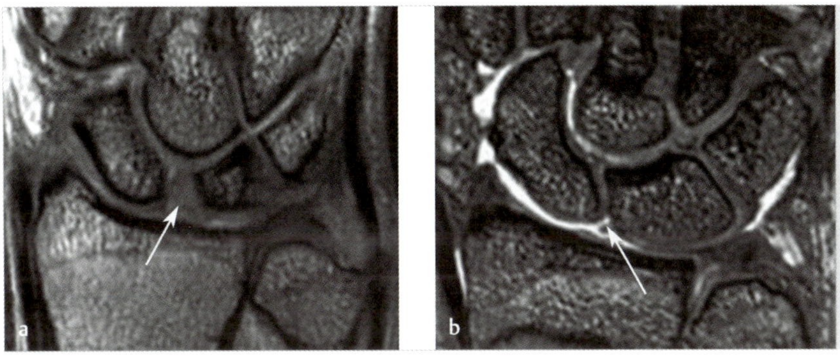

Fig. 9.5 Scapholunate ligament tear. **(a)** A coronal gradient-echo image of the wrist showing partial stretching of the scapholunate ligament with concurrent widening of the scapholunate interval (*arrow*). **(b)** A coronal gradient-echo image of the wrist showing a small perforation in the membranous portion of the scapholunate ligament (*arrow*). (Reproduced with permission from Brunton LM, Anderson MW, Chhabra AB. The wrist and hand. In: Khanna AJ, ed. MRI for orthopaedic surgeons. New York: Thieme; 2010:129–143.)

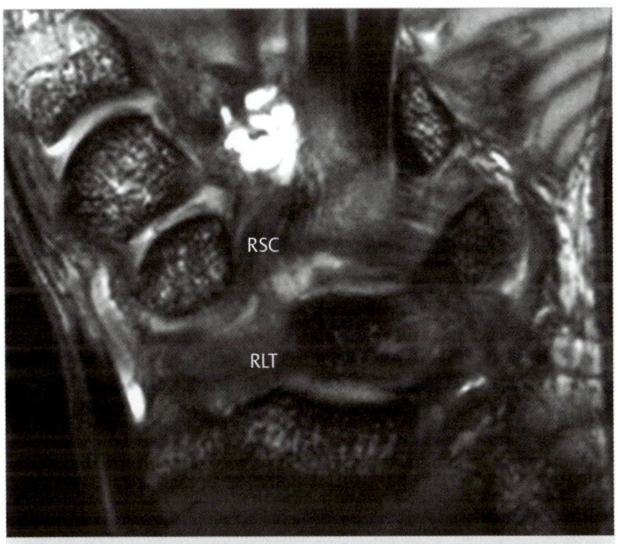

Fig. 9.6 A coronal gradient-echo image of the wrist showing the extrinsic ligaments comprising part of the volar wrist capsule, including the radioscaphocapitate (*RSC*) and radiolunotriquetral (*RLT*) ligaments. (Reproduced with permission from Brunton LM, Anderson MW, Chhabra AB. The wrist and hand. In: Khanna AJ, ed. MRI for orthopaedic surgeons. New York: Thieme; 2010:129–143.)

9.4.5 Thumb Ulnar Collateral Ligament Injury

The ulnar collateral ligament of the metacarpophalangeal joint is the primary stabilizer of the ulnar aspect of the thumb. Rupture of this ligament is common in skiers and results from forced abduction of the thumb. A Stener lesion describes displacement of the torn ligament to a position superficial to the aponeurosis of the adductor pollicis muscle, a conformation that inhibits ligament healing and is an indication for surgery. Although clinical presentation and stress radiography may be enough for the diagnosis of a torn ulnar collateral ligament, they cannot predict the presence of a Stener lesion. MRI helps guide surgical treatment of acute injuries by detecting Stener lesions and allowing measurement of ligament displacement, which has been used in predicting the success of nonoperative treatment (▶ Fig. 9.7).[30,31,32]

9.4.6 Tendon Injuries

Tendon pathology may occur as a result of acute trauma, chronic overuse, or inflammatory arthropathies such as rheumatoid arthritis (RA). The spectrum of pathology ranges from tendon thickening and various degrees of tendon or tendon sheath inflammation to frank tears. In patients with traumatic injury, partial or complete rupture of a hand or wrist tendon may be difficult to diagnose clinically. Although tenderness and localized swelling are often present, the degree of flexion or extension loss may be equivocal. The use of MRI and ultrasonography in this setting is evolving. Occasionally, ruptures of the extensor wrist tendons can be detected by MRI (▶ Fig. 9.8). On T2-weighted sequences, partial tendon tears typically show increased intrasubstance signal intensity (▶ Fig. 9.9), whereas complete tears show separation of the tendon ends with fluid tracking between its margins. Timely and accurate diagnosis has important clinical implications because early surgical repair

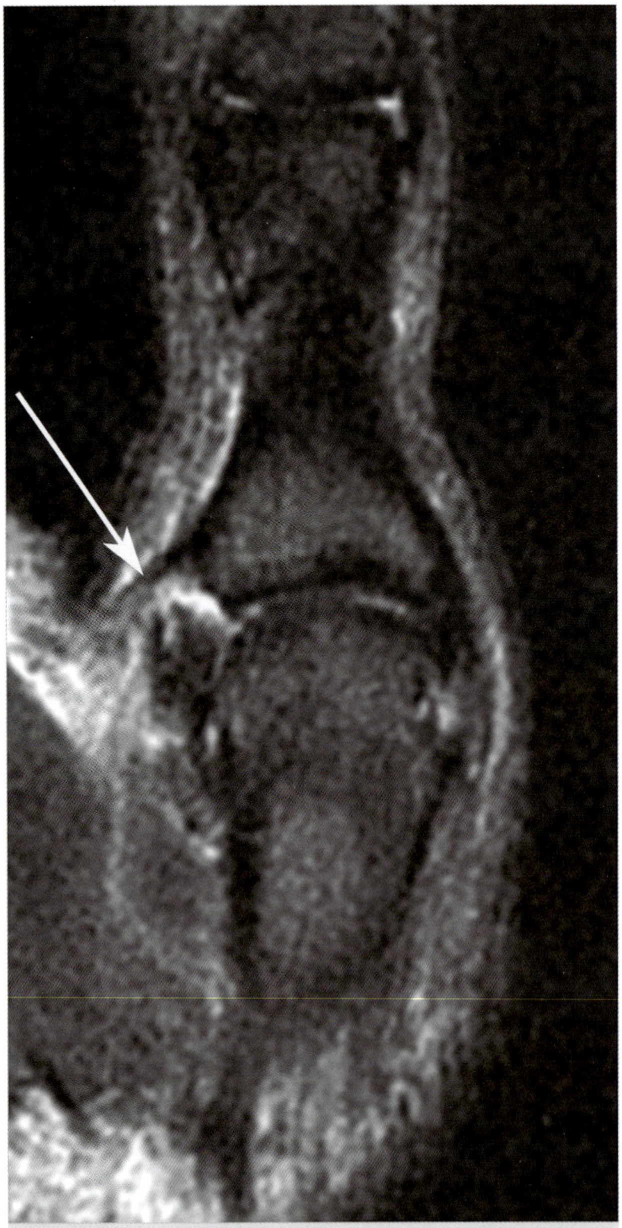

Fig. 9.7 A coronal oblique T2-weighted image of the thumb showing a complete rupture of the ulnar collateral ligament at the metacarpophalangeal joint with increased fluid emanating from the joint (*arrow*). (Reproduced with permission from Brunton LM, Anderson MW, Chhabra AB. The wrist and hand. In: Khanna AJ, ed. MRI for orthopaedic surgeons. New York: Thieme; 2010:129–143.)

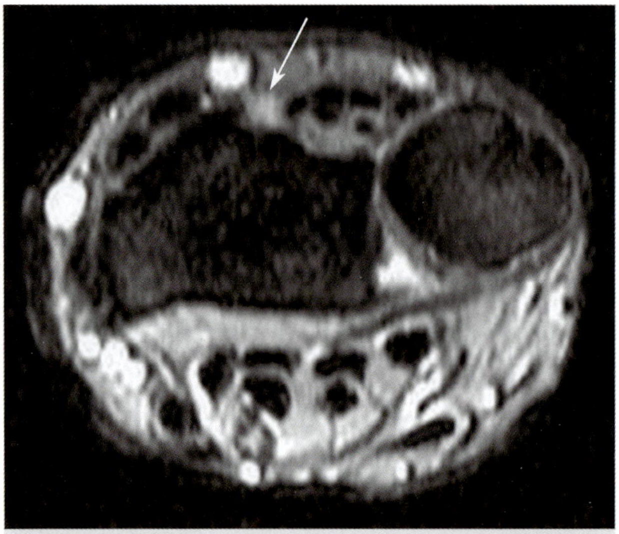

Fig. 9.8 An axial gradient-echo image of the wrist showing absence of the extensor pollicis longus tendon in the third extensor compartment, indicative of complete rupture (*arrow*). (Reproduced from Brunton LM, Anderson MW, Chhabra AB. The wrist and hand. In: Khanna AJ, ed. MRI for orthopaedic surgeons. New York: Thieme; 2010:129–143.)

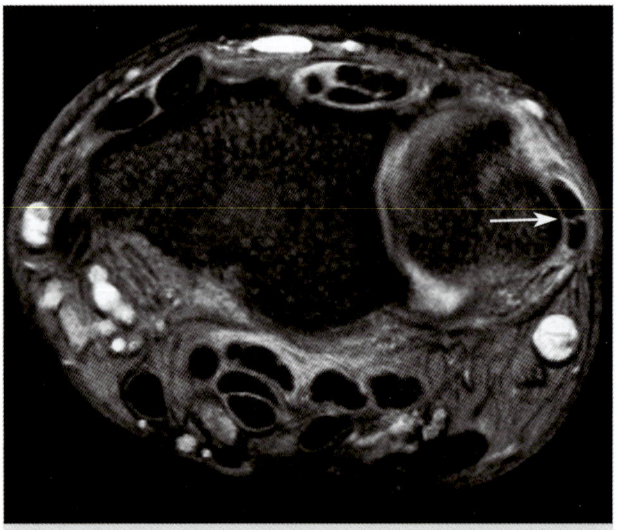

Fig. 9.9 An axial fat-suppressed T2-weighted image at the level of the distal radioulnar joint, showing subluxation of the extensor carpi ulnaris tendon and a high-signal-intensity split within the tendon, indicating a partial tear (*arrow*). (Reproduced with permission from Brunton LM, Anderson MW, Chhabra AB. The wrist and hand. In: Khanna AJ, ed. MRI for orthopaedic surgeons. New York: Thieme; 2010:129–143.)

provides the best outcome for zone-II flexor tendon tears comprising more than 50% of their width.[33] Similarly, identifying the location of the retracted tendon end after a zone-I flexor digitorum profundus avulsion injury (Jersey finger) is important for determining the appropriate treatment. Advances in image quality with sophisticated systems and MR tenography, in which contrast material is injected within the tendon sheath, have led to the detection of flexor pulley system injuries and concomitant bowstringing deformities of the flexor tendons.[1,34]

9.5 Degenerative Conditions

The wrist and hand are affected by various degenerative conditions, although the usefulness of MRI may be limited to evaluating ulnar impaction syndrome, tendon disorders, and carpal instability in select patients. Other common degenerative conditions in the hand and wrist such as first carpometacarpal joint and radiocarpal joint osteoarthritis are adequately imaged with conventional radiography.

9.5.1 Ulnar Impaction Syndrome

Ulnar variance relates to the relative lengths of the radius and ulna. In patients with ulnar positive variance, the relatively long ulna may abut the proximal carpal row when the wrist is ulnarly deviated, leading to ulnar-side wrist pain from excessive loading across the ulnar aspect of the wrist. Chronic impaction may lead to subchondral sclerosis or cyst formation of the proximal and ulnar portions of the lunate, the radial portion of the triquetrum, and/or the distal and radial portions of the ulnar head. Focal defects of the articular cartilage or increased marrow signal on T2-weighted images may be visualized (▶ Fig. 9.10). These findings can be differentiated from Kienböck disease because the signal changes are focal rather than diffuse, and the ulnar variance is usually positive rather than negative or neutral. MRI may also detect accompanying degenerative triangular fibrocartilage complex or lunotriquetral ligament tears.[35]

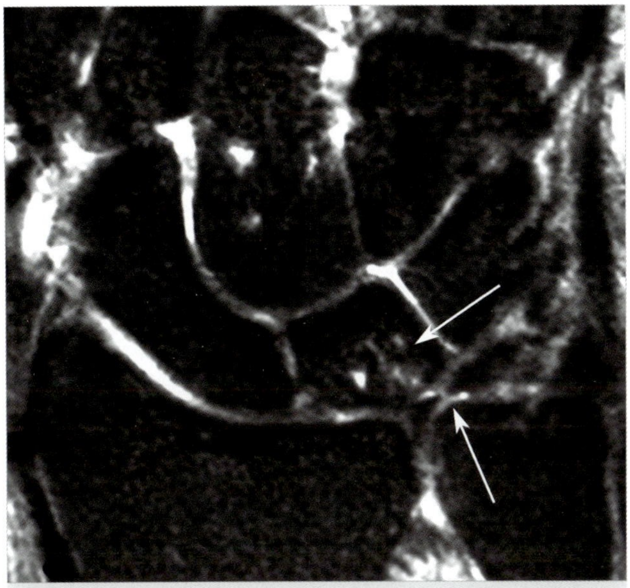

Fig. 9.10 A coronal short tau inversion recovery (STIR) image of the wrist showing focal edema and cystic changes at the proximal ulnar aspect of the lunate consistent with ulnar impaction syndrome (*top arrow*). A small perforation of the central portion of the triangular fibrocartilage complex is also shown (*bottom arrow*). (Reproduced with permission from Brunton LM, Anderson MW, Chhabra AB. The wrist and hand. In: Khanna AJ, ed. MRI for orthopaedic surgeons. New York: Thieme; 2010:129–143.)

9.5.2 Tendon Disorders

Pain and diminished function of the wrist and hand may be caused by various forms of tendon pathology, ranging from tendinosis to tenosynovitis to partial or complete tears. Although these conditions may result from simple overuse, other causes include inflammatory arthropathies, indolent infections, pigmented villonodular synovitis, gout, sarcoidosis, or amyloidosis.[36] Although tendon pathology is often self-limiting, MRI is excellent for assessing the spectrum of tendon pathology. MRI may show tendon thickening or thinning in patients with tendinosis. T2-weighted images may show distended tendon sheaths filled with high-signal-intensity fluid in patients with tenosynovitis (▶ Fig. 9.10). Occasionally, tiny foci of low signal intensity, called *rice bodies*, are seen within the fluid in patients with chronic tenosynovitis.

As an example, de Quervain tenosynovitis is a common inflammatory disorder of the first dorsal compartment. A spectrum of MRI findings may be seen, including thickening of the abductor pollicis longus and extensor pollicis brevis tendons, adjacent fluid collections, and increased intratendinous T2-weighted signal intensity (▶ Fig. 9.11). Similar findings are described for other commonly affected tendons, including the extensor carpi ulnaris, extensor carpi radialis longus, extensor

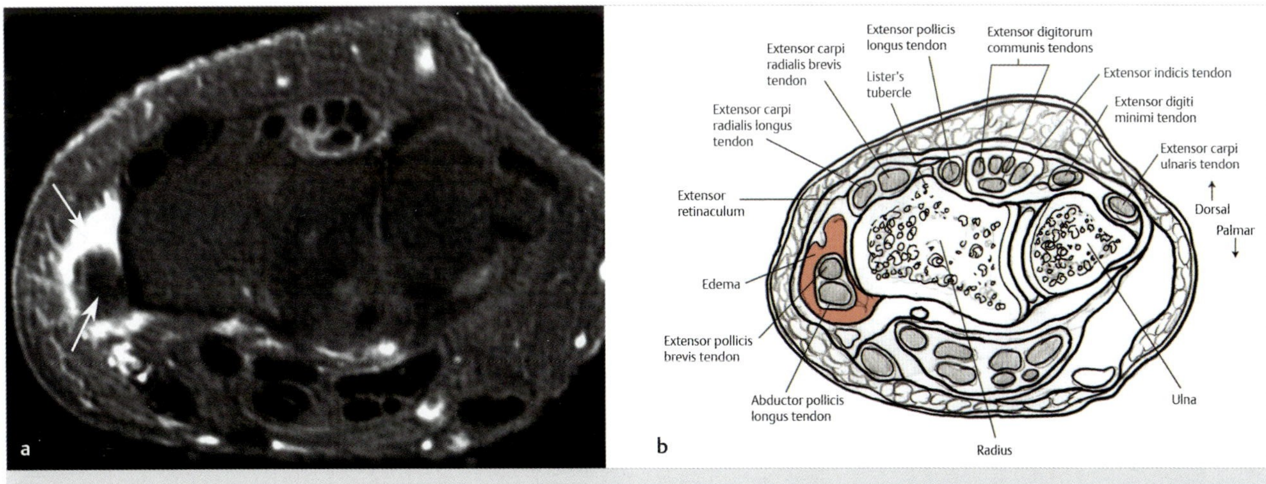

Fig. 9.11 De Quervain tenosynovitis. An axial fat-suppressed T2-weighted image (**a**) and illustration (**b**) showing thickening of the first compartment tendons and surrounding edema (*arrows on* **a**). (Reproduced with permission from Brunton LM, Anderson MW, Chhabra AB. The wrist and hand. In: Khanna AJ, ed. MRI for orthopaedic surgeons. New York: Thieme; 2010:129–143.)

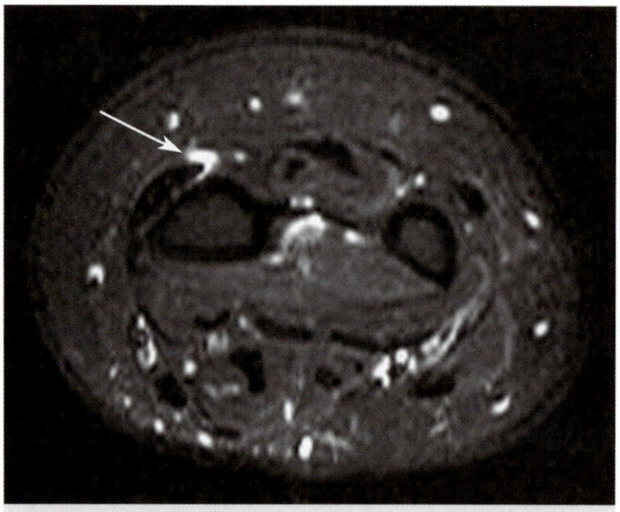

Fig. 9.12 Axial fat-suppressed T2-weighted image showing peritendinous fluid at the level where the tendons of the first and second extensor compartments cross, consistent with intersection syndrome from chronic overuse (*arrow*). (Reproduced with permission from Brunton LM, Anderson MW, Chhabra AB. The wrist and hand. In: Khanna AJ, ed. MRI for orthopaedic surgeons. New York: Thieme; 2010:129–143.)

pollicis longus, flexor carpi radialis, and flexor carpi ulnaris (▶ Fig. 9.12). Tendon subluxation or dislocation from chronic overuse may be detected on axial images. MRI may help differentiate chronic tenosynovitis and soft tissue masses such as giant cell tumor of the tendon sheath.

The clinician should keep in mind that when a tendon lies at approximately 55 degrees relative to the direction of the external magnetic field during scanning, artifactual increased intratendinous signal intensity may be observed on some imaging sequences secondary to the *magic angle phenomenon*, not to true pathology.[37,38] This phenomenon is recognized easily because the signal disappears and the tendon appears normal on heavily T2-weighted images. This phenomenon also is seen in the shoulder where the presence of the magic angle phenomenon may be mistaken for rotator cuff tendinopathy (see Chapter 7, The Shoulder).

Given that the clinical findings are typically diagnostic, MRI is not necessary for the diagnosis of stenosing tenosynovitis of the digits (trigger finger), although it may have a role in evaluating patients with postoperative recurrence or in ruling out other causes of symptoms such as tendon sheath tumor, rheumatoid synovitis, or volar plate pathology.

9.5.3 Carpal Instability

The most common pattern of carpal instability is dorsal-intercalated segment instability, often associated with disruption of the scapholunate and volar extrinsic carpal ligaments. Volar intercalated segment instability from lunotriquetral ligament deficiency is far less common. Clinically, carpal instabilities usually present as chronic wrist pain months to years after traumatic injury or secondary to inflammatory arthropathy. Physical examination findings are often equivocal, and standard lateral wrist radiographs may not always show abnormal carpal alignment. In patients with static carpal instability, the malalignment will be evident on sagittal images, and MRI may also detect associated abnormalities of the stabilizing carpal ligaments such as laxity, thickening, retraction, edema, or absence. MR arthrography and thin-section coronal gradient-echo images are the most useful for identifying the pathology of these structures. Perforations of the central portions of the interosseous ligaments may be asymptomatic and consistent with normal aging.[39]

9.6 Other Pathologic Conditions

MRI is useful in evaluating other pathologic conditions affecting the wrist and hand such as infections, osteonecrosis, RA, compression neuropathies, and soft tissue masses.

9.6.1 Infectious Conditions

Soft tissue abscesses within the hand or wrist typically show intermediate to low signal intensity on T1-weighted images and high signal intensity on T2-weighted images. A thick, enhancing wall is usually seen after the administration of intravenous contrast. MRI can evaluate the extent of soft tissue involvement and the presence or absence of osteomyelitis. An emergent MRI may be necessary in select patients with suspected necrotizing fasciitis, for which T2-weighted images may help confirm the diagnosis with increased signal intensity seen in the deep fascia, although this imaging finding is nonspecific. Given the need for urgent treatment of this condition, the clinician should also carefully evaluate for the presence of crepitus within the soft tissues and rapidly spreading erythema and induration. Prompt treatment of infectious processes in critically ill patients should never be delayed while awaiting an MRI study. MRI is of limited use in monitoring the progress of infections during the course of treatment because many of the changes observed on imaging resolve very slowly after successful treatment.[40]

9.6.2 Kienböck Disease

Idiopathic osteonecrosis of the lunate is known as Kienböck disease. This diagnosis must be considered in patients with subacute or chronic dorsal wrist pain of unknown cause. A strong association with negative ulnar variance exists, and the cause of the disorder may stem from chronic microtrauma secondary to increased shear stress on the lunate. Lichtman et al[41] defined four stages of Kienböck disease:

- Stage I: normal on conventional radiographs, changes in the lunate on MRI.
- Stage II: lunate sclerosis on conventional radiographs.
- Stage III: lunate collapse.
- Stage IV: pancarpal arthritis.

Early diagnosis by MRI is critical because nonoperative treatment and surgery are most successful in the initial stages of the disease, long before progression to lunate collapse or pancarpal arthritis.

In the first stage of Kienböck disease, MRI shows distinct changes in the lunate. On T1-weighted images, abnormally low lunate vascularity leads to diffuse low signal intensity of the bone marrow compared with the surrounding carpal bones (▸ Fig. 9.13). This diffuse involvement distinguishes Kienböck disease from focal T1-weighted signal loss secondary to ulnar impaction syndrome, fracture, or tumor. The findings on T2-weighted images have been correlated with prognosis, showing low signal intensity with complete marrow fibrosis and increased signal intensity with lunate revascularization. When stage-I Kienböck disease is diagnosed, patients are typically immobilized for up to 3 months, and follow-up MRI examinations are used to monitor the success of nonoperative treatment. Normalization of T1 and T2 signal intensity has also been observed on MRI postoperatively in patients undergoing surgery for Kienböck disease.[42]

MRI findings are similar in idiopathic osteonecrosis of the scaphoid, also known as Preiser disease, and other carpal bones. However, because of its relative rarity, Preiser disease has been less well-characterized. One study supports the possibility of two patterns of Preiser disease based on disparate MRI patterns of vascular impairment[43]:

- Type-1 variant, diffuse involvement of the scaphoid.
- Type-2 variant, only partial necrosis.

Another study describes stages rather than patterns of Preiser disease[44]: an initial stage with proximal osteonecrosis but unaltered overall scaphoid morphology, an advanced stage with pathologic fractures and volume loss of the proximal pole, and a final stage with the entire scaphoid involved. The recognition of these distinct imaging patterns has implications for treatment, and the clinical outcome may be less favorable for patients with more diffuse involvement.[43]

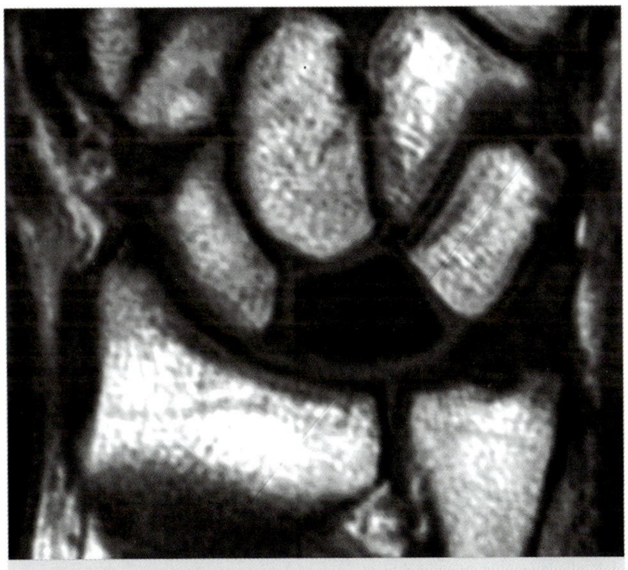

Fig. 9.13 Coronal T1-weighted image showing complete loss of normal marrow signal within the lunate, indicating necrosis (Kienböck disease). (Reproduced with permission from Brunton LM, Anderson MW, Chhabra AB. The wrist and hand. In: Khanna AJ, ed. MRI for orthopaedic surgeons. New York: Thieme; 2010:129–143.)

9.6.3 Posttraumatic Scaphoid Osteonecrosis

The tenuous retrograde blood supply of the scaphoid often results in delayed union, nonunion, and/or osteonecrosis of the proximal pole. These complications are minimized with the early diagnosis of a scaphoid fracture and the implementation of appropriate treatment. In patients with scaphoid nonunion, determination of bone viability is critical to subsequent management. Vascularity of the proximal fragment has been shown to be an important determinant of outcome after surgical reconstruction of a scaphoid nonunion.[45] Patients with proximal pole osteonecrosis may require vascularized bone grafting. Visual inspection of intraoperative punctate bleeding typically corresponds with viability of the proximal pole. Because conventional radiographs are unreliable for detecting bone vascularity, MRI can be used to assess the degree of osteonecrosis before surgery. Osteonecrosis is indicated by low signal intensity on T1-weighted images, in stark contrast to the high signal intensity of the marrow of the normal surrounding carpal bones (▸ Fig. 9.14). T2-weighted images have been shown to be unreliable for determining whether osteonecrosis is present.[46] Various authors have investigated the use of dynamic gadolinium-enhanced MRI in determining proximal pole viability and have not found it to add predictive value compared with unenhanced or standard enhanced images.[46,47]

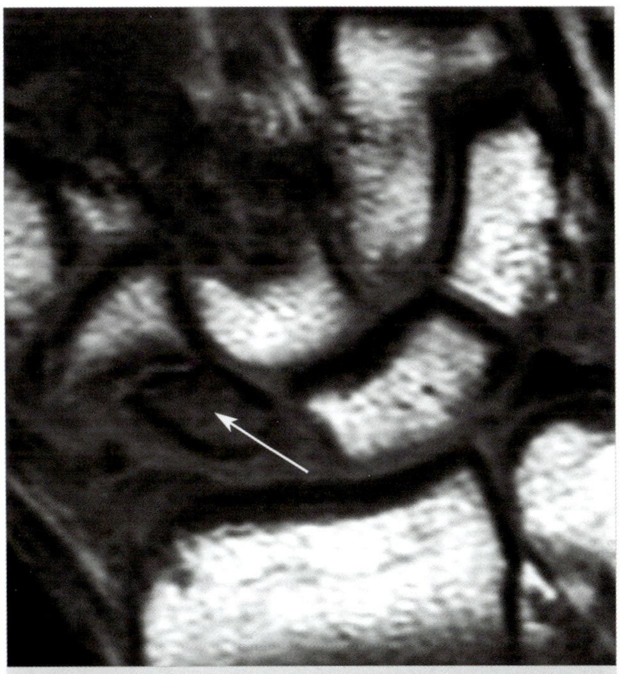

Fig. 9.14 A coronal T1-weighted image showing loss of normal marrow signal in the proximal pole of the scaphoid (*arrow*), indicative of posttraumatic osteonecrosis. (Reproduced with permission from Brunton LM, Anderson MW, Chhabra AB. The wrist and hand. In: Khanna AJ, ed. MRI for orthopaedic surgeons. New York: Thieme; 2010:129–143.)

9.6.4 RA

RA, the most common form of inflammatory arthritis, is characterized by inflammation of the synovial lining of joints and tendon sheaths. It frequently affects the hand and wrist early in the disease process. Although RA may become a severely disabling condition, recent clinical trials unequivocally support early intervention with aggressive pharmacologic therapy for the prevention of rapid joint erosion and the improvement of long-term outcomes.[48] The necessity for timely and accurate diagnosis is implicit within this strategy. For many patients, this diagnosis is achieved only by history, physical examination, laboratory data, and conventional radiographic findings. A more expeditious diagnosis of early RA, however, may be provided with MRI.

Several reports have shown the value of MRI in detecting bone erosion and active synovitis before changes are visible on conventional radiographs.[49,50] MRI bone edema in patients with early RA has also been associated with radiographic progression.[51] Contrast-enhanced images can be obtained to investigate a possible diagnosis of RA via MRI. Intense bilateral contrast enhancement in the wrist, metacarpophalangeal joint, or proximal interphalangeal joint suggests active synovitis and indicates inflammatory arthritis (▶ Fig. 9.15). In addition, adjacent bone edema or frank erosions can be detected (▶ Fig. 9.16). These imaging findings are nonspecific; therefore, the clinician must consider the entire clinical picture so that other diagnoses (e.g., systemic lupus erythematosus, scleroderma, polymyositis, dermatomyositis, Behçet disease, or mixed connective disease) are excluded.[52,53] Advanced techniques have been developed to quantify the volume of affected synovium and bone erosion with MRI. These methods may be useful in predicting disease progression and monitoring the response to treatment.[54]

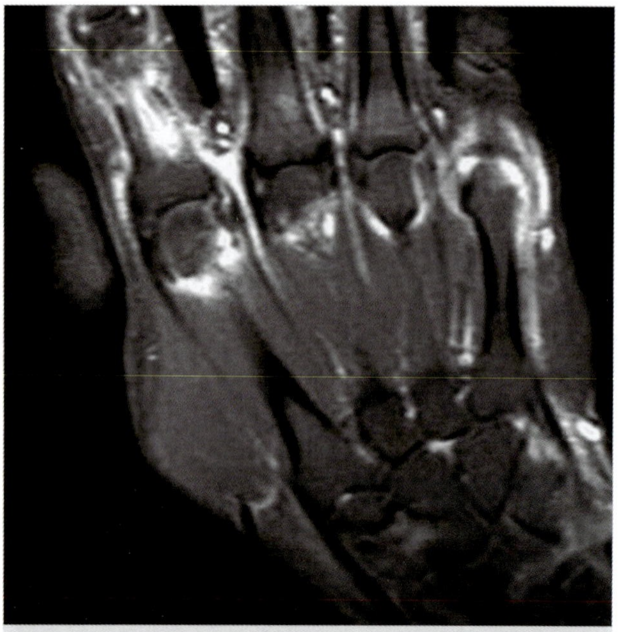

Fig. 9.15 A coronal fat-suppressed postgadolinium T1-weighted image showing diffuse high signal enhancement surrounding the metacarpophalangeal joints, consistent with synovitis from early rheumatoid arthritis (RA). Conventional radiographs were normal. (Reproduced with permission from Brunton LM, Anderson MW, Chhabra AB. The wrist and hand. In: Khanna AJ, ed. MRI for orthopaedic surgeons. New York: Thieme; 2010:129–143.)

9.6.5 Compression Neuropathies

The nerve branches in the hand and wrist most frequently affected by compression syndromes are the median nerve in the carpal tunnel and the ulnar nerve in Guyon canal. The superficial sensory branch of the radial nerve is affected much less commonly. Compression neuropathies may be triggered by intrinsic or extrinsic sources. Most patients are diagnosed by history and physical examination findings, which are then corroborated by electrodiagnostic testing. Although T2-weighted axial images may show increased intraneural signal because of nerve compression, MRI plays a primarily adjunctive role in evaluating compression neuropathies. Some patients present with atypical or equivocal clinical features or nerve conduction

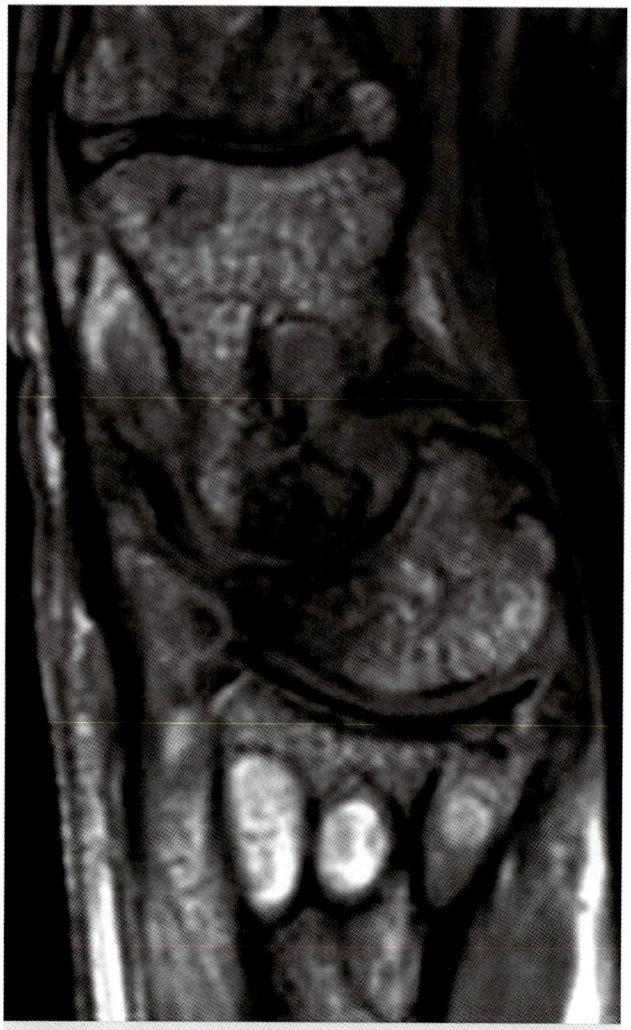

Fig. 9.16 A sagittal gradient-echo image of the wrist showing multiple subchondral cysts and periarticular erosions in the setting of advanced rheumatoid arthritis (RA). (Reproduced with permission from Brunton LM, Anderson MW, Chhabra AB. The wrist and hand. In: Khanna AJ, ed. MRI for orthopaedic surgeons. New York: Thieme; 2010:129–143.)

study results, and an MRI examination may be indicated for the investigation of atypical causes such as nerve sheath tumors or extrinsic space-occupying lesions. Another indication for MRI is recurrent symptoms after surgery in patients with incomplete decompression, excessive scarring, hematoma formation, or another space-occupying lesion, for whom additional treatment can be initiated accordingly (▶ Fig. 9.17).

In the evaluation of the median nerve at the carpal tunnel, T1-weighted and T2-weighted axial images are obtained to screen for obvious anatomic anomalies or pathologic findings. The median nerve is examined for changes in size, shape, or signal intensity. A predominant finding in patients with carpal tunnel syndrome is increased signal within the median nerve on T2-weighted images, which is related to chronic compression or ischemia. Other detectable abnormalities include bowing of the flexor retinaculum, deep palmar bursitis, tenosynovitis, or the presence of a space-occupying soft tissue mass. Intraneural lesions usually are well delineated. Although dynamic and motion studies of the median nerve in the carpal tunnel have been described, they are rarely used.[55]

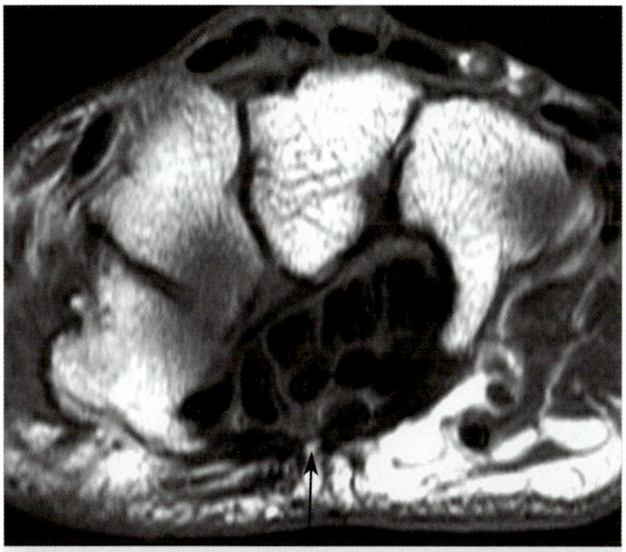

Fig. 9.17 A postoperative axial T1-weighted image at the level of the carpal tunnel showing incomplete release of the transverse carpal ligament (*arrow*). (Reproduced with permission from Brunton LM, Anderson MW, Chhabra AB. The wrist and hand. In: Khanna AJ, ed. MRI for orthopaedic surgeons. New York: Thieme; 2010:129–143.)

In the presence of ulnar nerve compression at the wrist, MRI may elucidate the cause when other diagnostic methods do not. Several causes include posttraumatic neuritis, occult fractures, pisotriquetral arthropathy, anatomic variants or ganglion cysts, and other soft tissue masses (▶ Fig. 9.18). Again, axial images are best for evaluating the ulnar nerve in Guyon canal. The information gained from MRI may help guide treatment decisions, with surgical decompression reserved for patients in whom an extrinsic source of compression is found.

In chronic cases of any nerve compression syndrome, MRI may show patterns of muscle atrophy consistent with denervation of the affected nerve. Denervated muscles typically show increased signal intensity on T1-weighted images, representing fatty replacement in the more chronic setting, or on fat-suppressed T2-weighted sequences, representing muscle edema in the more acute to subacute phases.

9.6.6 Soft Tissue Masses

Soft tissue masses occur commonly in the wrist and hand. Many of these lesions such as ganglia can be managed reliably without the use of advanced imaging. Nevertheless, MRI remains the standard for evaluating soft tissue masses of unclear clinical diagnoses. The primary role of MRI is in differentiating determinate from indeterminate lesions (see Chapter 19, Soft Tissue Tumors, and Chapter 20, Bone Tumors).[56] Determinate lesions may be diagnosed on MRI by a radiologist or clinician with a high degree of certainty on the basis of the imaging characteristics. Indeterminate lesions are those for which the radiologist or clinician is unable to provide a definitive diagnosis and which therefore warrant biopsy. Intravenous contrast may help in distinguishing solid and cystic lesions.

Benign solid lesions of the wrist and hand with characteristic MRI features include hemangioma, giant cell tumor of the tendon sheath, lipoma, Dupuytren disease, hamartoma, peripheral

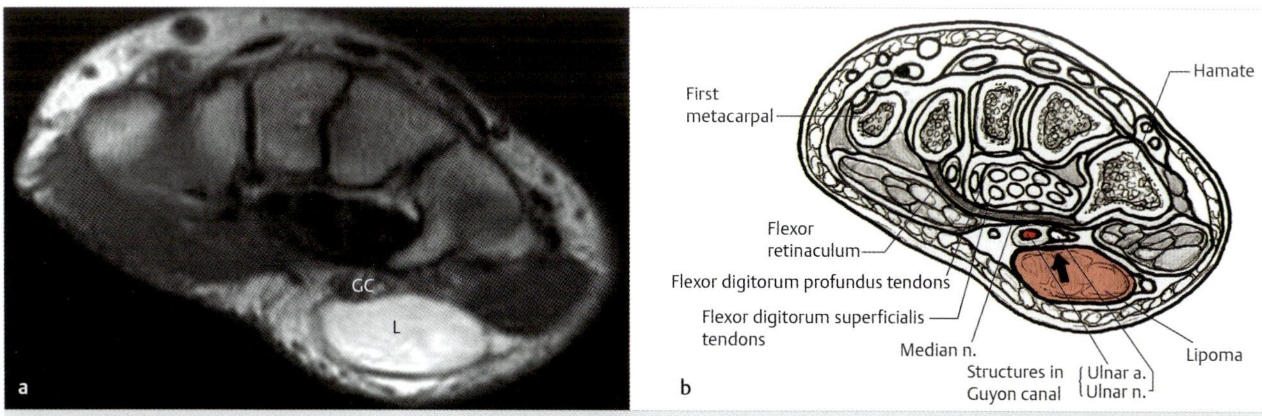

Fig. 9.18 Ulnar tunnel syndrome. An axial T1-weighted image **(a)** and illustration **(b)** showing a large well-circumscribed lipoma (*L*) compressing Guyon canal (GC). (Reproduced with permission from Brunton LM, Anderson MW, Chhabra AB. The wrist and hand. In: Khanna AJ, ed. MRI for orthopaedic surgeons. New York: Thieme; 2010:129–143.)

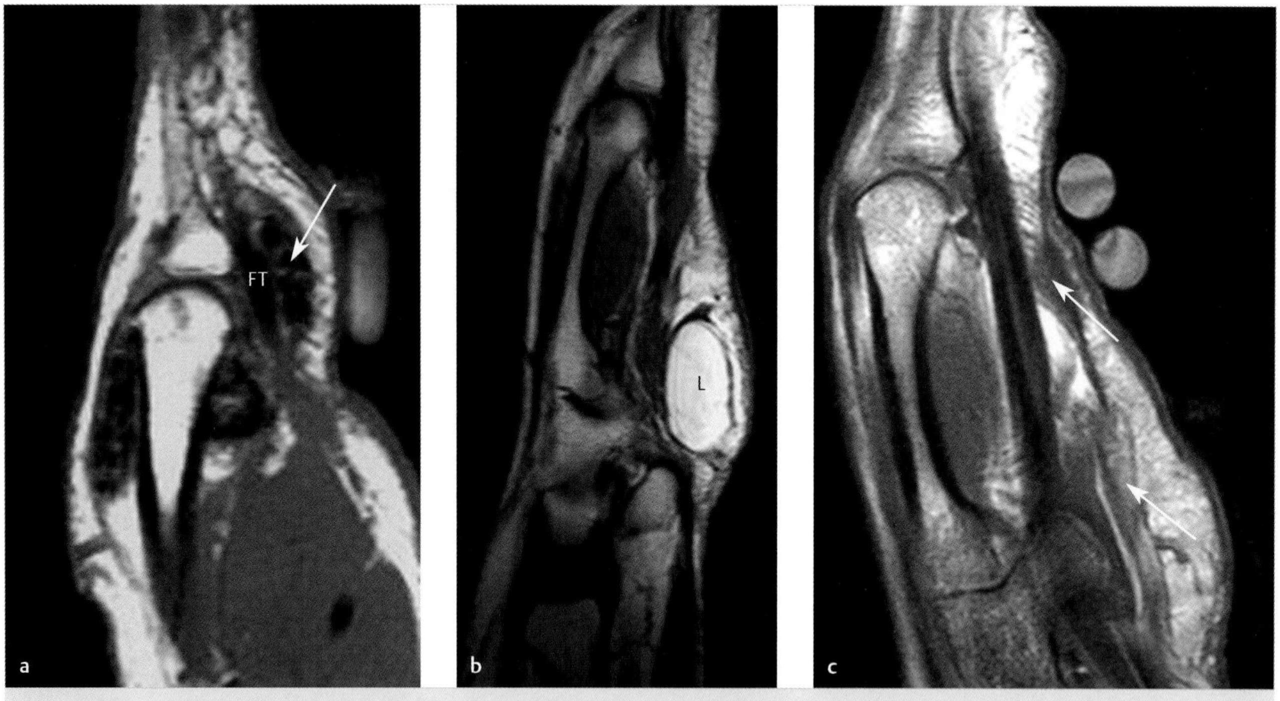

Fig. 9.19 Benign, soft tissue tumors of the hand. **(a)** Giant cell tumor of the tendon sheath. A sagittal T1-weighted image of the hand and digit depicting a solid mass (*arrow*) of mixed signal intensity originating from the underlying flexor tendon (*FT*). **(b)** Lipoma. A sagittal T1-weighted image showing a well-circumscribed lipoma (*L*) in the distal palm. Note how the signal characteristics of the lipoma match those of surrounding subcutaneous fat. **(c)** Dupuytren contracture. A sagittal T1-weighted image showing thickened palmar fascial bands (*bottom arrow*) and a fibrotic nodule just proximal to the metacarpophalangeal joint (*top arrow*) in a patient with Dupuytren disease. The circular structures are fiduciary markers that delineate the site of the patient's symptoms. (Reproduced with permission from Brunton LM, Anderson MW, Chhabra AB. The wrist and hand. In: Khanna AJ, ed. MRI for orthopaedic surgeons. New York: Thieme; 2010:129–143.)

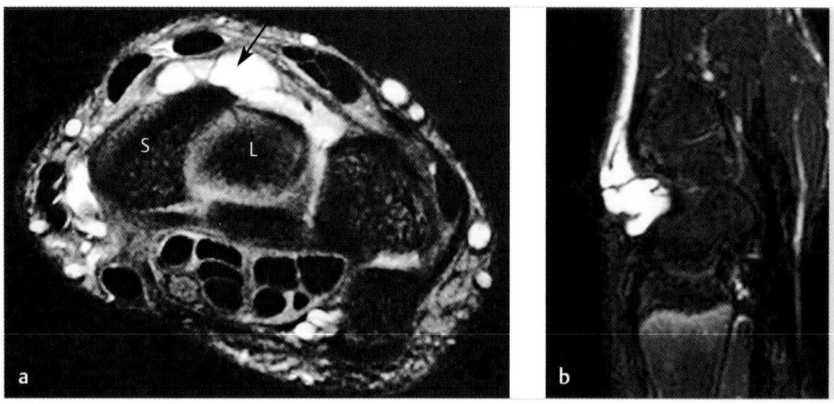

Fig. 9.20 Ganglion cyst. **(a)** An axial short tau inversion recovery (STIR) image of the wrist showing a multiloculated ganglion cyst (*arrow*) adjacent to the dorsal margin of the scapholunate articulation. *S*, scaphoid; *L*, lunate. **(b)** A sagittal STIR image depicting a dorsal ganglion cyst. (Reproduced with permission from Brunton LM, Anderson MW, Chhabra AB. The wrist and hand. In: Khanna AJ, ed. MRI for orthopaedic surgeons. New York: Thieme; 2010:129–143.)

nerve sheath tumor, and glomus tumor (▸ Fig. 9.19). Although malignant, soft tissue masses are rare in the hand and wrist, MRI may show irregular features or tissue necrosis that suggests a malignant process and requires additional evaluation before excision.[57] Many malignant lesions, however, have a nonaggressive appearance on MR images. The value of MRI in the assessment of bone malignancies is to identify and characterize the extent of soft tissue involvement.

Ganglion cysts usually can be diagnosed clinically with palpation and visualization. However, occult ganglions can cause chronic dorsal wrist pain or nerve compression. Conventional radiography is usually normal. MRI may help in differentiating ganglion cysts from synovitis in the chronically painful wrist. There are important differences between the two entities with regard to margins, shape, specific site of involvement, dimensions, internal structure, and contrast enhancement.[58] Ganglia have defined margins, a spherical shape, a septated, multilocular appearance, and wall enhancement (▸ Fig. 9.20), whereas synovitis shows diffuse margins, a crescentic shape, lack of septa, and diffuse enhancement.[58] Distinguishing these two diagnoses in the setting of chronic wrist pain has obvious implications for treatment because patients with findings of chronic synovitis typically undergo a more prolonged course of nonoperative treatment than do patients with ganglia. Approximately 30% of patients with radial-side ganglia may have associated pathology such as interosseous ligament tears that are detectable by MRI.[59]

9.7 Postoperative MRI Findings

Interpretation of postoperative MRI of the hand and wrist can be challenging because of the presence of postsurgical changes and, in some cases, orthopaedic hardware. If metal implants are present, special consideration is needed to reduce susceptibility artifacts, which cause signal void, pile-up, distortion, and loss of fat suppression. When using conventional MR sequences, FSE and STIR sequences produced with a high bandwidth and thin sections tend to be most resistant to metal artifact, whereas gradient-echo sequences should be avoided.[60] Newer multispectral MRI techniques specifically designed to reduce metal artifact, such as multiacquisition variable-resonance image combination (MAVRIC) and slice encoding for metal artifact correction (SEMAC), are highly effective.[61] Nonetheless, MRI has an established role in evaluating patients after hand and wrist surgery. After scaphoid fixation or vascularized bone grafting, MRI with or without gadolinium enhancement can be used to evaluate proximal pole viability.[62,63] In patients with recurrent or persistent symptoms after triangular fibrocartilage complex or intrinsic ligament repair, MRI can be used to evaluate the integrity of the repair and may show a persistent defect or a new tear.[64] After tendon repair or transfer, MRI can be used to detect tendon ruptures, peritendinous adhesions, and pulley injuries in patients with continued motion loss.[65] MRI can also be useful in patients with compressive neuropathy who have not improved after nerve release. After carpal tunnel release, MRI findings should include a complete defect in the flexor retinaculum and transverse carpal ligament with enlargement of the carpal tunnel and volar displacement of the flexor tendons and median nerve.[66] In patients with continued or recurrent symptoms, MRI may show incomplete release of the transverse carpal tunnel, a ganglion cyst or other structural lesion compressing the nerve, or structural or signal abnormalities within the nerve itself.

9.8 Common Clinical Questions

1. A 58-year-old man presents with ulnar-sided wrist pain that is especially bothersome during his golf swing. A T2-weighted MR image is shown below. What is the most likely cause of his discomfort?
   a) Scapholunate ligament injury.
   b) Triangular fibrocartilage complex injury.
   c) Pisotriquetral arthritis.
   d) Distal radioulnar arthritis.

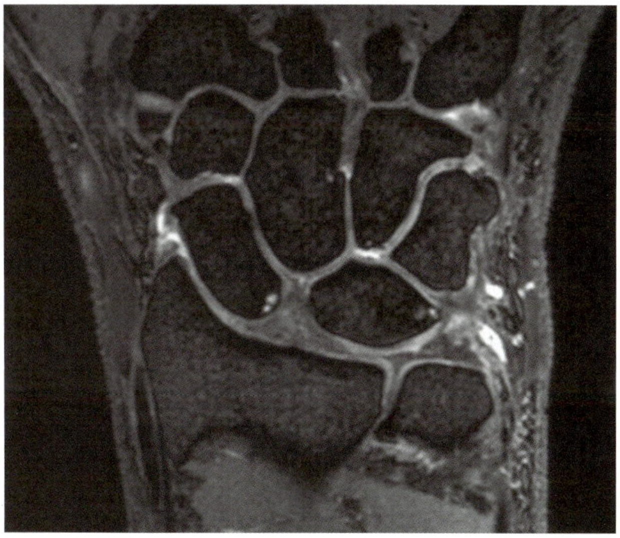

2. A 41-year-old woman presents for evaluation of a 10-year history of wrist pain. The pain has become worse over time. She denies any history of wrist injury. A T1-weighted MR image is shown. What is the most likely diagnosis?
   a) Preiser disease.
   b) Ulnar impaction syndrome.
   c) Kienböck disease.
   d) Scapholunate ligament avulsion.

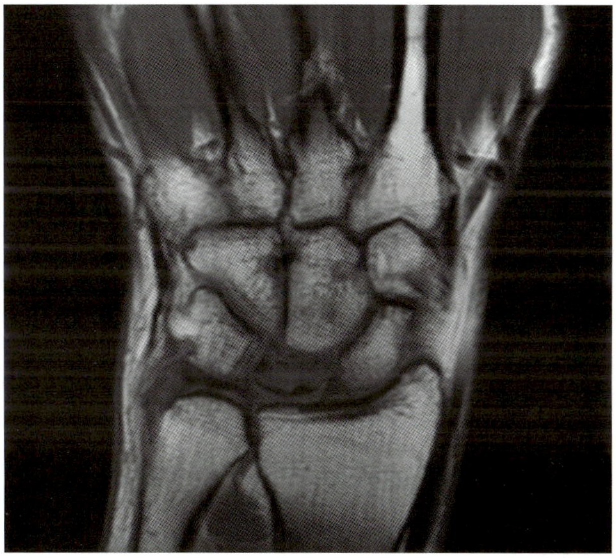

3. What imaging features characterize soft tissue abscesses of the hand?
   a) High signal intensity on T1-weighed images and low signal intensity on T2-weighted images.
   b) Low signal intensity on T1-weighted and T2-weighted images.
   c) High signal intensity on T1-weighted and T2-weighted images.
   d) Low signal intensity on T1-weighed images and high signal intensity on T2-weighted images.

4. In which of the following patients is an MRI most likely to be useful in making a diagnosis?
   a) A patient with numbness in the thumb, index finger, and middle finger and evidence of carpal tunnel syndrome on electrodiagnostic testing.
   b) A patient with numbness in the small and ring fingers and evidence of cubital tunnel syndrome on electrodiagnostic testing.
   c) A patient with a 0.5 × 0.5-cm dorsal wrist mass that is nonadherent to the overlying skin and transilluminates.
   d) A patient with numbness in the thumb, index finger, and middle finger that has recurred after carpal tunnel release with evidence of carpal tunnel syndrome on electrodiagnostic testing.

5. A 17-year-old boy has had persistent wrist pain since falling on an outstretched hand while skateboarding 7 months ago. This is the first time he has sought treatment. T1-weighted and T2-weighted precontrast MR images are shown below. Postcontrast images show uniform enhancement of the scaphoid. What is the diagnosis?
   a) Posttraumatic scaphoid osteonecrosis.
   b) Scaphoid fracture nonunion.
   c) Healed scaphoid fracture.
   d) Preiser disease.

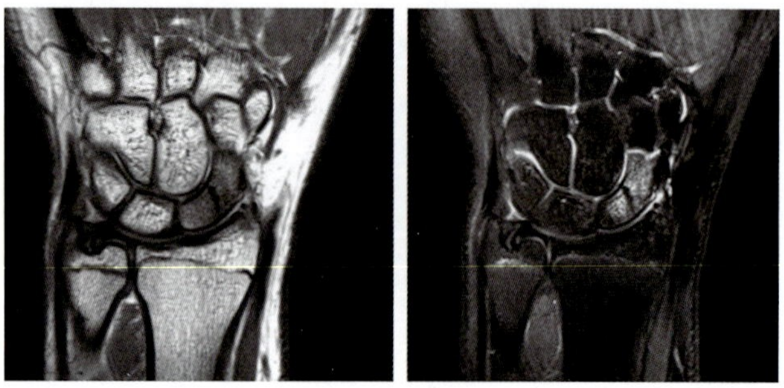

References

[1] Gupta P, Lenchik L, Wuertzer SD, Pacholke DA. High-resolution 3-T MRI of the fingers: review of anatomy and common tendon and ligament injuries. AJR Am J Roentgenol. 2015; 204(3):W314–23

[2] Bateni CP, Bartolotta RJ, Richardson ML, Mulcahy H, Allan CH. Imaging key wrist ligaments: what the surgeon needs the radiologist to know. AJR Am J Roentgenol. 2013; 200(5):1089–1095

[3] Palmer AK, Werner FW. The triangular fibrocartilage complex of the wrist: anatomy and function. J Hand Surg Am. 1981; 6(2):153–162

[4] Chhabra A, Soldatos T, Thawait GK, et al. Current perspectives on the advantages of 3-T MR imaging of the wrist. Radiographics. 2012; 32(3):879–896

[5] Saupe N, Prüssmann KP, Luechinger R, Bösiger P, Marincek B, Weishaupt D. MR imaging of the wrist: comparison between 1.5- and 3-T MR imaging: preliminary experience. Radiology. 2005; 234(1):256–264

[6] Stehling C, Langer M, Bachmann R, et al. Three-Tesla magnetic resonance imaging of the wrist: diagnostic performance compared to 1.5-T. J Comput Assist Tomogr. 2009; 33(6):934–939

[7] LiMarzi GM, O'Dell MC, Scherer K, Pettis C, Wasyliw CW, Bancroft LW. Magnetic resonance arthrography of the wrist and elbow. Magn Reson Imaging Clin N Am. 2015; 23(3):441–455

[8] Karl JW, Swart E, Strauch RJ. Diagnosis of occult scaphoid fractures: a cost-effectiveness analysis. J Bone Joint Surg Am. 2015; 97(22):1860–1868

[9] Mallee WH, Wang J, Poolman RW, et al. Computed tomography versus magnetic resonance imaging versus bone scintigraphy for clinically suspected scaphoid fractures in patients with negative plain radiographs. Cochrane Database Syst Rev. 2015(6):CD010023

[10] Brydie A, Raby N. Early MRI in the management of clinical scaphoid fracture. Br J Radiol. 2003; 76(905):296–300

[11] Hunter JC, Escobedo EM, Wilson AJ, Hanel DP, Zink-Brody GC, Mann FA. MR imaging of clinically suspected scaphoid fractures. AJR Am J Roentgenol. 1997; 168(5):1287–1293

[12] Murthy NS. The role of magnetic resonance imaging in scaphoid fractures. J Hand Surg Am. 2013; 38(10):2047–2054

[13] Lohman M, Kivisaari A, Vehmas T, et al. MR imaging in suspected acute trauma of wrist bones. Acta Radiol. 1999; 40(6):615–618

[14] Spence LD, Savenor A, Nwachuku I, Tilsley J, Eustace S. MRI of fractures of the distal radius: comparison with conventional radiographs. Skeletal Radiol. 1998; 27(5):244–249

[15] Futami T, Foster BK, Morris LL, LeQuesne GW. Magnetic resonance imaging of growth plate injuries: the efficacy and indications for surgical procedures. Arch Orthop Trauma Surg. 2000; 120(7–8):390–396

[16] Palmer AK. Triangular fibrocartilage complex lesions: a classification. J Hand Surg Am. 1989; 14(4):594–606

[17] Cooney WP. Evaluation of chronic wrist pain by arthrography, arthroscopy, and arthrotomy. J Hand Surg Am. 1993; 18(5):815–822

[18] Reinus WR, Hardy DC, Totty WG, Gilula LA. Arthrographic evaluation of the carpal triangular fibrocartilage complex. J Hand Surg Am. 1987; 12(4): 495–503

[19] Potter HG, Asnis-Ernberg L, Weiland AJ, Hotchkiss RN, Peterson MGE, McCormack RR, Jr. The utility of high-resolution magnetic resonance imaging in the evaluation of the triangular fibrocartilage complex of the wrist. J Bone Joint Surg Am. 1997; 79(11):1675–1684

[20] Iordache SD, Rowan R, Garvin GJ, Osman S, Grewal R, Faber KJ. Prevalence of triangular fibrocartilage complex abnormalities on MRI scans of asymptomatic wrists. J Hand Surg Am. 2012; 37(1):98–103

[21] Haims AH, Schweitzer ME, Morrison WB, et al. Limitations of MR imaging in the diagnosis of peripheral tears of the triangular fibrocartilage of the wrist. AJR Am J Roentgenol. 2002; 178(2):419–422

[22] Smith TO, Drew B, Toms AP, Jerosch-Herold C, Chojnowski AJ. Diagnostic accuracy of magnetic resonance imaging and magnetic resonance arthrography for triangular fibrocartilaginous complex injury: a systematic review and meta-analysis. J Bone Joint Surg Am. 2012; 94(9): 824–832

[23] Blazar PE, Chan PSH, Kneeland JB, Leatherwood D, Bozentka DJ, Kowalchick R. The effect of observer experience on magnetic resonance imaging interpretation and localization of triangular fibrocartilage complex lesions. J Hand Surg Am. 2001; 26(4):742–748

[24] Daunt N. Magnetic resonance imaging of the wrist: anatomy and pathology of interosseous ligaments and the triangular fibrocartilage complex. Curr Probl Diagn Radiol. 2002; 31(4):158–176

[25] Zlatkin MB, Chao PC, Osterman AL, Schnall MD, Dalinka MK, Kressel HY. Chronic wrist pain: evaluation with high-resolution MR imaging. Radiology. 1989; 173(3):723–729

[26] Andersson JK, Andernord D, Karlsson J, Fridén J. Efficacy of magnetic resonance imaging and clinical tests in diagnostics of wrist ligament injuries: a systematic review. Arthroscopy. 2015; 31(10):2014–20.e2

[27] Magee T. Comparison of 3-T MRI and arthroscopy of intrinsic wrist ligament and TFCC tears. AJR Am J Roentgenol. 2009; 192(1):80–85

[28] Scheck RJ, Kubitzek C, Hierner R, et al. The scapholunate interosseous ligament in MR arthrography of the wrist: correlation with non-enhanced MRI and wrist arthroscopy. Skeletal Radiol. 1997; 26(5):263–271

[29] Taljanovic MS, Malan JJ, Sheppard JE. Normal anatomy of the extrinsic capsular wrist ligaments by 3-T MRI and high-resolution ultrasonography. Semin Musculoskelet Radiol. 2012; 16(2):104–114

[30] Ahn JM, Sartoris DJ, Kang HS, et al. Gamekeeper thumb: comparison of MR arthrography with conventional arthrography and MR imaging in cadavers. Radiology. 1998; 206(3):737–744

[31] Harper MT, Chandnani VP, Spaeth J, Santangelo JR, Providence BC, Bagg MA. Gamekeeper thumb: diagnosis of ulnar collateral ligament injury using magnetic resonance imaging, magnetic resonance arthrography and stress radiography. J Magn Reson Imaging. 1996; 6(2):322–328

[32] Milner CS, Manon-Matos Y, Thirkannad SM. Gamekeeper's thumb: a treatment-oriented magnetic resonance imaging classification. J Hand Surg Am. 2015; 40(1):90–95

[33] Verdan CE. Half a century of flexor-tendon surgery. Current status and changing philosophies. J Bone Joint Surg Am. 1972; 54(3):472–491

[34] Hauger O, Chung CB, Lektrakul N, et al. Pulley system in the fingers: normal anatomy and simulated lesions in cadavers at MR imaging, CT, and US with and without contrast material distention of the tendon sheath. Radiology. 2000; 217(1):201–212

[35] Cerezal L, del Piñal F, Abascal F, García-Valtuille R, Pereda T, Canga A. Imaging findings in ulnar-sided wrist impaction syndromes. Radiographics. 2002; 22(1):105–121

[36] Berquist TH. Infection. In: Berquist TH, ed. MRI of the hand and wrist. Philadelphia, PA: Lippincott Williams & Wilkins; 2003:142–152

[37] Erickson SJ, Cox IH, Hyde JS, Carrera GF, Strandt JA, Estkowski LD. Effect of tendon orientation on MR imaging signal intensity: a manifestation of the "magic angle" phenomenon. Radiology. 1991; 181(2):389–392

[38] Peh WCG, Chan JHM. The magic angle phenomenon in tendons: effect of varying the MR echo time. Br J Radiol. 1998; 71(841):31–36

[39] Totterman SMS, Seo GS. MRI findings of scapholunate instabilities in coronal images: a short communication. Semin Musculoskelet Radiol. 2001; 5(3): 251–256

[40] Bierry G, Huang AJ, Chang CY, Torriani M, Bredella MA. MRI findings of treated bacterial septic arthritis. Skeletal Radiol. 2012; 41(12):1509–1516

[41] Lichtman DM, Mack GR, MacDonald RI, Gunther SF, Wilson JN. Kienböck's disease: the role of silicone replacement arthroplasty. J Bone Joint Surg Am. 1977; 59(7):899–908

[42] Nakamura R, Watanabe K, Tsunoda K, Miura T. Radial osteotomy for Kienböck's disease evaluated by magnetic resonance imaging. 24 cases followed for 1–3 years. Acta Orthop Scand. 1993; 64(2):207–211

[43] Kalainov DM, Cohen MS, Hendrix RW, Sweet S, Culp RW, Osterman AL. Preiser's disease: identification of two patterns. J Hand Surg Am. 2003; 28(5): 767–778

[44] Schmitt R, Fröhner S, van Schoonhoven J, Lanz U, Gölles A. Idiopathic osteonecrosis of the scaphoid (Preiser's disease): MRI gives new insights into etiology and pathology. Eur J Radiol. 2011; 77(2):228–234

[45] Cerezal L, Abascal F, Canga A, García-Valtuille R, Bustamante M, del Piñal F. Usefulness of gadolinium-enhanced MR imaging in the evaluation of the vascularity of scaphoid nonunions. AJR Am J Roentgenol. 2000; 174(1): 141–149

[46] Fox MG, Gaskin CM, Chhabra AB, Anderson MW. Assessment of scaphoid viability with MRI: a reassessment of findings on unenhanced MR images. AJR Am J Roentgenol. 2010; 195(4):W281–W286

[47] Larribe M, Gay A, Freire V, Bouvier C, Chagnaud C, Souteyrand P. Usefulness of dynamic contrast-enhanced MRI in the evaluation of the viability of acute scaphoid fracture. Skeletal Radiol. 2014; 43(12):1697–1703

[48] Quinn MA, Emery P. Potential for altering rheumatoid arthritis outcome. Rheum Dis Clin North Am. 2005; 31(4):763–772

[49] Rominger MB, Bernreuter WK, Kenney PJ, Morgan SL, Blackburn WD, Alarcon GS. MR imaging of the hands in early rheumatoid arthritis: preliminary results. Radiographics. 1993; 13(1):37–46

[50] Sugimoto H, Takeda A, Masuyama J, Furuse M. Early-stage rheumatoid arthritis: diagnostic accuracy of MR imaging. Radiology. 1996; 198(1):185–192

[51] Nakashima Y, Tamai M, Kita J, et al. Magnetic resonance imaging bone edema at enrollment predicts rapid radiographic progression in patients with early RA: results from the Nagasaki University Early Arthritis Cohort. J Rheumatol. 2016; 43(7):1278–1284

[52] Stomp W, Krabben A, van der Heijde D, et al. Are rheumatoid arthritis patients discernible from other early arthritis patients using 1.5 T extremity magnetic resonance imaging? A large cross-sectional study. J Rheumatol. 2014; 41(8):1630–1637

[53] Sugimoto H, Takeda A, Hyodoh K. Early-stage rheumatoid arthritis: prospective study of the effectiveness of MR imaging for diagnosis. Radiology. 2000; 216(2):569–575

[54] Taouli B, Guermazi A, Sack KE, Genant HK. Imaging of the hand and wrist in RA. Ann Rheum Dis. 2002; 61(10):867–869

[55] Brahme SK, Hodler J, Braun RM, Sebrechts C, Jackson W, Resnick D. Dynamic MR imaging of carpal tunnel syndrome. Skeletal Radiol. 1997; 26(8):482–487

[56] Papp DF, Khanna AJ, McCarthy EF, Carrino JA, Farber AJ, Frassica FJ. Magnetic resonance imaging of soft-tissue tumors: determinate and indeterminate lesions. J Bone Joint Surg Am. 2007; 89 Suppl 3:103–115

[57] Teh J, Whiteley G. MRI of soft tissue masses of the hand and wrist. Br J Radiol. 2007; 80(949):47–63

[58] Anderson SE, Steinbach LS, Stauffer E, Voegelin E. MRI for differentiating ganglion and synovitis in the chronic painful wrist. AJR Am J Roentgenol. 2006; 186(3):812–818

[59] el-Noueam KI, Schweitzer ME, Blasbalg R, et al. Is a subset of wrist ganglia the sequela of internal derangements of the wrist joint? MR imaging findings. Radiology. 1999; 212(2):537–540

[60] Ariyanayagam T, Malcolm PN, Toms AP. Advances in metal artifact reduction techniques for periprosthetic soft tissue imaging. Semin Musculoskelet Radiol. 2015; 19(4):328–334

[61] Johnson D, Stevens KJ, Riley G, Shapiro L, Yoshioka H, Gold GE. Approach to MR imaging of the elbow and wrist: technical aspects and innovation. Magn Reson Imaging Clin N Am. 2015; 23(3):355–366

[62] Dailiana ZH, Zachos V, Varitimidis S, Papanagiotou P, Karantanas A, Malizos KN. Scaphoid nonunions treated with vascularised bone grafts: MRI assessment. Eur J Radiol. 2004; 50(3):217–224

[63] Sakuma M, Nakamura R, Imaeda T. Analysis of proximal fragment sclerosis and surgical outcome of scaphoid non-union by magnetic resonance imaging. J Hand Surg [Br]. 1995; 20(2):201–205

[64] Trumble TE, Gilbert M, Vedder N. Isolated tears of the triangular fibrocartilage: management by early arthroscopic repair. J Hand Surg Am. 1997; 22(1):57–65

[65] Drapé JL, Silbermann-Hoffman O, Houvet P, et al. Complications of flexor tendon repair in the hand: MR imaging assessment. Radiology. 1996; 198(1): 219–224

[66] Momose T, Uchiyama S, Kobayashi S, Nakagawa H, Kato H. Structural changes of the carpal tunnel, median nerve and flexor tendons in MRI before and after endoscopic carpal tunnel release. Hand Surg. 2014; 19(2):193–198

Answers to Common Clinical Questions

1. Answer: b. The MRI shows a central perforation of the triangular fibrocartilage complex (TFCC). Although TFCC abnormalities can be found in asymptomatic individuals, this patient's history of ulnar-sided pain exacerbated by repetitive wrist pronation and supination (as occurs in golfing) is highly consistent with the diagnosis of a TFCC tear.
2. Answer: c. The MRI shows diffusely low signal intensity of the lunate compared with the surrounding carpal bones on T1-weighted imaging, consistent with the diagnosis of Kienböck disease.
3. Answer: d. Soft tissue abscesses within the hand typically are characterized by low signal intensity on T1-weighted images and high signal intensity on T2-weighted images.
4. Answer: d. Most patients with carpal tunnel and cubital tunnel syndrome are diagnosed on the basis of history and physical examination findings, which are corroborated by electrodiagnostic testing. Many ganglion cysts can also be diagnosed clinically. However, MRI is indicated in patients who have recurrent symptoms after undergoing carpal or cubital tunnel release to evaluate for incomplete decompression, excessive scarring, hematoma formation, or another space-occupying lesions.
5. Answer: b. This is a scaphoid fracture nonunion. Low signal intensity on T1-weighted and T2-weighted images would be suggestive of osteonecrosis. In this case, enhancement with the addition of contrast confirms scaphoid vascularity.

Part III

Lower Extremity

III

10 The Hip

Andrea M. Spiker, Michael K. Shindle, Marc J. Philippon, Bryan T. Kelly, Luis E. Moya, and Douglas N. Mintz

Abstract
The aim of this chapter is to provide a systematic approach to identifying pathologies of the hip. In this chapter we review hip anatomy in the sagittal, coronal and axial planes and describe the most common pathologic conditions seen in the hip. In addition, this chapter will detail MRI findings seen in a wide array of hip pathologies that physicians must be wary of. By the end of this chapter, the reader will be able to determine the ideal MRI technique required to diagnose a hip pathology and recognize characteristic findings associated with it.

Keywords: hip, magnetic resonance imaging (MRI), hip imaging, femoral-acetabular impingement, intra-articular hip pathology

10.1 Normal Anatomy

When evaluating the hip, it is helpful to divide the normal hip anatomy into four distinct layers: layer 1, the osteochondral layer; layer 2, the capsulolabral layer; layer 3, the muscular layer; and layer 4, the neural layer.[1] Magnetic resonance imaging (MRI) offers the ability to evaluate each of these layers in detail.

10.1.1 Sagittal Anatomy

The sagittal images of the hip allow visualization of the gluteus maximus, medius, and minimus muscles laterally; the short external rotator tendons as they insert on or near the greater trochanter; and as the hip joint comes into view, the cartilage of the acetabular weight-bearing dome, the iliopsoas anterior to the femoral head, and the anterior acetabular labrum. One can often also see the hamstring origin and the sciatic nerve, depending on the extent of the scan. When evaluating the anterior acetabular labrum for evidence of tear or degeneration, the sagittal view will provide the best visualization (▶ Fig. 10.1).

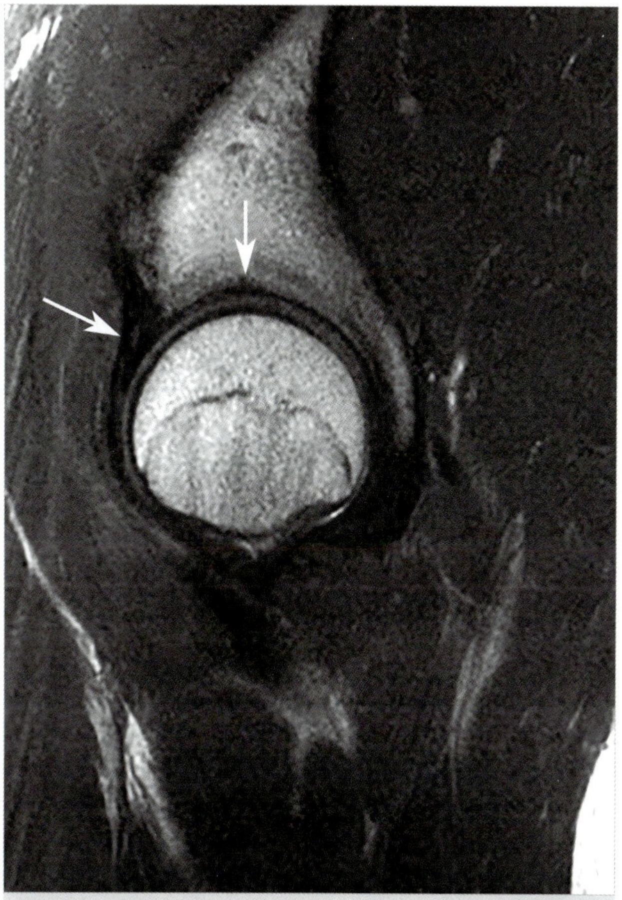

Fig. 10.1 A sagittal fast spin-echo (FSE) image of the hip showing a normal anterior labrum (*left arrow*) as a triangular focus of low signal and normal articular cartilage of the acetabulum (*top arrow*). (Source: © 2009 Hospital for Special Surgery, New York, NY.)

10.1.2 Coronal Anatomy

The coronal images demonstrate the pubic symphysis and the aponeurotic plate of the adductors anteriorly, the cartilage and acetabular labrum of the hip joint, the attachment of the gluteus medius and minimus tendons on the greater trochanter, and the hamstring origins from the ischial tuberosity posteriorly. The ligamentum teres, iliac wing (including abductor and sartorius origins), iliopsoas bursa, and rectus femoris origin can be identified. Coronal imaging gives the best view of the weight-bearing surface over the femoral head, as well as the lateral dome of the acetabulum and the superior labrum (▶ Fig. 10.2).

10.1.3 Axial Anatomy

Axial anatomy of the hip is useful to identify. From superior to inferior, it consists of the psoas and iliacus muscles, the iliopsoas tendon anterior to the femoral head, the acetabular labrum, and the sciatic nerve as it exits the sciatic notch. Axial imaging can demonstrate the pubis, the short external rotators, adductors, and rectus femoris and sartorius muscles and can rule out other causes of pelvic area pain, including obturator and inguinal hernias (▶ Fig. 10.3).

10.2 Specialized Pulse Sequences and Imaging Protocols

As with MRI of any anatomic region, accurate MRI assessment of the hip requires attention to technical detail. Traditionally, MRI of the hip performed for suspicion of osteonecrosis or an occult fracture used large fields of view, which provided poor in-plane resolution and little to no detail of the articular cartilage or labrum. More recently, improvements in MRI technology allow small fields of view and high spatial resolution. Survey images of the entire pelvis are still helpful for screening for other causes of pain such as the following:

- Muscle strains.
- Pelvic masses.
- Hernias.
- Spine and sacroiliac (SI) joint pathology.
- Occult fractures.

At the authors' institution, intermediate TE (proton-density) sequences are used in each plane with high resolution (512 × 320–384) and a maximum field of view of 20 cm. These are obtained in the sagittal and coronal planes and an oblique axial image through the femoral neck. Sometimes radial images through the femoral neck are added. Survey images of the pelvis using a coronal fat-suppressed sequence (usually inversion recovery) and an axial proton-density sequence are obtained.

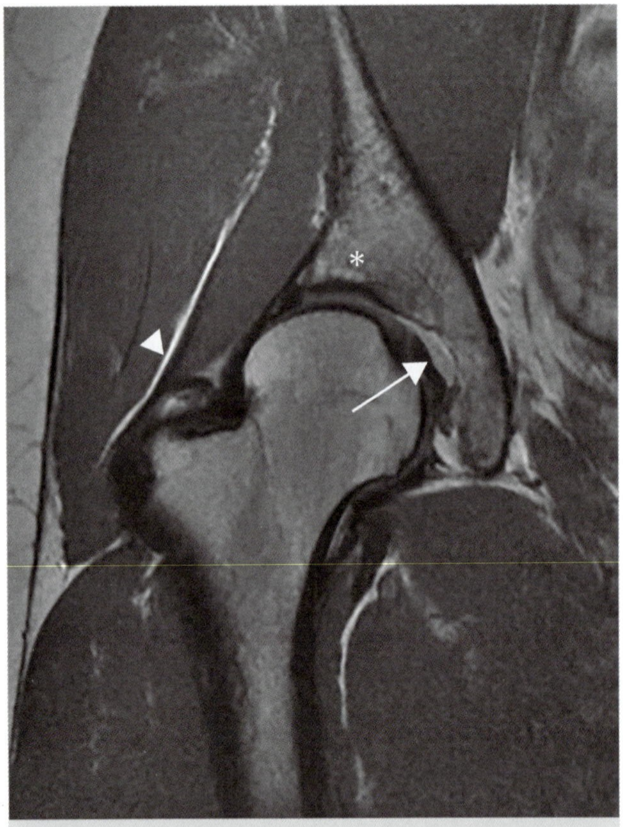

Fig. 10.2 A coronal fast spin-echo (FSE) of the hip showing a normal ligamentum teres (*arrow*), acetabular labrum (*asterisk*), and attachment of the gluteus minimus tendon (*arrow head*).

At the authors' institution, use of the intermediate TE sequence rather than T1-weighted and T2-weighted images is preferred for several reasons. First, T1 is poor for evaluating cartilage because there is no contrast between fluid and cartilage. Second, it is also poor for evaluating subtle muscle abnormalities, so another sequence in each plane would be required for a thorough evaluation, and yet a third to evaluate cartilage. The intermediate TE sequence eliminates this redundancy by allowing enough signal for excellent resolution and enough contrast to evaluate all structures (bone, ligament, tendon, muscle, and articular cartilage), as well as the quality of synovitis, if present. One can obtain this sequence in each plane and then add one fat-suppressed sequence to evaluate for subtle findings and to assess acuity.

Many authors advocate using MR arthrography of the hip for the evaluation of labral pathology and articular cartilage (see chapter 5, Articular Cartilage),[2,3,4] but this modality increases the cost and imaging time and makes MRI an invasive procedure.[5] Although noncontrast imaging has been shown to identify labral and chondral pathology and is becoming more popular as new technology allows detailed evaluation, many institutions in the United States and abroad continue to use MR arthrography to improve the visualization of intra-articular hip pathology, especially labral pathology.[6,7]

10.3 Systematic Approach to Image Review

Beginning with the fat-suppressed images, we look for areas of bone edema, as may be seen with a stress reaction or stress fracture of the femoral neck (▶ Fig. 10.11), osteonecrosis, subchondral fracture, or advanced arthrosis. Then we examine the greater trochanteric region for trochanteric bursitis. The remainder of the evaluation is done using proton-density images, with confirmation using the fat-suppressed images. First we look at the abductor insertions on the coronal images, and then we use both coronal and sagittal images to evaluate the labrum and articular cartilage. A torn labrum appears as a line of high signal interrupting the continuity of the otherwise low-signal triangle of labrum as it becomes confluent with the low-signal articular cartilage (▶ Fig. 10.4).

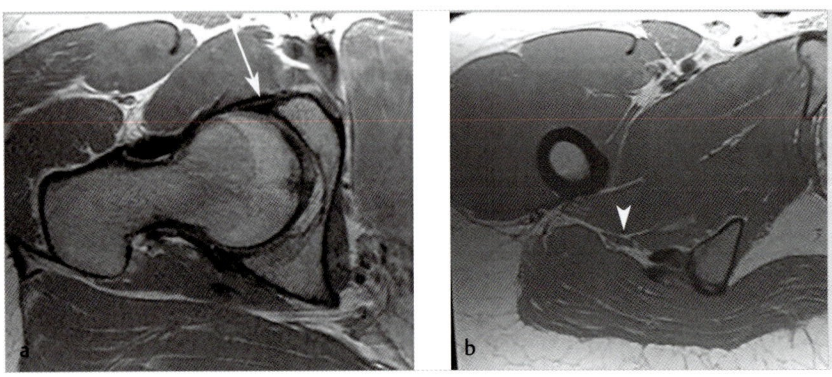

Fig. 10.3 An axial fast spin-echo (FSE) image of the hip demonstrating **(a)** the acetabular labrum (*arrow*) and **(b)** more distally, the sciatic nerve (*arrow head*).

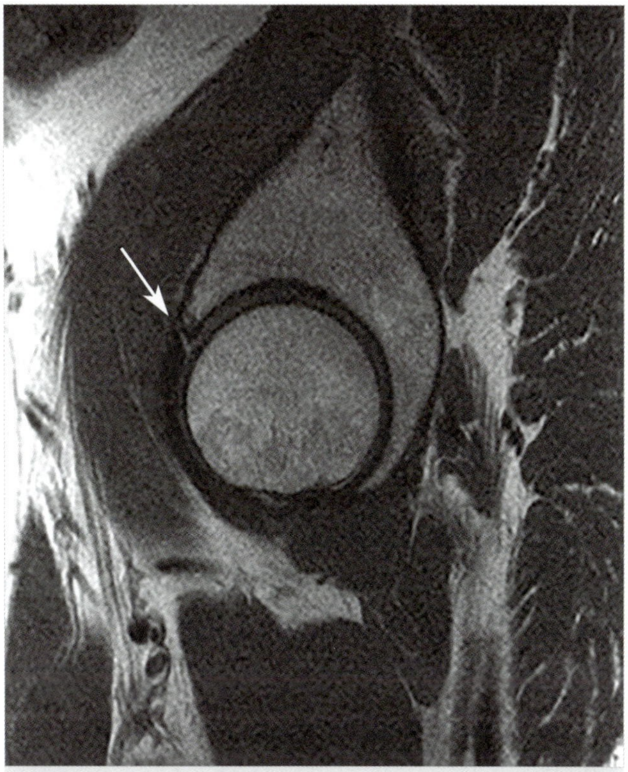

Fig. 10.4 A sagittal fast spin-echo (FSE) image of the hip showing a nondisplaced anterior labral tear (*arrow*). (Source: © 2009 Hospital for Special Surgery, New York, NY.)

Next we examine the ligamentum teres, the joint capsule, the shape of the femoral neck, and the presence/absence and quality of joint effusion. We then evaluate the extra-articular anatomy, including the spine, SI joints, hamstrings, muscles, pubis, and presence/absence of hernia. This survey also takes into account any extra-articular impingement and the global shape of the hip (i.e., acetabular under- or overcoverage).

10.4 Traumatic Conditions and the Athletic Hip

10.4.1 Acetabular Labral Tears

The fibrocartilaginous labrum (type I collagen) appears as a triangular, low signal structure that surrounds the rim of the acetabulum.[8] It is contiguous with the transverse acetabular ligament inferiorly. The labrum is thought to play an important role in maintaining hydrostatic fluid pressure in the joint,[9] and labral pathology is not only a cause of substantial hip pain (▶ Table 10.1) but is also associated with the development of osteoarthritis.[10] The labrum is thickest superiorly and posteriorly and widest anteriorly and superiorly. The joint capsule attaches to the acetabular rim adjacent to the labrum; however, at the superior aspect of the joint, the capsule inserts a few millimeters above the labrum, which creates a sublabral recess or sulcus.[11] Free nerve endings and nerve end organs have been identified in the labrum, most abundantly in the anterosuperior and posterosuperior zones, and they may be involved in pain and proprioception.[12,13] The blood supply to the acetabular labrum is poor overall but there are regional variations, with significantly more vascularity on the capsular side than the articular side.[14] Detachment of the posterior labrum should raise suspicion for a posterior subluxation event.

Most (75%) labral tears occur anterosuperiorly and on the articular side.[15] Labral tears are identified by the presence of increased signal intensity (often equivalent to that of synovial fluid) on fat-suppressed images through the substance of the labrum (▶ Fig. 10.4). Partial or complete detachment is characterized by fluid-matching signal undermining the attachment between the labrum and acetabulum. The presence of paralabral cysts should prompt careful inspection of the labrum to discern the often subtle splits that serve as the origin for these cysts (▶ Fig. 10.5). There is a high rate of asymptomatic labral tears (33–69%) found on MRI in young adults,[16,17] so diagnosis of a labral tear must be paired carefully with history and physical examination. In patients older than 50 years with hip pain, 73% have labral tears and 93% have some labral pathology,[18] whereas in pediatric patients (aged 2–18 y) the rate of asymptomatic labral tear is very low (1.4%).[19]

To optimize outcomes, the underlying cause of the labral injury must be identified. In addition to degenerative labral tears associated with arthritis, there are at least five causes of labral tears[20]:

- Femoroacetabular impingement (FAI).
- Traumatic labral injury (dislocation/subluxation).
- Atraumatic capsular laxity (hypermobility).
- Psoas impingement.
- Dysplasia.

Several classification systems have been used for labral tears, two of which are described here. In a cadaveric study, Seldes et al[15] determined histologically that there were two distinct types of tears (▶ Fig. 10.6):

- Detachment of the labrum from the hyaline cartilage at the transitional zone (type 1).
- Cleavage of variable depth within the substance of the labrum (type 2).

In another study, Lage et al[21] developed an arthroscopic classification based on morphology:

- Radial flap tear.
- Radial fibrillated tear.
- Longitudinal peripheral tear.
- Unstable tear.

Blankenbaker et al[22] found little correlation between MR arthrographic appearance of labral tears and the Lage arthroscopic classification and suggested that morphologic descriptions are the best way to describe tears on imaging. Ilizaliturri et al[23] described a zone method for classifying intra-articular pathology used during hip arthroscopy (▶ Fig. 10.7), which they found to be more reproducible than the clock-face method of describing tears at the time of surgery.

Two potential pitfalls may occur when interpreting noncontrast MRI and MR arthrography studies, potentially leading to an inaccurate diagnosis of a labral tear. First, there is a normal variant of the posteroinferior sublabral groove, which is a relatively common occurrence and typically seen on axial images.[11]

Table 10.1 Differential diagnosis of hip pain

Primary labral pathology	Nonmusculoskeletal causes
Femoroacetabular impingement	Genitourinary
Laxity	Spine
Trauma	Psoas muscle abscess
Dysplasia	Hernia
Degenerative	Endometriosis
	Ovarian cyst
	Peripheral vascular disease
Primary chondral	**Bone etiology**
Lateral impact	Subchondral fractures
Subluxation/dislocation	Other fractures
Osteonecrosis	
Loose bodies	
Degeneration	
Primary capsule	**Synovial proliferative disorders**
Laxity	Pigmented villonodular synovitis
Adhesive capsulitis	Synovial chondromatosis
Synovitis/inflammation	Chondrocalcinosis
Extra-articular	**Infectious/tumor/metabolic**
Snapping hip (internal/external)	Septic arthritis
Trochanteric bursitis	Osteomyelitis
Ischial bursitis	
Psoas bursitis/subiliacus bursitis	**Neoplasms**
Osteitis pubis	Benign bone and soft tissue
Core muscle injury (formerly sports hernia or athletic pubalgia)	Malignant bone and soft tissue
Deep gluteal syndrome	Paget disease
Sacroiliac joint	Primary hyperparathyroidism
Tendinitis	Metastatic bone disease
Hip flexor	
Adductor	
Abductor	
Gluteus medius tear Trochanteric impingement Hamstring strain/tear Calcific tendonitis	
Inflammatory	**Systemic**
Rheumatoid arthritis	Polyarticular
Reiter syndrome	Reflex sympathetic dystrophy
Psoriatic arthritis	Complex regional pain syndrome
Bursitis	Hormonal

Source: Reproduced with permission from Shindle MK, Ranawat AS, Kelly BT. Diagnosis and management of traumatic and atraumatic hip instability in the athletic patient. Clin Sports Med 2006;25:309–326. Reprinted by permission.

The clinician should recognize that this location is distinct from that of most labral tears. The second variant is a superior sublabral recess at the anterosuperior margin of the acetabulum, which has been described in the presence of mild acetabular dysplasia.[24]

The high prevalence of labral tears in the anterosuperior labrum is speculated to be secondary to decreased vascularity in this zone,[15,20] as well as the collagen content and fiber orientation in this area.[25] Kalhor et al[26] found that the blood supply to the labrum originates from the periacetabular vascular ring, which then travels toward the free edge of the labrum, traversing the osseolabral junction on the capsular side. These findings supported those of previous studies that identified the main blood supply to the acetabular labrum as located on the capsular surface.[14,15] In examination of fetal labra, Turker et al[25] found a parallel orientation of collagen fibers to the chondrolabral junction in the anterosuperior quadrants and a perpendicular orientation of denser collagen in the posterior inferior quadrant. Such studies have important implications for labral surgery in terms of determining the type and location of tears that would be amenable to successful repair, as well as avoiding detaching the labrum when performing a debridement or repair.

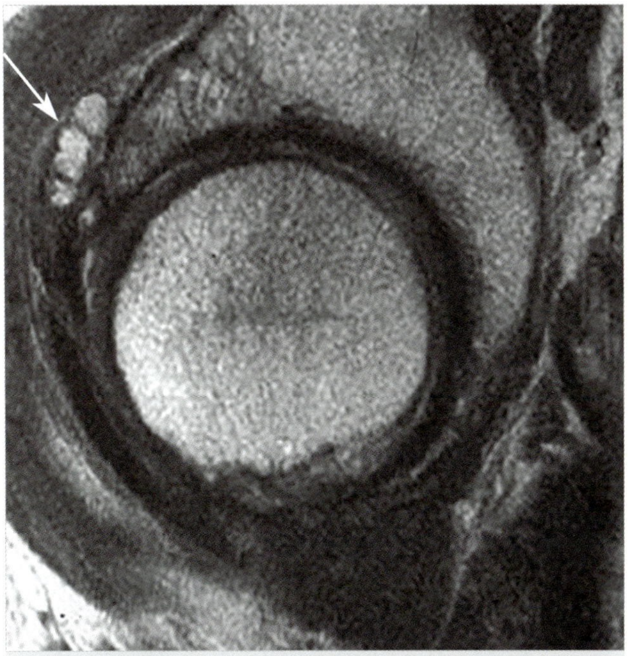

Fig. 10.5 A sagittal fast spin-echo (FSE) image of the hip showing paralabral cysts (*arrow*) associated with an anterior labral tear and full-thickness cartilage loss of the anterior acetabulum. (Source: © 2009 Hospital for Special Surgery, New York, NY)

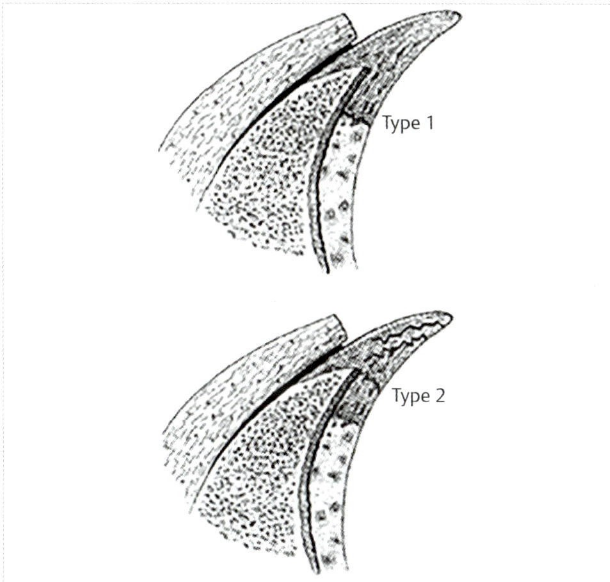

Fig. 10.6 Seldes type-1 and type-2 labral tears: detachment of the labrum from the hyaline cartilage at the transitional zone and cleavage of variable depth within the substance of the labrum, respectively. (Reproduced with permission from Seldes RM, Tan V, Hunt J, Katz M, Winiarsky R, Fitzgerald RH, Jr. Anatomy, histologic features, and vascularity of the adult acetabular labrum. Clin Orthop Relat Res. 2001(382):232–240.[15])

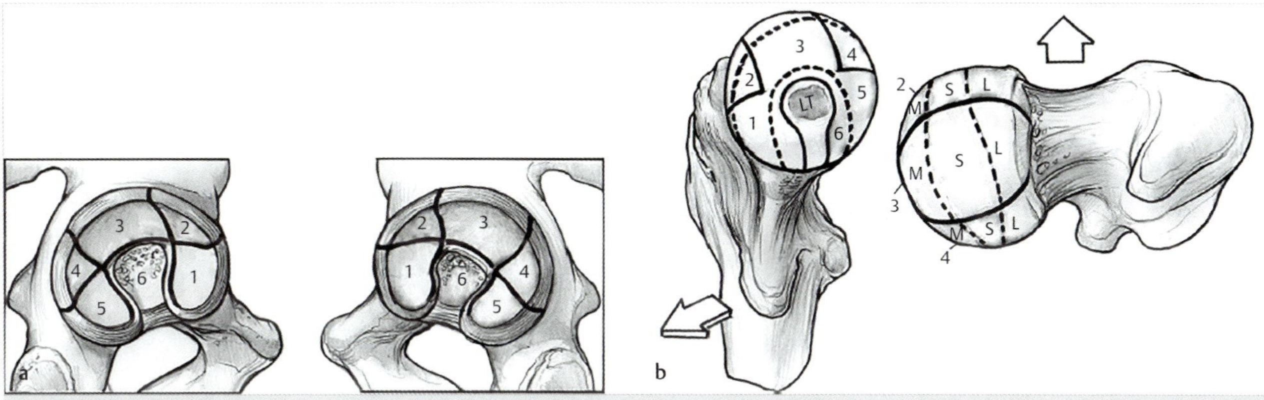

Fig. 10.7 Zone classification. **(a)** An artist's depiction of the left and right hemipelvis. The acetabulum has been subdivided into six zones: 1, anterior-inferior; 2, anterior-superior; 3, central-superior; 4, posterior-superior; 5, posterior-inferior; and 6, acetabular notch. **(b)** An artist's depiction of the left and right proximal femurs. (*Left*) The frontal view of the femoral head is divided into six zones around the acetabular fossa (there is a *dotted line* around the ligamentum teres [*LT*]): 1, anterior-inferior; 2, anterior-superior; 3, central-superior; 4, posterior-superior; 5, posterior-inferior; and 6, area around the ligamentum teres. (*Right*) The superior view shows the three subdivisions of zones 2, 3, and 4: medial (*M*), superior (*S*), and lateral (*L*). (Reproduced with permission from Ilizaliturri VM Jr, Byrd JWT, Sampson TG, et al. A geographic zone method to describe intra-articular pathology in hip arthroscopy: cadaveric study and preliminary report. Arthroscopy 2008;24:534–539.[23])

10.4.2 Femoroacetabular Impingement

Femoroacetabular impingement (FAI) is a well-described pathologic condition that is now understood to lead to hip degeneration and osteoarthritis through progressive chondral and labral injury.[27,28,29,30,31,32] FAI is caused by two main types of mechanism: "cam" and "pincer." Most FAI cases represent a combination of both mechanisms (▶ Fig. 10.8).[27] Although the cause of FAI is not completely understood, subclinical, slipped, capital femoral epiphysis has been theorized to lead to the femoral neck deformity,[33] and more recently it has been suggested that increased loading of the hip during late childhood and early adolescence plays a role in the development of the head-neck junction deformity.[34,35,36] A genetic component has also been suggested; Pollard et al[37] found that the siblings of a patient with FAI had a relative risk of 2.0 of having a rim deformity ($p = 0.001$) and a relative risk of 2.8 of having a cam deformity ($p < 0.00001$).

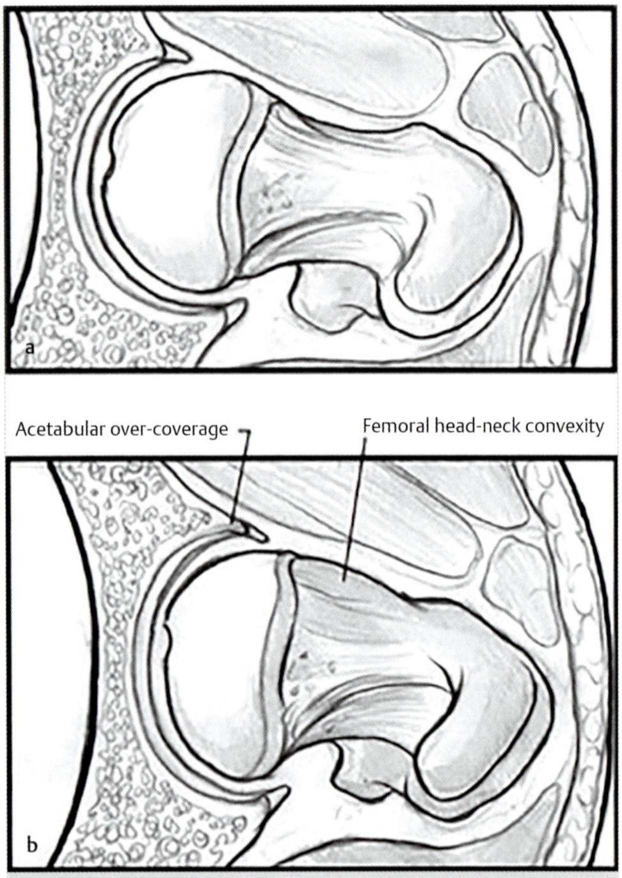

Fig. 10.8 Diagrammatic representation of (a) a normal acetabulum and femur morphology and (b) combined femoroacetabular impingement with reduced head-neck offset (cam mechanism) and excessive anterior overcoverage (pincer mechanism). (Reproduced with permission from Michael K. Shindle, Bryan T. Kelly, Luis E. Moya, and Douglas N. Mintz. The hip. In: Khanna AJ, ed. MRI for orthopaedic surgeons. New York: Thieme; 2010:147–163.)

Repetitive microtrauma from impingement during hip flexion and internal rotation leads to degeneration of the acetabular labrum and articular cartilage and is a source of hip pain.[29,31,32] MRI is an excellent modality to evaluate FAI because it permits early detection of the disease process and can identify labral tears, cartilage damage, subchondral cysts, and underlying subtle anatomic variations of the femoral head-neck junction or acetabulum associated with cam or pincer impingement. There is, however, a relatively high incidence of FAI in asymptomatic individuals, so careful correlation of MRI and clinical examination findings is warranted. A recent systematic review found the prevalence of asymptomatic cam deformity was 37% (55% in athletes, 23% in the general population); and the prevalence of asymptomatic pincer lesion was 67%.[38]

Cam-type FAI involves shear forces created by the nonspherical portion of the femoral head-neck junction impinging on the acetabulum, resulting in a characteristic pattern of cartilage loss over the anterosuperior weight-bearing portion of the acetabulum and, eventually, possible tear or detachment of the principally uninvolved labrum (▶ Fig. 10.9).[31,39] MRI can detect subtle anatomic variations of the femoral head-neck junction, labral pathology, adjacent cartilage damage, and subchondral cysts. Typical findings include any of the following[31,39]:

- High signal of the anterior joint margin extending to the tidemark.
- Intermediate-signal labral degeneration.
- Labral tears with a linear or diffuse increased signal intensity.
- Defects, fissures, or delamination in the articular cartilage.
- Femoral head/neck cysts.

Typical findings on fast spin-echo (FSE) may also include abnormal contour of the acetabular labrum and a cam lesion. Decreased offset of the femoral head-neck junction can be detected on conventional radiographs or MRI as a prominent lateral extension of the femoral head at the step-off to the adjacent femoral neck.[31] Other features that can be present on MRI are the following:

- Congruent but nonspherical head.
- Small head-to-neck ratio.
- Short neck.

As part of the multiplanar assessment of FAI, oblique axial MRI sequences can be helpful in defining the abnormal osseous neck-shaft offset. In those images, the segment prescription is parallel to the neck-shaft angle of a coronal image, passing directly through the center of the femoral head. The α angle, measured according to the method of Nötzli et al,[40] can help define the anterior margin of the waist of the femoral neck (▶ Fig. 10.10).

Pincer-type FAI involves contact between a normal femoral neck and an abnormal anterior acetabular rim secondary to focal or diffuse acetabular retroversion or protrusion of the femoral head into the pelvis (protrusio acetabuli or acetabular profunda). In this setting, the acetabular labrum fails first, which leads to degeneration and eventual ossification, worsening the overcoverage (retroversion). In patients with a retroverted acetabulum, axial MRI shows increased coverage of the anterior femoral head.[41] This is also observed on radiographs and computed tomography (CT) images. During flexion and internal rotation, the prominent anterolateral edge of the acetabulum leads to impingement and subsequent labral degeneration. Synovial fluid may penetrate into the subchondral bone and lead to subchondral cyst formation.[41,42,43] In addition, persistent anterior abutment can result in contrecoup cartilage lesions of the posteroinferior acetabulum. A pincer-type lesion could also result from focal superior acetabular retroversion. Overall, the pincer type has fewer chondral manifestations compared with the deep chondral lesions associated with cam impingement.[44,45] Intralabral ossification can be noted at the anterior and lateral margins of the hip joint.[39]

High rates of FAI are found in patients with hip instability, suggesting that FAI may predispose patients to hip instability because of the morphologic changes of the bone levering the femoral head posteriorly.[46,47] Although MRI has limitations in evaluating for hip instability, > 5-mm widening of the anterior hip joint recess and thinning to < 3 mm of the joint capsule lateral to the zona orbicularis on MR arthrography has been used as an indication of hip instability.[48]

10.4.3 Stress Fractures

Stress fractures, which result from cyclic mechanical stress, can be categorized into one of two groups: fatigue or insufficiency.

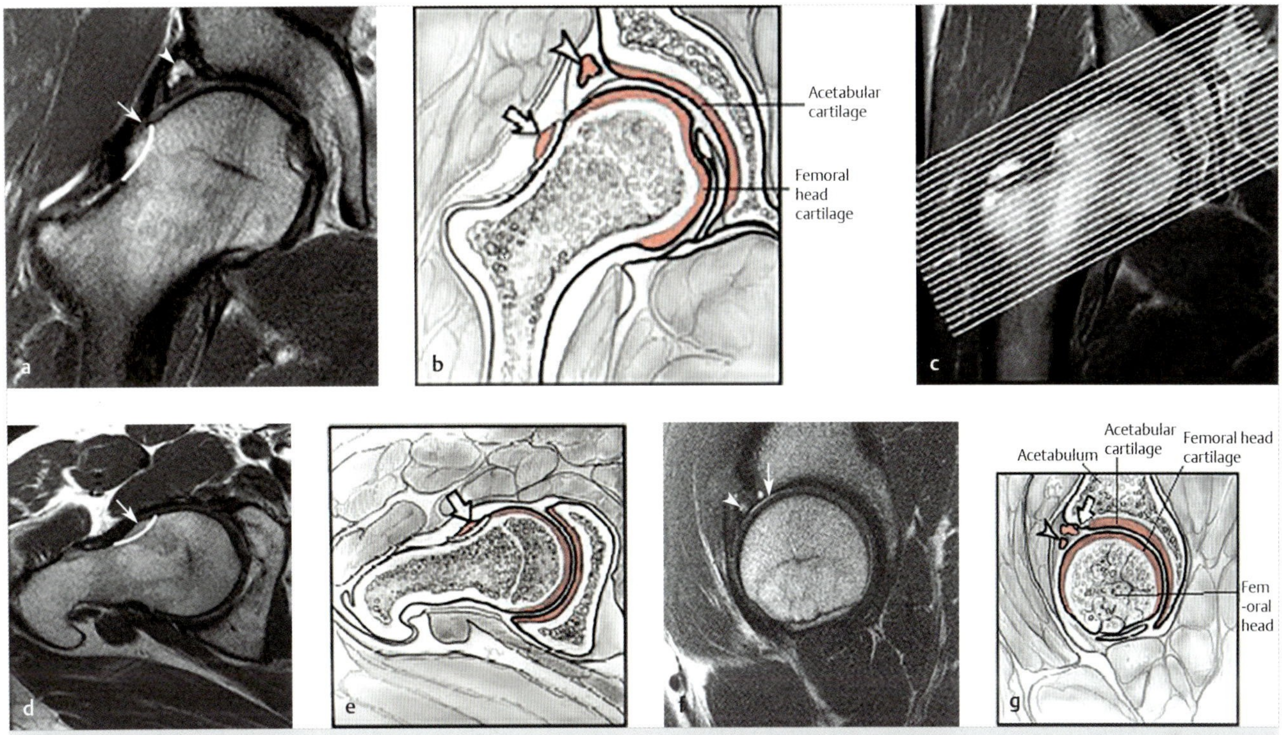

Fig. 10.9 Fast spin-echo (FSE) images and sketches of a 41-year-old patient with combined femoroacetabular impingement of the right hip. **(a)** The coronal with the labral tear and cam lesion **(b)** and associated artist's sketch. **(c)** The series prescription for the oblique axial sequence. **(d)** The oblique axial view **(e)** and associated artist's sketch **(f)** The sagittal MRI sequence **(g)** and associated artist's sketch. (Reproduced with permission from Shindle MK, Foo LF, Kelly BT, et al. Magnetic resonance imaging of cartilage in the athlete: current techniques and spectrum of disease. J Bone Joint Surg Am 2006;88:27–46.)

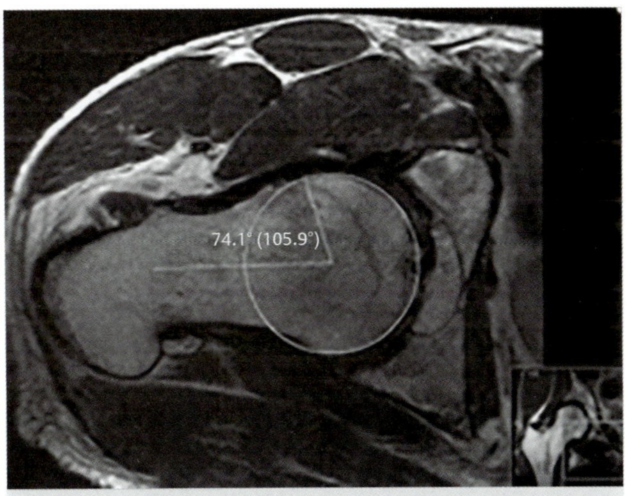

Fig. 10.10 An oblique axial fast spin-echo (FSE) image of the left hip showing an increased α angle in a nonspherical femoral head with a cam lesion. (Source: © 2009 Hospital for Special Surgery, New York, NY.)

Fatigue fractures are caused by abnormal stresses on normal bone; insufficiency fractures result from normal forces in abnormal bone. Military recruits and athletes are more susceptible than the general population to fatigue fractures, given that they occur in normal bone that is exposed to repetitive mechanical overload that overwhelms the physiologic remodeling process.[49] Insufficiency fractures occur more commonly in the elderly secondary to osteoporosis, osteomalacia, or other processes that weaken the bone, permitting osseous failure to occur with fewer loading cycles than in normal bone. Insufficiency fractures in the athletic population have also been described in female athletes, in association with the female athletic triad.[50] Stress fractures can occur on the compression (medial) or the tension (lateral) side of the femoral neck.[51] Compression stress fractures are more common and begin at the inferior cortex of the femoral neck. Tension stress fractures begin in the superior cortex, have a greater propensity to displace, and thus require more aggressive treatment.[52,53] A fracture line with a benign periosteal reaction may be visualized using conventional radiography or CT. Bone scintigraphy is more sensitive but not specific for the diagnosis of femoral neck stress fracture. MRI is both sensitive and specific to the presence of underlying bone marrow lesions, and a linear fracture line associated with the preservation of fatty marrow confirms a diagnosis of a stress fracture.[51,54] Fat-suppressed coronal images show a low signal line amid an area of increased signal intensity, indicating an acute or subacute fracture (▶ Fig. 10.11). MRI is also useful for excluding underlying lesions such as a tumor and marrow disorders that may be the cause of a pathologic stress fracture.

10.4.4 Traumatic Posterior Subluxation/ Dislocation/Lateral Impaction

Traumatic posterior hip dislocation most commonly occurs as a result of a motor vehicle accident when the hip and knee are flexed and the knee impacts the dashboard, producing a posteriorly directed force on the hip. Blanchard et al[55] found that in children who sustained traumatic hip dislocation, a consistent pattern of near complete avulsion of the posterior labrum occurred. In the acute setting, MRI may aid in the diagnosis of the following[56,57,58]:

- Femoral head contusions.
- Chondral injury.
- Labral disruption or entrapment.
- Capsular tear.
- Sciatic nerve injury.
- Intra-articular fragments.
- Ligamentum teres disruption.
- Nondisplaced fractures of the femoral head or acetabulum.

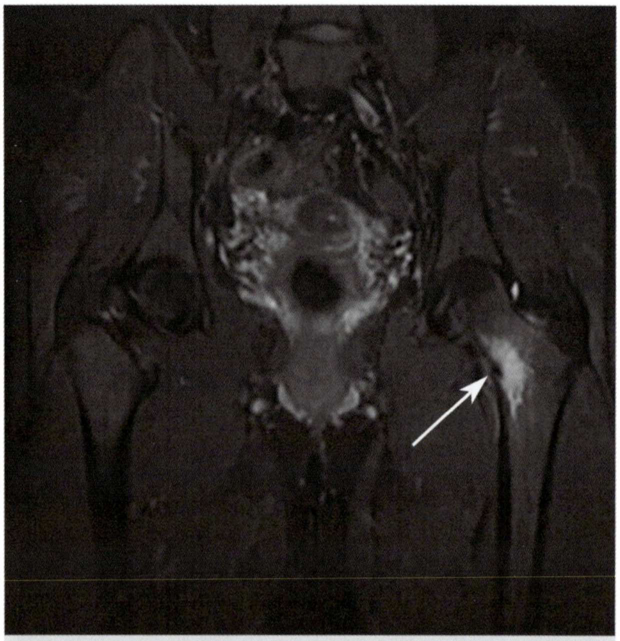

Fig. 10.11 A coronal fat-suppressed image obtained with a body coil technique, showing increased signal intensity (*arrow*) surrounding a stress fracture at the medial aspect of the left femoral neck. (Source: © 2009 Hospital for Special Surgery, New York, NY.)

Hip subluxation can occur with low-energy mechanisms such as a fall onto a flexed hip or knee, and because its presentation is often subtler than hip dislocation, it can be misdiagnosed as a hip strain or sprain. Hip subluxation can, however, lead to substantial morbidity if missed. Traumatic posterior subluxation can occur in contact sports such as football and may result in symptomatic cartilage/labral injury despite a lack of radiographic evidence of dislocation.[59] Hip translation associated with a subluxation event can result in anterior or posterior labrum or posterior wall displacement. The iliofemoral ligament and parafoveal cartilage can also be disrupted, typically during relocation of the hip joint (▶ Fig. 10.12). MRI is useful for monitoring sequelae of the subluxation, including osteonecrosis and femoral head edema (see section "Osteonecrosis").[59,60] Serial MRI can aid in determining when an athlete can return to sport. A direct blow to the greater trochanter in young, otherwise physically fit patients can result in an isolated chondral injury, as described by Byrd et al.[61] MRI can be used to determine the extent of chondral damage and the presence of osteochondral loose bodies.

10.4.5 Muscle Strains and Tears

The most frequent injuries about the groin and hip are muscle strains and tears. These injuries typically affect the myotendinous junction, which is the weakest point of the musculotendinous unit, but tendon avulsion from the osseous attachment can also occur.[62] The most commonly strained muscles around the hip joint are the following[62]:

- Hamstrings (biceps femoris, semimembranosus, and semitendinosus).
- Rectus femoris.
- Adductors.

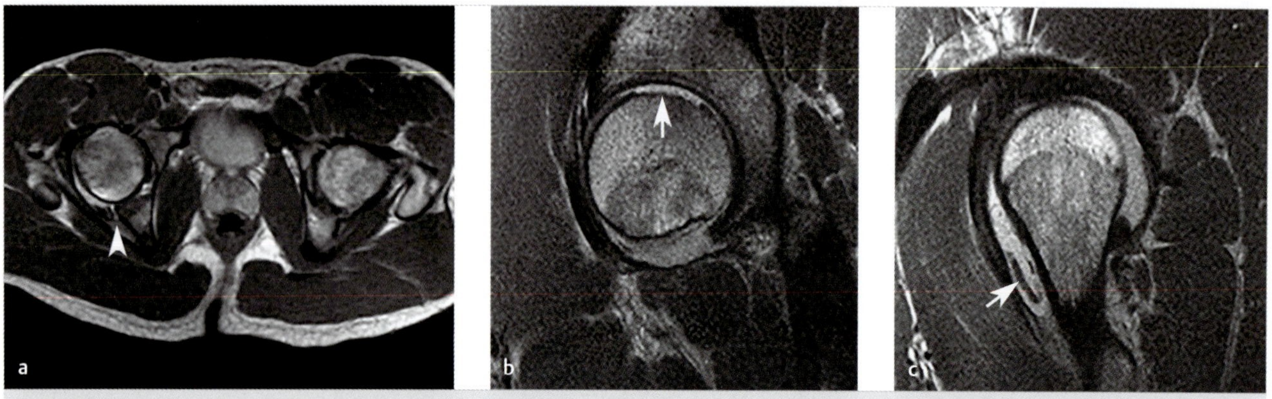

Fig. 10.12 Posterior hip subluxation. Axial body coil **(a)** and sagittal surface coil **(b,c)** fast spin-echo (FSE) images of the hip in an 18-year-old patient with sequelae of posterior hip subluxation. An intact right posterior hip capsule is seen, attached to a posterior wall fracture (**a**, *arrowhead*) and associated with a large, full-thickness chondral shear injury of the femoral head (**b**, *arrow*). Cartilaginous debris (**c**, *arrow*) is seen within the anteroinferior dependent recess of the joint. (Reproduced with permission from Shindle MK, Foo LF, Kelly BT, et al. Magnetic resonance imaging of cartilage in the athlete: current techniques and spectrum of disease. J Bone Joint Surg Am 2006;88:27–46.)

The adductor group is frequently involved, especially in hockey, soccer, and football players. Medial thigh or groin pain is the presenting symptom.[62] The MRI classification is based on the extent of disruption present: on fat-suppressed images, muscle avulsions and tears typically have high signal intensity in areas of hemorrhage or edema. First-degree strains have a minor degree of fiber disruption and a “feathery” pattern of increased signal intensity intermediate to T2-weighted images secondary to interstitial edema and hemorrhage that extends into the adjacent muscle fascicles. Second-degree strains have a partial tear without retraction and often also have a hematoma at the myotendinous junction. Third-degree strains have a complete rupture of the myotendinous unit.[63] Acute tendinous avulsion injuries of the rectus femoris origin at the anterior inferior iliac spine can be seen. This injury occurs most commonly after forceful extension of the hip (▶ Fig. 10.13).[64] Hamstring tears are typically partial-thickness tears, and the biceps femoris is the most frequently injured structure, followed by the semitendinosus and semimembranosus muscles. Injuries typically occur at the musculotendinous junction with the characteristic featherlike edema pattern described above.

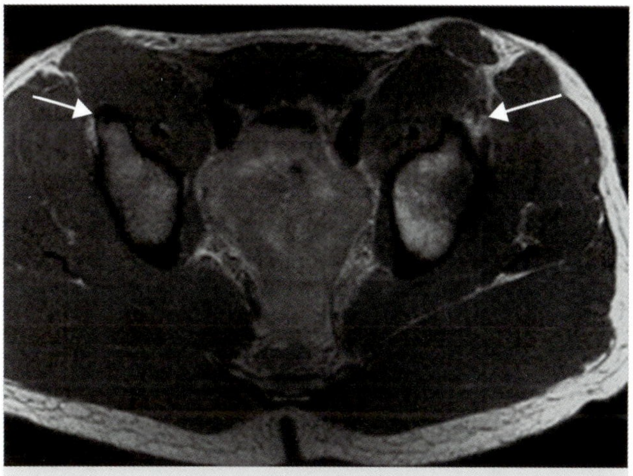

Fig. 10.13 An axial fast spin-echo (FSE) image obtained with a body coil technique, showing avulsion of the proximal portion of the rectus femoris from the patient’s left anterior inferior iliac spine (*left arrow*). A normal low-signal tendinous insertion is seen on the right (*right arrow*). (Source: © 2009 Hospital for Special Surgery, New York, NY.)

10.4.6 Apophyseal Avulsion

Apophyseal avulsion injuries characteristically occur in adolescents and are equivalent to muscle strains in adults. During running and jumping activities, the hamstring origins at the ischial tuberosity may be avulsed; these injuries have been referred to as hurdler’s fractures.[65] Apophyseal injuries of the pelvis may also involve the rectus femoris or sartorius muscles at the anteroinferior or anterosuperior iliac spines, respectively. In competitive sports that require kicking motions with extreme hip flexion, avulsions of the iliopsoas tendon off the lesser trochanter may be seen.

10.4.7 Athletic Pubalgia/Core Muscle Injury

The term “athletic pubalgia” describes a spectrum of activity-induced pain that occurs at the pubic symphysis. This can include osteitis pubis, adductor, or core muscle injuries.[66] MRI plays a central role in identifying the cause of symptoms in athletic pubalgia. Osteitis pubis is a noninfectious inflammation of the pubic symphysis, which is thought to be related to instability at the pubic symphysis resulting from ligamentous, muscular, or tendinous injury.[67] MRI will demonstrate bone marrow edema at the pubis, fluid within the pubic symphysis joint, or symphyseal widening[68] (▶ Fig. 10.14). Core muscle injuries, or rectus abdominis/adductor aponeurosis injuries, involve the insertion of the rectus abdominis, the origin of the adductor longus, and the periosteum of the pubic tubercle.[69] This injury has been referred to as sports hernia, Gilmore groin, pubic inguinal pain syndrome, or sportsmen’s groin.[70] MRI will demonstrate marrow edema at the pubis, a visible defect in the rectus abdominis anterior to the pubic tubercle, detachment of or fluid interspersed within the adductor longus tendon, or a cleft beneath the pubic bone indicating a lesion within the aponeurosis.[69] Injuries can also be present further posteriorly in the pubis and can extend to the adductor brevis.

10.4.8 Ligamentum Teres Tears

The ligamentum teres tightens in hip abduction, medial rotation, and lateral rotation. It is thought to prevent inferior, posterior, and anterior subluxation of the femoral head in abduction, medial rotation, and lateral rotation, respectively.[71] However, its contribution to overall hip function is debated. Tears of the

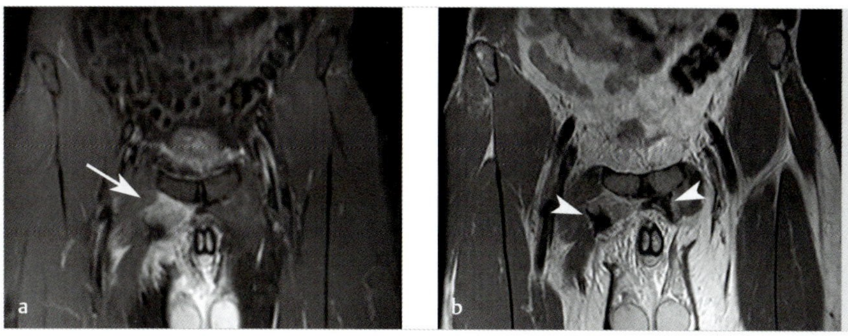

Fig. 10.14 Core muscle injury. **(a)** Right-sided edema at origin of adductor tendons on inversion recovery sequence (*arrow*). **(b)** Coronal proton-density sequence demonstrating the avulsed tendon on the patient’s right (*left arrowhead*) and the intact tendon on the left (*right arrowhead*).

ligamentum teres can be a source of hip pain, and some degree of tearing has been identified in 50 to 88% of patients undergoing hip surgery.[72,73] Chahla et al[73] found that the ligamentum teres was frayed or partially torn in 88% of patients undergoing hip arthroscopy and that it was fullytorn in only 1.5%. Complete tears of the ligamentum teres were associated with increased hip laxity and femoral head chondral defects. A higher incidence of atraumatic ligamentum teres tears has been found in athletes who repetitively load the ligament with excessive hip range of motion, such as professional ballet dancers.[74] Ligamentum teres hypertrophy has been noted in asymptomatic elite gymnasts.[75]

10.4.9 Greater Trochanteric Pain Syndrome

Greater trochanteric pain syndrome is a term that encompasses greater trochanteric bursitis, effusion, tears/tendinosis of the gluteus medius and minimus, and external coxa saltans (snapping hip). The major clinical findings are nonspecific, typically with tenderness localized to the lateral aspect of the hip or thigh. Clinically, distinguishing isolated bursal pathologic changes from tendon abnormalities or other soft tissue lesions is difficult; therefore, the differential diagnosis is broad and requires consideration of articular, periarticular, and distant processes as sources of lateral hip pain.[76]

Trochanteric Bursitis

The surface of the greater trochanter has four distinct facets:

- Anterior.
- Posterior.
- Lateral.
- Superoposterior.

The overlying trochanteric bursa is composed of three discrete parts[76]:

- Subgluteus maximus bursa.
- Subgluteus medius bursa.
- Subgluteus minimus bursa.

Excessive friction from the overlying iliotibial band (ITB) is the most likely cause but trochanteric bursitis is often a manifestation of underlying abductor tendon pathology. Thus, the presence of trochanteric bursitis should prompt careful attention to the underlying abductor tendons. Fat-suppressed MR sequences, particularly coronal and axial images, should be evaluated for bursal distention with high signal intensity (▶ Fig. 10.15a).

10.4.10 Abductor Tears

The gluteus medius inserts onto the superoposterior and lateral facets, and the gluteus minimus inserts onto the anterior facet of the greater trochanter. MRI evaluation of the hip in patients older than 40 years often reveals several pathologic processes, including some degree of the following[18,77,78]:

- Cartilage degeneration.
- Degenerative labral lesions.
- Extracapsular abnormalities (including abductor or iliopsoas tendinosis).

Abductor tears have been termed the "rotator cuff tears of the hip" and are highly prevalent in patients with osteoarthritis.[79,80] Coronal and axial MRI sequences should be evaluated for the presence or absence of such tears. Partial-thickness abductor tears show hyperintensity with abnormal morphology or alterations in tendon caliber and signal of the torn tendon fibers, and full-thickness tears show a fluid-filled gap with a retracted tendon (▶ Fig. 10.15b). Some patients have "intractable" symptoms of trochanteric bursitis despite multiple injections and nonoperative treatment. For such patients, MRI may be diagnostic for a gluteus medius or minimus rupture.[81]

10.4.11 Snapping Hip Syndrome (Coxa Saltans)

Snapping hip syndrome, or coxa saltans, is characterized by an audible or palpable snapping of the hip during flexion or extension, occasionally causing pain. The causes of coxa saltans have been divided into three categories[82]:

- Intra-articular.
- Internal (snapping of the iliopsoas tendon against an osseous ridge).
- External (snapping of the ITB or gluteus maximus muscle over the greater trochanter).

It is important to accurately determine the source of the snapping so the appropriate treatment can be given. MRI is useful

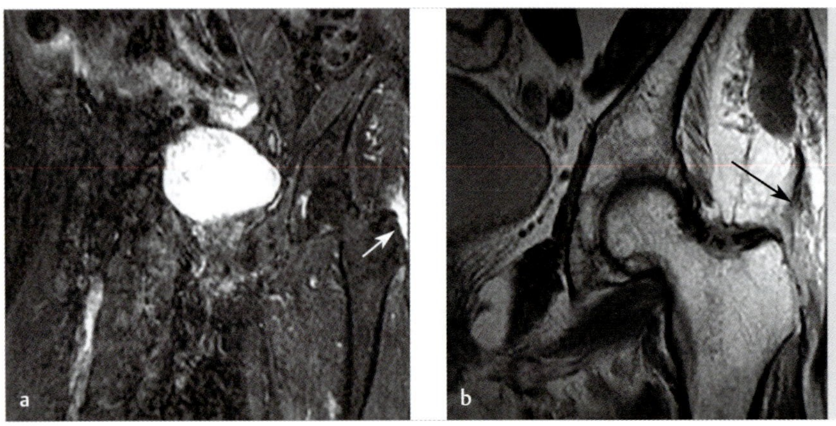

Fig. 10.15 Hip abductor tear. **(a)** A coronal fat-suppressed image of the hip showing a fluid-filled space that should be occupied by the left hip abductors, indicating a tear (*arrow*). **(b)** A fast spin-echo (FSE) image showing the tear with retraction of the gluteus medius tendon (*arrow*) with dehiscence of its insertion from the greater trochanter. (Source: © 2009 Hospital for Special Surgery, New York, NY.)

for excluding other intra- or extra-articular hip abnormalities but its role in diagnosing coxa saltans is limited because of its lack of dynamic capabilities. With internal coxa saltans, fat-suppressed images may display iliopsoas bursa fluid. With external coxa saltans, fat-suppressed images may show a high-signal ITB, trochanteric bursa, and anterior border of the gluteus maximus. Dynamic sonography of the hip is beneficial as an adjuvant to static MRI to confirm the diagnosis.

10.4.12 Deep Gluteal Syndrome

Deep gluteal syndrome (DGS) describes pain in the buttock area, hip, or posterior thigh and/or nondiscogenic radicular pain caused by entrapment of the sciatic nerve within the subgluteal space.[83] The sciatic nerve exits the pelvis through the greater sciatic notch. Although variations exist, the nerve is most often located immediately anterior to the piriformis muscle. Irritation of the piriformis musculotendinous unit can cause compression of the sciatic nerve,[84] which is a subtype of DGS often referred to as "piriformis syndrome." MRI may show an abnormal hypertrophic piriformis muscle and/or hyperintensity of the sciatic nerve on fat-suppressed images, a variant course of the nerve through the piriformis muscle, or a mass effect, resulting in displacement of the muscle from anterior to posterior with a loss of normal muscle striations.[64] Other sources of extrapelvic sciatic nerve compression include fibrous bands interposed with blood vessels, gluteal muscles, hamstring muscles, the ischial tuberosity, the gemelli-obturator internus complex, or quadratus femoris or ischiofemoral pathology.[83,85] MRI is useful to carefully evaluate the sciatic nerve and the structures that could be causing the patient's DGS.

10.5 Degenerative Conditions

10.5.1 Osteoarthritis

Osteoarthritis is characterized by articular cartilage loss with hip joint space narrowing; the incidence of this process increases with age. The hip is one of the most common sites for osteoarthritis,[86] and there are several conditions that lead to osteoarthritis, including the following[31]:

- FAI.
- Previous slipped capital femoral epiphysis.
- Developmental dysplasia of the hip.
- Legg-Calvé-Perthes disease.
- Trauma.
- Osteonecrosis.
- Paget disease.
- Other anatomic variants.

It is now well accepted that FAI is a precursor for the development of hip osteoarthritis.[27,28,29,30,31,32] The appearance of osteoarthritis on MRI is similar to that on conventional radiographs, including the following:

- Hypointense subchondral bone of the femoral head and acetabulum.
- Joint space narrowing (thinning of cartilage).
- Osteophyte formation.
- Subchondral cysts.
- Deformity of the femoral head or acetabulum.

Osteoarthritis may also be associated with labral tears, paralabral cysts, synovitis, or osteonecrosis of the femoral head.[87] With advancements in quantitative MRI, there is increased focus on evaluating articular cartilage thickness and ultrastructural integrity in the setting of FAI or prior hip injury.[88,89]

10.5.2 Dysplasia

Acetabular dysplasia describes acetabular undercoverage of the femoral head. Patients may experience hip instability as a result of increased forces on the secondary, soft tissue stabilizers of the hip joint, and abnormal forces on articular cartilage can lead to the development of osteoarthritis.[90,91,92,93] Hip dysplasia is classically diagnosed on the basis of an anteroposterior radiograph of the pelvis, in which the lateral center edge angle is < 25 degrees. Most dysplastic hips have a component of acetabular anteversion, but 15 to 20% have acetabular retroversion.[94,95] Acetabular retroversion has been associated with early osteoarthritis, and if there is concomitant femoral retroversion, the affect seems to be additive in leading to early osteoarthritis.[96] MRI can demonstrate cartilaginous and soft tissue changes that may be associated with dysplasia. These can include a hypertrophied labrum and/or ligamentum teres.[97]

10.6 Other Pathologic Conditions

10.6.1 Osteonecrosis

Osteonecrosis (also called avascular necrosis) of the femoral head is the cellular necrosis of the bone and bone marrow elements that comprise part or all of the femoral head. The cause of osteonecrosis is unknown, or "idiopathic," in up to 30% of cases[98] but some of the known predisposing causes including the following[99]:

- Corticosteroid use.
- Collagen vascular disease.
- Trauma (dislocation of the hip, femoral neck fracture).
- Hemoglobinopathies (e.g., sickle cell disease).

MRI has been shown to be more sensitive than conventional radiography, nuclear scintigraphy, or CT for the early detection of osteonecrosis.[99,100,101,102] Besides aiding in early detection, MRI is useful for differentiating osteonecrosis from other pathologic processes and for defining the extent of osteonecrosis, which is a predictor of the likelihood of femoral head collapse.[103,104] Although sometimes difficult, it is especially important to distinguish between osteonecrosis and subchondral insufficiency fractures. Subchondral insufficiency fractures often present as acute onset of severe pain, and MRI will show the fracture parallel and adjacent to the subchondral plate, following the contour of the femoral head.[39]

Osteonecrosis of the femoral head has a characteristic MRI appearance: a low-signal, crescent-shaped rim in a subchondral location that corresponds to the interface between normal and ischemic bone (▶ Fig. 10.16). A second rim of increased signal that is pathognomonic of osteonecrosis typically is present on fat-suppressed images.[101,103]

The presence of a band of low signal intensity on T1-weighted images or of the "double-line" sign on T2-weighted or fat-suppressed proton-density images is each reported to be an

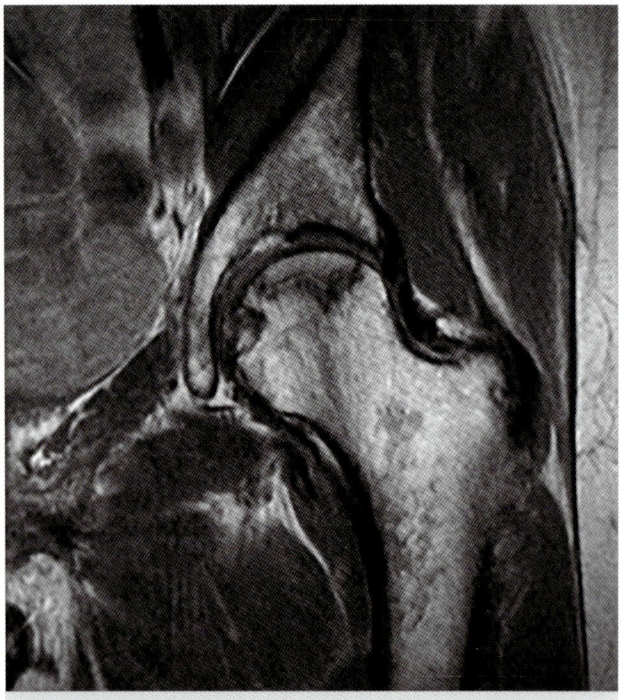

Fig. 10.16 A coronal fast spin-echo (FSE) image of the left hip showing a region of osteonecrosis at the weight-bearing surface of the femoral head with a classic serpentine line of demarcation from the adjacent normal bone. (Source: © 2009 Hospital for Special Surgery, New York, NY.)

early specific sign of nontraumatic osteonecrosis of the femoral head.[101,102] The double-line sign, which appears as a low-signal-intensity peripheral line and a parallel inner line of high signal intensity, can be observed in up to 80% of lesions.[31] These MRI abnormalities represent the reactive interface between necrotic and viable bone.[101,105] MRI may also show a joint effusion on fat-suppressed sequences.

In the presence of a posterior hip subluxation, MRI is useful for detecting osteonecrosis. In the acute setting, MRI is not an accurate predictor of osteonecrosis, and a repeat study should be obtained at 6 weeks. If there is no evidence of osteonecrosis, patients may safely return to sports activity. However, if there is evidence of osteonecrosis, patients are at increased risk for subsequent collapse and joint degeneration.[59]

Limited MRI examination of the hips (without extra time required for scout images) can be obtained to detect femoral head osteonecrosis and to quantify of the size of the lesion.[106] Several methods have been proposed to measure the extent of osteonecrosis for prognosis determination and treatment planning. Lafforgue et al[107] measured the α angle on the coronal T1-weighted images, selecting the largest area of necrosis and determining the angle formed at the center of the femoral head. An angle of > 75 degrees corresponded with a poor prognosis, and an angle of < 46 degrees corresponded to a satisfactory clinical response. Koo and Kim[108] measured the angle formed from the center of the femoral head on midcoronal and midsagittal MR images to quantify the size of the lesion objectively. Cherian et al[109] modified this method for quantifying the extent of osteonecrosis of the femoral head by using the coronal and sagittal MR images with maximal femoral head involvement. They concluded that that method was a reproducible and reliable way of determining the extent of osteonecrosis.

A low percentage of involvement of the femoral head weight-bearing surface has been well correlated with favorable outcomes in patients with early stages of the disease[107] and the unlikelihood of femoral head collapse after core decompressive surgery.[110] In one study, femoral head collapse did not occur when MRI showed that < 25% of the weight-bearing surface was involved.[110] However, when > 50% of the surface was involved, 87% of hips had femoral head collapse.[110]

MRI is also useful for identifying and localizing the necrotic lesion before performing a core decompression procedure. It is not uncommon to see cartilage loss and geode formation on the acetabular side as a result of osteonecrosis of the femoral head.[107] This finding is important because it may change the treatment approach—for example, total hip replacement rather than femoral head resurfacing or core decompression.

10.6.2 Idiopathic Transient Osteoporosis

Idiopathic transient osteoporosis is a rare and often unrecognized cause of hip pain that is usually seen in healthy young adults. The condition most commonly affects women in the third trimester of pregnancy and middle-aged men. Symptoms often present insidiously, with pain in the affected hip, and then progress to gait disturbance and functional disability. Transient osteoporosis of the hip should be considered after more common causes of hip pain (such as infection, stress fractures, or malignancy) are ruled out. Conventional radiographs typically show focal osteopenia of the femoral head and neck with loss of cortical continuity, although this finding may be subtle and is frequently missed. Fat-suppressed MR images show diffuse high signal intensity compatible with edema in the femoral head and proximal femoral neck and a small hip joint effusion, which are the classic findings of transient osteoporosis of the hip. However, this diffuse edema pattern may be related to a subtle subchondral fracture (▶ Fig. 10.17).[111,112] This entity can be differentiated from osteonecrosis of the hip, which shows signal changes at the weight-bearing surface of the femoral head and is not as diffuse as that seen with transient osteoporosis of the hip. Most cases resolve spontaneously within 6 to 12 months. However, subchondral fractures leading to femoral head collapse have been reported.[31,113] Therefore, patients should be treated with protected weight-bearing and monitored carefully with repeat MRI until the edema is resolved and the clinical symptoms subside.

10.7 Inflammatory Disorders

Rheumatoid arthritis (RA) is a systemic autoimmune inflammatory disorder that primarily affects the small joints of the hands and feet but may involve the larger weight-bearing joints, including the hip. Over the past decade, in concert with an increase in antirheumatic drug consumption, there has been a decrease in the number of RA patients undergoing hip replacements, indicating a decline in the effect of RA at the hip.[114] MRI is useful for evaluating erosions, effusion, and synovial pannus formation in patients who are affected at the hip.[115] The synovial proliferation is typically a mass-like prominence of tissue within the joint that is hyperintense on fat-suppressed sequences.[31] The pannus may be heterogeneous or homogeneous in appearance, and pannus hemorrhages can form with areas of low signal hemosiderin.[115] As with osteoarthritis, the MR findings of inflammatory arthritis correlate with the radiographic appearance, including any of the following[115]:

- Symmetric joint space narrowing.
- Periarticular erosions.
- Juxta-articular osteoporosis.
- Protrusio acetabuli.

Other findings may include the following[31]:

- Hyperintense joint effusion.
- Joint capsule distention.
- Hyperintense marrow edema.

Ankylosing spondylitis is another form of inflammatory arthritis. It most often involves the axial skeleton, and the hip is affected in 24 to 36% of patients, with 9 to 22% demonstrating radiographic evidence of hip arthritis.[116,117,118] Ankylosing spondylitis can have symmetric involvement in the hips but it can be distinguished from RA by its characteristic involvement of the SI joints when the hips are involved.[115] MRI is useful in identifying active inflammatory lesions of the spine and SI joints, which can aid in the diagnosis of this condition.[119]

10.8 Synovial Disorders

Synovial proliferative disorders are not uncommon, so careful scrutiny of the synovium on MRI is warranted. In the hip, negative intra-articular pressure and the tight capsule may result in more prominent erosions than those associated with synovial proliferative disorders in other joints such as the knee, which has several patulous synovial recesses.[31] Synovial chondromatosis is a monoarticular synovium-based cartilage metaplasia that commonly involves the hip joint.[31,120] MRI will show intracapsular fragments of intermediate signal intensity, and this can progress to a "cast" of synovium when the disease becomes confluent (▶ Fig. 10.18).[39] Ferro et al[121] found that patients with synovial chondromatosis do well after arthroscopic synovectomy.

Pigmented villonodular synovitis presents in either a nodular form or a diffuse form. Hemosiderin degradation products creates a low signal intensity that can be helpful in confirming the

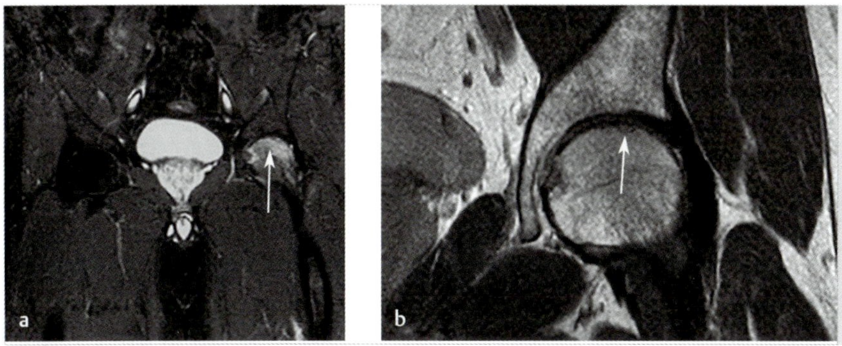

Fig. 10.17 Subchondral fractures of the hip. **(a)** A coronal fast spin-echo (FSE) image with fat suppression showing diffuse and extensive high signal of the left femoral head without a demarcated focus (*arrow*). Because there is no evidence of demarcation defining osteonecrosis, the diagnosis is consistent with transient osteoporosis of the hip. **(b)** Most cases of transient osteoporosis actually represent subchondral femoral head stress fractures, which can be appreciated on this coronal FSE image (*arrow*). (Source: © 2009 Hospital for Special Surgery, New York, NY.)

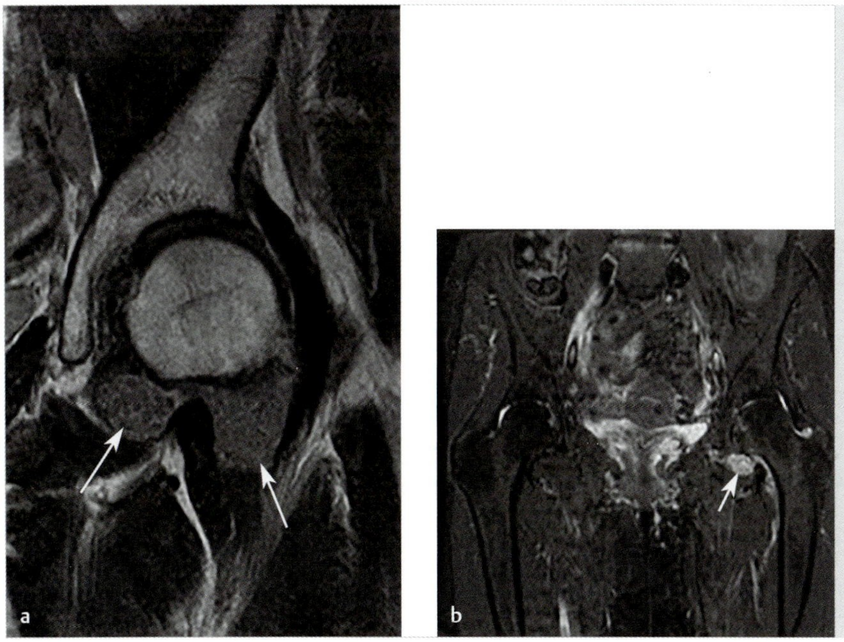

Fig. 10.18 Synovial osteochondromatosis. **(a)** A coronal fast spin-echo (FSE) image of the left hip showing synovial osteochondromatosis with cartilaginous bodies in the inferior capsule (*arrows*). **(b)** A coronal fat-suppressed FSE image of the pelvis also showing detached cartilaginous bodies (*arrow*). (Source: © 2009 Hospital for Special Surgery, New York, NY.)

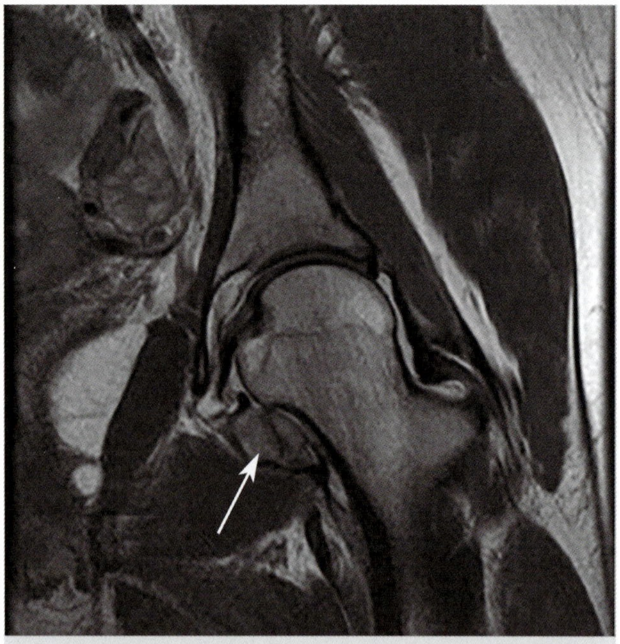

Fig. 10.19 Pigmented villonodular synovitis. A coronal fast spin-echo (FSE) image of the left hip showing pigmented villonodular synovitis with hemosiderin-laden synovium (*arrow*). (Source: © 2009 Hospital for Special Surgery, New York, NY.)

diagnosis (▶ Fig. 10.19).[122] In its nodular form, it is seen as an intermediate to low signal intensity focus of solitary, intracapsular soft tissue mass within the anteromedial recess or bare area.[31,39] The diffuse form may be characterized by rapid cartilage loss. MRI can help quantify the amount of intra- and extracapsular disease, which is helpful in preoperative planning.[39]

10.9 Postoperative MRI Findings

MRI evaluation of the hip after treatment for FAI with femoral osteochondroplasty, acetabular rim resection, and/or labral repair can aid in diagnosing the cause of persistent or recurrent pain after surgery. Considerations for postoperative MRI include using a gradient-echo sequence in patients with metallic implants[123] and accounting for normal postoperative changes in the bone and soft tissues.

The most common reason for revision surgery is residual structural deformity.[124] MRI can show any residual head-neck junction offset and the extent of femoral osteochondroplasty. Insufficiency fractures of the femoral neck after osteochondroplasty have been reported at an average of 4.4 weeks postoperatively and at a frequency of 1.9% at one institution.[125] These fractures are typically nondisplaced and can be seen on fat-suppressed MRI as a low-intensity signal line surrounded by bone edema.[123] Other postoperative sources of pain that can be identified on MRI include[123]:

- Intra-articular adhesions.
- Progressive joint degeneration.
- Retear of the labrum.
- Capsular incompetence.
- Heterotopic ossification.

Intra-articular adhesions typically occur between the labrum and the joint capsule or between the joint capsule and the site of femoral neck osteochondroplasty.[126] Assessing a retear of the acetabular labrum can be challenging because labral debridement will cause a persistent abnormal intralabral signal secondary to abnormally mobile water in the degenerative fibrocartilage. Blankenbaker et al[127] found that the diagnosis of recurrent tear was best achieved when MR arthrography demonstrated the following: a new line extending to the labral surface, a distorted or enlarged labrum, or a new paralabral cyst. They also found that after labral tear excision, labra appeared shortened on MRI. Capsular incompetence after surgery could be iatrogenic if the capsulotomies used in hip arthroscopy are not closed or it could be the result of capsular dehiscence. MRI will demonstrate an anterior capsular defect with fluid extravasation beneath the iliopsoas bursa.[123] Bedi et al[128] described the incidence of heterotopic ossification after hip arthroscopy as 4.7%, most often in male patients whose surgical procedure included a capsular cut and osteoplasty. Introducing indomethacin into the postoperative prophylaxis protocol reduced the incidence from 8.3% in patients receiving naproxen only to 1.8%.[128]

10.10 Brief High-Yield Review

- The normal hip anatomy can be divided into the osteochondral layer, the capsulolabral layer, the muscular layer, and the neural layer. Sagittal MRI is especially helpful in evaluation of the anterior acetabular labrum. Coronal MRI gives the best view of the weight-bearing cartilage layer of the acetabulum. Axial MRI allows for evaluation of the sciatic nerve.
- Most labral tears occur anterosuperiorly. There is a high incidence of asymptomatic tears, so a tear found on imaging must be clinically correlated.
- MRI is sensitive and specific in identifying stress fractures. Other conditions that may present with increased signal intensity in the femoral head/neck include transient osteoporosis of the hip, which appears as diffuse high signal intensity, or infection.
- Posterior hip subluxation/dislocation and lateral impaction can result in chondral and labral damage, as well as femoral head and sciatic nerve contusions or intra-articular fragments.
- Muscle strains and tears are the most frequent injuries around the groin and hip and can include injury to the hamstrings, adductors, abductors, and core muscles.
- Lateral hip pain can result from greater trochanter pain syndrome, which encompasses trochanteric bursitis, abductor tears, and snapping hip syndrome.
- DGS is a nondiscogenic pain syndrome resulting from entrapment of the sciatic nerve in the subgluteal space.
- FAI is caused by "cam," "pincer," or a combination of "cam" and "pincer." Repetitive microtrauma from impingement of these lesions leads to degeneration of the cartilage of the hip joint.
- MRI is the most sensitive method of imaging to diagnose osteonecrosis, or the necrosis of the bone and bone marrow elements, of the femoral head. The characteristic MRI finding is the "double-line" sign on T2-weighted or fat-suppressed proton-density images.

- Inflammatory conditions of the hip include ankylosing spondylitis and RA. Ankylosing spondylitis often has SI joint involvement. RA on MRI will present with a synovial proliferation. Other synovial proliferative disorders include synovial chondromatosis, which presents on MRI with intracapsular fragments of intermediate signal intensity, and pigmented villonodular synovitis, which is seen on MRI as nodular or diffuse intermediate to low signal, intracapsular, soft tissue masses.
- Postoperative MRI can be obtained to assess for recurrent or persistent pain after surgical treatment of FAI. MRI is useful to assess for residual structural deformity, new labral tears, insufficiency fractures of the femoral neck, capsular incompetence, or heterotopic ossification.

10.11 Common Clinical Questions

1. What is the best MRI sequence when looking for a labral tear?
   a) Coronal.
   b) Sagittal.
   c) Axial.

2. What is the prevalence of asymptomatic FAI?
   a) Asymptomatic CAM, 67%; asymptomatic pincer, 37%; asymptomatic labral tear, 15 to 35%.
   b) Asymptomatic CAM, 37%; asymptomatic pincer, 67%; asymptomatic labral tear, 33 to 69%.
   c) Asymptomatic CAM, 67%; asymptomatic pincer, 37%; asymptomatic labral tear, 55 to 79%.
   d) Asymptomatic CAM, 37%; asymptomatic pincer, 67%; asymptomatic labral tear, 55 to 79%.

3. How should I manage an athlete with suspected hip subluxation?
   a) If no edema on initial MRI, allow to return to sports when asymptomatic.
   b) If evidence of femoral head edema, proceed immediately to core decompression.
   c) Repeat MRI in 6 weeks and monitor femoral head edema with repeat MRI as needed; return to sports when edema has resolved.
   d) Monitor with radiographs alone to look for femoral head collapse.

4. What are MRI indications of athletic pubalgia?
   a) Bone marrow edema at the pubis.
   b) Fluid within the pubic symphysis joint.
   c) Widening of the pubic symphysis.
   d) Fluid beneath the pubic bone (within the aponeurosis).
   e) All of the above.

5. What are clinical and imaging findings associated with idiopathic transient osteoporosis? (choose all that apply)
   a) Most commonly in third trimester of pregnancy and in middle-aged men.
   b) Fat-suppressed MRI shows diffuse high-signal-intensity edema in the femoral head and proximal femoral neck and a small hip joint effusion.
   c) MRI shows focal signal changes at the weight-bearing surface of the femoral head.
   d) MRI shows low-signal, crescent-shaped rim in a subchondral location.

References

[1] Weber AE, Poultsides LA, O'Sullivan E, Kelly BT, Bedi A. Anatomical considerations and clinical examination. In: Kelly BT, Bedi A, Larson CM, O'Sullivan E, eds. Sports hip injuries: diagnosis and management. Thorofare, NJ: SLACK Incorporated; 2015:3–24

[2] Kassarjian A, Yoon LS, Belzile E, Connolly SA, Millis MB, Palmer WE. Triad of MR arthrographic findings in patients with cam-type femoroacetabular impingement. Radiology. 2005; 236(2):588–592

[3] Kramer J, Recht MP. MR arthrography of the lower extremity. Radiol Clin North Am. 2002; 40(5):1121–1132

[4] Schmid MR, Nötzli HP, Zanetti M, Wyss TF, Hodler J. Cartilage lesions in the hip: diagnostic effectiveness of MR arthrography. Radiology. 2003; 226(2): 382–386

[5] Potter HG, Foo LF. Magnetic resonance imaging of articular cartilage: trauma, degeneration, and repair. Am J Sports Med. 2006; 34(4):661–677

[6] Mintz DN, Hooper T, Connell D, Buly R, Padgett DE, Potter HG. Magnetic resonance imaging of the hip: detection of labral and chondral abnormalities using noncontrast imaging. Arthroscopy. 2005; 21(4):385–393

[7] Toomayan GA, Holman WR, Major NM, Kozlowicz SM, Vail TP. Sensitivity of MR arthrography in the evaluation of acetabular labral tears. AJR Am J Roentgenol. 2006; 186(2):449–453

[8] Kelly BT, Williams RJ, III, Philippon MJ. Hip arthroscopy: current indications, treatment options, and management issues. Am J Sports Med. 2003; 31(6): 1020–1037

[9] Ferguson SJ, Bryant JT, Ganz R, Ito K. An in vitro investigation of the acetabular labral seal in hip joint mechanics. J Biomech. 2003; 36(2):171–178

[10] McCarthy JC, Noble PC, Schuck MR, Wright J, Lee J. The Otto E. Aufranc Award: the role of labral lesions to development of early degenerative hip disease. Clin Orthop Relat Res. 2001(393):25–37

[11] Dinauer PA, Murphy KP, Carroll JF. Sublabral sulcus at the posteroinferior acetabulum: a potential pitfall in MR arthrography diagnosis of acetabular labral tears. AJR Am J Roentgenol. 2004; 183(6):1745–1753

[12] Alzaharani A, Bali K, Gudena R, et al. The innervation of the human acetabular labrum and hip joint: an anatomic study. BMC Musculoskelet Disord. 2014; 15:41

[13] Kim YT, Azuma H. The nerve endings of the acetabular labrum. Clin Orthop Relat Res. 1995(320):176–181

[14] Kelly BT, Shapiro GS, Digiovanni CW, Buly RL, Potter HG, Hannafin JA. Vascularity of the hip labrum: a cadaveric investigation. Arthroscopy. 2005; 21(1):3–11

[15] Seldes RM, Tan V, Hunt J, Katz M, Winiarsky R, Fitzgerald RH, Jr. Anatomy, histologic features, and vascularity of the adult acetabular labrum. Clin Orthop Relat Res. 2001(382):232–240

[16] Lee AJ, Armour P, Thind D, Coates MH, Kang AC. The prevalence of acetabular labral tears and associated pathology in a young asymptomatic population. Bone Joint J. 2015; 97-B(5):623–627

[17] Register B, Pennock AT, Ho CP, Strickland CD, Lawand A, Philippon MJ. Prevalence of abnormal hip findings in asymptomatic participants: a prospective, blinded study. Am J Sports Med. 2012; 40(12):2720–2724

[18] Jayakar R, Merz A, Plotkin B, Wang D, Seeger L, Hame SL. Magnetic resonance arthrography and the prevalence of acetabular labral tears in patients 50 years of age and older. Skeletal Radiol. 2016; 45(8):1061–1067

[19] Georgiadis AG, Seeley MA, Chauvin NA, Sankar WN. Prevalence of acetabular labral tears in asymptomatic children. J Child Orthop. 2016; 10(2):149–154

[20] Kelly BT, Weiland DE, Schenker ML, Philippon MJ. Arthroscopic labral repair in the hip: surgical technique and review of the literature. Arthroscopy. 2005; 21(12):1496–1504

[21] Lage LA, Patel JV, Villar RN. The acetabular labral tear: an arthroscopic classification. Arthroscopy. 1996; 12(3):269–272

[22] Blankenbaker DG, De Smet AA, Keene JS, Fine JP. Classification and localization of acetabular labral tears. Skeletal Radiol. 2007; 36(5):391–397

[23] Ilizaliturri VM, Jr, Byrd JWT, Sampson TG, et al. A geographic zone method to describe intra-articular pathology in hip arthroscopy: cadaveric study and preliminary report. Arthroscopy. 2008; 24(5):534–539

[24] Byrd JWT. Labral lesions: an elusive source of hip pain case reports and literature review. Arthroscopy. 1996; 12(5):603–612
[25] Türker M, Kılıçoğlu Ö, Göksan B, Bilgiç B. Vascularity and histology of fetal labrum and chondrolabral junction: its relevance to chondrolabral detachment tears. Knee Surg Sports Traumatol Arthrosc. 2012; 20(2):381–386
[26] Kalhor M, Horowitz K, Beck M, Nazparvar B, Ganz R. Vascular supply to the acetabular labrum. J Bone Joint Surg Am. 2010; 92(15):2570–2575
[27] Beck M, Kalhor M, Leunig M, Ganz R. Hip morphology influences the pattern of damage to the acetabular cartilage: femoroacetabular impingement as a cause of early osteoarthritis of the hip. J Bone Joint Surg Br. 2005; 87(7): 1012–1018
[28] Ganz R, Parvizi J, Beck M, Leunig M, Nötzli H, Siebenrock KA. Femoroacetabular impingement: a cause for osteoarthritis of the hip. Clin Orthop Relat Res. 2003(417):112–120
[29] Ito K, Minka MA, II, Leunig M, Werlen S, Ganz R. Femoroacetabular impingement and the cam-effect. A MRI-based quantitative anatomical study of the femoral head-neck offset. J Bone Joint Surg Br. 2001; 83(2):171–176
[30] McGuffin WS, Melkus G, Rakhra KS, Beaulé PE. Is the contralateral hip at risk in patients with unilateral symptomatic cam femoroacetabular impingement? A quantitative T1ρ MRI study. Osteoarthritis Cartilage. 2015; 23(8):1337–1342
[31] Stoller DW, Sampson T, Bredella M. The hip. In: Stoller DW, ed. Magnetic resonance imaging in orthopaedics and sports medicine. Philadelphia, PA: Lippincott Williams & Wilkins; 2007:41–304
[32] Tanzer M, Noiseux N. Osseous abnormalities and early osteoarthritis: the role of hip impingement. Clin Orthop Relat Res. 2004(429):170–177
[33] Leunig M, Casillas MM, Hamlet M, et al. Slipped capital femoral epiphysis: early mechanical damage to the acetabular cartilage by a prominent femoral metaphysis. Acta Orthop Scand. 2000; 71(4):370–375
[34] Agricola R, Heijboer MP, Ginai AZ, et al. A cam deformity is gradually acquired during skeletal maturation in adolescent and young male soccer players: a prospective study with minimum 2-year follow-up. Am J Sports Med. 2014; 42(4):798–806
[35] Johnson AC, Shaman MA, Ryan TG. Femoroacetabular impingement in former high-level youth soccer players. Am J Sports Med. 2012; 40(6):1342–1346
[36] Siebenrock KA, Wahab KHA, Werlen S, Kalhor M, Leunig M, Ganz R. Abnormal extension of the femoral head epiphysis as a cause of cam impingement. Clin Orthop Relat Res. 2004(418):54–60
[37] Pollard TC, Villar RN, Norton MR, et al. Genetic influences in the aetiology of femoroacetabular impingement: a sibling study. J Bone Joint Surg Br. 2010; 92(2):209–216
[38] Frank JM, Harris JD, Erickson BJ, et al. Prevalence of femoroacetabular impingement imaging findings in asymptomatic volunteers: a systematic review. Arthroscopy. 2015; 31(6):1199–1204
[39] Potter HG, Schachar J. High resolution noncontrast MRI of the hip. J Magn Reson Imaging. 2010; 31(2):268–278
[40] Nötzli HP, Wyss TF, Stoecklin CH, Schmid MR, Treiber K, Hodler J. The contour of the femoral head-neck junction as a predictor for the risk of anterior impingement. J Bone Joint Surg Br. 2002; 84(4):556–560
[41] Reynolds D, Lucas J, Klaue K. Retroversion of the acetabulum. A cause of hip pain. J Bone Joint Surg Br. 1999; 81(2):281–288
[42] Bredella MA, Stoller DW. MR imaging of femoroacetabular impingement. Magn Reson Imaging Clin N Am. 2005; 13(4):653–664
[43] Siebenrock KA, Schoeniger R, Ganz R. Anterior femoro-acetabular impingement due to acetabular retroversion. Treatment with periacetabular osteotomy. J Bone Joint Surg Am. 2003; 85(2):278–286
[44] Lavigne M, Parvizi J, Beck M, Siebenrock KA, Ganz R, Leunig M. Anterior femoroacetabular impingement: part I. Techniques of joint preserving surgery. Clin Orthop Relat Res. 2004(418):61–66
[45] Shindle MK, Voos JE, Heyworth BE, et al. Hip arthroscopy in the athletic patient: current techniques and spectrum of disease. J Bone Joint Surg Am. 2007; 89 Suppl 3:29–43
[46] Canham CD, Yen YM, Giordano BD. Does femoroacetabular impingement cause hip instability? A systematic review. Arthroscopy. 2016; 32(1):203–208
[47] Krych AJ, Thompson M, Larson CM, Byrd JW, Kelly BT. Is posterior hip instability associated with cam and pincer deformity? Clin Orthop Relat Res. 2012; 470(12):3390–3397
[48] Magerkurth O, Jacobson JA, Morag Y, Caoili E, Fessell D, Sekiya JK. Capsular laxity of the hip: findings at magnetic resonance arthrography. Arthroscopy. 2013; 29(10):1615–1622
[49] Armstrong DW, III, Rue JPH, Wilckens JH, Frassica FJ. Stress fracture injury in young military men and women. Bone. 2004; 35(3):806–816
[50] Anderson K, Strickland SM, Warren R. Hip and groin injuries in athletes. Am J Sports Med. 2001; 29(4):521–533
[51] Boden BP, Osbahr DC. High-risk stress fractures: evaluation and treatment. J Am Acad Orthop Surg. 2000; 8(6):344–353
[52] Devas MB. Stress fractures of the femoral neck. J Bone Joint Surg Br. 1965; 47 (4):728–738
[53] Egol KA, Koval KJ, Kummer F, Frankel VH. Stress fractures of the femoral neck. Clin Orthop Relat Res. 1998(348):72–78
[54] Fredericson M. Diagnosing tibial stress injuries in athletes. West J Med. 1995; 162(2):150
[55] Blanchard C, Kushare I, Boyles A, Mundy A, Beebe AC, Klingele KE. Traumatic, posterior pediatric hip dislocations with associated posterior labrum osteochondral avulsion: recognizing the acetabular "fleck" sign. J Pediatr Orthop. 2016; 36(6):602–607
[56] Berkes MB, Cross MB, Shindle MK, Bedi A, Kelly BT. Traumatic posterior hip instability and femoroacetabular impingement in athletes. Am J Orthop. 2012; 41(4):166–171
[57] Laorr A, Greenspan A, Anderson MW, Moehring HD, McKinley T. Traumatic hip dislocation: early MRI findings. Skeletal Radiol. 1995; 24(4):239–245
[58] Potter HG, Montgomery KD, Heise CW, Helfet DL. MR imaging of acetabular fractures: value in detecting femoral head injury, intraarticular fragments, and sciatic nerve injury. AJR Am J Roentgenol. 1994; 163(4): 881–886
[59] Moorman CT, III, Warren RF, Hershman EB, et al. Traumatic posterior hip subluxation in American football. J Bone Joint Surg Am. 2003; 85(7):1190–1196
[60] Shindle MK, Ranawat AS, Kelly BT. Diagnosis and management of traumatic and atraumatic hip instability in the athletic patient. Clin Sports Med. 2006; 25(2):309–326, ix–x
[61] Byrd JWT. Lateral impact injury. A source of occult hip pathology. Clin Sports Med. 2001; 20(4):801–815
[62] Palmer WE, Kuong SJ, Elmadbouh HM. MR imaging of myotendinous strain. AJR Am J Roentgenol. 1999; 173(3):703–709
[63] Bencardino JT, Kassarjian A, Palmer WE. Magnetic resonance imaging of the hip: sports-related injuries. Top Magn Reson Imaging. 2003; 14(2): 145–160
[64] Meislin R, Abeles A. Role of hip MR imaging in the management of sports-related injuries. Magn Reson Imaging Clin N Am. 2005; 13(4):635–640
[65] Pavlov H. Roentgen examination of groin and hip pain in the athlete. Clin Sports Med. 1987; 6(4):829–843
[66] Frank JS, Gambacorta PL, Eisner EA. Hip pathology in the adolescent athlete. J Am Acad Orthop Surg. 2013; 21(11):665–674
[67] Zoga AC, Mullens FE, Meyers WC. The spectrum of MR imaging in athletic pubalgia. Radiol Clin North Am. 2010; 48(6):1179–1197
[68] Kunduracioglu B, Yilmaz C, Yorubulut M, Kudas S. Magnetic resonance findings of osteitis pubis. J Magn Reson Imaging. 2007; 25(3):535–539
[69] Khan W, Zoga AC, Meyers WC. Magnetic resonance imaging of athletic pubalgia and the sports hernia: current understanding and practice. Magn Reson Imaging Clin N Am. 2013; 21(1):97–110
[70] Litwin DE, Sneider EB, McEnaney PM, Busconi BD. Athletic pubalgia (sports hernia). Clin Sports Med. 2011; 30(2):417–434
[71] Martin RL, Kivlan BR, Clemente FR. A cadaveric model for ligamentum teres function: a pilot study. Knee Surg Sports Traumatol Arthrosc. 2013; 21(7): 1689–1693
[72] Botser IB, Martin DE, Stout CE, Domb BG. Tears of the ligamentum teres: prevalence in hip arthroscopy using 2 classification systems. Am J Sports Med. 2011; 39 Suppl:117S–125S
[73] Chahla J, Soares EA, Devitt BM, et al. Ligamentum teres tears and femoroacetabular impingement: prevalence and preoperative findings. Arthroscopy. 2016; 32(7):1293–1297
[74] Mayes S, Ferris AR, Smith P, Garnham A, Cook J. Atraumatic tears of the ligamentum teres are more frequent in professional ballet dancers than a sporting population. Skeletal Radiol. 2016; 45(7):959–967
[75] Papavasiliou A, Siatras T, Bintoudi A, et al. The gymnasts' hip and groin: a magnetic resonance imaging study in asymptomatic elite athletes. Skeletal Radiol. 2014; 43(8):1071–1077
[76] Dwek J, Pfirrmann C, Stanley A, Pathria M, Chung CB. MR imaging of the hip abductors: normal anatomy and commonly encountered pathology at the greater trochanter. Magn Reson Imaging Clin N Am. 2005; 13(4):691–704, vii

[77] Chung CB, Robertson JE, Cho GJ, Vaughan LM, Copp SN, Resnick D. Gluteus medius tendon tears and avulsive injuries in elderly women: imaging findings in six patients. AJR Am J Roentgenol. 1999; 173(2):351–353

[78] Kingzett-Taylor A, Tirman PF, Feller J, et al. Tendinosis and tears of gluteus medius and minimus muscles as a cause of hip pain: MR imaging findings. AJR Am J Roentgenol. 1999; 173(4):1123–1126

[79] Bunker TD, Esler CNA, Leach WJ. Rotator-cuff tear of the hip. J Bone Joint Surg Br. 1997; 79(4):618–620

[80] Howell GED, Biggs RE, Bourne RB. Prevalence of abductor mechanism tears of the hips in patients with osteoarthritis. J Arthroplasty. 2001; 16(1):121–123

[81] LaBan MM, Weir SK, Taylor RS. "Bald trochanter" spontaneous rupture of the conjoined tendons of the gluteus medius and minimus presenting as a trochanteric bursitis. Am J Phys Med Rehabil. 2004; 83(10):806–809

[82] Jacobson T, Allen WC. Surgical correction of the snapping iliopsoas tendon. Am J Sports Med. 1990; 18(5):470–474

[83] Hernando MF, Cerezal L, Pérez-Carro L, Abascal F, Canga A. Deep gluteal syndrome: anatomy, imaging, and management of sciatic nerve entrapments in the subgluteal space. Skeletal Radiol. 2015; 44(7):919–934

[84] Papadopoulos EC, Korres DS, Papachristou G, Efstathopoulos N. Piriformis syndrome. Orthopedics. 2004; 27(8):797–799, 799, author reply 799

[85] O'Sullivan E, Antolak S, Martin HD. Nerve compression injuries about the hip and deep gluteal syndrome. In: Kelly BT, Bedi A, Larson CM, O'Sullivan E, eds. Sports hip injuries: diagnosis and management. Thorofare, NJ: SLACK Incorporated; 2015:153–170

[86] Felson DT. An update on the pathogenesis and epidemiology of osteoarthritis. Radiol Clin North Am. 2004; 42(1):1–9, v

[87] Sadro C. Current concepts in magnetic resonance imaging of the adult hip and pelvis. Semin Roentgenol. 2000; 35(3):231–248

[88] Blankenbaker DG, Tuite MJ. MR imaging of early hip joint degeneration. Magn Reson Imaging Clin N Am. 2011; 19(2):365–378

[89] Gold SL, Burge AJ, Potter HG. MRI of hip cartilage: joint morphology, structure, and composition. Clin Orthop Relat Res. 2012; 470(12):3321–3331

[90] Cooperman D. What is the evidence to support acetabular dysplasia as a cause of osteoarthritis? J Pediatr Orthop. 2013; 33 Suppl 1:S2–S7

[91] Klaue K, Durnin CW, Ganz R. The acetabular rim syndrome. A clinical presentation of dysplasia of the hip. J Bone Joint Surg Br. 1991; 73(3): 423–429

[92] Murphy SB, Ganz R, Müller ME. The prognosis in untreated dysplasia of the hip. A study of radiographic factors that predict the outcome. J Bone Joint Surg Am. 1995; 77(7):985–989

[93] Reijman M, Hazes JM, Pols HA, Koes BW, Bierma-Zeinstra SM. Acetabular dysplasia predicts incident osteoarthritis of the hip: the Rotterdam study. Arthritis Rheum. 2005; 52(3):787–793

[94] Fujii M, Nakashima Y, Yamamoto T, et al. Acetabular retroversion in developmental dysplasia of the hip. J Bone Joint Surg Am. 2010; 92(4): 895–903

[95] Kim WY, Hutchinson CE, Andrew JG, Allen PD. The relationship between acetabular retroversion and osteoarthritis of the hip. J Bone Joint Surg Br. 2006; 88(6):727–729

[96] Tönnis D, Heinecke A. Acetabular and femoral anteversion: relationship with osteoarthritis of the hip. J Bone Joint Surg Am. 1999; 81(12):1747–1770

[97] Atweh LA, Kan JH. Multimodality imaging of developmental dysplasia of the hip. Pediatr Radiol. 2013; 43 Suppl 1:S166–S171

[98] Assouline-Dayan Y, Chang C, Greenspan A, Shoenfeld Y, Gershwin ME. Pathogenesis and natural history of osteonecrosis. Semin Arthritis Rheum. 2002; 32(2):94–124

[99] Coleman BG, Kressel HY, Dalinka MK, Scheibler ML, Burk DL, Cohen EK. Radiographically negative avascular necrosis: detection with MR imaging. Radiology. 1988; 168(2):525–528

[100] Hauzeur JP, Pasteels JL, Schoutens A, et al. The diagnostic value of magnetic resonance imaging in non-traumatic osteonecrosis of the femoral head. J Bone Joint Surg Am. 1989; 71(5):641–649

[101] Mitchell DG, Steinberg ME, Dalinka MK, Rao VM, Fallon M, Kressel HY. Magnetic resonance imaging of the ischemic hip. Alterations within the osteonecrotic, viable, and reactive zones. Clin Orthop Relat Res. 1989 (244):60–77

[102] Totty WG, Murphy WA, Ganz WI, Kumar B, Daum WJ, Siegel BA. Magnetic resonance imaging of the normal and ischemic femoral head. AJR Am J Roentgenol. 1984; 143(6):1273–1280

[103] Hayes CW, Balkissoon AA. Magnetic resonance imaging of the musculoskeletal system. II. The hip. Clin Orthop Relat Res. 1996(322):297–309

[104] Shimizu K, Moriya H, Akita T, Sakamoto M, Suguro T. Prediction of collapse with magnetic resonance imaging of avascular necrosis of the femoral head. J Bone Joint Surg Am. 1994; 76(2):215–223

[105] Takatori Y, Kamogawa M, Kokubo T, et al. Magnetic resonance imaging and histopathology in femoral head necrosis. Acta Orthop Scand. 1987; 58(5): 499–503

[106] Khanna AJ, Yoon TR, Mont MA, Hungerford DS, Bluemke DA. Femoral head osteonecrosis: detection and grading by using a rapid MR imaging protocol. Radiology. 2000; 217(1):188–192

[107] Lafforgue P, Dahan E, Chagnaud C, Schiano A, Kasbarian M, Acquaviva PC. Early-stage avascular necrosis of the femoral head: MR imaging for prognosis in 31 cases with at least 2 years of follow-up. Radiology. 1993; 187(1):199–204

[108] Koo KH, Kim R. Quantifying the extent of osteonecrosis of the femoral head. A new method using MRI. J Bone Joint Surg Br. 1995; 77(6):875–880

[109] Cherian SF, Laorr A, Saleh KJ, Kuskowski MA, Bailey RF, Cheng EY. Quantifying the extent of femoral head involvement in osteonecrosis. J Bone Joint Surg Am. 2003; 85(2):309–315

[110] Beltran J, Herman LJ, Burk JM, et al. Femoral head avascular necrosis: MR imaging with clinical-pathologic and radionuclide correlation. Radiology. 1988; 166(1 Pt 1):215–220

[111] Beltran J, Opsha O. MR imaging of the hip: osseous lesions. Magn Reson Imaging Clin N Am. 2005; 13(4):665–676, vi

[112] Kalliakmanis AG, Pneumaticos S, Plessas S, Papachristou G. Transient hip osteoporosis. Orthopedics. 2006; 29(3):263–264

[113] Klontzas ME, Vassalou EE, Zibis AH, Bintoudi AS, Karantanas AH. MR imaging of transient osteoporosis of the hip: an update on 155 hip joints. Eur J Radiol. 2015; 84(3):431–436

[114] Pedersen AB, Mor A, Mehnert F, Thomsen RW, Johnsen SP, Nørgaard M. Rheumatoid arthritis: trends in antirheumatic drug use, C-reactive protein levels, and surgical burden. J Rheumatol. 2015; 42(12):2247–2254

[115] Koulouris G, Morrison WB. MR imaging of hip infection and inflammation. Magn Reson Imaging Clin N Am. 2005; 13(4):743–755

[116] Burki V, Gossec L, Payet J, et al. Prevalence and characteristics of hip involvement in spondyloarthritis: a single-centre observational study of 275 patients. Clin Exp Rheumatol. 2012; 30(4):481–486

[117] Chen HA, Chen CH, Liao HT, et al. Factors associated with radiographic spinal involvement and hip involvement in ankylosing spondylitis. Semin Arthritis Rheum. 2011; 40(6):552–558

[118] Vander Cruyssen B, Muñoz-Gomariz E, Font P, et al. ASPECT-REGISPONSER-RESPONDIA working group. Hip involvement in ankylosing spondylitis: epidemiology and risk factors associated with hip replacement surgery. Rheumatology (Oxford). 2010; 49(1):73–81

[119] Lee S, Lee JY, Hwang JH, Shin JH, Kim TH, Kim SK. Clinical importance of inflammatory facet joints of the spine in ankylosing spondylitis: a magnetic resonance imaging study. Scand J Rheumatol. 2016; 45(6):491–498

[120] Szypryt P, Twining P, Preston BJ, Howell CJ. Synovial chondromatosis of the hip joint presenting as a pathological fracture. Br J Radiol. 1986; 59(700): 399–401

[121] Ferro FP, Philippon MJ. Arthroscopy provides symptom relief and good functional outcomes in patients with hip synovial chondromatosis. J Hip Preserv Surg. 2015; 2(3):265–271

[122] Tyler WK, Vidal AF, Williams RJ, Healey JH. Pigmented villonodular synovitis. J Am Acad Orthop Surg. 2006; 14(6):376–385

[123] Dietrich TJ, Dora C, Pfirrmann CW. Postoperative imaging in femoroacetabular impingement. Semin Musculoskelet Radiol. 2013; 17(3):272–278

[124] Clohisy JC, Nepple JJ, Larson CM, Zaltz I, Millis M, Academic Network of Conservation Hip Outcome Research (ANCHOR) Members. Persistent structural disease is the most common cause of repeat hip preservation surgery. Clin Orthop Relat Res. 2013; 471(12):3788–3794

[125] Zingg PO, Buehler TC, Poutawera VR, Alireza A, Dora C. Femoral neck fractures after arthroscopic femoral neck osteochondroplasty for femoroacetabular impingement. Knee Surg Sports Traumatol Arthrosc. 2014; 22(4):926–931

[126] Beck M. Groin pain after open FAI surgery: the role of intraarticular adhesions. Clin Orthop Relat Res. 2009; 467(3):769–774

[127] Blankenbaker DG, De Smet AA, Keene JS. MR arthrographic appearance of the postoperative acetabular labrum in patients with suspected recurrent labral tears. AJR Am J Roentgenol. 2011; 197(6):W1118–22

[128] Bedi A, Zbeda RM, Bueno VF, Downie B, Dolan M, Kelly BT. The incidence of heterotopic ossification after hip arthroscopy. Am J Sports Med. 2012; 40(4): 854–863

Answers to Common Clinical Questions

1. Answer: b. Coronal imaging provides visualization of the superior labrum, but sagittal cuts best show the superior/anterior labrum, where most labral tears occur. Although MR arthrography is still used, we prefer T1 noncontrast imaging for the best visualization of labral pathology.
2. Answer: b: The prevalence of asymptomatic CAM lesions is 37%, asymptomatic pincer lesions is 67%, and asymptomatic labral tears in young adults is 33%–69%.
3. Answer: c. Initial MRI may not show evidence of subluxation, and the process may continue to evolve. Although there may be alternative approaches to treatment of hip subluxation, it is the authors' preference to repeat the MRI to monitor for femoral head edema resolution while keeping the patient non-weight-bearing and allowing return to sports when MRI shows resolution of edema.
4. Answer: e. Athletic pubalgia can manifest on MRI as involvement of the insertion of the rectus abdominis, the origin of the adductor longus, or the periosteum of the pubic tubercle.
5. Answer: a and b. These are clinical and MRI findings associated with idiopathic transient osteoporosis. c and d are associated with osteonecrosis of the femoral head.

11 The Knee

Miho J. Tanaka, Bashir Zikria, A. Jay Khanna, Andrew J. Cosgarea, and John D. Reeder

Abstract
The aim of this chapter is to provide an overview of the MRI techniques to evaluate knee pathology. MRI is a useful tool to assess acute knee trauma, characterize and grade meniscal and ligamentous tears. MR angiography can be used to detect vascular injuries after a knee dislocation, and patellar tendon ruptures. MRI may also detect degenerative (non-acute) and infectious pathology in the knee. In this chapter, we have provided a broad overview of various MRI findings in the knee.

Keywords: meniscal tear, MRI sequences, trauma, ligament tear, tendon rupture, degenerative knee disease, infection, postoperative findings

11.1 Specialized Pulse Sequences and Protocols

For magnetic resonance imaging (MRI) of the knee, the patient is positioned with the leg in comfortable external rotation. Sagittal, coronal, and axial imaging are obtained with fat-suppressed acquisition in at least one plane. To optimize spatial resolution, thinner segments are preferred, but the choice of segment thickness must be balanced with signal-to-noise and scan time constraints. In general, MRI systems with higher field strengths can achieve thinner segments with a better signal-to-noise ratio in less time than can units with lower field strength. For most spin-echo (SE) protocols designed for knee imaging, the effective segment thickness is 3 to 4 mm; that for gradient-echo imaging is 1 to 3 mm.

A typical low magnetic field strength protocol for knee imaging may include T1-weighted and T2-weighted sagittal acquisitions, a coronal short tau inversion recovery (STIR) sequence, and an axial fast spin-echo (FSE) T2-weighted sequence. A sagittal 3D gradient-echo sequence represents an additional option, particularly with low field strength systems; this high-resolution technique offers a relatively thin segment with a superior signal-to-noise ratio, useful for meniscal assessment. A high field strength approach to knee imaging may include the following sequences:

- Sagittal FSE proton-density fat-suppressed sequence to evaluate the following:
  - Menisci.
  - Articular cartilage.
  - Cruciate ligaments.
  - Extensor mechanism.
  - Articular fluid.
- Coronal FSE fat-suppressed T2-weighted sequence to assess the following:
  - Osseous injury.
  - Articular and meniscal cartilage.
  - Collateral supporting structures.
  - Fluid distribution.
- Sagittal T1-weighted sequence for the following:
  - Evaluate marrow and subcutaneous fat.
  - Detect heterotopic ossification.
  - Provide further evaluation of meniscal integrity.
- Axial FSE T2-weighted sequence primarily to assess the patellofemoral joint.

11.2 Traumatic Pathology

11.2.1 Acute Hemarthrosis

Acute knee trauma commonly presents with pain and hemarthrosis. Anterior cruciate ligament (ACL) tears are seen in more than 70% of acute hemarthroses.[1] Usually, ACL tears are associated with other injuries such as meniscal tears, osteochondral fractures, patellar dislocations, and ligament and tendon tears. MRI is commonly used to discern the etiology of an acute hemarthrosis, especially when the knee is too tender or the patient is too anxious for a thorough physical examination. MRI is especially helpful when conventional radiographs are negative. Typically, acute hemarthrosis appears as fluid within the joint with high signal intensity on T2-weighted images and intermediate signal intensity on T1-weighted images. Similar findings can be seen with inflammatory processes, resulting in a nontraumatic knee effusion, and the two processes may be differentiated by the clinician, based on the history and physical examination. The presence of blood in joint fluid causes a relatively brighter appearance on T1 imaging than that observed with nonhemorrhagic fluid because of the effect of methemoglobin. Hemosiderin deposition within joint fluid appears dark on all pulse sequences. This can occur with a variety of pathologies including chronic hemorrhage and pigmented villonodular synovitis (PVNS), a benign, progressive tumor that most commonly arises from the synovium of the knee or hip joint.

11.2.2 Meniscal Tears

Meniscal tears are a very common finding on MRI. Clinical suspicion of a meniscal tear is a common reason for ordering an MRI. Tears can be a source of pain and disability, or they can be incidental findings. The tears can range from intrasubstance degeneration that can be seen only on MRI to complete tears that allow fragments of the meniscus to flip or displace.

Meniscal tears are graded according to how they appear on MRI (▶ Table 11.1[2]; ▶ Fig. 11.1), and are best seen on T1-weighted, gradient-echo, and proton-density images. The

Table 11.1 Grading of meniscal tears

Grade	Grading of meniscal tears
1	Degenerative process; focal, globular intrasubstance increased signal; no extension to articular surface
2	Degenerative process; horizontal, linear intrasubstance increased signal; no extension to articular surface
3	Meniscal tear; increased signal extends to or communicates with at least one articular surface
4	Complex tear/macerated meniscus

Source: (Reproduced with permission from Khanna AJ, Cosgarea AJ, Mont MA, et al. Magnetic resonance imaging of the knee. Current techniques and spectrum of disease. J Bone Joint Surg Am. 2001; 83-A Suppl 2 Pt 2:128–141).[2] Reproduced by permission.

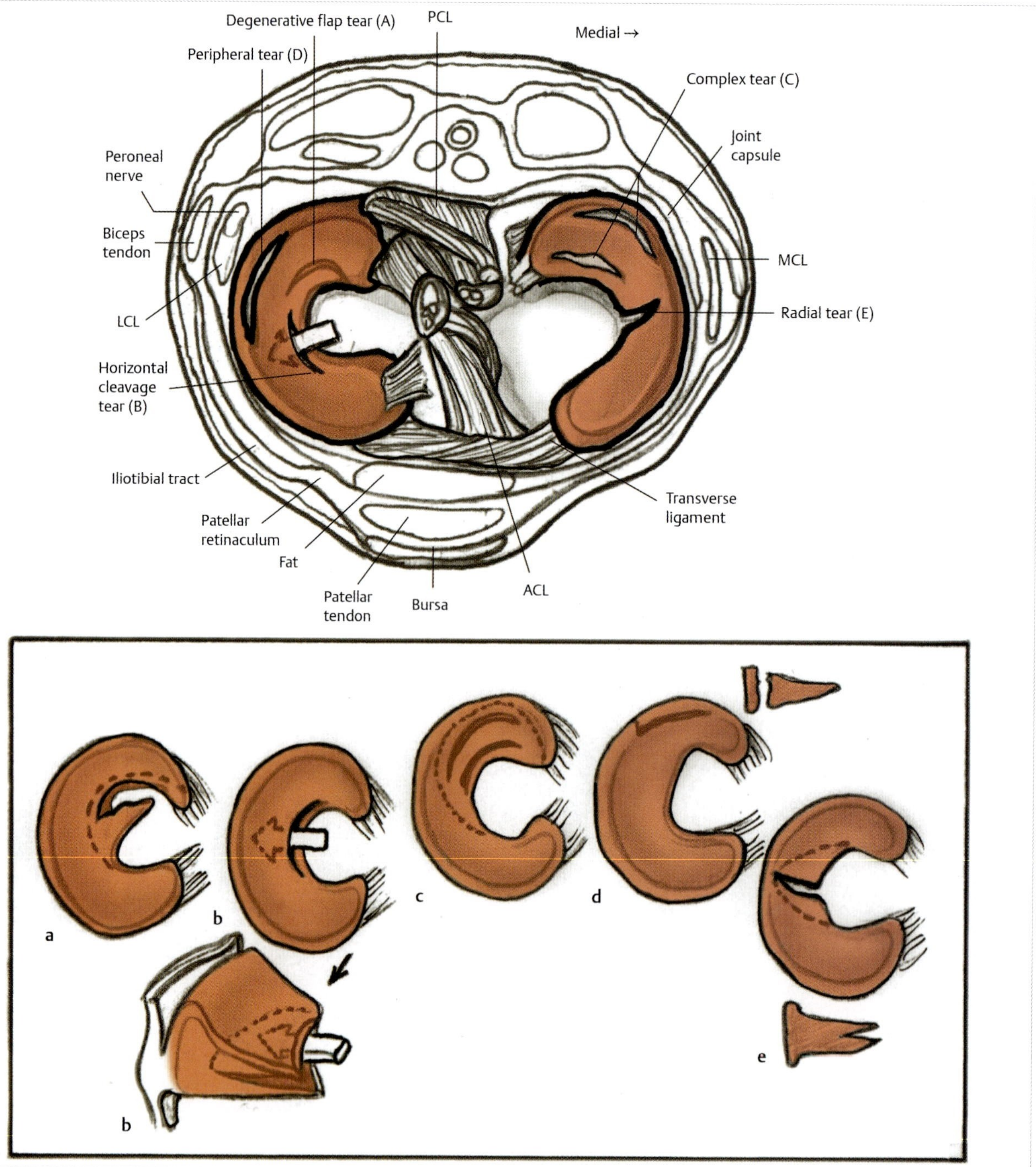

Fig. 11.1 Artist's sketch illustrating the morphology of meniscal tear patterns and relevant anatomy of the knee: **(a)** degenerative flap tear, **(b)** horizontal cleavage tear, **(c)** complex tear, **(d)** peripheral vertical longitudinal tear, and **(e)** vertical radial tear. Abbreviations: PCL, posterior cruciate ligament; LCL, lateral collateral ligament; MCL, medial collateral ligament; ACL, anterior cruciate ligament. (Reproduced with permission from Cascio BM, Khanna AJ, Glait SA, Cosgarea AJ, Johnson TS, Reeder JD. The Knee. In: Khanna AJ, ed. MRI for orthopaedic surgeons. New York: Thieme; 2010:164–201.)

menisci are low intensity on all sequences.[3,4,5,6,7,8,9,10] Most tears involve the medial meniscus, but most acute tears involve the lateral meniscus (► Table 11.2[2,11]). Special attention should be given to the menisci in the presence of a chronic ACL tear because associated meniscus tears are common. The medial meniscus is commonly torn in the chronically ACL-deficient knee because the meniscus plays a secondary stabilizing role to anterior tibial translation.

The types of meniscal tear morphologies have been well described (► Table 11.2[2,11]). In early publications on MRI

Table 11.2 Characteristics of meniscal tears on MRI

Meniscal tear morphology	Description	Appearance on MRI
Horizontal	Separates meniscus into superior (femoral) and inferior (tibial) fragments	Primarily horizontal signal on sagittal images
Vertical radial	Splits central margin of meniscus	Vertical signal oriented perpendicular to the curvature of the meniscus
Vertical longitudinal	Extends along length of meniscus; separates meniscus into inner and outer fragments	Vertical signal oriented parallel to the curvature of the meniscus
Bucket handle	Subtype of the longitudinal tear in which the displaced central fragment resembles a bucket handle	"Double-PCL" sign; displaced fragment often seen parallel to the PCL in the intercondylar notch on sagittal images
Complex	Combination of multiple planes; commonly horizontal and radial	Characteristics of each tear type or fragmented/ macerated
Meniscocapsular separation	Rupture of meniscus-capsule junction	Increased signal between the edge of the meniscus and the capsule

Abbreviations: MRI, magnetic resonance imaging; PCL, posterior cruciate ligament.
Source: Adapted from Khanna et al 2001,[2] combined with information from Kelley and Berquist 2006.[11]

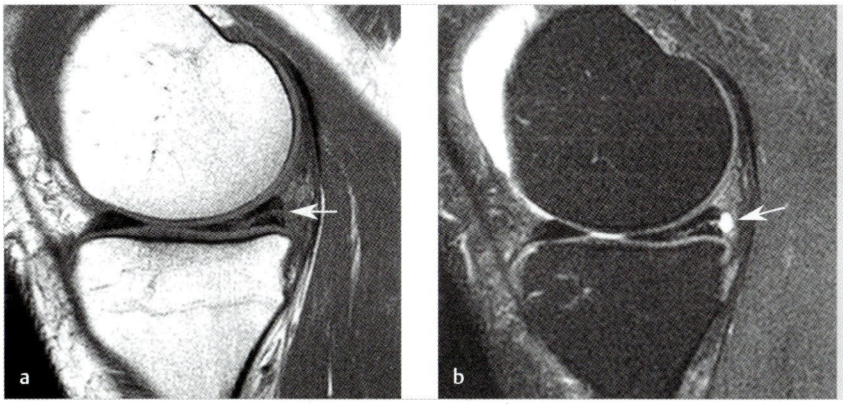

Fig. 11.2 Horizontal tear in the posterior horn of the medial meniscus. Sagittal T1-weighted **(a)** and fat-suppressed proton-density **(b)** images showing a horizontal tear (*arrow on each*) communicating with the undersurface of the meniscus. Note the small meniscal cyst posterior to the meniscus on the fat-suppressed proton-density image. (Reproduced with permission from Cascio BM, Khanna AJ, Glait SA, Cosgarea AJ, Johnson TS, Reeder JD. The Knee. In: Khanna AJ, ed. MRI for orthopaedic surgeons. New York: Thieme; 2010:164–201.)

evaluation of meniscal pathology, detection focused primarily on meniscal signal intensity patterns and their relationship to the meniscal surface.[12,13] Grade I and grade II[9] meniscal tears referred to increased intrameniscal signal that appeared punctate or linear, respectively, and were particularly evident on T1-weighted images. The grade III designation indicated that the signal intensity pattern communicated with the superior or inferior meniscal surface, and therefore most likely corresponded to an arthroscopically identifiable meniscal tear.[9] If grade II meniscal pathology was reported in an MRI interpretation as a grade II tear, it could create the erroneous impression that meniscal surface pathology existed. Although grade II intrameniscal signal can reflect the presence of a meniscal contusion or an intrameniscal tear, it may also denote myxoid internal meniscal degeneration, artifact (*magic angle effect* or truncation), or normal meniscal vascularity in a child or young adult.[14,15] This grading system also does not consider morphologic alterations in characterizing meniscal pathology. Because the morphology of a meniscal tear impacts its relative clinical significance and influences surgical planning, a more specific classification system, currently afforded wide acceptance, uses MRI findings to categorize tears as follows[13]:

- Horizontal.
- Vertical radial.
- Vertical longitudinal with/without flap displacement.
- Complex.

Horizontal tears divide the meniscus into superior and inferior components, identified on sagittal and coronal imaging series (▶ Fig. 11.2). The tear often communicates with the inferior meniscal surface; sometimes a concomitant meniscal cyst is identified, involving the perimeniscal soft tissue (▶ Fig. 11.3).

Vertical radial tears exhibit a linear signal pattern. They violate the superior and inferior meniscal surfaces and are oriented perpendicular to the meniscal axis of curvature.[16] As such, if a vertical radial tear involves the anterior or posterior portion of the meniscus, the tear will show a linear vertical configuration on coronal images (▶ Fig. 11.4a) and an abrupt truncation of the central meniscal contour on sagittal images (▶ Fig. 11.4b). With this type of tear, the change in meniscal morphology, appreciated in the imaging plane oriented parallel to the tear, is equally as important as the surface communication of linear abnormal meniscal signal intensity, noted in the imaging plane perpendicular to the axis of the tear. If the vertical radial tear involves the mid-body of the meniscus, a linear meniscal defect is noted on sagittal images (▶ Fig. 11.5a), and blunting or truncation of the central meniscal contour is observed on coronal images (▶ Fig. 11.5b). A commonly overlooked vertical radial tear occurs at the root of the posterior horn of the medial meniscus (▶ Fig. 11.6). This tear, particularly common in obese patients, destabilizes the meniscus, and medial extrusion of the meniscus is often identified on MRI.

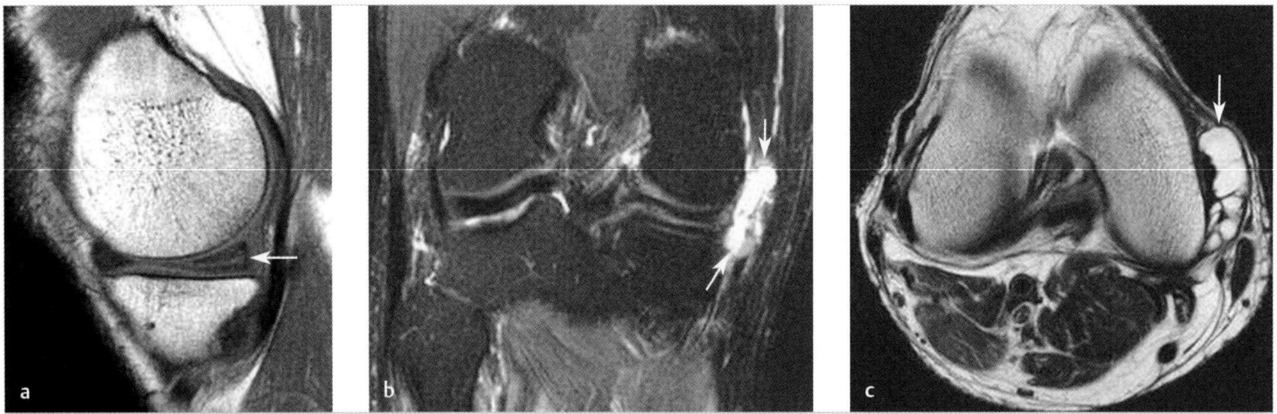

Fig. 11.3 Horizontal medial meniscal tear with large meniscal cyst in the right knee. **(a)** A sagittal T1-weighted image shows a horizontal tear (*arrow*) of the posterior horn of the medial meniscus. **(b)** A coronal fat-suppressed T2-weighted image shows a large meniscal cyst (*arrows*) extending medial to the medial compartment. **(c)** An axial T2-weighted image shows a multiloculated meniscal cyst (*arrow*). (Reproduced with permission from Cascio BM, Khanna AJ, Glait SA, Cosgarea AJ, Johnson TS, Reeder JD. The Knee. In: Khanna AJ, ed. MRI for orthopaedic surgeons. New York: Thieme; 2010:164–201.)

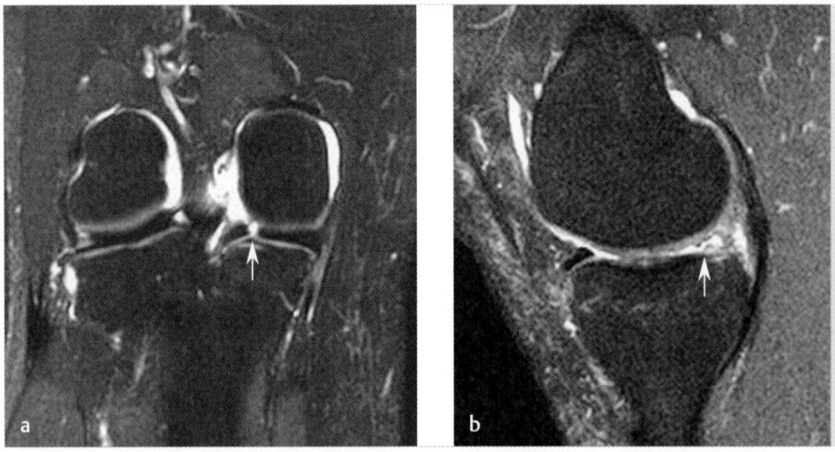

Fig. 11.4 Vertical radial meniscal tear in the posterior horn of the medial meniscus in the right knee. **(a)** A coronal fat-suppressed T2-weighted image shows a vertical defect (*arrow*) involving the posterior horn of the medial meniscus. **(b)** A sagittal fat-suppressed proton-density image, obtained in the plane of the tear, shows truncation (*arrow*) and abnormal signal intensity involving the posterior horn. Note the normal anterior horn. (Reproduced with permission from Cascio BM, Khanna AJ, Glait SA, Cosgarea AJ, Johnson TS, Reeder JD. The Knee. In: Khanna AJ, ed. MRI for orthopaedic surgeons. New York: Thieme; 2010:164–201.)

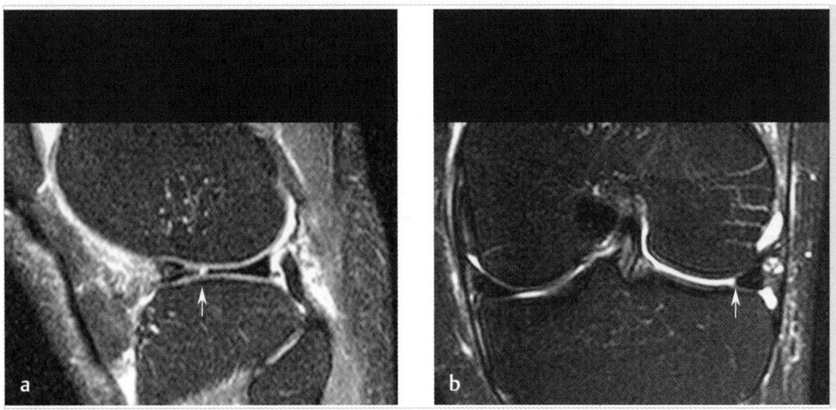

Fig. 11.5 Vertical radial meniscal tear in the mid-body lateral meniscus in the left knee. **(a)** A sagittal fat-suppressed proton-density image shows a vertical tear (*arrow*) of the central edge of the lateral meniscus, oriented perpendicular to the curvature of the meniscus. Note the superimposed horizontal tear of the anterior horn. **(b)** A coronal fat-suppressed T2-weighted image shows the same tear with truncation of the central meniscal margin (*arrow*). (Reproduced with permission from Cascio BM, Khanna AJ, Glait SA, Cosgarea AJ, Johnson TS, Reeder JD. The Knee. In: Khanna AJ, ed. MRI for orthopaedic surgeons. New York: Thieme; 2010:164–201.)

Chondromalacia and osseous stress injury are also frequently observed in association with these radial tears of the root of the posterior horn of the medial meniscus.[17]

Vertical longitudinal tears also exhibit a vertical signal orientation on MRI, but because the tear is oriented parallel to the axis of meniscal curvature, it is identified as a vertical linear signal intensity interfacing with the superior and inferior meniscal articular surfaces on sagittal and coronal imaging planes. Peripheral vertical longitudinal tears of the posterior horn of the medial meniscus and vertical longitudinal tears of the posterior horn of the lateral meniscus at the attachment of the meniscofemoral ligament are commonly associated with ACL tears (▶ Fig. 11.7). Displacement of a meniscal flap associated with a vertical longitudinal tear may occur, and unstable meniscal tears are more likely to be symptomatic and impair biomechanics; in such circumstances, surgical intervention usually is necessary to restore function.[18] Failure to address surgically the presence of a displaced meniscal flap or fragment represents a cause of persistent joint pain and

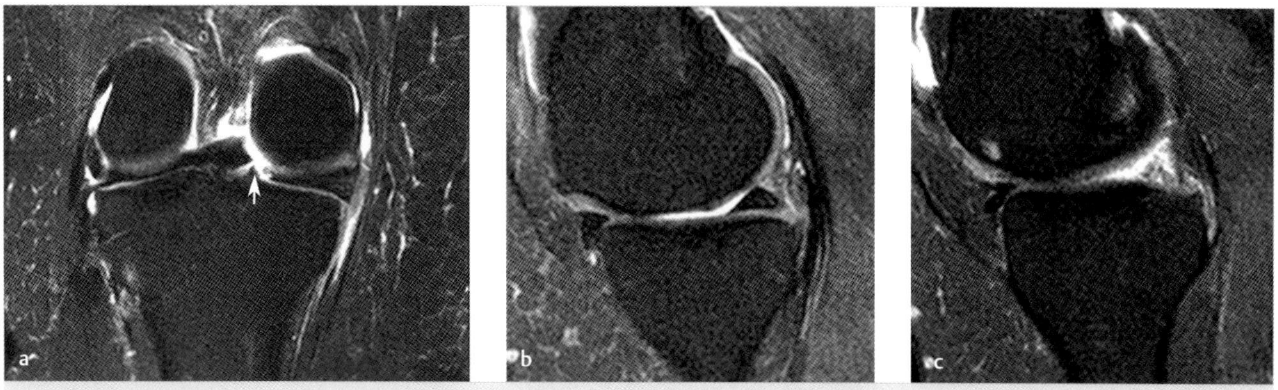

Fig. 11.6 Vertical radial tear of the meniscal root in the right knee. **(a)** A coronal fat-suppressed T2-weighted image shows a vertical radial defect (*arrow*) at the meniscal root. **(b)** A sagittal fat-suppressed proton-density image, obtained just medial to the tear, shows normal posterior horn morphology. **(c)** A sagittal fat-suppressed proton-density image, obtained in the plane of the tear, shows abrupt transition to markedly abnormal posterior meniscal morphology, corresponding to the meniscal root tear. (Reproduced with permission from Cascio BM, Khanna AJ, Glait SA, Cosgarea AJ, Johnson TS, Reeder JD. The Knee. In: Khanna AJ, ed. MRI for orthopaedic surgeons. New York: Thieme; 2010:164–201.)

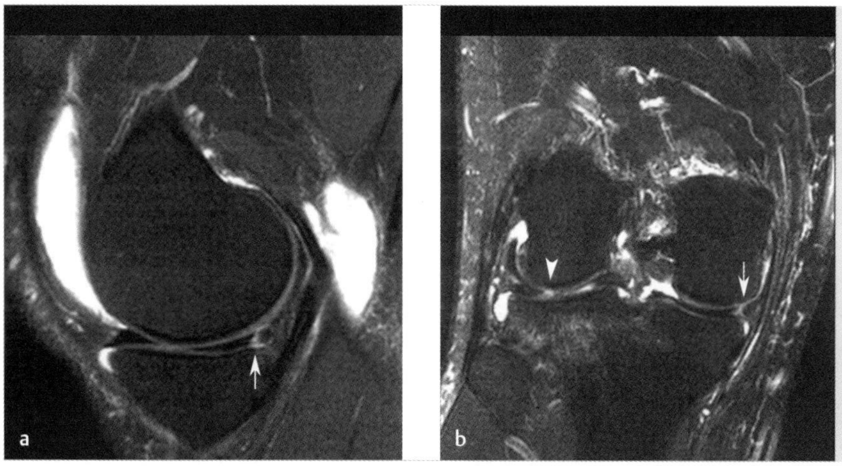

Fig. 11.7 Vertical longitudinal tear in the right knee. **(a)** A sagittal fat-suppressed proton-density image shows a peripheral vertical longitudinal tear (*arrow*) of the posterior horn of the medial meniscus. Note the effusion and Baker cyst. **(b)** A coronal fat-suppressed T2-weighted image shows the vertical longitudinal tear (*arrow*), propagating parallel to the meniscal curvature. Note the tear of the posterior horn of the lateral meniscus (*arrowhead*) with an adjacent lateral tibial plateau bone bruise in this patient with an acute anterior cruciate ligament (ACL) tear. (Reproduced with permission from Cascio BM, Khanna AJ, Glait SA, Cosgarea AJ, Johnson TS, Reeder JD. The Knee. In: Khanna AJ, ed. MRI for orthopaedic surgeons. New York: Thieme; 2010:164–201.)

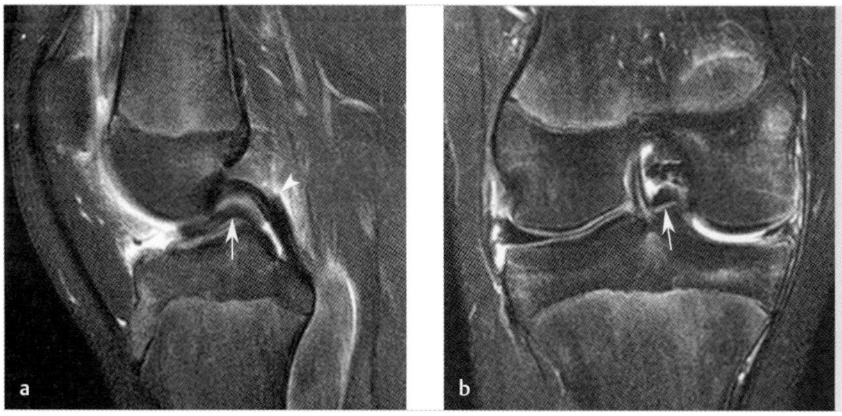

Fig. 11.8 Bucket-handle tear in the right knee. **(a)** A sagittal fat-suppressed proton-density image shows a meniscal flap (*arrow*), arising from the medial meniscus and displaced inferior to the posterior cruciate ligament (PCL) (*arrowhead*), exhibiting the double-PCL sign. **(b)** A coronal fat-suppressed T2-weighted image shows a centrally displaced meniscal flap (*arrow*) inferior to the PCL. Note the abnormal morphology of the nondisplaced medial meniscal remnant. (Reproduced with permission from Cascio BM, Khanna AJ, Glait SA, Cosgarea AJ, Johnson TS, Reeder JD. The Knee. In: Khanna AJ, ed. MRI for orthopaedic surgeons. New York: Thieme; 2010:164–201.)

dysfunction after arthroscopy.[19] Unstable meniscal tears may exhibit central or peripheral flap displacement. A typical bucket-handle tear represents a vertical longitudinal tear with central displacement of meniscal tissue. If the medial meniscus is involved, the flap is displaced inferior to the posterior cruciate ligament (PCL), creating the double-PCL sign[20] (▶ Fig. 11.8, ▶ Fig. 11.9). Bucket-handle tears of the lateral meniscus often exhibit anterior central displacement of a flap arising from the posterior horn of the meniscus (▶ Fig. 11.10). Displaced bucket-handle tears are a common cause of locked knee in an athlete. Posterior central flap displacement may also occur with a flap arising from the posterior horn of the medial meniscus and the displaced meniscal tissue positioned in the recess between the distal PCL and the medial meniscus (▶ Fig. 11.11). Meniscal tissue may also displace

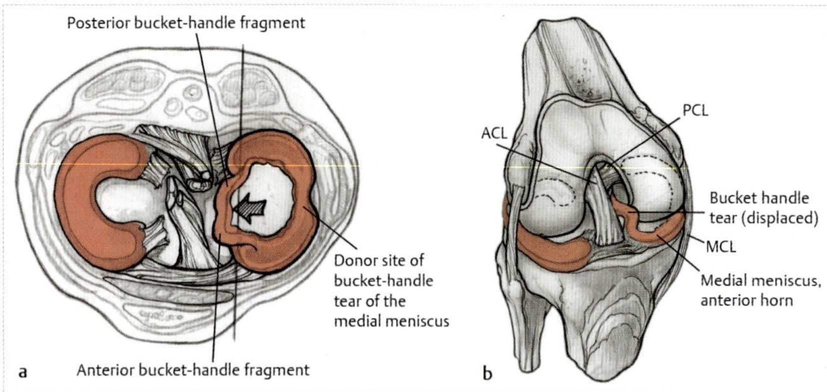

Fig. 11.9 Artist's sketches illustrating a displaced bucket-handle tear of the medial meniscus in the axial plane **(a)** and from an anterior perspective **(b)**. Abbreviations: PCL, posterior cruciate ligament; MCL, medial collateral ligament; ACL, anterior cruciate ligament. (Reproduced with permission from Cascio BM, Khanna AJ, Glait SA, Cosgarea AJ, Johnson TS, Reeder JD. The Knee. In: Khanna AJ, ed. MRI for orthopaedic surgeons. New York: Thieme; 2010:164–201.)

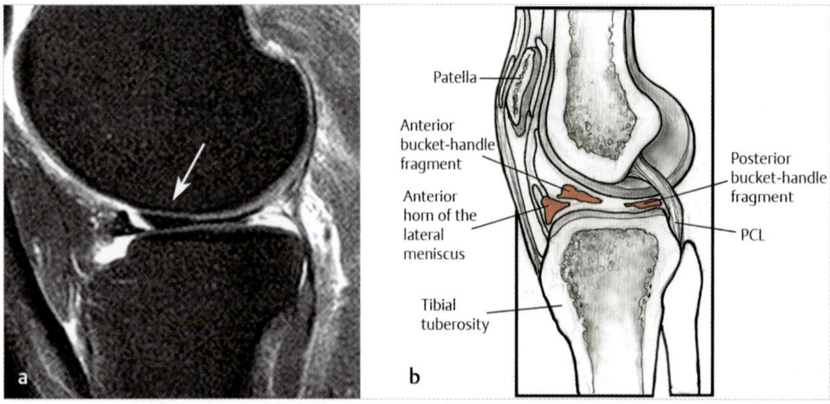

Fig. 11.10 A sagittal fat-saturated proton-density image **(a)** and artist's drawing **(b)** showing anterior displacement of the posterior horn of the lateral meniscus (*arrow*) with the displaced flap positioned just posterior to the anterior horn of the lateral meniscus. Abbreviations: PCL, posterior cruciate ligament. (Reproduced with permission from Cascio BM, Khanna AJ, Glait SA, Cosgarea AJ, Johnson TS, Reeder JD. The Knee. In: Khanna AJ, ed. MRI for orthopaedic surgeons. New York: Thieme; 2010:164–201.)

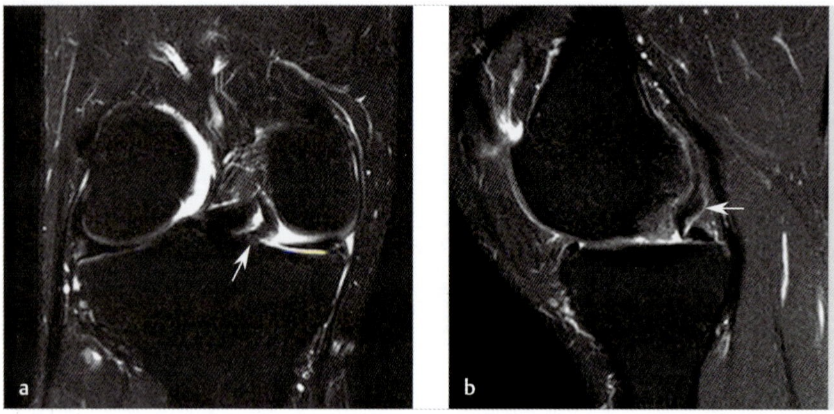

Fig. 11.11 Displaced meniscal tear in the right knee. Coronal fat-suppressed T2-weighted **(a)** and sagittal fat-suppressed proton-density **(b)** images show the posterior central displacement of a medial meniscal flap (*arrow on each*). (Reproduced with permission from Cascio BM, Khanna AJ, Glait SA, Cosgarea AJ, Johnson TS, Reeder JD. The Knee. In: Khanna AJ, ed. MRI for orthopaedic surgeons. New York: Thieme; 2010:164–201.)

peripherally into the recess between the capsule and the femoral condyle (▶ Fig. 11.12) or between the capsule and the tibial plateau (▶ Fig. 11.13). Although peripherally displaced tears are less likely than centrally displaced tears to result in locking, they tend to cause adjacent capsular inflammation and osseous stress reaction, contributing to pain related to the meniscal tear. Preoperative identification and localization of the displaced meniscal flap with MRI contribute to a more expeditious operative procedure.[10]

The designation of a tear as complex, based on MRI findings, implies that the tear exhibits multiple vectors or that the meniscus appears macerated and fragmented. These tears are usually unstable and, if chronic, are associated with chondromalacia and osseous stress reaction, also identified on MRI.

11.2.3 ACL Tears

ACL evaluation is one of the primary indications for MRI of the knee.[21] The patient usually describes a noncontact, twisting, or valgus injury to the knee with a planted foot and often describes sensing a "pop" inside the knee. The patient may experience a subsequent lack of quadriceps function because of the resulting effusion. Physical examination findings include a positive Lachman test and pivot shift. The patient's anxiety may

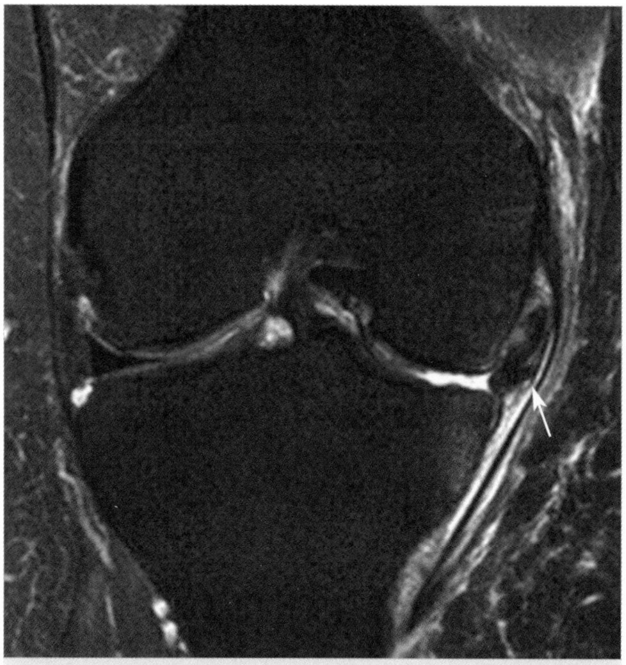

Fig. 11.12 This coronal fat-suppressed T2-weighted image of the right knee shows the peripheral superior displacement of a large meniscal flap (*arrow*), arising from the medial meniscus and extending into the recess medial to the medial femoral condyle. (Reproduced with permission from Cascio BM, Khanna AJ, Glait SA, Cosgarea AJ, Johnson TS, Reeder JD. The Knee. In: Khanna AJ, ed. MRI for orthopaedic surgeons. New York: Thieme; 2010:164–201.)

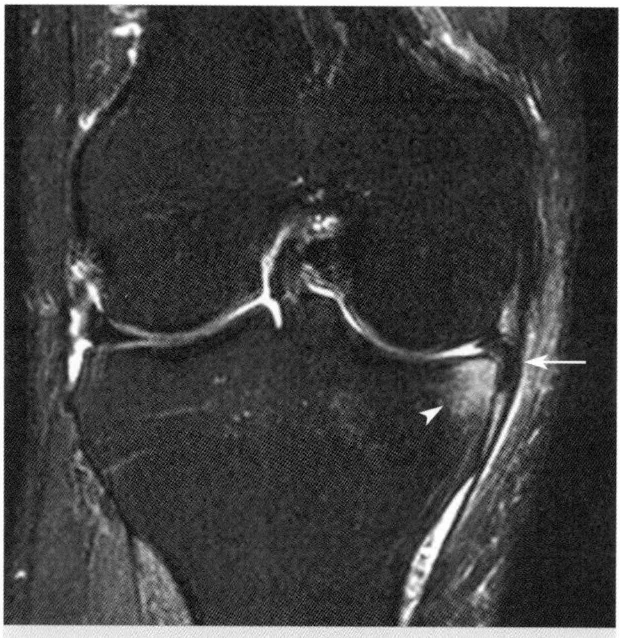

Fig. 11.13 This coronal fat-suppressed T2-weighted image of the right knee shows the peripheral inferior displacement of a meniscal flap (*arrow*), arising from the medial meniscus and extending into the recess medial to the medial tibial plateau. Note the adjacent osseous stress reaction (*arrowhead*) and pericapsular edema. (Reproduced with permission from Cascio BM, Khanna AJ, Glait SA, Cosgarea AJ, Johnson TS, Reeder JD. The Knee. In: Khanna AJ, ed. MRI for orthopaedic surgeons. New York: Thieme; 2010:164–201.)

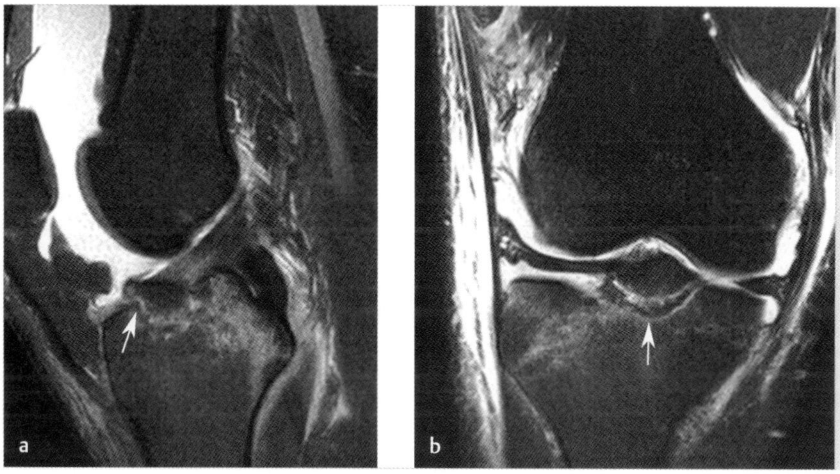

Fig. 11.14 Anterior cruciate ligament (ACL) avulsion. Sagittal fat-suppressed proton-density **(a)** and coronal fat-suppressed T2-weighted **(b)** images of the right knee show an avulsion (*arrow on each*) of the tibial attachment of the ACL. (Reproduced with permission from Cascio BM, Khanna AJ, Glait SA, Cosgarea AJ, Johnson TS, Reeder JD. The Knee. In: Khanna AJ, ed. MRI for orthopaedic surgeons. New York: Thieme; 2010:164–201.)

make the physical examination equivocal, increasing the importance of the MRI.

The adult ACL usually avulses from its femoral attachment or develops an intrasubstance tear. The tendon does not have to dissociate completely to become incompetent.[22] The presence of blood at the femoral avulsion can appear as a "pseudomass" because of volume averaging.[23] With skeletally immature patients, the ACL may remain intact and avulse a fragment of bone off of the tibial attachment (▶ Fig. 11.14). Treatment is determined by the degree of displacement, but it usually requires surgical fixation via arthroscopic or open techniques.

The signs of an ACL injury on MRI include abnormal ligament signal and loss of the normal orientation and continuity of the ligament (▶ Fig. 11.15). There are primary and secondary signs of ACL tears as visualized on MRI (summarized in ▶ Table 11.3[24,25,26]). MRI findings commonly associated with acute ACL injury include loss of ligament continuity and replacement of the ligament by a poorly marginated pseudomass that shows high signal on T2-weighted imaging and low signal on T1-weighted imaging (▶ Fig. 11.16). With both acute and chronic ACL tears, the ligament may appear abnormal in angulation, typically because of inferior displacement of the proximal portion of the ligament. Acute tears of the ACL are often accompanied by bone bruises involving the posterior aspect of the lateral tibial plateau, the anterolateral aspect of the lateral femoral condyle with impaction of the articular surface notch,

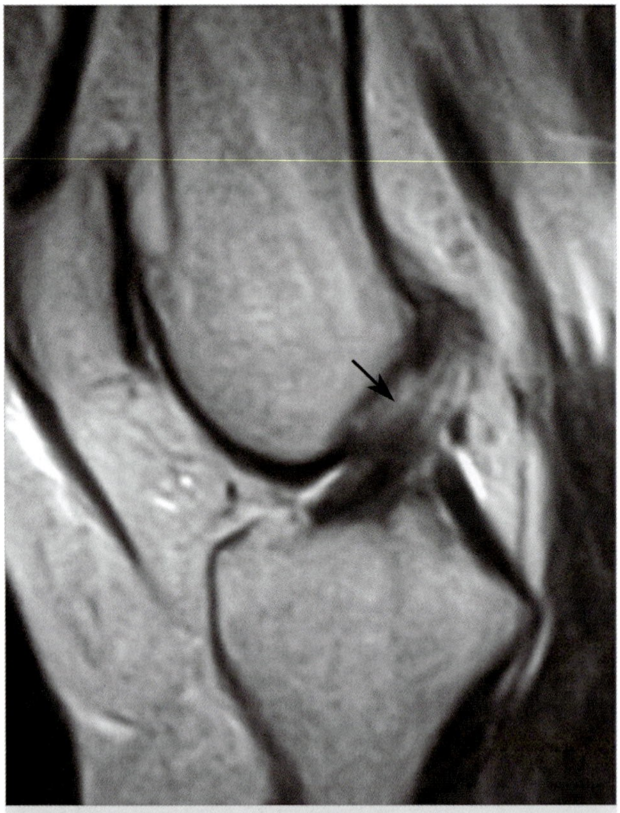

Fig. 11.15 This sagittal T2-weighted image shows a proximal anterior cruciate ligament (ACL) tear (*arrow*). (Reproduced with permission from Cascio BM, Khanna AJ, Glait SA, Cosgarea AJ, Johnson TS, Reeder JD. The Knee. In: Khanna AJ, ed. MRI for orthopaedic surgeons. New York: Thieme; 2010:164–201.)

and the posterior aspect of the medial tibial plateau (▶ Fig. 11.17). The osseous contusions are related to the initial pivot shift rotational stress (lateral injuries) and the subsequent abrupt return to normal alignment (medial plateau injury). Additional findings include anterior translation of the tibia, resulting in increased PCL flexion, popliteus muscle strain, peripheral tears of the posterior horn of the medial meniscus (▶ Fig. 11.18), and tears of the lateral meniscus associated with the attachment of the meniscofemoral ligament (▶ Fig. 11.19).

Other knee structures are also commonly injured at the time of ACL injury, and it is imperative that the MRI be evaluated for these concomitant injuries. These injuries, such as meniscus tears, bone bruises, and cartilage injuries, not only may need to be addressed surgically, but also aid in the diagnosis when the ACL tear is not obvious.[27]

A variety of other radiographic findings seen in association with ACL tears are considered secondary signs (▶ Table 11.3[24,25,26]). A relatively small avulsion fracture seen at the lateral tibial cortex (known as a Segond fracture) is caused by avulsion of the middle third of the lateral capsule[28] (▶ Fig. 11.20).

When the ACL tears, the posterior tibial plateau translates anteriorly, impacting the anterior aspect of the lateral femoral condyle in the region of the terminal sulcus. The resulting contusion leaves a bone bruise pattern in these two locations, best seen on T2-weighted images (▶ Fig. 11.17). This pathologic contact of the tibial and the femoral condyles may leave an

Table 11.3 Signs of an ACL tear on MRI

Primary signs
• Nonvisualization of ligament
• Complete disruption of a ligament segment
• Abnormal signal within ligament on T2-weighted images
• Alteration of normal linear configuration of ligament
• Alteration of normal angulation of ligament
Secondary signs
• Bone contusion (posterolateral and posteromedial tibia, lateral condyle of femur)
• Deepening of lateral femoral condyle notch or sulcus
• Anterior translation of tibia > 5 mm from posterior margin of femoral condyle
• Buckling of the PCL (decreased angle of the PCL)
• Segond fracture
• Meniscal tear
• Posterior horn medial meniscus and tear of the lateral meniscus at the meniscofemoral ligament attachment
• Posterior displacement of posterior horn of lateral meniscus

Abbreviations: ACL, anterior cruciate ligament; MRI, magnetic resonance imaging; PCL, posterior cruciate ligament.

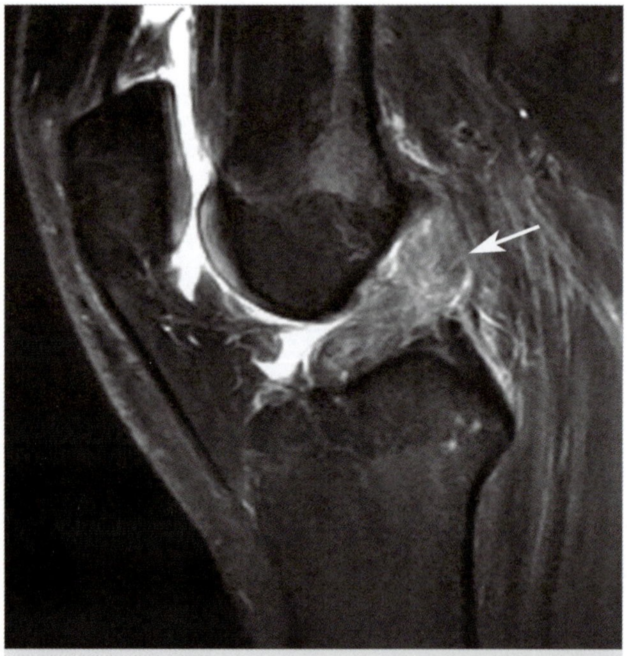

Fig. 11.16 This sagittal fat-suppressed proton-density image shows the pseudomass appearance (*arrow*) of an acute anterior cruciate ligament (ACL) tear. (Reproduced with permission from Cascio BM, Khanna AJ, Glait SA, Cosgarea AJ, Johnson TS, Reeder JD. The Knee. In: Khanna AJ, ed. MRI for orthopaedic surgeons. New York: Thieme; 2010:164–201.)

indentation or notch, also called a “deepened terminal sulcus,” particularly when the patient experiences repeated instability episodes. Another sign of chronic ACL insufficiency is buckling of the PCL, which suggests that the tibia is positioned in an anteriorly displaced position. Patients with chronic ACL insufficiency also frequently develop secondary degenerative changes, including partial- and full-thickness chondral lesions, peripheral osteophytes, and peaking of the tibial spines.

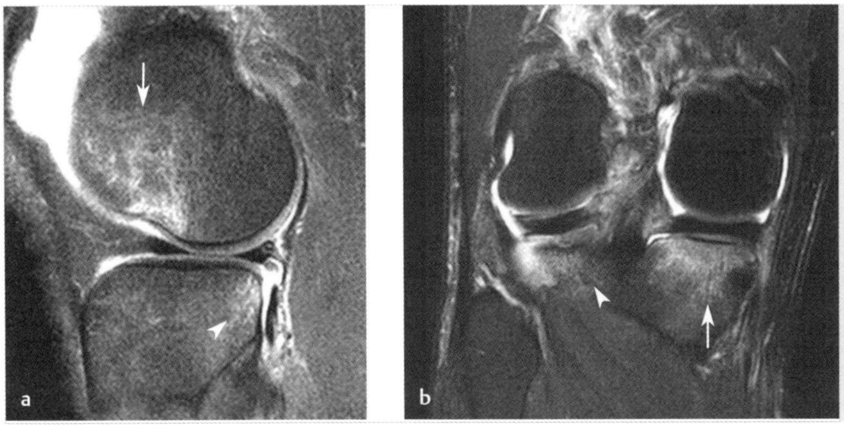

Fig. 11.17 Bone bruise pattern with anterior cruciate ligament (ACL) tear. **(a)** A sagittal fat-suppressed proton-density image shows a bone bruise (*arrow*) with osteochondral impaction involving the lateral femoral condyle and a bone bruise (*arrowhead*) involving the posterior aspect of the lateral tibial plateau. **(b)** A coronal fat-suppressed T2-weighted image of the right knee shows bone bruises involving the posterior aspect of the lateral tibial plateau (*arrowhead*) and medial tibial plateau (*arrow*). (Reproduced with permission from Cascio BM, Khanna AJ, Glait SA, Cosgarea AJ, Johnson TS, Reeder JD. The Knee. In: Khanna AJ, ed. MRI for orthopaedic surgeons. New York: Thieme; 2010:164–201.)

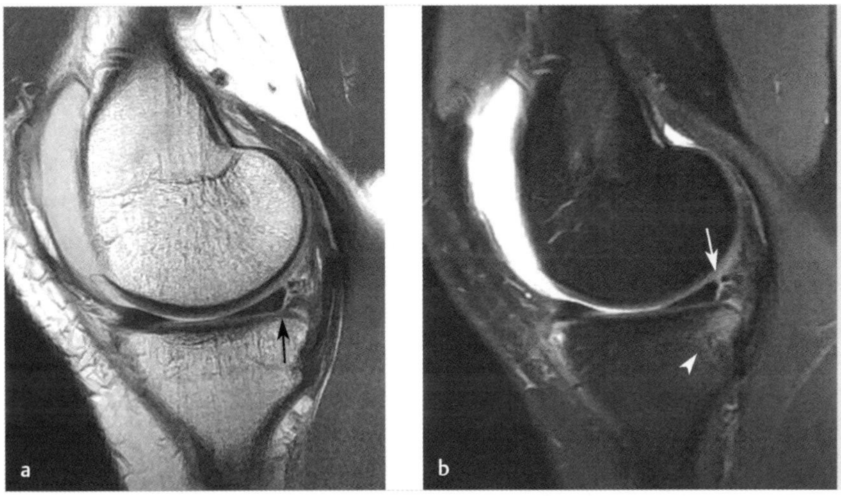

Fig. 11.18 Medial meniscal tear with anterior cruciate ligament (ACL) tear. Sagittal proton-density **(a)** and sagittal fat-suppressed T2-weighted **(b)** images show a peripheral tear (*arrow on each*) of the posterior horn of the medial meniscus. Note the bone bruise (*arrowhead on* **b**) of the posterior aspect of the medial tibial plateau. (Reproduced with permission from Cascio BM, Khanna AJ, Glait SA, Cosgarea AJ, Johnson TS, Reeder JD. The Knee. In: Khanna AJ, ed. MRI for orthopaedic surgeons. New York: Thieme; 2010:164–201.)

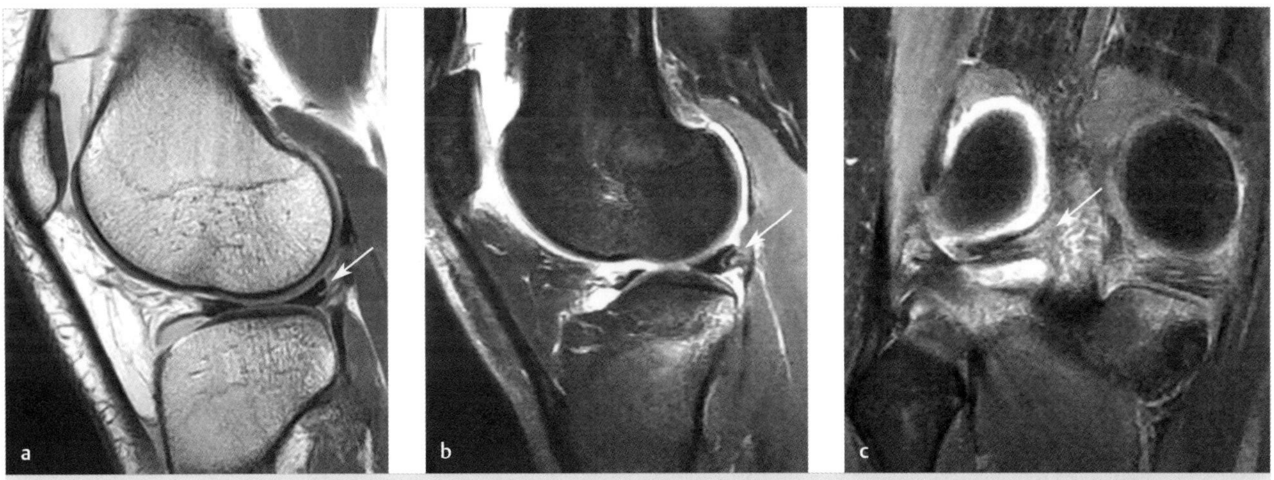

Fig. 11.19 Lateral meniscal tear with anterior cruciate ligament (ACL) tear. Sagittal proton-density **(a)**, sagittal fat-suppressed T2-weighted **(b)**, and coronal fat-suppressed T2-weighted **(c)** images of the right knee show a peripheral tear of the posterior horn of the lateral meniscus (*arrow on each*), associated with the attachment of the meniscofemoral ligament. Note the proximal tibial bone bruises, typical for an acute ACL injury. (Reproduced with permission from Cascio BM, Khanna AJ, Glait SA, Cosgarea AJ, Johnson TS, Reeder JD. The Knee. In: Khanna AJ, ed. MRI for orthopaedic surgeons. New York: Thieme; 2010:164–201.)

When evaluating the MRI study of a patient with ACL injury, multiple factors should be taken into consideration and included in the description of the MRI findings, including the location and degree of disruption of the ACL. In addition, the collateral ligaments, PCL, and secondary restraints (including the menisci) should be carefully reviewed. It is also important to review the status of the osseous structures and articular cartilage because injuries to these structures can also be treated at

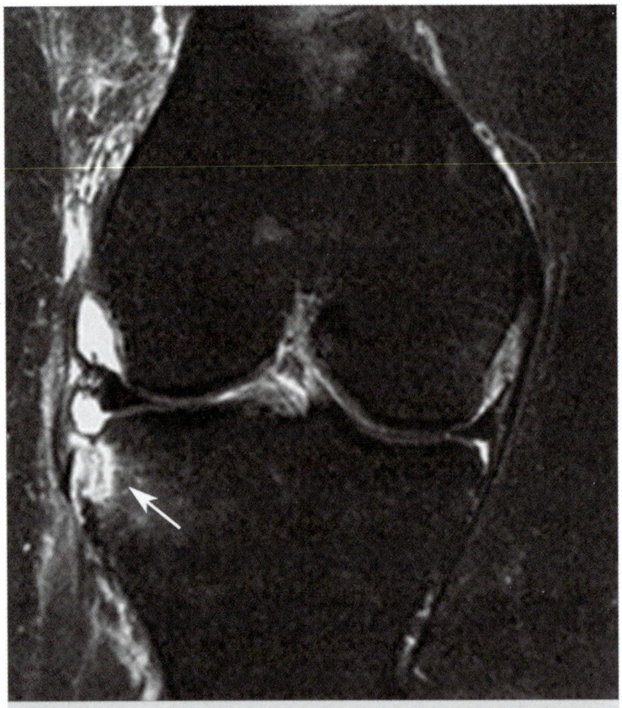

Fig. 11.20 This coronal fat-suppressed T2-weighted image of the right knee shows a Segond fracture (*arrow*) of the lateral aspect of the lateral tibial plateau at the capsular attachment in a patient with an acute anterior cruciate ligament (ACL) tear. (Reproduced with permission from Cascio BM, Khanna AJ, Glait SA, Cosgarea AJ, Johnson TS, Reeder JD. The Knee. In: Khanna AJ, ed. MRI for orthopaedic surgeons. New York: Thieme; 2010:164–201.)

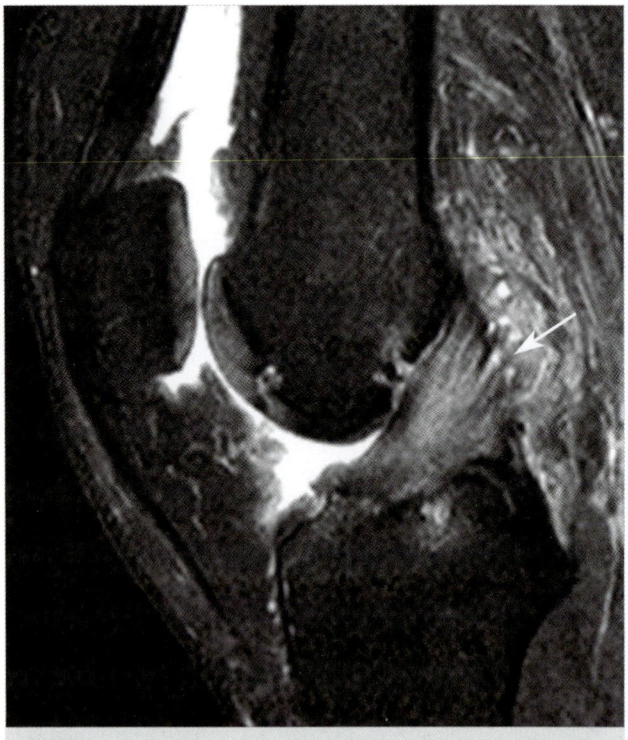

Fig. 11.21 This sagittal fat-suppressed proton-density image shows advanced degeneration (marked thickening) of the anterior cruciate ligament (ACL) (*arrow*). (Reproduced with permission from Cascio BM, Khanna AJ, Glait SA, Cosgarea AJ, Johnson TS, Reeder JD. The Knee. In: Khanna AJ, ed. MRI for orthopaedic surgeons. New York: Thieme; 2010:164–201.)

the time of ACL reconstruction and repair. Lastly, the condition of any tissues that might be used when reconstructing the ACL should be evaluated, and injury to them should be ruled out.

Chronic degeneration of the ACL should be differentiated from an acute ACL injury or tear. Patients with chronic degeneration often present with chronic knee discomfort and a vague, nonspecific knee pain. The process is thought to be secondary to repetitive low-energy microtrauma as opposed to a single high-energy event that might produce an acute ACL tear. Minimal to no instability is seen on physical examination. The MRI may show evidence of advanced degeneration of the ACL with thickening of the ligament and less increase in T2-weighted signal than that which is typically seen with an acute tear (▶ Fig. 11.21). Such patients also often have similar PCL involvement.

11.2.4 PCL Tears

The PCL is more robust and more consistently has lower signal on MRI than does the ACL. MRI is very sensitive for tears of the PCL because of its normal low signal (▶ Fig. 11.22). Any increased signal within the PCL on T2-weighted images is suspicious for injury.[29,30,31] The PCL can be torn partially, indicated by increased signal on T2 images with the ligament in continuity (▶ Fig. 11.23), or completely, visualized as a loss of continuity of the ligament. Bone bruises may be present, depending on the mechanism of injury. A blow to the proximal tibia from a dashboard during a motor vehicle accident can produce soft tissue edema and a bone contusion involving the tibial plateau, best seen on T2-weighted images. Bone bruises may be present on the anterior tibial plateaus and the femoral condyles if the PCL injury occurs from a hyperextension mechanism.

It is important to note evidence for avulsion injuries or multiple ligament injuries because both are indications for early operative repair (for avulsions) or reconstruction (for tears). A "reverse Segond" fracture on the medial side of the joint has been associated with PCL tears.[32] PCL tears can be graded according to the amount of laxity noted on the posterior drawer examination. Laxity grades of 2.5 or more usually are associated with other knee injuries, so a high index of suspicion is indicated when reviewing the MR images of such patients.[33]

The clinician can be alerted to the amount of PCL laxity by noting the resting position of the tibia in relation to the femur on midsagittal images (see ▶ Table 11.4[33] for a summary of one grading system for PCL laxity). The degree of posterior tibial subluxation relates to the severity of the PCL insufficiency. More severe PCL tears can benefit from reconstruction. As with ACL injuries, care should be taken to evaluate the MRI study for associated knee injuries.

11.2.5 Collateral Ligament Tears

Coronal images allow for optimal evaluation of collateral ligament injury. Collateral ligament injury can be classified as mild, moderate (▶ Fig. 11.24), or severe (▶ Fig. 11.25; ▶ Table 11.5[34,35]).[34] Injured ligaments should show varying amounts of increased signal

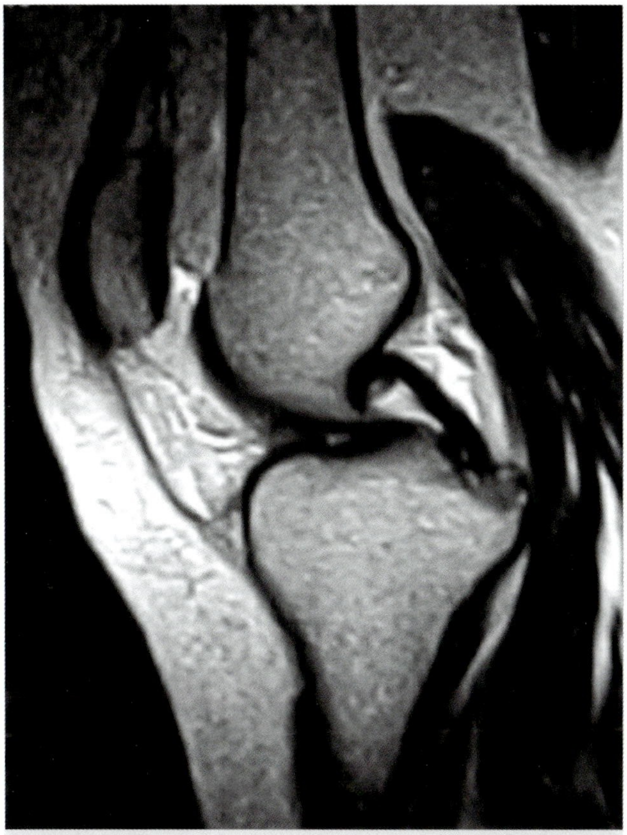

Fig. 11.22 This sagittal T2-weighted image shows a normal posterior cruciate ligament (PCL). Note the absence of signal within the PCL. (Reproduced with permission from Cascio BM, Khanna AJ, Glait SA, Cosgarea AJ, Johnson TS, Reeder JD. The Knee. In: Khanna AJ, ed. MRI for orthopaedic surgeons. New York: Thieme; 2010:164–201.)

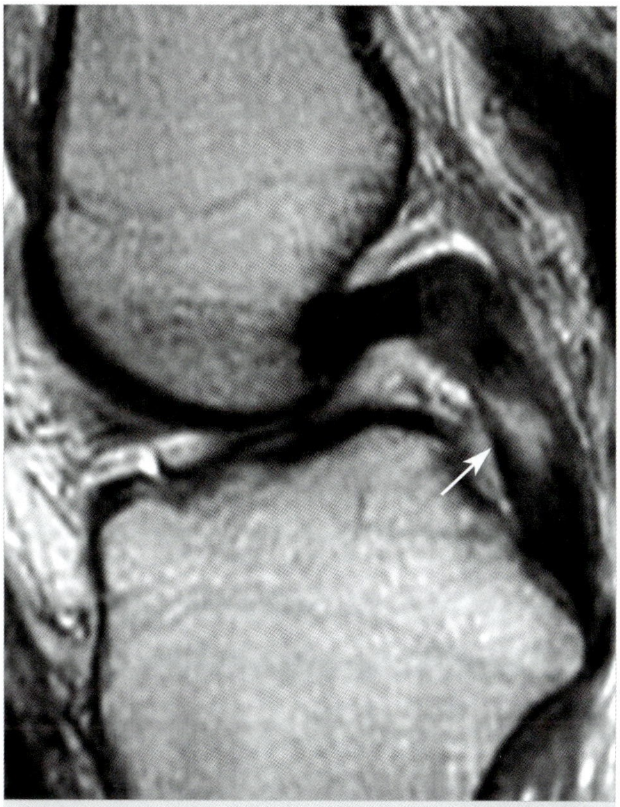

Fig. 11.23 This sagittal T2-weighted image shows thickening and abnormal signal intensity of the posterior cruciate ligament (PCL) (*arrow*), corresponding to a tear. (Reproduced with permission from Cascio BM, Khanna AJ, Glait SA, Cosgarea AJ, Johnson TS, Reeder JD. The Knee. In: Khanna AJ, ed. MRI for orthopaedic surgeons. New York: Thieme; 2010:164–201.)

Table 11.4 Grading of PCL laxity

Grade	Description of posterior drawer examination
1.0	3- to 5-mm difference in tibial step-off; tibial plateau prominence remaining anterior to femoral condyles
1.5	6- to 8-mm difference in tibial step-off; tibial and femoral condyles not yet flush
2.0	9- to 10-mm difference in tibial step-off; anterior tibia and femoral condyles flush with each other
2.5	11- to 13-mm difference in tibial step-off; anterior tibia is posterior to femoral condyles
3.0	> 13 mm difference in tibial step-off; anterior tibia is well posterior to femoral condyles; other ligamentous laxity most likely present

Abbreviation: PCL, posterior cruciate ligament.
Note: It is important to note evidence for avulsion injuries or multiple ligament injuries.

intensity on T2-weighted images based on severity of tissue damage.

In general, complete medial collateral ligament (MCL) tears are treated nonoperatively, whereas complete lateral collateral ligament (LCL) tears are addressed surgically with early repair and later reconstruction with allograft or autograft.

MCL injuries comprise part of the "terrible triad"; the other two components are ACL tears and medial meniscus tears. However, it has been found that lateral meniscus tears, rather than medial meniscus tears, are more common with acute ACL tears.[36]

11.2.6 Posterolateral Corner

The posterolateral corner of the knee is complex from an anatomic and, therefore, imaging standpoint. The variability of the posterolateral structures makes the images of this area of the knee even more difficult to interpret. The posterolateral corner structures resist varus and external rotation forces. The structures that comprise the posterolateral corner are the following:

- LCL.
- Arcuate ligament.
- Popliteal tendon.
- Lateral head of the gastrocnemius.
- Posterolateral capsule.
- Biceps tendon.
- Meniscofibular ligament.
- Popliteofibular ligament.
- Fabellofibular ligament (when the fabella is present).

Although the biceps tendon and LCL usually are identifiable, identifying the popliteofibular ligament is more difficult.[37] This difficulty could contribute to the incidence of missed posterolateral corner injuries. Coronal oblique images offer the best imaging for evaluating and diagnosing the posterolateral structures

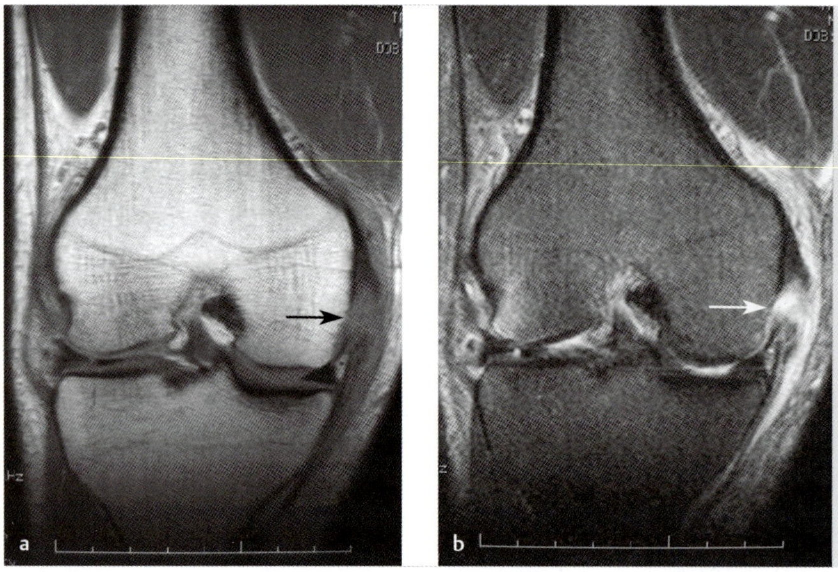

Fig. 11.24 Moderate medial collateral ligament (MCL) injury in the right knee. Coronal T1-weighted (a) and coronal fat-suppressed T2-weighted (b) images show a focal tear (*arrow on each*) of the proximal MCL. Note the corresponding impaction-related bone bruise of the lateral femoral condyle and the lateral meniscal tear. (Reproduced with permission from Cascio BM, Khanna AJ, Glait SA, Cosgarea AJ, Johnson TS, Reeder JD. The Knee. In: Khanna AJ, ed. MRI for orthopaedic surgeons. New York: Thieme; 2010:164–201.)

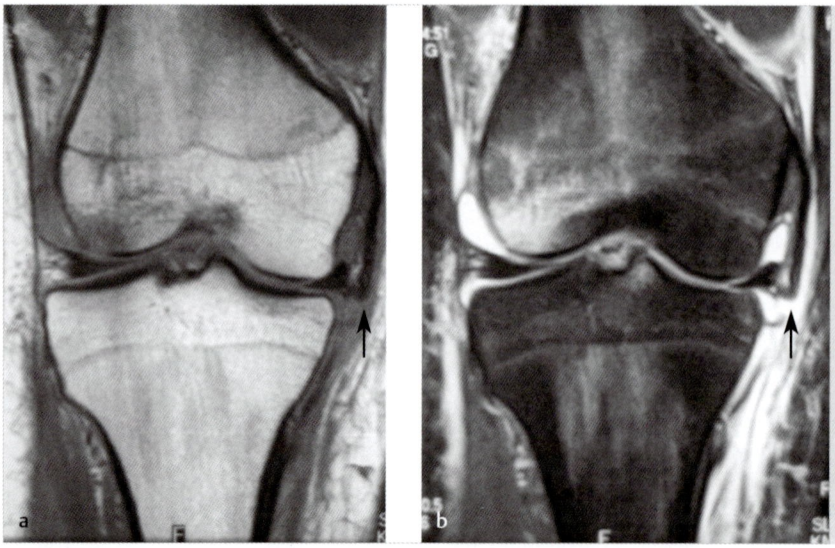

Fig. 11.25 Marked medial collateral ligament (MCL) injury in the right knee. Coronal T1-weighted (a) and fat-suppressed T2-weighted (b) images show a high-grade MCL injury (*arrow on each*). Note the marked lateral femoral condyle bone contusion. (Reproduced with permission from Cascio BM, Khanna AJ, Glait SA, Cosgarea AJ, Johnson TS, Reeder JD. The Knee. In: Khanna AJ, ed. MRI for orthopaedic surgeons. New York: Thieme; 2010:164–201.)

Table 11.5 Collateral ligament tears

Grade of tear	Description	MRI appearance
Mild	Ligament has some torn or stretched fibers	Periligamentous edema; ligament grossly intact, hematoma possible
Moderate	Incomplete tear with no laxity	Partial tear with edema, hematoma possible
Severe	Loss of ligament integrity, pathologic laxity	Complete tear, fibers not in continuity, considerable edema and hematoma

Abbreviation: MRI, magnetic resonance imaging.

(▶ Fig. 11.26). Specific attention should be given to including imaging through the entire fibular head. A high-energy varus injury to the knee can place tension on, and even rupture, the peroneal nerve after the posterolateral knee structures are torn. Careful attention should also be given to noting discontinuity or edema of the peroneal nerve.

The arcuate complex is composed of the LCL, arcuate ligament, and popliteus tendon. It provides posterolateral stability of the knee to varus and rotatory stress. The arcuate ligament is an inconsistent structure and is occasionally absent in individuals with large fabellae. Injury to this complex area of the knee is seen as increased signal intensity on T2-weighted images because of the underlying edema (▶ Fig. 11.27).

11.2.7 Posteromedial Corner

The posteromedial corner is composed of the deep and superficial MCLs, the posterior oblique ligament, and the oblique popliteal ligament. Damage to the posteromedial corner can cause valgus instability of the knee and increased anteromedial subluxation. The posterior oblique ligament is attached to the posterior horn of the medial meniscus. Some authors have advocated surgical repair of damage to this complex.[38] Coronal images (▶ Fig. 11.28) offer the best views of these structures. The femoral and tibial attachments of the structures should be evaluated carefully for increased signal on T2-weighted images, which indicates edema and injury.

11.2.8 Knee Dislocation

Knee dislocation is a serious injury that may lead to compartment syndrome and rhabdomyolysis, with resultant loss of limb and even life. Vascular injury occurs in as many as 50% of knee dislocations, whereas peroneal or tibial nerve injuries occur in up to 30%.[39,40] Although angiography is the standard for diagnosing vascular injuries associated with knee dislocations, MR angiography is less invasive and can play a valuable role . Care must be taken to evaluate for peroneal nerve or tibial nerve edema or discontinuity. A careful neurovascular examination is essential. As with many other diagnoses, the clinician has a substantial advantage over the radiologist, given that the clinician can correlate the clinical findings with the imaging findings to determine the most likely diagnosis with a high degree of certainty. Knee dislocations are associated with fractures, cartilage injury, and tears of the ACL, PCL, LCL, MCL, and posterolateral and posteromedial corners (▶ Fig. 11.29); imaging studies should be scrutinized carefully for the presence or absence of these findings.

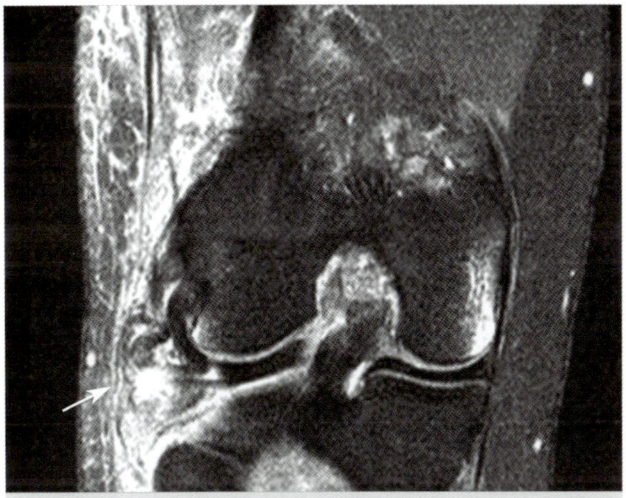

Fig. 11.26 This coronal fat-suppressed T2-weighted image of the right knee shows tears of the fibular collateral ligament (*arrow*) and biceps femoris tendon at the fibular head. Note the corresponding impaction injury of the medial femoral condyle. (Reproduced with permission from Cascio BM, Khanna AJ, Glait SA, Cosgarea AJ, Johnson TS, Reeder JD. The Knee. In: Khanna AJ, ed. MRI for orthopaedic surgeons. New York: Thieme; 2010:164–201.)

11.2.9 Extensor Mechanism

Traumatic injuries to the extensor mechanism include patellar dislocation, quadriceps tendon rupture, and patellar tendon rupture.[41]

Patellar Dislocation

Patellar dislocations occur through noncontact mechanisms such as rotation on a planted foot (e.g., as during batting in baseball) and through contact mechanisms (e.g., laterally directed force to the medial side of the patella). Patients can be first-time dislocators, which can imply acute trauma, or recurrent dislocators, implying chronicity. The MRI findings in the recurrent dislocator without a history of trauma may not be as definitive. The patella is usually already reduced by the time the MRI study is obtained, but it is frequently subluxated laterally. Images of acute patellar dislocations commonly show bone bruises of the lateral trochlea and the medial patella (▶ Fig. 11.30), which are injuries from the relocation event. When the patella displaces over the lateral femoral condyle, varying sizes of osteochondral fragments may be fractured from the patella or trochlea, or both. On MRI, these loose bodies may be found in the joint, and fluid–fluid levels may be seen. MRI typically reveals a rupture of the medial patellar retinaculum, including the medial patellofemoral ligament (▶ Fig. 11.31). Patterns of injury in the medial patellofemoral ligament may vary by the patient's age.[42,43] Noting the location of the medial patellofemoral ligament is important because it can guide decisions about repair or reconstruction and may help identify the optimal location for the incision. Edema may also be seen in the region of the vastus medialis oblique. The only clue for chronic dislocators may be an attenuation or laxity of the medial retinaculum and medial patellofemoral ligament. Large effusions are commonly seen on MRI of these injuries. MRI also can help the clinician determine risk factors for patellar dislocation. For instance, a hypoplastic lateral trochlea seen on axial images suggests instability secondary to insufficient osseous constraint.

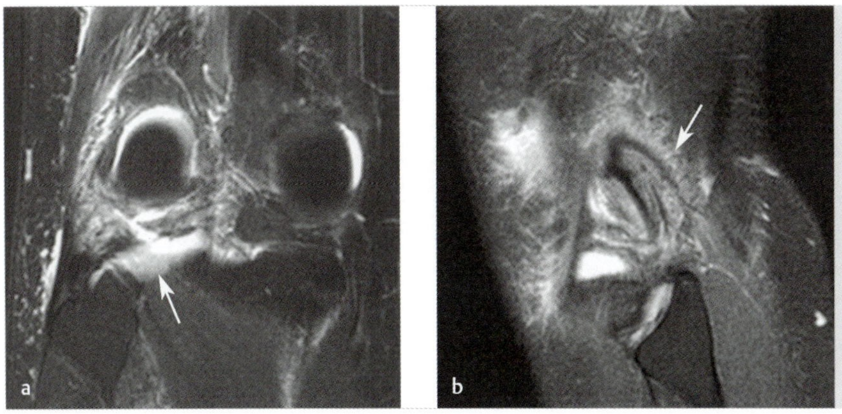

Fig. 11.27 Posterolateral corner injury in the right knee. Coronal fat-suppressed T2-weighted **(a)** and sagittal fat-suppressed proton-density **(b)** images of a patient with an acute anterior cruciate ligament (ACL) injury show marked soft tissue edema (*arrow on each*) involving the posterolateral corner of the knee. (Reproduced with permission from Cascio BM, Khanna AJ, Glait SA, Cosgarea AJ, Johnson TS, Reeder JD. The Knee. In: Khanna AJ, ed. MRI for orthopaedic surgeons. New York: Thieme; 2010:164–201.)

Identification of these predisposing factors assists with surgical planning and determination of prognosis, although bony morphology may be better assessed on computed tomography.[44]

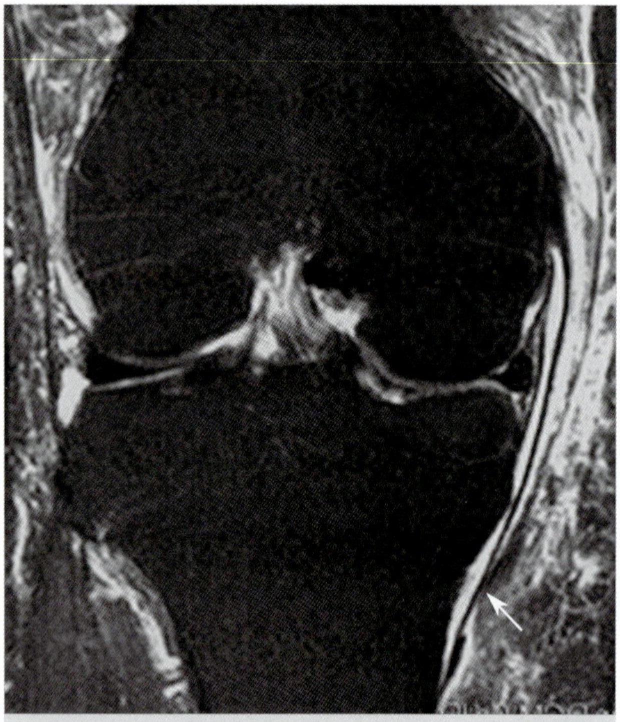

Fig. 11.28 This coronal fat-suppressed T2-weighted image of a patient with a medial collateral ligament (MCL) sprain in the right knee shows the deep and superficial (*arrow*) components of the MCL complex, separated by fluid and edema. (Reproduced with permission from Cascio BM, Khanna AJ, Glait SA, Cosgarea AJ, Johnson TS, Reeder JD. The Knee. In: Khanna AJ, ed. MRI for orthopaedic surgeons. New York: Thieme; 2010:164–201.)

Quadriceps and Patellar Tendon Ruptures

The quadriceps tendon has a laminated appearance on MRI because it is formed as a conjoined structure from four muscles. Understanding this concept allows the orthopaedic surgeon to avoid misreading the normal appearance of the quadriceps tendon as an intrasubstance injury or strain of the quadriceps tendon. Partial quadriceps tendon tears often are associated with increased T2-weighted signal, especially on fat-suppressed images, just anterior to the quadriceps tendon.

Patellar tendon ruptures (▸ Fig. 11.32) usually occur in young patients (< 50 y old), whereas quadriceps tendon ruptures (▸ Fig. 11.33) occur in older patients, in patients with comorbidities such as diabetes mellitus and obesity, and in patients on steroids. Sagittal images are ideal for visualizing both types of ruptures. Tendon discontinuity with patella alta is seen on T1-weighted sagittal images with patellar tendon rupture. Discontinuity of the tendon and patella baja can be seen in patients with quadriceps tendon rupture.[45] Both types of rupture show edema on T2-weighted images. It is helpful to differentiate an avulsion from an intratendinous failure because bone-to-tendon healing allows for a better prognosis. Although the diagnosis of quadriceps and patellar tendon rupture can frequently be made by history and physical examination (including palpation of a suprapatellar or infrapatellar defect), MRI may still provide valuable information regarding the presence or absence of other intra-articular injuries, such as cruciate ligament or meniscal tears, that may be treated at the time of ligament repair or reconstruction.

11.2.10 Muscle Strain

Muscle strains about the knee are common.[46] The biceps femoris (▸ Fig. 11.34) is by far the most commonly strained muscle

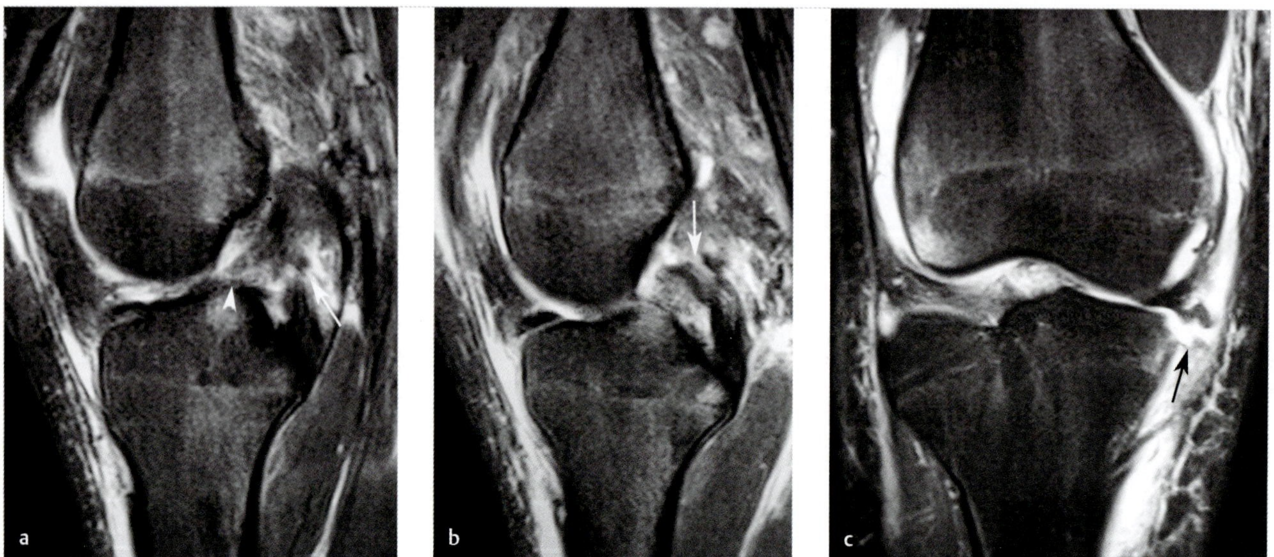

Fig. 11.29 Knee dislocation. **(a)** A sagittal fat-suppressed T2-weighted image of the right knee shows tears of the anterior cruciate ligament (ACL) (*arrowhead*) and posterior cruciate ligament (PCL) (*arrow*). **(b)** A sagittal fat-suppressed T2-weighted image shows a proximal PCL tear (*arrow*). **(c)** A coronal fat-suppressed T2-weighted image of the right knee shows severe medial collateral ligament (MCL) injury (*arrow*) and a lateral femoral condylar bone bruise. (Reproduced with permission from Cascio BM, Khanna AJ, Glait SA, Cosgarea AJ, Johnson TS, Reeder JD. The Knee. In: Khanna AJ, ed. MRI for orthopaedic surgeons. New York: Thieme; 2010:164–201.)

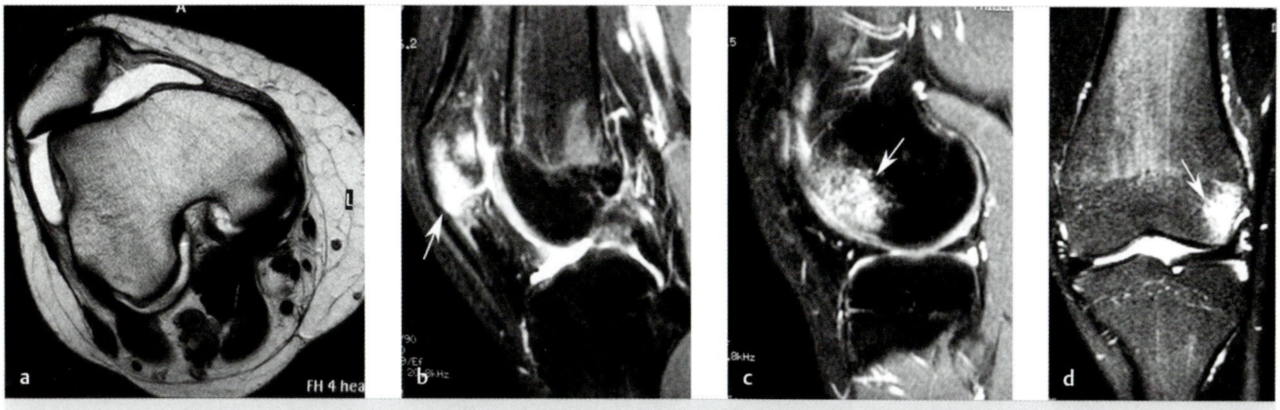

Fig. 11.30 Lateral patellar dislocation. **(a)** An axial T2-weighted image of the right knee shows lateral patellar subluxation and chondral injury involving the medial facet of the patella. **(b)** A sagittal fat-suppressed T2-weighted image shows a fracture and bone bruise of the patella (*arrow*). **(c)** A sagittal fat-suppressed T2-weighted image shows an impaction-related bone bruise of the anterolateral aspect of the lateral femoral condyle (*arrow*). **(d)** A coronal fat-suppressed T2-weighted image of the left knee shows a lateral femoral condylar bone bruise (*arrow*). (Reproduced with permission from Cascio BM, Khanna AJ, Glait SA, Cosgarea AJ, Johnson TS, Reeder JD. The Knee. In: Khanna AJ, ed. MRI for orthopaedic surgeons. New York: Thieme; 2010:164–201.)

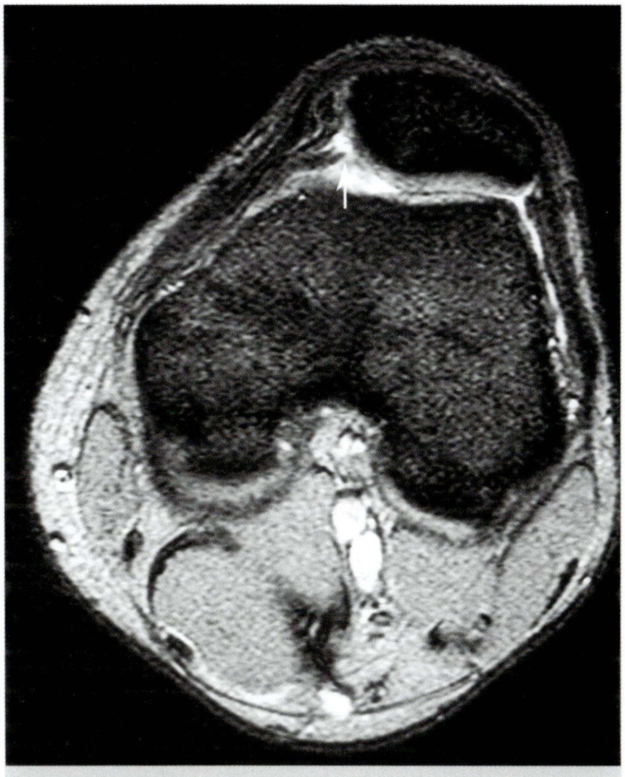

Fig. 11.31 This axial fat-suppressed T2-weighted image of the left knee shows a tear (*arrow*) of the medial patellar retinaculum at its patellar attachment. (Reproduced with permission from Cascio BM, Khanna AJ, Glait SA, Cosgarea AJ, Johnson TS, Reeder JD. The Knee. In: Khanna AJ, ed. MRI for orthopaedic surgeons. New York: Thieme; 2010:164–201.)

at the knee, followed by the semimembranosus and semitendinosus muscles.[47] A muscle strain is identified on MRI as a region of increased T2-weighted signal within the substance of the muscle without frank discontinuity of the muscle fibers. One-third of all strains involve multiple muscles.[46] The length of abnormal signal in the strained muscle is predictive of the athlete's ability to return to play.[48] Care must be taken to differentiate an avulsion from a strain, given that avulsions can require surgical intervention.

11.2.11 Loose Bodies

Loose bodies greater than 1 cm can be an indication for arthroscopic surgery. There are two typical sources for loose bodies:

- Osteophytes and degenerative cartilage debris in the osteoarthritic knee.
- Osteochondral fragments from acute trauma, such as when the patella dislocates.

The source of the loose body sometimes is recognizable; when it is, it offers valuable information. MRI is useful for locating chondral or osseous fragments in the knee, especially purely chondral and unmineralized lesions, which are not visible on conventional radiographs. Estimating the size of osteochondral fragments is important because the size can dictate what treatment options are available. Loose bodies are found most frequently in the suprapatellar pouch, the medial and lateral gutters, and the posterior compartments[49] (▸ Fig. 11.35). A good clue that allows for diagnosis of a loose body is identification of the osteochondral donor site. Multiple loose bodies seen on MRI without evidence of donor sites may suggest synovial osteochondromatosis, a benign proliferative disorder of the synovium.

MRI and MR arthrography can be used to evaluate loose bodies, which typically have low signal on T1-weighted and T2-weighted pulse sequences. Gradient-echo images are also frequently used, especially to help differentiate the diagnosis from PVNS. As with other diagnoses, it is important to correlate the MRI findings with those seen on conventional radiographs.

Meniscal ossicles, which may be mistaken for loose bodies, are typically located at the posterior horns of the menisci and, on MRI, appear as corticated structures with marrow signal characteristics on all sequences. Meniscal ossicles are rare and frequently asymptomatic. Their etiology and clinical significance are unclear.

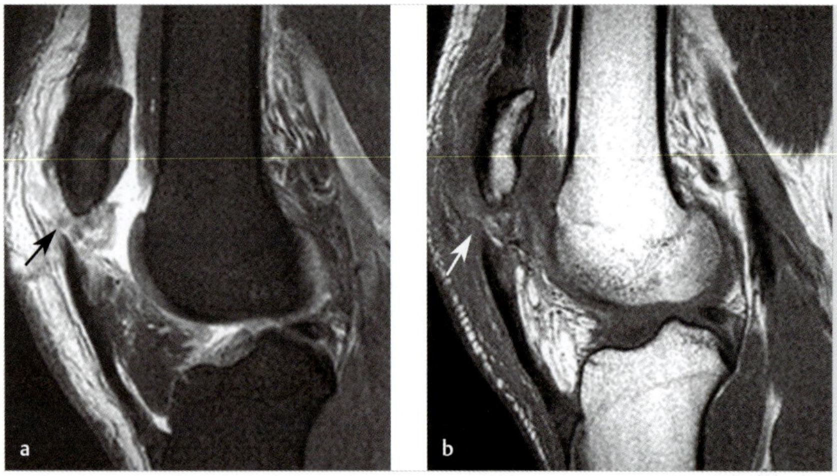

Fig. 11.32 Patellar tendon rupture. Sagittal fat-suppressed proton-density **(a)** and sagittal T1-weighted **(b)** images show a complete tear (*arrow on each*) of the proximal patellar tendon. (Reproduced with permission from Cascio BM, Khanna AJ, Glait SA, Cosgarea AJ, Johnson TS, Reeder JD. The Knee. In: Khanna AJ, ed. MRI for orthopaedic surgeons. New York: Thieme; 2010:164–201.)

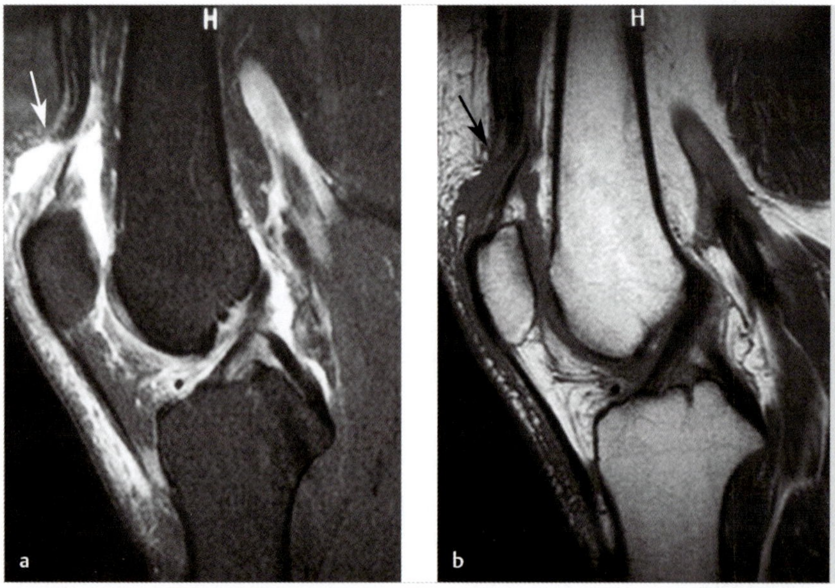

Fig. 11.33 Quadriceps tendon rupture. Sagittal fat-suppressed T2-weighted **(a)** and sagittal T1-weighted **(b)** images show a rupture of the quadriceps tendon (*arrow on each*). (Reproduced with permission from Cascio BM, Khanna AJ, Glait SA, Cosgarea AJ, Johnson TS, Reeder JD. The Knee. In: Khanna AJ, ed. MRI for orthopaedic surgeons. New York: Thieme; 2010:164–201.)

11.2.12 Hoffa Disease

Hoffa disease (fat pad disease) has been described in young athletes, usually after traumatic events.[11] Acutely, edema is found in the patellar fat pad and can cause pain. The fat pad may hypertrophy, and repetitive trauma and fibrosis can ensue (see section "Anterior Interval Scarring").

11.3 Degenerative (Nonacute) Pathology

11.3.1 Stress Fracture

Stress fractures about the knee are often missed because this diagnosis may not be considered.[50] There may be no changes on conventional radiographs, especially early in the progression and before the sclerosis seen in the healing phase occurs. MRI findings of an acute stress fracture include a low-signal-intensity line on T1-weighted images and a high-signal-intensity linear region on T2-weighted images because of the presence of surrounding edema (▶ Fig. 11.36). Although stress fractures of the femoral neck have more severe clinical consequences, stress fractures of the proximal tibia and distal femur must be identified early and treated appropriately.

11.3.2 Extensor Mechanism: Patellar Tendinosis

Also known as jumper's knee, patellar tendinosis is a common entity in patients participating in activities requiring explosive jumping motions, such as basketball, soccer, and volleyball. MR images may show variable amounts of focal thickening of the tendon and associated increased signal intensity on T2-weighted images (▶ Fig. 11.37).[51,52] These partial tears usually are located at the proximal aspect of the tendon just distal to the inferior pole of the patella. The diagnosis of patellar tendinosis is important because the inflammatory process and associated tendon degeneration may proceed to complete rupture.

11.3.3 Osteochondroses

Osgood-Schlatter Disease

Osgood-Schlatter disease is an osteochondrosis of the immature apophysis of the patellar insertion found commonly in adolescent males. The patella tendon insertion is tender to the touch. The adolescent can have severe pain with activity, especially with forceful extension of the flexed knee. MRI shows focal fragmentation of the patellar tendon insertion onto the tibia with associated edema (▶ Fig. 11.38). Patients are treated with activity modification, rest, and occasionally casting. Very rarely, surgery is necessary to remove recalcitrant, painful fragments.

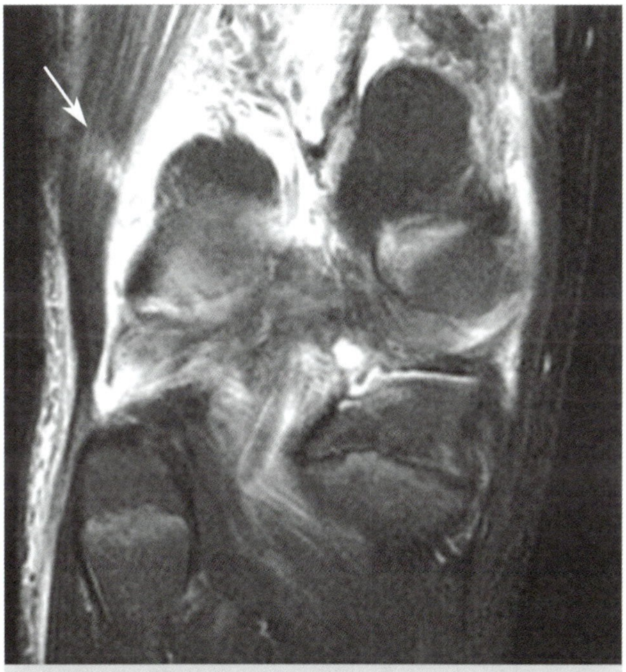

Fig. 11.34 This coronal fat-suppressed T2-weighted image of the right knee shows intramuscular edema (*arrow*), compatible with strain, involving the biceps femoris muscle. (Reproduced with permission from Cascio BM, Khanna AJ, Glait SA, Cosgarea AJ, Johnson TS, Reeder JD. The Knee. In: Khanna AJ, ed. MRI for orthopaedic surgeons. New York: Thieme; 2010:164–201.)

Sinding-Larsen-Johansson Disease

This entity, which is similar to but less common than Osgood-Schlatter disease, occurs at the inferior pole of the patella.

11.3.4 Discoid Meniscus

This entity occurs in approximately 5% of the population.[53,54,55] The lateral meniscus is much more commonly involved than is the medial meniscus.[56] Discoid menisci were first classified by Wantanabe et al[57] as follows:

- Grade I (complete).
- Grade II (incomplete).
- Grade III (Wrisberg or lateral meniscal variant, i.e., a meniscus that is not secured to the posterior tibia by coronary ligaments).

Monllau et al[58] described a fourth, ring-shaped type. Symptoms include a popping sensation in the knee and pain. Treatment includes arthroscopic contouring or stabilization of the discoid meniscus.

The discoid lateral meniscus is recognizable on sagittal and coronal MR images with central bridging of the anterior and posterior horns (▶ Fig. 11.39). Particularly on sagittal images obtained through the central portion of the lateral compartment, the normally separate triangular anterior and posterior meniscal horns are connected by fibrocartilaginous tissue. The discoid meniscus may show increased signal intensity on T1-weighted images because of internal myxoid degeneration, even in children and young adults.

11.3.5 Plicae

Plicae are synovial folds that are embryologic remnants. Usually four plicae are described (▶ Fig. 11.40):

- Suprapatellar.
- Infrapatellar.
- Lateral.
- Medial.

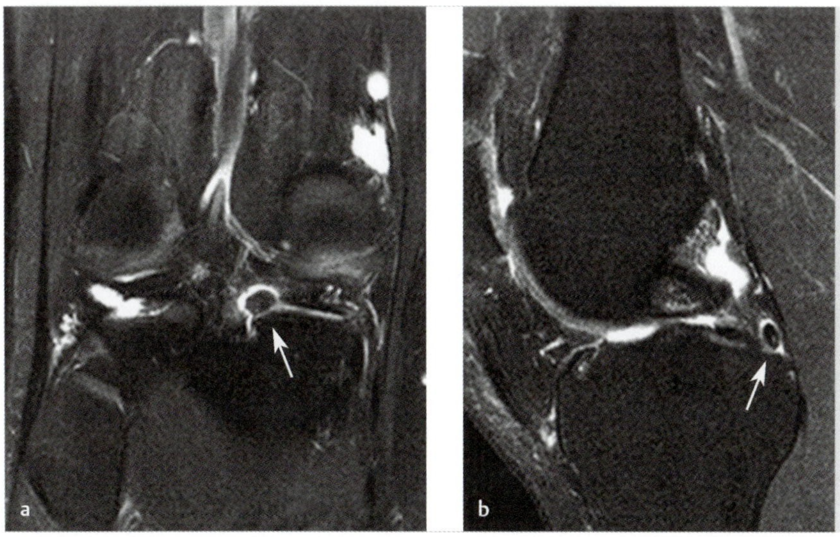

Fig. 11.35 Loose bodies. Axial fat-suppressed T2-weighted **(a)** and sagittal fat-suppressed proton-density **(b)** images of the right knee show a loose body (*arrow on each*) located within the recess lateral to the posterior horn of the medial meniscus. (Reproduced with permission from Cascio BM, Khanna AJ, Glait SA, Cosgarea AJ, Johnson TS, Reeder JD. The Knee. In: Khanna AJ, ed. MRI for orthopaedic surgeons. New York: Thieme; 2010:164–201.)

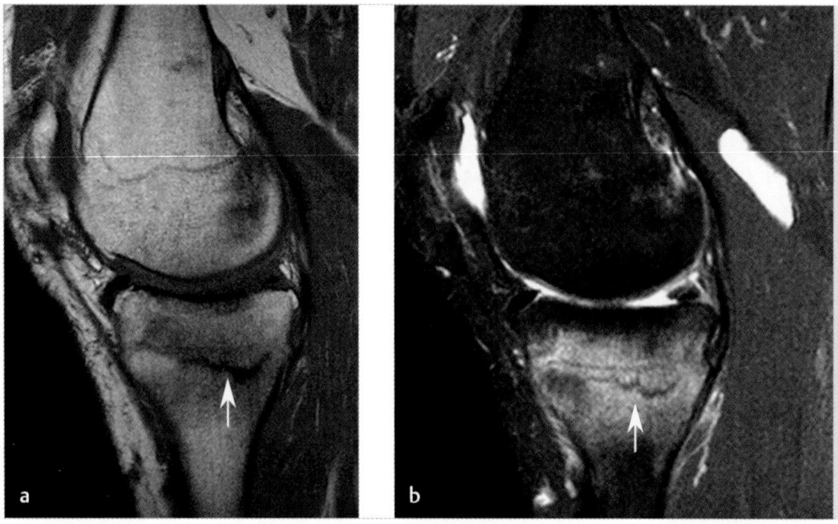

Fig. 11.36 Stress fracture. Sagittal T1-weighted **(a)** and fat-suppressed proton-density **(b)** images show a horizontal fracture (*arrow on each*) of the medial tibial metaphysis in a patient with a partial medial meniscectomy. Note the surrounding bone marrow edema pattern. (Reproduced with permission from Cascio BM, Khanna AJ, Glait SA, Cosgarea AJ, Johnson TS, Reeder JD. The Knee. In: Khanna AJ, ed. MRI for orthopaedic surgeons. New York: Thieme; 2010:164–201.)

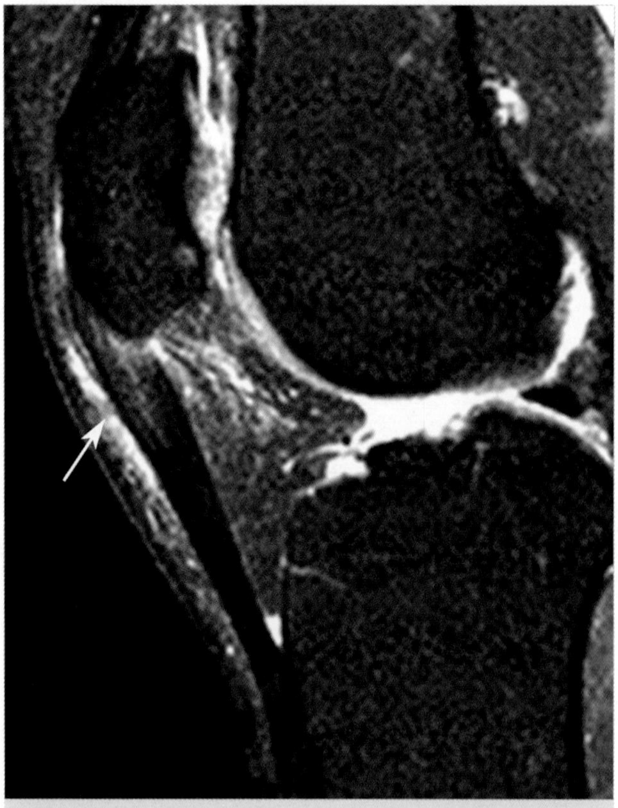

Fig. 11.37 This sagittal fat-suppressed proton-density image shows thickening and abnormal signal intensity (*arrow*) involving the proximal patellar tendon, indicative of a partial tear (jumper's knee). (Reproduced with permission from Cascio BM, Khanna AJ, Glait SA, Cosgarea AJ, Johnson TS, Reeder JD. The Knee. In: Khanna AJ, ed. MRI for orthopaedic surgeons. New York: Thieme; 2010:164–201.)

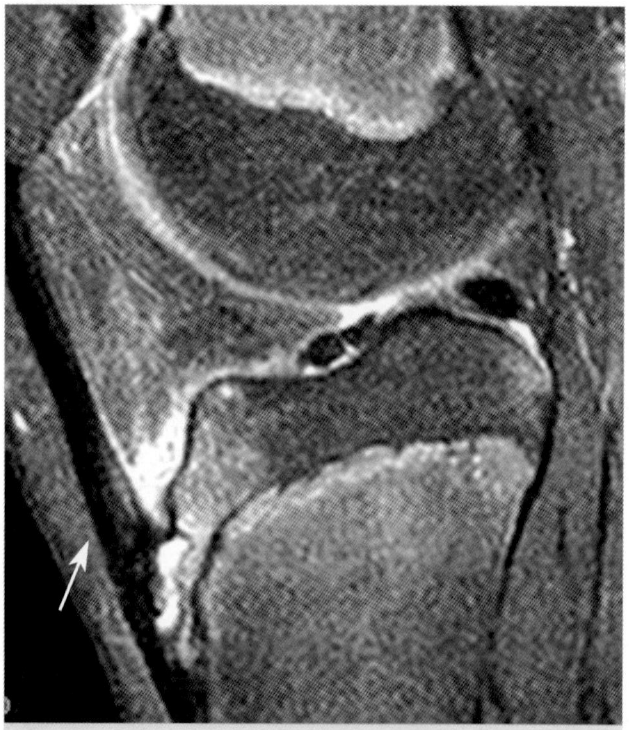

Fig. 11.38 This sagittal fat-suppressed proton-density image shows Osgood-Schlatter disease: thickening and abnormal signal intensity involving the distal patellar tendon (*arrow*); bone marrow edema and slight distraction of the tibial tubercle apophysis; and fluid accumulation and edema involving the deep infrapatellar bursa, posterior to the distal patellar tendon. (Reproduced with permission from Cascio BM, Khanna AJ, Glait SA, Cosgarea AJ, Johnson TS, Reeder JD. The Knee. In: Khanna AJ, ed. MRI for orthopaedic surgeons. New York: Thieme; 2010:164–201.)

Plicae are a common source of atraumatic, activity-associated pain in young, active individuals. The medial plica is the most commonly symptomatic source, and it may cause pain secondary to irritation and even abrasion of the medial femoral condyle at approximately 30 degrees of flexion as it rubs across the condyle (▶ Fig. 11.41). The patient typically presents with a sharp, pinching pain, usually on the anteromedial aspect of the knee proximal to the joint line, associated with activity requiring repetitive knee flexion such as running or bicycling. Well-developed and large plicae can present with a painful popping sensation in the knee. If nonoperative therapy fails to relieve symptoms, arthroscopic removal of the offending plica is indicated. Chondroplasty of the abraded cartilage, if identified, is also indicated.

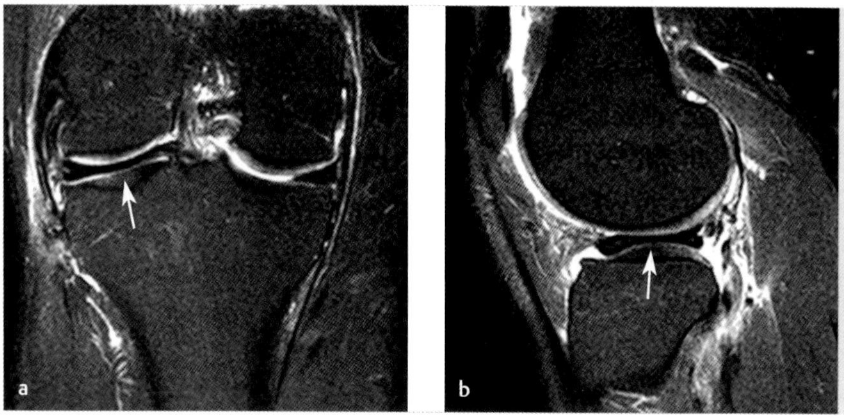

Fig. 11.39 Discoid lateral meniscus. Coronal fat-suppressed T2-weighted **(a)** and sagittal fat-suppressed proton-density **(b)** images of the right knee show central bridging (*arrow on each*) of the anterior and posterior horns of the lateral meniscus. (Reproduced with permission from Cascio BM, Khanna AJ, Glait SA, Cosgarea AJ, Johnson TS, Reeder JD. The Knee. In: Khanna AJ, ed. MRI for orthopaedic surgeons. New York: Thieme; 2010:164–201.)

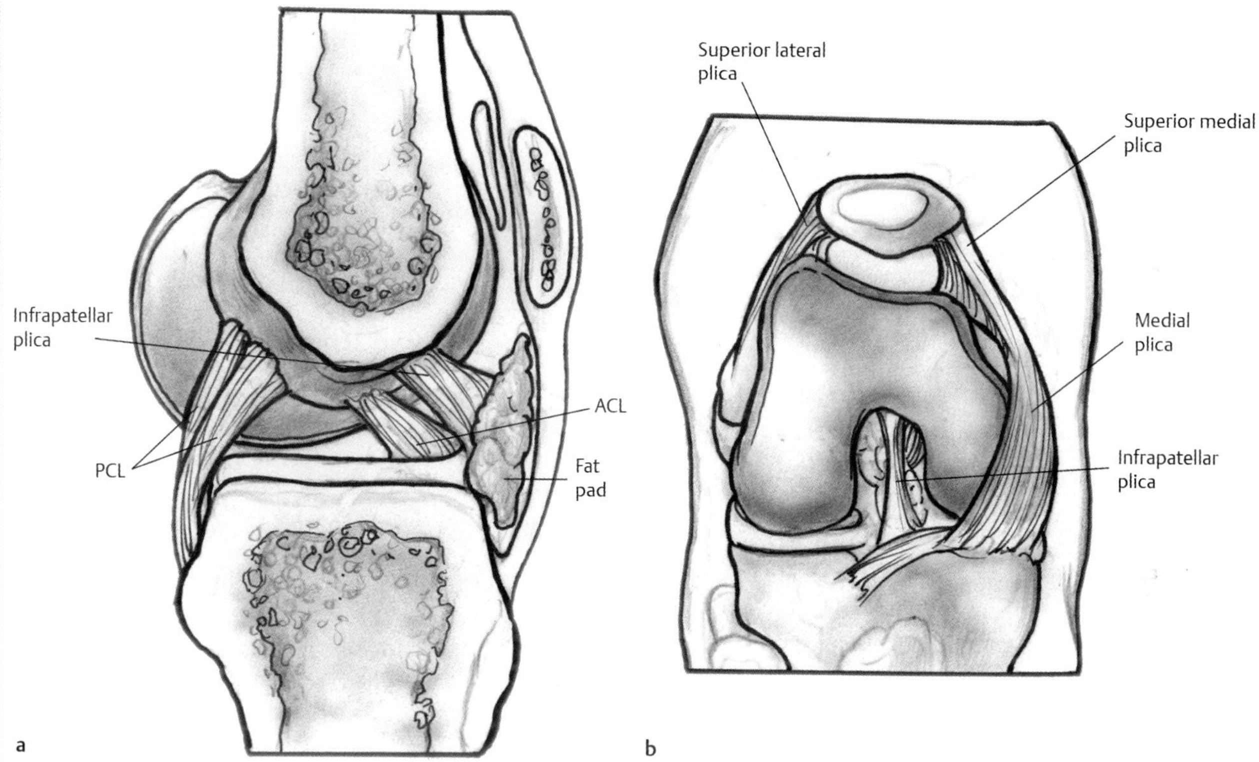

Fig. 11.40 Artist's sketch illustrating the location of superior, inferior, and medial plicae of the knee in the sagittal **(a)** and coronal **(b)** planes. Abbreviations: PCL, posterior cruciate ligament; ACL, anterior cruciate ligament. (Reproduced with permission from Cascio BM, Khanna AJ, Glait SA, Cosgarea AJ, Johnson TS, Reeder JD. The Knee. In: Khanna AJ, ed. MRI for orthopaedic surgeons. New York: Thieme; 2010:164–201.)

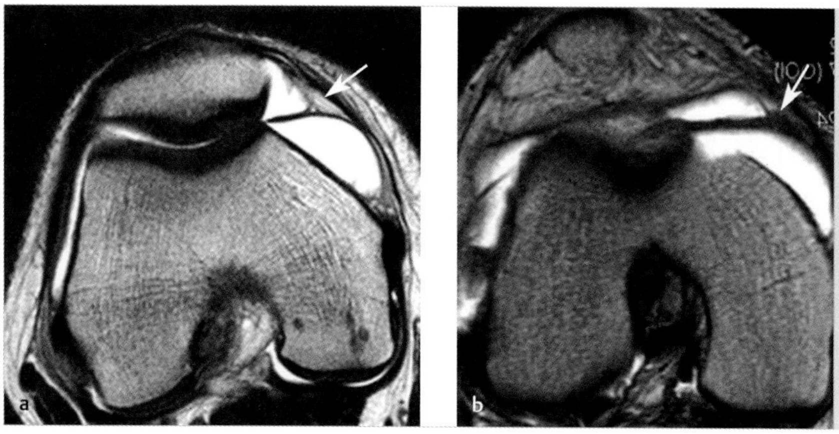

Fig. 11.41 Medial plica. **(a)** An axial T2-weighted image of the right knee showing a medial plica (*arrow*) with normal thickness. **(b)** An axial T2-weighted image of the right knee showing a medial plica (*arrow*) with thickening in a patient with plica syndrome. (Reproduced with permission from Cascio BM, Khanna AJ, Glait SA, Cosgarea AJ, Johnson TS, Reeder JD. The Knee. In: Khanna AJ, ed. MRI for orthopaedic surgeons. New York: Thieme; 2010:164–201.)

11.3.6 Bursitis

The pes anserine bursa lies over the tendinous attachment of the sartorius, gracilis, and semitendinosus tendons. The Voshell bursa is deep to the superficial MCL. T2-weighted MR images show fluid in inflamed bursae (▶ Fig. 11.42). Aspiration of the fluid is an option if a collection of fluid is identified. The physical examination is indispensable for this diagnosis because pain on palpation of the pes bursa is the sine qua non of bursitis. Bursae can become infected, which makes treating them more difficult. Saphenous neuritis is in the differential diagnosis for pain in the proximal, anteromedial knee. If the bursa does not appear to be inflamed on MRI when bursitis is the suspected diagnosis, then a repeat physical examination is warranted and a diagnostic injection can be considered.

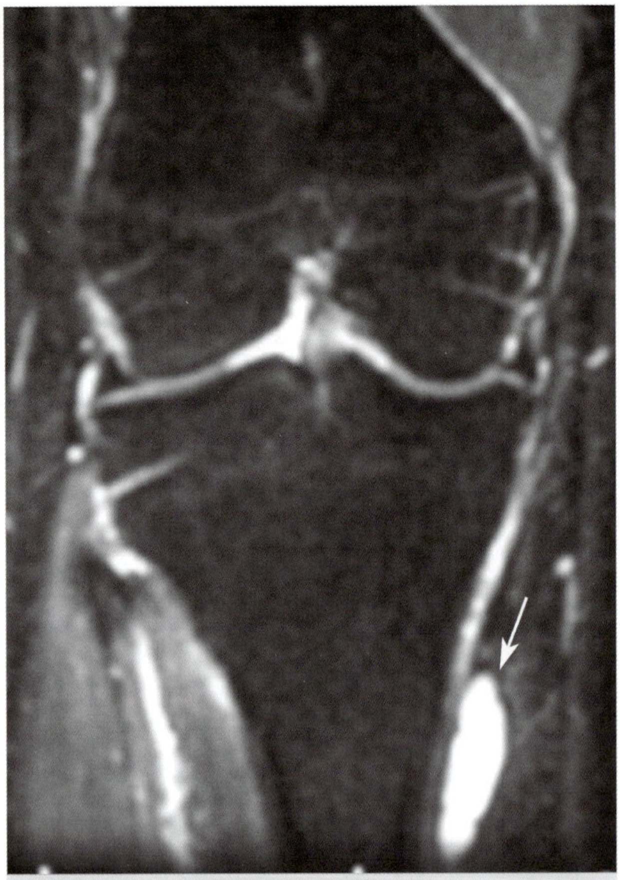

Fig. 11.42 This coronal fat-suppressed T2-weighted image of the right knee shows fluid accumulation within the bursa (*arrow*) associated with the insertion of the pes anserine tendons. (Reproduced with permission from Cascio BM, Khanna AJ, Glait SA, Cosgarea AJ, Johnson TS, Reeder JD. The Knee. In: Khanna AJ, ed. MRI for orthopaedic surgeons. New York: Thieme; 2010:164–201.)

Prepatellar bursitis (▶ Fig. 11.43) is a common clinical diagnosis that is seen in active individuals after an abrasion to the anterior aspect of the knee. MRI shows fluid in the prepatellar bursa. Aspiration and, rarely, surgical debridement are used to treat this condition. Similar to prepatellar bursitis, the infrapatellar bursa may also be affected.

11.3.7 ITB Syndrome

Iliotibial band (ITB) syndrome is a common cause of lateral knee pain in runners. Other conditions in the differential diagnosis for lateral knee pain include the following:

- LCL injury.
- Lateral meniscal tears and degeneration.
- Popliteal tendon and hamstring strains.

The presence or absence of each of these entities should be evaluated carefully, especially in patients presenting with lateral knee pain. The ITB is best seen on coronal and axial T2-weighted and fat-suppressed T2-weighted images. Edema is seen superficial to the lateral femoral epicondyle, involving the ITB. Small fluid collections, which are relatively poorly defined, and variable thickening of the ITB are often seen. The athlete has pain on palpation over the lateral femoral epicondyle. The classic Ober test is useful for diagnosing a tight ITB. If a tight ITB is found, then stretching is the first line of treatment. Activity modification, nonsteroidal anti-inflammatory medications, and modalities such as ultrasound are other options.

11.3.8 Osteonecrosis

Osteonecrosis (also known as avascular necrosis) in the knee is associated with many causative factors (▶ Table 11.6[59,60,61,62,63]); most often, they are atraumatic in nature (▶ Fig. 11.44). The most

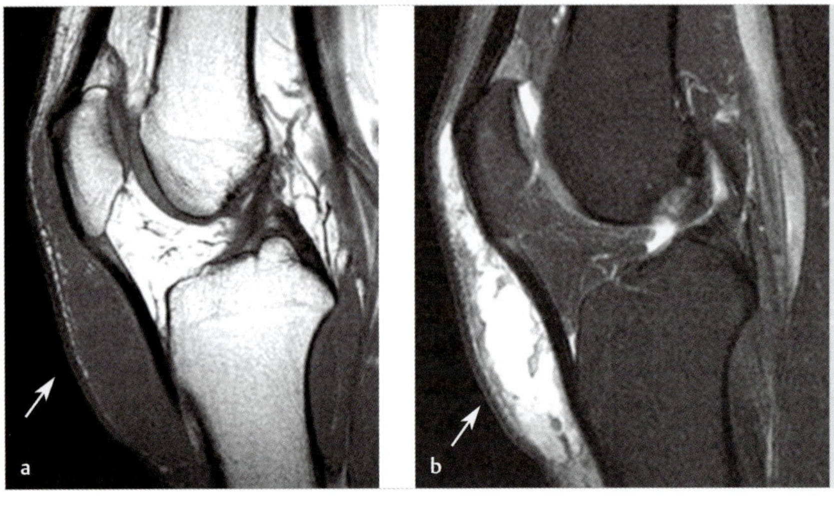

Fig. 11.43 Prepatellar bursitis. Sagittal T1-weighted **(a)** and fat-suppressed proton-density **(b)** images show distention of the prepatellar and superficial infrapatellar bursae (*arrow on each*). (Reproduced with permission from Cascio BM, Khanna AJ, Glait SA, Cosgarea AJ, Johnson TS, Reeder JD. The Knee. In: Khanna AJ, ed. MRI for orthopaedic surgeons. New York: Thieme; 2010:164–201.)

Table 11.6 Osteonecrosis

Parameter	SPONK	Atraumatic Osteonecrosis of the Knee[a]
Location	Medial femoral condyle	Multiple condyles, tibial involvement 20–30%
Distribution	Subcortical	Epiphyseal, metaphyseal, and diaphyseal common
Age	Usually > 60 y	Usually < 45 y
Bilateral knee involvement	< 1%	> 80%
Hip involvement	None	90%
Associated risk factors	Rare	> 80% (e.g., steroids, alcohol)
Pathogenesis	May represent microtrauma, osteoarthritis, or osteopenia	Multiple theories regarding etiology

[a]Synonym: secondary or steroid-associated osteonecrosis.

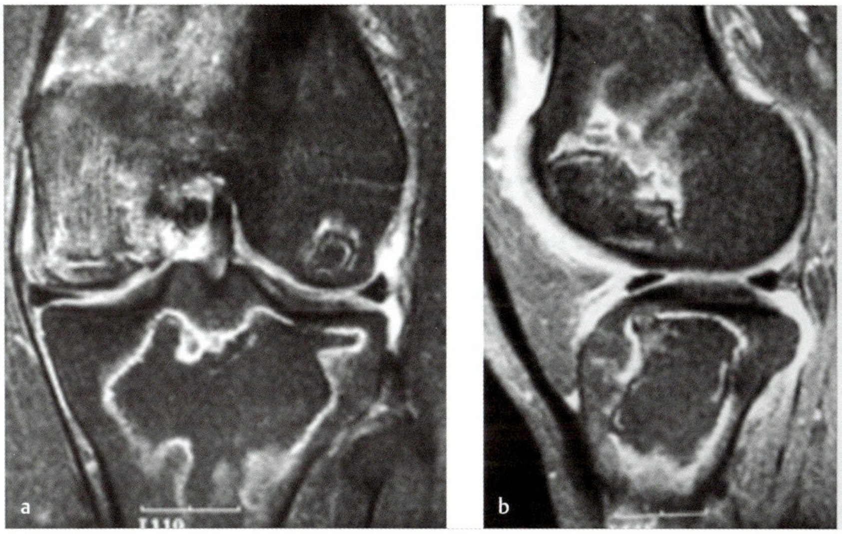

Fig. 11.44 Osteonecrosis. Sagittal T2-weighted **(a)** and proton-density **(b)** images of the left knee show findings typical for osteonecrosis of the distal femur. Note the extensive reactive and stress-related bone marrow edema, subchondral fracture and cyst formation involving the lateral femoral condyle. (Reproduced with permission from Khanna AJ, Cosgarea AJ, Mont MA, et al. Magnetic resonance imaging of the knee. Current techniques and spectrum of disease. J Bone Joint Surg Am. 2001; 83-A Suppl 2 Pt 2:128–141).

common atraumatic causes are alcohol abuse and steroid use, but others include the following:

- Gaucher disease.
- Sickle cell disease.
- Caisson disease.

The exact pathophysiology has not been elucidated, but it may involve an increase in intramedullary pressure. Bone death in the femur can involve the epiphysis, metaphysis, and diaphysis. Occurring less commonly than true bone infarcts, osteonecrosis can develop secondary to an insufficiency fracture of the subchondral bone.[59] This process, termed *SPONK*, usually occurs in female patients > 60 years old and involves the medial femoral condyle.[60] Lesions > 2.3 cm^2 have been found to lead to osteoarthritis.[61]

MRI is the most sensitive and specific imaging modality for the early detection of osteonecrosis (▶ Table 11.6[59,60,61,62,63]). Early diagnosis is an important consideration because patients usually do not feel pain until the joint surface collapses, and early detection may make it possible to prevent this collapse. MRI also can help distinguish osteonecrosis and SPONK. On MRI, SPONK appears as a wedge-shaped lesion in the epiphysis that can extend into the metaphysis and diaphysis. In contrast, atraumatic osteonecrosis shows a serpiginous zone demarcating the extent of the necrosis and bone marrow edema. There can be marrow conversion from red to fatty marrow. The fatty marrow shows high signal intensity on T1-weighted images.[64]

The lesion in SPONK is subchondral and usually involves collapse and flattening of the medial femoral condyle. It is important to distinguish between these two forms of osteonecrosis because the treatments differ.

11.3.9 Degenerative Joint Disease

Traditionally, much of the evaluation of degenerative knee disease is accomplished with conventional radiographs. In the past, when the findings and symptoms of degenerative knee disease were severe enough, patients were offered total joint arthroplasty. Currently, for active, physiologically young patients with unicompartmental disease, there are other options, including the following:

- High tibial osteotomy.
- Unicompartmental arthroplasty.
- Arthroscopy (for selected patients).

In the active patient with degenerative knee disease, there are findings on MRI that potentially can be addressed, at least temporarily, with less extensive procedures than total knee arthroplasty; these findings include the following:

- Scarring of the suprapatellar pouch.
- Complex meniscus tears with flap formation.
- Localized cartilage lesions.
- Scarring and adhesions of the infrapatellar fat pad.

Osteophyte formation is a common finding in degenerative disease and contributes to the painful loss of motion of the knee. Typically, flexion contractures occur, which substantially hinder a patient's gait. When flexion contractures occur because of a mechanical block to extension, identification of these offending osteophytes allows for planning for their surgical removal.

11.3.10 Degenerative Meniscus

Degenerative meniscus refers to a meniscus with complex tears and attenuation. Eventually, the meniscus can be extruded out of the compartment and into the medial or lateral gutter. Initially, primarily one compartment is affected, depending on the alignment of the knee. Because varus alignment is more common, the medial compartment, which receives most of the forces, usually is affected primarily. Typically, associated cartilage changes also occur.

It is useful to note whether the meniscus appears to have degenerated severely and is not functional, or is still essentially intact. This may correlate with the clinical presence of mechanical symptoms and can help with patient counseling and surgical planning.

11.3.11 Adhesion Formation

Part of the degenerative process is the formation of adhesions, especially in the suprapatellar pouch. Adhesions appear as dark gray or black bands on MRI. These bands can be seen in the suprapatellar pouch, usually on sagittal T2-weighted images, running from the quadriceps tendon posteriorly to the synovium on the anterior aspect of the femur. The adhesions are thought to affect the biomechanics of the knee adversely and are a source of ongoing investigation. Plicae and adhesions combine to decrease the volume of the knee joint and create pseudocompartments. If the steroid and anesthetic are injected into a pseudocompartment, then the painful areas of the knee are not exposed to the medications, which provides an explanation for why an injection into the knee may not relieve symptoms. Arthroscopic release of adhesions increases the volume of the knee joint and may restore more normal knee mechanics.[65]

11.3.12 Anterior Interval Scarring

The anterior interval of the knee is the space between the patellar tendon and the intermeniscal ligament. It usually is filled with a mobile, compliant fat pad. Surgery and senescent degeneration of the knee are associated with scarring and decreased compliance of this space. Physical examination of such patients reveals an immobile, noncompliant patellar tendon. If the patient complains of pain in the anterior aspect of the knee in the presence of fat pad scaring, then an excision or release of this scar tissue may be beneficial. Similar to suprapatellar adhesions, anterior interval scarring appears as linear bands. These bands begin on the patellar tendon and traverse the fat pad to insert on the anterior aspect of the proximal tibia, anterior to the ACL.

11.3.13 Baker (Popliteal) Cyst

A Baker cyst (▶ Fig. 11.45), a classic finding in degenerative knee disease, is a collection of fluid that has escaped from the joint posteromedially and rests between the medial head of gastrocnemius and semimembranosus. Although the term *Baker cyst* is commonly used to describe all popliteal or synovial cysts in the region of the knee, it should be noted that the term is intended for those cases in which the gastrocnemiosemimembranosus bursa is involved.[66] The typical MRI findings include a mass in the posterior fossa with uniform low signal on T1-weighted images and high signal on T2-weighted images. The walls of the cyst are well circumscribed.

These collections can decompress spontaneously into the lower leg. Operative treatment is not usually recommended, but when the cyst is present for an extended period of time, the contents may become gelatinous, and then open or arthroscopic intervention may be beneficial.

11.4 Infectious Conditions: Osteomyelitis and Septic Effusion

Osteomyelitis and septic effusion are common forms of infection involving the knee. MRI is the most sensitive and specific test for the presence of osteomyelitis.[67,68,69] Osteomyelitis causes an intense reaction of the surrounding tissue characterized by edema that is seen on T2-weighted images. A septic effusion can be seen on T2-weighted images as a fluid collection within the joint. Septic arthritis also causes associated bone marrow edema. The diagnosis can be confirmed with aspiration or biopsy, and surgical intervention and antibiotics usually are necessary for treatment. Periarticular

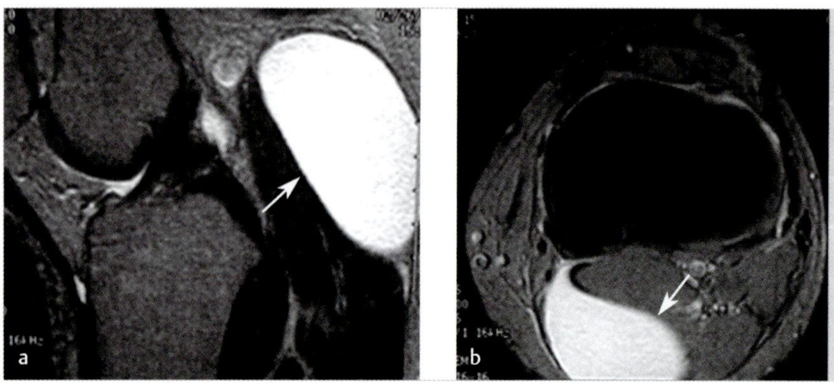

Fig. 11.45 Baker cyst. Sagittal **(a)** and axial **(b)** T2-weighted images show distension of the gastrocnemiosemimembranosus bursa (*arrow on each*). (Reproduced with permission from Cascio BM, Khanna AJ, Glait SA, Cosgarea AJ, Johnson TS, Reeder JD. The Knee. In: Khanna AJ, ed. MRI for orthopaedic surgeons. New York: Thieme; 2010:164–201.)

osteomyelitis involving the knee joint exhibits a bone marrow edema pattern, hyperintense relative to normal marrow on T2-weighted and STIR images and hypointense on T1-weighted images. Loss of the normally sharply defined low-signal-intensity cortical margin may occur with osteolysis secondary to infection. An intraosseous fluid collection, surrounded by edema, suggests the presence of focal bone abscess. Septic arthritis may simply exhibit features of a knee joint effusion, but frequently synovial thickening is observed, particularly conspicuous on contrast-enhanced fat-suppressed T1-weighted imaging. Also, a periarticular bone marrow edema pattern may be identified secondary to generalized hyperemia, independent of actual osseous infection.

11.5 Postoperative Findings

11.5.1 Postoperative Meniscus: Partial Meniscectomy, Repair, and Allograft Replacement

Surgical approaches to the treatment of meniscal tears include meniscal debridement or partial meniscectomy, meniscal repair, and meniscal allograft placement. These techniques are designed to stabilize the meniscus while maintaining its shock-absorbing and loading-force-distributing properties. The procedures share the clinical goals of pain relief, restoration of mechanical function, and prevention or mitigation of the development of chondromalacia and osteoarthritis.

With partial meniscectomy, as little meniscal tissue as possible is resected to stabilize the articular margin of the meniscus without excessively exposing the articular cartilage to unprotected impaction forces. Thus, on MRI, it is common to identify the presence of a small tear involving the meniscal remnant (► Fig. 11.46). The tear may be stable and asymptomatic. Also, because the process of meniscal debridement creates a new articular surface, intrameniscal MRI findings related to myxoid degeneration may abut the surgically recontoured articular margin, converting internal meniscal signal (noted on T1-weighted or proton-density images) into surface-communicating signal and potentially creating the false impression of a meniscal tear.[4] Although T2-weighted imaging and MR arthrography may be used to differentiate converted intrameniscal signal intensity from a true surface defect into which fluid can dissect, evidence of a surface tear does not necessarily translate to a clinically relevant cause of a patient's symptoms. However, if, after a conservative partial meniscectomy, a large tear involving the meniscal remnant is noted on MRI, its clinical significance probably is similar to that of a tear in a nondebrided meniscus. After partial meniscectomy, severe tears identified with MRI typically exhibit a complex signal pattern, flap, or fragment displacement or show progressive enlargement on serial postoperative MRI studies[70] (► Fig. 11.47).

Meniscal repairs, typically performed in the context of a vertical longitudinal tear, often continue to manifest abnormal signal, communicating with the meniscal articular surfaces despite successful stabilization of the meniscus (► Fig. 11.48).[4,70,71,72]

On serial follow-up MRI examinations, the apparent surface defect may remain, but if progressive development of adjacent chondromalacia or osseous stress reaction is not identified on subsequent postoperative studies and the morphology of the tear remains unchanged, surgical stabilization of the meniscus probably has been achieved (► Fig. 11.49). In the case of a displaced meniscal tear that has been repaired, the MRI study should reveal normal meniscal morphology and positioning but, again, the linear tear may remain evident. MR arthrography does not statistically improve accuracy in detecting postoperative meniscal tears and, like nonarthrographic techniques, cannot distinguish between residual and recurrent tears.[73] In addition, the penetration or imbibition of gadolinium contrast material in a repaired

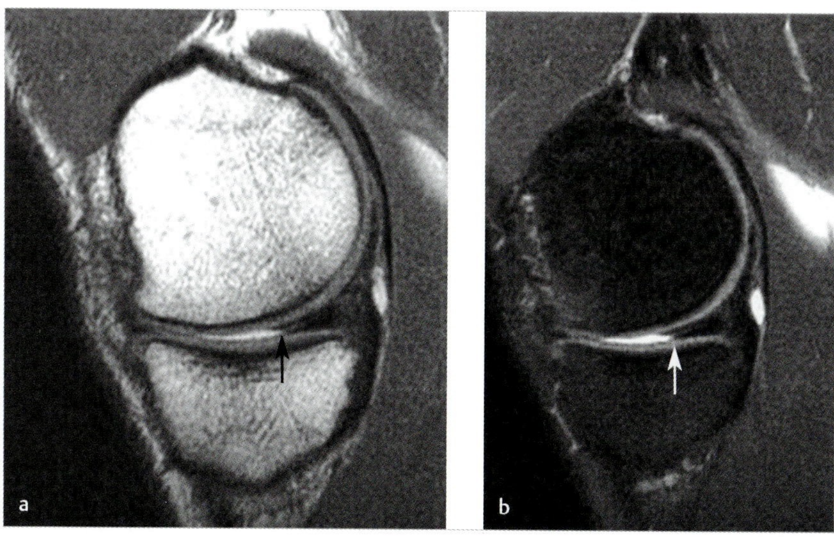

Fig. 11.46 Partial meniscectomy. Sagittal proton-density **(a)** and sagittal fat-suppressed T2-weighted **(b)** images show blunting of the anterior margin of the posterior horn of the medial meniscus, consistent with meniscal debridement. The small horizontal tear (*arrow*) is unlikely to be clinically symptomatic. (Reproduced with permission from Cascio BM, Khanna AJ, Glait SA, Cosgarea AJ, Johnson TS, Reeder JD. The Knee. In: Khanna AJ, ed. MRI for orthopaedic surgeons. New York: Thieme; 2010:164–201.)

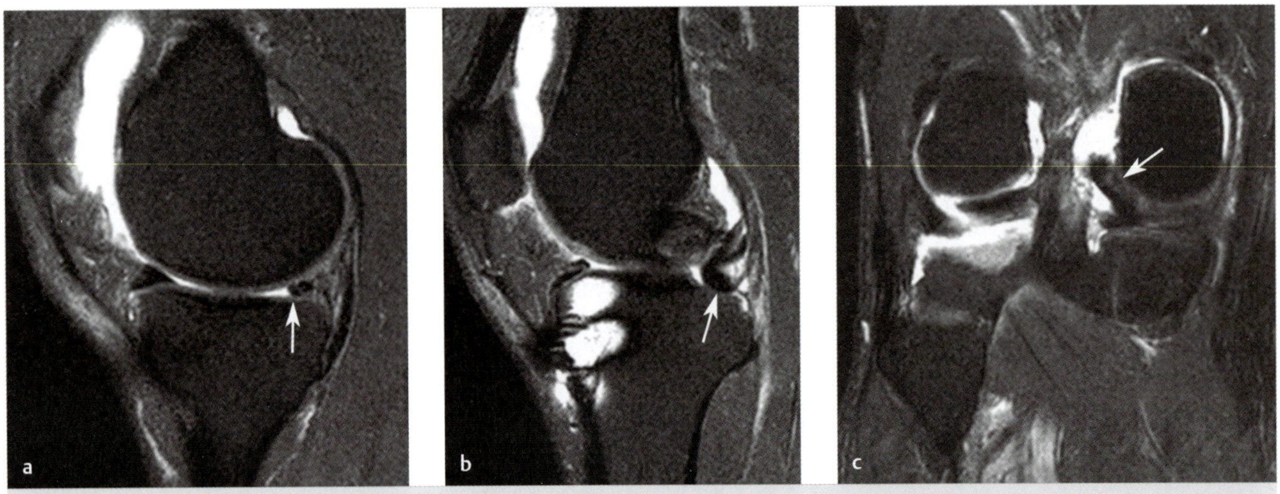

Fig. 11.47 Postoperative medial meniscus with displaced flap. **(a)** A sagittal fat-suppressed proton-density image shows decreased meniscal size (*arrow*), a finding that may simply reflect partial resection of the meniscus. **(b)** A sagittal fat-suppressed proton-density image, obtained lateral to the **(a)** image, shows posterior central displacement of a large meniscal flap, arising from the posterior horn remnant (*arrow*). **(c)** A fat-suppressed coronal T2-weighted image of the right knee shows central displacement of a large posterior medial meniscal flap (*arrow*). (Reproduced with permission from Cascio BM, Khanna AJ, Glait SA, Cosgarea AJ, Johnson TS, Reeder JD. The Knee. In: Khanna AJ, ed. MRI for orthopaedic surgeons. New York: Thieme; 2010:164–201.)

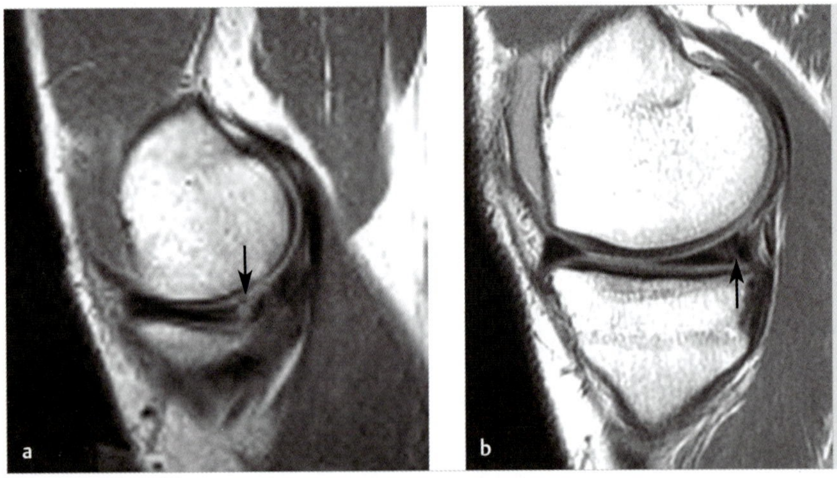

Fig. 11.48 Meniscal repair. **(a)** A preoperative sagittal T1-weighted image shows a peripheral vertical longitudinal tear (*arrow*) of the posterior horn of the medial meniscus. **(b)** A postoperative sagittal T1-weighted image in the same patient shows persistent signal communication with the articular surface of the meniscus (*arrow*). (Reproduced with permission from Cascio BM, Khanna AJ, Glait SA, Cosgarea AJ, Johnson TS, Reeder JD. The Knee. In: Khanna AJ, ed. MRI for orthopaedic surgeons. New York: Thieme; 2010:164–201.)

meniscal defect does not necessarily indicate that the tear is unstable or responsible for a patient's symptoms.

With meniscal allograft procedures, MRI is used to evaluate the positioning of the graft. A graft may be displaced by loading, shearing, or rotational forces that exceed its surgical attachments; by traction related to capsular adhesions or contracture; or by adjacent arthrofibrosis (▶ Fig. 11.50). On MRI, tears involving the meniscal allograft exhibit the same features as do tears in a native meniscus,[74] although the anterior one-third of grafts have been shown to have lower specificity and positive predictive value than the mid-body and posterior one-third.[75]

In summary, care must be taken when assessing the clinical significance of MRI findings after meniscal surgery. Most importantly, a meniscal tear involving a debrided or repaired meniscus, even when observed with MR arthrography, does not necessarily correlate with the presence of clinical symptoms or functional impairment. In a patient with knee pain and a history of meniscal surgery, the role of MRI includes evaluation of the knee for other potential symptom-producing pathology, especially chondromalacia, osseous stress injury, and osteonecrosis.[76,77]

11.5.2 ACL Reconstruction

The ACL graft is a low-signal-intensity structure that should run in continuity along approximately the same trajectory as the native ACL (▶ Fig. 11.51). Metallic screws can be identified on MRI by their very dark appearance. Ferromagnetic artifact is a major problem because it can conceal local pathology. Bioabsorbable

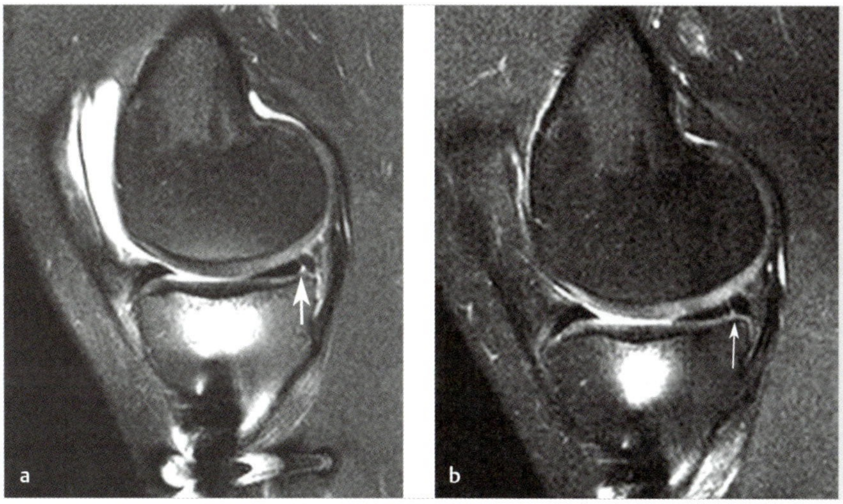

Fig. 11.49 Meniscal repair. (a) A sagittal fat-suppressed proton-density image, obtained after repair of a peripheral vertical longitudinal tear, shows persistent signal communication with the articular surface of the posterior horn of the medial meniscus (*arrow*). (b) A sagittal fat-suppressed proton-density image, obtained 1 year later in the same patient, shows stability of the meniscal signal pattern (*arrow*). (Reproduced with permission from Cascio BM, Khanna AJ, Glait SA, Cosgarea AJ, Johnson TS, Reeder JD. The Knee. In: Khanna AJ, ed. MRI for orthopaedic surgeons. New York: Thieme; 2010:164–201.)

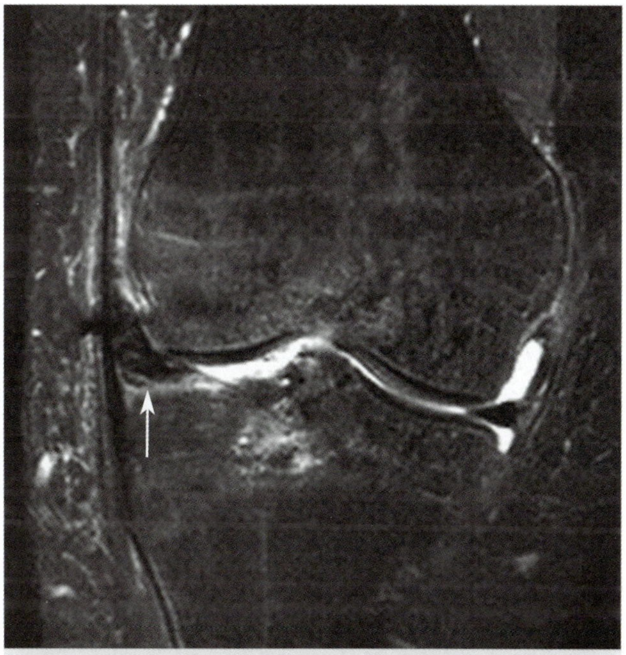

Fig. 11.50 This coronal fat-suppressed T2-weighted image of the right knee shows fibrous adherence of the meniscal allograft (*arrow*) to the iliotibial band (ITB) with lateral displacement of the allograft. (Reproduced with permission from Cascio BM, Khanna AJ, Glait SA, Cosgarea AJ, Johnson TS, Reeder JD. The Knee. In: Khanna AJ, ed. MRI for orthopaedic surgeons. New York: Thieme; 2010:164–201.)

interference screws and transfixion pins do not cause such artifact. Absorption of bioabsorbable implants varies but takes at least 1 year.[78] Cyst formation is a normal finding around these screws as they are absorbed.[79] Bone graft incorporation, which can take 3 years or more,[79] also can be seen on MRI.

MRI is useful in the evaluation of the patient who has had an ACL reconstruction or repair. The study should be evaluated for the following (▶ Fig. 11.52):

- Presence or absence of graft failure.
- Impingement.
- Arthrofibrosis.
- Placement and orientation of the graft, hardware, and tunnels.

Most ACL grafts are 8 to 10 mm wide, and the associated tunnel should not be more than 10 mm wide on MRI. Widening of the graft tunnel can be seen with chronic remodeling secondary to the presence of a ganglion cyst or other process, within the graft.

All of the potential sites of osseous impingement should be evaluated carefully, including the following:

- Intercondylar roof.
- Intra-articular entrance zones of the bone tunnels.
- Side walls of the intercondylar fossa.

The MRI findings in roof impingement include posterior bowing of the graft caused by contact of the graft against the roof, increased signal in the distal two-thirds of the graft, and placement of the tibial tunnel anterior to the slope of the intercondylar roof when the knee is in an extended position.[80]

11.5.3 Cyclops Lesion

The cyclops lesion results from granulation tissue overgrowth of remnant ACL. This entity, which can cause a painful block to full extension, is found anterior to the ACL graft and is easily seen on MRI (▶ Fig. 11.53). Patients with a cyclops lesion often also have associated anterior compartment degenerative changes, which should be evaluated carefully on the MRI study. Care should be taken to differentiate cyclops lesions from partial ACL graft tears.[81]

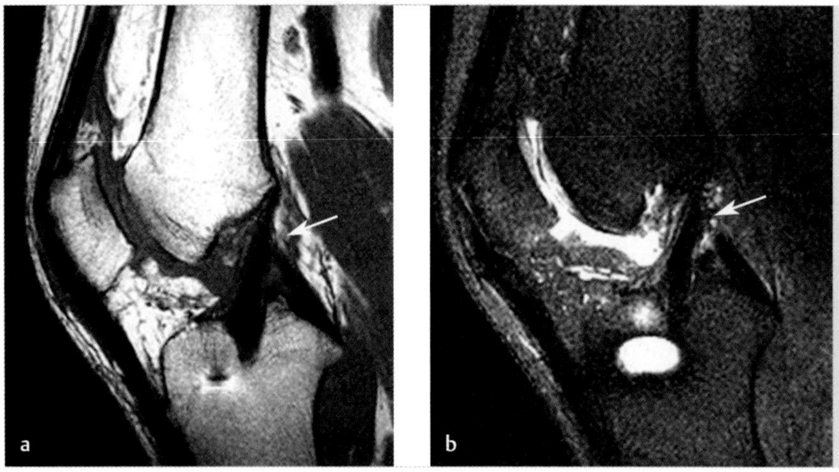

Fig. 11.51 Anterior cruciate ligament (ACL) reconstruction. Sagittal T1-weighted **(a)** and fat-suppressed proton-density **(b)** images show normal ACL graft trajectory (*arrow on each*). (Reproduced with permission from Cascio BM, Khanna AJ, Glait SA, Cosgarea AJ, Johnson TS, Reeder JD. The Knee. In: Khanna AJ, ed. MRI for orthopaedic surgeons. New York: Thieme; 2010:164–201.)

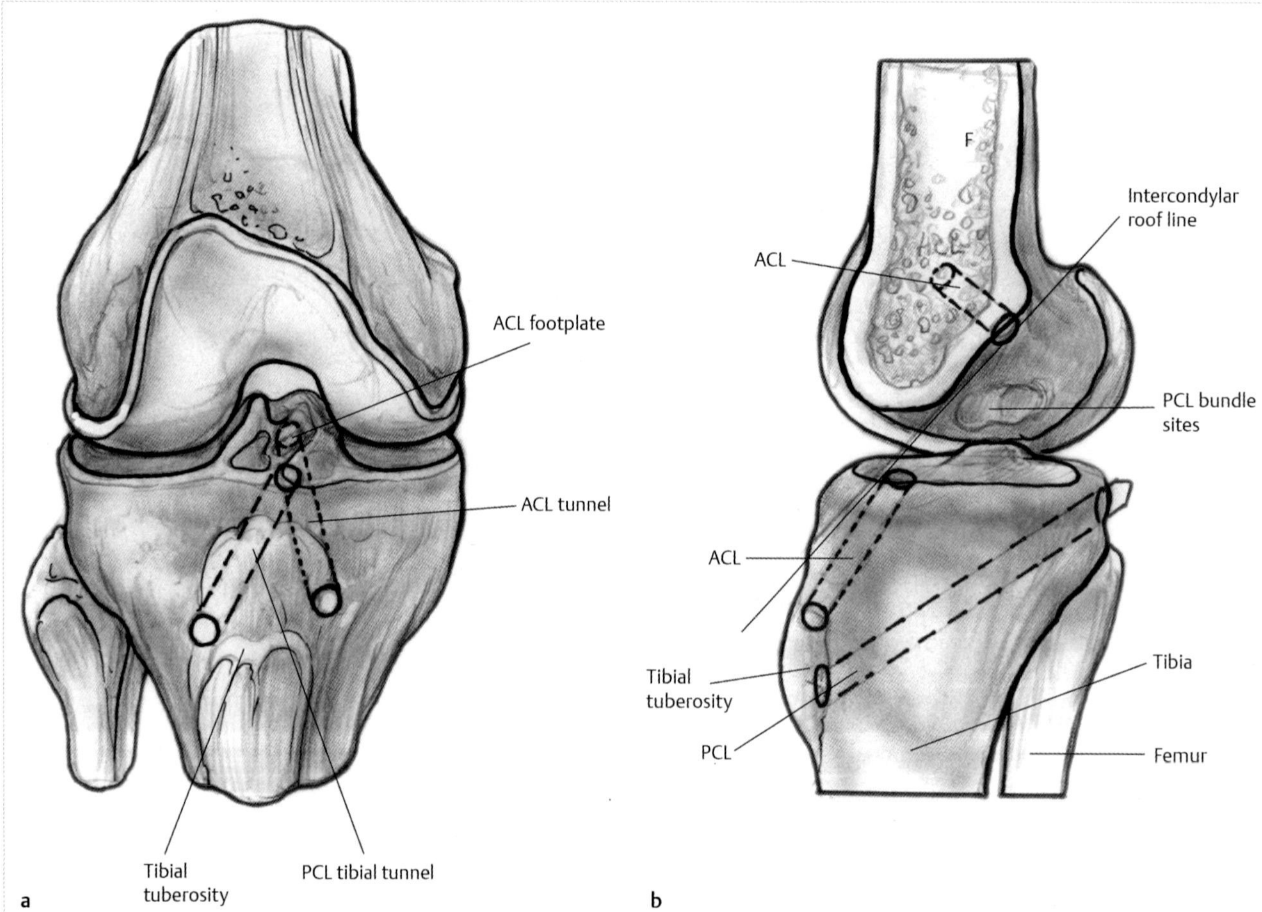

Fig. 11.52 Artist's sketches illustrating optimal anterior cruciate ligament (ACL) and posterior cruciate ligament (PCL) graft tunnel placement in the coronal **(a)** and sagittal **(b)** planes. (Reproduced with permission from Cascio BM, Khanna AJ, Glait SA, Cosgarea AJ, Johnson TS, Reeder JD. The Knee. In: Khanna AJ, ed. MRI for orthopaedic surgeons. New York: Thieme; 2010:164–201.)

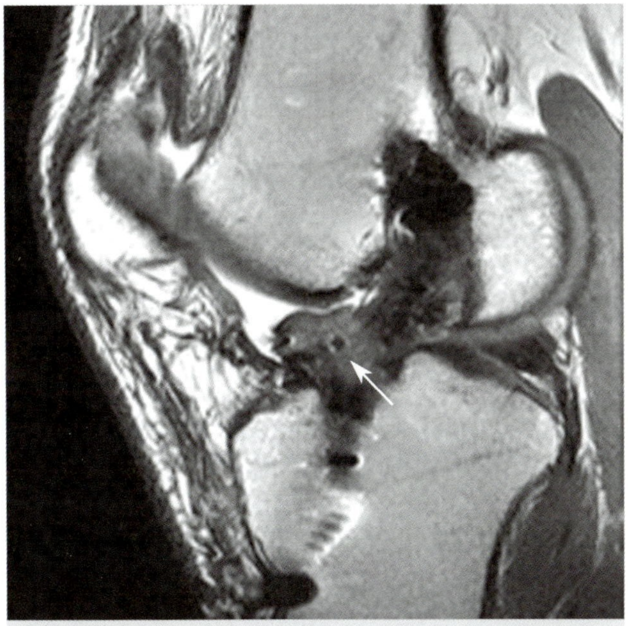

Fig. 11.53 This sagittal proton-density image shows focal arthrofi brosis, consistent with a cyclops lesion (*arrow*), anterior to an ACL graft. (Reproduced with permission from Cascio BM, Khanna AJ, Glait SA, Cosgarea AJ, Johnson TS, Reeder JD. The Knee. In: Khanna AJ, ed. MRI for orthopaedic surgeons. New York: Thieme; 2010:164–201.)

11.6 Summary

The workup of knee trauma typically begins with conventional radiographs. A number of traumatic pathologies, however, are better evaluated using MRI. This includes hemarthrosis, meniscal tears, ligament disruption, and extensor mechanism injury. Coronal and sagittal T1-weighted and T2-weighted images are the views of choice in most cases. Exceptions to this include posterolateral corner injuries which are best visualized using coronal oblique T2-weighted images.

MRI is not the preferred imaging modality for assessing degenerative knee disease, although it can help identify related issues within the joint. Loose chondral or osseous fragments, especially unmineralized lesions, may be visualized on MRI when not seen on conventional radiographs. In active patients with degenerative disease, MRI can be used to identify concomitant joint issues such as meniscal tears. These issues are typically easier to address and may temporarily reduce knee symptoms until an arthroplasty is required.

Although knee MRI is most commonly utilized in the setting of trauma, it can be used to assist in evaluating a host of additional pathologies including tumors, adhesions, infection, tendinitis, and stress fractures. MRI is the most specific and sensitive study for early detection of osteonecrosis. It can also be used to evaluate the status of previous surgeries including meniscectomy, meniscal repair, and ligament reconstruction. When evaluating any knee pathology with MRI, it is important to correlate the MRI findings with conventional radiographs, history, and physical exam findings.

11.7 Common Clinical Questions

1. Patella baja on sagittal MRI or lateral knee x-ray would correlate with which measurement and diagnosis?
   a) Insall-Salvati ratio of 1.4, quadriceps tendon rupture.
   b) Insall-Salvati ratio of 1.5, patellar tendon rupture.
   c) Insall-Salvati ratio of 0.5, quadriceps tendon rupture.
   d) Insall-Salvati ratio of 0.5, ACL rupture.
   e) Insall-Salvati ratio of 1.0, medial patellofemoral ligament rupture.

2. What type of meniscus pathology can result in a "Double-PCL" sign on MRI? On what image sequence is this evident?
   a) Bucket handle lateral meniscus tear, coronal images.
   b) Longitudinal lateral meniscus tear, sagittal images.
   c) Bucket handle lateral meniscus tear, sagittal images.
   d) Discoid meniscus, coronal images.
   e) Bucket handle medial meniscus tear, sagittal images.

3. What imaging sequence is best suited for evaluating posterolateral corner injuries of the knee?
   a) Coronal oblique T2-weighted images.
   b) Sagittal oblique T1-weighted images.
   c) Axial T2-weighted images.
   d) Sagittal oblique T2-weighted images.
   e) Axial oblique T2-weighted images.

4. Bakers cysts are fluid collections with low signal on T1-weighted imaging and high signal on T2-weighted images that are found between what knee structures?
   a) Medial meniscus, MCL.
   b) Medial head of the gastrocnemius, semimembranosus.
   c) Lateral head of the gastrocnemius, biceps femoris.
   d) MCL, semitendinosus.
   e) Popliteus, biceps femoris.

5. What is the typical pattern of bone bruising that can be seen on MRI in the setting of an acute ACL tear?
   a) Anteromedial aspect of the lateral femoral condyle, posterior aspect of the lateral tibial plateau.
   b) Posterolateral aspect of the lateral femoral condyle, anterior aspect of the lateral tibial plateau.
   c) Posterior aspect of the lateral femoral condyle, anterolateral aspect of the lateral tibial plateau.
   d) Anteromedial aspect of the medial femoral condyle, anterior aspect of the medial tibial plateau.
   e) Anterolateral aspect of the lateral femoral condyle, posterior aspect of the lateral tibial plateau.

References

[1] Hardaker WT, Jr, Garrett WE, Jr, Bassett FH, III. Evaluation of acute traumatic hemarthrosis of the knee joint. South Med J. 1990; 83(6):640–644

[2] Khanna AJ, Cosgarea AJ, Mont MA, et al. Magnetic resonance imaging of the knee. Current techniques and spectrum of disease. J Bone Joint Surg Am. 2001; 83-A Suppl 2 Pt 2:128–141

[3] Cheung LP, Li KC, Hollett MD, Bergman AG, Herfkens RJ. Meniscal tears of the knee: accuracy of detection with fast spin-echo MR imaging and arthroscopic correlation in 293 patients. Radiology. 1997; 203(2):508–512
[4] Deutsch AL, Mink JH, Fox JM, et al. Peripheral meniscal tears: MR findings after conservative treatment or arthroscopic repair. Radiology. 1990; 176(2): 485–488
[5] Justice WW, Quinn SF. Error patterns in the MR imaging evaluation of menisci of the knee. Radiology. 1995; 196(3):617–621
[6] Kaplan PA, Nelson NL, Garvin KL, Brown DE. MR of the knee: the significance of high signal in the meniscus that does not clearly extend to the surface. AJR Am J Roentgenol. 1991; 156(2):333–336
[7] Kornick J, Trefelner E, McCarthy S, Lange R, Lynch K, Jokl P. Meniscal abnormalities in the asymptomatic population at MR imaging. Radiology. 1990; 177(2):463–465
[8] Rubin DA, Paletta GA, Jr. Current concepts and controversies in meniscal imaging. Magn Reson Imaging Clin N Am. 2000; 8(2):243–270
[9] Stoller DW, Martin C, Crues JV, III, Kaplan L, Mink JH. Meniscal tears: pathologic correlation with MR imaging. Radiology. 1987; 163(3):731–735
[10] Wright DH, De Smet AA, Norris M. Bucket-handle tears of the medial and lateral menisci of the knee: value of MR imaging in detecting displaced fragments. AJR Am J Roentgenol. 1995; 165(3):621–625
[11] Kelley EA, Berquist TH. Knee. In: Berquist TH, ed. MRI of the musculoskeletal system. Philadelphia, PA: Lippincott Williams & Wilkins; 2006:303–429
[12] De Smet AA, Norris MA, Yandow DR, Quintana FA, Graf BK, Keene JS. MR diagnosis of meniscal tears of the knee: importance of high signal in the meniscus that extends to the surface. AJR Am J Roentgenol. 1993; 161(1):101–107
[13] Rubin DA. MR imaging of the knee menisci. Radiol Clin North Am. 1997; 35 (1):21–44
[14] Peterfy CG, Janzen DL, Tirman PFJ, van Dijke CF, Pollack M, Genant HK. "Magic-angle" phenomenon: a cause of increased signal in the normal lateral meniscus on short-TE MR images of the knee. AJR Am J Roentgenol. 1994; 163(1):149–154
[15] Turner DA, Rapoport MI, Erwin WD, McGould M, Silvers RI. Truncation artifact: a potential pitfall in MR imaging of the menisci of the knee. Radiology. 1991; 179(3):629–633
[16] Tuckman GA, Miller WJ, Remo JW, Fritts HM, Rozansky MI. Radial tears of the menisci: MR findings. AJR Am J Roentgenol. 1994; 163(2):395–400
[17] Costa CR, Morrison WB, Carrino JA. Medial meniscus extrusion on knee MRI: is extent associated with severity of degeneration or type of tear? AJR Am J Roentgenol. 2004; 183(1):17–23
[18] Vande Berg BC, Malghem J, Poilvache P, Maldague B, Lecouvet FE. Meniscal tears with fragments displaced in notch and recesses of knee: MR imaging with arthroscopic comparison. Radiology. 2005; 234(3):842–850
[19] Lecas LK, Helms CA, Kosarek FJ, Garret WE. Inferiorly displaced flap tears of the medial meniscus: MR appearance and clinical significance. AJR Am J Roentgenol. 2000; 174(1):161–164
[20] Vande Berg BC, Poilvache P, Duchateau F, et al. Lesions of the menisci of the knee: value of MR imaging criteria for recognition of unstable lesions. AJR Am J Roentgenol. 2001; 176(3):771–776
[21] Gentili A, Seeger LL, Yao L, Do HM. Anterior cruciate ligament tear: indirect signs at MR imaging. Radiology. 1994; 193(3):835–840
[22] Umans H, Wimpfheimer O, Haramati N, Applbaum YH, Adler M, Bosco J. Diagnosis of partial tears of the anterior cruciate ligament of the knee: value of MR imaging. AJR Am J Roentgenol. 1995; 165(4):893–897
[23] Cone RO III. Knee. Section B. Imaging sports-related injuries of the knee. In: DeLee JC, Drez D Jr, Miller MD, eds. DeLee and Drez's orthopaedic sports medicine: principles and practice. Philadelphia, PA: WB Saunders; 2003:1595–1652
[24] Graf BK, Cook DA, De Smet AA, Keene JS. "Bone bruises" on magnetic resonance imaging evaluation of anterior cruciate ligament injuries. Am J Sports Med. 1993; 21(2):220–223
[25] Robertson PL, Schweitzer ME, Bartolozzi AR, Ugoni A. Anterior cruciate ligament tears: evaluation of multiple signs with MR imaging. Radiology. 1994; 193(3):829–834
[26] Tung GA, Davis LM, Wiggins ME, Fadale PD. Tears of the anterior cruciate ligament: primary and secondary signs at MR imaging. Radiology. 1993; 188 (3):661–667
[27] McCauley TR, Moses M, Kier R, Lynch JK, Barton JW, Jokl P. MR diagnosis of tears of anterior cruciate ligament of the knee: importance of ancillary findings. AJR Am J Roentgenol. 1994; 162(1):115–119
[28] Goldman AB, Pavlov H, Rubenstein D. The Segond fracture of the proximal tibia: a small avulsion that reflects major ligamentous damage. AJR Am J Roentgenol. 1988; 151(6):1163–1167
[29] Gross ML, Grover JS, Bassett LW, Seeger LL, Finerman GA. Magnetic resonance imaging of the posterior cruciate ligament. Clinical use to improve diagnostic accuracy. Am J Sports Med. 1992; 20(6):732–737
[30] Sonin AH, Fitzgerald SW, Friedman H, Hoff FL, Hendrix RW, Rogers LF. Posterior cruciate ligament injury: MR imaging diagnosis and patterns of injury. Radiology. 1994; 190(2):455–458
[31] Sonin AH, Fitzgerald SW, Hoff FL, Friedman H, Bresler ME. MR imaging of the posterior cruciate ligament: normal, abnormal, and associated injury patterns. Radiographics. 1995; 15(3):551–561
[32] Escobedo EM, Mills WJ, Hunter JC. The "reverse Segond" fracture: association with a tear of the posterior cruciate ligament and medial meniscus. AJR Am J Roentgenol. 2002; 178(4):979–983
[33] Shelbourne KD, Rubinstein RA, Jr. Methodist Sports Medicine Center's experience with acute and chronic isolated posterior cruciate ligament injuries. Clin Sports Med. 1994; 13(3):531–543
[34] O'Donoghue DH. Treatment of acute ligamentous injuries of the knee. Orthop Clin North Am. 1973; 4(3):617–645
[35] Yao L, Dungan D, Seeger LL. MR imaging of tibial collateral ligament injury: comparison with clinical examination. Skeletal Radiol. 1994; 23 (7):521–524
[36] D'Amato MJ, Bach BR Jr. Knee. Section J: Anterior cruciate ligament injuries. Part 1: Anterior cruciate ligament reconstruction in the adult. In: DeLee JC, Drez D Jr, Miller MD, eds. DeLee and Drez's orthopaedic sports medicine: principles and practice. Philadelphia, PA: WB Saunders; 2003:2012–2067
[37] LaPrade RF, Gilbert TJ, Bollom TS, Wentorf F, Chaljub G. The magnetic resonance imaging appearance of individual structures of the posterolateral knee. A prospective study of normal knees and knees with surgically verified grade III injuries. Am J Sports Med. 2000; 28(2):191–199
[38] Hughston JC, Eilers AF. The role of the posterior oblique ligament in repairs of acute medial (collateral) ligament tears of the knee. J Bone Joint Surg Am. 1973; 55(5):923–940
[39] Green NE, Allen BL. Vascular injuries associated with dislocation of the knee. J Bone Joint Surg Am. 1977; 59(2):236–239
[40] Good L, Johnson RJ. The dislocated knee. J Am Acad Orthop Surg. 1995; 3(5): 284–292
[41] Sonin AH, Fitzgerald SW, Bresler ME, Kirsch MD, Hoff FL, Friedman H. MR imaging appearance of the extensor mechanism of the knee: functional anatomy and injury patterns. Radiographics. 1995; 15(2):367–382
[42] Felus J, Kowalczyk B. Age-related differences in medial patellofemoral ligament injury patterns in traumatic patellar dislocation: case series of 50 surgically treated children and adolescents. Am J Sports Med. 2012; 40(10): 2357–2364
[43] Petri M, von Falck C, Broese M, et al. Influence of rupture patterns of the medial patellofemoral ligament (MPFL) on the outcome after operative treatment of traumatic patellar dislocation. Knee Surg Sports Traumatol Arthrosc. 2013; 21(3):683–689
[44] Camp CL, Stuart MJ, Krych AJ, et al. CT and MRI measurements of tibial tubercle-trochlear groove distances are not equivalent in patients with patellar instability. Am J Sports Med. 2013; 41(8):1835–1840
[45] Zeiss J, Saddemi SR, Ebraheim NA. MR imaging of the quadriceps tendon: normal layered configuration and its importance in cases of tendon rupture. AJR Am J Roentgenol. 1992; 159(5):1031–1034
[46] De Smet AA, Best TM. MR imaging of the distribution and location of acute hamstring injuries in athletes. AJR Am J Roentgenol. 2000; 174(2):393–399
[47] Koulouris G, Connell D. Evaluation of the hamstring muscle complex following acute injury. Skeletal Radiol. 2003; 32(10):582–589
[48] Connell DA, Schneider-Kolsky ME, Hoving JL, et al. Longitudinal study comparing sonographic and MRI assessments of acute and healing hamstring injuries. AJR Am J Roentgenol. 2004; 183(4):975–984
[49] Brossmann J, Preidler KW, Daenen B, et al. Imaging of osseous and cartilaginous intraarticular bodies in the knee: comparison of MR imaging and MR arthrography with CT and CT arthrography in cadavers. Radiology. 1996; 200(2):509–517
[50] Capps GW, Hayes CW. Easily missed injuries around the knee. Radiographics. 1994; 14(6):1191–1210
[51] Yu JS, Petersilge C, Sartoris DJ, Pathria MN, Resnick D. MR imaging of injuries of the extensor mechanism of the knee. Radiographics. 1994; 14 (3):541–551
[52] Yu JS, Popp JE, Kaeding CC, Lucas J. Correlation of MR imaging and pathologic findings in athletes undergoing surgery for chronic patellar tendinitis. AJR Am J Roentgenol. 1995; 165(1):115–118
[53] Kato Y, Oshida M, Aizawa S, Saito A, Ryu J. Discoid lateral menisci in Japanese cadaver knees. Mod Rheumatol. 2004; 14(2):154–159

[54] Rao PS, Rao SK, Paul R. Clinical, radiologic, and arthroscopic assessment of discoid lateral meniscus. Arthroscopy. 2001; 17(3):275–277
[55] Rohren EM, Kosarek FJ, Helms CA. Discoid lateral meniscus and the frequency of meniscal tears. Skeletal Radiol. 2001; 30(6):316–320
[56] Berquist TH. Musculoskeletal imaging companion. Philadelphia, PA: Lippincott Williams & Wilkins; 2002
[57] Wantanabe M, Takeda S, Ikeuchi H. Atlas of arthroscopy. Berlin: Springer-Verlag; 1979
[58] Monllau JC, León A, Cugat R, Ballester J. Ring-shaped lateral meniscus. Arthroscopy. 1998; 14(5):502–504
[59] Yamamoto T, Bullough PG. Spontaneous osteonecrosis of the knee: the result of subchondral insufficiency fracture. J Bone Joint Surg Am. 2000; 82(6):858–866
[60] Ecker ML, Lotke PA. Spontaneous osteonecrosis of the knee. J Am Acad Orthop Surg. 1994; 2(3):173–178
[61] Rozing PM, Insall J, Bohne WH. Spontaneous osteonecrosis of the knee. J Bone Joint Surg Am. 1980; 62(1):2–7
[62] Ramnath RR, Kattapuram SV. MR appearance of SONK-like subchondral abnormalities in the adult knee: SONK redefined. Skeletal Radiol. 2004; 33 (10):575–581
[63] Yates PJ, Calder JD, Stranks GJ, Conn KS, Peppercorn D, Thomas NP. Early MRI diagnosis and non-surgical management of spontaneous osteonecrosis of the knee. Knee. 2007; 14(2):112–116
[64] Vande Berg BC, Gilon R, Malghem J, Lecouvet F, Depresseux G, Houssiau FA. Correlation between baseline femoral neck marrow status and the development of femoral head osteonecrosis in corticosteroid-treated patients: a longitudinal study by MR imaging. Eur J Radiol. 2006; 58(3):444–449
[65] Millett PJ, Steadman JR. The role of capsular distention in the arthroscopic management of arthrofibrosis of the knee: a technical consideration. Arthroscopy. 2001; 17(7):E31
[66] Lindgren PG, Willén R. Gastrocnemio-semimembranosus bursa and its relation to the knee joint. I. Anatomy and histology. Acta Radiol Diagn (Stockh). 1977; 18(5):497–512
[67] Bancroft LW. MR imaging of infectious processes of the knee. Magn Reson Imaging Clin N Am. 2007; 15(1):1–11
[68] Kapoor A, Page S, Lavalley M, Gale DR, Felson DT. Magnetic resonance imaging for diagnosing foot osteomyelitis: a meta-analysis. Arch Intern Med. 2007; 167(2):125–132
[69] Pineda C, Vargas A, Rodríguez AV. Imaging of osteomyelitis: current concepts. Infect Dis Clin North Am. 2006; 20(4):789–825
[70] Farley TE, Howell SM, Love KF, Wolfe RD, Neumann CH. Meniscal tears: MR and arthrographic findings after arthroscopic repair. Radiology. 1991; 180 (2):517–522
[71] Davis KW, Tuite MJ. MR imaging of the postoperative meniscus of the knee. Semin Musculoskelet Radiol. 2002; 6(1):35–45
[72] Lim PS, Schweitzer ME, Bhatia M, et al. Repeat tear of postoperative meniscus: potential MR imaging signs. Radiology. 1999; 210(1):183–188
[73] White LM, Schweitzer ME, Weishaupt D, Kramer J, Davis A, Marks PH. Diagnosis of recurrent meniscal tears: prospective evaluation of conventional MR imaging, indirect MR arthrography, and direct MR arthrography. Radiology. 2002; 222(2):421–429
[74] Potter HG, Rodeo SA, Wickiewicz TL, Warren RF. MR imaging of meniscal allografts: correlation with clinical and arthroscopic outcomes. Radiology. 1996; 198(2):509–514
[75] Kim JM, Kim JM, Jeon BS, et al. Comparison of postoperative magnetic resonance imaging and second-look arthroscopy for evaluating meniscal allograft transplantation. Arthroscopy. 2015; 31(5):859–866
[76] Brahme SK, Fox JM, Ferkel RD, Friedman MJ, Flannigan BD, Resnick DL. Osteonecrosis of the knee after arthroscopic surgery: diagnosis with MR imaging. Radiology. 1991; 178(3):851–853
[77] Dandy DJ, Jackson RW. Meniscectomy and chondromalacia of the femoral condyle. J Bone Joint Surg Am. 1975; 57(8):1116–1119
[78] Cossey AJ, Kalairajah Y, Morcom R, Spriggins AJ. Magnetic resonance imaging evaluation of biodegradable transfemoral fixation used in anterior cruciate ligament reconstruction. Arthroscopy. 2006; 22(2):199–204
[79] Macarini L, Murrone M, Marini S, Mocci A, Ettorre GC. [MRI in ACL reconstructive surgery with PDLLA bioabsorbable interference screws: evaluation of degradation and osteointegration processes of bioabsorbable screws]. Radiol Med (Torino). 2004; 107(1–2):47–57
[80] Watanabe BM, Howell SM. Arthroscopic findings associated with roof impingement of an anterior cruciate ligament graft. Am J Sports Med. 1995; 23(5):616–625
[81] Simpfendorfer C, Miniaci A, Subhas N, Winalski CS, Ilaslan H. Pseudocyclops: two cases of ACL graft partial tears mimicking cyclops lesions on MRI. Skeletal Radiol. 2015; 44(8):1169–1173

Answers to Common Clinical Questions

1. Answer: c. The Insall-Salvati ratio is determined by dividing the length of the patellar tendon (measured from the inferior pole of the patella to the tendon insertion on the tibia) by the length of the patella (measured from the superior pole to the inferior pole). A normal ratio is between 0.8-1.2. When the quadriceps tendon is ruptured, the superior soft tissue attachment to the patella is disrupted and the patella translates inferiorly resulting in patella baja. With inferior translation of the patella, the measurement for the patellar tendon length decreases and thus our resulting Insall-Salvati ratio also decreases.
2. Answer: e. A bucket handle tear of the meniscus occurs when a vertical longitudinal tear displaces centrally, potentially causing symptoms of locking within the knee. When the medial meniscus is involved, the medial fragment of the tear displaces inferiorly to the PCL. On sagittal imaging, the displaced fragment can often be seen parallel to the PCL in the intercondylar notch which creates the "Double-PCL" sign.
3. Answer: a. Posterolateral corner injuries of the knee are difficult to diagnose due to complex and variable anatomy in the area. This is makes it especially troublesome to obtain clear imaging. The best images to evaluate and diagnose posterolateral corner injuries are coronal oblique T2-weighted images. Injury to the posterolateral corner will show increased signal intensity on T2-weighted images due to underlying edema.
4. Answer: b. Bakers cysts are common finding in patients with degenerative knee disease. They occur when fluid leaks out of the joint capsule posteromedially and accumulates between the medial head of the gastrocnemius and the semimembranosus. These posterior fossa masses are well circumscribed on MRI and are typically treated non-operatively.
5. Answer: e. Acute ACL tears typically occur during a noncontact twisting injury in which the knee is forced into a valgus position with a planted foot. The resulting pattern of bone bruising seen on MRI is a result of the initial pivot shift rotation stress which causes lateral sided bone bruising. Bruising is typically seen in the anterolateral aspect of the lateral femoral condyle and the posterior aspect of the medial tibial plateau. Additional bruising may also be seen in the posterior aspect of the medial tibial plateau due to a subsequent return to normal alignment after the initial injury.

12 The Foot and Ankle

Casey Jo Humbyrd, Shadpour Demehri, Delaram Shakoor, Rebecca Cerrato, and James R. Ficke

Abstract

This chapter introduces the reader to the anatomy and orthopaedic conditions of the foot and ankle. The text focuses on common pathology and provides a useful reference for all, from experienced radiologists to novice surgeons. Particular focus is given to sports conditions of the foot and ankle, with information on differentiating normal anatomy from injuries. The variety of MRI diagnostic tools is discussed, especially as important to surgical techniques. The chapter also highlights postsurgical imaging techniques.

Keywords: Achilles tendon, ankle, bone marrow edema, foot, fractures, ligaments, osteochondral lesions, soft-tissue disorders, sprains, tendons

12.1 Imaging of the Normal Anatomy

12.1.1 Osseous Structures

The ankle and foot have complex anatomy, including several small osseous structures, supporting ligaments, and tendons. The ankle joint complex comprises three distinct articulations, which enable ankle/hindfoot motion: the tibiotalar, talocalcaneal (subtalar), and talocalcaneonavicular (transverse-tarsal) joints. The subtalar joint is a uniaxial joint with three separate articulation facets on the superior aspect of the calcaneus. The distal tibiofibular joint is regarded as the core part of the tibiotalar joint, but it is sometimes considered a distinct joint.[1] The foot can be divided into three functional and anatomic regions. The hindfoot consists of the talus and the calcaneus, which is connected to the midfoot by the talonavicular joint and the calcaneocuboid joint, also known as the Chopart or midtarsal joint.[2] The midfoot contains the cuboid, navicular, and three cuneiforms. The midfoot bones form lateral and medial longitudinal arches, as well as the transverse arch, which collectively creates a half-dome.[3] Metatarsal and sesamoid bones, as well as phalanges, constitute the forefoot. The Lisfranc or tarsometatarsal joint separates the forefoot from the midfoot.[4]

12.1.2 Ligaments

The ankle and tarsal bones are embraced by multiple ligaments, which stabilize and support their articulations. They are observed as linear low-signal-intensity structures on T1- and T2-weighted images, as well as intermediate-weighted proton-density (PD) magnetic resonance imaging (MRI) sequences.[5] These structures are highly prone to pathology, and injured ligaments appear as disrupted or irregular structures with signal alterations, which are best visualized on fluid-sensitive sequences. These structures can be categorized into the following five complexes according to their position and anatomy: lateral collateral ligament complex, distal tibiofibular syndesmosis, medial collateral ligament complex, plantar calcaneonavicular ligament, and the sinus tarsi.

The lateral collateral ligament complex includes the anterior talofibular ligament (ATFL), calcaneofibular ligament (CFL), and posterior talofibular ligament (PTFL). The primary function of the lateral collateral ligament complex is to restrain movement of the talus and calcaneus in relation to the tibia and fibula, and they are considered the primary lateral stabilizer of the ankle joint.[6] Sprains of the ankle during plantar flexion and inversion are associated with lateral collateral ligament complex injury and represent > 20% of sport-related injuries and 85% of pathologies associated with ankle sprain.[7] CFL is best viewed in the oblique coronal plane, whereas the axial view is ideal for detection of ATFL and PTFL pathologies (▶ Fig. 12.1).

The distal tibiofibular syndesmosis is a ligamentous complex consisting of anterior, transverse, and posterior tibiofibular ligaments and the interosseous ligament. It is best displayed in axial and oblique coronal planes. The syndesmosis unites the distal aspect of the tibia and fibula and is commonly injured after dorsiflexion and external rotation, which can lead to ankle instability, pain, and ultimately secondary osteoarthritis.[8]

The medial collateral ligament complex, also known as the deltoid ligament, works as the main stabilizer of the axially loaded ankle. The deep layer of this ligament is intra-articular and acts synergistically with the superficial layer to stabilize the ankle by preventing valgus, rotational, and pronation forces on the talus. The deep layer, which is covered by synovium, includes anterior and posterior deep tibiotalar ligaments, whereas the tibionavicular, tibiocalcaneal, tibiospring, and posterior superficial tibiotalar ligaments form the superficial layer. The deltoid ligament stabilizes the talocalcaneonavicular joint and assists the posterior tibialis tendon in stabilizing the medial plantar arch. Both layers of the deltoid ligament and their various components are well visualized on coronal and axial MR images. Deltoid injuries are more common than previously thought and are usually associated with lateral ligament injuries. Although several conditions can lead to deltoid pathology, most patients report multiple episodes of ankle sprain, and the single mechanism of injury that leads to deltoid pathology is still unidentified.[9]

The plantar calcaneonavicular ligament, also known as the spring ligament complex, connects the calcaneus and navicular bones. This ligament plays a critical role in the stability of the midfoot and medial plantar arch by supporting the talar head. It consists of the following three components: the superomedial (SM), medioplantar oblique, and inferoplantar longitudinal bands. The SM and oblique medioplantar bands are best seen on coronal and axial MR images, whereas the inferoplantar band is best visualized on sagittal and axial images.[10]

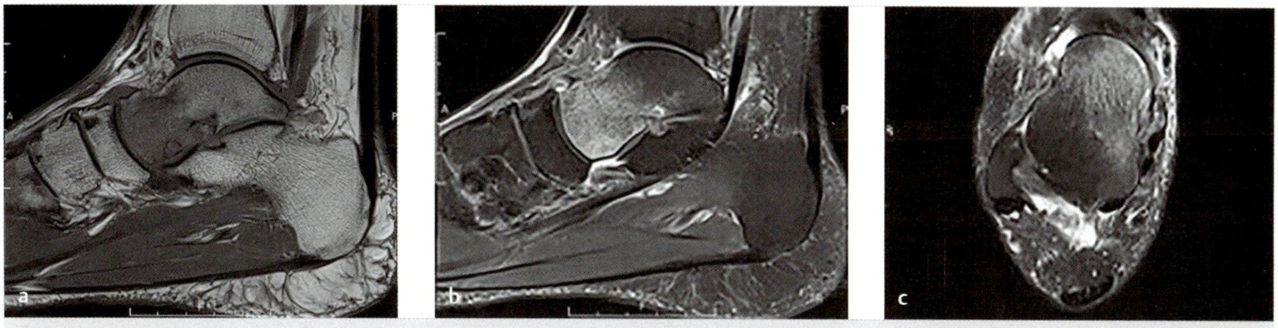

Fig. 12.1 Talus bone contusion. **(a)** Sagittal T1-weighted image showing a talar neck and head contusion. Note the low signal within the talar head and neck with an ill-defined margin. No definitive fracture line is visualized. **(b)** Sagittal T2-weighted image of the same patient showing high signal within the talar head and neck region signifying edema within the bone marrow. **(c)** Axial T2-weighted image showing the high signal within the medial portion of the talar head and neck region. The cortex is intact.

The sinus tarsi is defined as a recess between the calcaneus and talus, which is open to the lateral aspect of the hindfoot. This nonosseous structure separates the posterior facet of the subtalar joint from the anterior and middle facets. It includes neurovascular structures, as well as interosseous talocalcaneal and cervical ligaments, fat, and the extensor retinaculum. The sinus tarsi ligaments assist in maintaining the medial plantar arch by stabilizing the talus and the calcaneus.[10]

12.1.3 Tendons

Several tendons cross the ankle joint and are clustered into four groups according to location. The anterior tibial tendon, extensor digitorum longus tendon, and extensor hallucis longus tendon form the anterior compartment. Peroneus longus and peroneus brevis tendons pass under the lateral malleolus. Achilles and plantaris tendons are in the posterior compartment. On the medial side, the posterior tibial tendon (PTT) and flexor digitorum longus tendon (FDLT) pass under the medial malleolus; the flexor hallucis longus tendon (FHLT) lies under the sustentaculum tali. Ankle tendons are best visualized in axial MRI planes, and an oblique coronal plane is an alternative to observe lateral and medial tendons along their course under the lateral and medial malleoli.[11]

12.2 Specialized Pulse Sequence and Imaging Protocols

To obtain ankle MRI with adequate spatial resolution for diagnosis of injuries in small ankle structures, one must perform several sequences, including T1-, T2-, and intermediate-weighted PD and fast spin-echo (FSE) sequences with and without fat suppression.[12] For axial, coronal, and sagittal plane images of the ankle, the patient lies in the supine position with the ankle in neutral position. Foot imaging requires oblique planes, which are obtained perpendicular and parallel to the long axis of metatarsal bones. The patient lies in a supine position with the ankle in 20-degree plantar flexion to attain better visualization of the CFL and the fat plane between peroneal tendons and to reduce the magic angle effect (MAE).[13]

With recent advancements in magnet strength and MRI protocols, there have been marked improvements in contrast-to-noise and signal-to-noise ratios, which lead to high spatial resolution optimized for foot and ankle imaging.[14] Although high spatial resolution is required for maintaining diagnostic accuracy, overall imaging time is also a major concern. Therefore, application of parallel imaging technology and phased array coils are associated with reduced scan time, which prevents motion artifacts and allows for more in protocol design.[14] Furthermore, 3D imaging techniques substantially shorten scan time. 3D imaging has the capability of multiplanar reformation using small isotropic voxels with image quality that has comparable accuracy to that of 2D FSE sequence in detecting ligamentous injuries, as well as damage of other small structures.[15,16] Despite the recent developments in MRI techniques, imaging of thin, incongruent articular surface cartilage of the tibiotalar joint still poses a major challenge.[17,18] However, application of 2D FSE and fluid-sensitive sequences, including T2-weighted and PD-weighted sequences, has provided satisfactory results in evaluating articular cartilage defects of the talus dome.[19] Furthermore, with the advent of ultra-high-field scanners with 3D reconstruction, as well as advanced imaging sequences such as T1-weighted ρ MR sequences, T2 mapping, and sodium imaging, there may be promising results for early detection of cartilage defects of the tibiotalar joint.[17,20,21]

PD-weighted and T2-weighted images with fat suppression are used to detect subtle bone marrow signal alteration related to numerous conditions, including contusion, edema, malignancy, and infection. In the background of dark, normal fatty marrow, an abnormal high-intensity signal suggests pathology.[22] Postoperative MRI can be challenging because of the presence of metallic objects, which obscure MRI findings. Among conventional pulse sequences, the FSE sequence is considered the best option to reduce metallic artifacts. However, novel imaging methods, including multiacquisition variable-resonance image combination (MAVRIC) and slice-encoding for metal artifact correction (SEMAC), have shown promising results in reducing metal artifacts.[23]

MR arthrography (MRA) is another minimally invasive technique that enhances the potential of conventional MRI in viewing musculoskeletal pathologies. Direct MRA involves injection of a mixture of 0.1 to 0.2 mL of gadolinium with 10 mL of normal saline into the joint, until the joint capsule is appropriately distended. Imaging protocol sequence is performed in axial, coronal, and sagittal planes, and the choice of sequences depends on the MR device and the radiologist's preference. However, T1-weighted SE with and without fat saturation and T2-weighted SE with fat suppression should be included to track the location and distribution of the intra-articular gadolinium. Indirect MRA is an alternative technique that requires intravenous administration of a gadolinium-containing contrast agent followed by light exercise. Although this technique does not require direct injection, several uncontrolled variables affect the degree of articular enhancement, resulting in inconsistent image quality.[24,25] Direct MRA improves the accuracy of MRI in evaluating ankle instability and ligamentous injuries. Furthermore, it enhances visualization of intra-articular structures, expanding MRI capabilities in assessing ankle impingement syndromes and identifying synovial disorders, intra-articular fibrosis, and loose bodies. It also provides excellent delineation of articular surfaces, which aids in accurate discrimination of different stages of osteochondral and cartilaginous lesions. It is currently the optimal modality to diagnose adhesive capsulitis or "frozen ankle," confirming the associated diminished joint space volume during intravenous gadolinium administration.[24]

12.3 Systemic Approach to Image Review

Currently, MRI serves a key role in the assessment of soft tissue disorders of the ankle and foot and is also used for early detection of a vast array of osseous-related pathologies in this anatomic location.[22] According to the American College of Radiology appropriateness criteria guideline, MRI is the next best step after conventional radiography in the setting of suspicious pathology and ankle pain persisting for > 6 weeks.[19,26]

12.3.1 Axial and Coronal Planes

Axial and coronal MR images provide optimal visualization of most foot and ankle structures, including ligaments and tendons. Increased signal intensity, irregular contour, thickening, and an abnormal course of ligament are signs of pathology.[27] PD FSE sequences with and without fat saturation are currently being used to detect lateral ligament injury.[6,28] ATFL and PTFL tears are detected at the tip of the fibula, which appears as a C-shaped concave structure on axial images. The ATFL is a distinct thickening of the capsule approximately 16 mm long and 7 mm in diameter. It is composed of two or three bands, which are separated by fat planes. Unlike the ATFL, the PTFL is a multifasciculated structure in which short anterior and long posterior bands are the thickest. The CFL has a diameter of approximately 5 mm with a mean length of 25 mm and is located close to peroneal tendons. Because of the oblique course of the CFL, an oblique coronal plane parallel to the long axis of the ligament has been regarded as superior in assessment of CFL. Obliteration of surrounding fat or presence of fluid in the peroneal tendon sheath may indicate CFL injury.[28]

In axial images with PD-weighted and T2-weighted FSE sequences with and without fat suppression, the anterior tibiofibular ligament and its posterior counterpart are visualized as striated structures with heterogeneous intensity. The fibula appears as a D-shaped structure at the same level at which we can observe the tibial plafond and talar dome. Joint fluid extension into the tibiofibular space or lateral gutter and fibrofatty tissue prolapse are indirect signs of syndesmosis injury.[29,30] Within the deltoid ligament complex, its posterior superficial tibiotalar ligament and tibionavicular ligament are shown in only half of studies, and the anterior tibiotalar ligament is very thin and may not be detected. The oblique coronal plane has been shown to be helpful for superior depiction of the anterior tibiotalar and tibionavicular ligaments. The posterior deep tibiotalar ligament is the strongest and thickest component of the medial collateral ligament and like the PTFL appears heterogeneous on MRI. The absence of its normal striations is considered a sign of acute or chronic injury. Other components may have variable intensity on MRI, and tears of the deltoid ligament should be confirmed by further signs, including altered shape and course. PD-weighted and T2-weighted FSE sequences with and without fat suppression are also used for the assessment of medial capsuloligament complex injuries.[9,31]

The SM band of the spring ligament is separated from the PTT by a 1- to 3-mm space containing loose connective tissue. A ligament diameter of > 4 mm or < 2 mm is considered abnormal. On T2-weighted images, the presence of fluid in the adjacent talonavicular joint leads to enhanced visualization of spring ligament recess and shows a bright signal, which should be differentiated from ligament injury. Spring ligament pathology is depicted in all planes with PD-weighted and T2-weighted sequences; however, the coronal planes are optimal for assessment.[10]

The routine protocol of MRI on Lisfranc injuries includes obtaining axial T1-weighted, PD fat-saturated images along with coronal and sagittal T2-weighted fat-saturated images. The coronal plane is also the best to visualize the integrity of Lisfranc ligaments, which appear as homogeneous or striated structures with low-to-intermediate intensity.[32,33]

Of the medial flexor tendons, at the level of retromalleolar groove and tarsal tunnel, the PTT appears as the largest and most medial. It always appears as an ovoid structure with low signal intensity, with the exception of its insertion to the navicular bone, which appears mildly heterogeneous. A small amount of fluid around the PTT is normal; however, fluid with > 2-mm thickness or a circumferential nature indicates PTT tenosynovitis. Thick PTT with normal or heterogeneous signal intensity suggests tendinopathy, which frequently occurs at its insertion site. MR images with T2-weighted and PD-weighted FSE sequences with and without fat saturation are the modality of choice to assess PTT pathology and further ankle tendons.[34] The PTT, FDLT, and posterior tibialis neurovascular structures lie in a fibro-osseous tunnel called the tarsal tunnel. The tarsal tunnel is located posterior to the medial malleolus, deep to the flexor retinaculum. Entrapment of the posterior tibial nerve by space-occupying lesions, including ganglion cyst or lipoma, is detected easily by using MRI and leads to posterior ankle pain.[27] The FHLT and FDLT also appear as low-signal-intensity structures, and a small amount of fluid in their sheath is normal. However, an increase in tendon size or a signal intensity change should prompt the evaluation for tendinosis or tear.[35]

The Achilles tendon appears homogeneously dark on all sequences. On axial images, it is detected as a flat or slightly concave structure with a normal diameter of < 6 mm. An increase in its diameter or a round shape indicates tendinosis. High, heterogeneous T2-weighted signal intensity within the tendon suggests a partial tear, which may be accompanied by edema and hemorrhage in Kager fat pad in acute conditions. The altered signal in partial tears tends to occur in the posterior part, whereas tendinosis has a central signal-intensity change. Discontinuity and retraction of torn parts of the tendon suggest a complete tear. Inflammation in the paratendon is often detected by irregular or linear zones of altered signal intensity in Kager fat pad.[35,36]

The anterior tibial tendon and extensor hallucis longus tendon are the most anteromedial structures at the ankle joint level, whereas the extensor digitorum longus tendon lies more laterally. Presence of fluid in their sheaths implies the possibility of tenosynovitis, whereas fusiform thickening and altered signal intensity on T1-weighted and PD-weighted images indicates the possibility of partial tear or tendinosis.[37] MAE is a well-known artifact of MRI that occurs when evaluating certain structures, particularly peroneal tendons and the extensor hallucis longus tendon in foot and ankle imaging. To avoid misinterpretation, abnormal findings should not be solely relied on signal intensity, and shape and configuration of these tendons should also be assessed for optimal diagnosis. One should also use other sequences, including T2-weighted sequences, and reconfirm such abnormal signal intensity in all available sequences.[37,38]

12.3.2 Sagittal Planes

In addition to axial and coronal images, sagittal images can provide useful data on the longitudinal course of ankle, soft tissue structures. For example, plantar fascia thickening (> 4 mm) and hyperintensity, which occur in plantar fasciitis, are seen easily on sagittal images.[34,36] Sagittal planes are also used to detect pathologies of osseous structures. Detection of a low-density line in the talar dome on T1-weighted images and a high-density T2-weighted signal line that outlines the avascular region confirms the diagnosis.[39] Regarding osteochondral fracture of the talus, sagittal images also provide useful information on the integrity of overlying articular cartilage. On T1-weighted MR images, osteochondral lesions (OCLs) appear hypointense. On T2-weighted images, OCLs appear as a hyperintense line at the base exhibiting detachment.[19,40]

In summary, MRI has been recognized as the modality of choice for the evaluation of ankle and foot disorders.[22] However, the advantages of robust diagnostic information provided by this modality may be hampered by its overuse. Thorough evaluation of ligament integrity on MRI requires the MRI plane to be parallel to the long axis of the ligaments, and consistent MRI protocols are mandated to reproduce reliable findings.[41] Because of the complex anatomy of the ankle and foot, MRI can produce false-positive results[19,38]; therefore, diagnosis and treatment should not rely solely on MRI findings. MRI data should be used to supplement information from history and physical examination findings to devise a well-informed treatment plan.[19,38]

12.4 Traumatic Conditions

Injuries to the bone are represented on MRI as "bone marrow edema" (BME) and occur on a spectrum ranging from a mild bone contusion to stress fractures. BME is seen as an area within the trabecular bone that is hypointense on T1-weighted images compared with skeletal muscle, but hyperintense on T2-weighted, fat-suppressed, and short tau inversion recovery (STIR) images (▶ Fig. 12.1a–c).[42] It represents edema, hemorrhage, and infarction caused by microscopic fracture of the trabecular bone. BME typically occurs with acute injuries; however, it is also associated with chronic joint pain in athletes caused by repetitive stresses.[43] BME can also occur in patients who are asymptomatic. One study[44] found BME in up to 88% of professional runners. Furthermore, many conditions such as osteomyelitis, bone tumors, osteonecrosis, and osteoporosis can cause BME, which is detectable on MRI; therefore, imaging results must correlate with a thorough history and physical examination to diagnose BME.[45] Some injuries produce certain patterns of BME. For example, approximately 27% of inversion ankle sprains result in contusions of the medial talus. Such subchondral bone lesions may represent elastic deformation of the articular cartilage with resultant disruption of the underlying trabecular microarchitecture.[46]

12.5 Stress Fractures

BME typically resolves within 8 to 12 weeks. However, continued repetitive stress to the area may result in a stress fracture. MRI is useful when there is high clinical suspicion for fracture on conventional radiographs—as many as 20% of injuries are missed on conventional radiographs alone.[43] MRI allows detection of these injuries weeks earlier than does conventional radiography. On radiographs, changes are typically not visible until 10 to 14 days after initial injury, and approximately 50% of bone density must be affected to appear.[45] As with contusions, early changes show increased signal intensity on fluid-sensitive (T2-weighted, fat-suppressed, and STIR) sequences (▶ Fig. 12.2a, b). Further progression of the stress reaction allows visualization on T1-weighted images as a dark area on a white background. In more advanced stress fractures, a distinct fracture line can be seen on T1- and T2-weighted images, appearing as an area of

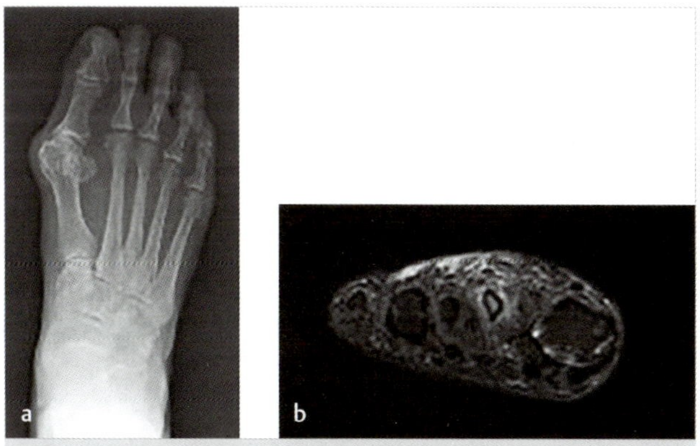

Fig. 12.2 Second metatarsal stress fracture. **(a)** Anteroposterior (AP) radiograph of a patient with 2 weeks of severe forefoot pain and swelling. **(b)** Coronal short tau inversion recovery (STIR) sequence of the patient's foot showing increased signal intensity within the second metatarsal and surrounding periosseous edema.

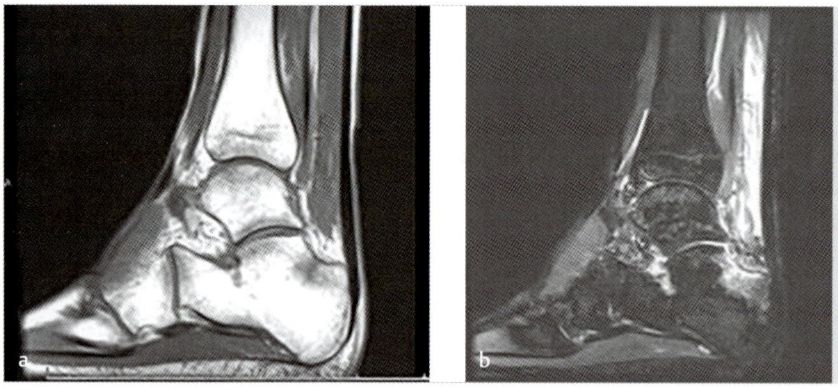

Fig. 12.3 Calcaneal stress fracture. **(a)** Sagittal T1-weighted image of a calcaneal stress fracture showing a fracture line perpendicular to the normal trabecular cancellous stress lines. **(b)** Sagittal T2-weighted image of the calcaneus with marrow edema along the superior region of the body.

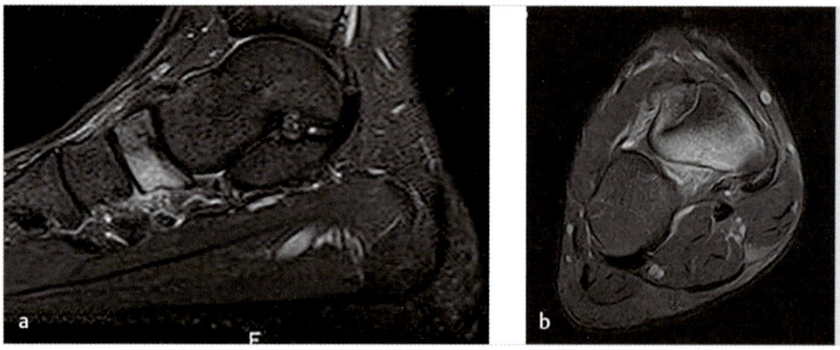

Fig. 12.4 Navicular stress fracture. **(a)** Sagittal short tau inversion recovery (STIR) sequence of an 18-year-old basketball player's foot with 3 months of progressive foot pain showing severe marrow edema in the navicular. **(b)** Coronal T2-weighted image of the same patient showing a sclerotic fracture extending to the dorsal cortex with surrounding marrow edema.

low signal intensity perpendicular to the trabecular lines (▶ Fig. 12.3a, b).[45,47] Below is a grading system recently modified by Nattiv et al[48]:

- Grade 1: Mild marrow or periosteal edema on T2-weighted images; T1-weighted images normal.
- Grade 2: Moderate marrow or periosteal edema; T1-weighted images normal (differs from grade 1 in degree of edema).
- Grade 3: Severe marrow or periosteal edema on T1- and T2-weighted images; no fracture line visible.
- Grade 4: Severe marrow or periosteal edema on T1- and T2-weighted images, plus visible fracture line on either sequence.

Metatarsals are the most common site for stress fractures, followed by the calcaneus; other common locations include the navicular (▶ Fig. 12.4a, b) and the cuboid.[45,47]

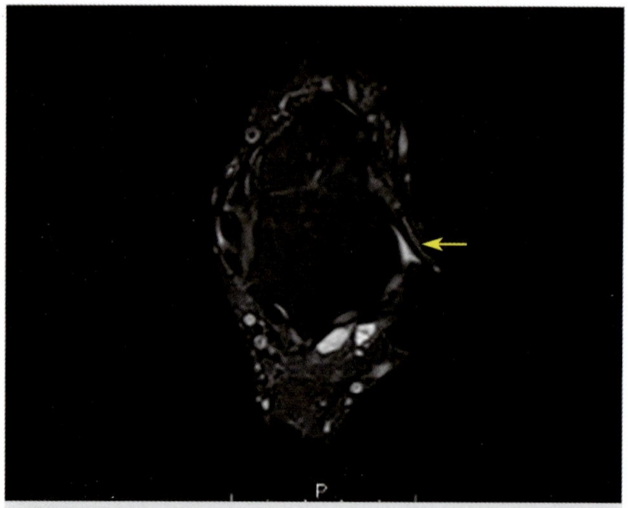

Fig. 12.5 Axial T2-weighted image of an ankle at the level of the inferior fibula. Normal well-defined fibers of the anterior talofibular ligament (ATFL) are seen extending from the fibula to the neck of the talus (*arrow*).

12.5.1 Ankle Sprains

Ankle trauma accounts for 10 to 30% of all sports injuries, of which ankle sprains are the most prevalent—approximately 2 million occur each year in the United States alone.[49] Typically, a thorough physical examination combined with radiography to rule out fracture is sufficient. However, MRI is helpful for diagnosing associated pathology that occurs with ankle sprains such as osteochondritis dissecans lesions or loose bodies, other tendon injuries, and involvement of the syndesmosis.[47,50,51]

The ligaments of the ankle are best evaluated in the axial and coronal planes using thin (3-mm) cuts with the foot in mild plantar flexion. Approximately 20 degrees of plantar flexion decrease the MAE of the peroneal tendons and allow better visualization of the CFL.[49] Normally, ligaments appear on MRI as low-signal-intensity structures between two bones, surrounded by fat signal (▶ Fig. 12.5). Acute injury shows intraligamentous disruption or detachment, wavy striation or thinning, and increased signal on T2-weighted images representing edema or hemorrhage. This is seen within 2 weeks after trauma. Chronic ligament injury does not have the increased T2 signal as seen in acute injury because the edema and hemorrhage have resorbed, typically by 4 weeks. At 15 to 28 days after injury, the ligament may be absent on MRI or appear heterogeneous or wavy/thickened/thinned. Decreased fat signal is seen on T1- and T2-weighted images because of scarring or synovial proliferation. After 7 weeks, any ligamentous defect will have closed, resulting in a thin hypoplastic- or thick hyperplastic-appearing ligament.[49,50,52] The following MRI grading system has been proposed for ligament injuries[50,53]:

- Grade 0: Normal.
- Grade 1 (low-grade sprain): Periligamentous high signal/edema on PD-weighted sequences and no discontinuity of fibers.
- Grade 2 (partial disruption): Partial discontinuity but preserved remnant fibers.
- Grade 3 (complete disruption): Complete discontinuity.
- Grade 4 (scar tissue): Thinned or thickened ligament without discontinuity or periligamentous edema.

Lateral Ankle Sprains

Lateral ankle sprains are the most common ligament injury in the foot and ankle. Injury to the lateral ankle ligamentous complex occurs during forced plantar flexion and inversion of the ankle, resulting in elongation and eventual tearing of the ATFL, followed predictably by the CFL, then the PTFL. Hence, the ATFL is most commonly injured with up to 75% involvement, followed by the ATFL in combination with the CFL in approximately half of injuries. The PTFL is the least commonly injured, occurring in < 10% of patients, and is extremely rare in isolation.[50,54,55] More than two-thirds of patients with lateral ankle sprains have associated pathology on MRI—most commonly bone bruising (70%), but also deltoid ligament injury (up to 50%) and acute lateral OCLs of the talus in approximately 8% of patients.[50,54] In addition, avulsion fractures of lateral ankle ligaments occur in up to 26% of severe sprains.[56]

The ATFL is best seen on axial or axial-oblique T1-weighted or high-resolution PD MRI. It appears as a flat, thin, homogeneous band of low signal intensity arising from the anterior margin of the lateral malleolus and attaches distally to the talar neck. With the foot positioned in slight plantar flexion, the ATFL follows an anteromedial course, positioned at a 45-degree angle to the coronal plane of the tibia. ATFL tears are often associated with a rupture of the anterolateral joint capsule, and joint fluid may be seen in the soft tissues surrounding this area (▶ Fig. 12.6). In chronic injuries, scar tissue can form within the anterolateral gutter and give a triangular appearance on MRI, resulting in the name "meniscoid lesion" because of its similar appearance to the meniscus in the knee (▶ Fig. 12.7). This can cause anterolateral ankle impingement.[49,52]

The CFL is best seen on coronal images, although it can be seen in the axial plane, as well (▶ Fig. 12.8). On T1-weighted sequences, it appears as a low-signal, thin, homogeneous structure deep to the peroneal tendons, coursing posteroinferiorly from the inferior lateral malleolus to the lateral aspect of the calcaneus. When torn, it appears as indistinct, heterogeneous fibers, frequently thickened with obliteration of the surrounding fat

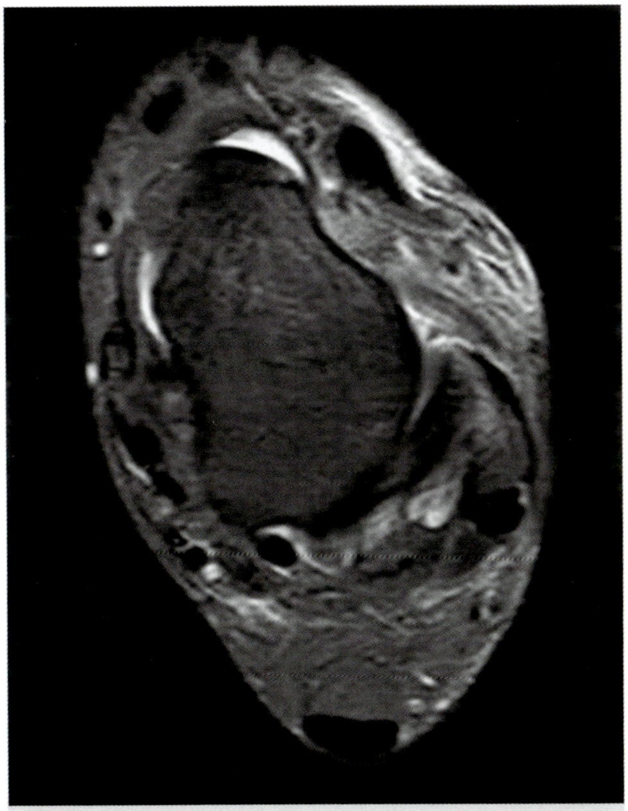

Fig. 12.6 Axial STIR-weighted image of the ankle. No ligament is seen at the expected location of the attachment of the anterior talofibular ligament (ATFL).

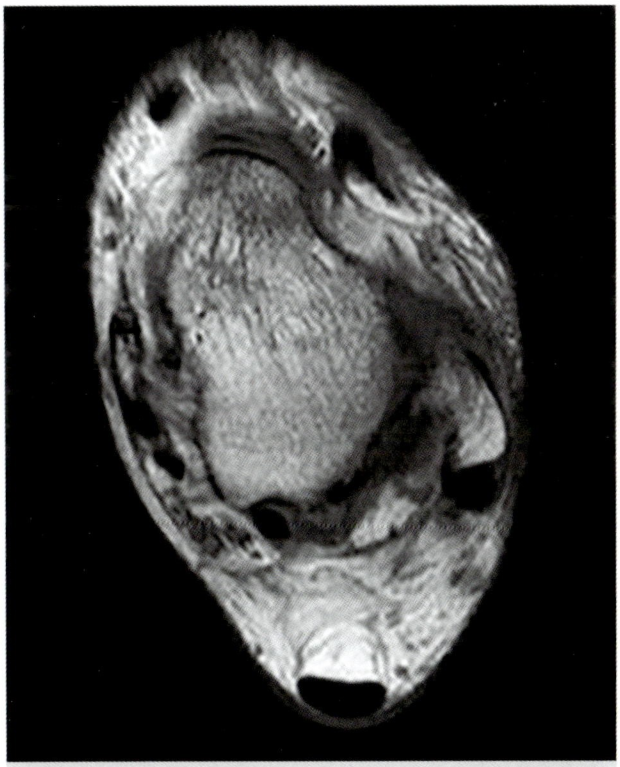

Fig. 12.7 Axial T1-weighted image of the ankle in a patient with chronic lateral ankle instability. Poorly defined fibers extend anteriorly from the fibula, representing a grade-III tear.

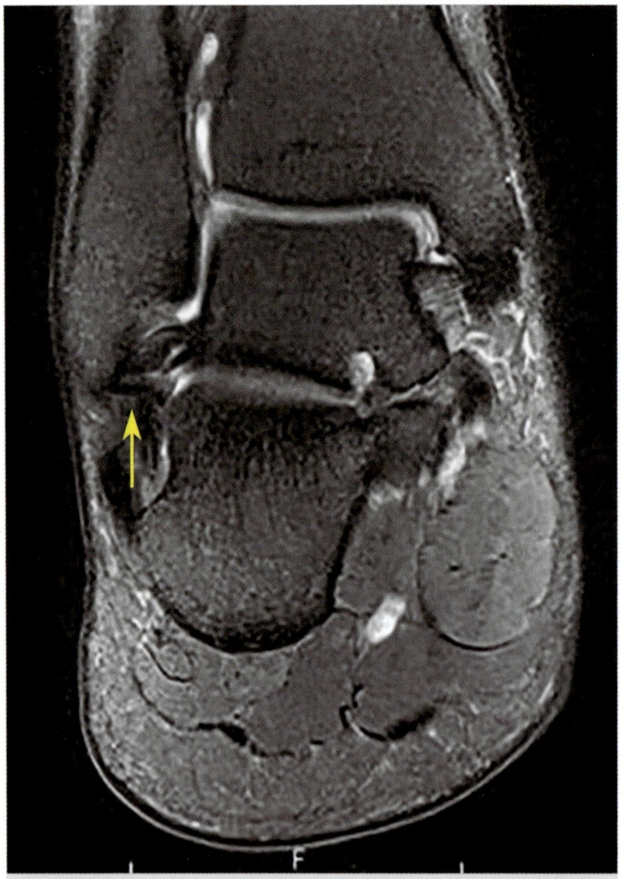

Fig. 12.8 Coronal proton-density (PD) pulse image of a normal calcaneofibular ligament (CFL) ligament (*arrow*).

planes. Because of the proximity of the superior peroneal retinaculum, this can appear thickened or show fluid within the peroneal tendon sheath with CFL tearing.[13,49]

Similar to the CFL, the PTFL is best seen on axial or coronal imaging. It appears as a heterogeneous wide, fan-shaped ligament traveling from the deep portion of the lateral malleolus to its attachment on the mid-posterior talus, following an inferomedial course (▶ Fig. 12.9). It is intracapsular but extrasynovial. Injury produces high T2 signal within the ligament, which becomes irregular and wavy.[49]

Medial Ankle Sprains

Injuries to the deltoid ligament are rare in isolation but frequently are associated with other injuries, particularly lateral ligament injuries (they occur in up to half of all lateral ankle sprains[50]) and lateral malleolus fractures. Although not recommended to differentiate between operative and nonoperative supination–external rotation ankle fractures,[57] physical examination alone is inadequate to detect such fractures. As with lateral ankle ligaments, axial and coronal image sequences are most useful for imaging the deltoid ligament complex. The three portions of the deltoid ligament complex that are routinely visualized on MRI are the tibiospring and tibionavicular ligaments in the superficial layer and the posterior tibiotalar ligament in the deep layer.[55] The deep deltoid

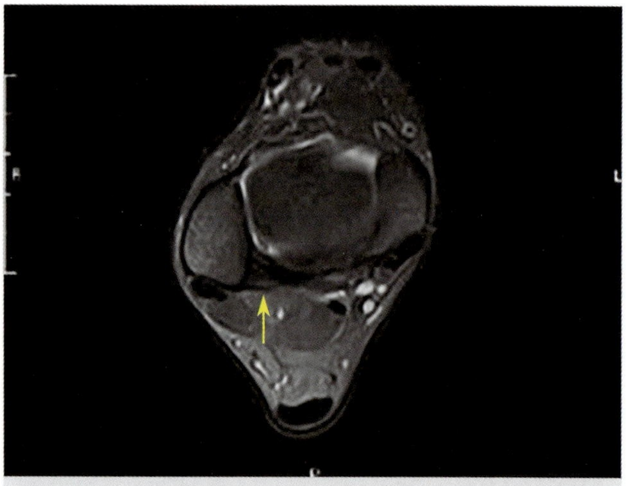

Fig. 12.9 Axial T2-weighted image at the level of the ankle joint showing the normal morphology of the posterior talofibular ligament (PTFL) (*arrow*).

ligament appears striated because of fat tissue on T1-weighted and intermediate-weighted imaging sequences. The superficial portion has low signal intensity on all sequences (▶ Fig. 12.10a, b). Lower-grade sprains show loss of the striated appearance of the deep deltoid ligament on T1- and intermediate-weighted image sequences. In more severe injuries, ligament disruption appears as increased signal on fat-saturated images (▶ Fig. 12.11a, b).[9] Subcutaneous edema on the medial side of the ankle is more indicative of deltoid ligament disruption.[47]

12.5.2 Syndesmotic Injuries

Although the true prevalence of syndesmotic injuries is unknown, it is estimated that they occur in up to 20% of ankle sprains. They are much more common in contact sports such as hockey and football, representing 31 to 74% of ankle sprains.[58,59] Time to return-to-play is substantially greater with syndesmotic injury than with pure lateral ankle sprains, underscoring the importance of establishing a correct diagnosis on presentation. Radiographs may not show medial clear space widening or lateral subluxation of the talus; therefore, if clinical suspicion warrants further imaging studies, MRI may be considered. MRI can show syndesmotic ligament injury with 93 to 100% sensitivity and 96 to 100% specificity.[50,59] Isolated syndesmotic disruption is rare but occurs; most commonly, it is associated with deltoid injury or proximal fibular fracture. Most injuries occur through forced external rotation or hyperdorsiflexion mechanisms, resulting in disruption of the anterior inferior tibiofibular ligament (AITFL), followed by the posterior inferior tibiofibular ligament (PITFL).[49,59] The AITFL and PITFL are seen on two or more sequential axial or coronal images at the level of the ankle joint (▶ Fig. 12.12). The AITFL is trapezoidal, has multiple bands, and has several anatomic variations, making its evaluation on MRI challenging. The PITFL is triangular and inserts broadly onto the tibia. Injury to the syndesmotic ligamentous complex has many presentations on MRI, including

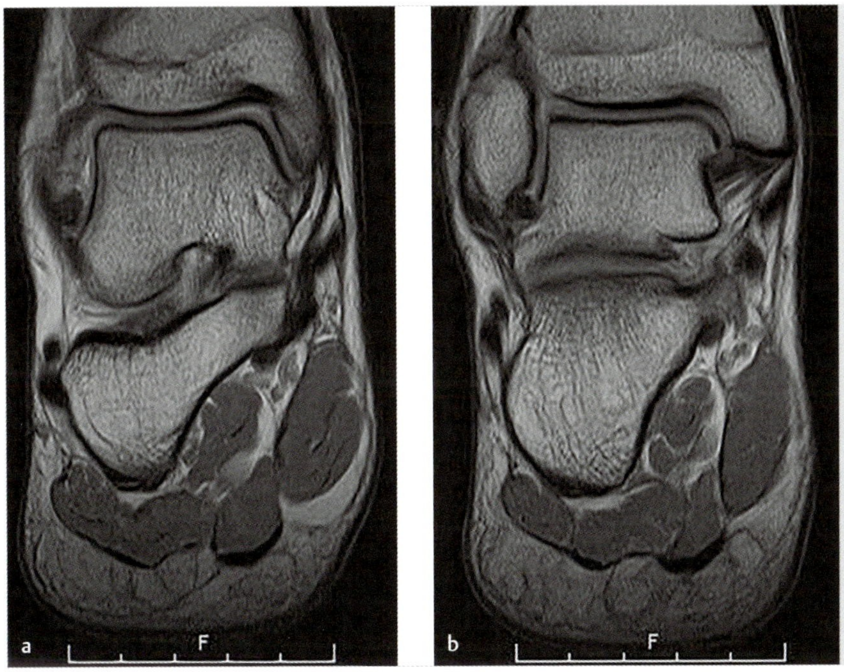

Fig. 12.10 Normal deltoid ligament. **(a)** Coronal T1-weighted image showing the normal low-signal appearance of the superficial deltoid layer. **(b)** Coronal proton-density (PD) pulse image of the deep deltoid fibers showing the normal striated pattern.

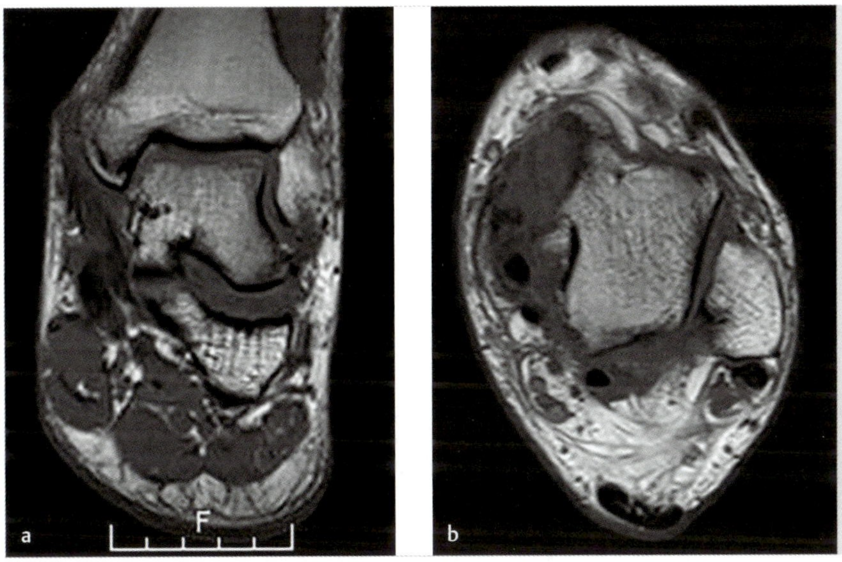

Fig. 12.11 **(a)** Coronal T1-weighted image of an ankle with chronic deltoid insufficiency. The normal low signal intensity of the superficial fibers has been replaced with thickened, amorphous scar. **(b)** Axial T1-weighted image of the same patient showing thickened deep deltoid fibers.

fibular shortening or lateral subluxation, diastasis between the tibia and fibula, and increased fluid signal with blurring, waviness, or disruption of the ligaments on edema-specific sequences (▶ Fig. 12.13a, b).[8,12,49,60] It should be noted that proximal extent of the disruption is not indicative of recovery time.[58]

12.5.3 OCLs of the Ankle

OCLs of the ankle (also commonly referred to as osteochondritis dissecans) are injuries to the articular surface with or without involvement of its underlying subchondral bone.[60] They are seen frequently in association with ankle trauma and occur in up to 50% of ankle sprains and fractures.[61] Conventional radiography fails to detect between 30 and 50% of lesions, leading to missed diagnoses.[60]

The talus is most frequently involved; however, injuries to the tibial plafond occur and should not be overlooked.[62] Classically, talar dome lesions were described as occurring posteromedially or anterolaterally. However, more recent research showed talar dome lesions occurring more centrally, with the medial side more affected than the lateral side.[62]

Because of the limited reliability of conventional radiography in diagnosing OCLs, MRI has become a standard imaging technique for evaluating patients with a history of ankle trauma and continued ankle pain and swelling. MRI has been shown to have

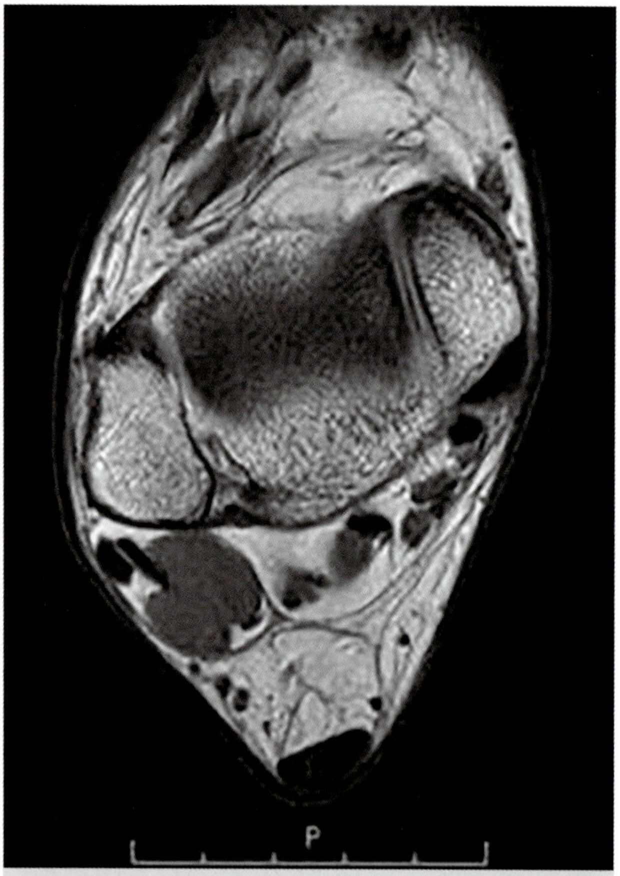

Fig. 12.12 Axial T1-weighted image of an ankle with an intact syndesmosis. The anterior inferior tibiofibular ligament (AITFL) and posterior inferior tibiofibular ligament (PITFL) are seen.

96% sensitivity and specificity for detecting OCLs.[63] T2-weighted sequences are recommended to evaluate the depth of cartilage damage; however, the true size of the lesion may be overestimated because of the presence of bony edema (see section "Traumatic Conditions").[60,61] OCLs may be seen in all imaging planes; however, the sagittal and coronal planes are most frequently used for localization and preoperative planning (▶ Fig. 12.14a, b). Multiple classification schemes have been created that attempt to delineate stable from unstable OCLs. Unstable lesions show fluid surrounding the fragment and are sometimes associated with cystic changes beneath it, which appear bright on T2-weighted images (▶ Fig. 12.15). There are also newer cartilage-specific sequences that have been helpful for postoperative evaluation of OCL healing, the most common being T2-weighted mapping.[60]

12.6 Degenerative Conditions

12.6.1 Tendon Disorders

MRI is the optimal imaging technique to evaluate tendon disorders. Tendons are susceptible to various pathologies, including rupture, inflammatory disorders (synovitis and tendinitis), and degeneration (tendinosis). Tendons are best evaluated when the image is perpendicular to the course of the tendon.[64,65,66] In the ankle and hindfoot, the tendons are best seen in the axial views because their course is perpendicular to imaging. In contrast, coronal views are most useful in evaluating tendons in the forefoot and midfoot.

Imaging of tendons in the foot and ankle may be complicated by the MAE. This effect occurs when imaging is performed on well-ordered collagen fibers (as in a tendon), and images are obtained at an oblique angle (55 degrees) on

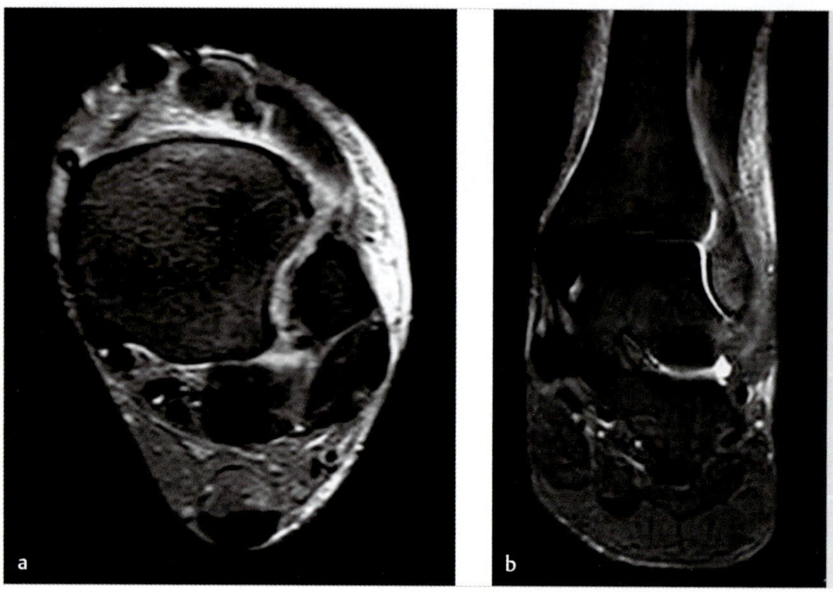

Fig. 12.13 Acute syndesmotic injury. **(a)** Axial short tau inversion recovery (STIR)-weighted image showing a disrupted anterior inferior tibiofibular ligament (AITFL) with surrounding subcutaneous, soft tissue edema. **(b)** Coronal T2-weighted image of the same patient showing continuous high signal intensity from the lateral gutter, ankle joint, and into the syndesmosis resembling the Greek letter lambda. This is a predictor of syndesmotic instability.

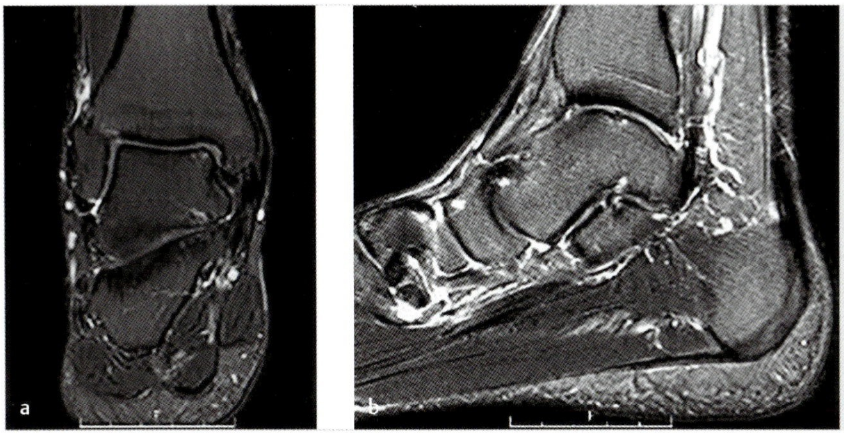

Fig. 12.14 Talus osteochondritis dissecans. **(a)** Coronal T2-weighted image of a medial talar dome osteochondral lesion (OCL) with osseous edema. **(b)** Sagittal T2-weighted image of the same medial talar dome OCL showing irregularity of the subchondral bone and overlying cartilage.

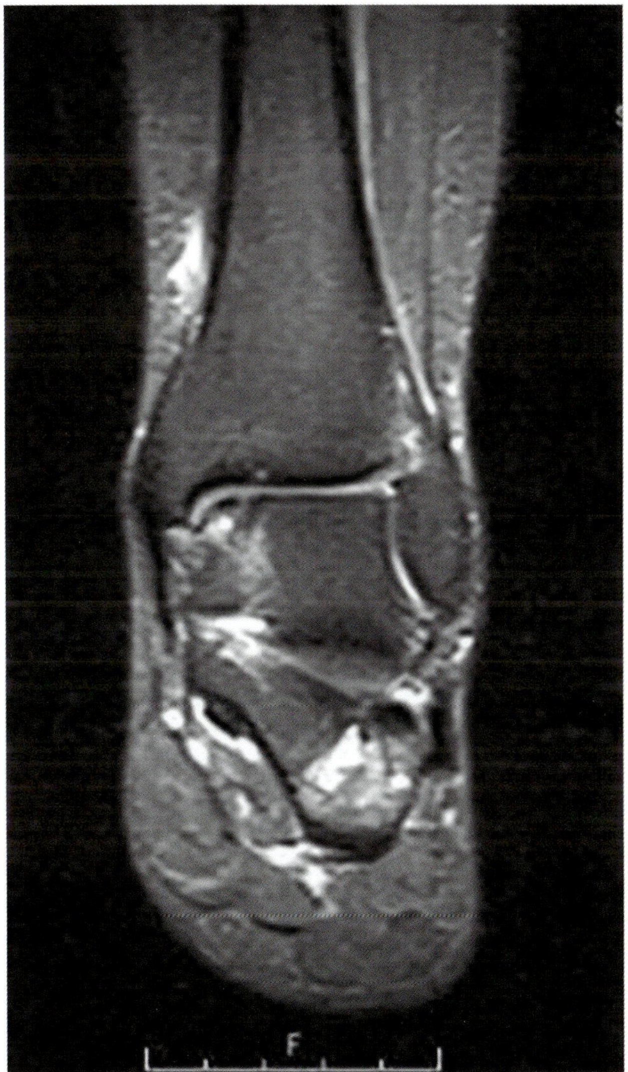

Fig. 12.15 Coronal T2-weighted image of an ankle with a medial talar osteochondral lesion (OCL) with increased signal surrounding the defect reflecting an unstable fragment.

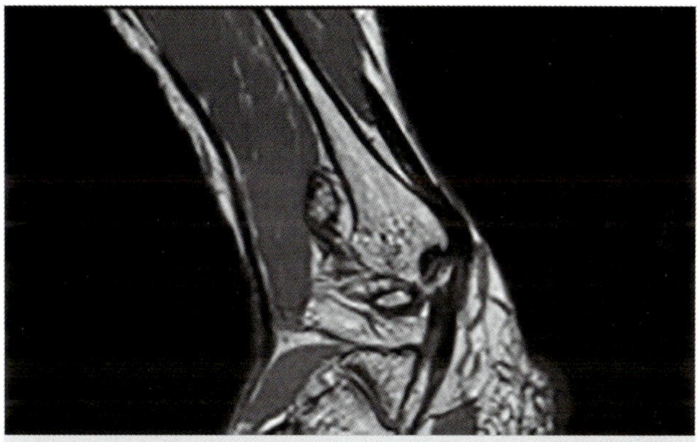

Fig. 12.16 T1-weighted sagittal image showing the magic angle effect (MAE) of the peroneus longus as it passes behind the distal fibula.

T1-weighted imaging.[67] When captured at this oblique angle, abnormal signal intensity is seen on the T1-weighted images. This phenomenon is not seen on T2-weighted imaging; therefore, T2-weighted images serve as a control to confirm that imaging represents pathology rather than artifact (▶ Fig. 12.16). The MAE is often seen in the PTT and peroneal tendons as they course behind the malleoli. It is exceedingly important to verify that any pathology visualized on T1-weighted imaging is also present on T2-weighted imaging when reviewing tendons at oblique angles.

Achilles Tendon Disorders

The Achilles tendon is the largest tendon in the body and has a broad spectrum of clinical and imaging pathology. The pathologies can be grouped broadly into those involving structures adjacent to the tendon, including retrocalcaneal bursitis and paratenonitis, and those involving the tendon such as tendinosis and rupture (▶ Fig. 12.17a, b).

Retrocalcaneal bursitis can be caused by mechanical impingement of the soft tissue from a Haglund deformity (posterosuperior process of the calcaneus) or from a systemic

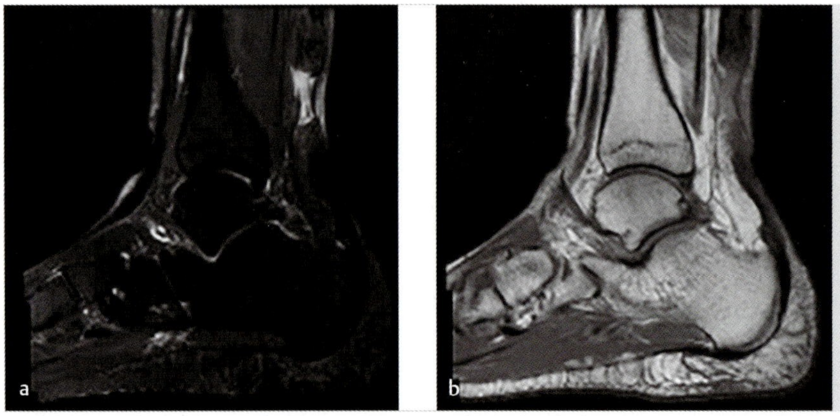

Fig. 12.17 (a) T1-weighted and (b) T2-weighted sagittal images showing an Achilles tendon rupture with preexisting tendinosis.

inflammatory disease. The normal retrocalcaneal bursa measures 6 mm proximal-to-distal and 2 mm anterior-to-posterior and is visible on MRI.[68] When the retrocalcaneal bursa is inflamed, sagittal MRI will show decreased signal intensity on T1-weighted images and increased signal intensity on T2-weighted images.

The Achilles tendon lacks a sheath. Instead, it has a thin, vascular membrane called a paratenon. For this reason, edema surrounding the tendon is referred to as paratenonitis or peritendinitis.[69] On MRI, the paratenon will appear thickened and hyperintense on fat-suppressed T2-weighted and STIR images. There will also be a loss of the normal sharp interface between the Achilles and surrounding soft tissues, but the tendon itself will maintain its normal intrasubstance appearance.[47]

The term "Achilles tendinitis" is now thought to be a misnomer because the tendon appears to experience a degenerative process rather than an inflammatory process. The degenerative process of tendinosis results in disorganization of the collagen fibers, myxoid degeneration, and microscopic intrasubstance tearing.[70] Tendinosis is related to the normal aging process and will present in all individuals to some degree. It can also occur from repetitive strain or overuse, commonly in running athletes.[71] Symptoms are thought to occur when degenerative changes advance to intrasubstance or partial tears.[68]

There are two categories of Achilles tendinosis: insertional and noninsertional. Insertional tendinosis occurs at the insertion of the tendon onto the calcaneus, whereas noninsertional tendinosis occurs at the vascular watershed area 3 to 6 cm proximal to the insertion.[47,70]

On MRI, the tendon appears thickened, leading to a convex rather than concave appearance on axial images.[72] This thickening can be diffuse, fusiform, or occasionally nodular.[68] Mucoid degeneration is seen as an intermediate signal.[69] There is a loss of the sharp tendon interface with surrounding tissues. Tendon hypertrophy can best be seen on axial and sagittal T1-weighted images. This imaging also shows heterogeneity of the substance. T2-weighted imaging should be evaluated to visualize the intratendinous edema and splitting.[47]

PTT Dysfunction

PTT dysfunction is caused by degeneration, inflammatory disorders, structural issues, or trauma. Loss of normal PTT function leads to a flatfoot deformity. At the microscopic level, the tendon has tears and collagen disorganization. There is myxoid degeneration and increased mucin content seen histologically.[73] On examination, patients have pain to the medial ankle, flattening of the normal arch, forefoot abduction, and hindfoot valgus. The disease is staged according to clinical and radiographic findings.[74]

Weight-bearing radiographs are the "gold standard" for diagnosis. Arthritis of the hindfoot develops in stage-III disease; whereas, stage-IV disease is defined by the development of ankle valgus or arthritis.[74] In these patients, MRI is not typically indicated because treatment requires arthrodesis because of bony deformity. However, in earlier stages of the disease, MRI can be a useful adjunct. It is the optimal modality to show inflammation and tears of the tendon. The PTT is typically two to three times the caliber of the FDLT. In a normal tendon, there should be less than 1 to 2 mm of surrounding synovial fluid.[75] A healthy tendon will show a homogeneous signal on T1- and T2-weighted images.

PTT tears most commonly occur by the medial malleolus or 2 to 3 cm proximal to the tendon insertion on the navicular.[76,77] Tendon tears are most readily identified on T2-weighted and fat-suppressed axial images, which show changes in signal and morphology (▶ Fig. 12.18). The insertion of the tendon onto the navicular should also be evaluated with axial and sagittal imaging.

Some patients have pain at the insertion of the tendon caused by an accessory navicular (▶ Fig. 12.19). In these patients, T2-weighted and fat-suppressed images may show edema within the navicular or within the synchondrosis.[47]

A classification for PTT tears as seen on MRI has been described.[76] In type-I tears, the tendon has interstitial tearing, as well as hypertrophy and scar formation. The tendon becomes thickened and may be four to five times the size of the flexor digitorum longus. Type-II tears have decreased diameter because of their increased severity. The longitudinal splits cause the tendon to attenuate to one-half to one-third of its original thickness. Type-III tears show complete rupture of the tendon, with retraction of the stump and a gap.

Peroneal Tendon Disorders

Peroneal tendons are the primary evertors of the foot. They are prone to injury because of their location and trajectory, and the

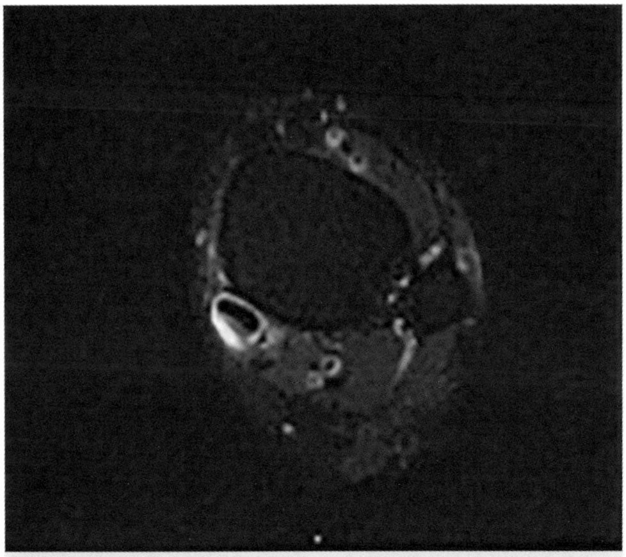

Fig. 12.18 T2-weighted axial image showing posterior tibial tendinosis in a patient with underlying rheumatoid arthritis.

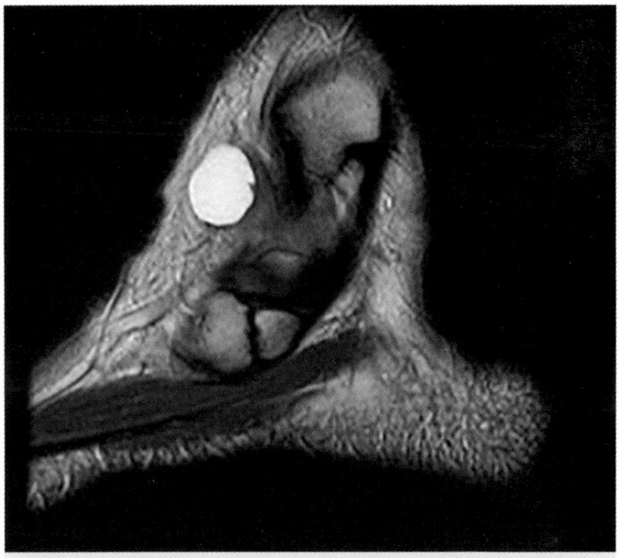

Fig. 12.19 Sagittal T1-weighted image showing an accessory navicular. A ganglion cyst of the anterior ankle is incidentally seen.

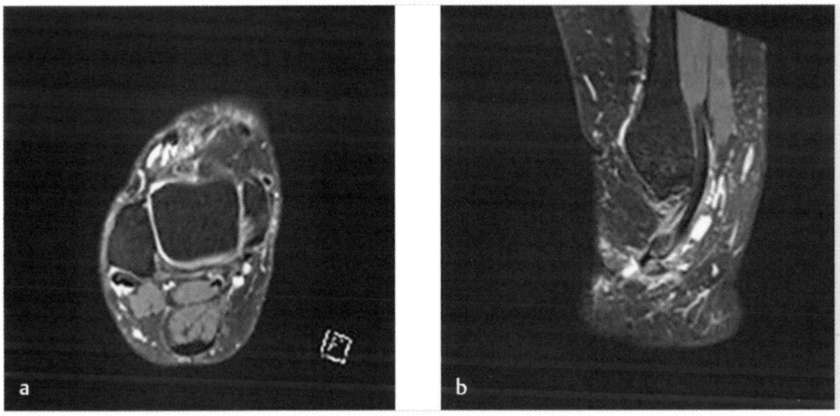

Fig. 12.20 (a) Axial T2-weighted and (b) sagittal T2-weighted images showing peroneal tenosynovitis.

pathology generally corresponds to the location. In addition to tenosynovitis and tears, peroneal tendons are at risk for subluxation or dislocation. MRI is an effective tool for defining the location and type of peroneal pathology (▶ Fig. 12.20a, b). It is also imperative to consider that 33% of asymptomatic individuals have peroneal pathology on MRI.[38]

Tenosynovitis and tears can be acute or chronic. They often occur behind the retrofibular groove posterior to the fibula. This pathology is best seen on axial images.[66] There is typically some amount of fluid observed in the peroneal sheaths, but it may be considered pathological and appear as tenosynovitis when the fluid is larger than the tendon or if there is complexity to the fluid.[47] Chronic tendinopathy may be visualized on MRI and is defined by tendon thickening and increased signal intensity.

Acute peroneal tendon ruptures are uncommon but do occur. They are often associated with trauma, corticosteroid use, and inflammatory arthropathy. Acute tears are best visualized on axial images. The tendon will appear irregular on T1-weighted images with increased fluid within the sheath and soft tissue on T2-weighted images (▶ Fig. 12.21).

Chronic peroneal tendon tears are much more common than acute injuries. One proposed mechanism for injury is chronic abrasion along the posterolateral ridge of the fibula as a result of instability.[78] Another mechanism is compression of the peroneus brevis by the longus against the posterior fibula. In chronic tears, axial images will show an irregular appearance and fluid within the sheath. The retrofibular groove should be evaluated because flat or convex grooves are associated with increased likelihood of injury. Spurring of the lateral edge of the fibula is also associated with injury.[66,75,79,80]

Chronic peroneal tendon subluxation and instability are associated with flat or convex fibular grooves and attenuation of the superior peroneal retinaculum. This type of pathology is best

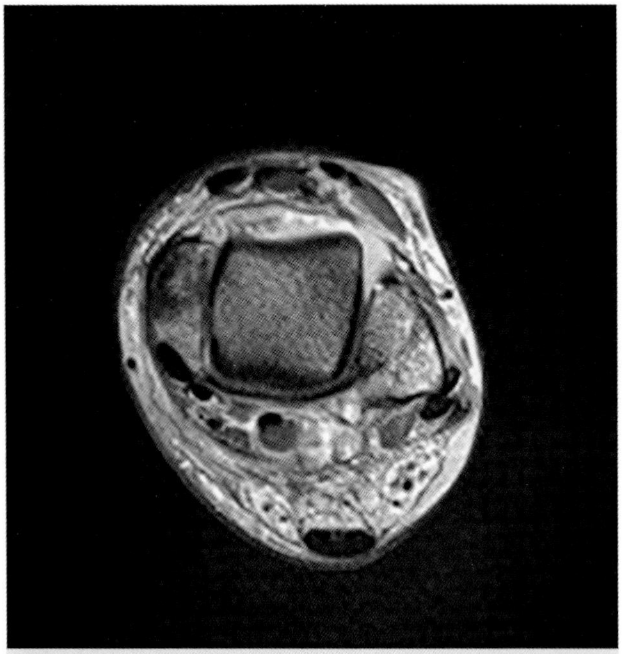

Fig. 12.21 Axial T1-weighted image showing acute peroneal dislocation. The peroneal retinaculum is disrupted.

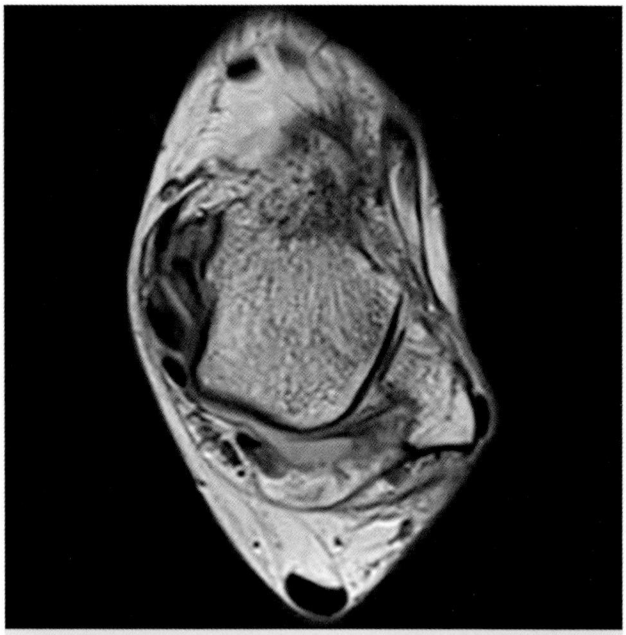

Fig. 12.22 Axial T1-weighted image showing chronic peroneal tendon dislocation in a patient with Ehlers-Danlos syndrome. The peroneal retinaculum is distended but intact over the dislocated tendon.

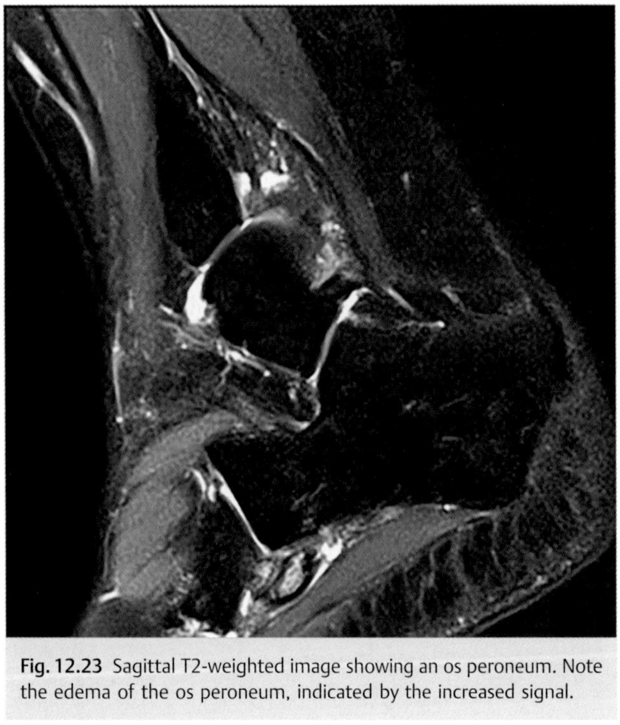

Fig. 12.23 Sagittal T2-weighted image showing an os peroneum. Note the edema of the os peroneum, indicated by the increased signal.

visualized on axial images.[75,79,80] Occasionally, frank dislocation of the peroneal tendons can be seen, with the tendon lateral to the distal fibula (▶ Fig. 12.22).

Mass affect from overcrowding in the posterior fibular space has also been proposed as a mechanism of tendon subluxation. This can be caused by a low-lying peroneus brevis muscle belly, ganglion cyst, or accessory peroneus quartus muscle, which is present in 10 to 20% of individuals (more commonly in men).[79,81] This accessory muscle runs posterior to the longus and brevis and may insert directly on the tendons, calcaneus, or cuboid. It is best seen in T1-weighted axial images as a tendon separate from the longus and brevis.

Most peroneal tendon pathology occurs proximal to the tip of the fibula, but more distal pathology is possible. Tenosynovitis and tearing may occur beyond the fibula or at the insertion points. The peroneal tubercle on the lateral calcaneus can be a site of impingement. This is an issue in patients with hindfoot valgus such as that which occurs with a pes planus deformity. It is also common in patients who sustained a calcaneus fracture with malunion.

The distal peroneus brevis may have tenosynovitis at the insertion onto the fifth metatarsal. Distal peroneus longus pathology can present as painful os peroneum syndrome.[82] These patients have pain in the lateral foot proximal to the insertion of the base of the fifth metatarsal at the level of the cuboid. The pain is secondary to tenosynovitis or tearing of the longus tendon. If the tendon ruptures, the associated os peroneum will retract, often proximal to the calcaneocuboid joint. This may be seen on conventional radiographs as a fragmented or retracted os peroneum. On MRI, edema and fragmentation of the bone of the os peroneum are visible, as well as fluid and edema in the peroneus longus tendon sheath (▶ Fig. 12.23).

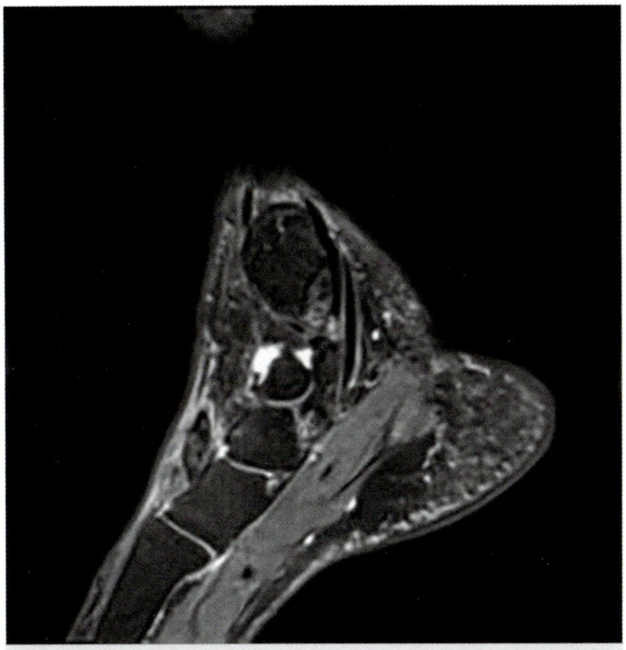

Fig. 12.24 Sagittal T2-weighted image showing tendinitis of the anterior tibial tendon as it inserts on to the dorsal midfoot.

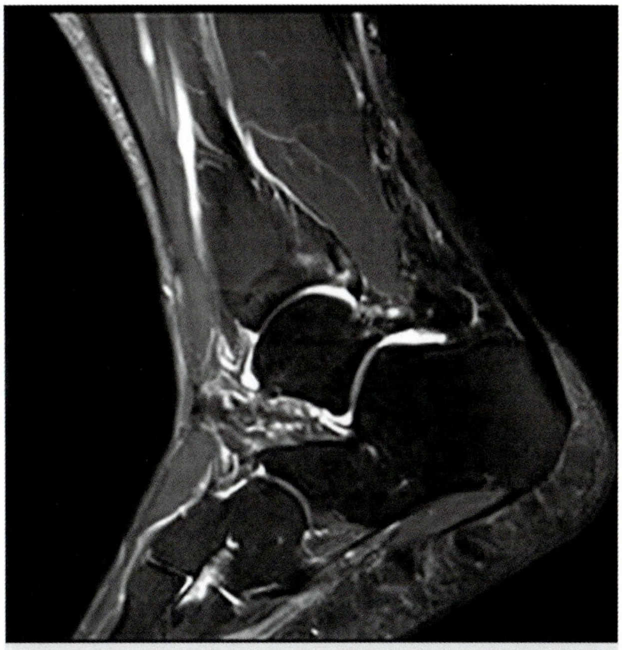

Fig. 12.25 Sagittal T2-weighted image showing an asymptomatic Os trigonum.

Anterior Tibial Tendon Disorders

Compared with pathology of the Achilles tendon, PTT, and peroneal tendon, pathology of the anterior tibial tendon is much less common. Tendinitis may occur secondary to systemic inflammatory disease, including gout and rheumatoid arthritis. It may also occur from overuse. Acute anterior tibial tendon tears are associated with trauma or laceration. Spontaneous ruptures have been reported in association with inflammatory disease, diabetes, vascular disorders, and steroid injections.[83] Chronic attritional tears can occur in elderly individuals.

Patients with a rupture present with anterior ankle pain, soft tissue swelling, and weakness of ankle dorsiflexion. Tendinitis presents with soft tissue edema on axial and sagittal T2-weighted images. Tendinosis appears on T1- and T2-weighted images as hypertrophy, heterogeneous signal changes with the tendon substance, and longitudinal splitting.[64,84] In complete rupture, the tendon will be discontinuous and fluid will be seen in the intervening space. This can best be seen on sagittal images. In addition, the SM limb of the extensor retinaculum may appear thickened and enhanced with contrast. These findings are associated with tibialis anterior tendon rupture (▸ Fig. 12.24).[83]

12.6.2 FHL and Posterior Impingement (Os Trigonum)

Pathology to the FHL is notably less common than other posterior ankle pathologies, particularly of the Achilles tendon. Nevertheless, tenosynovitis of the FHLT does occur, most often at the posterior ankle joint at the level of the talus. These injuries are most commonly seen in athletes who frequently plantarflex the ankle such as kicking athletes and ballet dancers who dance en pointe.[85] These injuries are typically subacute and related to overuse. They may overlap with posterior ankle impingement syndrome, whereby a prominent posterior process of the talus or an Os trigonum is impinging with plantarflexion. When this occurs, the posterior process or Os trigonum becomes trapped between the tibia and calcaneus with plantarflexion. This impaction creates osseous edema and inflammation. It may contribute to tenosynovitis and tearing in the FHL. On examination, passive plantarflexion of the ankle will reproduce the pain. In addition, dorsiflexion of the great toe may reproduce posterior ankle pain, indicating involvement of the FHLT.

Radiography is the optimal initial imaging modality for the diagnosis of posterior impingement. A radiograph in maximum plantarflexion can be useful, especially in ballet dancers, to show impingement occurring dynamically in the posterior ankle. MRI will show fluid and soft tissue signal posteriorly around the Os trigonum. This fluid may extend into the posterior ankle and subtalar joints.[47] There may also be fluid between the Os trigonum and posterior talus at the site of the fibrous synchondrosis, best seen on T2-weighted axial and sagittal images (▸ Fig. 12.25). Edema can also be seen in the posterior tibial and dorsal calcaneus from the repeated impaction stresses present with impingement.

The FHLT sheath can be enlarged and fluid filled. Loculation or ganglion cysts may be present. Although not as common as in other tendons, tearing may be present, and a partial tear will be appreciated by intratendinous signal change.[47]

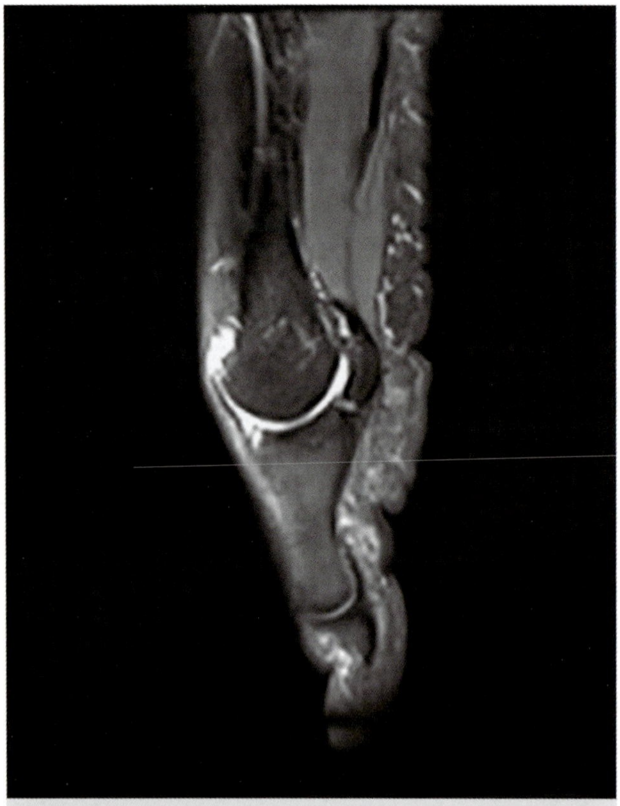

Fig. 12.26 Sagittal T2-weighted image showing a high-grade, partial-thickness tear of the great toe plantar plate.

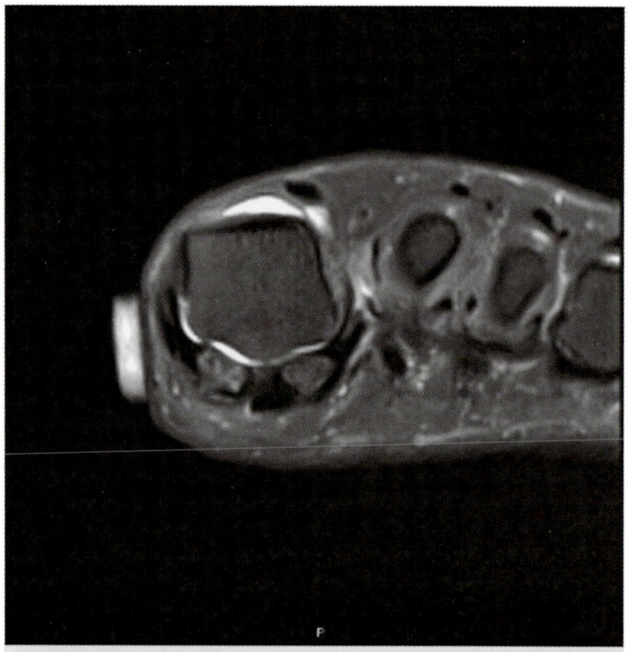

Fig. 12.27 Coronal T2-weighted image showing partial avascular necrosis of the tibial sesamoid. The normal fibular sesamoid is also seen.

12.6.3 Plantar Plate Injuries

Injuries to the first metatarsophalangeal joint have become more common with the introduction of artificial playing surfaces and more flexible athletic shoes. These injuries include fractures of the sesamoids and injuries to the plantar capsular ligaments of the metatarsophalangeal joint (i.e., "turf toe" injuries).[86] The classic mechanism of injury is a hyperextension force at the first metatarsophalangeal joint.

These structures are quite small and were difficult to fully visualize before the availability of higher-resolution images such as those obtained with a 3-T magnet. The presence of fluid as seen on T2-weighted images around the plantar capsule or thickening of the capsule as a result of injury may be the only pathologic signs visible on MRI with lower magnet strength.[87] With newer imaging modalities, the first metatarsophalangeal joint may be better visualized, and the capsuloligamentous complex may be fully visualized as a thickened plantar capsule of low signal intensity on T1- and T2-weighted images (▶ Fig. 12.26).[88] The flexor hallucis tendon runs plantar to the plantar plate between the two sesamoids. It should have a slightly lower signal intensity than the capsule. In addition to the soft tissue anatomy, the bony articulation of the joint should be evaluated for edema indicating a contusion or an articular cartilage abnormality indicating an OCL.

Sesamoid injuries may be acute or chronic. Patient history is key to differentiating between acute and chronic sesamoid injuries because a stress fracture will appear identical to an acute fracture on MRI.[87] Both will show edema and signal changes within the sesamoid, and possibly a fracture line (▶ Fig. 12.27).

It is also important to evaluate the presence of a bipartite sesamoid from an acute fracture. A CT scan is sometimes needed to differentiate acute injuries from a bipartite sesamoid. Edema around the sesamoid indicates an acute injury.

12.7 Postoperative MRI Findings

Conventional radiography remains the most common imaging modality used after surgery. However, MRI may be used for foot and ankle pathology, especially after a soft tissue or cartilage procedure.

12.7.1 Tendon Repair

Surgical repair of tendons often includes surgical reconnection of the apposed tendon ends or transfer of another tendon to fill the role of the torn tendon. The healing that occurs in the first month of tendon repair is well documented. It begins with granulation tissue in the anastomosis (week 1); increased vascularization of the paratenon (week 2); formation of collagen fibrils (week 3); and finally, resolution of the edema (week 4).[89] If a tendon rupture is treated nonoperatively, the muscle will retract, which often requires grafting or tendon transfer.[90]

Early after surgical repair, the tendon will appear thickened, and signal heterogeneity from the suture material may be seen.[89] Later, the main findings are tendon thickening and signal heterogeneity.[91]

If a tendon is transferred, the new, nonanatomic trajectory of the tendon should be evaluated. A common tendon transfer in Achilles tendon reconstruction is an FHLT transfer, in which the FHLT is rerouted into the calcaneus. Another common tendon transfer is an FDLT transfer to treat posterior tibial tendinitis. In this case, postoperative imaging will show the FDLT routed into the medial navicular. MRI can also be helpful before planned tendon transfer surgery in evaluating the quality and potential pathology of a tendon to be transferred.

For any postoperative imaging modality, comparison with preoperative images is of paramount importance. This allows new tears to be diagnosed (best seen as high signal on T2-weighted images) and anatomy to be fully evaluated (best evaluated on T1-weighted images). In addition, postoperative infections resulting in abscesses or osteomyelitis can be well evaluated by comparing images before and after contrast administration.

12.7.2 Lateral Ankle Ligament Reconstruction

Surgical reconstruction is used to treat patients with chronic lateral ankle instability and pain after an ankle sprain. There are various treatment options for these injuries, and understanding the potential treatment options is important for comprehending postoperative imaging.[92] The modified Brostrom-Gould procedure involves the surgical reconstruction of the ATFL and CFL.[93] Depending on surgeon preference, the reconstruction may include suture alone within the ligament or suture anchors placed in the distal fibula at the footprint of the ligament. These suture anchors can be seen as osseous tunnels.

There are also several surgical procedures characterized by nonanatomic anastomosis and osseous tunnels.[94] In the modified Evans procedure, the peroneus tendon is transected, passed through a fibular tunnel, and then anastomosed at the site of transection.[94] The Watson-Jones procedure also reroutes the peroneus brevis tendon through two fibular tunnels and a tarsal tunnel, with re-anastomosis distally. In this procedure, the proximal tendon is transferred to the peroneus longus. The Chrisman-Sook procedure splits the peroneus brevis and reroutes it through the fibula and calcaneus.[94] In all of these cases, osseous tunnels can be seen, and the integrity of the lateral tendons, as well as their new pathways, can be evaluated and defined. Comparison with preoperative imaging can be helpful to better understand the surgical procedure performed.

12.7.3 Other Foot and Ankle Surgical Procedures

There are many other common foot and ankle procedures that may be evaluated with MRI. Plantar fasciotomy will show a thickened area of plantar fascia with indistinct margins and a lack of edema, which characterizes plantar fascia.[95] MRI will show scarring of the fat and fascia medial to the tibial nerve, visible as areas of low T1 signal.[96] CT scans are often used to document fusion after an attempted arthrodesis, but MRI can also be used to assess the extent of bridging bone between the bony fusion sites. MRI can also be used to assess for secondary, soft tissue complications such as infection or tendon injury.

MRI of OCLs has been well characterized. Surgical treatment often includes drilling of the lesion, also called microfracture or bone marrow stimulation. In the successful treatment of these lesions, the low-intensity areas in T1-weighted images will typically decrease. In addition, the high signal seen in T2-weighted images, showing edema, will decrease or disappear with resolution of the patient's symptoms (▶ Fig. 12.28).[97] Comparison imaging is crucial in evaluating postoperative MRI for OCLs.

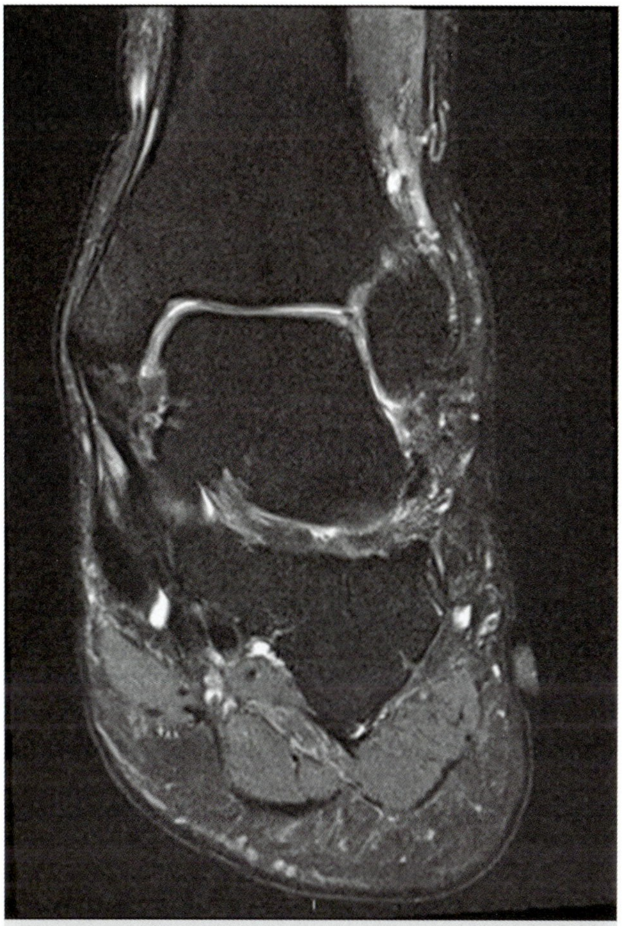

Fig. 12.28 Coronal T2-weighted image showing a surgically treated lateral osteochondral lesion (OCL) of the talus. There is no significant edema surrounding the OCL.

12.8 Common Clinical Questions

1. True/False. Conventional radiography has a high rate of missed diagnosis for osteochondral lesions of the talus.

2. True/False. The magic angle effect occurs when imaging is performed on well-ordered collagen fibers and images are obtained at an oblique angle on T2-weighted imaging.

3. The distal tibiofibular complex, also called the syndesmosis, unites the distal tibia and fibula. It is most commonly injured by which mechanism?
   a) Plantarflexion and internal rotation.
   b) Plantarflexion and external rotation.
   c) Dorsiflexion and external rotation.
   d) Dorsiflexion and internal rotation.
   e) Dorsiflexion and inversion.

4. Bone marrow edema occurs within trabecular bone and is hypointense on T1-weighted images compared with skeletal muscle but hyperintense on T2-weighted images. Which of the following conditions can lead to bone marrow edema?
   a) Stress fracture.
   b) Osteomyelitis.
   c) Osteonecrosis.
   d) Osteoporosis.
   e) All of the above.

5. A convex fibular groove is associated with which of the following conditions?
   a) CFL ankle sprain.
   b) Anterolateral ankle impingement.
   c) Posterior tibial tendon dysfunction.
   d) Peroneal subluxation.
   e) Osteochondral lesions of the talus.

References

[1] Brockett CL, Chapman GJ. Biomechanics of the ankle. Orthop Trauma. 2016; 30(3):232–238

[2] Christman RA. Radiographic anatomy of the foot and ankle-part 2: the greater tarsus. J Am Podiatr Med Assoc. 2014; 104(5):493–503

[3] Fraser JJ, Feger MA, Hertel J. Midfoot and forefoot involvement in lateral ankle sprains and chronic ankle instability. Part 1: anatomy and biomechanics. Int J Sports Phys Ther. 2016; 11(6):992–1005

[4] Christman RA. Radiographic anatomy of the foot and ankle—part 3: the lesser tarsus. J Am Podiatr Med Assoc. 2014; 104(6):633–643

[5] Martella I, Azzali E, Milanese G, et al. MRI in acute ligamentous injuries of the ankle. Acta Biomed. 2016; 87 Suppl 3:13–19

[6] Boonthathip M, Chen L, Trudell D, Resnick D. Lateral ankle ligaments: MR arthrography with anatomic correlation in cadavers. Clin Imaging. 2011; 35 (1):42–48

[7] Ngai SS, Tafur M, Chang EY, Chung CB. Magnetic resonance imaging of ankle ligaments. Can Assoc Radiol J. 2016; 67(1):60–68

[8] Croft S, Furey A, Stone C, Moores C, Wilson R. Radiographic evaluation of the ankle syndesmosis. Can J Surg. 2015; 58(1):58–62

[9] Chhabra A, Subhawong TK, Carrino JA. MR imaging of deltoid ligament pathologic findings and associated impingement syndromes. Radiographics. 2010; 30(3):751–761

[10] Omar H, Saini V, Wadhwa V, Liu G, Chhabra A. Spring ligament complex: Illustrated normal anatomy and spectrum of pathologies on 3 T MR imaging. Eur J Radiol. 2016; 85(11):2133–2143

[11] Kong A, Cassumbhoy R, Subramaniam RM. Magnetic resonance imaging of ankle tendons and ligaments: part I—anatomy. Australas Radiol. 2007; 51(4): 315–323

[12] Srikhum W, Nardo L, Karampinos DC, et al. Magnetic resonance imaging of ankle tendon pathology: benefits of additional axial short-tau inversion recovery imaging to reduce magic angle effects. Skeletal Radiol. 2013; 42(4): 499–510

[13] Rosenberg ZS, Beltran J, Bencardino JT. From the RSNA refresher courses. MR imaging of the ankle and foot. Radiographics. 2000; 20 Suppl 1:S153–S179

[14] Shapiro L, Harish M, Hargreaves B, Staroswiecki E, Gold G. Advances in musculoskeletal MRI: technical considerations. J Magn Reson Imaging. 2012; 36(4):775–787

[15] Gao F, Zhang R, Zhou D, Wang X, Huang K, Zhang J. A target field design of open multi-purpose RF coil for musculoskeletal MR imaging at 3 T. Magn Reson Imaging. 2016; 34(8):1064–1070

[16] Park HJ, Lee SY, Park NH, et al. Three-dimensional isotropic T2-weighted fast spin-echo (VISTA) ankle MRI versus two-dimensional fast spin-echo T2-weighted sequences for the evaluation of anterior talofibular ligament injury. Clin Radiol. 2016; 71(4):349–355

[17] Theysohn JM, Kraff O, Maderwald S, et al. MRI of the ankle joint in healthy non-athletes and in marathon runners: image quality issues at 7.0 T compared to 1.5 T. Skeletal Radiol. 2013; 42(2):261–267

[18] Zbýň Š, Brix MO, Juras V, et al. Sodium magnetic resonance imaging of ankle joint in cadaver specimens, volunteers, and patients after different cartilage repair techniques at 7 T: initial results. Invest Radiol. 2015; 50 (4):246–254

[19] Gatlin CC, Matheny LM, Ho CP, Johnson NS, Clanton TO. Diagnostic accuracy of 3.0 Tesla magnetic resonance imaging for the detection of articular cartilage lesions of the talus. Foot Ankle Int. 2015; 36(3):288–292

[20] Cha JG, Yi JS, Han JK, Lee YK. Comparison of quantitative cartilage T2 measurements and qualitative MR imaging between professional ballet dancers and healthy volunteers. Radiology. 2015; 276(1):199–206

[21] Crema MD, Roemer FW, Marra MD, et al. Articular cartilage in the knee: current MR imaging techniques and applications in clinical practice and research. Radiographics. 2011; 31(1):37–61

[22] Chhabra A, Soldatos T, Chalian M, Carrino JA, Schon L. Current concepts review: 3 T magnetic resonance imaging of the ankle and foot. Foot Ankle Int. 2012; 33(2):164–171

[23] Gutierrez LB, Do BH, Gold GE, et al. MR imaging near metallic implants using MAVRIC SL: initial clinical experience at 3 T. Acad Radiol. 2015; 22 (3):370–379

[24] Cerezal L, Llopis E, Canga A, Rolón A. MR arthrography of the ankle: indications and technique. Radiol Clin North Am. 2008; 46(6):973–994

[25] Haller J, Bernt R, Seeger T, Weissenbäck A, Tüchler H, Resnick D. MR-imaging of anterior tibiotalar impingement syndrome: agreement, sensitivity and specificity of MR-imaging and indirect MR-arthrography. Eur J Radiol. 2006; 58(3):450–460

[26] DeSmet AA, Dalinka MK, Alazraki N, et al. Chronic ankle pain. American College of Radiology. ACR Appropriateness Criteria. Radiology. 2000; 215 Suppl:321–332

[27] Wong GNL, Tan TJ. MR imaging as a problem solving tool in posterior ankle pain: a review. Eur J Radiol. 2016; 85(12):2238–2256

[28] Park HJ, Cha SD, Kim SS, et al. Accuracy of MRI findings in chronic lateral ankle ligament injury: comparison with surgical findings. Clin Radiol. 2012; 67(4):313–318

[29] Clanton TO, Ho CP, Williams BT, et al. Magnetic resonance imaging characterization of individual ankle syndesmosis structures in asymptomatic and surgically treated cohorts. Knee Surg Sports Traumatol Arthrosc. 2016; 24(7):2089–2102

[30] Muratli HH, Biçimoğlu A, Celebi L, Boyacigil S, Damgaci L, Tabak AY. Magnetic resonance arthrographic evaluation of syndesmotic diastasis in ankle fractures. Arch Orthop Trauma Surg. 2005; 125(4):222–227

[31] Mengiardi B, Pfirrmann CW, Vienne P, Hodler J, Zanetti M. Medial collateral ligament complex of the ankle: MR appearance in asymptomatic subjects. Radiology. 2007; 242(3):817–824

[32] Crim J. MR imaging evaluation of subtle Lisfranc injuries: the midfoot sprain. Magn Reson Imaging Clin N Am. 2008; 16(1):19–27, v

[33] Siddiqui NA, Galizia MS, Almusa E, Omar IM. Evaluation of the tarsometatarsal joint using conventional radiography, CT, and MR imaging. Radiographics. 2014; 34(2):514–531

[34] Chhabra A, Soldatos T, Chalian M, et al. 3-Tesla magnetic resonance imaging evaluation of posterior tibial tendon dysfunction with relevance to clinical staging. J Foot Ankle Surg. 2011; 50(3):320–328

[35] Tall MA, Thompson AK, Greer B, Campbell S. The pearls and pitfalls of magnetic resonance imaging of the lower extremity. J Orthop Sports Phys Ther. 2011; 41(11):873–886

[36] Rosenberg ZS, Zanetti M. Imaging of the foot and ankle. In: Hodler J, von Schulthess GK, Zollikofer CL, eds. Musculoskeletal diseases: diagnostic imaging and interventional techniques. New York, NY: Springer; 2005:39–47

[37] Ng JM, Rosenberg ZS, Bencardino JT, Restrepo-Velez Z, Ciavarra GA, Adler RSUS. US and MR imaging of the extensor compartment of the ankle. Radiographics. 2013; 33(7):2047–2064

[38] O'Neil JT, Pedowitz DI, Kerbel YE, Codding JL, Zoga AC, Raikin SM. Peroneal tendon abnormalities on routine magnetic resonance imaging of the foot and ankle. Foot Ankle Int. 2016; 37(7):743–747

[39] Chen H, Liu W, Deng L, Song W. The prognostic value of the hawkins sign and diagnostic value of MRI after talar neck fractures. Foot Ankle Int. 2014; 35 (12):1255–1261

[40] Zanon G, DI Vico G, Marullo M. Osteochondritis dissecans of the talus. Joints. 2014; 2(3):115–123

[41] Duncan D, Mologne T, Hildebrand H, Stanley M, Schreckengaust R, Sitler D. The usefulness of magnetic resonance imaging in the diagnosis of anterolateral impingement of the ankle. J Foot Ankle Surg. 2006; 45(5):304–307

[42] Baker JC, Hoover EG, Hillen TJ, Smith MV, Wright RW, Rubin DA. Subradiographic foot and ankle fractures and bone contusions detected by MRI in elite ice hockey players. Am J Sports Med. 2016; 44(5):1317–1323

[43] Sadineni RT, Pasumarthy A, Bellapa NC, Velicheti S. Imaging patterns in MRI in recent bone injuries following negative or inconclusive plain radiographs. J Clin Diagn Res. 2015; 9(10):TC10–TC13

[44] Kornaat PR, Van de Velde SK. Bone marrow edema lesions in the professional runner. Am J Sports Med. 2014; 42(5):1242–1246

[45] Dodson NB, Dodson EE, Shromoff PJ. Imaging strategies for diagnosing calcaneal and cuboid stress fractures. Clin Podiatr Med Surg. 2008; 25(2): 183–201, vi

[46] Alanen V, Taimela S, Kinnunen J, Koskinen SK, Karaharju E. Incidence and clinical significance of bone bruises after supination injury of the ankle. A double-blind, prospective study. J Bone Joint Surg Br. 1998; 80(3):513–515

[47] Morrison WB. Magnetic resonance imaging of sports injuries of the ankle. Top Magn Reson Imaging. 2003; 14(2):179–197

[48] Nattiv A, Kennedy G, Barrack MT, et al. Correlation of MRI grading of bone stress injuries with clinical risk factors and return to play: a 5-year prospective study in collegiate track and field athletes. Am J Sports Med. 2013; 41(8):1930–1941

[49] Nazarenko A, Beltran LS, Bencardino JT. Imaging evaluation of traumatic ligamentous injuries of the ankle and foot. Radiol Clin North Am. 2013; 51 (3):455–478

[50] Roemer FW, Jomaah N, Niu J, et al. Ligamentous injuries and the risk of associated tissue damage in acute ankle sprains in athletes: a cross-sectional MRI study. Am J Sports Med. 2014; 42(7):1549–1557

[51] van Putte-Katier N, van Ochten JM, van Middelkoop M, Bierma-Zeinstra SM, Oei EH. Magnetic resonance imaging abnormalities after lateral ankle trauma in injured and contralateral ankles. Eur J Radiol. 2015; 84(12): 2586–2592

[52] Hodgson RJ, O'Connor PJ, Grainger AJ. Tendon and ligament imaging. Br J Radiol. 2012; 85(1016):1157–1172

[53] Thormeyer JR, Leonard JP, Hutchinson M. Syndesmotic injuries in athletes, an international perspective on topics in sports medicine and sports injury. In: Dr. Zaslav KR, ed. InTech. doi:10.5772/25764. https://www.intechopen.com/books/an-international-perspective-on-topics-in-sports-medicine-and-sports-injury/syndesmotic-injuries-in-athletes. Accessed on January 29, 2017

[54] Khor YP, Tan KJ. The anatomic pattern of injuries in acute inversion ankle sprains: a magnetic resonance imaging study. Orthop J Sports Med. 2013; 1 (7):2325967113517078

[55] Perrich KD, Goodwin DW, Hecht PJ, Cheung Y. Ankle ligaments on MRI: appearance of normal and injured ligaments. AJR Am J Roentgenol. 2009; 193 (3):687–695

[56] Haraguchi N, Toga H, Shiba N, Kato F. Avulsion fracture of the lateral ankle ligament complex in severe inversion injury: incidence and clinical outcome. Am J Sports Med. 2007; 35(7):1144–1152

[57] Nortunen S, Lepojärvi S, Savola O, et al. Stability assessment of the ankle mortise in supination-external rotation-type ankle fractures: lack of additional diagnostic value of MRI. J Bone Joint Surg Am. 2014; 96(22):1855–1862

[58] Howard DR, Rubin DA, Hillen TJ, et al. Magnetic resonance imaging as a predictor of return to play following syndesmosis (high) ankle sprains in professional football players. Sports Health. 2012; 4(6):535–543

[59] Uys HD, Rijke AM. Clinical association of acute lateral ankle sprain with syndesmotic involvement: a stress radiography and magnetic resonance imaging study. Am J Sports Med. 2002; 30(6):816–822

[60] van Bergen CJ, Gerards RM, Opdam KT, Terra MP, Kerkhoffs GM. Diagnosing, planning and evaluating osteochondral ankle defects with imaging modalities. World J Orthop. 2015; 6(11):944–953

[61] O'Loughlin PF, Heyworth BE, Kennedy JG. Current concepts in the diagnosis and treatment of osteochondral lesions of the ankle. Am J Sports Med. 2010; 38(2):392–404

[62] Elias I, Raikin SM, Schweitzer ME, Besser MP, Morrison WB, Zoga AC. Osteochondral lesions of the distal tibial plafond: localization and morphologic characteristics with an anatomical grid. Foot Ankle Int. 2009; 30(6):524–529

[63] Verhagen RA, Maas M, Dijkgraaf MG, Tol JL, Krips R, van Dijk CN. Prospective study on diagnostic strategies in osteochondral lesions of the talus. Is MRI superior to helical CT? J Bone Joint Surg Br. 2005; 87(1):41–46

[64] Khoury NJ, el-Khoury GY, Saltzman CL, Brandser EA. Rupture of the anterior tibial tendon: diagnosis by MR imaging. AJR Am J Roentgenol. 1996; 167(2): 351–354

[65] Khoury NJ, el-Khoury GY, Saltzman CL, Brandser EA. MR imaging of posterior tibial tendon dysfunction. AJR Am J Roentgenol. 1996; 167(3):675–682

[66] Khoury NJ, el-Khoury GY, Saltzman CL, Kathol MH. Peroneus longus and brevis tendon tears: MR imaging evaluation. Radiology. 1996; 200(3):833–841

[67] Erickson SJ, Cox IH, Hyde JS, Carrera GF, Strandt JA, Estkowski LD. Effect of tendon orientation on MR imaging signal intensity: a manifestation of the "magic angle" phenomenon. Radiology. 1991; 181(2):389–392

[68] Pierre-Jerome C, Moncayo V, Terk MR. MRI of the Achilles tendon: a comprehensive review of the anatomy, biomechanics, and imaging of overuse tendinopathies. Acta Radiol. 2010; 51(4):438–454

[69] Gonzalez FM, Morrison WB. Magnetic resonance imaging of sports injuries involving the ankle. Top Magn Reson Imaging. 2015; 24(4):205–213

[70] Puddu G, Ippolito E, Postacchini F. A classification of Achilles tendon disease. Am J Sports Med. 1976; 4(4):145–150

[71] Kvist M. Achilles tendon injuries in athletes. Sports Med. 1994; 18(3):173–201

[72] Jahss MH. Tendon disorders of the foot and ankle. In: Jahss MH, ed. Disorders of the foot & ankle medical and surgical management. Philadelphia, PA: WB Saunders; 1991:1461–1513

[73] Mosier SM, Lucas DR, Pomeroy G, Manoli A, II. Pathology of the posterior tibial tendon in posterior tibial tendon insufficiency. Foot Ankle Int. 1998; 19 (8):520–524

[74] Bluman EM, Title CI, Myerson MS. Posterior tibial tendon rupture: a refined classification system. Foot Ankle Clin. 2007; 12(2):233–249, v

[75] Schweitzer ME, Eid ME, Deely D, Wapner K, Hecht P. Using MR imaging to differentiate peroneal splits from other peroneal disorders. AJR Am J Roentgenol. 1997; 168(1):129–133

[76] Rosenberg ZS, Cheung Y, Jahss MH, Noto AM, Norman A, Leeds NE. Rupture of posterior tibial tendon: CT and MR imaging with surgical correlation. Radiology. 1988; 169(1):229–235

[77] Schweitzer ME, Karasick D. MR imaging of disorders of the posterior tibialis tendon. AJR Am J Roentgenol. 2000; 175(3):627–635

[78] Sobel M, Geppert MJ, Olson EJ, Bohne WH, Arnoczky SP. The dynamics of peroneus brevis tendon splits: a proposed mechanism, technique of diagnosis, and classification of injury. Foot Ankle. 1992; 13(7):413–422

[79] Major NM, Helms CA, Fritz RC, Speer KP. The MR imaging appearance of longitudinal split tears of the peroneus brevis tendon. Foot Ankle Int. 2000; 21(6):514–519

[80] Rosenberg ZS, Beltran J, Cheung YY, Colon E, Herraiz F. MR features of longitudinal tears of the peroneus brevis tendon. AJR Am J Roentgenol. 1997; 168(1):141–147

[81] Cheung YY, Rosenberg ZS, Ramsinghani R, Beltran J, Jahss MH. Peroneus quartus muscle: MR imaging features. Radiology. 1997; 202(3):745–750

[82] Sobel M, Pavlov H, Geppert MJ, Thompson FM, DiCarlo EF, Davis WH. Painful os peroneum syndrome: a spectrum of conditions responsible for plantar lateral foot pain. Foot Ankle Int. 1994; 15(3):112–124

[83] Lee MH, Chung CB, Cho JH, et al. Tibialis anterior tendon and extensor retinaculum: imaging in cadavers and patients with tendon tear. AJR Am J Roentgenol. 2006; 187(2):W161–8

[84] Mengiardi B, Pfirrmann CWA, Vienne P, et al. Anterior tibial tendon abnormalities: MR imaging findings. Radiology. 2005; 235(3):977–984

[85] Sammarco GJ, Cooper PS. Flexor hallucis longus tendon injury in dancers and nondancers. Foot Ankle Int. 1998; 19(6):356–362

[86] Coker TP, Arnold JA, Weber DL. Traumatic lesions of the metatarsophalangeal joint of the great toe in athletes. Am J Sports Med. 1978; 6(6):326–334

[87] Crain JM, Phancao JP, Stidham K. MR imaging of turf toe. Magn Reson Imaging Clin N Am. 2008; 16(1):93–103, vi

[88] Tewes DP, Fischer DA, Fritts HM, Guanche CA. MRI findings of acute turf toe. A case report and review of anatomy. Clin Orthop Relat Res. 1994(304):200–203

[89] Bergin D, Morrison WB. Postoperative imaging of the ankle and foot. Radiol Clin North Am. 2006; 44(3):391–406

[90] Platt MA. Tendon repair and healing. Clin Podiatr Med Surg. 2005; 22(4): 553–560, vi

[91] Reinig JW, Dorwart RH, Roden WC. MR imaging of a ruptured Achilles tendon. J Comput Assist Tomogr. 1985; 9(6):1131–1134

[92] Alparslan L, Chiodo CP. Lateral ankle instability: MR imaging of associated injuries and surgical treatment procedures. Semin Musculoskelet Radiol. 2008; 12(4):346–358

[93] DiGiovanni BF, Partal G, Baumhauer JF. Acute ankle injury and chronic lateral instability in the athlete. Clin Sports Med. 2004; 23(1):1–19, v

[94] Chien AJ, Jacobson JA, Jamadar DA, Brigido MK, Femino JE, Hayes CW. Imaging appearances of lateral ankle ligament reconstruction. Radiographics. 2004; 24(4):999–1008

[95] Woelffer KE, Figura MA, Sandberg NS, Snyder NS. Five-year follow-up results of instep plantar fasciotomy for chronic heel pain. J Foot Ankle Surg. 2000; 39 (4):218–223

[96] Recht MP, Donley BG. Magnetic resonance imaging of the foot and ankle. J Am Acad Orthop Surg. 2001; 9(3):187–199
[97] Higashiyama I, Kumai T, Takakura Y, Tamail S. Follow-up study of MRI for osteochondral lesion of the talus. Foot Ankle Int. 2000; 21(2):127–133

Answers to Common Clinical Questions

1. Answer: True. Conventional radiography fails to detect between 30 and 50% of lesions, leading to missed diagnosis.[60]
2. Answer: False. The magic angle effect occurs when imaging is performed on well-ordered collagen fibers and images are obtained at an oblique angle (55 degrees) on T1-weighted imaging.[67]
3. Answer: c. The syndesmosis is commonly injured after dorsiflexion and external rotation. This type of force can also create ankle fractures. Syndesmosis injuries can lead to instability, pain, and ultimately secondary osteoarthritis.[8]
4. Answer: e. Bone marrow edema represents edema, hemorrhage, and infarction caused by microscopic fracture of the trabecular bone. It is present in all of the above conditions.[43,44,45]
5. Answer: d. Chronic peroneal tendon subluxation and instability are associated with flat or convex fibular grooves and attenuation of the superior peroneal retinaculum. This pathology can best be visualized on axial images.[75,78,79]

Part IV

Neurological Imaging

IV

13 Normal Spine MRI Anatomy

Majd Marrache, Swati Deshmukh, John A. Carrino, Jason D. Dunleavy, and A. Jay Khanna

Abstract

The aim of this chapter is to describe the standard anatomy of the spine and its appearance on MRI. In this chapter we provide a detailed description of elements in the spine with the most ideal sequence required to provide optimal evaluation. In addition, we examine the normal anatomy of the cervical, thoracic, lumbar and sacral spine in the axial, sagittal and coronal planes on MRI. By the end of the chapter, the reader will have a firm grasp of spine anatomy and its appearance on MRI.

Keywords: spine anatomy, magnetic resonance imaging, MRI, cervical spine, thoracic spine, lumbar spine

13.1 Normal Anatomy

In order to effectively evaluate a magnetic resonance imaging (MRI) of the spine, it is crucial to have a basic understanding of its normal anatomy and radiographic appearance using MRI imaging. The figures and line drawings serve to highlight the structures with which the spine specialist or radiologist should be familiar before interpreting an imaging examination of the spine. Fully understanding the normal MRI appearance of the spine will enhance the clinician's understanding of the relevant pathologic conditions and facilitate recognition and differentiation of the subtle regional anatomic alterations that represent various pathologic conditions.

13.2 General Spine Anatomy

The spinal column is composed of a series of vertebrae, ligaments, and articulations. Functions of the spinal column include providing protection to the spinal cord and nerve roots and serving as a flexible support structure for the cranium, thorax, abdomen, and pelvis. There are three primary and five secondary ossification centers of the vertebrae. Primary ossification centers include: one ossification center for the vertebral body (centrum), which develops by the eighth week of life, and one ossification center for each vertebral arch, which develops by the seventh or eighth week.[1] Secondary ossification centers that develop after birth are seen at the tips of the transverse process, spinous process, and ring apophysis.[2] The spinal column shows a longitudinal growth pattern during childhood and adolescence, with approximately 75% of its length attributed to the height of the vertebral bodies and 25% to the height of disks.[3]

The spinal column is typically composed of 7 cervical vertebrae, 12 thoracic vertebrae, 5 lumbar vertebrae, the sacrum, and the coccyx. The spine (C2 through the sacrum) includes three different types of joints:

- Intervertebral disks.
- Facet joints (zygapophyseal joints).
- Fibrous joints.

The intervertebral disks represent fibrocartilaginous symphyses between vertebrae. The facet joints are synovial joints between the superior and inferior articular processes. The fibrous joints include the ligamentum flavum, interspinous ligaments, and supraspinous ligaments.

13.2.1 Vertebral Bodies

The normal spine has a natural S-shaped curve on lateral view. The cervical and lumbar spine contribute to normal spine lordosis while the thoracic spine contributes to the normal spine kyphosis.[4] The superior and inferior end plates should be intact and parallel to one another in the absence of vertebral compression fractures, other fractures, tumors, or infection. A limbus vertebra is a defect within a vertebral body caused by intraosseous disk herniation[5] (▶ Fig. 13.1). The most common location is within the anterior superior corner of the vertebral body.

The subaxial cervical vertebral bodies all have a similar appearance (▶ Fig. 13.2), whereas the atlas (C1) and axis (C2) have a unique anatomy. The atlas has no vertebral body, giving it a ring-like appearance, and the axis has an odontoid process (also known as dens).[6] Each of the lumbar vertebral bodies also has a similar appearance (▶ Fig. 13.3), as do the thoracic vertebral bodies (▶ Fig. 13.4). The anterior and posterior longitudinal ligaments, seen along the vertebral bodies, help stabilize the vertebra and have low signal intensity.[7] The midline of the posterior vertebral bodies provides an entry site to the basivertebral veins.[8] The spinal and radicular arteries course around the cord's anterior, posterior, and lateral aspects within the vertebral canal[9] (▶ Fig. 13.5). Increased fat intensity signal on T2-weighted MRI can decrease the sensitivity in the evaluation of neoplastic and infiltrative processes; thus, fat-suppression techniques can be used to nullify marrow signal and improve visualization of pathologies.[10,11]

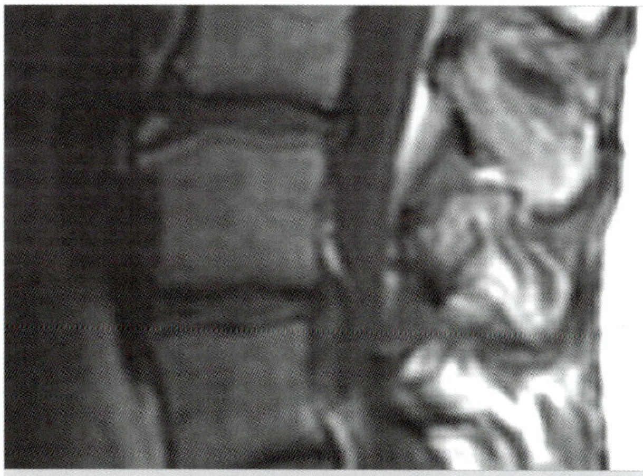

Fig. 13.1 A sagittal T1-weighted image of the lumbar spine shows a normal variant limbus vertebra. A limbus vertebra is a defect within a vertebral body caused by intraosseous disk herniation, most commonly within the anterior superior corner of the vertebral body. (Reproduced with permission from, Normal Spine MRI Anatomy. In: Khanna AJ, ed. MRI Essentials for the Spine Specialist. 1st Edition. New York: Thieme; 2014.)

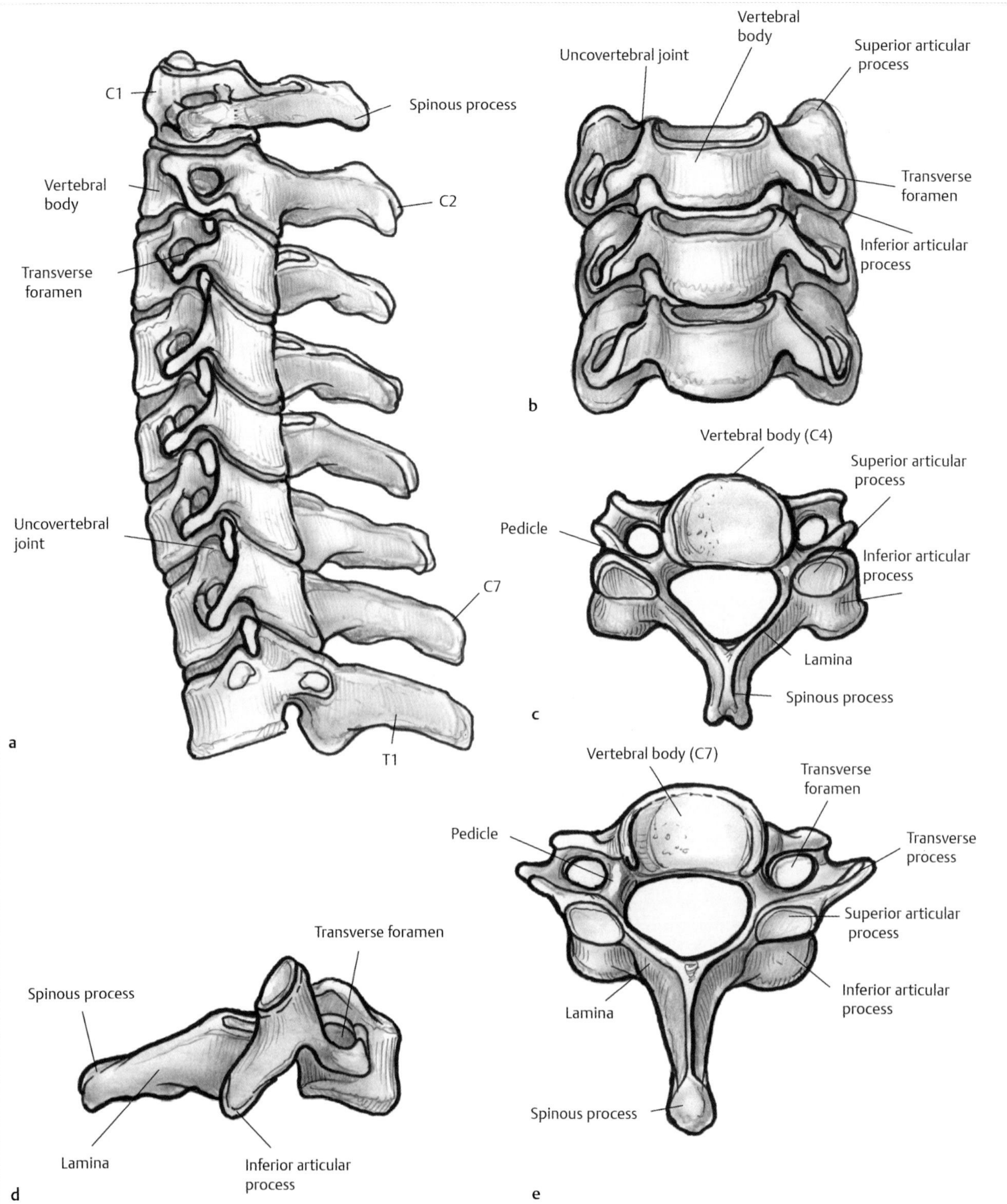

Fig. 13.2 Artist's sketches of the cervical vertebral bodies: **(a)** lateral vertebral bodies from C1–T1, **(b)** anteroposterior (AP) vertebral bodies from C4 to C7, **(c)** axial vertebral body at C4, **(d)** lateral vertebral body at C7, and **(e)** axial vertebral body at C7. (Reproduced with permission from, Normal Spine MRI Anatomy. In: Khanna AJ, ed. MRI Essentials for the Spine Specialist. 1st Edition. New York: Thieme; 2014.)

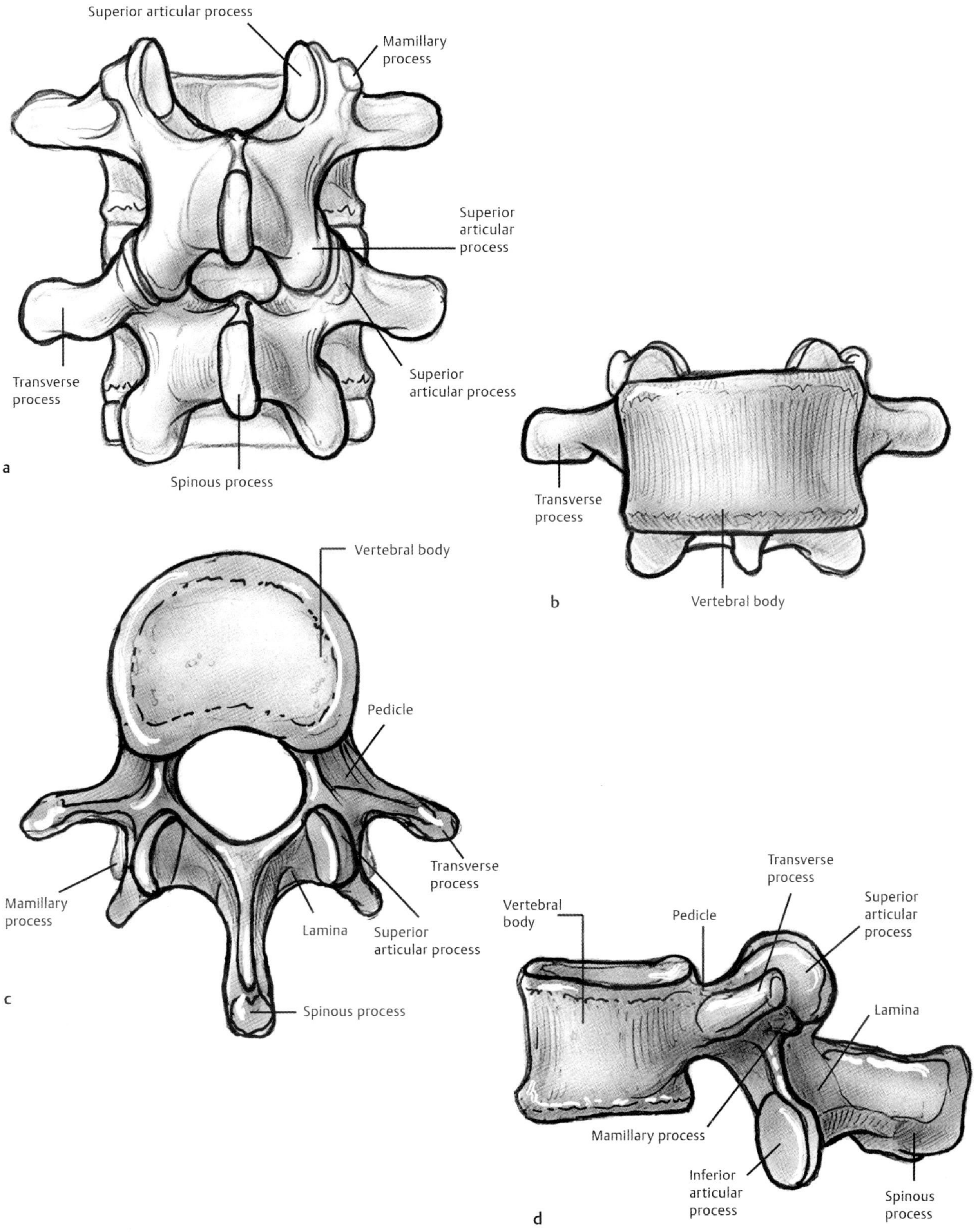

Fig. 13.3 Artist's sketches of the L3 and L4 lumbar vertebral bodies: **(a)** posterior, **(b)** anterior, **(c)** axial, and **(d)** lateral views. (Reproduced with permission from, Normal Spine MRI Anatomy. In: Khanna AJ, ed. MRI Essentials for the Spine Specialist. 1st Edition. New York: Thieme; 2014.)

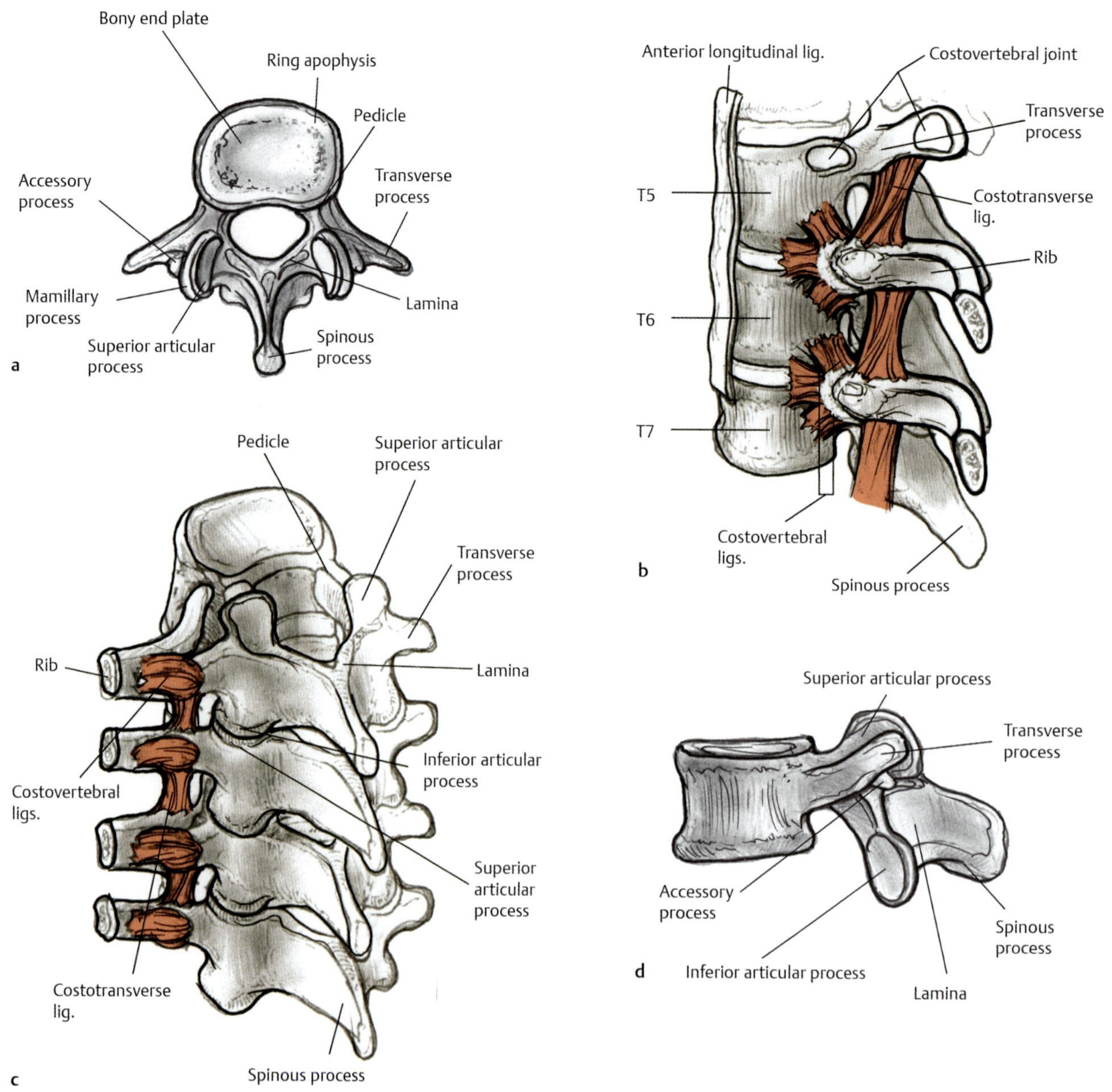

Fig. 13.4 Artist's sketches of the osseous structures of the thoracic spine, the costovertebral joints, and the costotransverse and costovertebral ligaments: **(a)** axial, **(b)** lateral, **(c)** posterior oblique, and **(d)** lateral views. (Reproduced with permission from, Normal Spine MRI Anatomy. In: Khanna AJ, ed. MRI Essentials for the Spine Specialist. 1st Edition. New York: Thieme; 2014.)

13.2.2 Intervertebral Disks

Intervertebral disks are present between each of the vertebral bodies from the axis to the sacrum.[12] They are immensely strong fibrocartilaginous structures that form the strongest bond between adjacent vertebrae.[13] The normal discovertebral complex has three structurally distinct components:

- Cartilaginous end plate.
- Annulus fibrosus.
- Nucleus pulposus.

Overall, the intervertebral disks show intermediate signal intensity on T1-weighted images and high signal intensity on T2-weighted images. The normal annulus fibrosus is hypointense

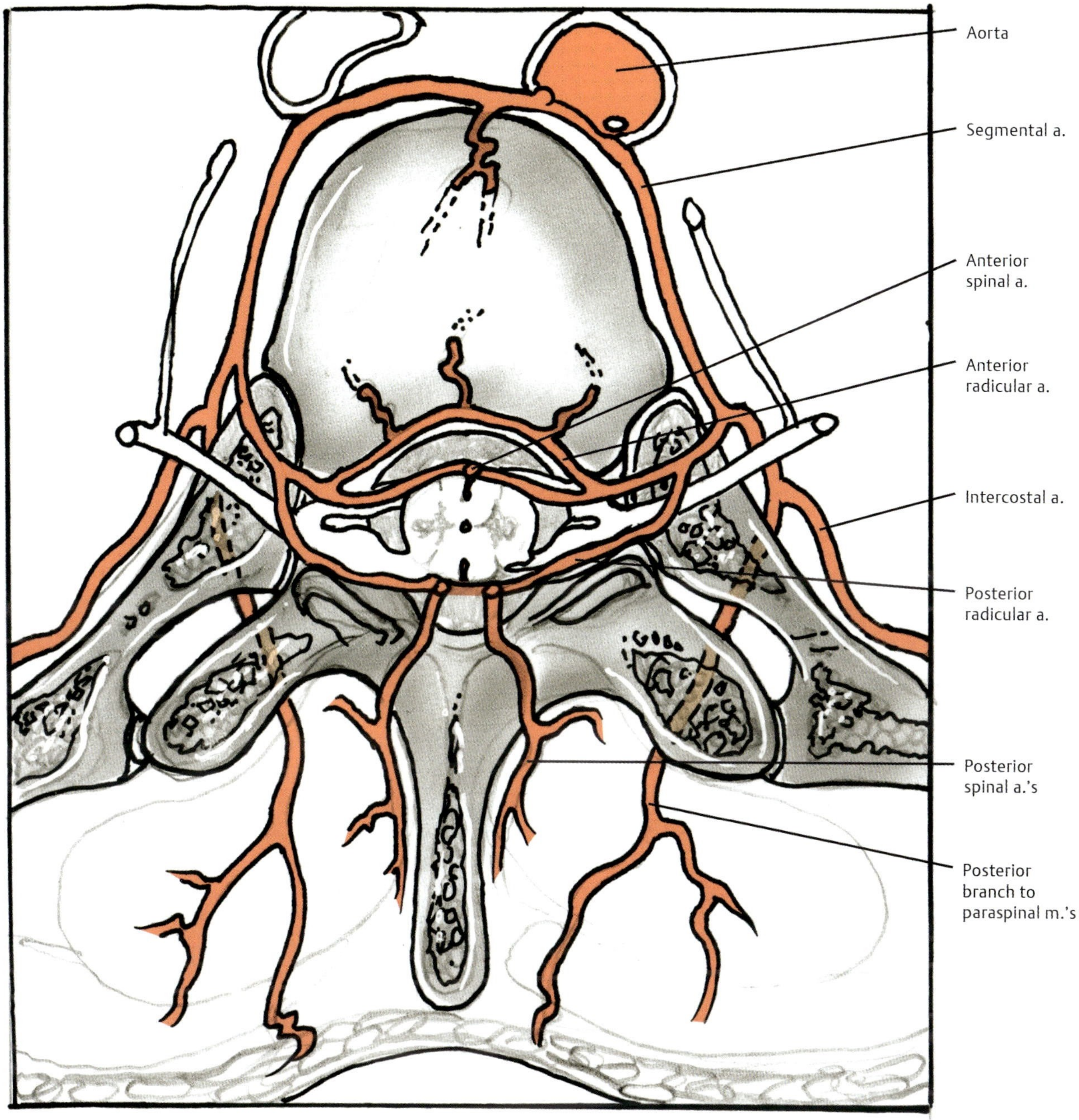

Fig. 13.5 A 3D artist's sketch (axial view) of the spinal, intercostal, and other arteries that supply the thoracic spine. (Reproduced with permission from, Normal Spine MRI Anatomy. In: Khanna AJ, ed. MRI Essentials for the Spine Specialist. 1st Edition. New York: Thieme; 2014.)

on T2-weighted images.[14] In comparison, the nucleus pulposus, which is composed of a proteoglycan matrix and type-II collagen, appears hyperintense on T2-weighted images and hypointense on T1-weighted images.[15]

As the disk degenerates and as patients age, the signal intensity of the nucleus pulposus decreases on T2-weighted images, and the structure becomes dark on all pulse sequences.[16] Additional pulse sequences, such as fat-suppressed T2-weighted images, are useful for accentuating fluid and edema, which may help in delineating spine pathology.[10,17]

End plates superiorly and inferiorly sandwich the nucleus pulposus. The end plate is a flat, osseous disk with a slightly

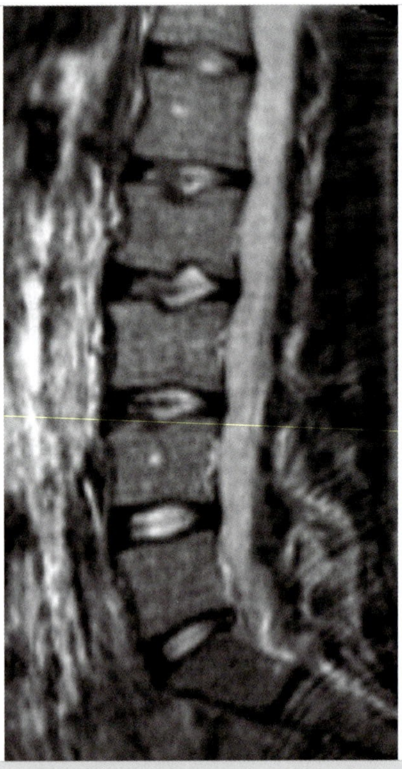

Fig. 13.6 A sagittal T2-weighted image shows multiple Schmorl nodes in the lumbar spine. A Schmorl node results from protrusion of the cartilage of intervertebral disks through the vertebral end plate and into the adjacent vertebra. (Reproduced with permission from, Normal Spine MRI Anatomy. In: Khanna AJ, ed. MRI Essentials for the Spine Specialist. 1st Edition. New York: Thieme; 2014.)

elevated rim secondary to the attached ring apophysis, which produces a central depression in the end plate that is occupied by hyaline cartilage. A Schmorl node results from herniation of the nucleus pulposus through the vertebral end plate and into the adjacent vertebra[18] (▶ Fig. 13.6).

The annulus fibrosus is composed of collagen fibers, proteoglycans, and elastic fibers.[19] Type-I collagen forms Sharpey fibers that are attached to the ring apophysis periosteum.[19,20] The annulus also blends with the anterior and posterior longitudinal ligaments. Unlike the lumbar spine, the annulus fibrosus of the cervical spine consists of a crescentic mass of collagen anteriorly, providing a thicker anterior annulus.[21] The annulus fibrosus is essentially deficient posterolaterally.[21] Intervertebral disks in the lumbar spine are thicker than those in the thoracic spine with the disk height gradually increasing inferiorly except at L5–S1. The posterior margin is concave in the upper lumbosacral spine and straight or convex at L4–L5 and L5–S1. The posterior margin should project no more than 1 mm beyond the end plate.

T1-weighted images provide optimal evaluation of anatomy, fracture lines, and other osseous detail. In addition, the use of

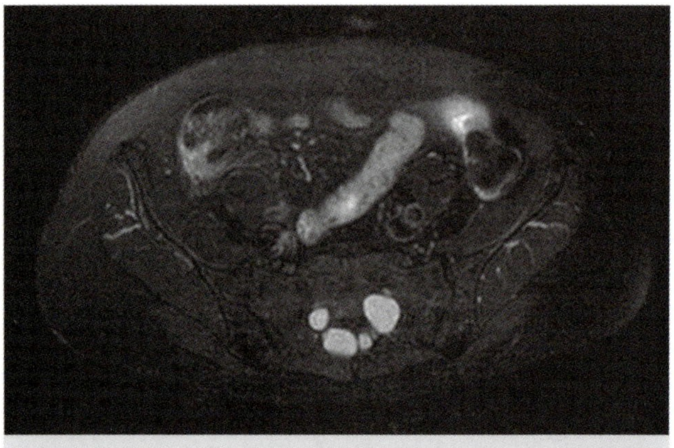

Fig. 13.7 An axial fat-suppressed T2-weighted image shows multiple Tarlov cysts in the sacrum. Tarlov cysts are extradural cerebrospinal fluid (CSF)-filled sacs that occur in the S1–S4 region of the spine and are often asymptomatic. (Reproduced with permission from, Normal Spine MRI Anatomy. In: Khanna AJ, ed. MRI Essentials for the Spine Specialist. 1st Edition. New York: Thieme; 2014.)

T1-weighted images is favorable when delineating the relationships of the vertebral bodies, intervertebral disks, central canal, and posterior elements. Special attention should be given to the posterior aspect of the disk on sagittal and axial T2-weighted images to evaluate for disk protrusion, extrusion, sequestration, or other pathology that may be contributing to central canal or neural foraminal stenosis.

13.2.3 Epidural Space

The epidural space in the spinal canal is the true space between the dura and bone extending from the foramen magnum to the caudal hiatus[22] Contents include epidural fat, nerves, blood vessels, the ligamentum flavum, and the posterior longitudinal ligament. The dura extends caudally to S2 and has lateral outpouchings to the nerve roots. At L5–S1, the thecal sac enlarges, and usually no epidural fat is seen on MRI. Tarlov cysts are common extradural cerebrospinal fluid (CSF)-filled sacs that occur in the sacral region of the spinal cord and are often asymptomatic[23,24] (▶ Fig. 13.7).

13.2.4 Cerebrospinal Fluid (CSF)

Similar to other fluids, CSF has low signal intensity on T1-weighted images and high signal intensity on T2-weighted images.[25] On sagittal and axial images, CSF is seen surrounding the spinal cord in the cervical, thoracic, and lumbar spine and around the cauda equina in the lower lumbar spine. Thus, T2-weighted images provide a myelographic appearance that allows for the detection of spinal stenosis. A potential pitfall spine specialists or radiologists should be aware of is the possibility for imaging artifacts relating to CSF flow.[26] These

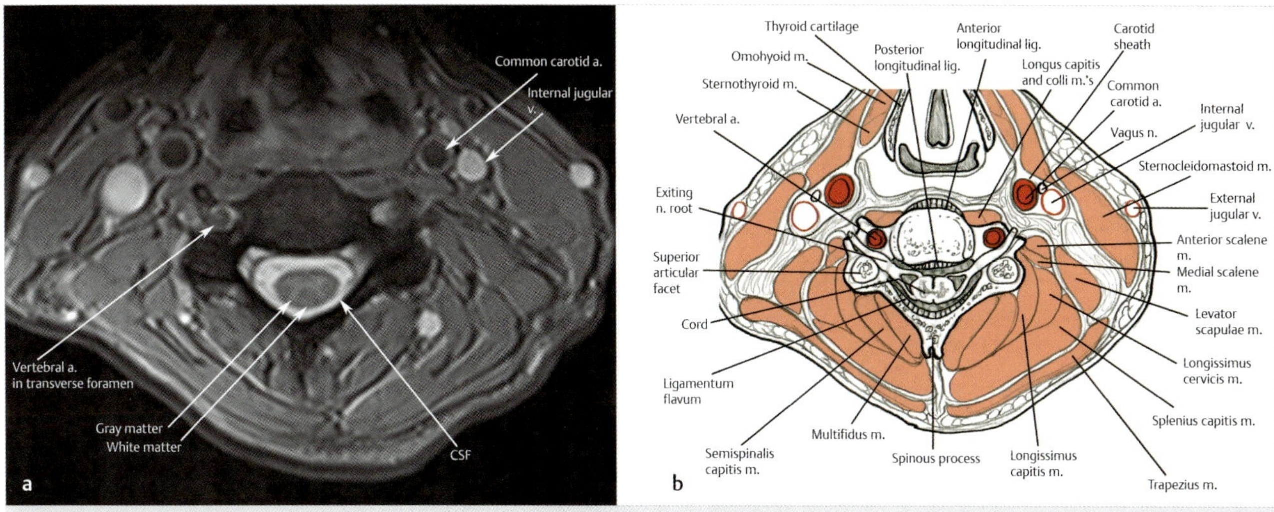

Fig. 13.8 This **(a)** axial T2-weighted image and **(b)** artist's sketch clearly define the gray and white matter of the cervical spinal cord, the cerebrospinal fluid (CSF) within the subarachnoid space, and epidural fat. Normal flow voids are seen within the carotid and vertebral arteries. (Reproduced with permission from, Normal Spine MRI Anatomy. In: Khanna AJ, ed. MRI Essentials for the Spine Specialist. 1st Edition. New York: Thieme; 2014.)

artifacts are most commonly seen in the thoracic spine and can be mistaken for tumors or arteriovenous fistulas.[26,27]

13.2.5 Spinal Cord

As noted above, the sagittal T2-weighted images provide a myelographic effect that allows the evaluation of spinal cord morphology and the presence of extrinsic compression. The cord should have homogeneous signal intensity in the absence of intrinsic pathology.[28] The central gray matter can be faintly identified on T2-weighted images. Specialized sequences obtained with high-field magnets enable detailed evaluation of central gray matter (▶ Fig. 13.8). The spinal cord should terminate at or above the L1–L2 level in adults.

13.2.6 Ligaments

Important ligaments include the transverse ligament, ligamentum flavum, anterior and posterior ligaments.[29] The ligaments should have low signal intensity on all pulse sequences. Thus, in cases of ligamentous disruption a focus of hyperintensity is present on MRI.[29] The transverse ligament can be seen posterior to the odontoid process (▶ Fig. 13.9) and is best visualized on axial images. The ligamentum flavum connects the lamina of adjacent vertebrae and is seen as a hypointense band posterior to the dura.[30] The ligamentum flavum blends with capsules of facet joints. In the cervical spine, the ligamentum flavum is typically 1.5 mm in thickness. In the lumbar spine, the ligamentum flavum is 4 to 6 mm in thickness. The ligamentum flavum may also calcify and lead to osseous spur formation and resultant neuroforaminal stenosis.[31,32] In addition, spinal stenosis can result from the hypertrophy of the ligamentum flavum.[33]

The anterior longitudinal ligament extends along the anterior surface of the spine from the anterior margin of the foramen magnum to S1. The anterior longitudinal ligament is broad, thick, and adherent to the anterior vertebral bodies. It is loosely attached to the intervertebral disks. Although deep fibers span one intervertebral articulation, superficial fibers span up to four articulations. The anterior longitudinal ligament is broad in the cervical spine, narrower in the thoracic spine, and the broadest in the lumbar spine.[34] The low signal on MRI blends with the peripheral portion of the annulus fibrosus and cortical bone.

The posterior longitudinal ligament extends from the body of the axis to the sacrum, merging superiorly with the tectorial membrane.[35] The posterior longitudinal ligament is thin, attached to the posterior vertebral cortex via the midline septum, and defines the anterior margin of the anterior epidural space at the midline (▶ Fig. 13.10). The anterior epidural space is not apparent at the disk level because the posterior longitudinal ligament fuses to the disks. Visualization of these structures may be limited with MRI because of partial volume averaging with the adjacent vertebral body.[36] The posterior longitudinal ligament is attached to the intervertebral disks and margins of the adjacent vertebral bodies. There is no attachment at the center of the vertebral bodies. Deep fibers extend between adjacent vertebrae, whereas superficial fibers bridge three to four bodies. Ossification of the posterior longitudinal ligament can result in stenosis and myelopathy.[37] The posterior longitudinal ligament, like most ligaments, has low signal on both T1- and T2-weighted images.

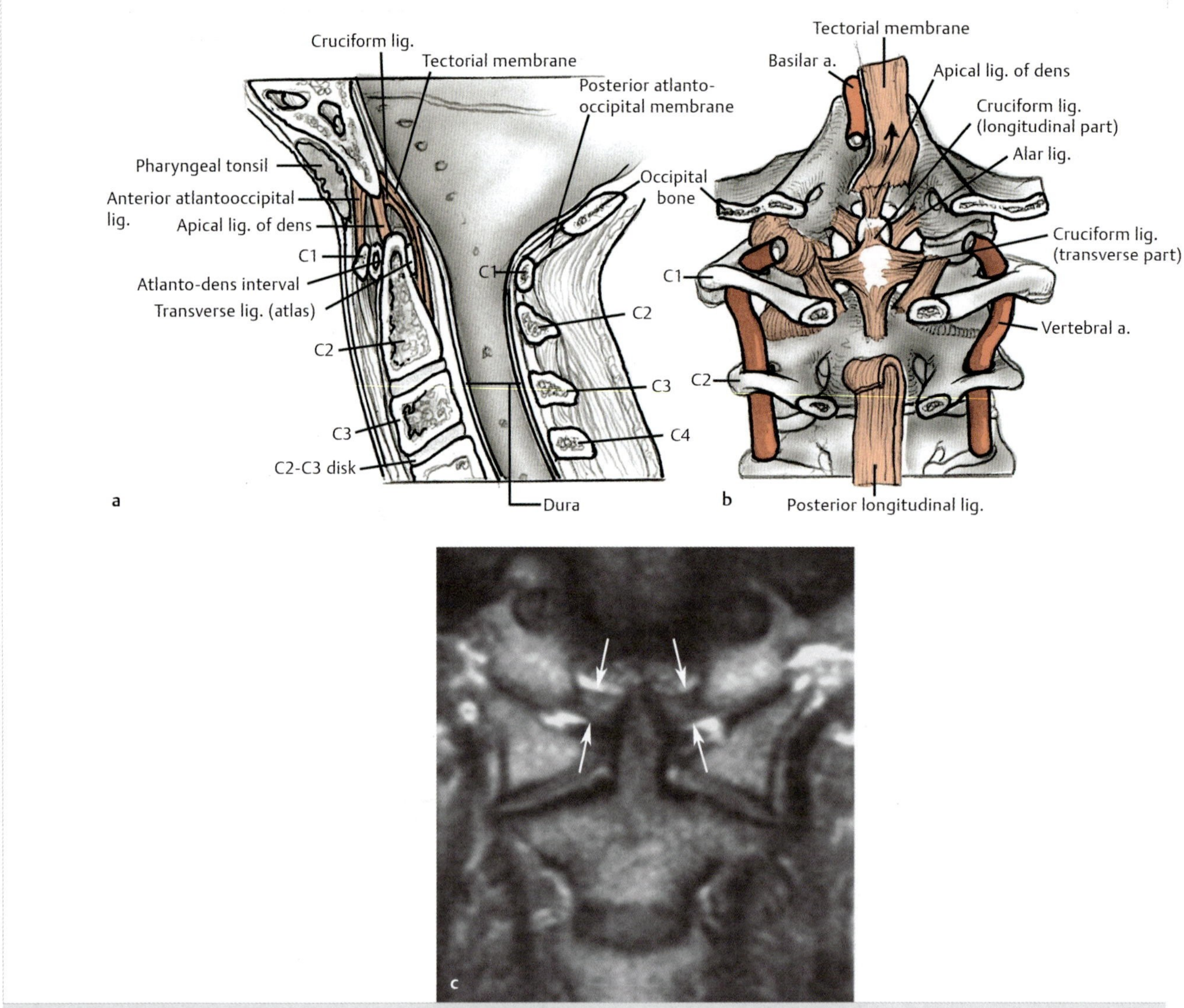

Fig. 13.9 These **(a)** sagittal and **(b)** posteroanterior artist's sketches showing the ligamentous structures of the skull base and cervical spine, including the alar ligament, cruciform ligament, and atlantooccipital ligaments. **(c)** A coronal T1-weighted image shows the alar ligaments (*arrows*). (Reproduced with permission from, Normal Spine MRI Anatomy. In: Khanna AJ, ed. MRI Essentials for the Spine Specialist. 1st Edition. New York: Thieme; 2014.)

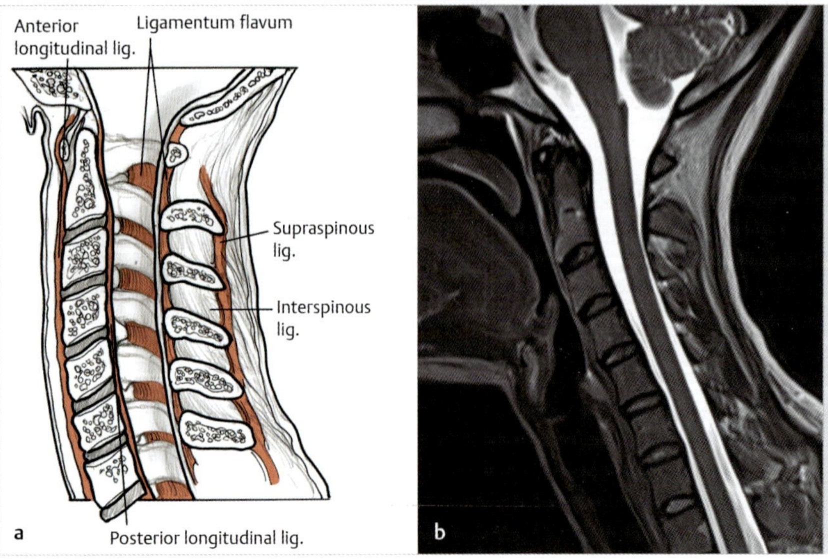

Fig. 13.10 This **(a)** sagittal T2-weighted image and **(b)** artist's sketch (lateral view) show the midsagittal ligaments of the cervical spine. (Reproduced with permission from, Normal Spine MRI Anatomy. In: Khanna AJ, ed. MRI Essentials for the Spine Specialist. 1st Edition. New York: Thieme; 2014.)

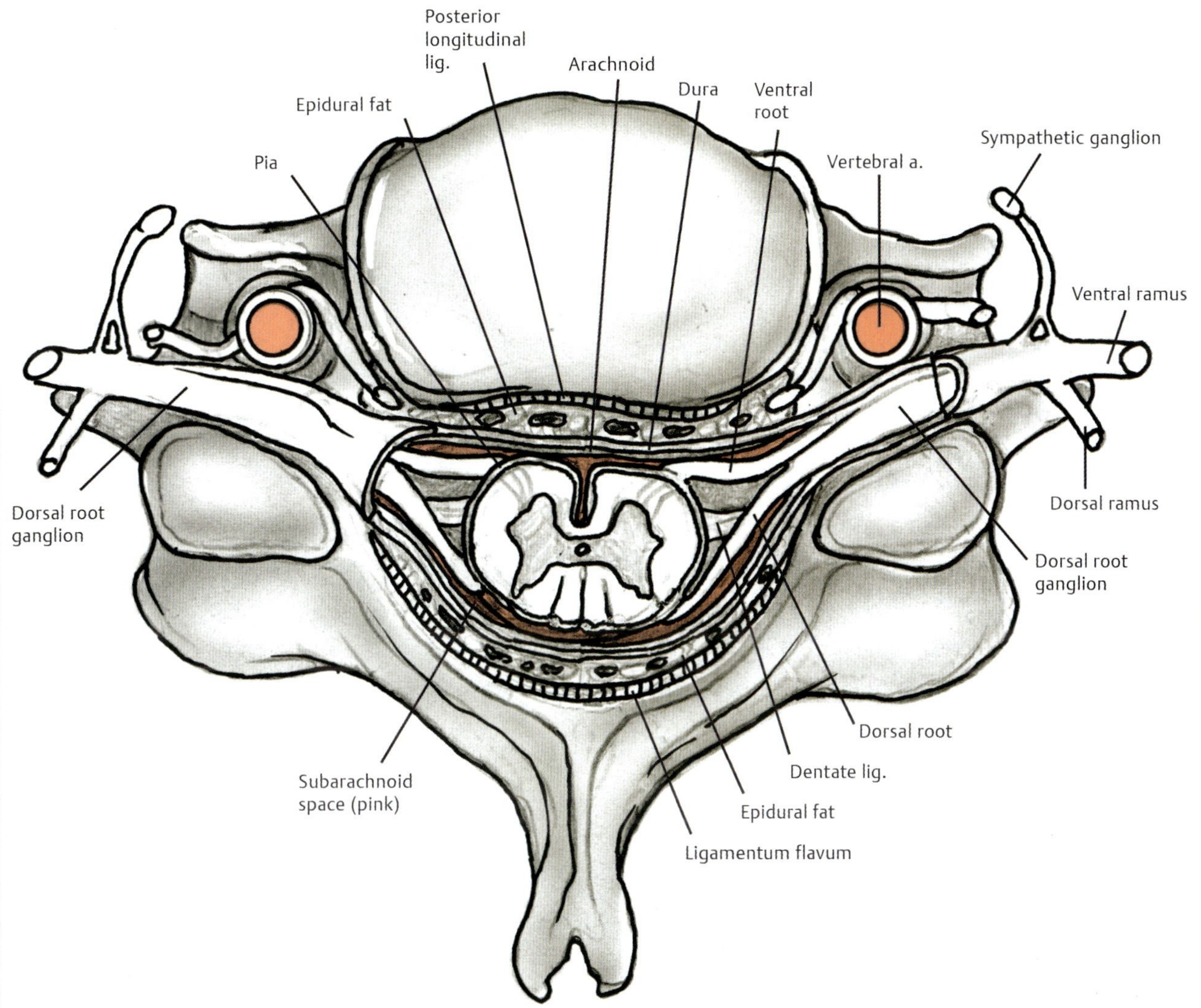

Fig. 13.11 An axial artist's sketch shows various anatomic structures around the spinal cord. (Reproduced with permission from, Normal Spine MRI Anatomy. In: Khanna AJ, ed. MRI Essentials for the Spine Specialist. 1st Edition. New York: Thieme; 2014.)

13.2.7 Roots and Foramina

The neuroforamina or neural canals are bordered anteriorly by the vertebral bodies and disks, posteriorly by the facet joint and articular processes, and superiorly and interiorly by pedicles. Nerve roots exit the spine laterally through the neuroforamen. The dorsal and ventral nerve roots can be identified within the neural foramina on the parasagittal images and the axial images. The nerve roots join around the intervertebral foramen to form a mixed nerve with motor and sensory fibers. The exiting nerve root is located just posterior to the vertebral artery in the cervical spine (▶ Fig. 13.11). Additional neural structures, including the sympathetic chain, are located in and around the cervical vertebral bodies (▶ Fig. 13.12). C1–C7 cervical nerve roots exit above the similarly numbered vertebral bodies, while C8 exits below the C7 vertebral body. It should be noted that the C2 nerve root exits the spine above the C2 pedicle and runs parallel to the C1–C2 facet joint (▶ Fig. 13.13). The 12 thoracic and 5 lumbar nerve roots exit below the similarly numbered vertebrae. The nerve roots have intermediate signal intensity and are surrounded by high-signal-intensity fat on T1-weighted images and by high-signal-intensity CSF on T2-weighted images. Common nerve sheaths are common at L4, L5, S1, and S2; one should be wary of the potential of nerve sheaths mimicking a disk herniation on MRI.[38] On gadolinium-enhanced MRI, there is

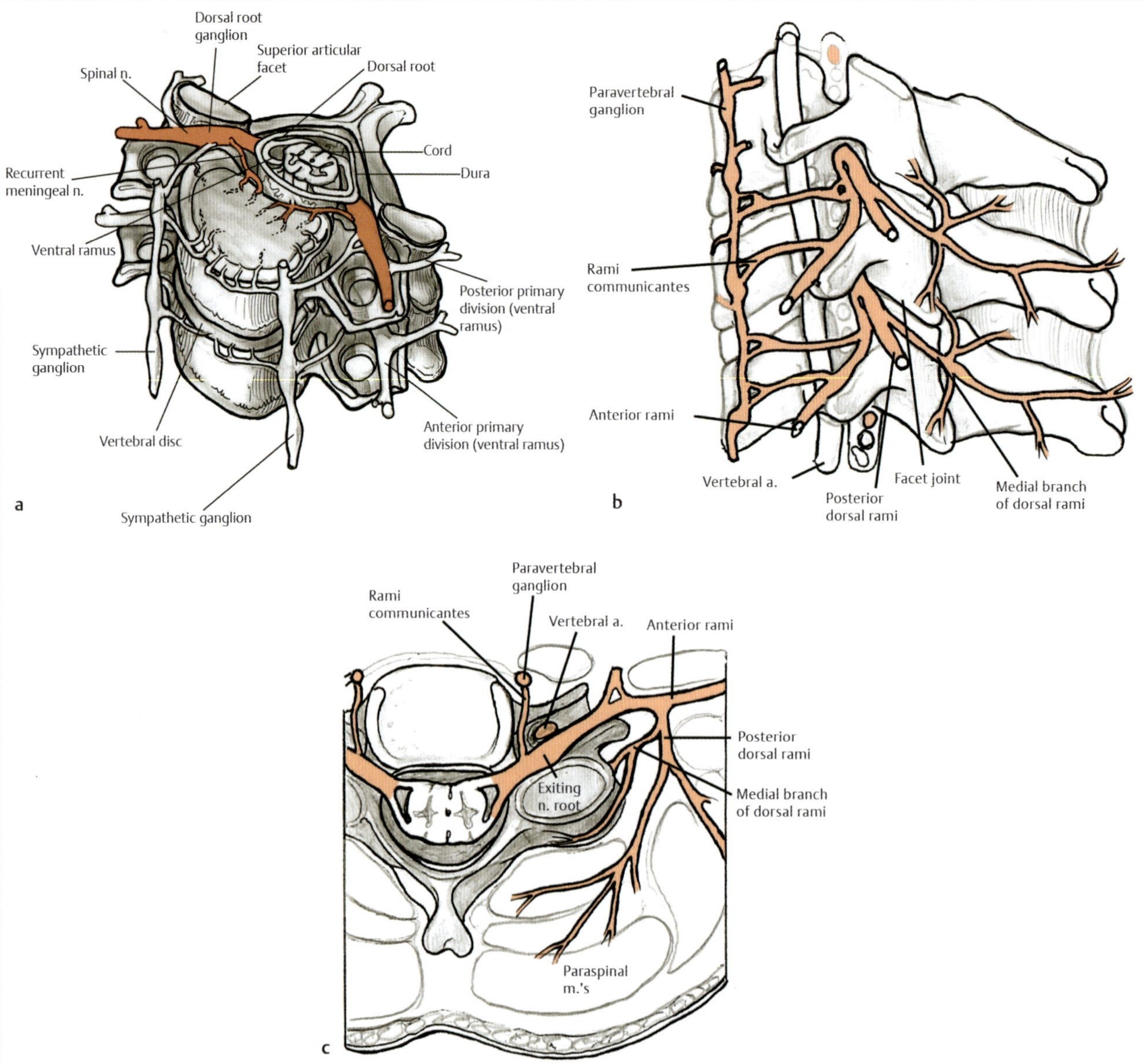

Fig. 13.12 Artist's sketches of the neural structures in and around the cervical spine from the **(a)** anterosuperior, **(b)** lateral, and **(c)** axial perspectives. (Reproduced with permission from, Normal Spine MRI Anatomy. In: Khanna AJ, ed. MRI Essentials for the Spine Specialist. 1st Edition. New York: Thieme; 2014.)

normal enhancement of the dorsal root ganglion. The normal conus medullaris ends around the level of the inferior end plate of L1 in adults.

13.2.8 Facet Joints

The facet joint is the articulation of the inferior articular process of the posterior elements of a vertebra with the superior articular process of the posterior elements of the next vertebra (▶ Fig. 13.14). It is a synovial-type joint that consists of a capsule, synovium, menisci, and hyaline (articular) cartilage lining the reciprocating surfaces. Facet joint pathologies could be a potential source of low back pain.[39,40] Because the term "facet" actually represents only the articular cartilage surface of the joint, a more appropriate term is zygapophyseal joint or "z-joint."

The anatomy of the zygapophyseal joint is oriented differently throughout the spine because of varying biomechanical stress. In the cervical spine, the zygapophyseal joint is oriented in a transverse/oblique plane (20- to 78-degree inclination

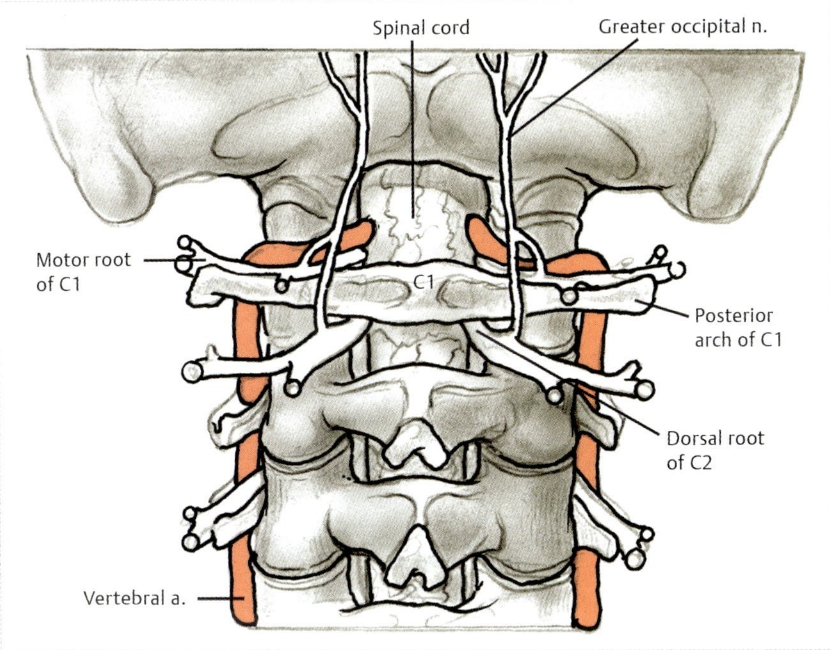

Fig. 13.13 A posterior 3D artist's sketch of the upper cervical spine shows the location of the vertebral artery relative to the posterior arch of C1 and the exit of the C2 nerve root above the pedicle of C2. (Reproduced with permission from, Normal Spine MRI Anatomy. In: Khanna AJ, ed. MRI Essentials for the Spine Specialist. 1st Edition. New York: Thieme; 2014.)

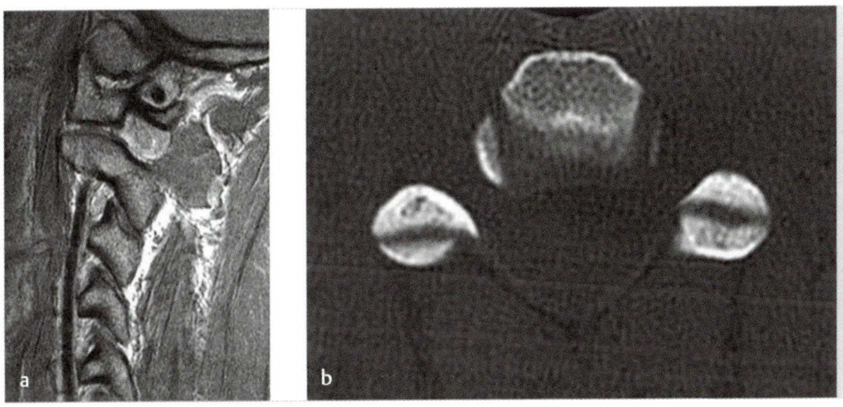

Fig. 13.14 Facet joints in the cervical spine. The facet joint is the articulation of the inferior articular process of the posterior elements of a vertebra with the superior articular process of the posterior elements of the next vertebra. **(a)** Parasagittal T1-weighted magnetic resonance (MR) and **(b)** axial computed tomography (CT) images show normal facet joints in the cervical spine. (Reproduced with permission from, Normal Spine MRI Anatomy. In: Khanna AJ, ed. MRI Essentials for the Spine Specialist. 1st Edition. New York: Thieme; 2014.)

angle in the sagittal plane).[41] In the thoracic spine, the zygapophyseal joint is oriented coronal (55–80 degrees in the sagittal plane).[41,42] In the lumbar spine, the zygapophyseal joint is typically oriented in the sagittal/oblique plane with a 82- to 86-degree inclination angle in the sagittal plane.[41]

13.2.9 Vascular Structures

Normal vascular anatomy is important to recognize when evaluating MRI studies of the spine and spinal cord (even when evaluating for nonvascular diagnoses) (▶ Fig. 13.15). The superior cord is supplied by the anterior spinal artery and two posterior spinal arteries that originate from the vertebral arteries.[43] Spinal radicular arteries supply the vertebrae, meninges, and spinal cord. Radicular arteries arise from the vertebral, deep cervical, posterior intercostal, lumbar, and lateral sacral arteries. Radicular arteries enter through the neuroforamina and divide into anterior and posterior branches (▶ Fig. 13.16).

The anterior spinal artery supplies the entire spinal cord, except for the dorsal column. The three major regions supplied are: the cervicothoracic, the midthoracic, and the thoracolumbar spinal cord (▶ Fig. 13.5, ▶ Fig. 13.17). There are

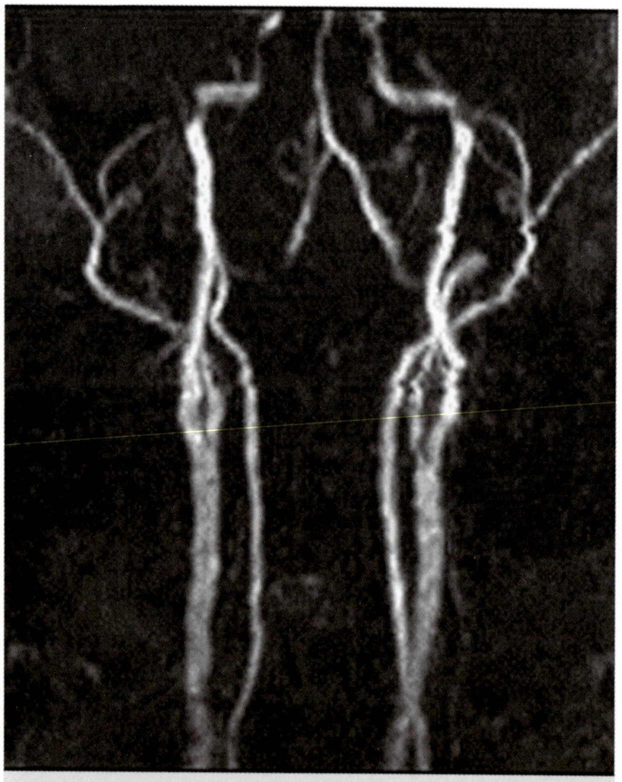

Fig. 13.15 This 2D time-of-flight sequence shows the normal vascular anatomy of the upper cervical spine. (Reproduced with permission from, Normal Spine MRI Anatomy. In: Khanna AJ, ed. MRI Essentials for the Spine Specialist. 1st Edition. New York: Thieme; 2014.)

watershed areas at the margins of each region where adequate collateral flow is not always available. Disabling consequences can ensue an infarction of the watershed areas in the case of systemic hypotension or compromise of a major radiculomedullary feeding vessel.[44,45]

There are several major radiculomedullary arteries that merit additional attention. The C3 radiculomedullary artery arises from the vertebral artery. The C6 radiculomedullary artery, or the artery of cervical enlargement, arises from the thyrocervical or costocervical trunk. The T4–T5 radiculomedullary artery arises from the intercostal artery. The T9–L1 radiculomedullary artery, also known as the artery of lumbar enlargement or the artery of Adamkiewicz, arises from an intercostal or lumbar artery.[43] The artery of Adamkiewicz has a "hairpin loop" configuration because of the differential growth of the spinal cord. In 85% of cases, the artery of Adamkiewicz arises from the left T9–L2 levels.[46] In the other 15% of cases, the artery of Adamkiewicz arises from T5 to T8.[46]

The posterior spinal artery originates from the vertebral artery or the posteroinferior cerebellar artery. Posterior arteries are smaller and more uniform in caliber than the anterior spinal artery (▶ Fig. 13.18). The two posterior spinal arteries are connected by frequent intercommunications across the dorsal surface of the spinal cord. There is infrequent intercommunication along the lateral surfaces of the cord between the posterior spinal arteries and the anterior spinal artery through the circumferential pial arterial plexus.

Venous drainage is compartmentalized into three groups: internal venous plexus, external venous plexus, and basivertebral plexus.[8] Venous drainage occurs via the external vertebral plexus and subsequently the internal vertebral plexus via basivertebral veins (▶ Fig. 13.19). The basivertebral plexus has a Y-shaped appearance on axial images. The cord and vertebral plexi drain via radicular and intervertebral veins through neuroforamina into the vertebral vein, ascending lumbar veins, and azygous system (▶ Fig. 13.20).

On gadolinium-enhanced MRI, there is normal enhancement of the vessels of the epidural plexus and the basivertebral venous plexus.

13.2.10 Muscles

The paraspinal muscles are the group of superficial and deep muscles that run adjacent to the spine (▶ Fig. 13.21). They help support the spine to maintain posture and stability.[35] In addition, paraspinal muscles assist with motion of individual bones and of the core as a whole. Muscles of the spine are arranged in layers. The superficial or extrinsic paraspinal muscles include the trapezius, latissimus dorsi, levator scapulae, rhomboid minor, and rhomboid major. The deep muscles of the cervical, thoracic, and lumbar spine include the splenius capitis, splenius cervicis, erector spinae, semispinalis, multifidus, rotatores, interspinalis, and intertransverse. Suboccipital deep muscles include the rectus capitis, oblique capitis superior, and oblique capitis inferior. Prevertebral deep muscles include the rectus capitis, longus colli, longus capitis, scalene, and psoas.[35] The paraspinal muscles should be evaluated by MRI to assess for asymmetry, atrophy, and/or pathology.

13.3 Cervical Spine

13.3.1 Anatomy

The occiput is labeled as C0. The occipital bone is a broad, flat bone that encircles the cerebellum as it gives rise to the pons and medulla in the posterior fossa. The sphenoid bone also contributes to the anterior aspect of the posterior fossa. The clivus is the portion of the sphenoid bone that meets the occipital bone. The foramen magnum is the opening at the base of the skull. It is defined anteriorly by the basion, posteriorly by the opisthion, and laterally by the occipital condyles. The occipital condyles contain the hypoglossal nerve as it courses anteriorly to exit the hypoglossal foramen. The external occipital protuberance is the attachment site of the ligamentum nuchae and the trapezius muscle. The inion, a term sometimes used as a synonym for the external occipital protuberance, is actually the highest point of the external occipital protuberance. The external occipital protuberance corresponds internally with the

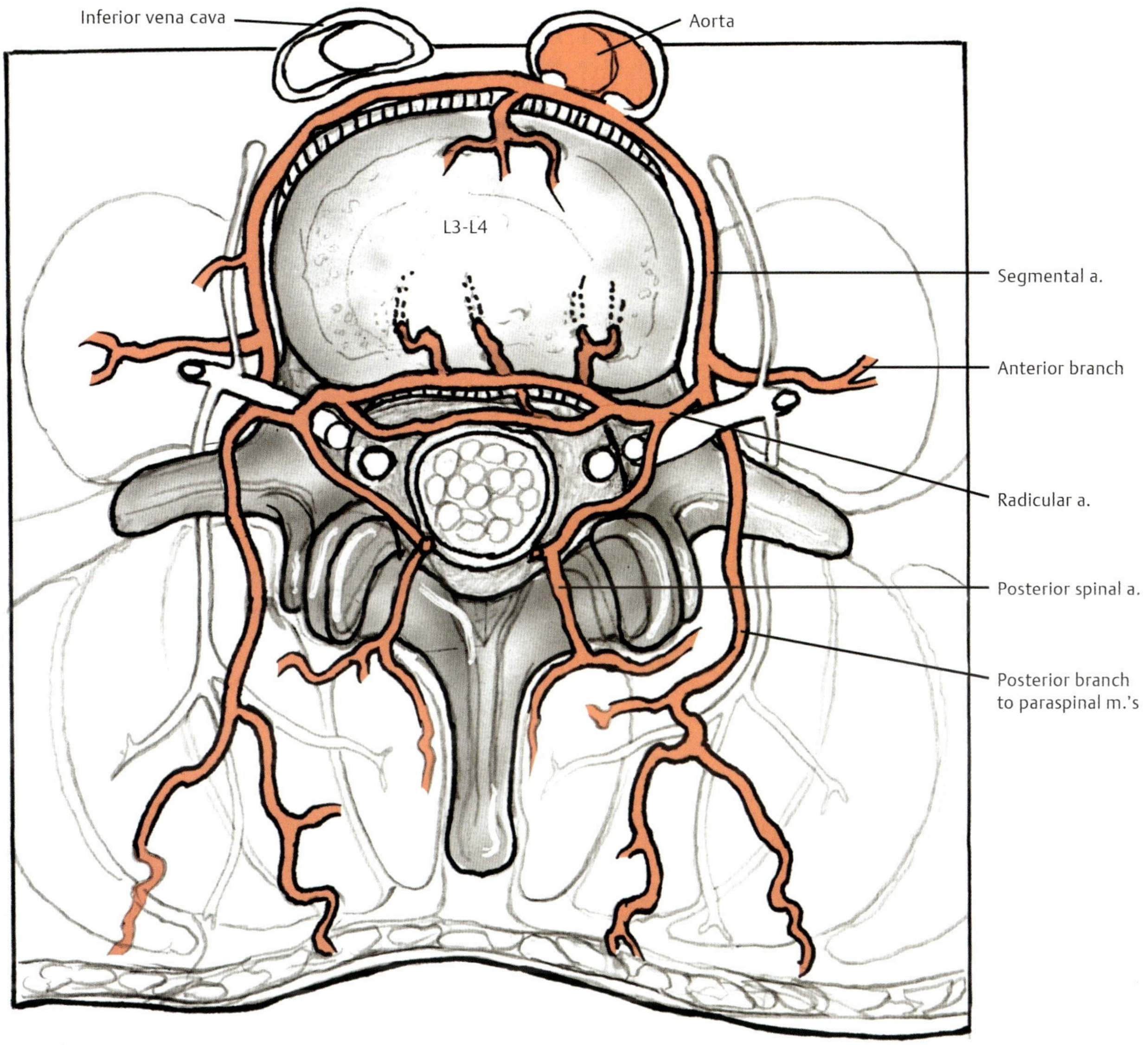

Fig. 13.16 An artist's sketch of the arterial vasculature of the lumbar spine (axial perspective at the L3–L4 level). The spinal radicular arteries supply the vertebrae, meninges, and spinal cord and enter via the neural foramina. (Reproduced with permission from, Normal Spine MRI Anatomy. In: Khanna AJ, ed. MRI Essentials for the Spine Specialist. 1st Edition. New York: Thieme; 2014.)

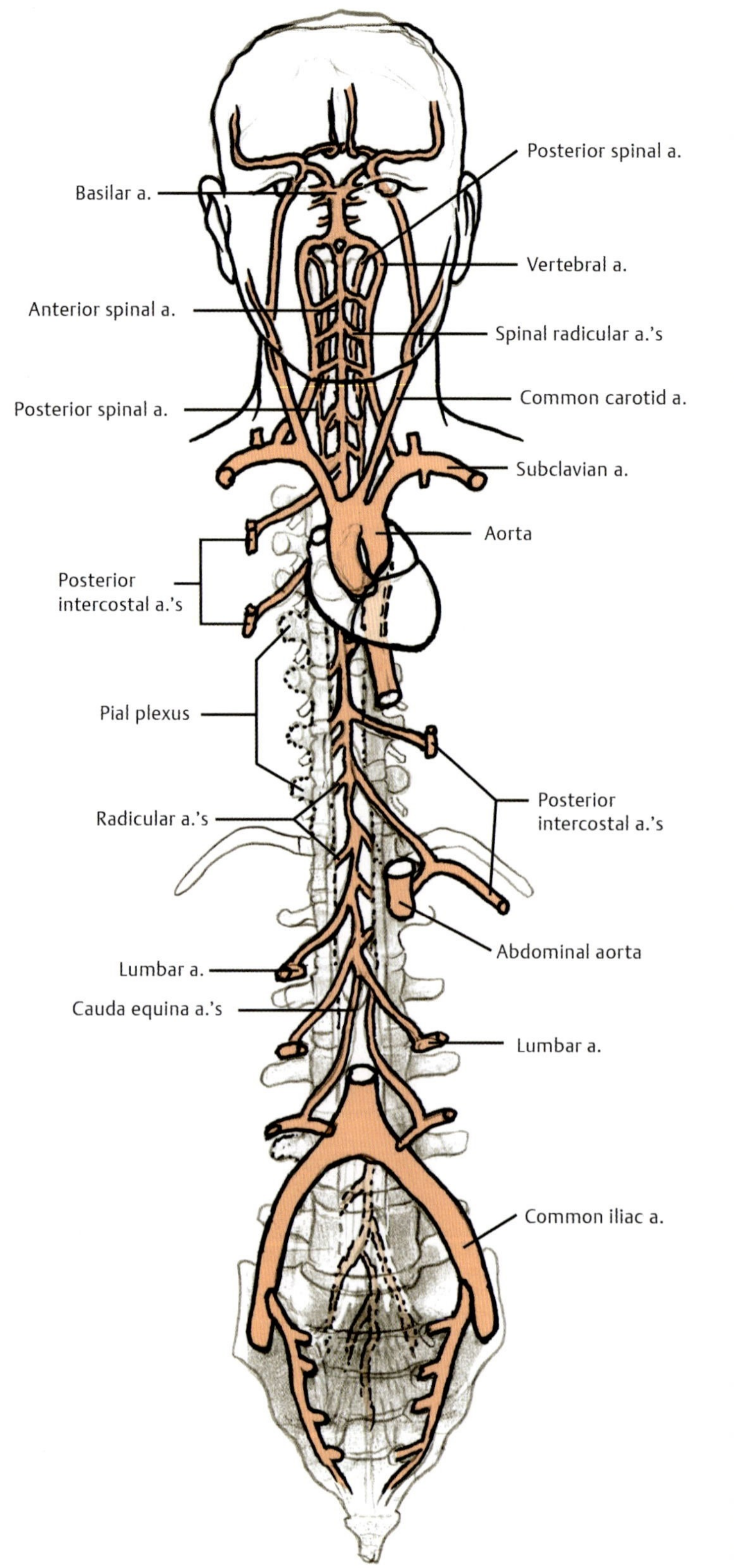

Fig. 13.17 An artist's sketch of the arterial vasculature of the spine from an anterior perspective. (Reproduced with permission from, Normal Spine MRI Anatomy. In: Khanna AJ, ed. MRI Essentials for the Spine Specialist. 1st Edition. New York: Thieme; 2014.)

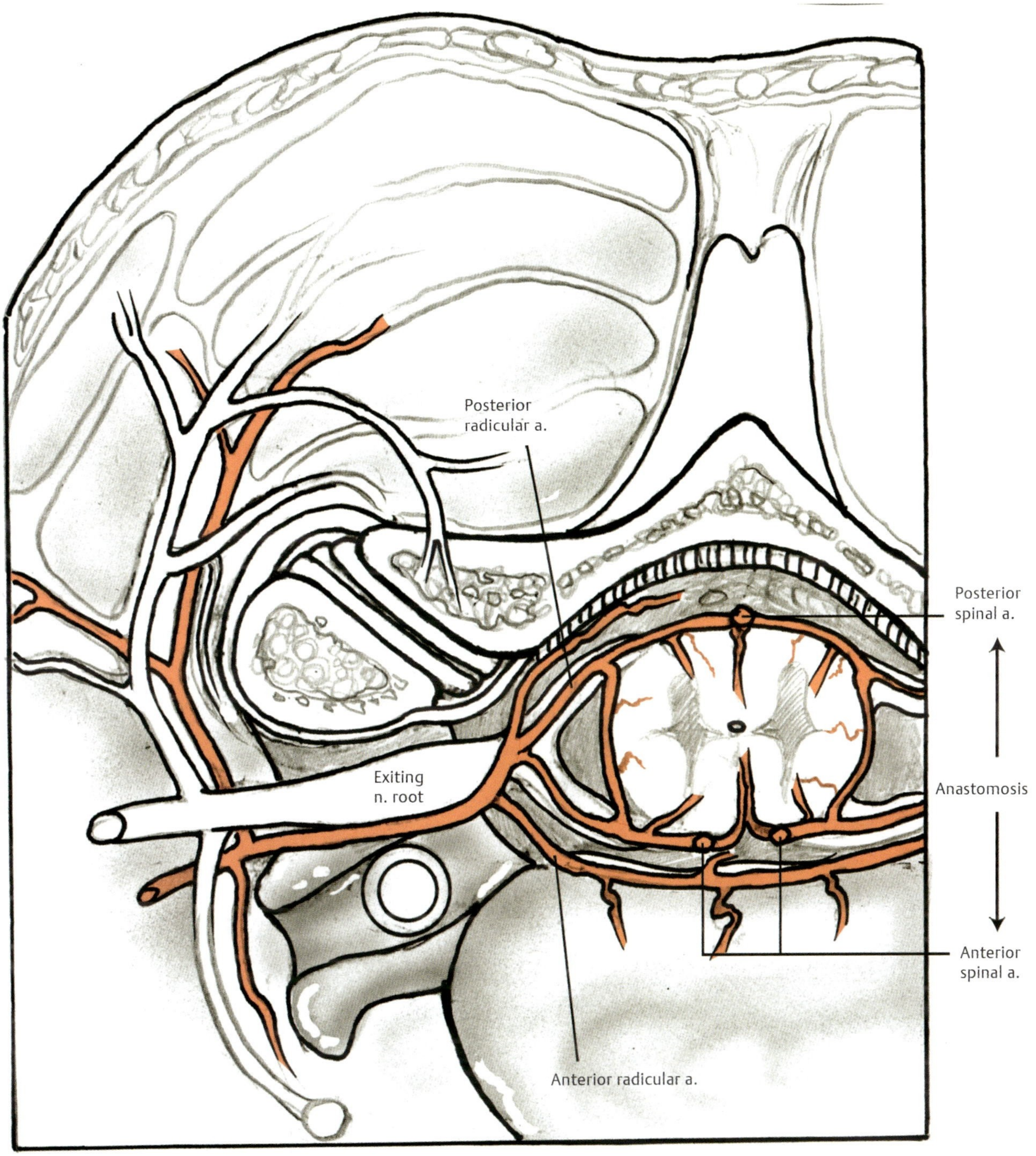

Fig. 13.18 An artist's sketch depicts the anastomoses between the posterior spinal artery and the anterior spinal artery. (Reproduced with permission from, Normal Spine MRI Anatomy. In: Khanna AJ, ed. MRI Essentials for the Spine Specialist. 1st Edition. New York: Thieme; 2014.)

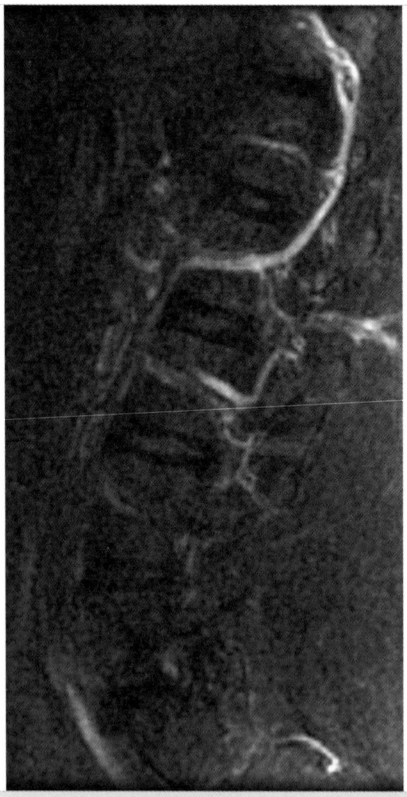

Fig. 13.19 A sagittal fat-suppressed T2-weighted image shows venous drainage in the spine. (Reproduced with permission from, Normal Spine MRI Anatomy. In: Khanna AJ, ed. MRI Essentials for the Spine Specialist. 1st Edition. New York: Thieme; 2014.)

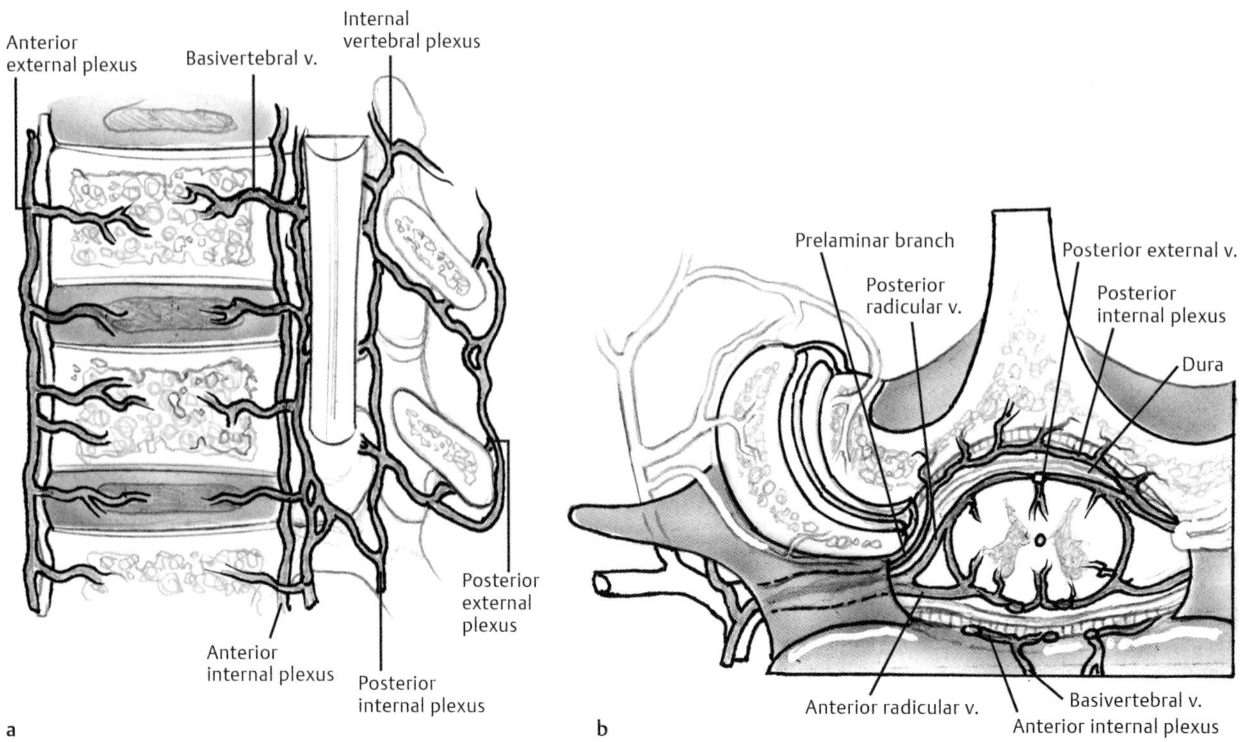

Fig. 13.20 Artist's sketches detail the venous drainage of the spine from **(a)** sagittal and **(b)** axial perspectives. (Reproduced with permission from, Normal Spine MRI Anatomy. In: Khanna AJ, ed. MRI Essentials for the Spine Specialist. 1st Edition. New York: Thieme; 2014.)

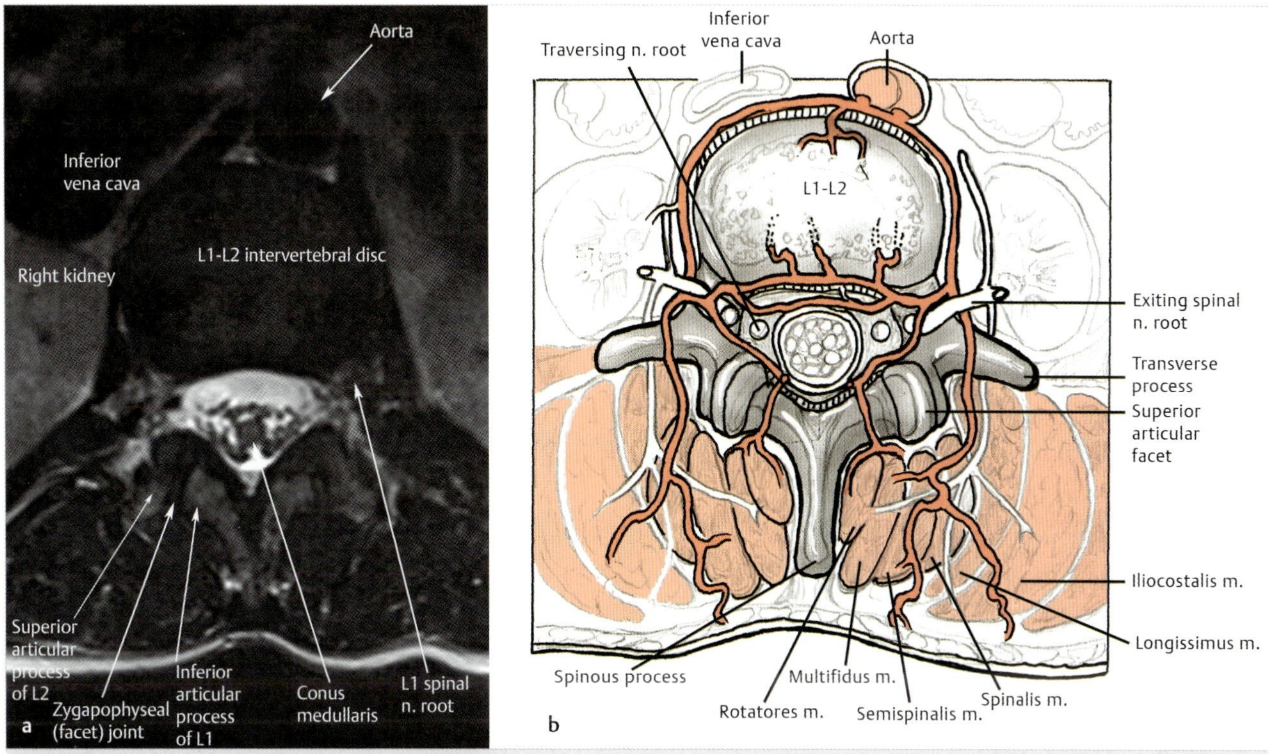

Fig. 13.21 This **(a)** axial T2-weighted image and **(b)** artist's sketch of the normal anatomic location of the paraspinal muscles and other neurovascular structures. These views at the level of the L1–L2 intervertebral disk show the conus medullaris and the L1 spinal nerve root, as well as the superior and inferior articular processes of the L1–L2 facet joint. (Reproduced with permission from, Normal Spine MRI Anatomy. In: Khanna AJ, ed. MRI Essentials for the Spine Specialist. 1st Edition. New York: Thieme; 2014.)

confluences of the sinuses. Other important external landmarks include the superior and inferior nuchal lines, which are attachment sites for cervical musculature. The rectus capitis posterior major, obliquus capitis inferior, and obliquus capitis superior form the borders of the suboccipital triangle.[6] The suboccipital triangle contains the vertebral artery, suboccipital nerve, and suboccipital venous plexus.

C1, also known as the atlas, is a unique ring-shaped structure that lacks a vertebral body. It is, instead, composed of two lateral masses, a short anterior arch, a longer posterior arch, and grooves for the vertebral artery. The right and left lateral masses are connected by the anterior and posterior arches. The lateral masses of C1 articulate inferiorly via facet joints with C2 (▶ Fig. 13.22). The dens, or odontoid process of C2, articulates with the anterior arch of C1 (▶ Fig. 13.23). The C0–C1 articulation is termed the atlantooccipital joint and is a cup-shaped configuration (▶ Fig. 13.24). In addition to primary stabilization from the morphology of the joint, ligamentous-stabilizing structures are present and include joint capsules, anterior and posterior atlantooccipital membranes, and C0–C2 ligaments. The primary motion of the atlantooccipital joint is flexion-extension by which the occipital condyles glide in the sockets of the atlas. Lateral flexion is constrained by the contralateral alar ligament that spans from the dens to the occipital condyles medially.

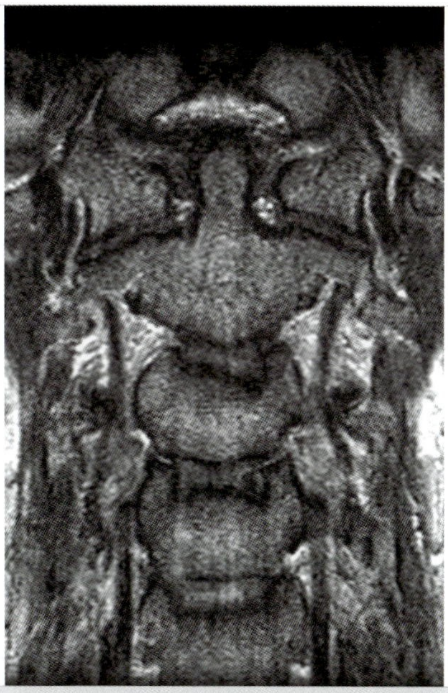

Fig. 13.22 A coronal T1-weighted image shows the normal anatomic articulation of the lateral masses of C1 and C2. (Reproduced with permission from, Normal Spine MRI Anatomy. In: Khanna AJ, ed. MRI Essentials for the Spine Specialist. 1st Edition. New York: Thieme; 2014.)

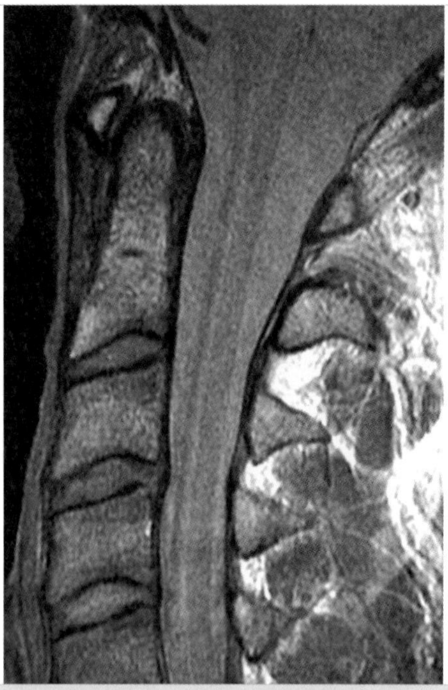

Fig. 13.23 A sagittal T1-weighted image shows the normal articulation of the anterior arch of C1 and the odontoid process of C2. (Reproduced with permission from, Normal Spine MRI Anatomy. In: Khanna AJ, ed. MRI Essentials for the Spine Specialist. 1st Edition. New York: Thieme; 2014.)

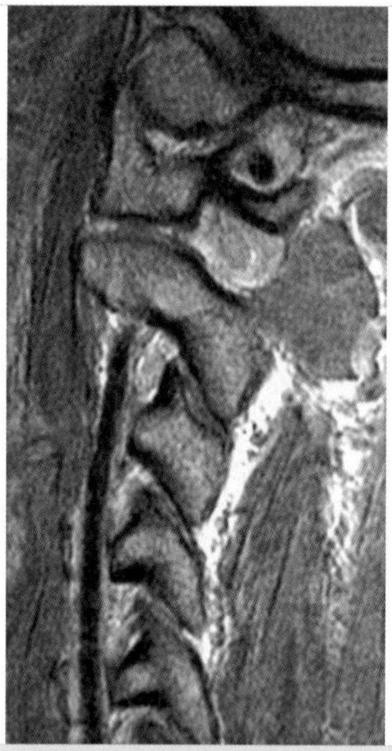

Fig. 13.24 A sagittal T1-weighted image shows the cup-shaped configuration of the craniocervical joint; the subaxial facet joints are also well visualized. (Reproduced with permission from, Normal Spine MRI Anatomy. In: Khanna AJ, ed. MRI Essentials for the Spine Specialist. 1st Edition. New York: Thieme; 2014.)

C2 is termed the axis. The dens, or the odontoid process, is a protuberance from the axis. An os odontoideum is a variant in which the dens is separate from the body of the axis (▶ Fig. 13.25). The cause of os odontoideum is unknown and may be a congenital failure of fusion secondary to trauma.[47] The C1–C2 articulation is termed the "atlantoaxial joint." There are paired lateral articulations and a midline medial articulation. The lateral atlantoaxial joint is formed between the lateral masses of the atlas and the superior articular surface of the axis. The median atlantoaxial joint is formed between the dens and the anterior arch of the atlas. These joints may communicate in total or in part, as appreciated on T2-weighted and contrast-enhanced MR images. The primary movement of the atlantoaxial joint is axial rotation. Flexion-extension is limited by the transverse ligament and the tectorial membrane. Lateral bending is limited by the contralateral alar ligament.

In addition to the alar ligament, there are several other key ligaments of the craniocervical junction (▶ Fig. 13.9). The transverse or horizontal cruciform ligament is the largest and strongest of the craniocervical junction ligaments. It passes posterior to the odontoid process and attaches at the lateral tubercles of the atlas, serving as the primary stabilizer of the atlantoaxial joint.[48] The apical ligament attaches the tip of the odontoid to the basion and has uncertain biomechanical function. The tectorial membrane is dorsal to the cruciform ligament and is contiguous with the posterior longitudinal ligament inferiorly and the dura of the clivus superiorly. The anterior and posterior atlantooccipital membranes attach the atlas to the foramen

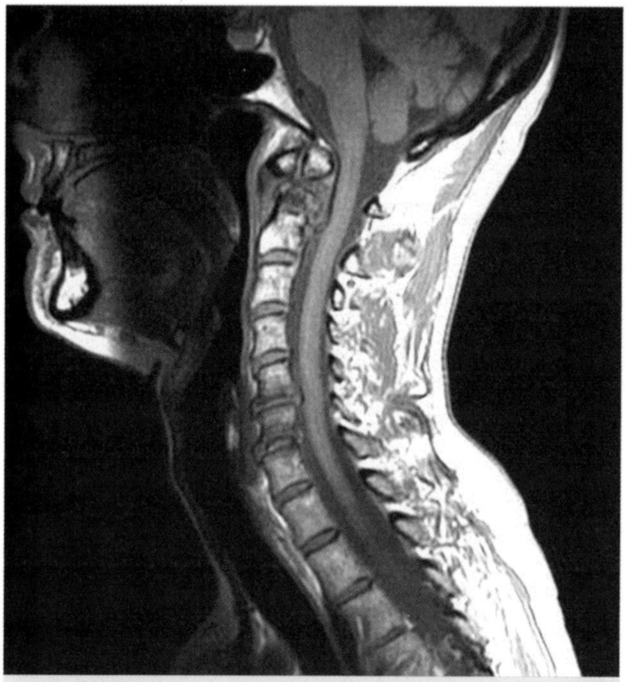

Fig. 13.25 A sagittal T1-weighted image shows an os odontoideum, often a normal variant where the dens is separate from the body of the axis. (Reproduced with permission from, Normal Spine MRI Anatomy. In: Khanna AJ, ed. MRI Essentials for the Spine Specialist. 1st Edition. New York: Thieme; 2014.)

magnum. The posterior atlantooccipital membrane plays a role in cervicogenic headaches.[49]

The cervical vertebrae of C3–C7 are small but relatively broad. They contain a large triangular vertebral foramen and short bifid spinous processes. There is a raised lip on the upper surface of the vertebral body. The vertebral arteries ascend in the bilateral foramen transversarium at C6 and rise toward C1. They pass lateral to the C1–C2 joint and pierce the dura above the C1 arch.

13.3.2 Sagittal MRI

The T1-weighted and T2-weighted sagittal images should be reviewed first to evaluate the spinal anatomy (▶ Fig. 13.26). The midsagittal image from the cervicomedullary to cervicothoracic junctions is a good anatomic screen of the cervical vertebral bodies, intervertebral disks, spinal cord, thecal sac, and posterior elements. To find the midsagittal image, the sagittal series should be reviewed for the image that best shows the entire cervical spinal cord and the odontoid process, basion, opisthion, midbrain, and fourth ventricle.

Sequential evaluation of the sagittal series away from the midsagittal image allows for assessment of facet joints and neural foramina (▶ Fig. 13.27). The foramina have an oblique orientation to the sagittal plane, which can cause distortion and lead to artifactual narrowing. T1-weighted images are somewhat limited because they afford poor differentiation of the vertebral body, the annular-posterior longitudinal ligament complex, and the CSF in the adjacent thecal sac.[50] However, exceptional resolution of the spinal cord and CSF within the spinal canal can be seen on T1-weighted images.[51] The posterior longitudinal ligament, a disk herniation, an osseous spur, and CSF all appear as a low-intensity signal on T1-weighted sagittal images.[50] The CSF-extradural interface is well defined on T2-weighted images, and a myelographic appearance is produced on T2-weighted sagittal images because of the high signal intensity of CSF. The intervertebral disks show intermediate signal intensity on T1-weighted images and high signal intensity on T2-weighted and gradient-echo images.

The cervical vertebral body has bright signal intensity on T1-weighted images because of the presence of normal fatty bone marrow. Normal cervical spine lordosis should be observed. The AP diameter of the canal tapers from the first to third

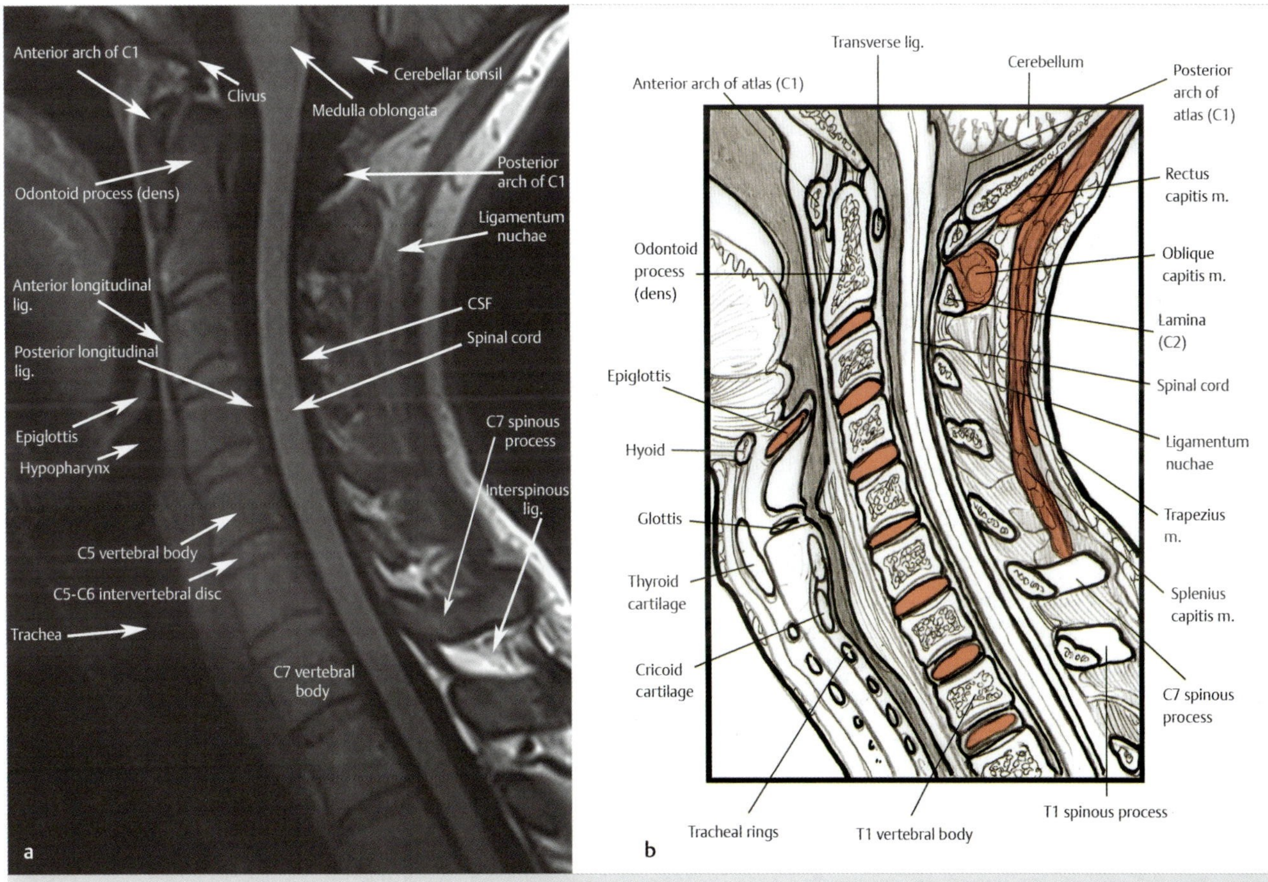

Fig. 13.26 This **(a)** sagittal T1-weighted midline image and **(b)** artist's sketch of the cervical spine depict the cervical cord, cerebrospinal fluid (CSF), and the anterior and posterior longitudinal ligaments, as well as the anterior and posterior elements of the cervical spine and the intervertebral disks. (Reproduced with permission from, Normal Spine MRI Anatomy. In: Khanna AJ, ed. MRI Essentials for the Spine Specialist. 1st Edition. New York: Thieme; 2014.)

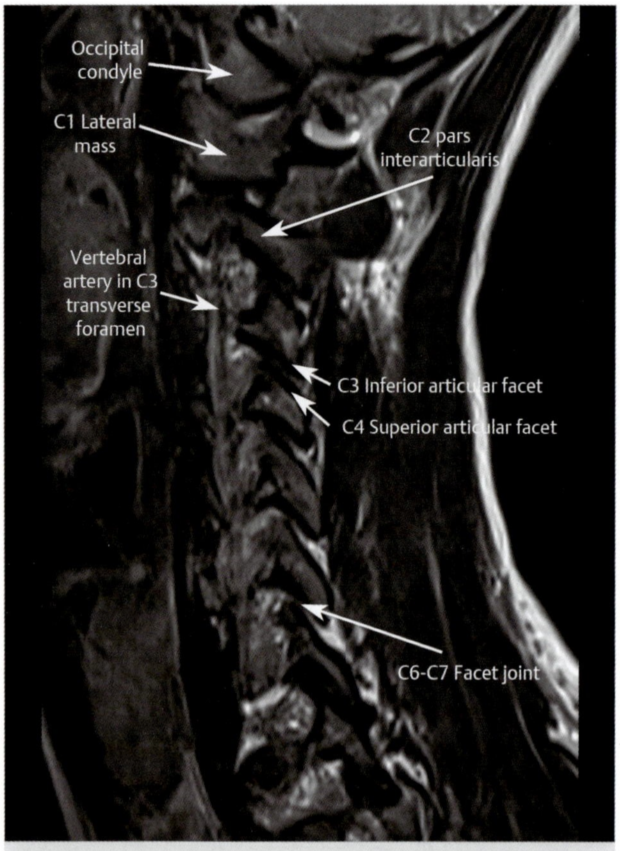

Fig. 13.27 A sagittal T2-weighted paramidline image of the cervical spine shows the vertebral artery in long axis coursing through the transverse foramina of the cervical spine. The facet joints are most easily evaluated in the parasagittal plane, as shown here. (Reproduced with permission from, Normal Spine MRI Anatomy. In: Khanna AJ, ed. MRI Essentials for the Spine Specialist. 1st Edition. New York: Thieme; 2014.)

cervical levels and then is relatively constant. Parasagittal images show the short cervical pedicles. The anterior and posterior longitudinal ligaments are depicted as low-signal-intensity linear structures along the vertebral bodies.[36,52] Often, a small cortical defect is seen in the midportion of the posterior vertebral body; this defect represents a vascular channel and is a normal finding.

13.3.3 Axial MRI

Evaluation of the cervical spine MR images in the axial plane requires the correct identification of the spinal level, which can be accomplished by using the localizing sagittal images or by evaluating signal-intensity differences between the intervertebral disks and vertebral bodies and sequentially numbering the levels caudal to the odontoid process. Given the potential risk of wrong-level surgery,[53,54] special care should be taken to identify the level by using a combination of these two labeling techniques. In addition, most imaging workstations have tools that enable the vertebral bodies to be identified using the numbering techniques just mentioned, which facilitates rapid localization on the midsagittal images while evaluating the associated axial images. The sagittal and axial images can often be linked on viewing stations and with image-viewing software to enable definitive localization of pathology in the sagittal and axial planes.

Cervical spine anatomy and anatomic pathology are well visualized on axial T1-weighted images; T2-weighted images have good CSF-to-cord contrast (▶ Fig. 13.8), which enables evaluation of spinal cord or nerve root compression.[36,52] Knowledge of the location of the various spinal tracts (▶ Fig. 13.28) can help a clinician correlate the clinical and radiographic findings in a patient with known or suspected spinal cord injury. When a more sensitive assessment of the spinal cord signal characteristics is required, axial T2-weighted images are

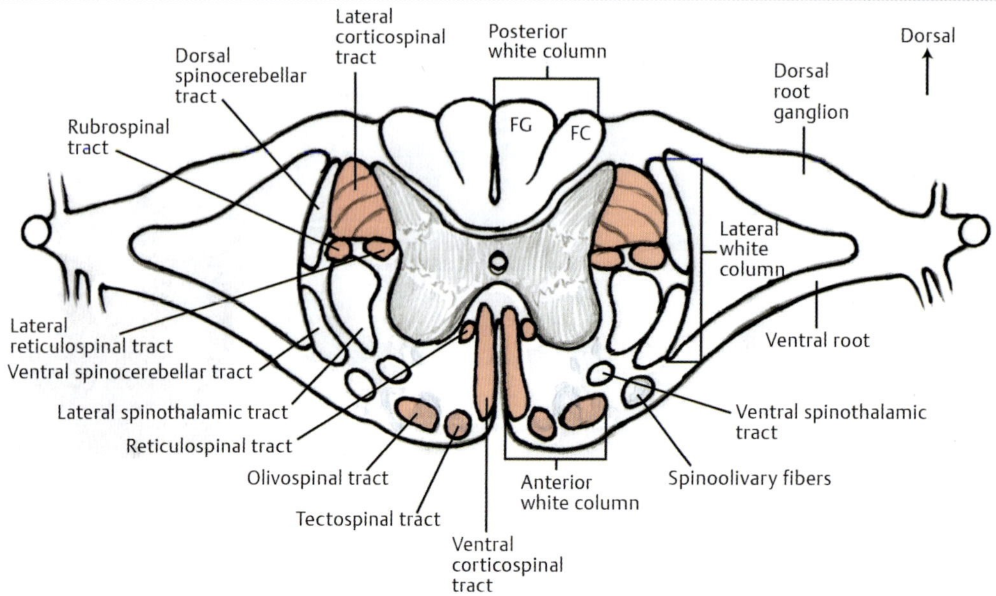

Fig. 13.28 Artist's axial sketch shows spinal cord anatomy, including the various spinal cord tracts. FC, fasciculus cuneatus; FG, fasciculus gracilis. (Reproduced with permission from, Normal Spine MRI Anatomy. In: Khanna AJ, ed. MRI Essentials for the Spine Specialist. 1st Edition. New York: Thieme; 2014.)

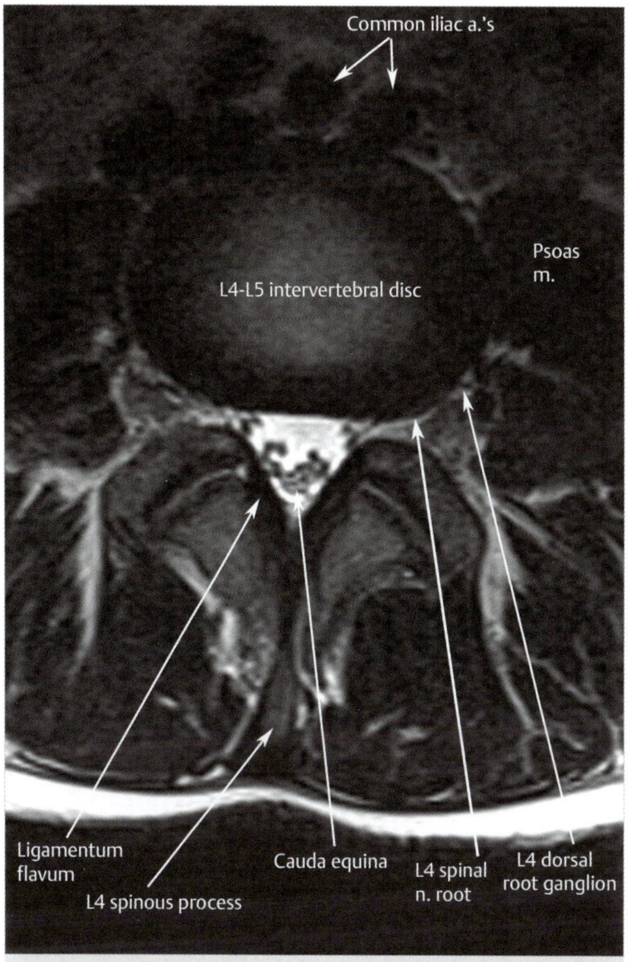

Fig. 13.29 An axial T2-weighted image of the lumbar spine at the L4–L5 level shows the cauda equina, L4 spinal nerve root, and L4 dorsal nerve root ganglion. Normal flow voids are seen within the common iliac arteries, just below the aortic bifurcation. (Reproduced with permission from, Normal Spine MRI Anatomy. In: Khanna AJ, ed. MRI Essentials for the Spine Specialist. 1st Edition. New York: Thieme; 2014.)

favorable due to their smaller field of view. Neural foramina are best depicted with gradient-echo and T2-weighted images and should be evaluated on axial and parasagittal images. Evaluation of the neural foramina in the axial and sagittal planes improves with experience and training, especially with patients who have scoliosis or poor positioning in the scanner, which can cause each neural foramen to be visualized on different parasagittal or axial images. Sagittal images are helpful in evaluating signal abnormalities in the spinal cord because one image can show a long segment of the spinal cord. Care should be taken to evaluate the axial T2-weighted images and to recognize the normal shape and size of the central canal and the neural foramina. Specifically, the three primary contributors to cervical spinal stenosis (disk pathology, facet arthropathy, and ligamentum flavum hypertrophy) should be noted, and their combined contribution to the degree of central and foraminal stenosis should be assessed.[55,56] The anterior border of the neural foramen is the disk, and the posterior border is the facet joint (▶ Fig. 13.29). It is important to note the location and course of the vertebral arteries on the axial images. Aberrant vertebral arteries should be identified preoperatively, especially if a cervical corpectomy is being considered. Furthermore, the vertebral arteries should show normal hypointense pulsation signal. As with any radiographic study, in addition to the structures detailed previously, all imaged structures should also be evaluated for potential pathology or incidental findings. For instance, lymph nodes in the neck should be evaluated for size and the presence of a normal fatty hilum. The thyroid should also be evaluated for size and to exclude large nodules.

13.3.4 Coronal MRI

Coronal images show the craniocervical spine articulations, intervertebral disks, uncinate processes, atlantooccipital joints, and lateral atlantoaxial joints.[36] Although the sagittal and axial images provide enough information for diagnosis in most cases, coronal images may be especially valuable for evaluating the craniocervical junction or assessing for spinal pathologies in patients with coronal plane deformities such as scoliosis.[57] Coronal plane MR images, along with conventional radiographs, also facilitate evaluation of the rarely occurring cervical scoliosis because the entire scoliotic spine can be included within a single imaging plane.

13.4 Thoracic Spine

Thoracic spine MRI is obtained less frequently than MRI of lumbar or cervical spine. Anatomic structures that make the thoracic spine unique are the costocentral joint and the costotransverse joint. The costocentral joint and the costotransverse joint connect the vertebral body to the rib head and the transverse process to the proximal rib, respectively.[58] The thoracic intervertebral disks are fairly uniform in shape and size. The facet joints are coronally oriented.

13.5 Lumbar Spine

13.5.1 Anatomy

The lumbar vertebrae are the largest segments of the spinal column. The fifth lumbar vertebra should have the largest body. Apart from its size, the lumbar vertebrae can be distinguished by the absence of transverse foramena and costal facets.[35] The spinal foramen is commonly triangular in shape. The transverse processes are thin and long. The superior articular facets are often vertical and concave, whereas the inferior articular facets are often vertical and convex.

13.5.2 Sagittal MRI

Sagittal imaging of the lumbar spine is usually obtained with T1-weighted and T2-weighted pulse sequences (▶ Fig. 13.30, ▶ Fig. 13.31). The T1-weighted images are best used for evaluating the anatomic detail of the lumbar spine. The midsagittal

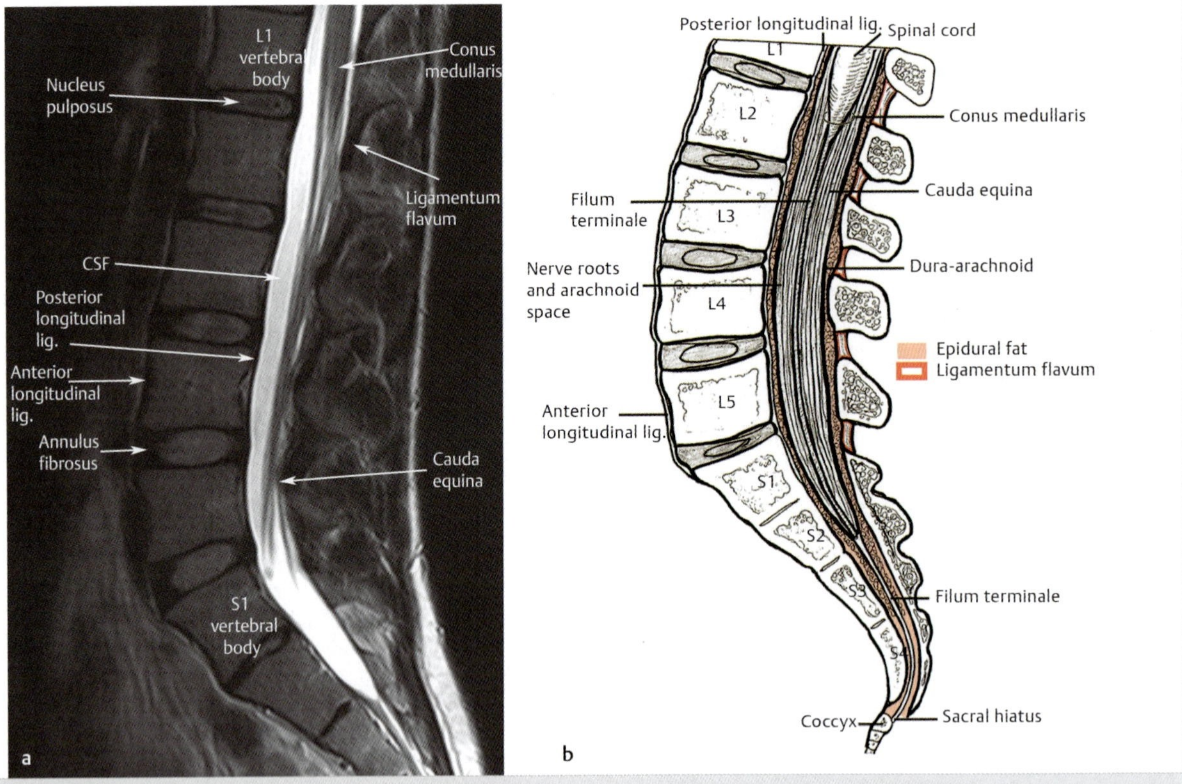

Fig. 13.30 This **(a)** sagittal T2-weighted midline image and **(b)** artist's sketch of the lumbar spine show the conus medullaris and other important structures as identified. The posterior longitudinal ligament, intervertebral disks, and vertebral bodies are better differentiated on the T2-weighted images than on T1-weighted images. (Reproduced with permission from, Normal Spine MRI Anatomy. In: Khanna AJ, ed. MRI Essentials for the Spine Specialist. 1st Edition. New York: Thieme; 2014.)

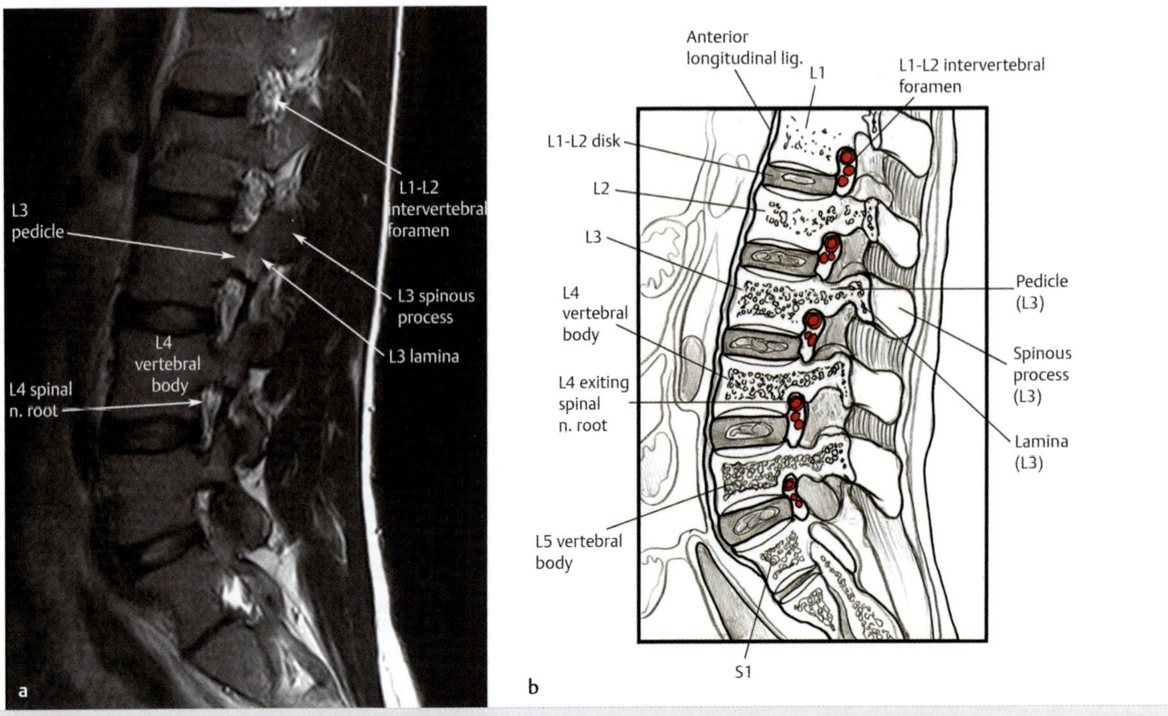

Fig. 13.31 This **(a)** parasagittal T2-weighted image and **(b)** artist's sketch of the lumbar spine show the neural foramina and exiting nerve roots at multiple levels. (Reproduced with permission from, Normal Spine MRI Anatomy. In: Khanna AJ, ed. MRI Essentials for the Spine Specialist. 1st Edition. New York: Thieme; 2014.)

image should be evaluated first. This image shows the full profile of the sacrum and most of the lumbar vertebral bodies, spinal cord, and cauda equina in patients without substantial scoliosis. After evaluating the midsagittal image, the sagittal images are sequentially evaluated toward each side to assess the facet joints and neural foramina. The sagittal images can be concurrently evaluated with the axial sequence to confirm laterality. The bright signal from CSF on T2-weighted images provides a myelographic effect. Advanced MRI techniques such as CSF flow sequence coupled with T2-weighted images allows for better depiction of cystic lesions in the spinal cord.[59] T1-weighted gradient-echo images assist by providing improved evaluation of end plate and osteophyte anatomy and differentiation of the anterior and posterior longitudinal ligaments from the cortical bone.

13.5.3 Axial MRI

Similar to cervical axial MRI images, when evaluating axial MR images of the lumbar spine it is imperative to accurately identify the level at which the pathology exists. This can be achieved by using the localizing sagittal image. In addition, each level can be identified by starting at the sacrum and numbering each vertebral body from L5 to L1. In complex cases where severe pathology is present at multiple levels, it may also be helpful to use the spine-labeling tool discussed previously in the section on the cervical spine. This tool is frequently available on imaging workstations, often with imaging software that includes studies provided on a CD/DVD or via Internet connection. Costal facets and the iliolumbar ligament could potentially serve as anatomical landmarks for T12 and L5 on axial images, respectively.[60] On axial images, the difference in signal intensity between the intervertebral disks and vertebral bodies allows for the distinction between vertebral levels. Accurate and consistent evaluation of the axial images requires more experience and training than does the evaluation of the sagittal images. Care should be taken to evaluate the axial T2-weighted images and recognize the normal shape and size of the central canal and the neural foramina (▶ Fig. 13.32). Specifically, the degree of contribution of the three primary contributors to spinal stenosis (disk pathology, facet arthropathy, and ligamentum flavum hypertrophy) should be noted, and their combined contribution to the degree of central and foraminal stenosis should be carefully assessed (▶ Fig. 13.33). Hypertrophy of the superior articular process can narrow the neural foramen and lead to lumbar foraminal stenosis. Thus, the relationship between the superior articular process from the caudal level and the exiting nerve root should be evaluated.[61,62] The extraforaminal zone should also be studied at each level to rule out far-lateral disk pathology. The psoas muscles are seen adjacent to the vertebral bodies in the lumbar spine (▶ Fig. 13.33), and the major vessels (including the aorta and vena cava) are seen anterior to

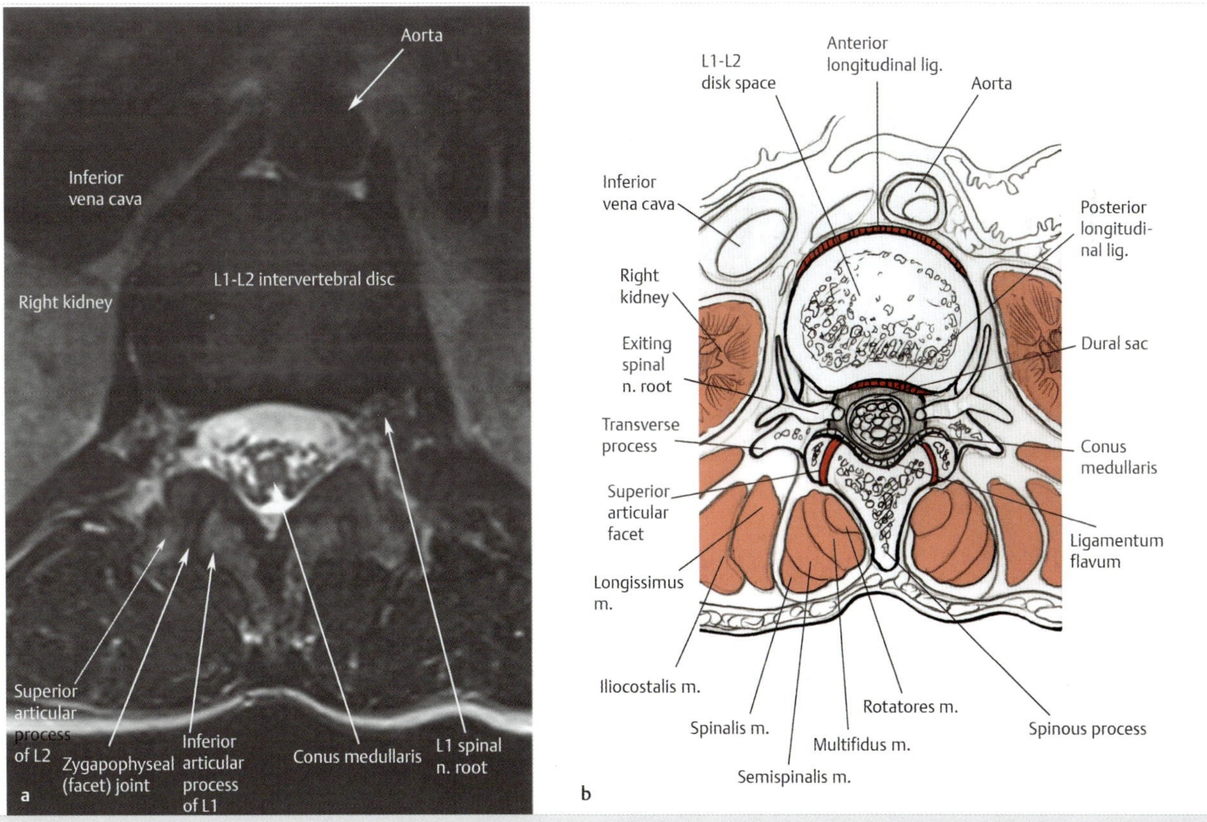

Fig. 13.32 This **(a)** axial T2-weighted image and **(b)** artist's sketch of the spine at the level of the L1–L2 intervertebral disk show the conus medullaris and the L1 spinal nerve root, as well as the superior and inferior articular processes of the L1–L2 facet joint. (Reproduced with permission from, Normal Spine MRI Anatomy. In: Khanna AJ, ed. MRI Essentials for the Spine Specialist. 1st Edition. New York: Thieme; 2014.)

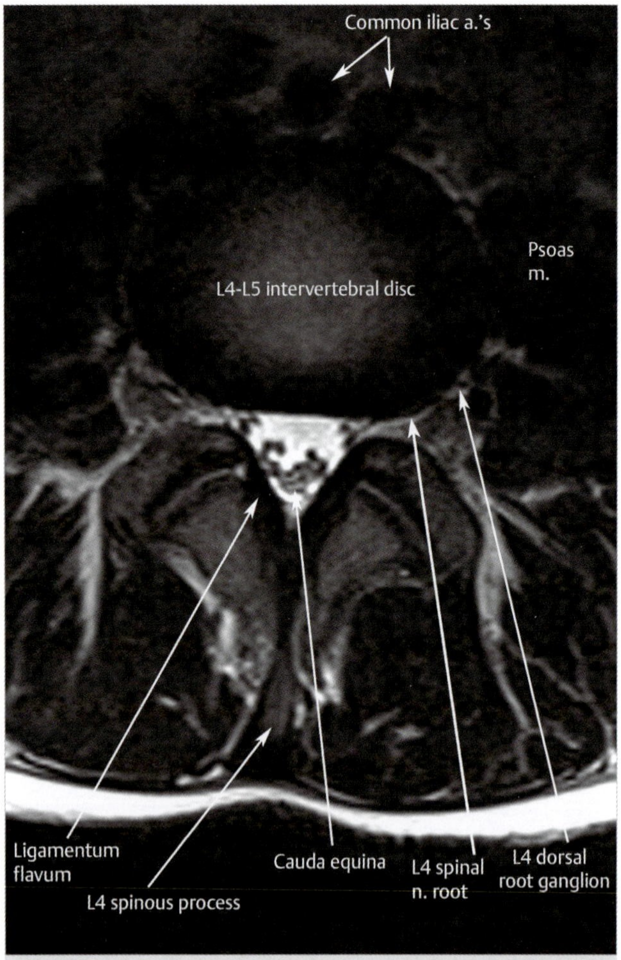

Fig. 13.33 An axial T2-weighted image at the level of the L4–L5 intervertebral disk shows the cauda equina, L4 spinal nerve root, and L4 dorsal root ganglion. Normal flow voids are seen within the common iliac arteries, just below the aortic bifurcation. (Reproduced with permission from, Normal Spine MRI Anatomy. In: Khanna AJ, ed. MRI Essentials for the Spine Specialist. 1st Edition. New York: Thieme; 2014.)

the vertebral bodies. Along with the spine, these structures should also be evaluated for pathologic processes such as aneurysm, thrombosis, and infection.

13.5.4 Coronal MRI

Coronal images provide a clear evaluation of the general alignment and anatomy of the lumbar spine, enabling the identification of the vertebrae and intervertebral disks. As with the cervical spine, coronal plane MR images of the lumbar spine, along with conventional radiographs, also facilitate evaluation of lumbar scoliosis. Because lordosis increases toward the caudal aspect of the lumbar spine, it is impossible to obtain one image that visualizes the entire spinal canal and its contents. The coronal plane images can be used to evaluate spinal alignment and transitional anatomy at the lumbosacral junction. In addition, the use of coronal short tau inversion recovery (STIR) sequence could aid in diagnosing etiologies of low back pain not elucidated by other MRI techniques.[47,63]

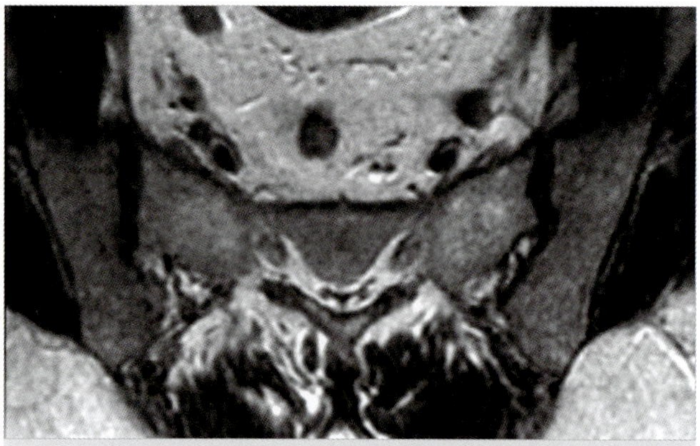

Fig. 13.34 An axial T1-weighted image shows the normal appearance of the sacroiliac joints. (Reproduced with permission from, Normal Spine MRI Anatomy. In: Khanna AJ, ed. MRI Essentials for the Spine Specialist. 1st Edition. New York: Thieme; 2014.)

13.6 Sacrum and Coccyx

The sacrum is a block of bone at the base of the vertebral column that consists of the fusion of S1–S5. It supports the spine and transmits load. The sacrum forms the posterior wall of the pelvis and is normally triangular in shape with broad cephalad tapers. There are anterior and posterior foramina. The coccyx articulates with the sacrum inferiorly and represents the fusion of four rudimentary vertebrae. The term "sacrum" literally translates to "holy bone."[64]

The sacroiliac joint has a small range of motion with essentially passive movements (▶ Fig. 13.34). There are no associated muscles that execute active movements. The axis of movement passes obliquely across the pelvis. With flexion, the axis passes backward from the pubic symphysis to the sciatic notch. With extension, the axis passes from the pubic symphysis through the pelvis between the ischium and the coccyx.

The sacroiliac joint shows sequential changes with age. In the embryo phase, the sacroiliac joint is a strip of mesenchyme that undergoes cavitation. During the first decade of life, the joint enlarges but remains flat. During the second decade, there is corrugation of joint surfaces. Osteophytes develop in the fifth and sixth decades, and large interdigitating osteophytes can develop during the eighth decade.[65]

13.7 Common Clinical Questions

1. The facet joints are synovial joints between the superior and inferior articular processes. True or false?

2. The spinal column typically comprises 7 cervical vertebrae, 13 thoracic vertebrae, 5 lumbar vertebrae, the sacrum, and the coccyx. True or false?

3. The most common location for a limbus vertebra is the:
   a) Anterior superior corner.
   b) Anterior inferior corner.
   c) Posterior superior corner.
   d) Posterior inferior corner.

4. Normal ligaments are bright on T1-weighted images. True or false?

5. Which pulse sequence provides a "myelographic" view of the spine and best allows for the assessment of spinal stenosis?
   a) Sagittal T1-weighted images.
   b) Sagittal T2-weighted images.
   c) Sagittal gradient-echo images.
   d) Coronal T1-weighted images.
   e) Sagittal postcontrast T1-weighted images.

References

[1] Bess S, Line B. Embryology and anatomy: spine/spinal cord. In: Akbarnia BA, Yazici M, Thompson GH, eds. The growing spine: management of spinal disorders in young children. Berlin, Heidelberg: Springer; 2016:3–13

[2] Perez-Cruet MJ, Fessler RG, Wang MY, eds. Anatomy of the spine: an overview. In: An anatomic approach to minimally invasive spine surgery. 2nd ed. Thieme Medical Publishers, Inc.; 2018. doi:10.1055/b-005-145242

[3] DeSai C, Agarwal A. Anatomy, back, vertebral column. In: StatPearls. Treasure Island (FL): StatPearls Publishing; 2019. http://www.ncbi.nlm.nih.gov/books/NBK525969/. Accessed April 29, 2019

[4] Roussouly P, Pinheiro-Franco JL. Sagittal parameters of the spine: biomechanical approach. Eur Spine J. 2011; 20 Suppl 5:578–585

[5] Huang P-Y, Yeh L-R, Tzeng W-S, et al. Imaging features of posterior limbus vertebrae. Clin Imaging. 2012; 36(6):797–802

[6] Dodwad S-NM, Khan SN, An HS. Cervical spine anatomy. In: Textbook of the cervical spine. Philadelphia, PA: Elsevier/Saunders; 2015:3–21

[7] Kumar Y, Hayashi D. Role of magnetic resonance imaging in acute spinal trauma: a pictorial review. BMC Musculoskelet Disord. 2016; 17:310

[8] Griessenauer CJ, Raborn J, Foreman P, Shoja MM, Loukas M, Tubbs RS. Venous drainage of the spine and spinal cord: a comprehensive review of its history, embryology, anatomy, physiology, and pathology. Clin Anat. 2015; 28(1):75–87

[9] Miyasaka K, Asano T, Ushikoshi S, Hida K, Koyanagi I. Vascular anatomy of the spinal cord and classification of spinal arteriovenous malformations. Interv Neuroradiol. 2000; 6 Suppl 1:195–198

[10] Delfaut EM, Beltran J, Johnson G, Rousseau J, Marchandise X, Cotten A. Fat suppression in MR imaging: techniques and pitfalls. Radiographics. 1999; 19 (2):373–382

[11] Lee S, Choi DS, Shin HS, Baek HJ, Choi HC, Park SE. FSE T2-weighted two-point Dixon technique for fat suppression in the lumbar spine: comparison with SPAIR technique. Diagn Interv Radiol. 2018; 24(3):175–180

[12] Shapiro IM, Risbud MV. Introduction to the structure, function, and comparative anatomy of the vertebrae and the intervertebral disc. In: Shapiro IM, Risbud MV, eds. The intervertebral disc: molecular and structural studies of the disc in health and disease. Vienna: Springer; 2014:3–15

[13] Bowles RD, Setton LA. Biomaterials for intervertebral disc regeneration and repair. Biomaterials. 2017; 129:54–67

[14] Klein JP. A practical approach to spine imaging. Continuum (Minneap Minn). 2015; 21 1 Spinal Cord Disorders:36–51

[15] Kasdan RB, Howard JL. Neuroimaging of spinal diseases: a pictorial review. Semin Neurol. 2008; 28(4):570–589

[16] Suthar P, Patel R, Mehta C, Patel N. MRI evaluation of lumbar disc degenerative disease. J Clin Diagn Res. 2015; 9(4):TC04–TC09

[17] Bloem JL, Reijnierse M, Huizinga TWJ, van der Helm-van Mil AHM. MR signal intensity: staying on the bright side in MR image interpretation. RMD Open. 2018; 4(1):e000728

[18] Kyere KA, Than KD, Wang AC, et al. Schmorl's nodes. Eur Spine J. 2012; 21 (11):2115–2121

[19] Smith LJ, Fazzalari NL. The elastic fibre network of the human lumbar anulus fibrosus: architecture, mechanical function and potential role in the progression of intervertebral disc degeneration. Eur Spine J. 2009; 18(4): 439–448

[20] Eyre DR, Muir H. Types I and II collagens in intervertebral disc. Interchanging radial distributions in annulus fibrosus. Biochem J. 1976; 157(1):267–270

[21] Mercer S, Bogduk N. The ligaments and annulus fibrosus of human adult cervical intervertebral discs. Spine. 1999; 24(7):619–626, discussion 627–628

[22] Mathis JM, Shaibani A, Wakhloo AK. Spine anatomy. In: Mathis JM, Golovac S, eds. Image-guided spine interventions. New York, NY: Springer; 2010:1–27

[23] Jiang W, Hu Z, Hao J. Management of symptomatic Tarlov cysts: a retrospective observational study. Pain Physician. 2017; 20(5):E653–E660

[24] Murphy KJ, Nussbaum DA, Schnupp S, Long D. Tarlov cysts: an overlooked clinical problem. Semin Musculoskelet Radiol. 2011; 15(2):163–167

[25] Lisanti C, Carlin C, Banks KP, Wang D. Normal MRI appearance and motion-related phenomena of CSF. AJR Am J Roentgenol. 2007; 188(3):716–725

[26] Elliott JM, Flynn TW, Al-Najjar A, Press J, Nguyen B, Noteboom JT. The pearls and pitfalls of magnetic resonance imaging for the spine. J Orthop Sports Phys Ther. 2011; 41(11):848–860

[27] Larsen DW, Teitelbaum GP, Norman D. Cerebrospinal fluid flow artifact. A possible pitfall on fast-spin-echo MR imaging of the spine simulating intradural pathology. Clin Imaging. 1996; 20(2):140–142

[28] Smith SA, Pekar JJ, Van Zijl PCM. Chapter 6—Advanced MRI strategies for assessing spinal cord injury. In: Verhaagen J, McDonald JW, eds. Handbook of clinical neurology. Vol. 109. Spinal cord injury. Elsevier; 2012:85–101

[29] Goldberg AL, Kershah SM. Advances in imaging of vertebral and spinal cord injury. J Spinal Cord Med. 2010; 33(2):105–116

[30] Okuda T, Fujimoto Y, Tanaka N, Ishida O, Baba I, Ochi M. Morphological changes of the ligamentum flavum as a cause of nerve root compression. Eur Spine J. 2005; 14(3):277–286

[31] Hasegawa T, An HS, Haughton VM, Nowicki BH. Lumbar foraminal stenosis: critical heights of the intervertebral discs and foramina. A cryomicrotome study in cadavera. J Bone Joint Surg Am. 1995; 77(1):32–38

[32] Nowicki BH, Haughton VM, Schmidt TA, et al. Occult lumbar lateral spinal stenosis in neural foramina subjected to physiologic loading. AJNR Am J Neuroradiol. 1996; 17(9):1605–1614

[33] Park J-B, Lee J-K, Park S-J, Riew KD. Hypertrophy of ligamentum flavum in lumbar spinal stenosis associated with increased proteinase inhibitor concentration. J Bone Joint Surg Am. 2005; 87(12):2750–2757

[34] Rios JC, Naidich TP, Daniels DL, et al. The normal spinal column: overview and cervical spine. In: Imaging of the spine. Philadelphia, PA: Elsevier/Saunders; 2011:45–74

[35] Standring S, ed. Gray's Anatomy : The Anatomical Basis of Clinical Practice. Forty-first edition. Elsevier Limited; 2016.

[36] White ML. Cervical spine: MR imaging techniques and anatomy. Magn Reson Imaging Clin N Am. 2000; 8(3):453–470

[37] Temin N, Galper M, Small JE. Ossification of the posterior longitudinal ligament. In: Neuroradiology: spectrum and evolution of disease. Philadelphia, PA: Elsevier; 2019:189–199

[38] Dietemann J-L, Bogorin A, Abu Eid M, et al. Tips and traps in neurological imaging: imaging the perimedullary spaces. Diagn Interv Imaging. 2012; 93 (12):985–992

[39] Perolat R, Kastler A, Nicot B, et al. Facet joint syndrome: from diagnosis to interventional management. Insights Imaging. 2018; 9(5):773–789

[40] Saravanakumar K, Harvey A. Lumbar zygapophyseal (facet) joint pain. Rev Pain. 2008; 2(1):8–13

[41] Jaumard NV, Welch WC, Winkelstein BA. Spinal facet joint biomechanics and mechanotransduction in normal, injury and degenerative conditions. J Biomech Eng. 2011; 133(7):071010

[42] Pal GP, Routal RV, Saggu SK. The orientation of the articular facets of the zygapophyseal joints at the cervical and upper thoracic region. J Anat. 2001; 198(Pt 4):431–441

[43] Thron AK. Arterial blood supply. In: Thron AK, ed. Vascular anatomy of the spinal cord: radioanatomy as the key to diagnosis and treatment. Cham: Springer International Publishing; 2016:9–83

[44] Masson C, Pruvo JP, Meder JF, et al. Study Group on Spinal Cord Infarction of the French Neurovascular Society. Spinal cord infarction: clinical and magnetic resonance imaging findings and short term outcome. J Neurol Neurosurg Psychiatry. 2004; 75(10):1431–1435

[45] Salvador de la Barrera S, Barca-Buyo A, Montoto-Marqués A, Ferreiro-Velasco ME, Cidoncha-Dans M, Rodriguez-Sotillo A. Spinal cord infarction: prognosis and recovery in a series of 36 patients. Spinal Cord. 2001; 39 (10):520–525

[46] Lazorthes G, Gouaze A, Zadeh JO, Santini JJ, Lazorthes Y, Burdin P. Arterial vascularization of the spinal cord. Recent studies of the anastomotic substitution pathways. J Neurosurg. 1971; 35(3):253–262

[47] Romeo V, Cavaliere C, Sorrentino C, et al. Clinical impact of coronal-STIR sequence in a routine lumbar spine MR imaging protocol to investigate low back pain. Medicine (Baltimore). 2018; 97(23):e10789

[48] Ramieri A, Domenicucci M, Miscusi M, Costanzo G. Functional anatomy and biomechanics of the cervical spine. In: Menchetti PPM, ed. Cervical spine: minimally invasive and open surgery. Cham: Springer International Publishing; 2016:11–25

[49] Nash L, Nicholson H, Lee ASJ, Johnson GM, Zhang M. Configuration of the connective tissue in the posterior atlanto-occipital interspace: a sheet plastination and confocal microscopy study. Spine. 2005; 30(12):1359–1366

[50] Kaiser JA, Holland BA. Imaging of the cervical spine. Spine. 1998; 23(24): 2701–2712

[51] Stone J. Imaging techniques in the adult spine. In: Imaging of the spine. Philadelphia, PA: Elsevier/Saunders; 2011:3–21

[52] Khanna AJ, Carbone JJ, Kebaish KM, et al. Magnetic resonance imaging of the cervical spine. Current techniques and spectrum of disease. J Bone Joint Surg Am. 2002; 84-A Suppl 2:70–80

[53] Hsiang J. Wrong-level surgery: a unique problem in spine surgery. Surg Neurol Int. 2011; 2:47

[54] Palumbo MA, Bianco AJ, Esmende S, Daniels AH. Wrong-site Spine Surgery. J Am Acad Orthop Surg. 2013; 21(5):312–320

[55] Leonardi M, Boos N. Degenerative disorders of the cervical spine. In: Boos N, Aebi M, eds. Spinal disorders: fundamentals of diagnosis and treatment. Berlin, Heidelberg: Springer; 2008:429–479

[56] Rahman S, Than K, Park P, Marca FL. Cervical spondylotic myelopathy. In: Textbook of the cervical spine. Philadelphia, PA: Elsevier/Saunders; 2015:135–145

[57] Dewan AK, Malloy JP, Khanna AJ. Magnetic resonance imaging of the cervical spine. In: Textbook of the cervical spine. Philadelphia, PA: Elsevier/Saunders; 2015:86–104

[58] Saker E, Graham RA, Nicholas R, et al. Ligaments of the costovertebral joints including biomechanics, innervations, and clinical applications: a comprehensive review with application to approaches to the thoracic spine. Cureus. 2016; 8(11):e874

[59] Vargas MI, Delattre BMA, Boto J, et al. Advanced magnetic resonance imaging (MRI) techniques of the spine and spinal cord in children and adults. Insights Imaging. 2018; 9(4):549–557

[60] Jagannathan D, Indiran V, Hithaya F, Alamelu M, Padmanaban S. Role of anatomical landmarks in identifying normal and transitional vertebra in lumbar spine magnetic resonance imaging. Asian Spine J. 2017; 11(3):365–379

[61] Lim T-H, Choi SI, Cho HR, et al. Optimal cut-off value of the superior articular process area as a morphological parameter to predict lumbar foraminal stenosis. Pain Res Manag. 2017; 2017:7914836

[62] Barry M, Livesley P. Facet joint hypertrophy: the cross-sectional area of the superior articular process of L4 and L5. Eur Spine J. 1997; 6(2):121–124

[63] Gupta R, Mittal P, Mittal A, Mittal K, Gupta S, Kaur R. Additional merit of coronal STIR imaging for MR imaging of lumbar spine. J Craniovertebr Junction Spine. 2015; 6(1):12–15

[64] Sugar O. How the sacrum got its name. JAMA. 1987; 257(15):2061–2063

[65] Vleeming A, Schuenke MD, Masi AT, Carreiro JE, Danneels L, Willard FH. The sacroiliac joint: an overview of its anatomy, function and potential clinical implications. J Anat. 2012; 221(6):537–567

Answers to Common Clinical Questions

1. Answer: True. The facet joint is formed by the articulation between the superior articular process from the caudal vertebral body and the inferior articular process from the cranial vertebral body. It is a synovial joint.
2. Answer: False. The spinal column typically comprises 7 cervical vertebrae, 12 (not 13) thoracic vertebrae, 5 lumbar vertebrae, the sacrum, and the coccyx.
3. Answer: a. The most common location for a limbus vertebra is within the anterior superior corner of the vertebral body.
4. Answer: False. Normal ligaments should have low signal intensity on all pulse sequences.
5. Answer: b. Sagittal T2-weighted images provide a view of the spine and spinal cord that is similar to that seen with a conventional or CT myelogram in terms of contrast between the spinal cord (low signal) and CSF (high signal). This contrast allows for the optimal detection of spinal stenosis in the sagittal and axial planes.

14 The Occipitocervical Junction

Colin Haines, A. Jay Khanna, John A. Carrino, Shih-Chun Lin, and Joseph R. O'Brien

Abstract

Magnetic resonance imaging (MRI) enables assessment of the occipitocervical junction (OCJ). T1-weighted sequences show normal anatomy, whereas T2-weighted sequences highlight cerebrospinal fluid (CSF) and edema. Many measures created for use with conventional radiographs are now used on MRI. On midsagittal sequences, Wackenheim clivus baseline, McRae line, McGregor line, and Ranawat criteria are used to assess superior migration of C2. Midsagittal sequences show malformations of the hindbrain, occipital condyles, and odontoid process. Axial sequences help identify OCJ malformations, including ring defects of C1 or C2. Coronal images illustrate the cerebellar tonsils, alar and apical ligaments, atlantooccipital joint, and atlantoaxial joint.

Tumors are well assessed with MRI and are classified as extradural, intradural-extramedullary, or intramedullary. Posterior lesions are primary, whereas anterior masses usually represent metastases. Aggressive lesions typically show osseous erosions, soft tissue masses, or hypervascularity; benign or slow-growing tumors typically cause less soft tissue mass effect. A tumor's vascularity is apparent on MR angiography and often evident on T1-weighted and T2-weighted sequences.

Trauma is well assessed by MRI. On T2-weighted sequences, edema is apparent with osseous or ligamentous disruption. Vertebral artery injury can be seen on MRI or MR angiography.

Special measurements can aid in traumatic diagnoses. Midsagittal images can be used to calculate the Powers ratio and Harris technique for atlantooccipital dissociation or the atlantoaxial interval for C1–C2 instability. Coronal images are used to diagnose transverse ligament disruption by calculating the rule of Spence. Axial and sagittal images are used to correlate neurologic compression in traumatic and nontraumatic settings.

Keywords: lesion, magnetic resonance angiography, magnetic resonance imaging, occipitocervical junction, trauma, tumors

The occipitocervical junction (OCJ), also termed the "craniovertebral junction," refers to the articulations among the occiput (C0), atlas (C1), and axis (C2). The OCJ is highly mobile, with approximately 50% of cervical flexion-extension and rotation coming from the C0–C1 and C1–C2 articulations, respectively.[1] This region's strong capsuloligamentous attachments, rather than its intervertebral disks, are the basis of its stability.[2] An understanding of occipitocervical craniometry adds value to the diagnosis of abnormality at the OCJ. Treating abnormal conditions involving the OCJ requires a thorough understanding of osseous, ligamentous, and neurovascular anatomy (see Chapter 13, Normal Spine MRI Anatomy). Most orthopaedic surgeons without advanced training in spine surgery have limited experience in evaluating and treating abnormalities in this area. However, the ability to recognize the most common abnormalities in this region is important so the patient can be referred for treatment if needed.

14.1 Occipitocervical Craniometry

The OCJ can be imaged with conventional radiography, MRI, and CT to evaluate abnormal conditions.[3,4,5,6,7] Although normal relationships were defined originally with radiographs,[6,8,9,10] many of these relationships and lines are also used with MRI (▶ Table 14.1; ▶ Fig. 14.1), which offers better clarity and accuracy.[7,11]

The Wackenheim clivus baseline helps diagnose superior migration of the odontoid. The line is formed by creating a line along the rostral surface of the clivus[10]; protrusion of the odontoid tip superior posterior to this line is considered abnormal. The clivus canal angle is formed by intersecting the Wackenheim line and a line connecting the posterior vertebral bodies. In extension, 180 degrees is normal; in flexion, 150 degrees is normal. This measurement has been useful for documenting postsurgical correction of atlantoaxial dissociation.[12] The Chamberlain line is drawn between the hard palate and the opisthion (posterior lip of the foramen magnum), with > 3 mm of dens protrusion indicating abnormality.[8] Use of this line can be limited by the difficulty of identifying the hard palate and the margin of the opisthion on the lateral radiograph. The McGregor line is drawn from the hard palate to the most inferior point on the midline occipital curve.[9] If the odontoid process rises > 4.5 mm above this line, it is considered abnormal.[9] Difficulty in identifying the hard palate can limit the use of this line but using the occiput can be easier than using the opisthion. The McRae line is drawn from the opisthion to the basion (anterior lip of the foramen magnum), and any rostral odontoid elevation above this line is abnormal.[13,14] Identification of the opisthion can be difficult on the lateral radiograph. The Ranawat criterion is calculated by measuring the distance between the center of the pedicle of C2 and the C1 transverse axis.[15] In men, < 15 mm is abnormal; in women, < 13 mm is abnormal.[15]

Platybasia is measured by drawing a Welcher basal angle[16] (▶ Fig. 14.2). This condition, originally described by Virchow[17] to denote flattening of the skull base, is associated with basilar invagination or occipitalization of the atlas. Welcher basal angle is created from a line parallel to the clivus as it intersects a line along the surface of the sphenoid. The normal range is 125 to 143 degrees, and platybasia exists when the basal angle is > 143 degrees.

It is important to note that the previously mentioned radiographic parameter has a sensitivity or negative predictive value of > 90% on conventional radiographs alone.[7] Therefore, it is recommended that any suggestion of cranial settling on conventional radiographs be investigated with MRI or CT.[7]

14.2 MRI Anatomy and Imaging Protocols

MRI has enabled the detailed study of the normal anatomy[18,19] and the pathology[7,20] of the OCJ. The widespread use of MRI for

Table 14.1 Anatomic relationships and lines for use with MRI, CT imaging, and conventional radiography

Eponym	Parameters	Abnormality
Wackenheim clivus baseline	Tangent drawn along the superior surface of the clivus	Dens should be below line
Clivus canal angle	Angle formed between Wackenheim line and the posterior vertebral body line	Normal ranges are 180 degrees in extension to 150 degrees in flexion. An angle of < 150 degrees is considered abnormal
Chamberlain line	Between the hard palate and opisthion	Protrusion of the dens > 3 mm above this line is considered abnormal
McRae line	From the basion to the opisthion	Protrusion of the dens above this line is considered abnormal
McGregor line	From the hard palate to the most caudal point on the midline occipital curve	Odontoid process rising > 4.5 mm above this line is considered abnormal
Ranawat criterion	Distance between the center of the pedicle of C2 and the transverse axis of C1	Measurement of < 15 mm in males and < 13 mm in females is abnormal
Welcher basal angle	Tangent to the clivus as it intersects a tangent to the sphenoid bone	The normal range is 125–143 degrees. Platybasia exists when the basal angle is > 143 degrees

Abbreviations: CT, computed tomography; MRI, magnetic resonance imaging.

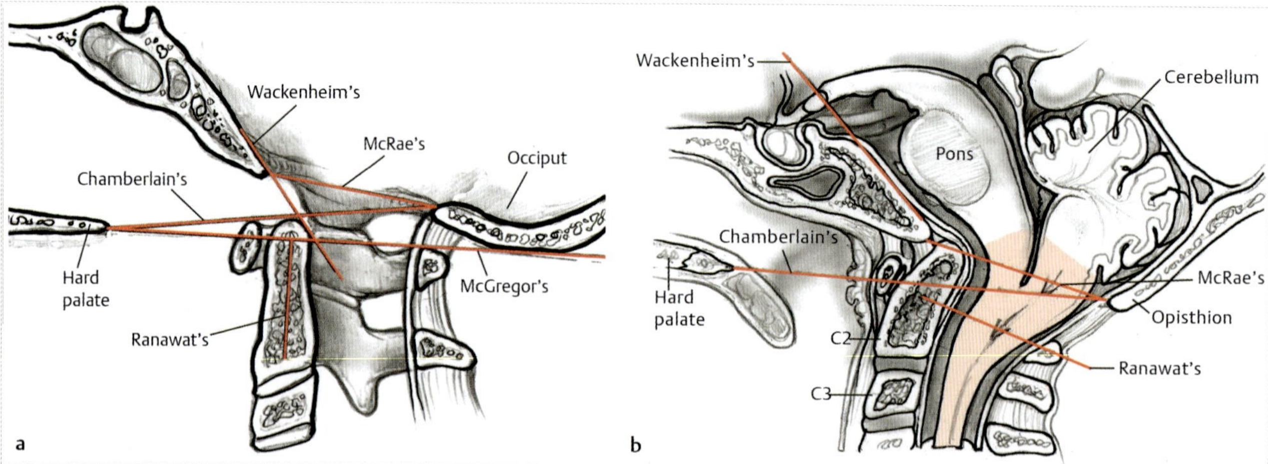

Fig. 14.1 Lines and measurements for evaluating basilar invagination. **(a)** Illustration of a case of normal relationships at the occipitocervical junction (OCJ). **(b)** Illustration of basilar invagination and Chiari type-II malformation. (Reproduced with permission from, Haines CM, Khanna AJ, Carrino JA, Lin SD, O'Brien JR. The Occipitocervical Junction. In: Khanna AJ, ed. MRI Essentials for the Spine Specialist. 1st Edition. New York: Thieme; 2014.)

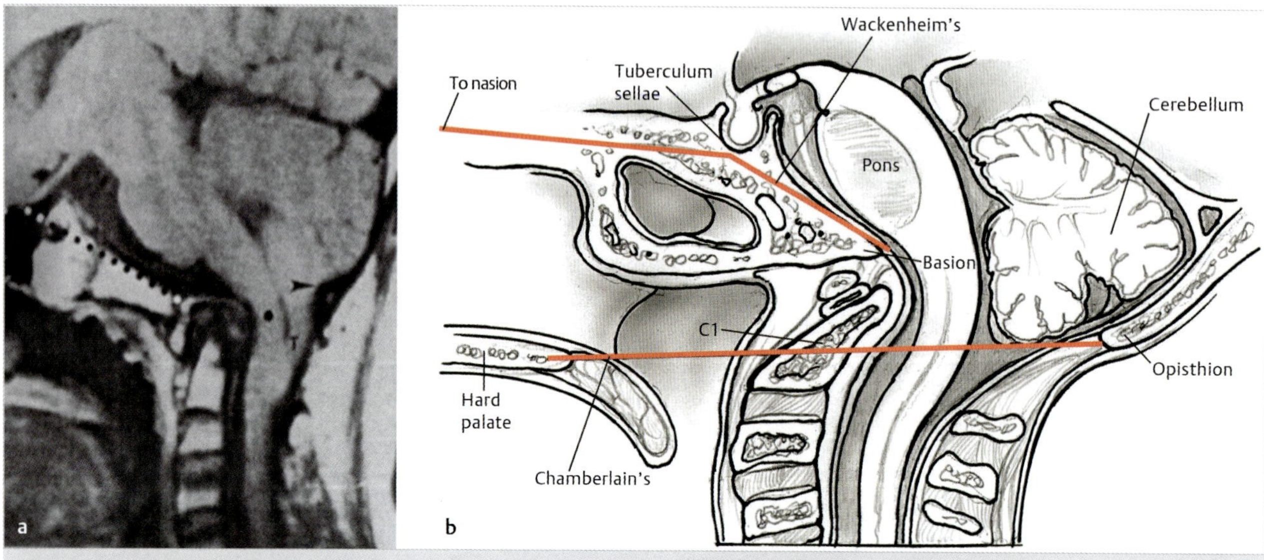

Fig. 14.2 **(a)** Sagittal T1-weighted image *(dotted line,* Wackenheim clivus baseline). **(b)** Illustration of platybasia. Welcher angle measures 160 degrees in this case; the normal measurement is 125–143 degrees. (Figure part a: Reproduced with permission, from Smoker WRK. MR imaging of the craniovertebral junction. Magn Reson Imaging Clin N Am 2000;8(3):635–650.)

studying this area has resulted in part from its ability to image directly in the sagittal and coronal planes.[21] Detailed study of the OCJ required using polytomography or thin-section CT imaging with coronal and sagittal reconstructions rather than images obtained directly in the coronal or sagittal planes.[22] MRI produces images in which cortical bone has a low signal on T1-weighted and T2-weighted images. However, low signal intensity does not limit the usefulness of MRI in studying the OCJ. Specialized pulse sequences can be used to evaluate the particular details of the OCJ anatomy.[18,23]

Many authors have reported difficulty in visualizing the alar ligaments with standard MRI protocols,[2,24,25,26] and others have reported abnormal signals in healthy volunteers.[27,28] Krakenes et al[18] developed an MRI protocol that addresses the need for accurate visualization of the craniovertebral ligaments by using intermediate-weighted sequences with 2-mm sections obtained with a standard 1.5-T coil with the patient's head in the neutral position. Their protocol has been validated by recent studies that visualize the normal ligaments of the OCJ (▶ Fig. 14.3).[23,29]

The gross anatomy of the OCJ is displayed precisely on high signal-to-noise T1-weighted images.[30] Gated T2-weighted images produce high signal from CSF, edema, and parenchymal lesions while minimizing CSF pulsation artifact.[30] For instance, myelomalacia from spinal cord compression is best visualized on T2-weighted images.

Sagittal images are ideally suited for evaluating the brainstem, fourth ventricle, and upper cervical spine.[30] Sagittal and parasagittal sections are taken from one occipital condyle to the other.[18] Craniometry measurements can be made from sagittal MRIs.[7] For instance, midsagittal MRIs can be used to measure the atlantoaxial interval, the posterior space available for the cord, or basilar impression using the Wackenheim line. The presence or absence of pannus at the C1–C2 articulation also can be delineated on sagittal images (▶ Fig. 14.4; ▶ Fig. 14.5). Parasagittal images can detail the C0–C1 and C1–C2 articulations. The sagittal and parasagittal images are also useful for mapping the vertebral artery anatomy, which is essential for planning surgical procedures at the C1 and C2 levels.

Coronal images are useful for evaluating the cerebellar tonsils and the C0–C1 and C1–C2 articulations. Coronal sections are taken from the anterior arch of the atlas to its posterior arch.[18] Coronal images show the lateral masses of C1 and the apical and alar ligaments.

Axial sections, typically obtained from the foramen magnum to the base of the dens,[18] provide detailed information about the cross-sectional anatomy of the OCJ. In particular, they are useful for characterizing the space available for the cord, atlantoaxial subluxation, and vertebral artery anatomy within C1 and C2. Correlating axial images with sagittal or coronal localizing images is vital when evaluating the OCJ to confirm the level (occiput vs. C1 vs. C2) that is being evaluated.

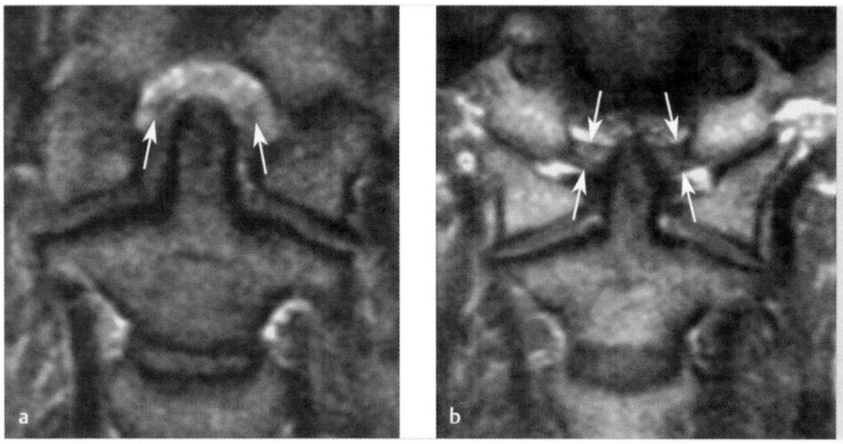

Fig. 14.3 The intact alar ligaments (*arrows*) in a normal spine are difficult to identify on **(a)** a coronal T2-weighted image but are more easily visualized on **(b)** a specialized intermediate-weighted image. (Reproduced with permission from, Haines CM, Khanna AJ, Carrino JA, Lin SD, O'Brien JR. The Occipitocervical Junction. In: Khanna AJ, ed. MRI Essentials for the Spine Specialist. 1st Edition. New York: Thieme; 2014.)

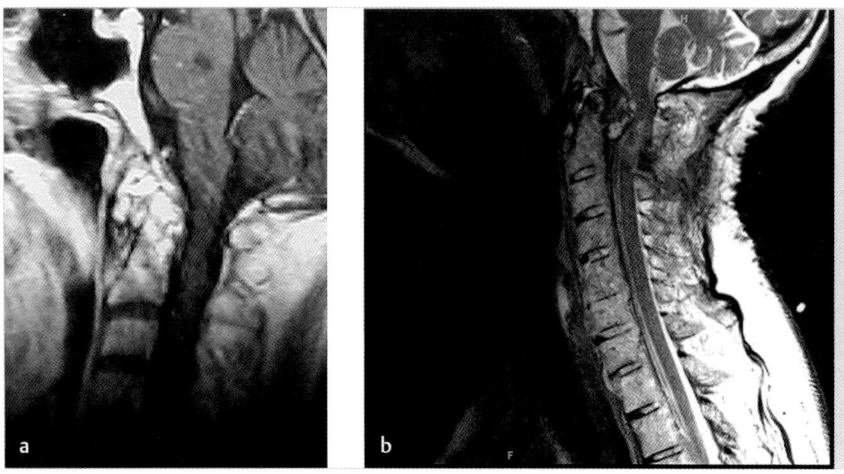

Fig. 14.4 C1–C2 pannus formation. **(a)** A sagittal T1-weighted image shows a large pannus in the atlantodens interval in a patient with rheumatoid arthritis (RA) and cranial settling. **(b)** A sagittal T2-weighted image of a patient with a large pannus posterior to the odontoid shows it is causing cord compression. (Reproduced with permission from, Haines CM, Khanna AJ, Carrino JA, Lin SD, O'Brien JR. The Occipitocervical Junction. In: Khanna AJ, ed. MRI Essentials for the Spine Specialist. 1st Edition. New York: Thieme; 2014.)

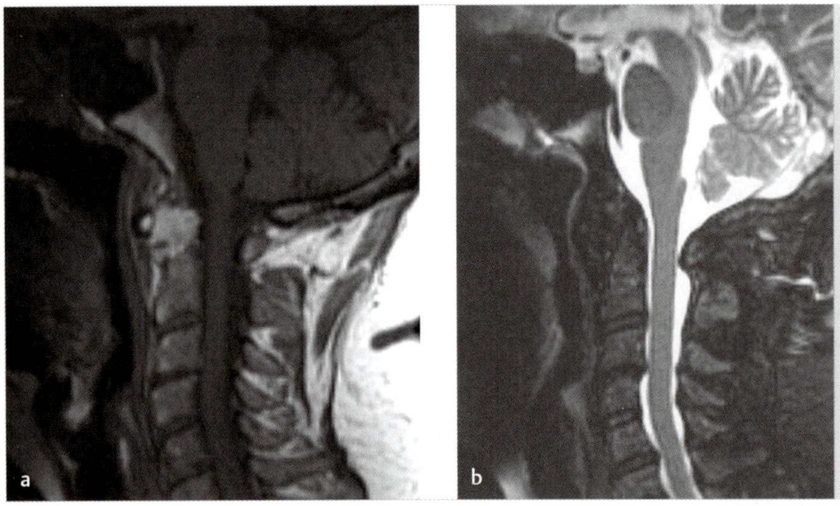

Fig. 14.5 These sagittal **(a)** T1-weighted and **(b)** short tau inversion recovery (STIR) images of a patient with rheumatoid arthritis (RA) and large pannus formation in which the pannus has caused substantial osseous erosion. (Reproduced with permission from, Haines CM, Khanna AJ, Carrino JA, Lin SD, O'Brien JR. The Occipitocervical Junction. In: Khanna AJ, ed. MRI Essentials for the Spine Specialist. 1st Edition. New York: Thieme; 2014.)

14.3 Pathology of the OCJ

OCJ abnormality can result in compression of neural elements and odontoid elevation. Conditions affecting the OCJ can be classified as primary/congenital or acquired.

14.3.1 Primary/Congenital Conditions

When congenital conditions result in brainstem compression, use of the term "basilar invagination" is appropriate.[2,24,25,26,27,28,29,30]

Congenital Anomalies of the Occiput

Anomalies of the occiput can result from failure of formation (often referred to as "hypoplasia") or of segmentation.[13,31,32,33] Failures of formation include basioccipital and occipital condyle hypoplasia.[2,22,23,24,25,26,27,28,29,30,31,32,33] Basioccipital hypoplasia is associated with a shortened clivus from poor development of the sclerotomes (▶ Fig. 14.6).[33,34] This condition has a wide range of clinical severity, although it is often associated with basilar invagination, which can be best seen with the Chamberlain line.[22] In occipital condyle hypoplasia, the deformity is usually bilateral; however, unilateral cases have been reported.[22,35] Shortened, flat condyles result in basilar invagination, and notably, the atlantooccipital joint axis angle seen on coronal MRI is widened. Clinically, this condition can result in limited atlantooccipital joint motion.

Failure of segmentation at the OCJ can result in atlantooccipital assimilation, which can be partial or complete (▶ Fig. 14.7).[22,36] The incidence in the general population has been reported to be 0.08 to 2.76%,[36,37] and sagittal MRI scans often show a comma-shaped basion.[22] This finding is often discovered incidentally on imaging after patients present with neck pain after minor trauma.[13,14,36] Approximately half of patients with C0–C1 assimilation progress to subsequent atlantoaxial instability and early onset myelopathy.[13,14,33,38,39,40] Families of children with atlantooccipital assimilation should be educated on the natural history of the disease and the warning signs of myelopathy.[36]

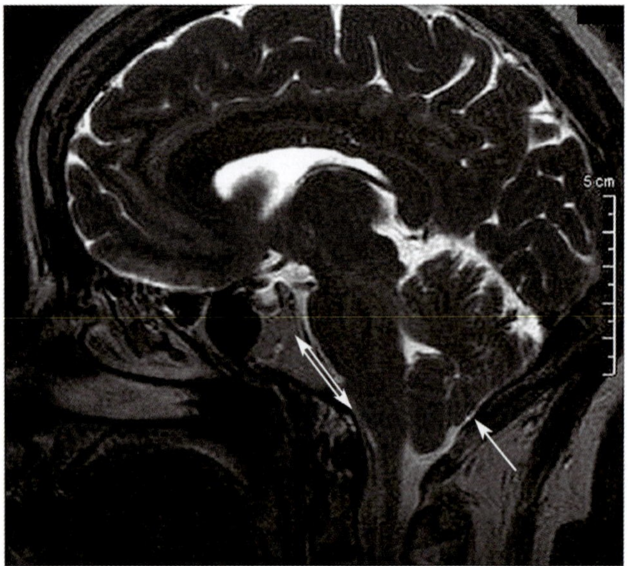

Fig. 14.6 A sagittal T2-weighted image shows basioccipital hypoplasia with Chiari type-I malformation (*single arrow*) and a shortened clivus (*double arrow*). (Reproduced with permission from Noudel R, Jovenin N, Eap C, Scherpereel B, Pierot L, Rousseaux P. Incidence of basioccipital hypoplasia in Chiari malformation type I: comparative morphometric study of the posterior cranial fossa. J Neurosurg 2009;111:1046–1052.)

Congenital Anomalies of the Atlas

Rachischisis is the developmental failure of the atlas.[22] In normal development, the posterior arch fuses with the lateral masses at 3 to 4 years of age, and the anterior arch fuses with the lateral masses at 6 to 8 years of age. In contrast to failure of segmentation, failure of formation of the atlas is rarely associated with basilar invagination.[22,41] Posterior atlas arch clefts are the most common pattern seen, with an incidence of 4% in autopsy specimens.[42,43] Most of these clefts are midline; only 3% are at the sulcus for the vertebral artery.[42,43] Anterior arch clefts are rarer, with an incidence of 0.1% of autopsy specimens[42,43];

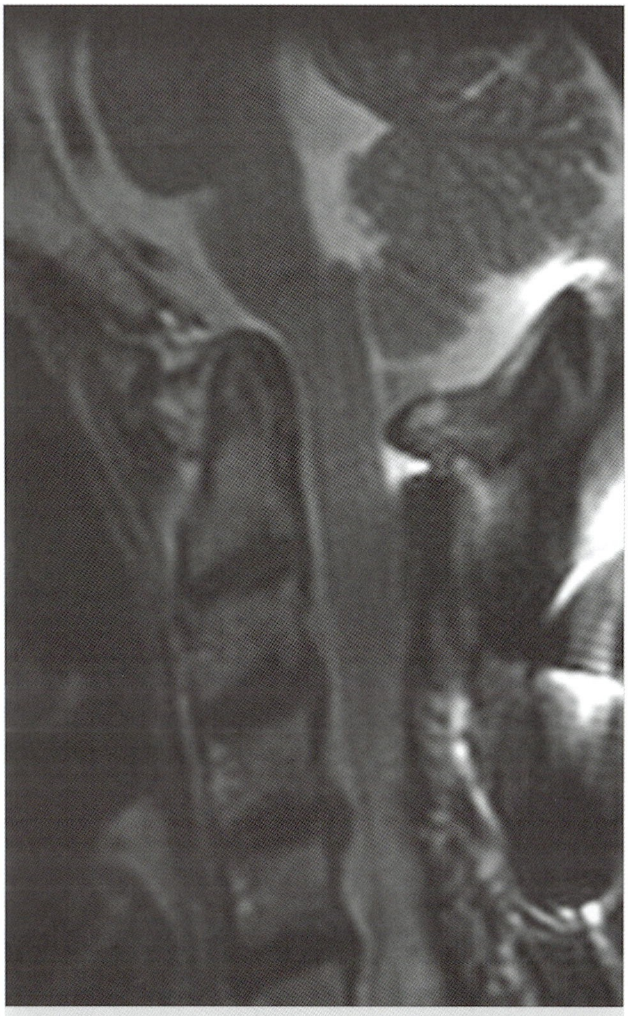

Fig. 14.7 A sagittal T2-weighted image shows atlantooccipital assimilation. The basion is more curved than normal, and there is superior migration of the odontoid process. (Reproduced with permission from, Haines CM, Khanna AJ, Carrino JA, Lin SD, O'Brien JR. The Occipitocervical Junction. In: Khanna AJ, ed. MRI Essentials for the Spine Specialist. 1st Edition. New York: Thieme; 2014.)

they can be associated with posterior clefts and can mimic a Jefferson fracture.[43] Well-corticated margins and the lack of a posterior tubercle suggest an arch defect.[22,42,43,44] In contrast, a defect with increased MRI signal intensity on fluid-sensitive sequences is more indicative of a Jefferson fracture. It is important to note that the midline physis closes at 4 years of age.[40,45] Overall, axial MRI views best illustrate C1 defects.

Congenital Anomalies of the Axis

Congenital anomalies of the axis are usually confined to the odontoid process and are rarely associated with basilar invagination[21] but can result in atlantoaxial instability.[46] To clarify the formation anomalies, a review of the physiologic axis development is detailed.[47]

Failure of fusion of the terminal ossicle is associated with a Bergman ossicle,[22] which can be confused with a type-I odontoid fracture[48] and is of little clinical significance. Fusion of the dentocentral synchondrosis normally occurs at 6 years of age.[49] Failure of fusion or fracture of the dentocentral synchondrosis is associated with an os odontoideum (▶ Fig. 14.8). This term refers to an ossicle that is above the body of C2. The anterior arch of C2 is rounded and hypertrophic, and the body of C2 has a well-corticated, convex upper margin.[22] Atlantoaxial instability is a hallmark of this disorder.[22,46] It is associated with congenital diseases involving abnormalities of connective tissue such as Down syndrome, spondyloepiphyseal dysplasia, and Morquio syndrome.[50] Odontoid aplasia is extremely rare and is associated with atlantoaxial instability.[22,46]

Although diagnosis of fusion failures of C2 can be made on the basis of radiographs, MRI provides more detailed information.[51] Coronal and sagittal cuts are most valuable for differentiating fusion failures from acute fractures. Fractures lack cortication on T1-weighted images and show edema on T2-weighted and fat-suppressed T2-weighted images.

Chiari Malformations

A type-I Chiari malformation[52,53] is defined as a defect in the cerebellum with a downward displacement of the tonsils > 5 mm below the plane of the foramen magnum; however, some authors have referred to downward displacement from 3 to 5 mm as a borderline diagnosis according to clinical parameters (▶ Fig. 14.9; ▶ Fig. 14.10).[54,55] Associated conditions include basilar invagination in 50%, atlantooccipital assimilation in 10%, and Klippel-Feil syndrome in 5%.[54,55] Midsagittal images most consistently show the downward tonsil displacement and decreased CSF content in the retrocerebellar space.[56]

A type-II Chiari malformation results from dysgenesis of the hindbrain.[22] It is almost always associated with myelomeningocele and can present with multiple anatomic anomalies, including hydrocephalus, hypoplasia of intracranial structures (e.g., falx cerebri and corpus callosum), and downward displacement of posterior fossa content (e.g., inferior cerebellar vermis, fourth ventricle, and medulla).[42] It is not associated with atlantooccipital assimilation or basilar invagination.[22]

A type-III Chiari malformation, which is a herniated hindbrain into a high cervical encephalocele, occurs rarely.[22,57] A type-IV Chiari malformation involves cerebellar hypoplasia without cerebellar herniation.

Klippel-Feil Syndrome

Klippel-Feil syndrome is classically described as a triad of a low posterior hairline, short neck, and limited neck mobility in association with congenital cervical fusions.[58] For the diagnosis to be made, there must be failure of segmentation of at least two cervical vertebrae.[59] Accelerated degeneration of adjacent levels and increased susceptibility to cord injury after minor trauma have been reported.[59,60] Coronal and sagittal images are most useful in diagnosing the lack of segmentation.

14.3.2 Acquired Conditions

Acquired conditions cause abnormality by softening the skull base, thereby potentiating odontoid elevation. Many disease processes can cause elevation of the odontoid process, including osteogenesis imperfecta, Paget disease, rickets, osteomalacia, rheumatoid arthritis (RA), and ankylosing spondylitis. "Basilar

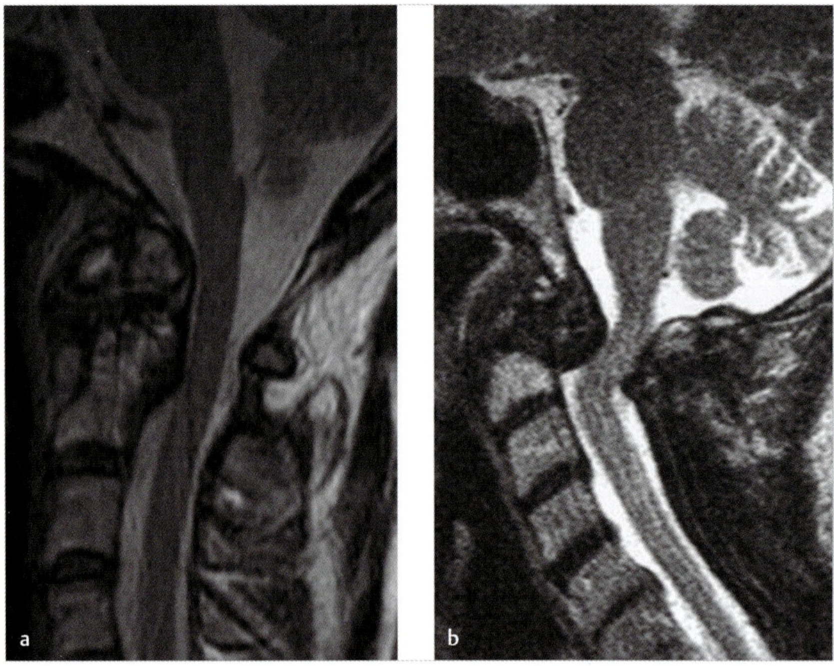

Fig. 14.8 Os odontoideum versus chronic odontoid fracture. **(a)** A sagittal T2-weighted image of an os odontoideum. An os is often round and does not preserve the shape of the dens but a chronic odontoid fracture, as seen on **(b)** a sagittal T2-weighted image, typically retains the typical anatomic architecture of the odontoid. (Reproduced with permission from, Haines CM, Khanna AJ, Carrino JA, Lin SD, O'Brien JR. The Occipitocervical Junction. In: Khanna AJ, ed. MRI Essentials for the Spine Specialist. 1st Edition. New York: Thieme; 2014.)

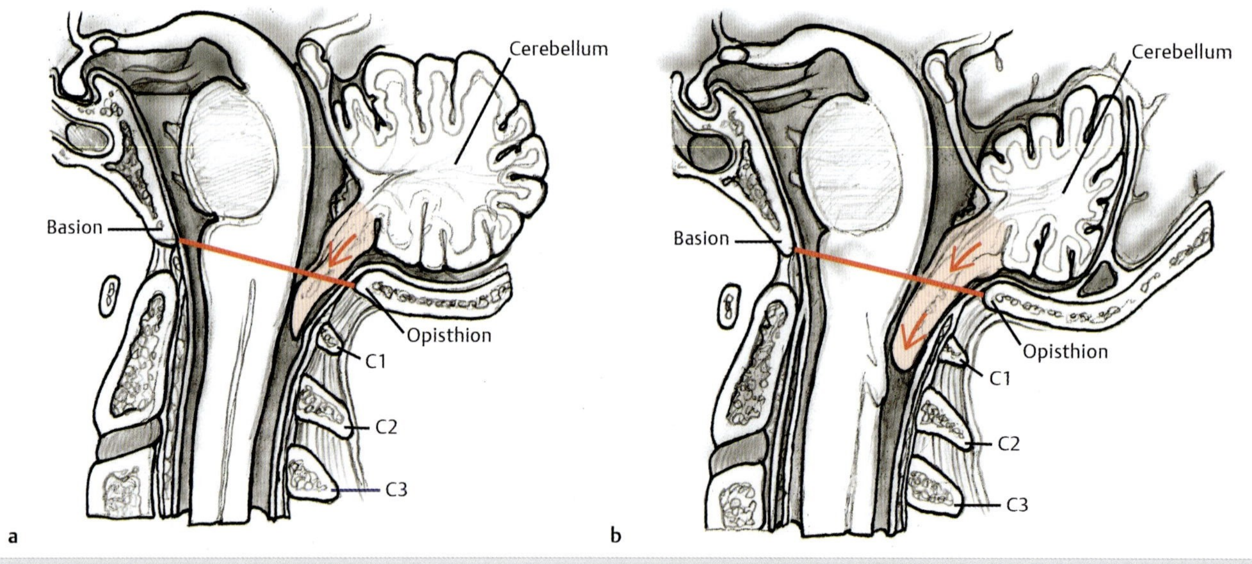

Fig. 14.9 Illustrations show the typical features of **(a)** type-I and **(b)** type-II Chiari malformations. (Reproduced with permission from, Haines CM, Khanna AJ, Carrino JA, Lin SD, O'Brien JR. The Occipitocervical Junction. In: Khanna AJ, ed. MRI Essentials for the Spine Specialist. 1st Edition. New York: Thieme; 2014.)

impression" is the term used to denote the odontoid's superior migration in the setting of acquired skull-base softening.[22,30]

Basilar Impression

It is useful to review certain terms related to craniocervical instability. Cranial settling differs from basilar invagination and basilar impression. Cranial settling is vertical subluxation of the odontoid caused by a loss of supporting ligamentous structures.[21] This condition can occur with RA or psoriatic arthritis. Basilar invagination results from a loss of skull height secondary to congenital abnormalities.[21] Basilar impression results from skull-base softening secondary to an acquired condition such as Paget disease.

RA/Cranial Settling

RA is a systemic disease that causes inflamed synovial joints. The synovial joints develop a pannus that generates enzymatic erosion of supporting ligamentous structures.[61,62] In the cervical spine, this condition can affect the craniocervical junction and the subaxial cervical spine.[61,62,63,64] Most commonly, atlantoaxial instability develops secondary to erosion of the ligaments at the OCJ.[61,62] As the disease progresses,

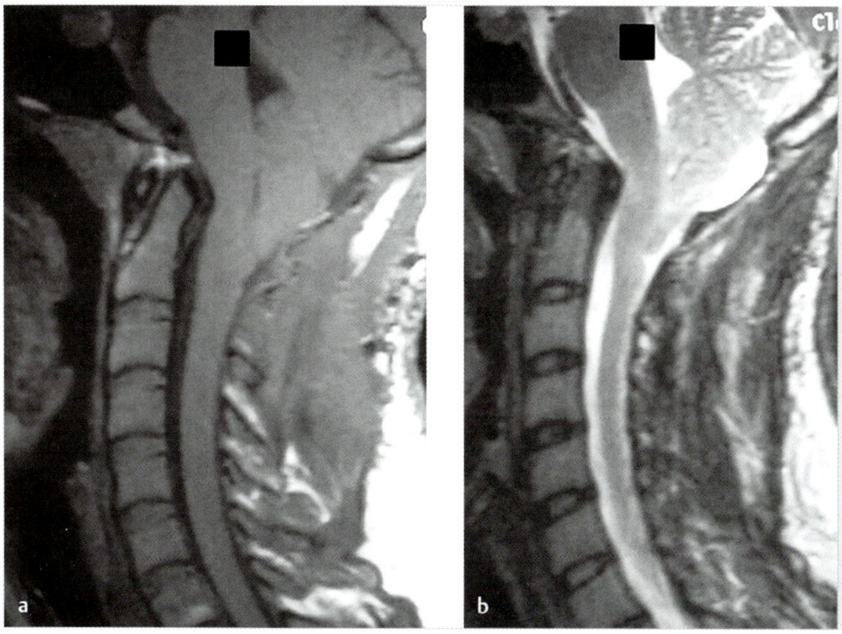

Fig. 14.10 These sagittal **(a)** T1-weighted and **(b)** T2-weighted images of a patient with a type-I Chiari malformation who has undergone a suboccipital decompression procedure. (Reproduced with permission from, Haines CM, Khanna AJ, Carrino JA, Lin SD, O'Brien JR. The Occipitocervical Junction. In: Khanna AJ, ed. MRI Essentials for the Spine Specialist. 1st Edition. New York: Thieme; 2014.)

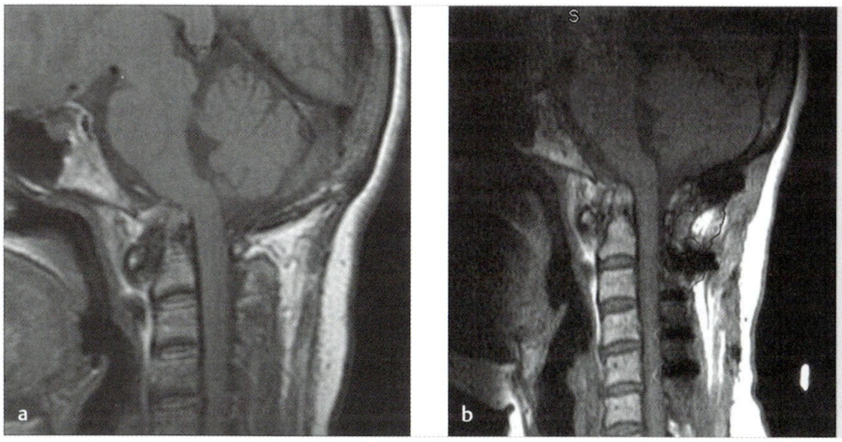

Fig. 14.11 Cranial settling. **(a)** A sagittal T1-weighted image shows cranial settling in a patient with rheumatoid arthritis. **(b)** A sagittal T1-weighted image with metal suppression after instrumented reduction from the occiput to C5, which resulted in decreased brainstem compression. (Reproduced with permission from, Haines CM, Khanna AJ, Carrino JA, Lin SD, O'Brien JR. The Occipitocervical Junction. In: Khanna AJ, ed. MRI Essentials for the Spine Specialist. 1st Edition. New York: Thieme; 2014.)

erosion of the lateral masses of C1, the occipital condyles, and facets of C2 occurs resulting in cranial settling (▶ Fig. 14.11).[22,61,62] After the odontoid begins to occupy a more rostral position, it compresses the brainstem and vertebrobasilar system. This abnormal process is postulated by some as the cause of sudden death in patients with advanced RA.[22,61,62,65] It is important to note that, in contrast to other disorders, the C1 arch migrates with the skull base to lie in a more caudal position.[22] In some cases, it has been reported to be as inferior as the C2–C3 disk space.[4,59,60,66] Because of the erosion of the osseous structures that takes place, the method of Redlund-Johnell and Pettersson[6] can be used to gauge settling. This technique uses the vertical distance from the McRae line to the C2–C3 disk space to gauge cranial settling. Boden and colleagues[61,62] reported on the use of MRI to measure the space available for the cord as a technique for predicting recovery after cervical stabilization for patients with RA and atlantoaxial instability. A cord space or space available for the cord > 14 mm on MRI was associated with better clinical outcomes than was a space < 10 mm, which was associated with a poor prognosis.[61,62]

14.3.3 Neoplasms

The neoplastic abnormalities that can affect the craniocervical junction are similar to neoplasms that affect the rest of the spine (see Chapter 21, Tumors of the Spine). As with the rest of the spine, tumors of the OCJ can be located within one of the three following compartments:

- Extradural.
- Intradural-extramedullary.
- Intramedullary.

Osseous neoplastic lesions within this region can be divided into primary and metastatic lesions, which is a critical distinction when applying a treatment paradigm. Imaging of this region is best performed with a combination of conventional radiography, CT, and MRI. Although the imaging modalities can help narrow the differential diagnosis, biopsy is the only method for definitive diagnosis.

Primary Osseous/Extradural Tumors

The primary osseous tumors in this region are as follows:

- Hemangioma.
- Chondroblastoma.
- Osteoid osteoma.
- Osteoblastoma.
- Chordoid rest.
- Aneurysmal bone cyst.
- Giant cell tumor.
- Chordoma.
- Various sarcomas.

The differential diagnosis of these primary bone tumors can be narrowed according to the tumor's location and imaging characteristics (▶ Fig. 14.12). Most primary tumors of the spine originate within the posterior elements (i.e., pedicles, facets, pars, lamina, and spinous processes). Hemangiomas, chordoid rests, chordomas, and giant cell tumors are more likely to be located anteriorly and to arise from the midline. Chondroblastomas, osteoid osteomas, and osteoblastomas tend to arise from the posterior elements of the spine.

Hemangiomas, chordoid rests, and chordomas are most frequently slow-growing tumors, and the bone tends to show evidence of remodeling. Chordoid rests and chordomas tend to have a bright "bubbly" appearance on T2-weighted MRI sequences, and in most cases they arise within the vertebral body.[67] The distinction between a chordoid rest and a chordoma largely depends on the lesion's size and clinical history. Hemangiomas also tend to be anteriorly located. They have a spiculated "wagon-wheel" appearance, with clearly defined margins. Aggressive or atypical hemangiomas can lose this characteristic appearance if they grow to considerable size.[68,69]

In contrast, more aggressive tumors typically exhibit varying degrees of osseous erosion. Giant cell tumors are often hypodense on T1-weighted and T2-weighted images and frequently enhance on T1-weighted images with contrast administration. MRI of giant cell tumors typically shows lytic lesions.[70] Sarcomas usually have an invasive appearance on MRI, as evidenced by cortical destruction and infiltration of the surrounding tissues. They tend to be anteriorly located and have a varying degree of soft tissue involvement.

Osteoid osteomas and osteoblastomas appear similar on imaging studies but they are distinguished according to size as follows: lesions < 1.5 cm are termed osteoid osteomas; larger lesions are called osteoblastomas. Both lesions have areas of blastic and clastic activity, giving a characteristic target appearance on CT imaging or a central sclerotic area surrounded by a hypodense area contained within a calcified margin.[71] If MR angiography is performed, it may show hypervascularity in the surrounding musculature that might suggest a more aggressive appearance of the lesion (e.g., osteosarcoma) but in reality, the hypervascularity is a reactive

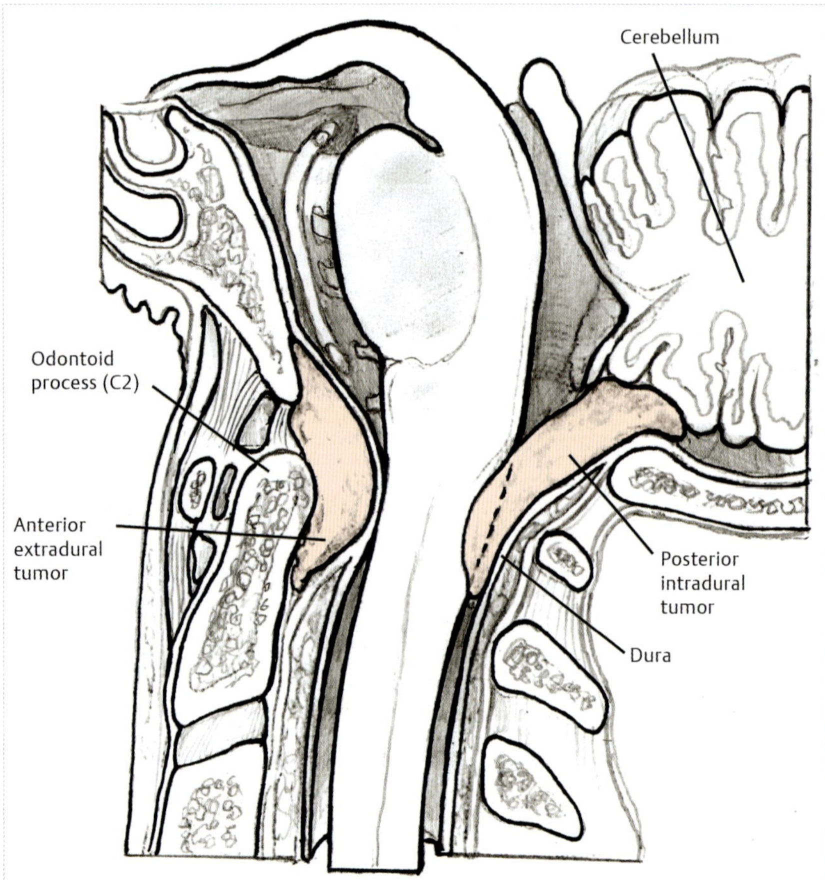

Fig. 14.12 Illustration shows anterior extradural and posterior intradural tumors at the occipitocervical junction (OCJ). (Reproduced with permission from, Haines CM, Khanna AJ, Carrino JA, Lin SD, O'Brien JR. The Occipitocervical Junction. In: Khanna AJ, ed. MRI Essentials for the Spine Specialist. 1st Edition. New York: Thieme; 2014.)

phenomenon and still compatible with the benign diagnosis of osteoid osteoma.[72]

Aneurysmal bone cysts are characterized by a slowly growing lesion with sclerotic boundaries on conventional radiographs or CT. On MRI, a thin expansile rim and fluid-fluid levels on T2-weighted imaging, representing areas of hemorrhage in different stages of evolution, can help confirm the diagnosis of aneurysmal bone cyst.[73] Multiple septate and small lobulations are usually present on T2-weighted images but may be imperceptible on T1-weighted sequences.[74]

Lesions that metastasize to the osseous spine often appear aggressive on imaging studies. They are often anteriorly located and show substantial osseous destruction. Compared with metastasis to other levels of the spine, epidural extension of the tumor at the level of the OCJ is unusual. Spinal cord compression seen with these lesions usually is the result of overt instability and osseous compression rather than epidural extension of the tumor. The apical, transverse, posterior longitudinal, and nuchal ligaments are very thick in this region, which prevents direct compression from epidural extension.[75]

Intradural-Extramedullary Tumors

Intradural-extramedullary abnormality in this region is also similar to that of other levels of the spine. These lesions are best characterized using MRI (T1-weighted, T2-weighted, and post-contrast T1-weighted sequences). Tumors seen in this region are the following:

- Meningioma.
- Hemangiopericytoma.
- Schwannoma.
- Neurofibroma.
- Metastatic disease (less commonly).

Meningiomas and hemangiopericytomas tend to be hypointense to isointense on T1-weighted and T2-weighted MRI, and they enhance strongly with contrast administration. These tumors typically produce a "dural tail," which appears as an epidural extension of the tumor, beyond the main bulk of the tumor, in the subdural space along the dura.[76,77,78] Although this finding can be seen with schwannomas and neurofibromas, its presence suggests a meningioma or hemangiopericytoma. These lesions tend to display substantial vascularity on MR angiography (hemangiopericytomas are very vascular lesions). Schwannomas and neurofibromas usually have a less midline location and typically extend toward (and sometimes through) the neural foramen (▶ Fig. 14.13).[67,70,79] They originate from the nerve root, which explains the eccentric nature. Appearance of these lesions can vary but it often resembles that of meningiomas without a dural tail. A spinal fluid space between the tumor and the spinal cord at either end of the tumor can suggest a nerve sheath tumor as opposed to meningioma in the differential diagnosis.

Intramedullary Tumors

The intramedullary abnormalities that can be found at the OCJ are as follows:

- Ependymoma.
- Hemangioblastoma.
- Glial tumor.
- Vascular lesion (i.e., cavernous malformation or arteriovenous malformation).
- Metastatic disease (less common).

Ependymomas arise from the ependymal layer of the central canal and are slow-growing lesions. They are usually centrally located, grow rostrally and caudally, and frequently have an associated syrinx. They are usually hypointense on T1-weighted and T2-weighted MRI sequences, and they homogeneously enhance with contrast administration (▶ Fig. 14.14).[80,81] Hemangioblastomas are also commonly hypointense on T1-weighted and T2-weighted MRI sequences and enhance with contrast administration. They are usually seen to be eccentric in location within the spinal cord and often have a large syrinx associated with them. Areas of hemorrhage of different ages may be seen surrounding the tumor and can markedly vary the appearance of these tumors on MRI.[82]

Angiography can be useful in showing the vascularity of the tumor and the location of the arterial feeders and draining veins.[83]

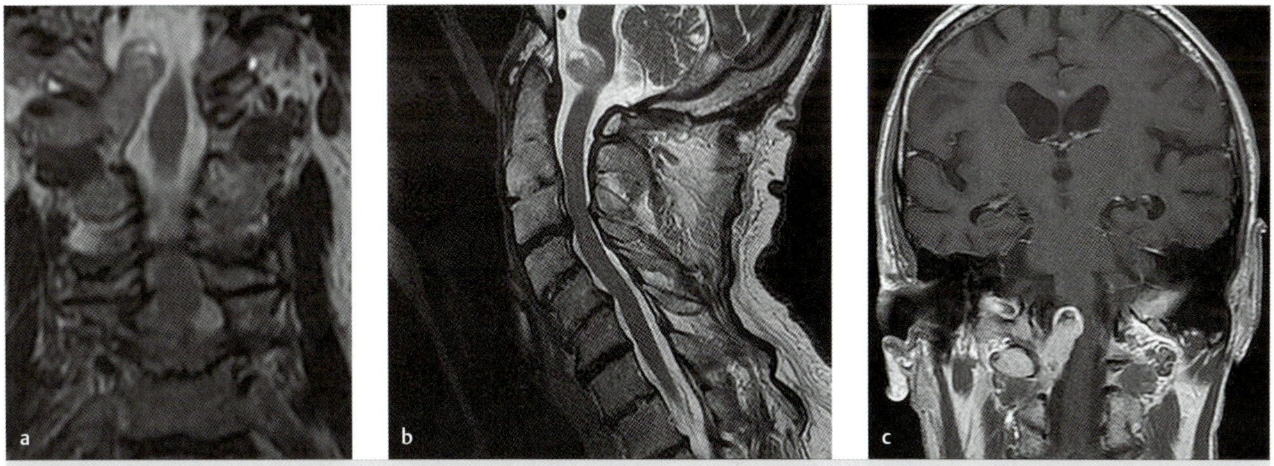

Fig. 14.13 These (a) coronal T2-weighted, (b) sagittal T2-weighted, and (c) coronal postgadolinium T1-weighted images show a schwannoma at C2 extending into the foramen magnum. (Reproduced with permission from, Haines CM, Khanna AJ, Carrino JA, Lin SD, O'Brien JR. The Occipitocervical Junction. In: Khanna AJ, ed. MRI Essentials for the Spine Specialist. 1st Edition. New York: Thieme; 2014.)

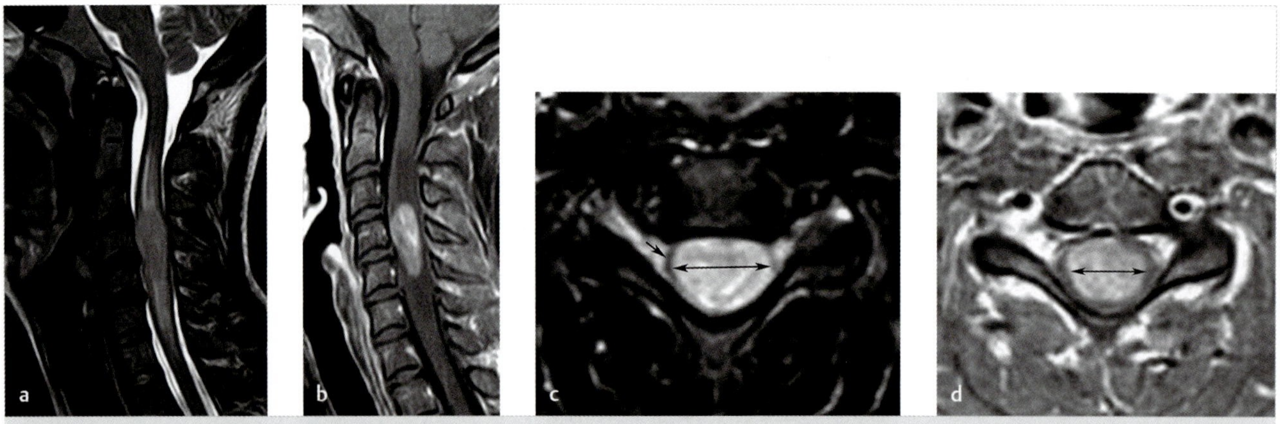

Fig. 14.14 Cervical ependymoma. **(a)** A sagittal T2-weighted image shows a large cervical ependymoma centered at C4–C5 but with cord signal change extending from C2 to C7. **(b)** A sagittal postgadolinium T1-weighted image shows that the tumor is located at C4–C5 and that the signal change extended from C2 to C7 shown in **(a)** represents edema proximal and distal to the lesion. **(c)** An axial T2-weighted image shows that the lesion (between *arrowheads*) is located within the spinal cord, which is seen as a thin sliver of low signal intensity surrounding the lesion (*arrow*). **(d)** An axial postgadolinium T1-weighted image shows similar findings with enhancement of the tumor. (Reproduced with permission from, Haines CM, Khanna AJ, Carrino JA, Lin SD, O'Brien JR. The Occipitocervical Junction. In: Khanna AJ, ed. MRI Essentials for the Spine Specialist. 1st Edition. New York: Thieme; 2014.)

Glial tumors can arise anywhere within the spinal cord substance. Unlike ependymomas, glial tumors usually do not have an associated syrinx or distinct margins on imaging studies. The cord has a swollen appearance (increased diameter) in the region of the tumor. These tumors are visualized best on T2-weighted imaging, and the degree of contrast enhancement usually correlates with the grade of the tumor. Given the imaging characteristics of glial tumors, these lesions can be difficult to distinguish from transverse myelitis and spinal cord signal change secondary to myelopathy and ischemia.[71]

Metastasis typically spreads to the vertebral bodies. However, intramedullary tumor spread can occur. Edema within the cord is commonly seen on fluid-sensitive MRI sequences. Cystic changes, as well as hemorrhage, may be noted for metastases within the spinal cord.[84]

The MRI characteristics of the multitude of tumors that can be seen at the OCJ can be used to generate and then narrow a differential diagnosis. Subsequently, a definitive diagnosis is made with an open or percutaneous (usually image-guided) biopsy. The tissue diagnosis, along with the location of the tumor, alteration in regional anatomy, degree of stenosis, presence or absence of instability, and degree of neural compromise can help guide the surgical or nonsurgical treatment. For patients treated surgically, MRI characteristics can help select the approach and assist with preoperative planning and postoperative follow-up.

14.4 Miscellaneous

14.4.1 Down Syndrome

Down syndrome is caused by trisomy 21. Among the disorders associated with Down syndrome, ligamentous laxity figures prominently. Atlantoaxial and atlantooccipital instabilities have also been described.[85,86,87,88,89,90,91,92] Although flexion-extension conventional radiographs can be used to detect atlantoaxial instability in children with Down syndrome[93] and are used widely as screening tools,[94,95] surgical decision making should be based on neural impingement seen on MRI.[92] Flexion-extension MRI can also be used to evaluate for stenosis in patients with Down syndrome, like it is used for patients with known or suspected instability secondary to more conventional degenerative stenosis (▶ Fig. 14.15).[96] It is important to note that patients with Down syndrome have increased incidence of os odontoideum and hypoplasia of the arch of the atlas than does the general population.[22,30,97]

14.4.2 Trauma to the OCJ

In a study of 34,069 patients with blunt trauma, 2.4% had trauma to the cervical spine.[94] Of those patients with cervical fracture, 34% had an injury to the OCJ.[94] Recognizing OCJ trauma is crucial because of the devastating effects of injury to this anatomic area.[98,99,100]

In 2007, the Spine Trauma Study Group provided a consensus statement on measurement techniques for upper cervical spine injuries.[101] Many of the techniques reviewed were developed for studying patients with cranial settling associated with RA.[13,14] Different measurement techniques are recommended in the setting of OCJ trauma.[101]

Occipitocervical Trauma

Occipitocervical dislocation can be a devastating injury (▶ Fig. 14.16).[98,99,100] Postmortem studies show that approximately one-third of individuals who die as a result of traffic accidents have this injury.[98,99,102] Delays in diagnosis averaging 2 days after the injury, correlating with worse neurologic outcomes, have been reported.[103] In addition, even without frank dislocation, the C0–C1 junction may be injured, as indicated by postmortem studies.[98,99,104] Therefore, familiarity with the advanced imaging appearance of the ligaments is vital for the practicing spine surgeon.[18,23,105,106,107]

Atlantoaxial dissociation can also be the result of a traumatic event (▶ Fig. 14.17).[108,109] It is associated with odontoid fractures or osseous displacement in the sagittal plane. T2-weighted

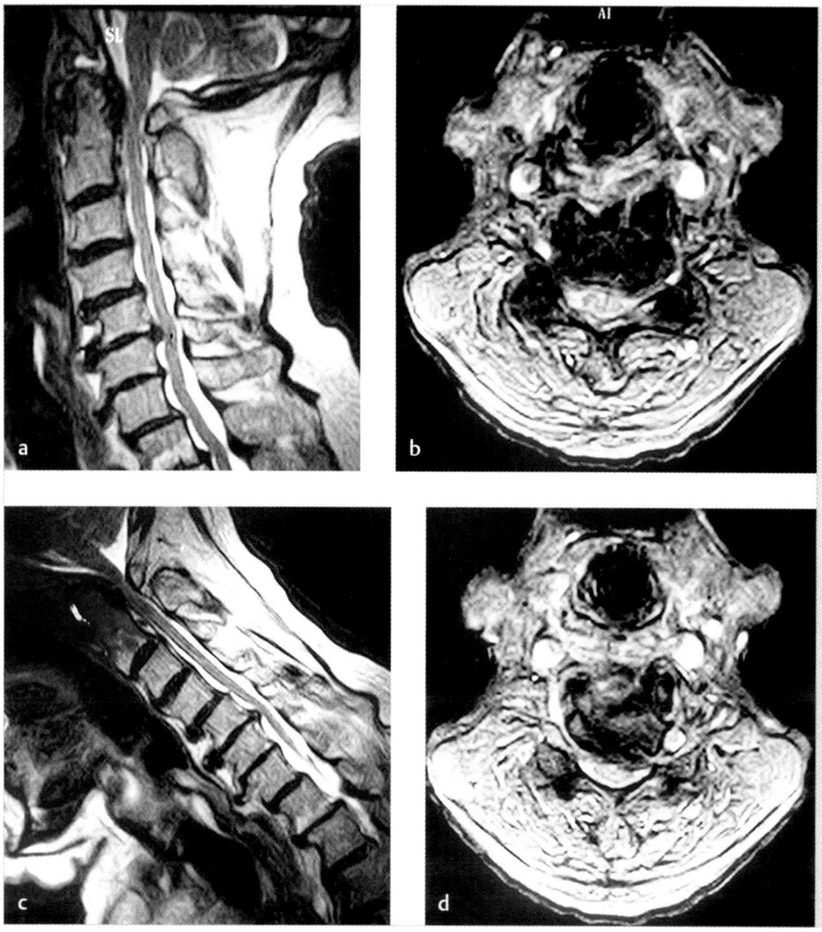

Fig. 14.15 A dynamic magnetic resonance imaging (MRI) sequence in a patient with atlantoaxial instability. **(a)** Sagittal T2-weighted and **(b)** axial T2-weighted images in extension show only mild cord compression, whereas **(c)** sagittal T2-weighted and **(d)** axial T2-weighted images in flexion show severe cord compression and widening of the anterior atlantodens interval. (Reproduced with permission from, Haines CM, Khanna AJ, Carrino JA, Lin SD, O'Brien JR. The Occipitocervical Junction. In: Khanna AJ, ed. MRI Essentials for the Spine Specialist. 1st Edition. New York: Thieme; 2014.)

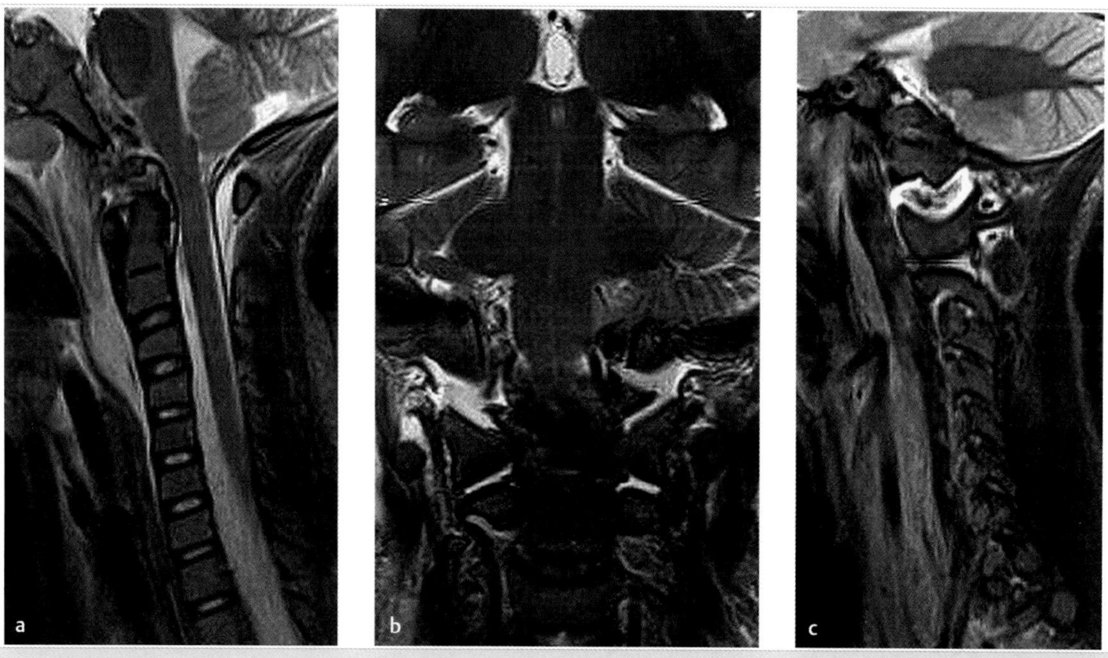

Fig. 14.16 These **(a)** midsagittal, **(b)** coronal, and **(c)** parasagittal T2-weighted images show atlantooccipital dissociation. The midsagittal image shows an increased distance between the basion and tip of the odontoid, whereas the coronal and parasagittal images show edema in the C0–C1 joint. (Reproduced with permission from, Haines CM, Khanna AJ, Carrino JA, Lin SD, O'Brien JR. The Occipitocervical Junction. In: Khanna AJ, ed. MRI Essentials for the Spine Specialist. 1st Edition. New York: Thieme; 2014.)

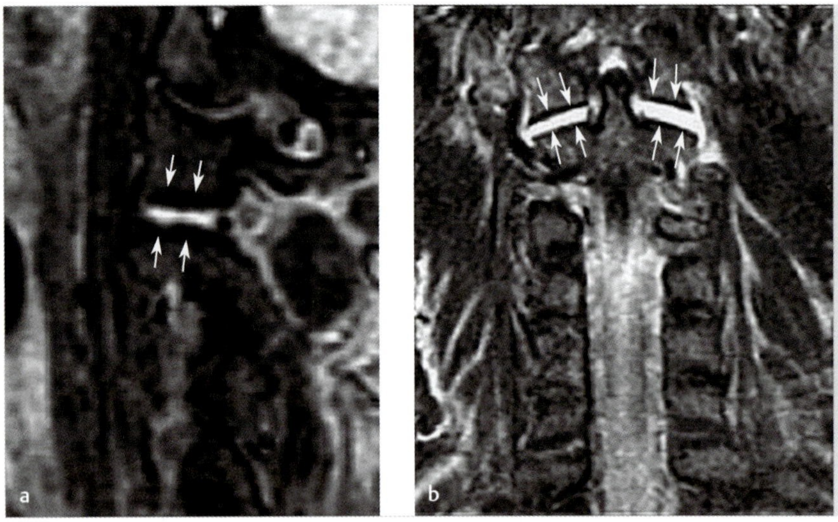

Fig. 14.17 These (a) sagittal T2-weighted and (b) coronal T2-weighted images of atlantoaxial dissociation show edema and distraction (*arrows* on each) through the C1–C2 joint. (Reproduced with permission from, Haines CM, Khanna AJ, Carrino JA, Lin SD, O'Brien JR. The Occipitocervical Junction. In: Khanna AJ, ed. MRI Essentials for the Spine Specialist. 1st Edition. New York: Thieme; 2014.)

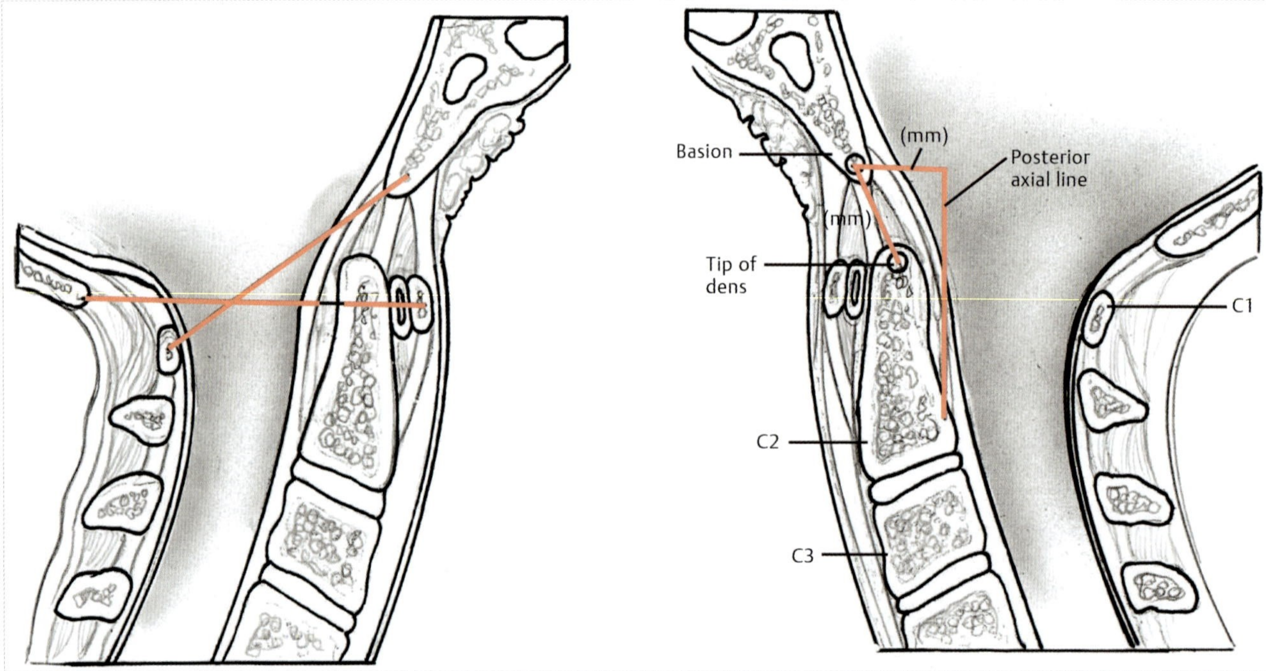

Fig. 14.18 Illustration depicts the Harris technique, which is used to evaluate the relationship between the occiput and cervical spine in cases of known or suspected atlantooccipital dissociation. (Reproduced with permission from, Haines CM, Khanna AJ, Carrino JA, Lin SD, O'Brien JR. The Occipitocervical Junction. In: Khanna AJ, ed. MRI Essentials for the Spine Specialist. 1st Edition. New York: Thieme; 2014.)

sequences are most useful in identifying a transverse ligament injury or osseous edema, which often accompanies the dissociation. Adjuvant dynamic MRI can also be helpful in illustrating the transverse ligament injury.

The Harris technique is useful in the radiographic diagnosis of atlantooccipital dislocation (▶ Fig. 14.18). To use this tool, one calculates the basion-dental interval and the basion-posterior axial line interval on midsagittal MRI sequences.[90] Measurements > 12 mm for the basion-dental interval and basion-posterior axial line interval are abnormal and suggestive of a dislocation. The Powers ratio has also been used to calculate injury (▶ Fig. 14.19).[110] The distance from the basion to the posterior arch is divided by the distance from the anterior arch to the opisthion. A value of 1 is considered normal. If the value is > 1, an anterior dislocation must be suspected, and if it is < 1, the potential for posterior dislocation exists.[110] However, the Harris technique has been shown to be better than the Powers ratio for diagnosing dislocation.[101]

Occipital condyle injuries have been classified on the basis of osseous versus ligamentous involvement.[111] Large osseous fragments have been noted to be more stable and have a greater chance at healing with nonoperative immobilization.[112,113]

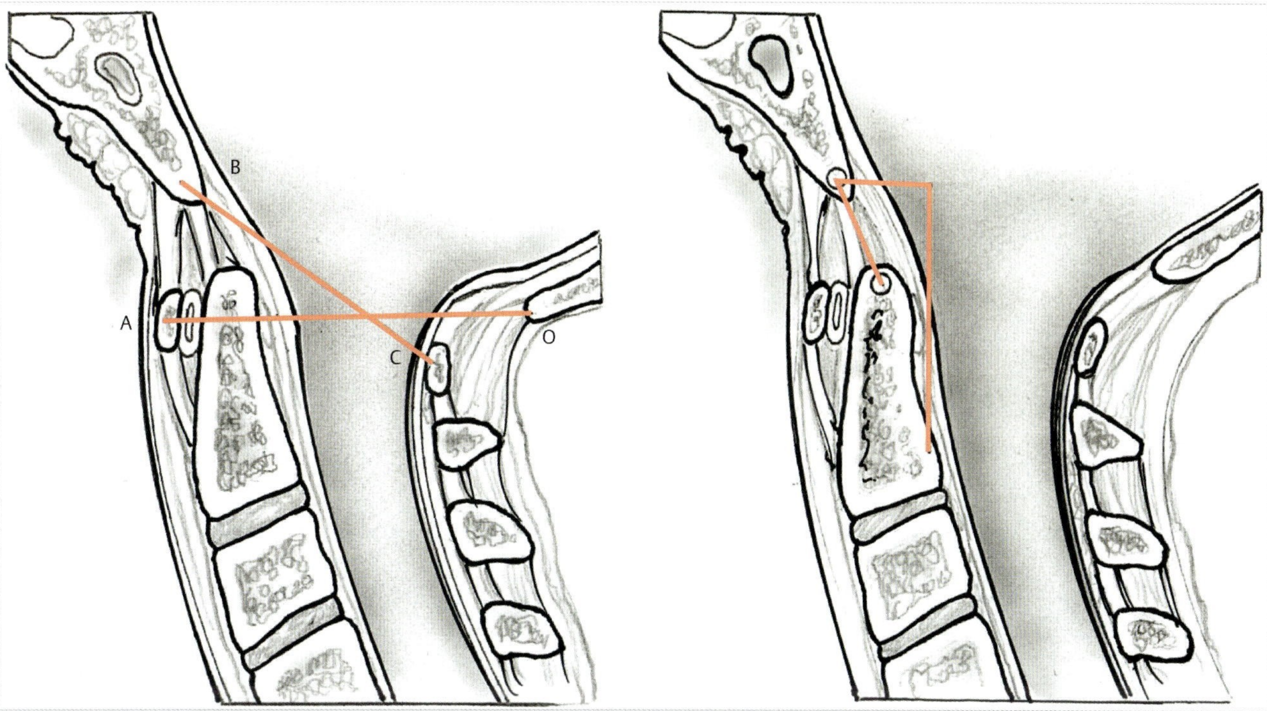

Fig. 14.19 Illustration depicts the Powers ratio, which, like the Harris technique, is used to evaluate the relationship between the occiput and cervical spine in cases of known or suspected atlantooccipital dissociation. A, anterior arch of C1; B, basion; C, posterior arch of C1; O, opisthion. (Reproduced with permission from, Haines CM, Khanna AJ, Carrino JA, Lin SD, O'Brien JR. The Occipitocervical Junction. In: Khanna AJ, ed. MRI Essentials for the Spine Specialist. 1st Edition. New York: Thieme; 2014.)

Although characterizing occipital condyle fractures is best performed with parasagittal and coronal CT images,[111] MRI will highlight the fracture and also the associated ligamentous injuries.

Trauma to the Atlas

An axial load to the OCJ at the atlas can result in burst fractures, which were originally described by Jefferson.[114] The injury is typically visualized on open-mouth odontoid radiographs or coronal CT images.[101,115,116] On open-mouth radiography, the rule of Spence[114] indirectly measures the integrity of the transverse ligament, which is paramount for stability. However, axial T2-weighted images can directly assess transverse ligament injury, including avulsion injuries (▶ Fig. 14.20).

Trauma to the Axis

C2 is the most commonly fractured cervical spine level.[94,117,118] Of cervical fractures secondary to blunt trauma, 24% involve C2 and one-third are odontoid fractures.[94] Fractures occur in a bimodal incidence as follows: one spike in the young and one in the elderly.[118] Elderly patients tend to have odontoid fractures that are posteriorly displaced. Fracture morphology, important in determining healing potential, can be best illustrated on lateral cervical radiography or CT,[101] whereas MRI can assess neural compression and also provide insight regarding the age of the fracture (▶ Fig. 14.21).

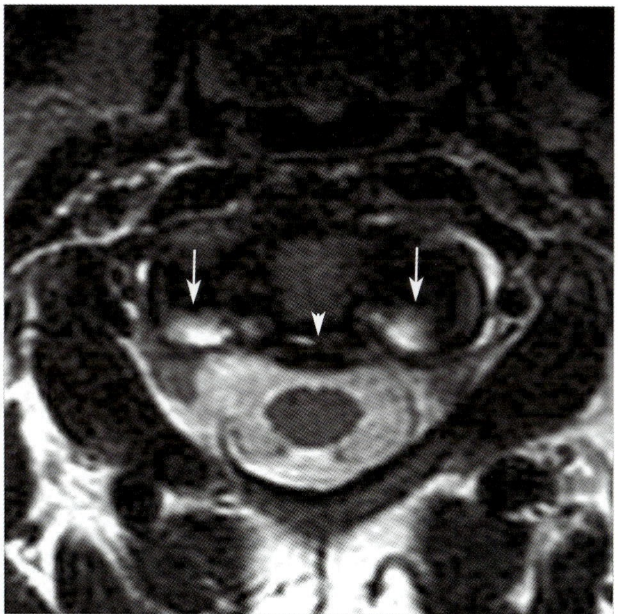

Fig. 14.20 An axial T2-weighted image shows prominence and edema at the insertion site of the transverse ligament *(arrowhead)* on the lateral masses of C1 (*arrows*). (Reproduced with permission from, Haines CM, Khanna AJ, Carrino JA, Lin SD, O'Brien JR. The Occipitocervical Junction. In: Khanna AJ, ed. MRI Essentials for the Spine Specialist. 1st Edition. New York: Thieme; 2014.)

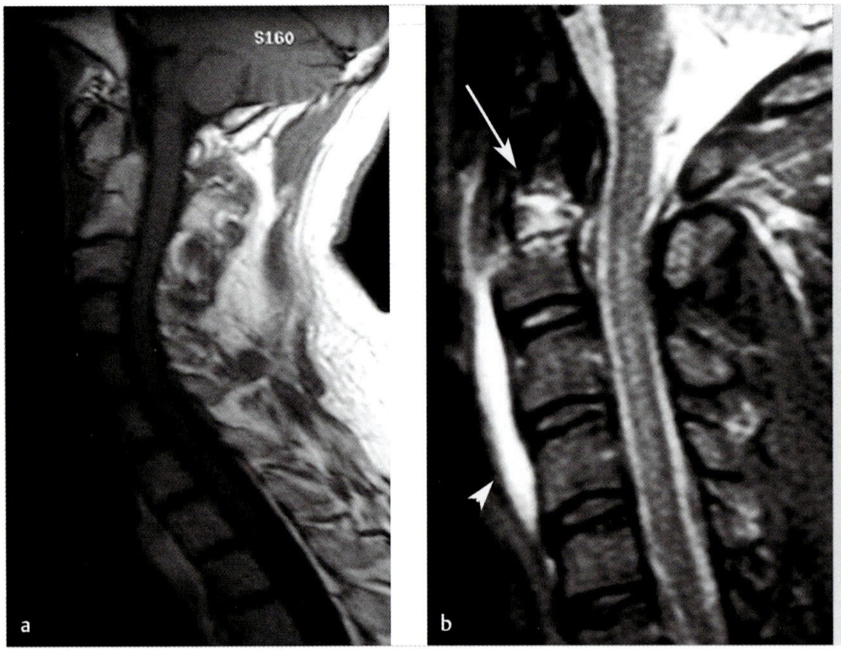

Fig. 14.21 Sagittal **(a)** T1-weighted and **(b)** T2-weighted images of at type-II odontoid fracture (*arrow*). Note the osseous and paravertebral edema or hematoma (*arrowhead*), which indicates an acute or subacute fracture. (Reproduced with permission from, Haines CM, Khanna AJ, Carrino JA, Lin SD, O'Brien JR. The Occipitocervical Junction. In: Khanna AJ, ed. MRI Essentials for the Spine Specialist. 1st Edition. New York: Thieme; 2014.)

Traumatic Spondylolisthesis of the Axis

Levine and Edwards[119] were the first to describe thoroughly the clinical and radiographic findings of traumatic spondylolisthesis of the axis. Treatment is guided by the fracture displacement and angulation, which are typically best viewed on CT images but also evident on MRI.[101,119] MRI is obtained to evaluate for cord or nerve compression.

14.5 Common Clinical Questions

1. All of the following radiographic measurements are useful for detecting cranial settling, except:
   a) Wackenheim clivus line.
   b) Chamberlain line.
   c) Welcher basal angle.
   d) Ranawat criteria.
   e) McGregor line.

2. Which of the following defines cranial settling?
   a) Acquired loss of ligamentous support resulting in upward migration of the odontoid.
   b) Acquired skull softening resulting in upward migration of the odontoid.
   c) Congenital loss of skull height resulting in an elevated odontoid.

3. Which of the following is true of a type-II Chiari malformation?
   a) It most commonly results in death.
   b) It occurs when the hindbrain herniates into an encephalocele.
   c) It is the inferior herniation of the cerebellar vermis, fourth ventricle, and medulla.
   d) It is the downward herniation of the cerebellar tonsils only.
   e) It is associated with basilar invagination.

4. All of the following are true about atlantooccipital dissociation, except:
   a) This injury is associated with high mortality.
   b) Diagnosis is typically delayed.
   c) The Harris technique is useful in diagnosis.
   d) The rule of Spence is useful in diagnosis.
   e) The Powers ratio is useful in diagnosis.
5. From the following list, which is seen earliest on MRI in a rheumatoid spine?
   a) Pannus formation in the subaxial spine.
   b) Pannus formation between C1 and C2.
   c) Cranial settling.
   d) Posterior ligamentous complex laxity.
   e) Occipital condyle erosion.

References

[1] White AA, III, Panjabi MM. The clinical biomechanics of the occipitoatlantoaxial complex. Orthop Clin North Am. 1978; 9(4):867–878
[2] Barnsley L, Lord SM, Wallis BJ, Bogduk N. The prevalence of chronic cervical zygapophysial joint pain after whiplash. Spine. 1995; 20(1):20–25, discussion 26
[3] Benke M, Yu WD, Peden SC, O'Brien JR. Occipitocervical junction: imaging, pathology, instrumentation. Am J Orthop. 2011; 40(10):E205–E215
[4] Kauppi M, Sakaguchi M, Konttinen YT, Hämäläinen M. A new method of screening for vertical atlantoaxial dislocation. J Rheumatol. 1990; 17(2): 167–172
[5] Pellicci PM, Ranawat CS, Tsairis P, Bryan WJ. A prospective study of the progression of rheumatoid arthritis of the cervical spine. J Bone Joint Surg Am. 1981; 63(3):342–350
[6] Redlund-Johnell I, Pettersson H. Radiographic measurements of the craniovertebral region. Designed for evaluation of abnormalities in rheumatoid arthritis. Acta Radiol Diagn (Stockh). 1984; 25(1):23–28
[7] Riew KD, Hilibrand AS, Palumbo MA, Sethi N, Bohlman HH. Diagnosing basilar invagination in the rheumatoid patient. The reliability of radiographic criteria. J Bone Joint Surg Am. 2001; 83(2):194–200
[8] Chamberlain WE. Basilar impression (platybasia). A bizarre developmental anomaly of the occipital bone and upper cervical spine with striking and misleading neurologic manifestations. Yale J Biol Med. 1939; 11 (5):487–496

[9] McGreger M. The significance of certain measurements of the skull in the diagnosis of basilar impression. Br J Radiol. 1948; 21(244):171–181

[10] Wackenheim A. Roentgen diagnosis of the craniovertebral region. New York: Springer-Verlag; 1974

[11] Lopez AJ, Scheer JK, Leibl KE, Smith ZA, Dlouhy BJ, Dahdaleh NS. Anatomy and biomechanics of the craniovertebral junction. Neurosurg Focus. 2015; 38(4):E2

[12] Srivastava SK, Aggarwal RA, Nemade PS, Bhosale SK. Single-stage anterior release and posterior instrumented fusion for irreducible atlantoaxial dislocation with basilar invagination. Spine J. 2016; 16(1):1–9

[13] McRAE DL. Bony abnormalities in the region of the foramen magnum: correlation of the anatomic and neurologic findings. Acta Radiol. 1953; 40 (2–3):335–354

[14] McRae DL, Barnum AS. Occipitalization of the atlas. Am J Roentgenol Radium Ther Nucl Med. 1953; 70(1):23–46

[15] Ranawat CS, O'Leary P, Pellicci P, Tsairis P, Marchisello P, Dorr L. Cervical spine fusion in rheumatoid arthritis. J Bone Joint Surg Am. 1979; 61(7): 1003–1010

[16] Taveras M, Wood EH. Congenital anomalies. In Part I: The skull. In: Diagnostic neuroradiology. Baltimore, MD: Williams & Wilkins; 1976:45–65

[17] Virchow R. Erklarung der Abbildungen. In: Untersuchungen uber die Entwickelung des Schn++delgrundes. Berlin: Druck und Verlag von Georg Reimer; 1857:123–128

[18] Krakenes J, Kaale BR, Rorvik J, Gilhus NE. MRI assessment of normal ligamentous structures in the craniovertebral junction. Neuroradiology. 2001; 43(12):1089–1097

[19] Nidecker AE, Shen PY. Magnetic resonance imaging of the craniovertebral junction ligaments: normal anatomy and traumatic injury. J Neurol Surg B Skull Base. 2016; 77(5):388–395

[20] Tassanawipas A, Mokkhavesa S, Chatchavong S, Worawittayawong P. Magnetic resonance imaging study of the craniocervical junction. J Orthop Surg (Hong Kong). 2005; 13(3):228–231

[21] Lee BCP, Kneeland JB, Deck MDF, Cahill PT. Posterior fossa lesions: magnetic resonance imaging. Radiology. 1984; 153(1):137–143

[22] Smoker WRK. MR imaging of the craniovertebral junction. Magn Reson Imaging Clin N Am. 2000; 8(3):635–650

[23] Krakenes J, Kaale BR. Magnetic resonance imaging assessment of craniovertebral ligaments and membranes after whiplash trauma. Spine. 2006; 31(24):2820–2826

[24] Schmidt P, Mayer TE, Drescher R. Delineation of alar ligament morphology: comparison of magnetic resonance imaging at 1.5 and 3 Tesla. Orthopedics. 2012; 35(11):e1635–e1639

[25] Willauschus WG, Kladny B, Beyer WF, Glückert K, Arnold H, Scheithauer R. Lesions of the alar ligaments. In vivo and in vitro studies with magnetic resonance imaging. Spine. 1995; 20(23):2493–2498

[26] Wilmink JT, Patijn J. MR imaging of alar ligament in whiplash-associated disorders: an observer study. Neuroradiology. 2001; 43(10):859–863

[27] Pfirrmann CW, Binkert CA, Zanetti M, Boos N, Hodler J. MR morphology of alar ligaments and occipitoatlantoaxial joints: study in 50 asymptomatic subjects. Radiology. 2001; 218(1):133–137

[28] Roy S, Hol PK, Laerum LT, Tillung T. Pitfalls of magnetic resonance imaging of alar ligament. Neuroradiology. 2004; 46(5):392–398

[29] Kaale BR, Krakenes J, Albrektsen G, Wester K. Head position and impact direction in whiplash injuries: associations with MRI-verified lesions of ligaments and membranes in the upper cervical spine. J Neurotrauma. 2005; 22(11):1294–1302

[30] Ross JS. Cervicomedullary and craniovertebral junctions. In: Modic MT, Masaryk TJ, Ross JS, eds. Magnetic resonance imaging of the spine. St. Louis, MO: Mosby-Year Book; 1994:191–215

[31] Garber JN. Abnormalities of the atlas and axis vertebrae-congenital and traumatic. J Bone Joint Surg Am. 1964; 46(8):1782–1791

[32] Macalister A. Notes on the development and variations of the atlas. J Anat Physiol. 1893; 27(Pt 4):519–542

[33] VanGilder JC, Menezes AH, Dolan KD. The craniovertebral junction and its abnormalities. Mount Kisco, NY: Futura Publishing; 1987

[34] Nager GT. Cephaloceles. Laryngoscope. 1987; 97(1):77–84

[35] Kunicki J, Ciszek B. The clinical anatomy and the occipital condyle variants. (letter). Clin Anat. 2005; 18(8):646–647, author reply 648

[36] Gholve PA, Hosalkar HS, Ricchetti ET, Pollock AN, Dormans JP, Drummond DS. Occipitalization of the atlas in children. Morphologic classification, associations, and clinical relevance. J Bone Joint Surg Am. 2007; 89(3):571–578

[37] Gopal K, Choudhary AK, Agarwal J, Ali S. Morphological status of assimilated atlas vertebra with occipital bone and its clinical significance. 2017; 3(2): 420–424

[38] Guille JT, Sherk HH. Congenital osseous anomalies of the upper and lower cervical spine in children. J Bone Joint Surg Am. 2002; 84(2):277–288

[39] Sherk HH. Lesions of the atlas and axis. Clin Orthop Relat Res. 1975(109): 33–41

[40] Von Torklus D, Gehl W. The upper cervical spine. Regional anatomy, pathology and traumatology. A systematic radiologic atlas and textbook. New York: Grune & Stratton; 1972

[41] Nishikawa K, Ludwig SC, Colón RJ, Fujimoto Y, Heller JG. Cervical myelopathy and congenital stenosis from hypoplasia of the atlas: report of three cases and literature review. Spine. 2001; 26(5):E80–E86

[42] Chambers AA, Gaskill MF. Midline anterior atlas clefts: CT findings. J Comput Assist Tomogr. 1992; 16(6):868–870

[43] Gehweiler JA, Jr, Daffner RH, Roberts L, Jr. Malformations of the atlas vertebra simulating the Jefferson fracture. AJR Am J Roentgenol. 1983; 140 (6):1083–1086

[44] de Zoete A, Langeveld UA. A congenital anomaly of the atlas as a diagnostic dilemma: a case report. J Manipulative Physiol Ther. 2007; 30(1):62–64

[45] Hosalkar HS, Gerardi JA, Shaw BA. Combined asymptomatic congenital anterior and posterior deficiency of the atlas. Pediatr Radiol. 2001; 31(11): 810–813

[46] Hensinger RN, Fielding JW. The cervical spine. In: Morrissy RT, ed. Lovell and Winter's pediatric orthopaedics. Philadelphia, PA: JB Lippincott; 1990:703–739

[47] Copley LA, Dormans JP. Cervical spine disorders in infants and children. J Am Acad Orthop Surg. 1998; 6(4):204–214

[48] Anderson LD, D'Alonzo RT. Fractures of the odontoid process of the axis. J Bone Joint Surg Am. 1974; 56(8):1663–1674

[49] Cokluk C, Aydin K, Rakunt C, Iyigun O, Onder A. The borders of the odontoid process of C2 in adults and in children including the estimation of odontoid/ body ratio. Eur Spine J. 2006; 15(3):278–282

[50] David KM, McLachlan JC, Aiton JF, et al. Cartilaginous development of the human craniovertebral junction as visualised by a new three-dimensional computer reconstruction technique. J Anat. 1998; 192(Pt 2):269–277

[51] Arvin B, Fournier-Gosselin MP, Fehlings MG. Os odontoideum: etiology and surgical management. Neurosurgery. 2010; 66(3) Suppl:22–31

[52] Batzdorf U. Pathogenesis and development theories. In: Anson JA, Benzel EC, Awad IA, eds. Syringomyelia and the chiari malformations. Park Ridge, IL: American Association of Neurological Surgeons; 1997:35–40

[53] Schenk M, Ruggieri PM. Imaging of syringomyelia and the Chiari malformations. In: Anson JA, Benzel EC, Awad IA, eds. Syringomyelia and the Chiari malformations. Park Ridge, IL: American Association of Neurological Surgeons; 1997:41–56

[54] Aboulezz AO, Sartor K, Geyer CA, Gado MH. Position of cerebellar tonsils in the normal population and in patients with Chiari malformation: a quantitative approach with MR imaging. J Comput Assist Tomogr. 1985; 9 (6):1033–1036

[55] Barkovich AJ, Wippold FJ, Sherman JL, Citrin CM. Significance of cerebellar tonsillar position on MR. AJNR Am J Neuroradiol. 1986; 7(5):795–799

[56] Milhorat TH, Chou MW, Trinidad EM, et al. Chiari I malformation redefined: clinical and radiographic findings for 364 symptomatic patients. Neurosurgery. 1999; 44(5):1005–1017

[57] Castillo M, Quencer RM, Dominguez R. Chiari III malformation: imaging features. AJNR Am J Neuroradiol. 1992; 13(1):107–113

[58] Pang D, Pollack IF. Spinal cord injury without radiographic abnormality in children: the SCIWORA syndrome. J Trauma. 1989; 29(5):654–664

[59] Ulmer JL, Elster AD, Ginsberg LE, Williams DW, III. Klippel-Feil syndrome: CT and MR of acquired and congenital abnormalities of cervical spine and cord. J Comput Assist Tomogr. 1993; 17(2):215–224

[60] Nagib MG, Maxwell RE, Chou SN. Identification and management of high-risk patients with Klippel-Feil syndrome. J Neurosurg. 1984; 61(3):523–530

[61] Boden SD. Rheumatoid arthritis of the cervical spine. Surgical decision making based on predictors of paralysis and recovery. Spine. 1994; 19(20): 2275–2280

[62] Boden SD, Dodge LD, Bohlman HH, Rechtine GR. Rheumatoid arthritis of the cervical spine. A long-term analysis with predictors of paralysis and recovery. J Bone Joint Surg Am. 1993; 75(9):1282–1297

[63] Dreyer SJ, Boden SD. Natural history of rheumatoid arthritis of the cervical spine. Clin Orthop Relat Res. 1999(366):98–106

[64] Reiter MF, Boden SD. Inflammatory disorders of the cervical spine. Spine. 1998; 23(24):2755–2766

[65] Oda T, Fujiwara K, Yonenobu K, Azuma B, Ochi T. Natural course of cervical spine lesions in rheumatoid arthritis. Spine. 1995; 20(10):1128–1135
[66] Goel A. Treatment of basilar invagination by atlantoaxial joint distraction and direct lateral mass fixation. J Neurosurg Spine. 2004; 1(3):281–286
[67] Ross JS, Brant-Zawadzki M, Moore KR, Crim J, Chen MZ, Katzman GL. Part IV: Neoplasms, cysts, and other masses. In: Ross JS, Brant-Zawadzki M, Moore KR, et al, eds. Diagnostic imaging: spine. Salt Lake City: Amirsys; 2004:IV-1-2-IV-2-32
[68] Baudrez V, Galant C, Vande Berg BC. Benign vertebral hemangioma: MR-histological correlation. Skeletal Radiol. 2001; 30(8):442–446
[69] Yochum TR, Lile RL, Schultz GD, Mick TJ, Brown CW. Acquired spinal stenosis secondary to an expanding thoracic vertebral hemangioma. Spine. 1993; 18 (2):299–305
[70] Murphey MD, Nomikos GC, Flemming DJ, Gannon FH, Temple HT, Kransdorf MJ. From the archives of AFIP. Imaging of giant cell tumor and giant cell reparative granuloma of bone: radiologic-pathologic correlation. Radiographics. 2001; 21(5):1283–1309
[71] Osborn AG. Cysts, tumors, and tumorlike lesions of the spine and spinal cord. In: Osborn AG, ed. Diagnostic neuroradiology. St. Louis, MO: Mosby; 1994:876–918
[72] Liu PT, Chivers FS, Roberts CC, Schultz CJ, Beauchamp CP. Imaging of osteoid osteoma with dynamic gadolinium-enhanced MR imaging. Radiology. 2003; 227(3):691–700
[73] Boriani S, De Iure F, Campanacci L, et al. Aneurysmal bone cyst of the mobile spine: report on 41 cases. Spine. 2001; 26(1):27–35
[74] Munk PL, Helms CA, Holt RG, Johnston J, Steinbach L, Neumann C. MR imaging of aneurysmal bone cysts. AJR Am J Roentgenol. 1989; 153(1):99–101
[75] Fourney DR, York JE, Cohen ZR, Suki D, Rhines LD, Gokaslan ZL. Management of atlantoaxial metastases with posterior occipitocervical stabilization. J Neurosurg. 2003; 98(2) Suppl:165–170
[76] Akhaddar A, Chakir N, Amarti A, et al. Thoracic epidural hemangiopericytoma. Case report. J Neurosurg Sci. 2002; 46(2):89–92, discussion 92
[77] Cohen-Gadol AA, Zikel OM, Koch CA, Scheithauer BW, Krauss WE. Spinal meningiomas in patients younger than 50 years of age: a 21-year experience. J Neurosurg. 2003; 98(3) Suppl:258–263
[78] Naderi S. Spinal meningiomas. Surg Neurol. 2000; 54(1):95
[79] Conti P, Pansini G, Mouchaty H, Capuano C, Conti R. Spinal neurinomas: retrospective analysis and long-term outcome of 179 consecutively operated cases and review of the literature. Surg Neurol. 2004; 61(1):34–43, discussion 44
[80] Lowe GM. Magnetic resonance imaging of intramedullary spinal cord tumors. J Neurooncol. 2000; 47(3):195–210
[81] Sun B, Wang C, Wang J, Liu A. MRI features of intramedullary spinal cord ependymomas. J Neuroimaging. 2003; 13(4):346–351
[82] Murota T, Symon L. Surgical management of hemangioblastoma of the spinal cord: a report of 18 cases. Neurosurgery. 1989; 25(5):699–707, discussion 708
[83] Sciubba DM, Mavinkurve GG, Gailloud P, et al. Preoperative imaging of cervical spine hemangioblastomas using three-dimensional fusion digital subtraction angiography. Report of two cases. J Neurosurg Spine. 2006; 5(1): 96–100
[84] Rykken JB, Diehn FE, Hunt CH, et al. Intramedullary spinal cord metastases: MRI and relevant clinical features from a 13-year institutional case series. AJNR Am J Neuroradiol. 2013; 34(10):2043–2049
[85] Brooke DC, Burkus JK, Benson DR. Asymptomatic occipito-atlantal instability in Down syndrome (trisomy 21). Report of two cases in children. J Bone Joint Surg Am. 1987; 69(2):293–295
[86] El-Khoury GY, Clark CR, Dietz FR, Harre RG, Tozzi JE, Kathol MH. Posterior atlantooccipital subluxation in Down syndrome. Radiology. 1986; 159(2): 507–509
[87] French HG, Burke SW, Roberts JM, Johnston CE, II, Whitecloud T, Edmunds JO. Upper cervical ossicles in Down syndrome. J Pediatr Orthop. 1987; 7(1): 69–71
[88] Gabriel KR, Mason DE, Carango P. Occipito-atlantal translation in Down's syndrome. Spine. 1990; 15(10):997–1002
[89] Georgopoulos G, Pizzutillo PD, Lee MS. Occipito-atlantal instability in children. A report of five cases and review of the literature. J Bone Joint Surg Am. 1987; 69(3):429–436
[90] Harris JH, Jr, Carson GC, Wagner LK. Radiologic diagnosis of traumatic occipitovertebral dissociation: 1. Normal occipitovertebral relationships on lateral radiographs of supine subjects. AJR Am J Roentgenol. 1994; 162(4): 881–886
[91] Hungerford GD, Akkaraju V, Rawe SE, Young GF. Atlanto-occipital and atlanto-axial dislocations with spinal cord compression in Down's syndrome: a case report and review of the literature. Br J Radiol. 1981; 54 (645):758–761
[92] Karol LA, Sheffield EG, Crawford K, Moody MK, Browne RH. Reproducibility in the measurement of atlanto-occipital instability in children with Down syndrome. Spine. 1996; 21(21):2463–2467, discussion 2468
[93] Bernini FP, Elefante R, Smaltino F, Tedeschi G. Angiographic study on the vertebral artery in cases of deformities of the occipitocervical joint. Am J Roentgenol Radium Ther Nucl Med. 1969; 107(3):526–529
[94] Goldberg W, Mueller C, Panacek E, Tigges S, Hoffman JR, Mower WR, NEXUS Group. Distribution and patterns of blunt traumatic cervical spine injury. Ann Emerg Med. 2001; 38(1):17–21
[95] Wiesel SW, Rothman RH. Occipitoatlantal hypermobility. Spine. 1979; 4(3): 187–191
[96] Romano A, Albertini G, Guida D, et al. A cervical flexion-extension MRI study in Down syndrome. Indian J Pediatr. 2015; 82(4):349–353
[97] Browd S, Healy LJ, Dobie G, et al. Morphometric and qualitative analysis of congenital occipitocervical instability in children: implications for patients with Down syndrome. J Neurosurg. 2006; 105(1) Suppl:50–54
[98] Adams VI. Neck injuries: I. Occipitoatlantal dislocation: a pathologic study of twelve traffic fatalities. J Forensic Sci. 1992; 37(2):556–564
[99] Adams VI. Neck injuries: III. Ligamentous injuries of the craniocervical articulation without occipito-atlantal or atlanto-axial facet dislocation. A pathologic study of 21 traffic fatalities. J Forensic Sci. 1993; 38(5):1097–1104
[100] Ahuja A, Glasauer FE, Alker GJ, Jr, Klein DM. Radiology in survivors of traumatic atlanto-occipital dislocation. Surg Neurol. 1994; 41(2):112–118
[101] Bono CM, Vaccaro AR, Fehlings M, et al. Spine Trauma Study Group. Measurement techniques for upper cervical spine injuries: consensus statement of the Spine Trauma Study Group. Spine. 2007; 32(5):593–600
[102] Alker GJ, Jr, Oh YS, Leslie EV. High cervical spine and craniocervical junction injuries in fatal traffic accidents: a radiological study. Orthop Clin North Am. 1978; 9(4):1003–1010
[103] Bellabarba C, Mirza SK, West GA, et al. Diagnosis and treatment of craniocervical dislocation in a series of 17 consecutive survivors during an 8-year period. J Neurosurg Spine. 2006; 4(6):429–440
[104] Saternus KS, Thrun C. [Traumatology of the alar ligaments]. Aktuelle Traumatol. 1987; 17(5):214–218
[105] Chaput CD, Walgama J, Torres E, et al. Defining and detecting missed ligamentous injuries of the occipitocervical complex. Spine. 2011; 36(9): 709–714
[106] Radcliff K, Kepler C, Reitman C, Harrop J, Vaccaro A. CT and MRI-based diagnosis of craniocervical dislocations: the role of the occipitoatlantal ligament. Clin Orthop Relat Res. 2012; 470(6):1602–1613
[107] Roy AK, Miller BA, Holland CM, Fountain AJ, Jr, Pradilla G, Ahmad FU. Magnetic resonance imaging of traumatic injury to the craniovertebral junction: a case-based review. Neurosurg Focus. 2015; 38(4):E3
[108] Hall GC, Kinsman MJ, Nazar RG, et al. Atlanto-occipital dislocation. World J Orthop. 2015; 6(2):236–243
[109] Pissonnier ML, Lazennec JY, Renoux J, Rousseau MA. Trauma of the upper cervical spine: focus on vertical atlantoaxial dislocation. Eur Spine J. 2013; 22(10):2167–2175
[110] Powers B, Miller MD, Kramer RS, Martinez S, Gehweiler JA, Jr. Traumatic anterior atlanto-occipital dislocation. Neurosurgery. 1979; 4(1):12–17
[111] Anderson PA, Montesano PX. Morphology and treatment of occipital condyle fractures. Spine. 1988; 13(7):731–736
[112] Hanson JA, Deliganis AV, Baxter AB, et al. Radiologic and clinical spectrum of occipital condyle fractures: retrospective review of 107 consecutive fractures in 95 patients. AJR Am J Roentgenol. 2002; 178(5):1261–1268
[113] Young WF, Rosenwasser RH, Getch C, Jallo J. Diagnosis and management of occipital condyle fractures. Neurosurgery. 1994; 34(2):257–260, discussion 260–261
[114] Jefferson G. Fracture of the atlas vertebra. Br J Surg. 1920; 7:407–422
[115] Lee C, Woodring JH. Unstable Jefferson variant atlas fractures: an unrecognized cervical injury. AJNR Am J Neuroradiol. 1991; 12(6):1105–1110
[116] Lee TT, Green BA, Petrin DR. Treatment of stable burst fracture of the atlas (Jefferson fracture) with rigid cervical collar. Spine. 1998; 23(18):1963–1967
[117] Horlyck E, Rahbek M. Cervical spine injuries. Acta Orthop Scand. 1974; 45 (6):845–853
[118] Ryan MD, Henderson JJ. The epidemiology of fractures and fracture-dislocations of the cervical spine. Injury. 1992; 23(1):38–40
[119] Levine AM, Edwards CC. The management of traumatic spondylolisthesis of the axis. J Bone Joint Surg Am. 1985; 67(2):217–226

Answers to Common Clinical Questions

1. Answer: c. The Wackenheim clivus line, Chamberlain line, Ranawat criteria, and McGregor line can all be used to evaluate for cranial settling (▶ Fig. 14.1). The Welcher basal angle is useful for detecting platybasia.
2. Answer: a. Cranial settling differs from basilar invagination and basilar impression. Cranial settling is vertical subluxation of the odontoid caused by a loss of supporting ligamentous structures. This condition can occur with RA or psoriatic arthritis. Basilar impression results from skull-base softening secondary to an acquired condition such as Paget disease. Basilar invagination results from a loss of skull height secondary to congenital abnormalities.
3. Answer: c. A type-II Chiari malformation results from dysgenesis of the hindbrain. It involves herniation of the inferior cerebellar vermis, fourth ventricle, and medulla and is associated with myelomeningocele. It is not associated with atlantooccipital assimilation or basilar invagination.
4. Answer: d. The rule of Spence is used to evaluate integrity of the transverse ligament, typically with Jefferson burst fractures. Atlantooccipital dissociation is associated with high mortality, and diagnosis is typically delayed. The Harris technique and the Powers ratio can be used to diagnose atlantooccipital dissociation.
5. Answer: b. Pannus formation between C1 and C2 is an early finding of RA that can be seen on MRI of the cervical spine. The other findings tend to occur in patients with more advanced RA.

15 The Cervical Spine

Lukas P. Zebala, Jacob M. Buchowski, Aditya R. Daftary, Joseph R. O'Brien, John A. Carrino, and A. Jay Khanna

Abstract
The typical magnetic resonance imaging (MRI) protocol for evaluating degenerative cervical spine abnormalities includes T2-weighted and T1-weighted images in sagittal and axial planes. However, imaging protocols vary among institutions and should be modified when specific diagnoses such as trauma, infection, or tumor are being considered.

The initial evaluation of patients with known or suspected cervical spine injury begins with conventional radiographs and/or computed tomographic (CT) imaging, which provide greater osseous detail and may show fractures or details that are not detected with conventional radiography. MRI provides soft tissue visualization that is superior to that of conventional radiography and CT and is useful for assessing spinal cord injury, ligamentous injury, degree of spinal stenosis, and fractures. MRI is also useful for evaluating obtunded patients and those with cervical spine injury, neurologic deficits, or unreliable physical examinations.

MRI is the preferred initial advanced imaging modality for evaluating symptomatic cervical spine degeneration and is highly sensitive and specific for detecting cervical degenerative changes. However, radiographic and MRI abnormalities do not always correlate with symptomatic degenerative lesions and, thus, it is important to correlate MRI findings with the patient's history and physical examination. Degenerative conditions that can be evaluated on cervical spine MRI include disk displacement, disk degeneration, and spinal stenosis.

Although the most common indication for MRI of the cervical spine is the evaluation of degenerative conditions, MRI is also frequently used to evaluate patients with Chiari malformations, infectious conditions, spinal tumors, inflammatory processes involving the spinal cord, and various arthritides.

Keywords: cervical spine, infection, magnetic resonance imaging, trauma, tumor

15.1 Specialized Pulse Sequences and Imaging Protocols

As with the lumbar spine and other regions in the musculoskeletal system, imaging protocols of the cervical spine for specific indications can vary among institutions. However, the standard magnetic resonance imaging (MRI) of the cervical spine for degenerative abnormalities usually includes the following pulse sequences:

- Sagittal T1-weighted spin-echo (SE).
- Sagittal T2-weighted fast spin-echo (FSE).
- Axial gradient-echo.
- Axial T2-weighted FSE.

A detailed discussion of all the imaging sequences used in the cervical spine is beyond the scope of this chapter; however, salient features of commonly used sequences are discussed.

T1-weighted images are useful in identifying fracture lines. Because they are sensitive to the presence of gadolinium contrast, T1-weighted images are also used for contrast-enhanced imaging, which is helpful in assessing neoplasms, infections, and the postoperative spine. Typically, fat-suppressed postgadolinium T1-weighted images are used to make lesions more conspicuous. T2-weighted images are sensitive to water (and thus edema) and are useful in identifying areas of potential abnormality. However, care must be taken when interpreting bone marrow edema because it may be seen in various conditions, including infection, inflammation, trauma, and degeneration. Although edema may focus attention toward an abnormality, many of these conditions can coexist, so additional analysis is required before making conclusions. FSE is now routinely used to acquire T2-weighted images at speeds up to 64 times faster than conventional SE T2-weighted images. Sometimes, the differentiation of fat, water, and lesions can be difficult, especially on T2-weighted FSE images, and therefore fat suppression is used to make these areas more conspicuous. This sequence can be obtained by applying a fat-suppression pulse to produce fat-suppressed T2-weighted images or by obtaining a short tau inversion recovery (STIR) sequence. Visualizing edema is helpful in identifying ligamentous injuries, and such visualization is best achieved with STIR or fat-suppressed T2-weighted images.[1] T2-weighted images are also most sensitive for evaluating the cord parenchyma for lesions and edema, which are seen as abnormally bright signal, although the sagittal orientation is subject to linear bright artifact within the cord (Gibbs phenomenon). For this reason, axial T2-weighted images are useful for detecting cord abnormalities and confirming lesions suspected on sagittal T2-weighted images.

Gradient-echo images are very susceptible to magnetic artifacts; this important characteristic makes them useful for detecting small areas of hemorrhage such as with cervical spine trauma and vascular malformations. However, these images can also overestimate the degree of canal and foraminal stenosis secondary to artifact from the adjacent bone. Because of the rapidity with which gradient-echo images are acquired, studies can be obtained with higher resolution than that required for other pulse sequences and even as a 3D volume set, which provides isotropic voxels and enables reformations in multiple planes. This volume set can then allow characterization of the cervical foramina in the appropriate oblique plane.

For the evaluation of vascular structures in the neck, MR angiography can be obtained without contrast, using 2D or 3D time-of-flight or phase-contrast imaging. These sequences create contrast between flowing and stationary structures. Phase-contrast imaging may also provide flow-velocity information. Time-of-flight imaging shows fat or subacute thrombus as bright signal and may be useful in detecting small, subtle thrombi. The 3D techniques require more time and are slightly less sensitive to slow flow states than are 2D techniques. Gadolinium-enhanced MR angiography may also be obtained and is extremely accurate.

15.2 Traumatic Conditions

Although the cervical spine is injured in only 2 to 3% of blunt-trauma accidents,[2] the potential for instability and critical neurologic injury makes prompt identification and treatment of cervical spine injuries important. Patients with suspected cervical spine injury should be evaluated initially with conventional radiographs (anteroposterior [AP], lateral, and open-mouth odontoid views). Computed tomographic (CT) imaging offers greater osseous detail than does conventional radiography and may show fractures or details that are not detected with radiography. CT is especially helpful in assessing fractures of the occipital condyles and cervicothoracic junction, where osseous overlap on conventional radiographs makes fracture detection difficult. MRI provides soft tissue visualization superior to that of conventional radiography or CT and is useful for the assessment of spinal cord injury, ligamentous injury, degree of spinal stenosis, and additional fracture evaluation. Occult fractures not visible on conventional radiographs or CT images may be detected by the presence of vertebral body edema on MR images. Although MRI is extremely sensitive in identifying cervical spine fractures, the characteristics of these fractures and the exact appearance of the osseous components can be challenging; CT may be a better choice for assessing such details. In addition, MRI is useful for the evaluation of obtunded patients or those with cervical spine injury, neurologic deficits, or an unreliable physical examination.[3,4,5,6,7]

MRI is indicated when neurologic deficit, vascular injury, or soft tissue injury is suspected in the setting of trauma. It is also useful in assessing posttraumatic sequelae.[8] Use of MRI to evaluate spinal gunshot injuries is controversial. Theoretically, a ferrous gunshot fragment may become mobile but most bullets are nonferrous; therefore, such patients can usually be imaged safely. Unfortunately, the material composition of a gunshot fragment is seldom known. Therefore, MRI remains controversial and dependent on clinical need.[9,10]

There are obstacles to obtaining MRI studies in the trauma setting, especially with regard to cervical spine trauma, because patients may have clinically significant neurologic deficits. These obstacles include the following:

- Lack of availability of MRI capabilities on an urgent basis.
- MR incompatibility of some ventilators, traction devices, and other equipment.
- Lack of clinical access to patients during the imaging study.

MRI protocols vary by institution, but commonly used sequences in trauma evaluation include the following[11]:

- Sagittal T1-weighted images to assess the alignment of the cervical spine, vertebral body integrity, fractures, and spinal cord caliber.
- Sagittal T2-weighted images to assess for the presence of cord edema, compression, and spondylotic changes.
- Sagittal STIR images to assess for the presence of paraspinal ligamentous injury and bone marrow edema.
- Axial T1-weighted and T2-weighted images to assess for the presence of posterior element fractures, to evaluate for spinal stenosis, to define disk abnormality, and to confirm the precise location of abnormalities detected on sagittal images.
- Sagittal T2-weighted gradient-echo images (at some institutions) to assess for the presence of acute spinal cord hemorrhage and disk herniation (high signal in the disk even with severe osseous degeneration, which enables differentiation between bone fragments and disk herniation).

Table 15.1 Evaluation of cervical spine trauma

Anatomy	Evaluation
Spinal column/ vertebral bodies	Alignment
	Vertebral body fracture
	Posterior element fracture
	Edema
	Degenerative change
Ligaments	Anterior longitudinal ligament
	Posterior longitudinal ligament
	Interspinous and supraspinous ligaments
	Ligamentum flavum
	Edema/rupture
Spinal cord	Edema
	Hemorrhage
	Compression
	Syrinx
Epidural space	Hematoma
	Disk herniation
	Osseous fragment
Vascular	Vertebral artery

Source: Reproduced with permission from, Takhtani D, Melhelm ER. MR imaging in cervical spine trauma. Magn Reson Imaging Clin N Am. 2000;8:615–634. Modified with permission.

Regardless of the institutional MRI protocol, a systematic approach (see Chapter 3, A Systematic Approach to the Review of Spine MRI Studies) for the evaluation of cervical spine MRI should be used to avoid missing pathologic conditions (▶ Table 15.1). In addition, it is essential that the MRI findings be interpreted in conjunction with other imaging modalities, including conventional radiographs with flexion and extension views if clinically indicated and CT (see Chapter 4, Correlation of MRI with Other Imaging Modalities).

15.2.1 Classification of Cervical Spine Trauma

Cervical spine injuries can be classified according to the mechanism of injury. Although the Allen-Ferguson classification system originally described six categories of fracture based on the suspected position of the spine at the time of injury and the dominant mechanism of spinal failure (i.e., vertical compression, compressive flexion, distractive flexion, lateral flexion, compressive extension, and distractive extension) (▶ Fig. 15.1),[12] the classification scheme is simplified here into three broad categories:

- Hyperflexion.
- Hyperextension.
- Axial loading.

In many instances, the mechanism of injury can be difficult to determine from an analysis of the clinical situation (in the absence

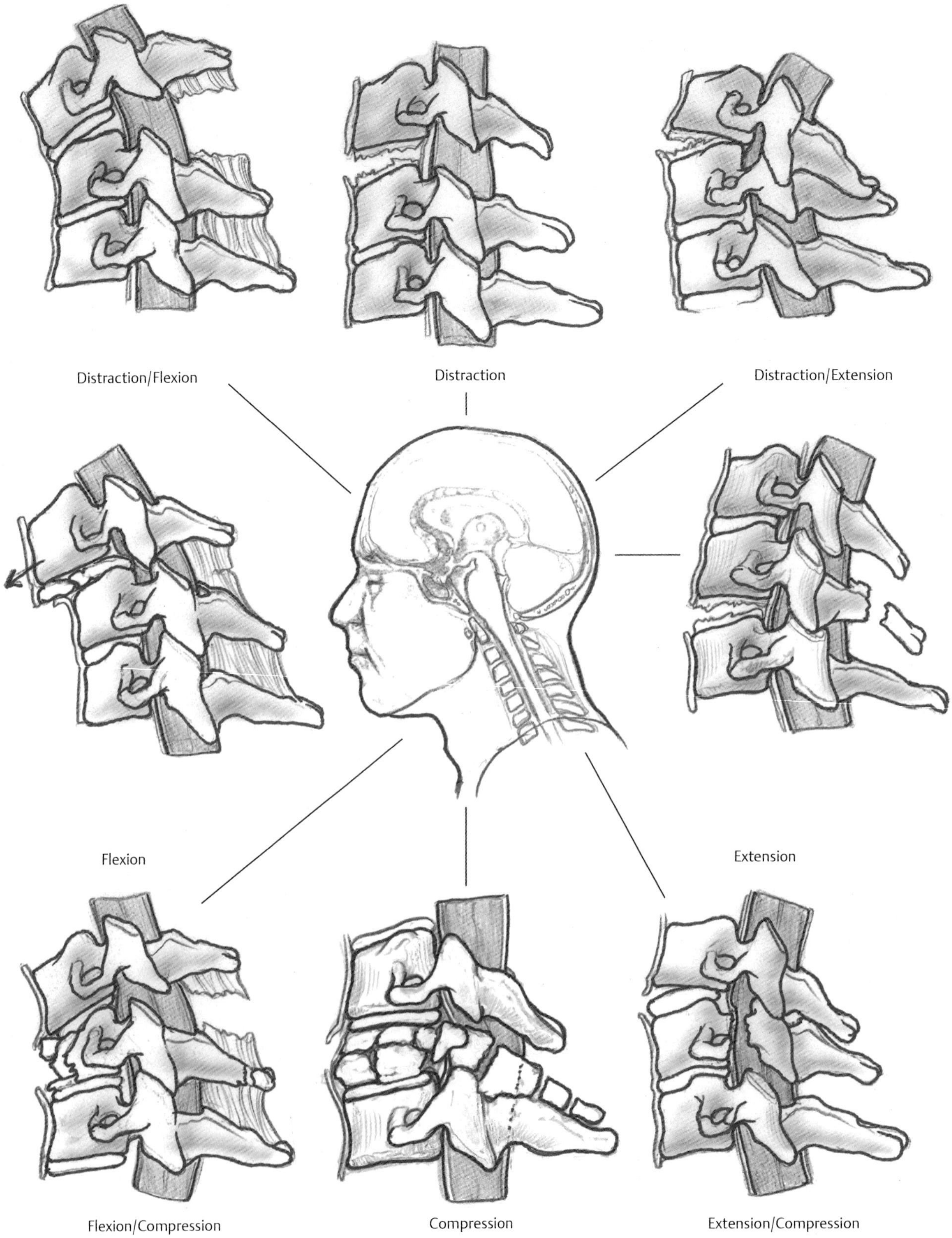

Fig. 15.1 An illustration of the Allen-Ferguson mechanistic classification system for subaxial cervical spine fractures. (Reproduced with permission from Chapman JR, Anderson PA. Cervical spine trauma. In: Frymoyer J, Ducker TB, Hadler NM et al, eds. The adult spine: principles and practice. 2nd ed. Philadelphia, PA: Lippincott-Raven; 1997:1245–1295.)

of imaging findings). Therefore, clinicians may choose to classify cervical spine injuries broadly, as follows:

- Secondary to blunt trauma.
- Secondary to penetrating trauma.

Table 15.2 Subaxial cervical spine injury classification system scale

Injury characteristic	Points
Morphology	
No abnormality	0
Compression	1
Burst	+ 1
Distraction (e.g., facet perch, hyperextension)	3
Rotation/translation (e.g., facet dislocation, unstable teardrop, or advanced-stage flexion-compression injury)	4
Neurologic status	
Intact	0
Root injury	1
Complete cord injury	2
Incomplete cord injury	3
Continuous cord compression in setting of neuro deficit (neuro modifier)	+ 1
Discoligamentous complex integrity	
Intact	0
Indeterminate (e.g., isolated interspinous widening, MRI signal change only)	1
Disrupted (e.g., widening of disk space, facet perch, or dislocation)	2

Source: Reproduced with permission from, Vaccaro AR, Hulbert RJ, Patel AA, et al; Spine Trauma Study Group. The subaxial cervical spine injury classification system. A novel approach to recognize the importance of morphology, neurology, and integrity of the disco-ligamentous complex. Spine (Phila Pa 1976). 2007;32:2365–2374. Modified with permission.

In addition, cervical spine injuries can be classified according to the region of injury within the occipitocervical spine:

- Occipitocervical junction (OCJ).
- Suboccipital cervical spine (C1–C2).
- Subaxial cervical spine (C3–C7).[13]

More recently, the Subaxial Cervical Spine Injury Classification (SLIC) system has been developed to evaluate injuries according to fracture morphology, neurologic injury, and the integrity of the discoligamentous complex (▶ Table 15.2).[14,15,16] A systematic evaluation of these three components can be used to guide the treatment of patients with cervical spine fractures.

Hyperflexion Injuries

Flexion-compression injuries range from minor anterior compression of the anterosuperior end plate (▶ Fig. 15.2) to a severe teardrop or quadrangular fracture. These injuries are associated with retrolisthesis, kyphosis, and circumferential soft-tissue disruption. The radiographic evaluation of flexion-compression injuries includes examination for the following:

- Anterior and middle column compromise.
- Loss of vertebral body height.
- Translation.
- Angulation.
- Posterior element competence.

Whereas conventional radiographs and CT scans can help evaluate fracture pattern, alignment, angulation, and translation, MRI can assist with the determination of treatment options for such patients because it facilitates the assessment of spinal cord compression and posterior element compromise.

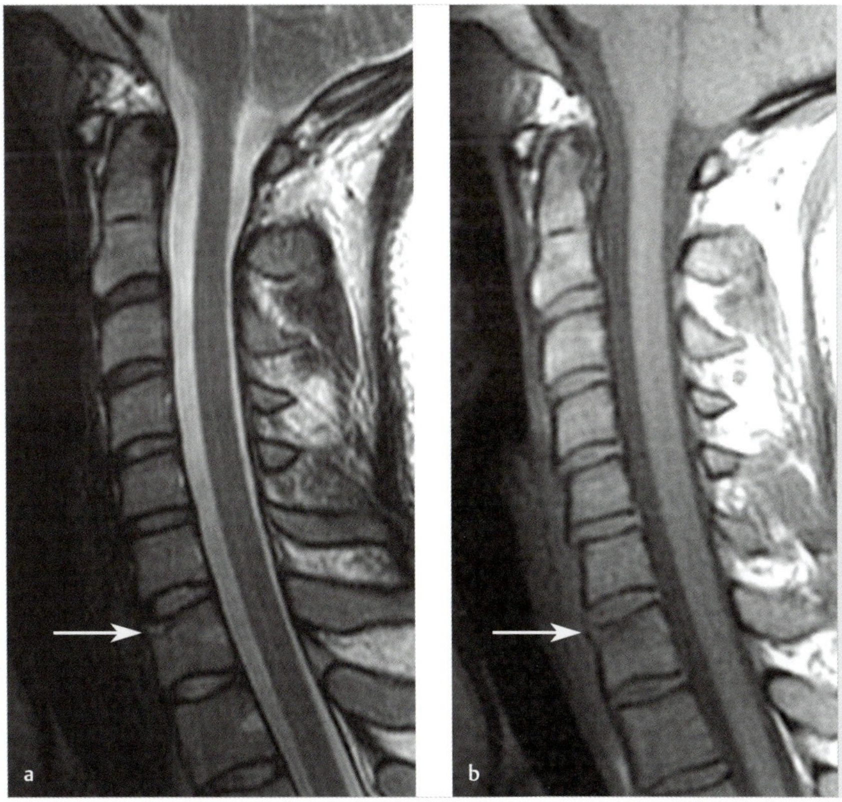

Fig. 15.2 C7 vertebral compression fracture. Sagittal **(a)** T2-weighted and **(b)** T1-weighted images show the fracture (*arrow on* each) with minimal loss of height. (Reproduced with permission from, Zebala LP, Buchowski JM, Daftary AR, et al. The cervical spine. In: Khanna AJ, ed. MRI Essentials for the Spine Specialist. New York: Thieme; 2014:111–154.)

Flexion-distraction forces can lead to facet subluxations, dislocations, or fracture-dislocations. These injuries represent a spectrum of osteoligamentous abnormality, ranging from the purely ligamentous dislocation to fractures of the facet and lateral mass. MRI helps assess the compromise of posterior musculature, interspinous ligaments, ligamentum flavum, and facet capsules that is often seen with flexion-distraction injuries.[17] The role of MRI in the treatment for patients who present with bilateral cervical facet dislocations (▶ Fig. 15.3) without neurologic compromise is the subject of substantial debate among researchers and spine surgeons.[17,18,19] Treatment options include MRI before attempting closed reduction or surgery; closed reduction with traction while monitoring the patient's neurologic examination; and surgery via anterior, posterior, or combined approaches.[17,18,19] One of the purposes of obtaining an MRI study before the reduction of bilateral facet dislocations is to rule out the possibility of an extruded disk fragment, which may displace into the spinal canal during closed reduction (▶ Fig. 15.4).

Most flexion injuries are well visualized on MRI, and MRI is particularly effective for the assessment of the following[11]:

- Alignment.
- Fractures.
- Ligamentous injury.
- Cord abnormalities.
- Acute disk herniations.
- The cause of anterior subluxation, chronic degenerative changes, or hyperflexion sprain.

Facet joint injuries may be seen on parasagittal or axial images, which show increased signal on T2-weighted images secondary to edema from facet capsule tears.[11,20,21,22] Injury to posterior ligaments may be seen as areas of hyperintensity on T2-weighted images, especially fat-suppressed T2-weighted or STIR images (▶ Fig. 15.5).

Hyperextension Injuries

Cervical spine extension injury is associated with the posterior translation or rotation of a vertebral body in the sagittal

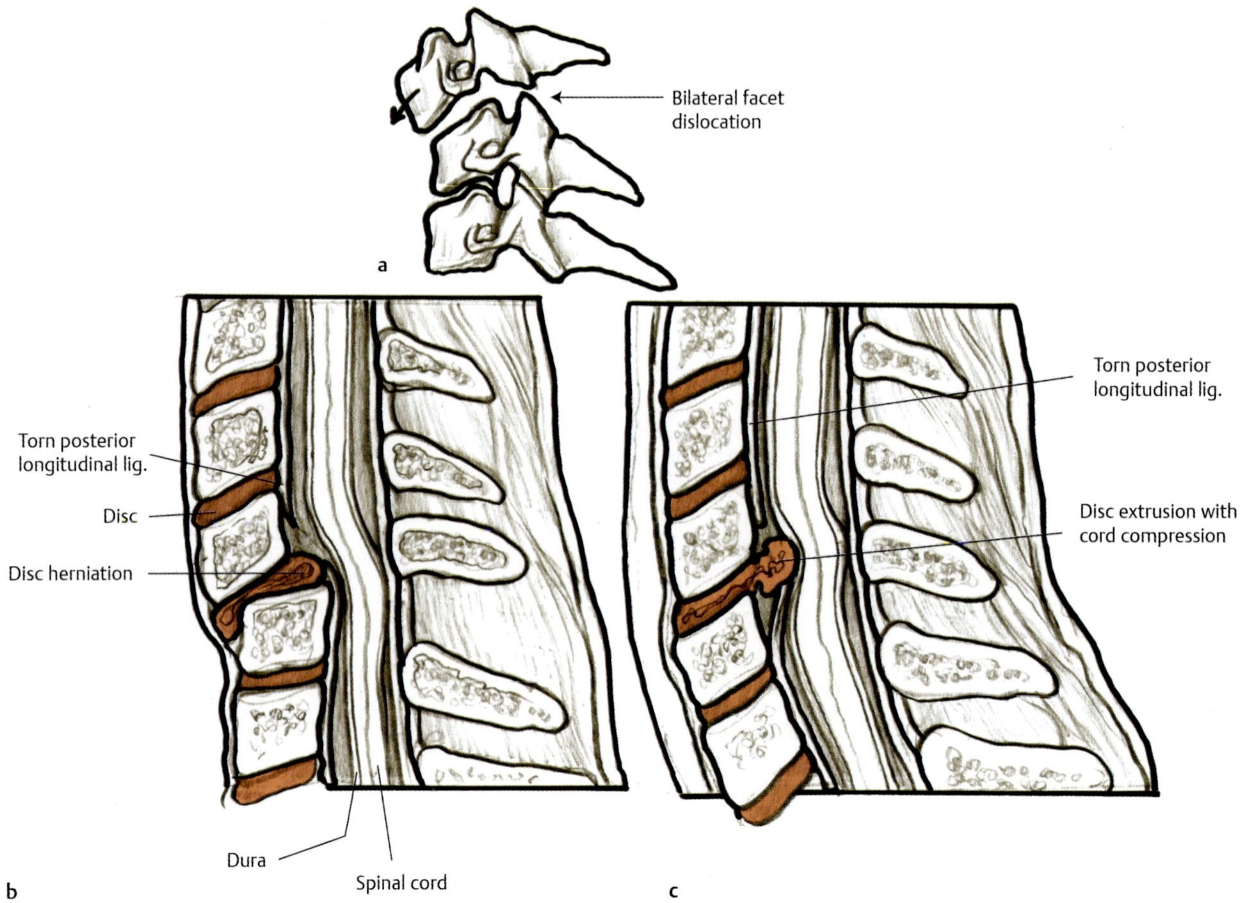

Fig. 15.3 Illustration of the abnormality in bilateral facet dislocation. **(a)** A lateral view of osseous structures shows that the facets are perched, and that additional translation will lead to complete dislocation. **(b)** A lateral view before reduction shows ~50% translation of the superior vertebral body relative to the inferior one and displacement of the intervertebral disk. **(c)** A lateral view after reduction shows that the intervertebral disk has displaced into the spinal canal and compressed the spinal cord during the reduction maneuver. (Reproduced with permission from, Zebala LP, Buchowski JM, Daftary AR, et al. The cervical spine. In: Khanna AJ, ed. MRI Essentials for the Spine Specialist. New York: Thieme; 2014:111–154.)

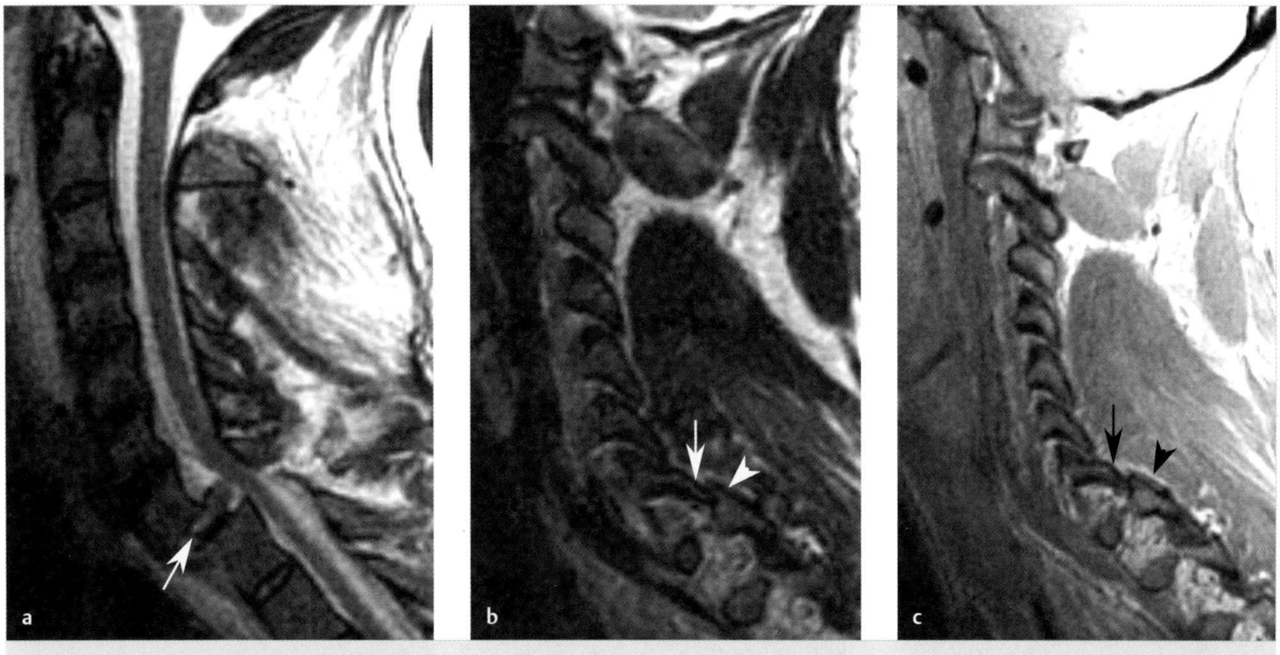

Fig. 15.4 Bilateral cervical facet dislocation. **(a)** A sagittal T2-weighted image shows anterior translation of C7 over T1 with an associated disk extrusion (*arrow*) and cord compression. **(b)** Parasagittal T2-weighted and **(c)** gradient-echo images show the inferior articular process of C7 (*arrow* on each) displaced anterior to the superior articular process of T1 (*arrowhead* on each). (Reproduced with permission from, Zebala LP, Buchowski JM, Daftary AR, et al. The cervical spine. In: Khanna AJ, ed. MRI Essentials for the Spine Specialist. New York: Thieme; 2014:111–154.)

plane.[5,11,23] Hyperextension injuries often are produced by rear-impact motor vehicle collisions or direct facial trauma.

In cervical spine hyperextension injuries, potential findings include the following[5,11,20,22,23]:

- Tear(s) of the anterior longitudinal ligament.
- Avulsion of the intervertebral disk from an adjacent vertebral body.
- Horizontal intervertebral disk rupture (▶ Fig. 15.6).

More severe and potentially unstable hyperextension injuries may be associated with the following[5]:

- Prevertebral hematoma.
- Widening of the disk space.
- Posterior ligament complex edema.
- Herniated disk.

Elderly patients with spondylosis and kyphosis of the cervical spine may experience spinal cord injury without fracture or ligamentous injury because of posterior infolding of the ligamentum flavum on a spinal canal already narrowed by posterior vertebral osteophytes.[5]

Whiplash injuries often show no associated osseous injury on standard radiographs or CT images, and flexion-extension radiographs may be nondiagnostic because of poor excursion secondary to pain. However, MRI is of limited value for the assessment of whiplash; several studies have failed to show positive MRI findings in the absence of neurologic symptoms.[21,24,25] In contrast, patients with a fused cervical spine secondary to ankylosing spondylitis or diffuse idiopathic skeletal hyperostosis may benefit from an MRI examination to assess for acute fracture, instability, or neurologic compromise. In such patients, the fused cervical spine acts like a long-bone fracture, and even minimally displaced fractures may be unstable.[26]

Finally, MRI can be used to assess intervertebral disk injury and subtle fractures caused by any of the aforementioned mechanisms.[11,20,21,22,27] Intervertebral disk injury may range from tear(s) of the outer annulus fibrosus (seen as increased T2-weighted signal in the outer annular fibers) to frank intervertebral disk herniation. The identification of an annular tear on MRI does not indicate acute traumatic injury and can be seen in asymptomatic individuals.[28,29] Intervertebral disk separation from the adjacent vertebral body may be seen as a horizontal hyperintense T2-weighted signal.[11,20,22] Subtle fractures such as vertebral end plate fractures may be best visualized with MRI, which can show osseous edema and hemorrhage not visible on conventional radiographs or CT images.[11,20,22]

Axial Load Injuries

Axial load injuries are caused by the axial transmission of force through the skull, through the occipital condyles, and into the spine. This force transmission can cause a Jefferson burst fracture or burst fractures of the subaxial cervical spine. MRI is useful for the assessment of C1 compression fractures and associated abnormalities such as lateral mass displacement on coronal images, atlantodental interval increase on sagittal images, and transverse ligament disruption on axial images.[11] For burst fractures, MRI is useful for diagnosing associated spinal cord injury caused by an acute herniated disk or retropulsion of osseous fragments (▶ Fig. 15.7). Because a purely axial force subjects the posterior capsuloligamentous structures to compression only, these posterior structures should remain intact.[11,23] However, during the traumatic event, there often is some degree of spine flexion that

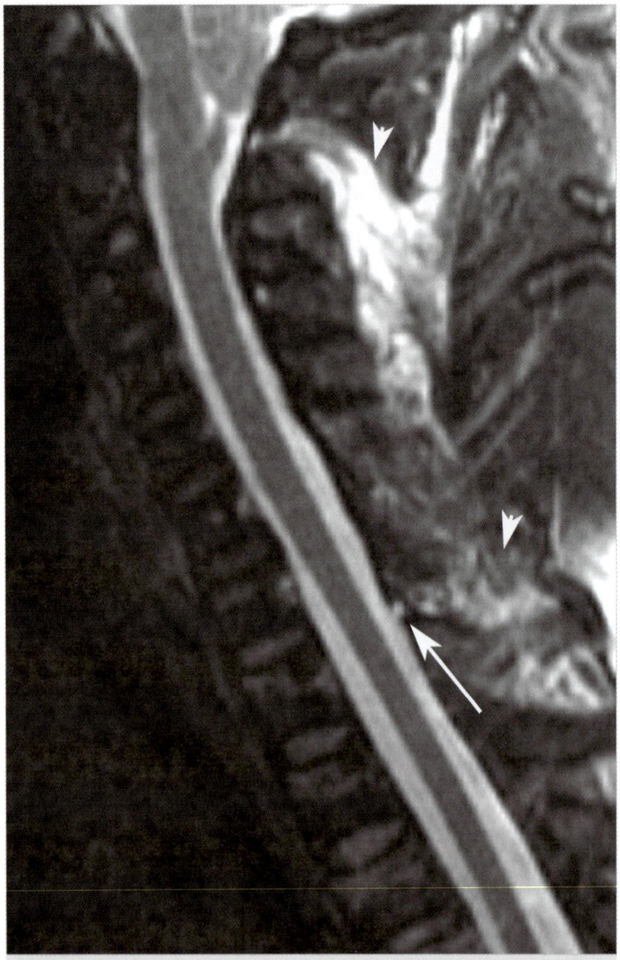

Fig. 15.5 A sagittal short tau inversion recovery (STIR) image shows edema in the supraspinous ligament region (*arrowhead*) and interspinous region at C6–C7 and C7–T1, with a small, focal region of increased T2-weighted signal in the ligamentum flavum at the C7–T1 level (*arrow*) compatible with a partial tear. (Reproduced with permission from, Zebala LP, Buchowski JM, Daftary AR, et al. The cervical spine. In: Khanna AJ, ed. MRI Essentials for the Spine Specialist. New York: Thieme; 2014:111–154.)

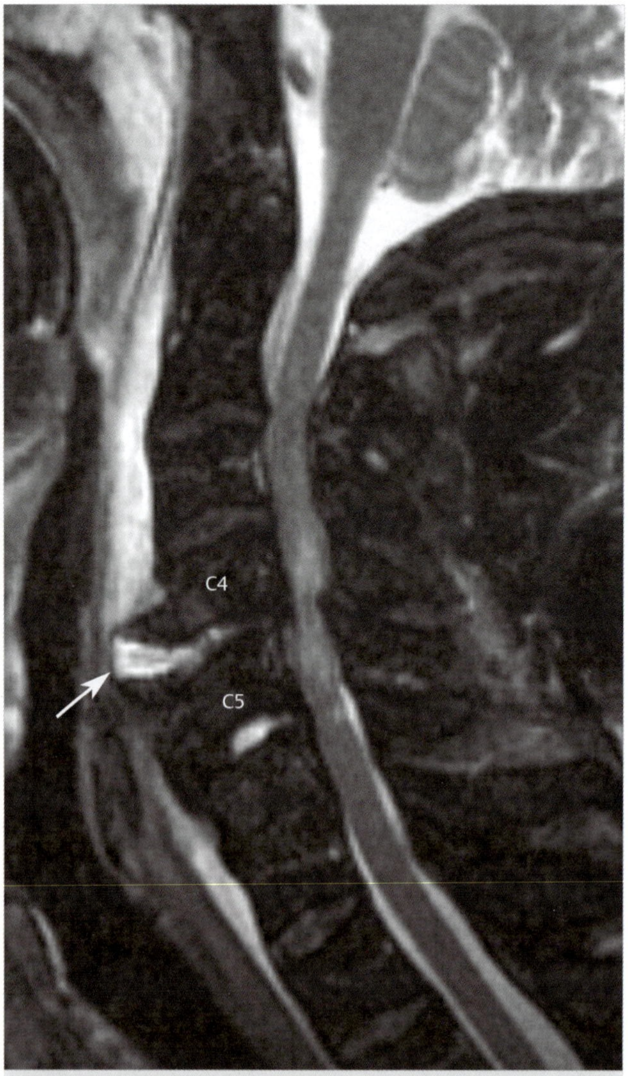

Fig. 15.6 A sagittal short tau inversion recovery (STIR) image shows an intervertebral disk rupture at C4–C5 (*arrow*) in a patient who sustained a hyperextension injury to the cervical spine. Note the associated prevertebral hematoma and the severe multilevel degenerative stenosis with associated cord signal change. (Reproduced with permission from, Zebala LP, Buchowski JM, Daftary AR, et al. The cervical spine. In: Khanna AJ, ed. MRI Essentials for the Spine Specialist. New York: Thieme; 2014:111–154.)

may cause injury to the posterior spinal elements, which can be detected on MRI.[23] It is important to scrutinize the fat-suppressed T2-weighted and other images carefully for evidence of injury to the posterior ligamentous and osseous structures because such injury will lead to consideration of posterior arthrodesis, in addition to the anterior decompression and arthrodesis that is often performed for patients with cervical burst fractures.

15.2.2 OCJ Injuries

Although injury to the OCJ occurs in a small percentage of blunt-trauma patients (0.8% in one study[30]), recognition of such injuries is crucial because of their devastating effects (see Chapter 14, The Occipitocervical Junction, for a detailed discussion of occipitocervical craniotomy and the various measurement techniques for evaluation of occipitocervical abnormality).[31,32,33,34] It is important to keep in mind that MRI studies of the OCJ should be reviewed in conjunction with conventional radiographic and CT imaging.

Atlantooccipital Dissociation

Atlantooccipital dissociation is any separation of the atlantooccipital articulation. The skull may displace anteriorly, posteriorly, or superiorly, and the displacement may be complete (dislocation) or partial (subluxation). Atlantooccipital dissociation can be a devastating injury.[31,32,33,34] The primary injury is to the ligaments that provide structural support to the cervicocranial junction. Even without frank dislocation, the occiput–C1 junction may be injured, as indicated by postmortem studies.[31,32] Although this injury may be fatal, improvements in resuscitative and medical treatments have increased survival rates. CT imaging may be used to assess associated fractures or relationships among the basion, dens, occipital condyles, and atlas in conjunction with atlantooccipital dissociation, whereas MRI is better at detecting injury to

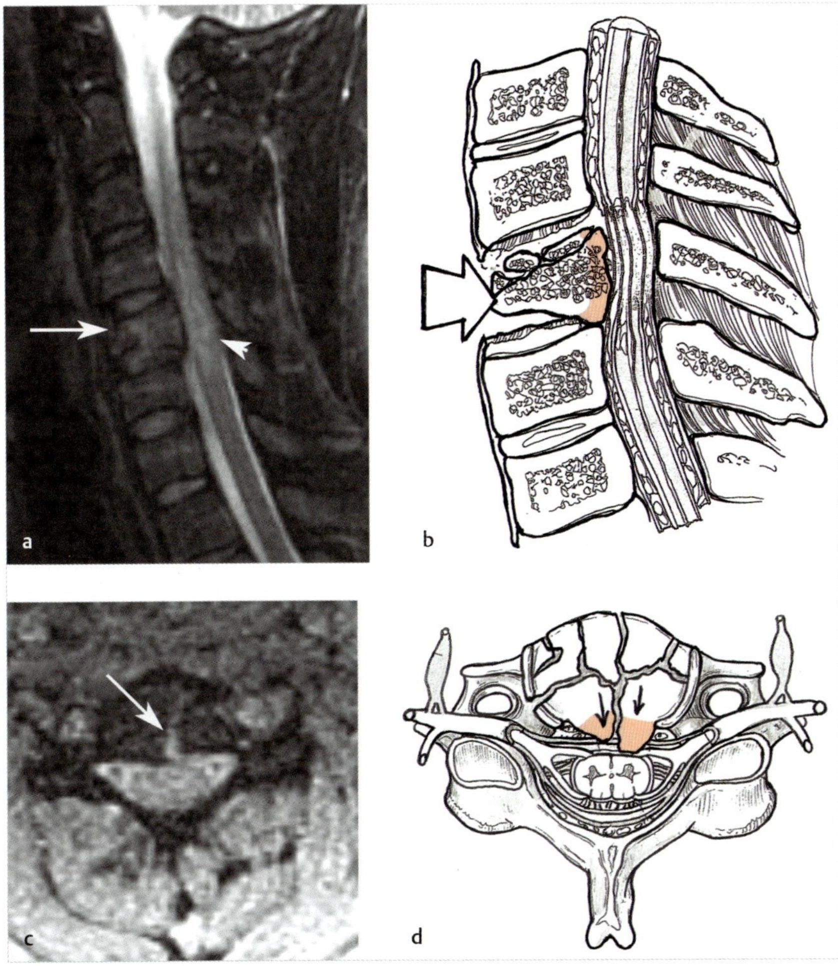

Fig. 15.7 Cervical burst fracture. **(a)** A sagittal fat-suppressed T2-weighted image and **(b)** corresponding illustration showing a C5 burst fracture (*arrow* on each) with moderate loss of height, retropulsion, and spinal cord contusion (*arrowhead* on **a**). **(c)** An axial T2-weighted gradient-echo image and **(d)** corresponding illustration showing the sagittal split component of the fracture (*arrows* on each). (Figure part **a**, **c**: Reproduced with permission from, Zebala LP, Buchowski JM, Daftary AR, et al. The cervical spine. In: Khanna AJ, ed. MRI Essentials for the Spine Specialist. New York: Thieme; 2014:111–154.)

the cervicocranial ligaments (e.g., transverse, apical, cruciate, atlantooccipital membrane and capsular ligaments, tectorial membrane), brainstem, or spinal cord.[11,22,35]

Trauma to the Atlas

Axial load to the OCJ at the atlas may cause a burst fracture of the atlas. The injury is visualized on open-mouth odontoid radiographs or coronal CT images.[36,37] As indicated by the cadaver study of Spence et al,[38] combined overhang of the lateral masses of C1 over C2 of $\geq$ 6.9 mm is associated with transverse ligament rupture and indicates an unstable Jefferson burst fracture. Axial T2-weighted images can be evaluated to identify or rule out injury to the transverse ligament. These images should be scrutinized for increased T2-weighted signal in or along the course of the transverse ligament. The ligament should also be evaluated for regions of discontinuity.

Trauma to the Axis

C2 is the most commonly fractured cervical spine level.[30] In the elderly, odontoid fractures tend to be displaced posteriorly. Fracture location, displacement, and angulation are important factors that assist with clinical decision-making. Lateral cervical radiographs and CT scans can be used to characterize such fractures and evaluate the osseous detail. MRI can assist in the evaluation of these fractures by providing assessment of the degree of edema at the fracture site (► Fig. 15.8). This information provides insight into the age of the fracture (acute, subacute, or chronic), which can be used to guide treatment. Sagittal and axial T2-weighted images should also be evaluated carefully to determine the degree of neural compression from a displaced fracture or underlying degenerative changes.

Atlantoaxial Dissociation

Atlantoaxial dissociation may be caused by distraction with superior migration of the atlas away from the axis or by odontoid fractures with anterior or posterior displacement of C1 relative to C2. MRI clearly depicts the associated abnormality seen with atlantoaxial dissociation[11] and is very useful for detecting ligamentous and spinal cord injury. The relationship of the atlas to the axis is clearly visible with MRI. The integrity of the transverse ligament should be evaluated along with the approximate size of the anterior atlantodens interval. This measurement is more frequently evaluated on flexion and extension lateral cervical spine radiographs (► Fig. 15.9).

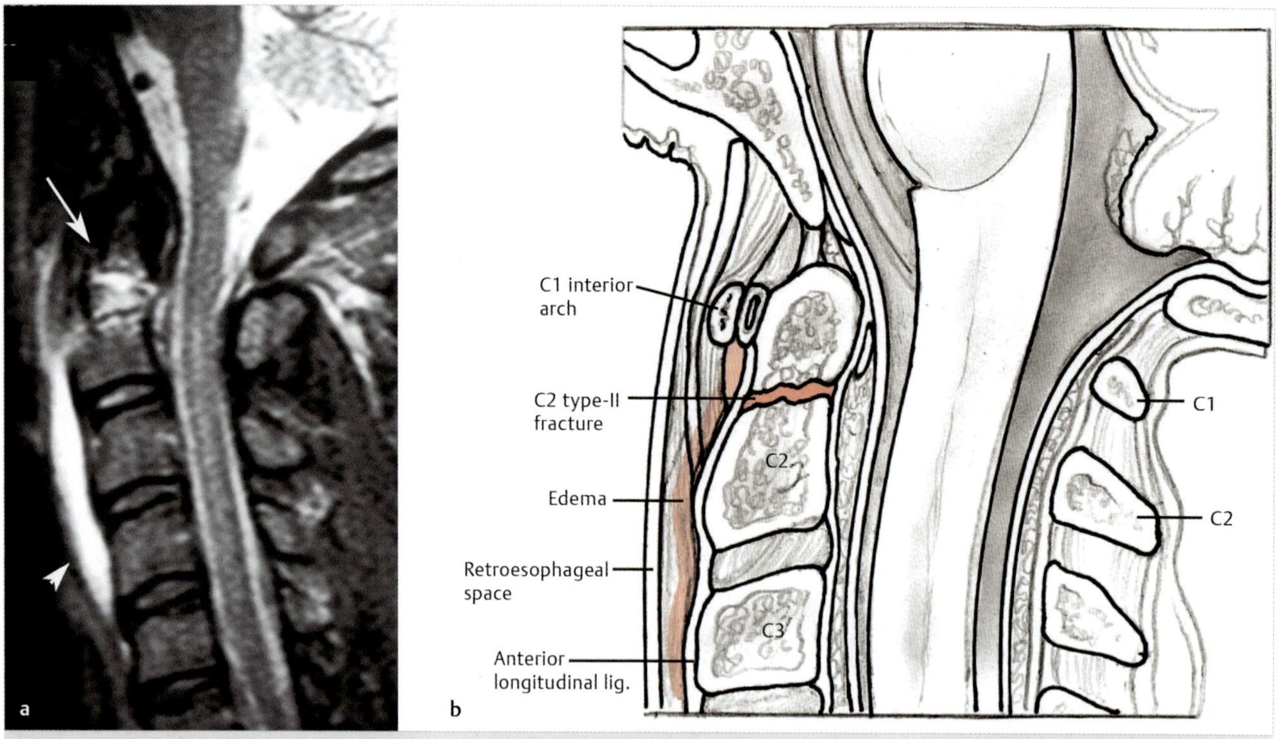

Fig. 15.8 Type-II odontoid fracture. **(a)** A sagittal T2-weighted image and **(b)** corresponding illustration of a type-II odontoid fracture show edema at the fracture site (*arrow on* **a**), indicating an acute or subacute fracture. Note the prevertebral edema or hematoma (*arrowhead* on a). (Reproduced with permission from, Zebala LP, Buchowski JM, Daftary AR, et al. The cervical spine. In: Khanna AJ, ed. MRI Essentials for the Spine Specialist. New York: Thieme; 2014:111–154.)

15.2.3 Vertebral Artery Injury

Vertebral artery injury is associated with blunt cervical trauma, with an incidence as high as 11%.[39] This potentially devastating injury may occur with cervical spine fractures extending into the transverse foramen but it is usually associated with unilateral or bilateral facet dislocations.[22,40,41] MR angiography may be used to assess vertebral artery patency, especially with such fractures.[22] MR angiography may show areas of vascular stenosis or occlusion. Flowing blood creates a signal void on axial SE images and is seen as a bright signal on gradient-echo images; merging the data from these two modalities can help determine the status of blood flow in the vertebral arteries (▶ Fig. 15.10).[22,42]

The types of vertebral artery injuries are thrombosis, dissection,[1] and transection (rare). MR angiography shows vertebral artery thrombosis as the absence of flow-related enhancement on images in the expected course of the vertebral artery and as an acute thrombus in the foramen transversarium, dissection as a tapering of the vessel, and transection as a focal discontinuity of the vessel. Major clues to vascular injury include changes in vessel caliber, loss of the normal rounded shape, increase in caliber from proximal to distal (except at the carotid bulb), or the presence of an extraluminal thrombus or a slit or dark band through the lumen.

15.2.4 Penetrating Trauma

Penetrating injury to the cervical spine can be caused by projectiles (e.g., bullets) or puncture mechanisms. Missiles can cause spinal cord injury by direct penetration, displacement of bone fragments into the spinal canal, compression of the spinal cord, or a blast effect. The osseous architecture of the spine often protects the spinal cord from direct injury from a stabbing mechanism because the lamina and spinous processes can deflect the penetrating object into the paraspinal soft tissues. MRI is useful for assessing the location, extent, and type of cord injury from penetrating trauma.

15.2.5 Characterization of Spinal Cord Injury

The severity of spinal cord injury depends on the characteristics of the traumatic event, including the amount, duration, and location of the applied force and the underlying health of the spinal cord. Spinal cord insult may range from a concussive injury (purely functional and reversible) to complete transection (irreversible). Spinal cord concussive injury often has no MRI evidence of edema (increased T2-weighted signal), or the edema is transient and resolves with time.[11] Spinal cord contusion is a more severe injury and may be caused by transient compression or stretching of the spinal cord. Spinal cord compression may show injury characteristics similar to those of spinal contusion but it can be associated with a specific compressive lesion such as disk herniation (▶ Fig. 15.11) or an osseous fragment.

Injury to a spinal cord segment may cause an increase in cord diameter because of swelling, edema, or hemorrhage. Characterization of an injured spinal cord segment using MRI is based on the degree of swelling, edema, or hemorrhage, each of which may

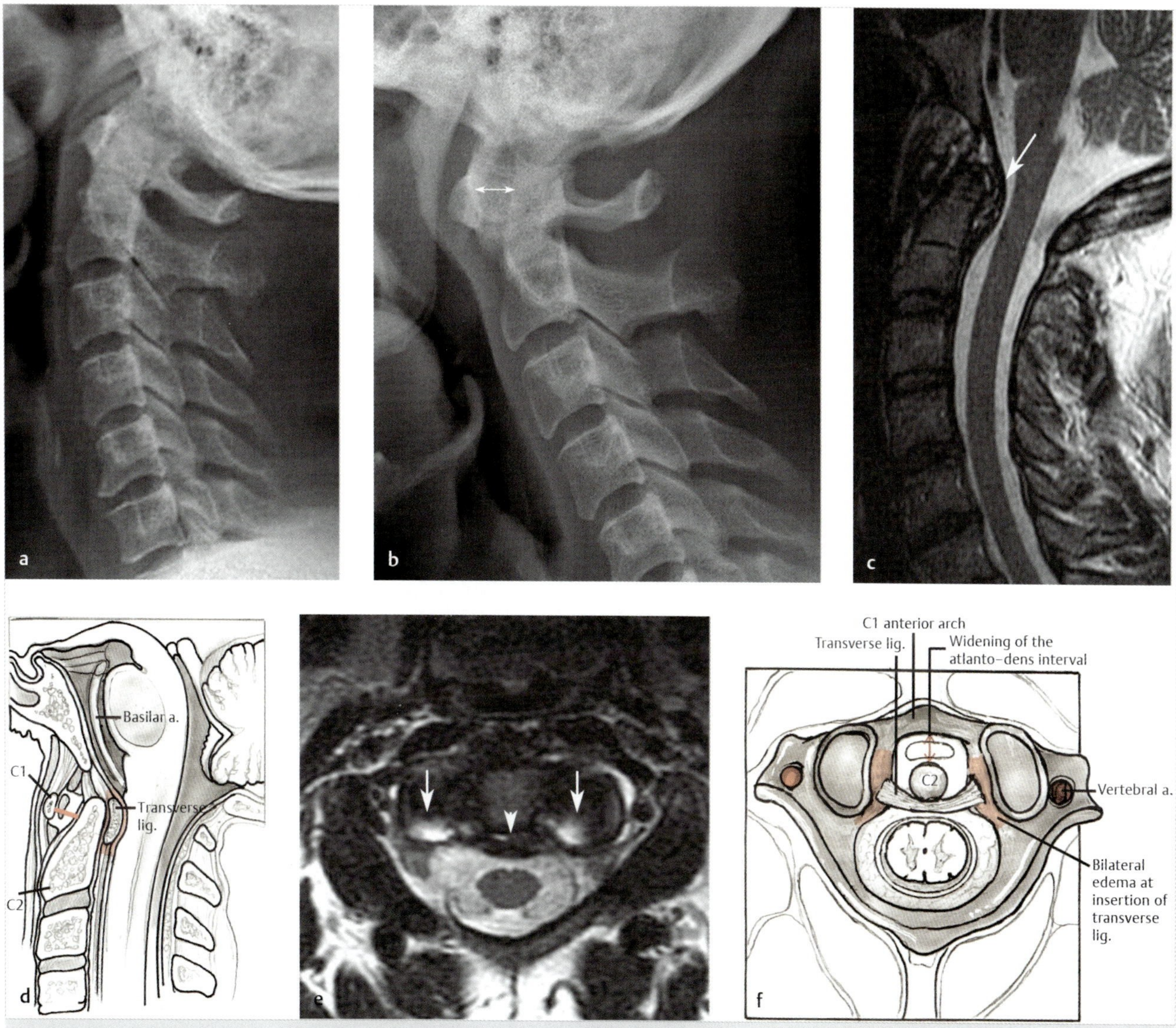

Fig. 15.9 Atlantoaxial instability, **(a)** lateral extension, and **(b)** flexion radiographs show instability at the C1–C2 level with widening of the anterior atlantodens interval on the flexion radiograph (*arrow* on **b**) relative to the extension radiograph. **(c)** A sagittal T2-weighted image (*arrow*) and **(d)** corresponding illustration showing prominence of the transverse ligament. **(e)** An axial T2-weighted image (*arrowhead*) and **(f)** corresponding illustration showing that prominence and edema at the insertion site of the transverse ligament on the lateral masses of C1. (Reproduced with permission from, Zebala LP, Buchowski JM, Daftary AR, et al. The cervical spine. In: Khanna AJ, ed. MRI Essentials for the Spine Specialist. New York: Thieme; 2014:111–154.)

have a different pattern of signal changes on various pulse sequences.[6,43] On T2-weighted images, edema and acute hemorrhage are seen as bright signal, whereas chronic hemorrhage is seen as darker signal. Gradient-echo images show dark areas that are larger than the abnormality seen on T2-weighted images. This enlargement, or "blooming," is the result of the magnetic susceptibility artifact from methemoglobin.[6] The anatomic location, morphology, and length of the spinal cord lesion are important factors in determining the degree of neurologic loss. Initial neurologic deficit and potential for recovery are related directly to the extent of spinal cord damage by hemorrhage or edema.[6] Evidence of parenchymal hemorrhage on MRI may predict worse functional outcomes or neurologic recovery than is associated with a spinal cord injury with predominantly edematous changes.[6]

Highly T2-weighted images offer a myelographic effect for the assessment of spinal cord compression. These images should be evaluated carefully in the sagittal and axial planes for regions of effacement of the ventral or dorsal cerebrospinal fluid (CSF) spaces, which indicate spinal stenosis and cord compression. Trauma patients who have underlying degenerative or congenital stenosis are at increased risk for spinal cord injury because of the decrease in cross-sectional area available for the spinal cord.

Clinical and experimental evidence has shown that surgical decompression of stenotic areas has a beneficial effect on neurologic recovery, which makes prompt identification of stenotic areas and distinguishing these areas from simple contusions important.[11] In addition, MRI assessment of cervical spine fractures in obtunded patients or patients who are uncooperative may identify disk herniations that may cause spinal cord compression and iatrogenic or progressive neurologic injury during fracture reduction.[23,44,45]

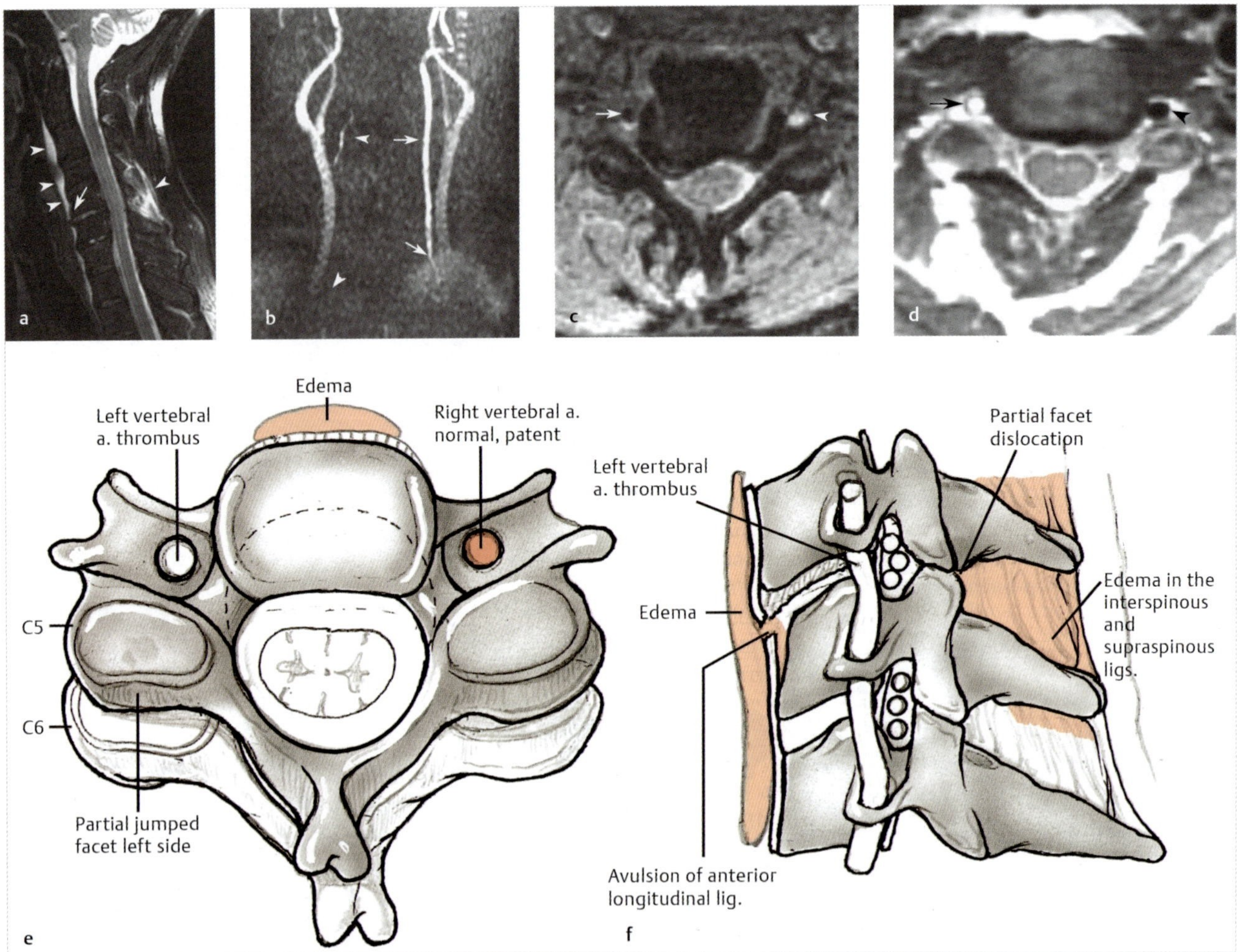

Fig. 15.10 Vertebral artery injury after unilateral facet dislocation at C5–C6 without spinal cord injury. **(a)** A sagittal T2-weighted image shows an injured disk at C5–C6 with increased signal intensity in the disk and probable avulsion of the anterior longitudinal ligament (*arrow*). Prevertebral edema (*small arrowheads*) and edema in the posterior paraspinal musculature (*large arrowhead*) are present. **(b)** A magnetic resonance (MR) angiogram (anterior view) from a 2D time-of-flight acquisition shows absence of signal intensity in the expected course of the right vertebral artery (*arrowheads*). Note the normal course of the left vertebral artery (*arrows*). **(c)** An axial image from a 3D gradient-echo acquisition shows an oval area of low signal intensity in the right foramen transversarium (*arrow*), corresponding to a thrombus in the right vertebral artery. Note the normal flow-related enhancement in the left foramen transversarium (*arrowhead*). **(d)** An axial fast spin-echo (FSE) image obtained at a similar level to that in **c** shows a high-signal-intensity thrombus (*arrow*) in the right foramen transversarium, indicative of a thrombosed vertebral artery. Note the normal flow void of the left vertebral artery in the left foramen transversarium (*arrowhead*). Illustration of the **(e)** sagittal and **(f)** axial planes show the displacement that leads to vertebral artery injury in this scenario. (Figure part **a**, **b**, **c**, and **d**: Reproduced with permission from Torina PJ, Flanders AE, Carrino JA, et al. Incidence of vertebral artery thrombosis in cervical spine trauma: correlation with severity of spinal cord injury. Am J Neuroradiol. 2005;26:2645–2651.) (Figure part **e**, **f**: Reproduced with permission from, Zebala LP, Buchowski JM, Daftary AR, et al. The cervical spine. In: Khanna AJ, ed. MRI Essentials for the Spine Specialist. New York: Thieme; 2014:111–154.)

15.2.6 Characterization of Cervical Spine Instability

White et al[46] defined cervical spine instability as the inability to maintain a normal association between vertebral segments while under a physiologic load. Cervical spine instability may be caused by damage to the osseous and/or ligamentous structures. Conventional radiographs and CT scans often provide the best assessment of osseous injuries. Ligamentous injury contributing to cervical spine instability may be assessed with flexion and extension lateral cervical spine radiographs and by physical examination. MRI can also be used to evaluate for ligamentous injury; the sensitivity for detection of such injuries is greatest within 24 to 72 hours after injury.[20,22,47,48] Important ligaments to assess include the following[23]:

- Anterior longitudinal ligament.
- Posterior longitudinal ligament.
- Posterior column ligament complex (supraspinous ligament, interspinous ligament, and ligamentum flavum), which has been recognized as an important restraint to spinal instability (especially kyphosis).[24,49]
- Transverse ligament.

MRI characteristics of ligamentous injury include increased T2-weighted signal (from edema) within the ligamentous and other posterior structures (▶ Fig. 15.12) or loss of ligament continuity

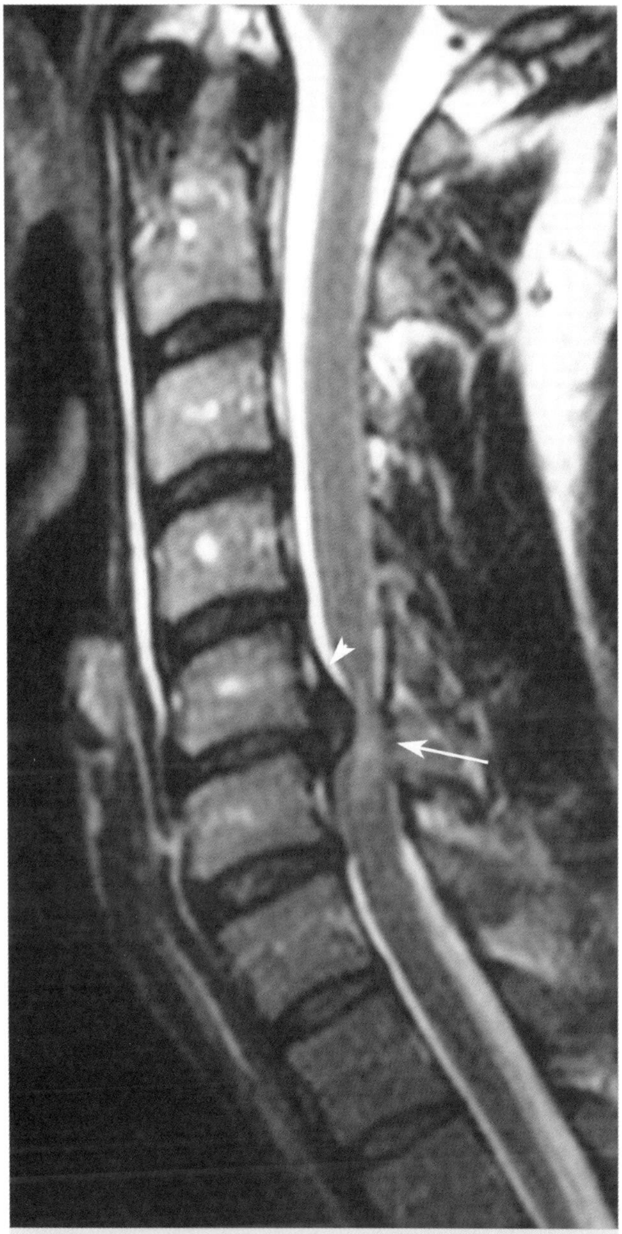

Fig. 15.11 A sagittal T2-weighted image shows a large central disk extrusion at the C5–C6 level with associated increased cord signal intensity (*arrow*) compatible with myelomalacia. Note the elevation of the posterior longitudinal ligament (*arrowhead*). (Reproduced with permission from, Zebala LP, Buchowski JM, Daftary AR, et al. The cervical spine. In: Khanna AJ, ed. MRI Essentials for the Spine Specialist. New York: Thieme; 2014:111–154.)

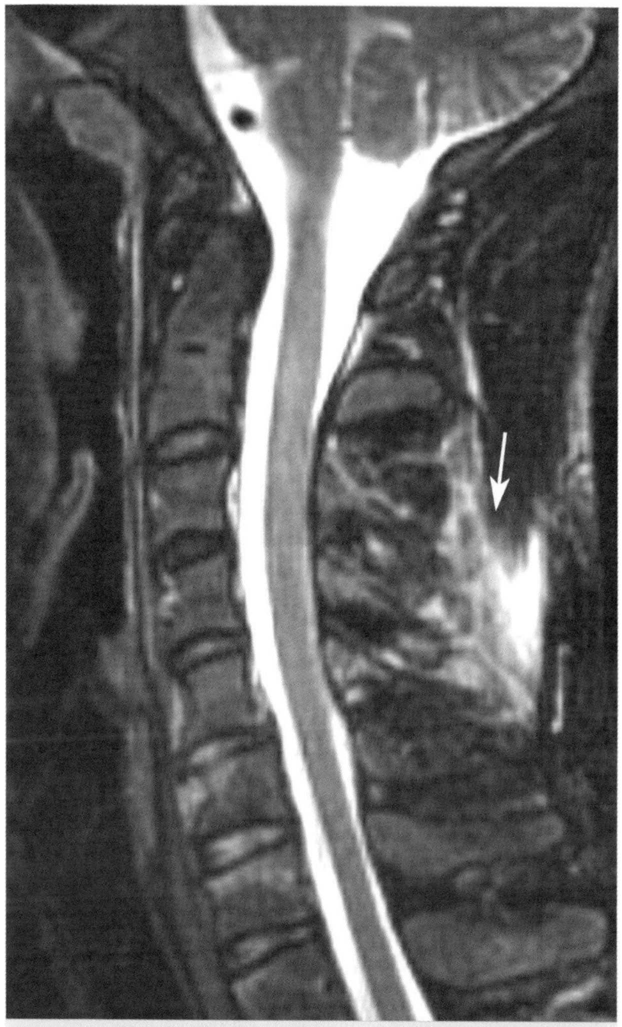

Fig. 15.12 A sagittal short tau inversion recovery (STIR) image of a patient who sustained a hyperflexion injury to the cervical spine shows increased signal intensity within the region of the supraspinous and interspinous ligaments from C3 to C6 (*arrow*). These findings are compatible with injury to the posterior ligamentous structures. (Reproduced with permission from, Zebala LP, Buchowski JM, Daftary AR, et al. The cervical spine. In: Khanna AJ, ed. MRI Essentials for the Spine Specialist. New York: Thieme; 2014:111–154.)

(normally a low-intensity continuous signal). Ligamentous injury is best assessed on STIR or fat-suppressed T2-weighted images.[23] A ligament strain, without complete disruption, may be seen as an elongated or redundant ligament on sagittal MR images. Despite the capability of MRI to detect ligamentous injury, not all MRI-detected ligamentous injuries cause spinal instability or warrant treatment.[23,25] For example, minor motor vehicle accidents that cause acute whiplash injury of the cervical spine without fracture do not need emergent MRI evaluation for ligamentous injury and may only be treated symptomatically.[25]

With the increasing availability of flexion-extension (kinematic) cervical spine MRI, a dynamic assessment of cervical spinal instability and associated stenosis can be obtained.[50] Although such information provides insight into the degree of spinal instability, it is most useful for the evaluation of patients with degenerative disorders of the cervical and lumbar spine (▸ Fig. 15.13).[51,52] Patients who have sustained severe trauma to the cervical spine are likely to be immobilized. After a period of immobilization and after frank instability of the cervical spine has been ruled out with patient-controlled flexion-extension cervical spine radiographs, a kinematic cervical spine MRI study can be considered. The information obtained from such kinematic studies can be used to guide surgical treatment and may enable the surgeon to decide among anterior, posterior, or combined surgical approaches.

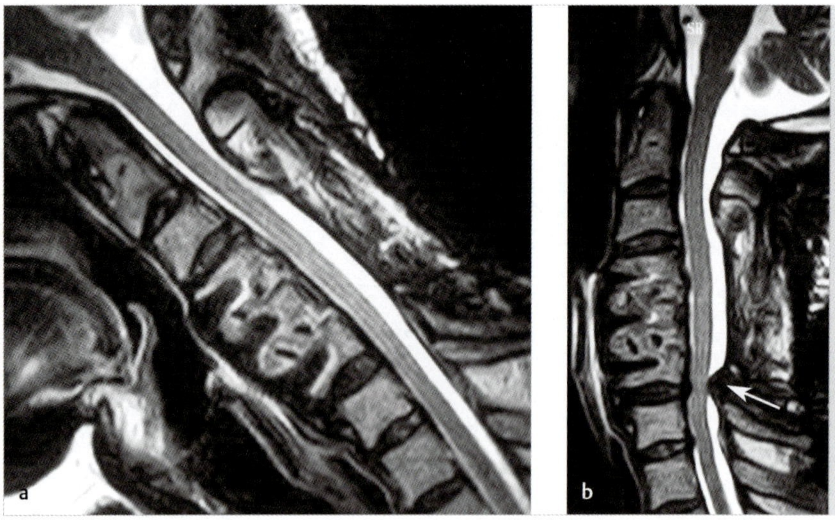

Fig. 15.13 Sagittal T2-weighted images of a patient after C4–C6 anterior cervical decompression and arthrodesis with allograft and plate. **(a)** Image obtained in flexion on an open, upright magnetic resonance (MR) system shows no substantial stenosis. **(b)** Image obtained in extension shows moderate stenosis at the C6–C7 level secondary to buckling of the ligamentum flavum (*arrow*) and disk bulge. (Reproduced with permission from, Zebala LP, Buchowski JM, Daftary AR, et al. The cervical spine. In: Khanna AJ, ed. MRI Essentials for the Spine Specialist. New York: Thieme; 2014:111–154.)

15.3 Degenerative Conditions

Degenerative changes of the cervical spine are common after the fourth decade of life.[53] Cervical spine degeneration may be asymptomatic or have acute or insidious onset of symptoms; it may cause pain, stiffness, radiculopathy, myelopathy, and even permanent disability. Degenerative abnormality may affect multiple areas in the cervical spine, including the following:

- Intervertebral disks.
- Facet joints.
- Uncovertebral joints of Luschka.
- Ligaments.
- Paravertebral musculature.

Because these elements are linked biomechanically, a single cervical spine level may have multiple degenerative abnormalities and cause adjacent-level degenerative changes. Conventional radiographs are often the initial screening studies for evaluating cervical spine degeneration and may guide the selection of more advanced imaging techniques.[54] MRI is usually the preferred initial advanced imaging modality for the evaluation of symptomatic cervical spine degeneration; it has a reported sensitivity and specificity of 91% for the detection of cervical degenerative changes.[54,55] Despite this high sensitivity and specificity, it is important to understand that radiographic and MRI abnormalities do not always correlate with a symptomatic degenerative lesion.[56] Boden et al[53] reported that almost 60% of their asymptomatic patients > 40 years old had cervical spine degenerative disk disease on MRI.

Although one should always correlate the patient's history and physical examination with the imaging findings (see Chapter 3, A Systematic Approach to the Review of Spine MRI Studies), this practice is especially important when evaluating the MRI studies of a patient with a suspected cervical or lumbar spine degenerative disorder. One should know whether a patient has neck pain, radiculopathy, myelopathy, or a more focal neurologic deficit.[57] The laterality and level of the symptoms should also be assessed, and this information should be considered, along with the imaging findings, when choosing among nonoperative and surgical treatment options.

15.3.1 Degenerative Disk Disease

An intervertebral disk is composed of an outer annulus fibrosus, an inner nucleus pulposus, and superior and inferior cartilaginous end plates. The structural composition of the intervertebral disk changes with age: the water content of the nucleus pulposus and annulus fibrosus decreases from ~90% during the first year of life to 70 to 75% during the eighth decade.[20,58,59] The remainder of the nucleus pulposus consists of proteoglycans and collagen that attract water, which creates pressure that enables the nucleus pulposus to resist axial loading. The collagen fibers in the annulus are abundant anteriorly but deficient posterolaterally, creating a potentially weak area at risk for degenerative tears and disk herniation.[59] The posterior longitudinal ligament reinforces this deficient area.[59]

With advancing age, the proteoglycan composition of the intervertebral disk changes and water is lost, diminishing the disk's ability to support load. The nucleus pulposus is replaced with more fibrous structures and blends with the adjacent annulus fibrosus into amorphous fibrocartilaginous tissue.[55] Disk desiccation leads to bulging of the annulus fibrosus and loss of disk height, causing increased stress transfer to adjacent facet and uncovertebral joints.[55] This increased stress propagates osteocartilaginous hypertrophy and osteophyte formation. In addition, the loss of intervertebral disk elasticity exposes these small vertebral joints to increased motion and instability, furthering their degeneration. Nerve root compression may occur secondary to the decreased width and height of the adjacent neural foramina caused by disk height loss, annulus bulging, and uncinate process and facet hypertrophy. On MRI, a normal intervertebral disk has intermediate signal intensity on T1-weighted images and high signal intensity on T2-weighted sequences, whereas disk desiccation has low signal intensity on T1- and T2-weighted images (▶ Fig. 15.14).[54,55]

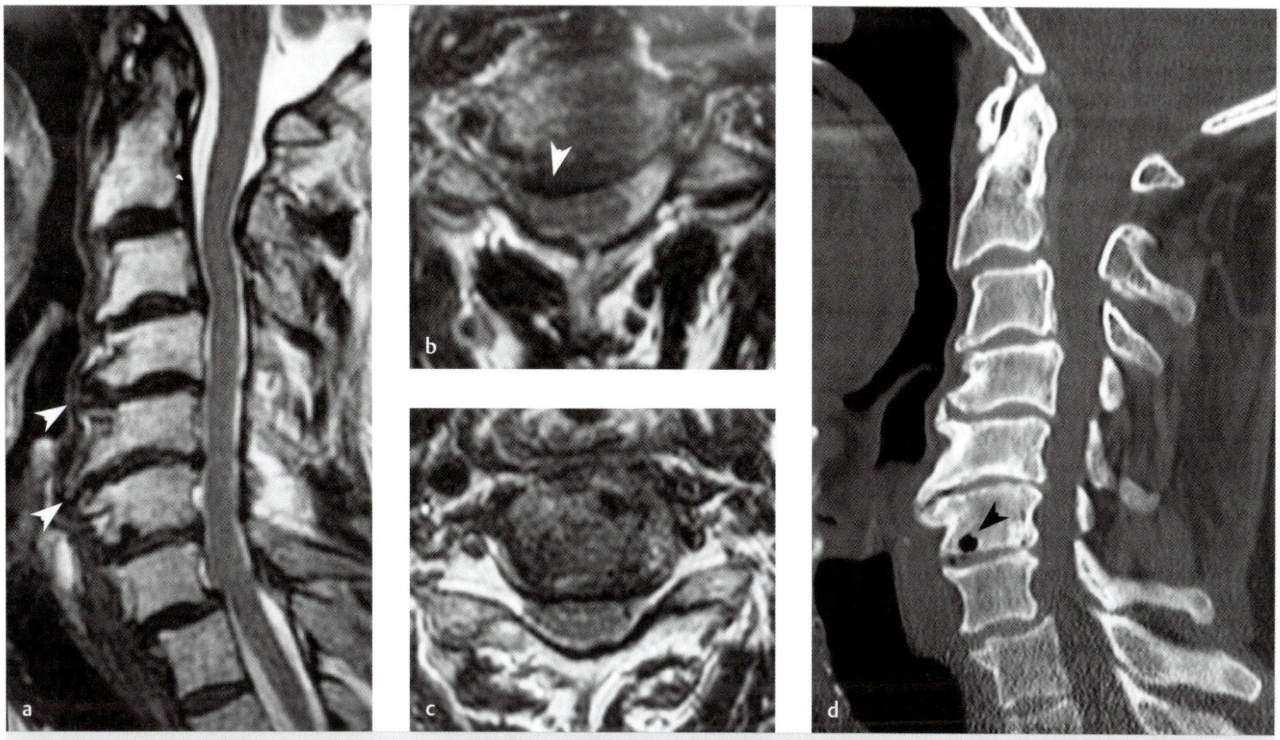

Fig. 15.14 Multilevel degenerative disk disease. **(a)** A sagittal T2-weighted image shows multilevel degenerative disk disease as evidenced by the loss of the normal high signal intensity within the disks. Note the degenerative spondylolisthesis at C2–C3, C3–C4 (subtle), and C7–T1, and the multilevel anterior osteophyte formation (*arrowheads*). There is also a loss of the normal cervical lordosis. **(b)** An axial T2-weighted image at the C3–C4 level shows a right paracentral disk bulge (*arrowhead*), causing moderate stenosis with asymmetric cord compression. **(c)** An axial T2-weighted image at the C5–C6 level shows moderate central stenosis. **(d)** A sagittal reconstructed computed tomographic (CT) image also shows multilevel degenerative disk disease and provides improved osseous detail that complements the information seen on the magnetic resonance (MR) images. Note the gas-containing subchondral cyst at the inferior end plate of C6 (*arrowhead*) and the multilevel anterior osteophyte formation. (Reproduced with permission from, Zebala LP, Buchowski JM, Daftary AR, et al. The cervical spine. In: Khanna AJ, ed. MRI Essentials for the Spine Specialist. New York: Thieme; 2014:111–154.)

As the disk degenerates and desiccates, degenerative changes also affect the annulus fibrosus and cause deamination of and change in the architecture of the concentric annular fibers.[20] These changes may lead to annular tears. Discogenic pain may be associated with transverse, radial, or complete tears.[55] On T2-weighted images, tears are seen as areas of high signal intensity within the annulus (▶ Fig. 15.15).[54,55] A weakened annulus fibrosus may lead to a spectrum of intervertebral disk abnormality according to the extent of annulus bulging and disk herniation (▶ Table 15.3). The findings of degenerative disk disease on MRI should be correlated with the degenerative changes seen on cervical spine radiographs. The degree of vertebral body endplate sclerosis can be best evaluated on radiographs, and oblique radiographs will best show foraminal stenosis secondary to osteophyte formation.

15.3.2 Disk Displacement

Along with the degenerative disk disease and normal aging process described in the preceding paragraphs, elevated pressures within the nucleus pulposus and compromise of the structural integrity of the annulus fibrosus can lead to migration of disk material toward the neural elements and produce the clinical findings of radiculopathy or myelopathy. Patients with large central disk herniations usually present with symptoms of myelopathy, whereas those with posterolateral disk herniations usually present with radiculopathy.

Disk herniations most commonly occur at the levels with greatest motion (C5–C6 and C6–C7) and may be classified as follows:

- Central (compression of the medial portion of the spinal cord) (▶ Fig. 15.16).
- Posterolateral (compression of the lateral portion of spinal cord and nerve root) (▶ Fig. 15.17).
- Lateral (compression of the nerve root only) (▶ Fig. 15.18).

The nomenclature used to describe cervical disk displacements varies widely among radiologists and clinicians. Although a task force has provided formal guidelines for the description of lumbar disk abnormality (see Chapter 16, The Lumbar and Thoracic Spine),[60] similar guidelines have not been adopted widely for the cervical spine. The terms *bulge, protrusion, extrusion,* and *sequestration* are commonly used to describe cervical disk abnormality (▶ Table 15.3). The anatomy of the cervical facet joints, which are located more laterally than those in the lumbar spine, essentially makes them the posterior wall of the intervertebral nerve root canals, and there is no subarticular recess in the cervical spine. Thus, disk herniation positions in the cervical spine are described as central, paracentral (left or right), foraminal, or far lateral.

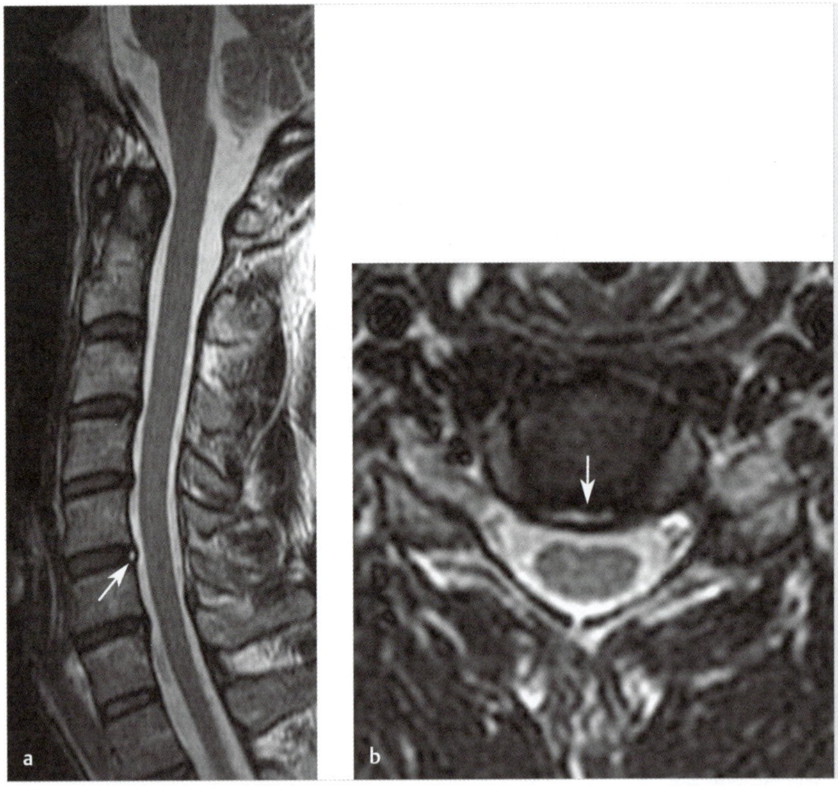

Fig. 15.15 Annular tear. **(a)** Sagittal and **(b)** axial T2-weighted images show a high-intensity zone in the posterior annulus at C5–C6 (*arrow* on each). This finding is compatible with an annular tear that may be responsible for the patient's discogenic neck pain. (Reproduced with permission from, Zebala LP, Buchowski JM, Daftary AR, et al. The cervical spine. In: Khanna AJ, ed. MRI Essentials for the Spine Specialist. New York: Thieme; 2014:111–154.)

Table 15.3 Intervertebral disk abnormality

Disk abnormality	MRI findings
Bulge	Symmetric extension of annulus beyond confines of adjacent end plates
Protrusion	Focal area of disk material that extends beyond vertebral margin but remains contained within the outer annular fibers
Extrusion	Herniation of nucleus pulposus beyond confines of annulus with disk attached to remainder of nucleus pulposus by a narrow pedicle
Sequestration	Portion of disk fragment entirely separated from parent disk

Source: Reproduced with permission from, Khanna AJ, Carbone JJ, Kebaish KM, et al. Magnetic resonance imaging of the cervical spine. J Bone Joint Surg Am. 2002;84:70–80. Modified with permission.

With regard to the size of the disk abnormality, the degree of mass effect on adjacent neural structures can be more important than the size of the disk abnormality itself. For example, a small protrusion in a patient with developmental spinal stenosis is more likely to produce symptoms than a similar protrusion in a patient with a capacious spinal canal.

In addition to evaluation of the level, direction, and configuration of disk displacement, the MRI study should be scrutinized for the presence or absence of areas of calcium deposition, anterior or posterior osteophyte formation, and vertebral end-plate changes.[54,55,61,62] These findings should be correlated with the findings seen on lateral and oblique cervical spine radiographs.

Additional scrutiny of the imaging findings enables the surgeon to determine whether a cervical disk protrusion can be classified as a "soft" (well-hydrated) or "hard" (poorly hydrated) disk (▶ Fig. 15.19). This information may help in determining whether an anterior or posterior approach is chosen when treating a patient with unilateral cervical radiculopathy. Such a

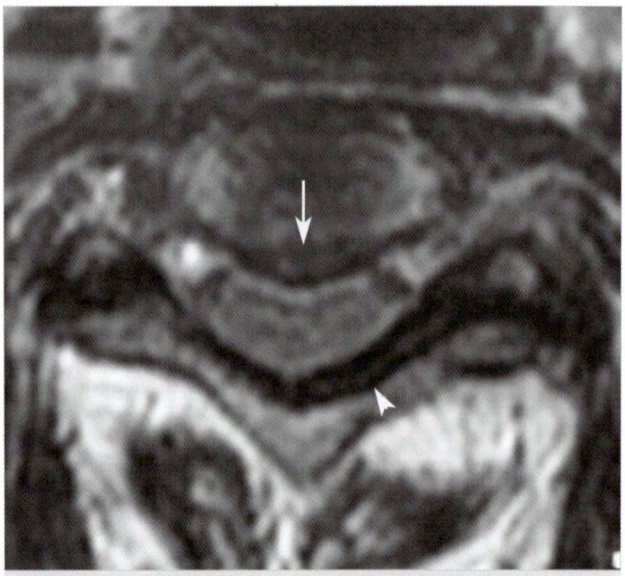

Fig. 15.16 An axial T2-weighted image at the C5–C6 level shows a central disk bulge (*arrow*) with moderate stenosis. The disk bulge and ligamentum flavum hypertrophy (*arrowhead*) act to produce effacement of the ventral and dorsal cerebrospinal fluid (CSF) spaces and deformity of the spinal cord. (Reproduced with permission from, Zebala LP, Buchowski JM, Daftary AR, et al. The cervical spine. In: Khanna AJ, ed. MRI Essentials for the Spine Specialist. New York: Thieme; 2014:111–154.)

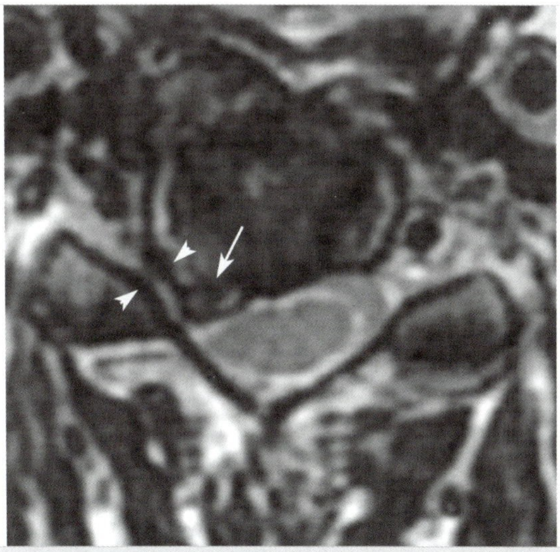

Fig. 15.17 An axial T2-weighted image at the C5–C6 level shows a right posterolateral disk protrusion with associated uncovertebral joint hypertrophy (*arrow*), which produces mild deformity of the right side of the spinal cord and severe foraminal stenosis (between *arrowheads*). Note the normal size of the neural foramen on the left side. (Reproduced with permission from, Zebala LP, Buchowski JM, Daftary AR, et al. The cervical spine. In: Khanna AJ, ed. MRI Essentials for the Spine Specialist. New York: Thieme; 2014:111–154.)

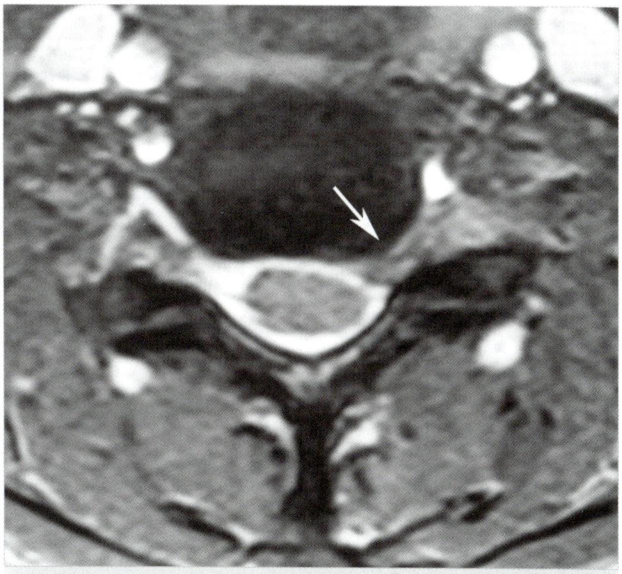

Fig. 15.18 An axial T2-weighted image at the C5–C6 level shows a lateral or foraminal disk protrusion (*arrow*) on the left side, which produces severe foraminal stenosis and compresses the nerve root. Note that the signal is different from that of the bone. (Reproduced with permission from, Zebala LP, Buchowski JM, Daftary AR, et al. The cervical spine. In: Khanna AJ, ed. MRI Essentials for the Spine Specialist. New York: Thieme; 2014:111–154.)

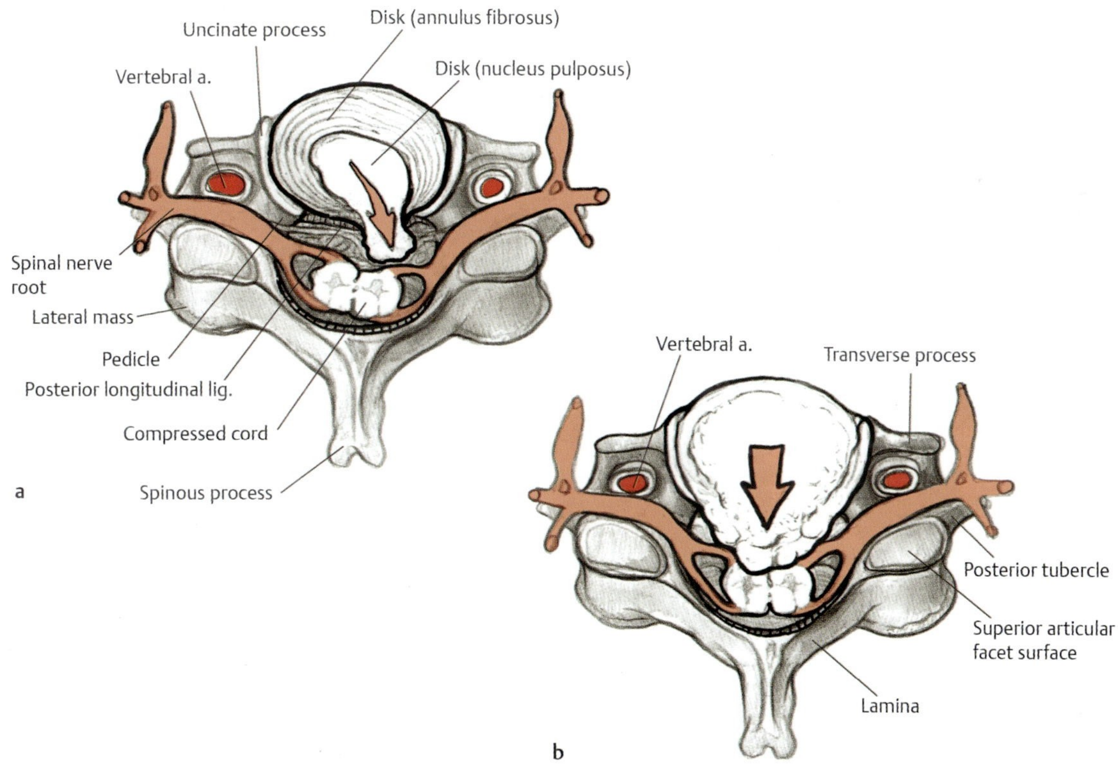

Fig. 15.19 Axial illustrations show the difference between soft and hard disk abnormality in the subaxial cervical spine. **(a)** A left posterolateral disk protrusion (*arrow*) causing mild deformity of the cord and compression of the exiting nerve root. **(b)** Moderate central stenosis secondary to a large, central disk protrusion with an associated osteophyte complex (*arrow*); the osteophyte creates most of the stenosis. (Reproduced with permission from, Zebala LP, Buchowski JM, Daftary AR, et al. The cervical spine. In: Khanna AJ, ed. MRI Essentials for the Spine Specialist. New York: Thieme; 2014:111–154.)

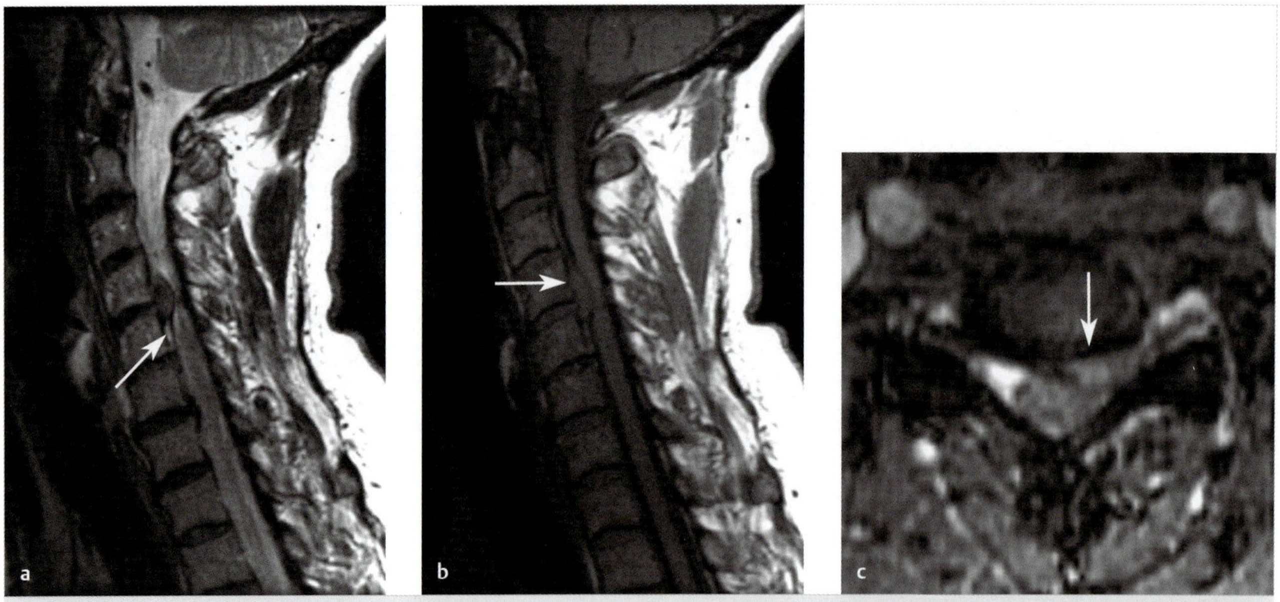

Fig. 15.20 Cervical disk extrusion. **(a)** A sagittal T2-weighted image shows a large disk extrusion at the C4–C5 level (*arrow*) that has migrated proximally, tenting the posterior longitudinal ligament. **(b)** A sagittal T1-weighted image shows the disk extrusion at the C4–C5 level (*arrow*) that is isointense to the intervertebral disk. **(c)** An axial T2-weighted image shows a left paracentral disk extrusion (*arrow*), which produces severe foraminal stenosis and deformity on the left side of the cord. (Reproduced with permission from, Zebala LP, Buchowski JM, Daftary AR, et al. The cervical spine. In: Khanna AJ, ed. MRI Essentials for the Spine Specialist. New York: Thieme; 2014:111–154.)

determination can be made by reviewing the images for increased T2-weighted signal within the displaced disk, which would be expected in a patient with a soft disk herniation. Conversely, a hard disk herniation shows low signal on T2-weighted images and may also show associated osteophytes on gradient-echo and other pulse sequences. This combination of hard disk disease and associated osteophytes is often referred to as a disk-ridge complex and may preclude the performance of a posterior keyhole foraminotomy and diskectomy in patients with unilateral radiculopathy.

The findings on MR images should be used to differentiate cervical disk disease and protrusions from ossification of the posterior longitudinal ligament. On most MR images showing cervical stenosis secondary to disk displacement (▶ Fig. 15.11, ▶ Fig. 15.14), the abnormality and stenosis are based at the level of the disk, and stenosis is seen only behind the vertebral body in cases of disk extrusion and migration (▶ Fig. 15.20). Conversely, MRI in patients with ossification of the posterior longitudinal ligament shows stenosis at the level of the disk and along the course of the posterior longitudinal ligament, which runs along the posterior aspect of the vertebral bodies (▶ Fig. 15.21).[63]

In patients with suspected ossification of the posterior longitudinal ligament, CT imaging can be obtained to rule in or rule out this diagnosis, given that it provides optimal visualization of calcification and osseous detail. The importance of this differentiation lies in the fact that anterior decompression for patients with ossification of the posterior longitudinal ligament can be difficult and is associated with increased rates of durotomy and bleeding. Therefore, surgeons may prefer to proceed with posterior decompression even though the primary compression is located ventral to the spinal cord.

15.3.3 Spinal Stenosis

The term *spinal stenosis* describes the compression of the neural elements in the spinal canal, lateral recesses, or neural foramina (▶ Fig. 15.22). Spinal stenosis can develop from congenital or acquired causes (▶ Table 15.4); patients can also develop degenerative stenosis superimposed on preexisting congenital stenosis (▶ Fig. 15.23).

Foraminal stenosis may be caused by a disk herniation or uncovertebral or facet joint hypertrophy. Central canal stenosis is usually caused by a combination of two or more of the following (▶ Fig. 15.24):

- Disk bulge or herniation.
- Uncovertebral joint osteophyte formation.
- Ligamentum flavum hypertrophy.
- Facet arthrosis.
- Thickening, calcification, or ossification of the posterior longitudinal ligament or other structures.

On MRI, central canal stenosis is characterized by compression of the thecal sac, best seen on sagittal and axial T2-weighted images. Such images provide a "myelographic effect," in which the CSF is seen as bright signal anterior and posterior to the spinal cord on sagittal images and circumferentially around the spinal cord on axial images. Effacement, discontinuity, or displacement of this CSF space is seen in patients with focal and concentric spinal stenosis.

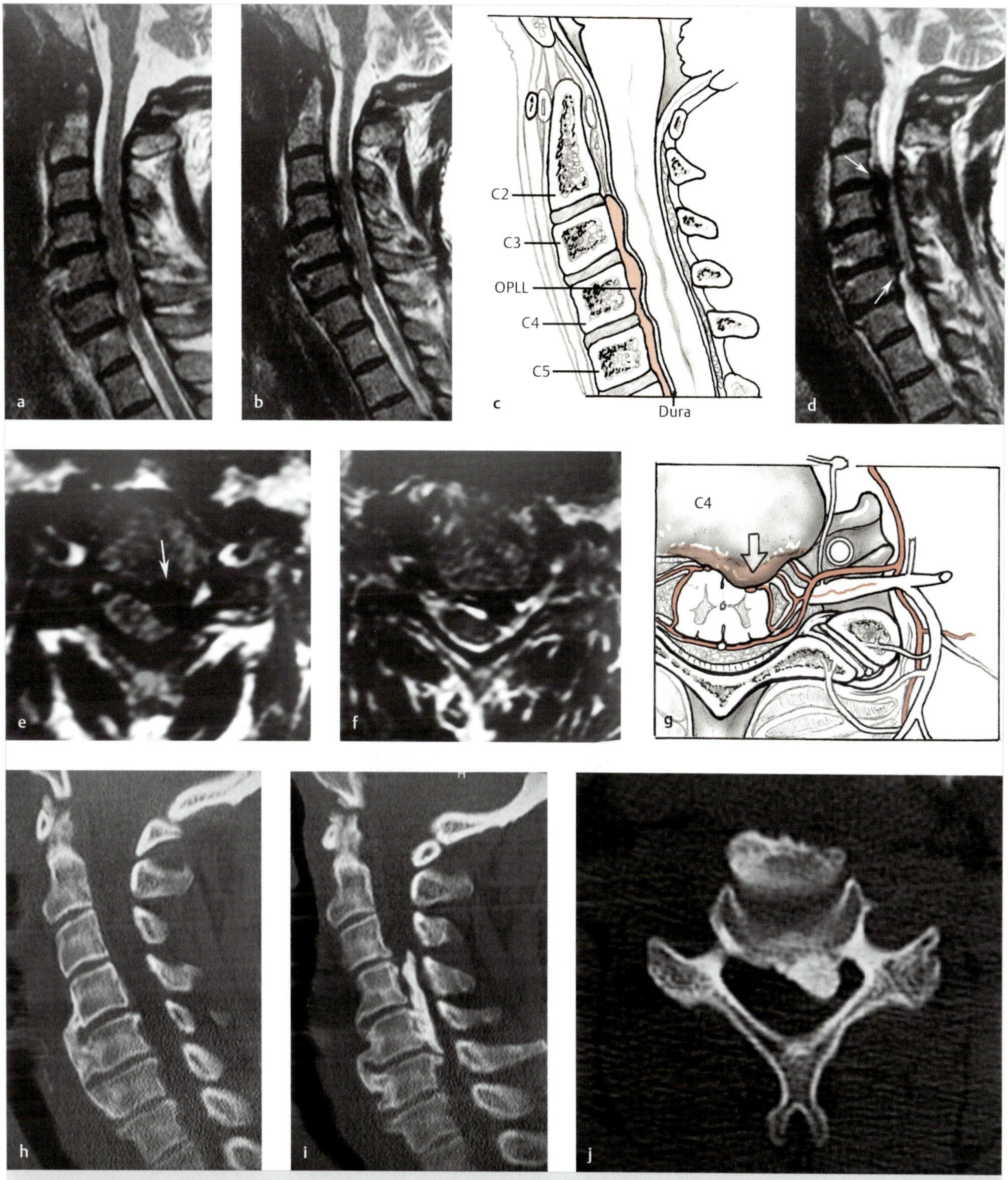

Fig. 15.21 Ossification of the posterior longitudinal ligament (OPLL). **(a)** A midline sagittal T2-weighted image shows multilevel degenerative disk disease and moderate stenosis from C3–C4 to C6–C7. The stenosis appears to be centered at the level of the disk spaces on this midline image. **(b)** A parasagittal T2-weighted image, obtained a few millimeters lateral to the midline, suggests that the posterior longitudinal ligament is thickened and that the stenosis is present at the level of the vertebral bodies and disks from C3 to C7. **(c)** A parasagittal T2-weighted image, obtained farther from the midline, shows that the posterior longitudinal ligament is markedly hypertrophied and nearly fills the spinal canal *(between arrows)* **(d)** A parasagittal reconstructed computed tomographic (CT) image, obtained at the same level as **c.** **(e)** Corresponding illustration showing ossification of the posterior longitudinal ligament extending from C3–C4 to C5–C6. (Reproduced with permission from, Zebala LP, Buchowski JM, Daftary AR, et al. The cervical spine. In: Khanna AJ, ed. MRI Essentials for the Spine Specialist. New York: Thieme; 2014:111–154.)

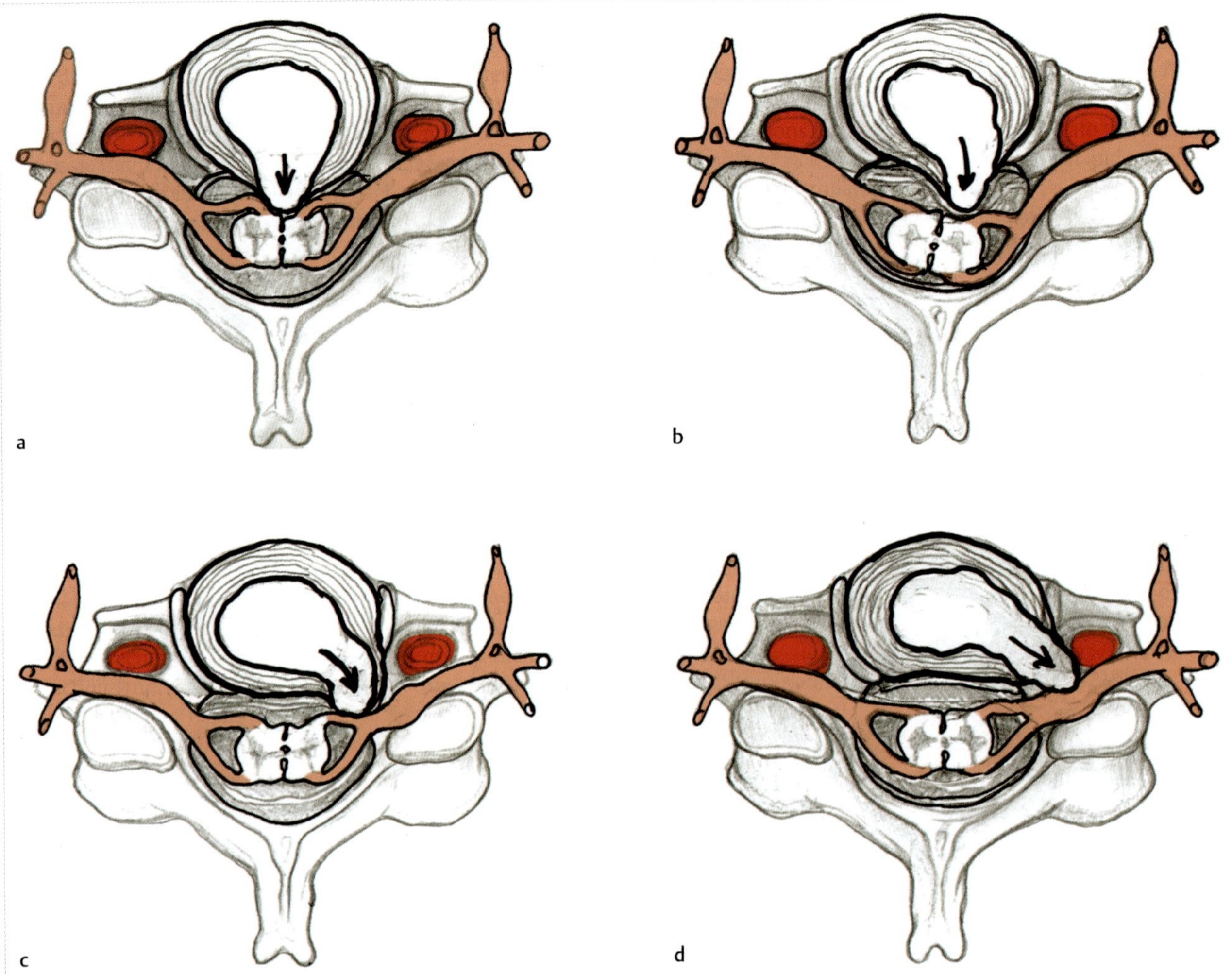

Fig. 15.22 Illustration showing four types of disk herniation in the cervical spine: (a) central, (b) posterolateral, (c) lateral recess, and (d) foraminal. (Reproduced with permission from, Zebala LP, Buchowski JM, Daftary AR, et al. The cervical spine. In: Khanna AJ, ed. MRI Essentials for the Spine Specialist. New York: Thieme; 2014:111–154.)

Table 15.4 Acquired and congenital factors associated with spinal stenosis

Type	Factor
Acquired	Intervertebral disk abnormality
	Uncovertebral joint hypertrophy
	Facet joint hypertrophy
	Ligamentous origin (ligamentum flavum hypertrophy/ ossification, ossification of the posterior longitudinal ligament, diffuse idiopathic skeletal hyperostosis)
	Spondylosis
	Metabolic causes
	Postinflammatory abnormality
	Spondylolisthesis
	Postoperative abnormality
	Neoplasm
Congenital	Idiopathic stenosis with short pedicles
	Skeletal growth disorders
	Down syndrome
	Achondroplasia
	Mucopolysaccharidosis
	Scoliosis

The degree of central canal stenosis can range from mild encroachment on the ventral subarachnoid space to severe compression and flattening of the spinal cord with myelomalacia. MRI findings may or may not correspond to the severity and duration of the compression.[54] Early changes of spinal cord compression can be seen as cord edema (high-signal areas on T2-weighted images)[64]; progressive compression may cause spinal cord necrosis and atrophy (▶ Fig. 15.25), cystic degeneration, and syrinx formation (low signal on T1-weighted and high signal on T2-weighted images).[54]

Given that most cervical spine MRI studies are obtained to evaluate for the presence, location, and degree of degenerative cervical spinal stenosis, one should use a systematic approach to the evaluation of these studies. The authors' suggested approach for the evaluation of a cervical spine MRI study (see Chapter 3, A Systematic Approach to the Review of Spine MRI Studies) includes a critical evaluation of the degree of spinal cord and nerve root compression on sagittal, parasagittal, and axial T2-weighted images. Midline sagittal T2-weighted images provide a global view of the levels and degree of effacement of the CSF column and spinal cord compression, whereas parasagittal images enable visualization of

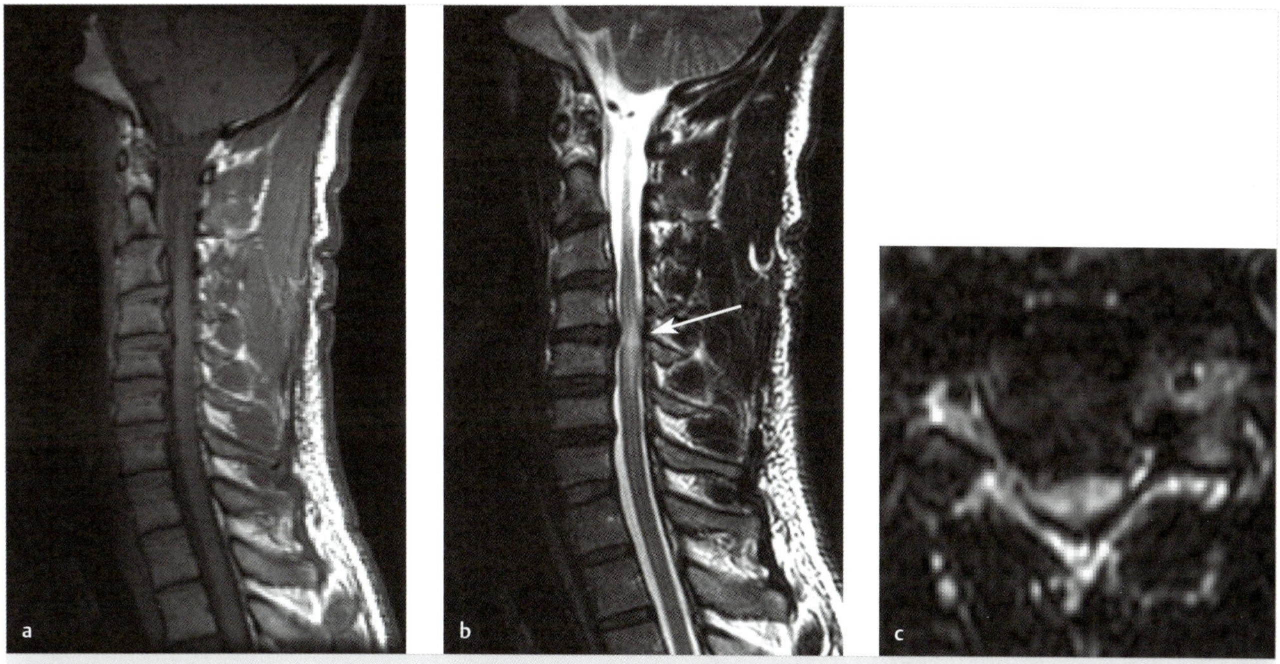

Fig. 15.23 Degenerative stenosis superimposed on congenital stenosis. **(a)** A sagittal T1-weighted image shows a developmentally shortened AP dimension of the spinal canal. **(b)** A sagittal T2-weighted image shows a small disk bulge at the C4–C5 level that causes spinal cord signal abnormality, representing spondylotic myelomalacia *(arrow)*. **(c)** An axial T2-weighted image shows moderate to severe central canal stenosis. (Reproduced with permission from, Zebala LP, Buchowski JM, Daftary AR, et al. The cervical spine. In: Khanna AJ, ed. MRI Essentials for the Spine Specialist. New York: Thieme; 2014:111–154.)

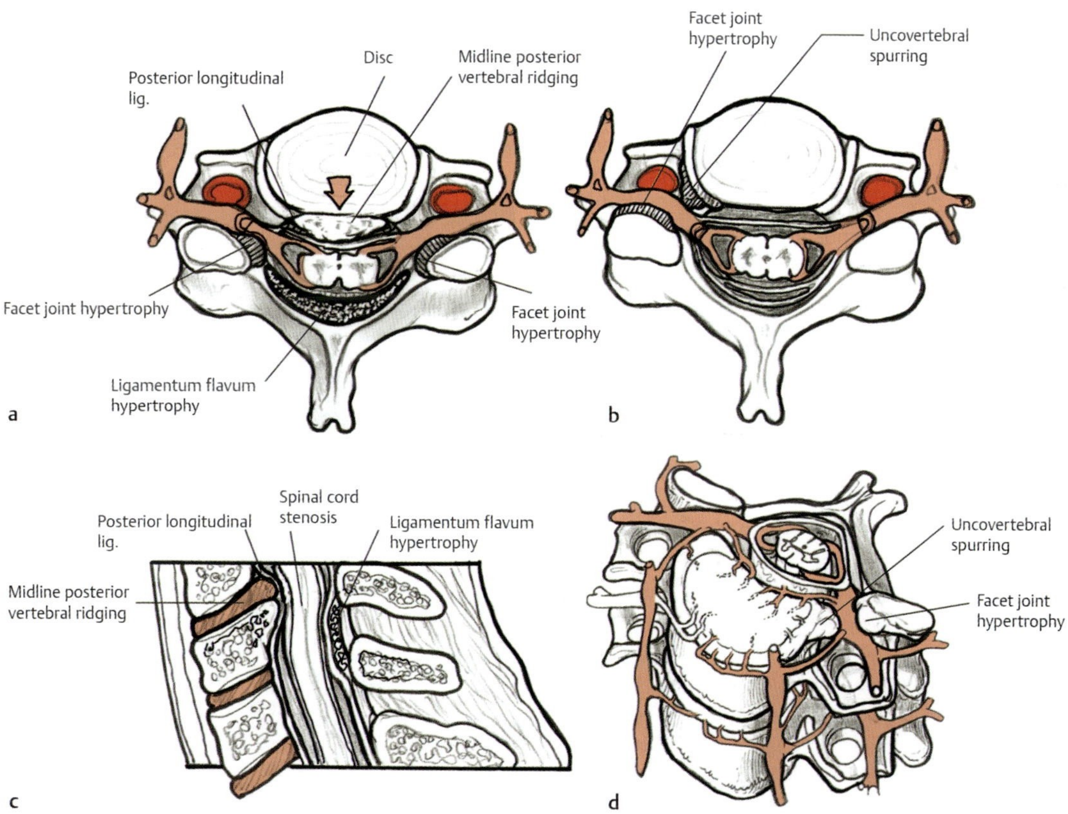

Fig. 15.24 Illustration showing various potential contributors to cervical spinal stenosis: central disk bulge, facet joint hypertrophy, and ligamentum flavum hypertrophy. **(a)** An axial view shows central stenosis. **(b)** An axial view shows foraminal stenosis. **(c)** A lateral view shows central stenosis with cord compression. **(d)** A 3D superolateral view shows foraminal stenosis. (Reproduced with permission from, Zebala LP, Buchowski JM, Daftary AR, et al. The cervical spine. In: Khanna AJ, ed. MRI Essentials for the Spine Specialist. New York: Thieme; 2014:111–154.)

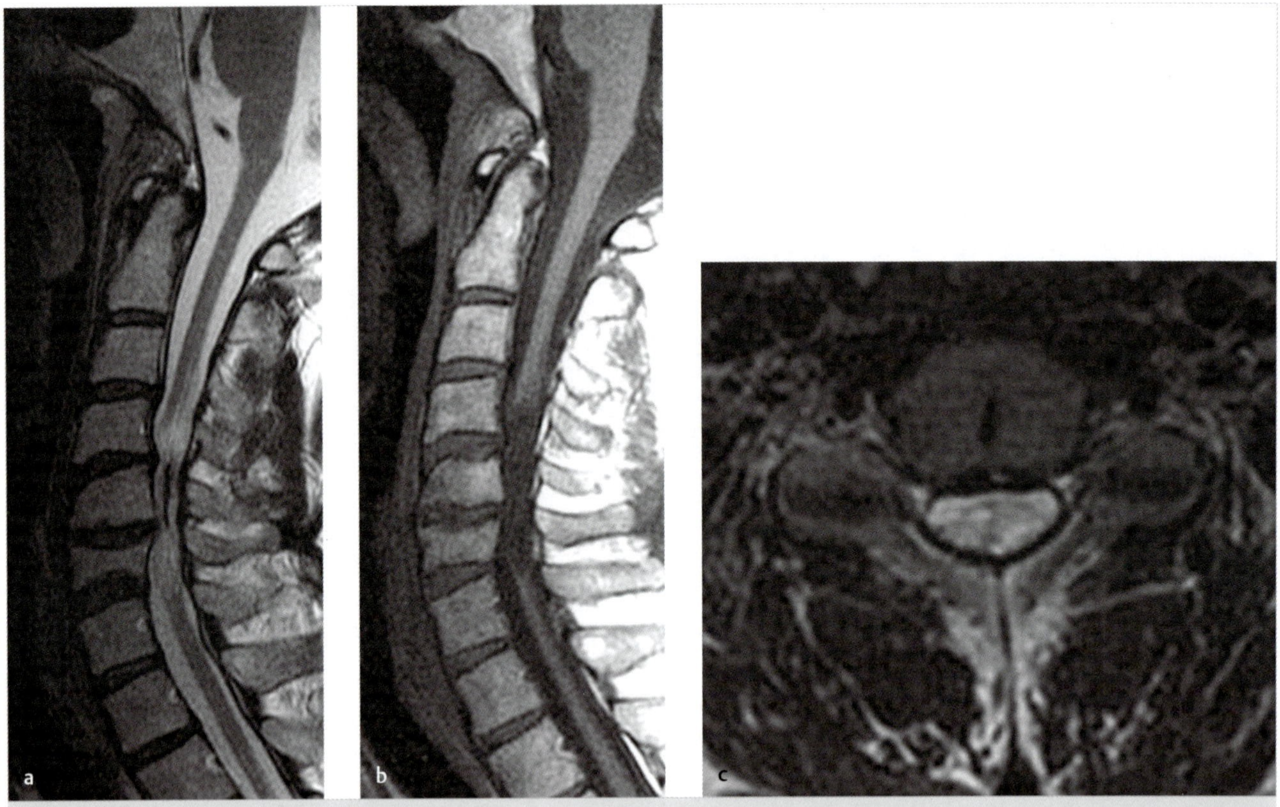

Fig. 15.25 Spinal cord atrophy. **(a)** A sagittal T2-weighted image shows moderate-severe stenosis at C4–C6, with resultant atrophy of the spinal cord at the level of C5 and regions of cord edema proximal and distal to the region of atrophy. **(b)** A sagittal T1-weighted image shows a segment of low signal intensity within the spinal cord from C4–C5 to C6–C7. **(c)** An axial T2-weighted image at the C4–C5 level shows atrophy of the spinal cord and indistinct margins between the spinal cord and the surrounding cerebrospinal fluid (CSF). (Reproduced with permission from, Zebala LP, Buchowski JM, Daftary AR, et al. The cervical spine. In: Khanna AJ, ed. MRI Essentials for the Spine Specialist. New York: Thieme; 2014:111–154.)

lateral recess and foraminal stenosis (▶ Fig. 15.26). The information from these images should be correlated with that from the axial images, which show the same abnormality in an orthogonal plane.

There are several objective measures of cervical spinal stenosis. Relative stenosis is defined as an AP canal diameter of < 13 mm, and absolute stenosis is defined as an AP canal diameter of < 10 mm. The Torg or Pavlov ratio is calculated by dividing the AP canal diameter by the AP vertebral body diameter, with a ratio < 0.8 defined as stenotic.[65] This ratio is often used to evaluate for congenital stenosis in athletes. Although such definitions are well known, most clinicians and radiologists typically grade the degree of spinal stenosis using the terms *mild, moderate,* and *severe,* and gradations such as *moderate-severe.* The authors use the following terms and definitions (▶ Fig. 15.27):

- Mild: stenosis occupying less than one-third of normal canal dimension, in which the ventral and dorsal CSF spaces are partially effaced by disk bulging, ligamentum flavum hypertrophy, and facet arthropathy; no mass effect on the cord.
- Moderate: stenosis occupying between one-third and two-thirds of normal canal dimension; findings similar to those of mild stenosis but with compression and minimal flattening and deformity of the spinal cord.
- Severe: stenosis occupying more than two-thirds of normal canal dimension, with very pronounced flattening and deformity of the spinal cord that is obvious on sagittal and axial T2-weighted images.

15.3.4 Rheumatoid Arthritis

Rheumatoid arthritis (RA) is a systemic disease that causes inflammation of synovial joints. The synovial joints develop pannus secondary to erosion of supporting ligamentous structures and the associated instability.[66,67,68] In the cervical spine, this condition may affect the craniocervical junction, as well as the subaxial cervical spine, as described subsequently.[66,67,68,69,70] Most commonly, atlantoaxial instability develops secondary to erosion of the ligaments at the OCJ.[66,67] As the disease progresses, erosion of the lateral masses of C1, the occipital condyles, and facets of C2 occurs, causing cranial settling.[66,67,68] As the odontoid process begins to occupy a more rostral position, it compresses the brainstem and vertebrobasilar system. This pathologic process is postulated by some as the cause of sudden death in those with advanced RA.[66,67,68,71] In contrast to other disorders, the C1 arch migrates with the skull base to lie in a more caudal position.[68] In some cases, it has been reported to be as inferior as the C2–C3 disk space.[66,67,68,72] Two studies

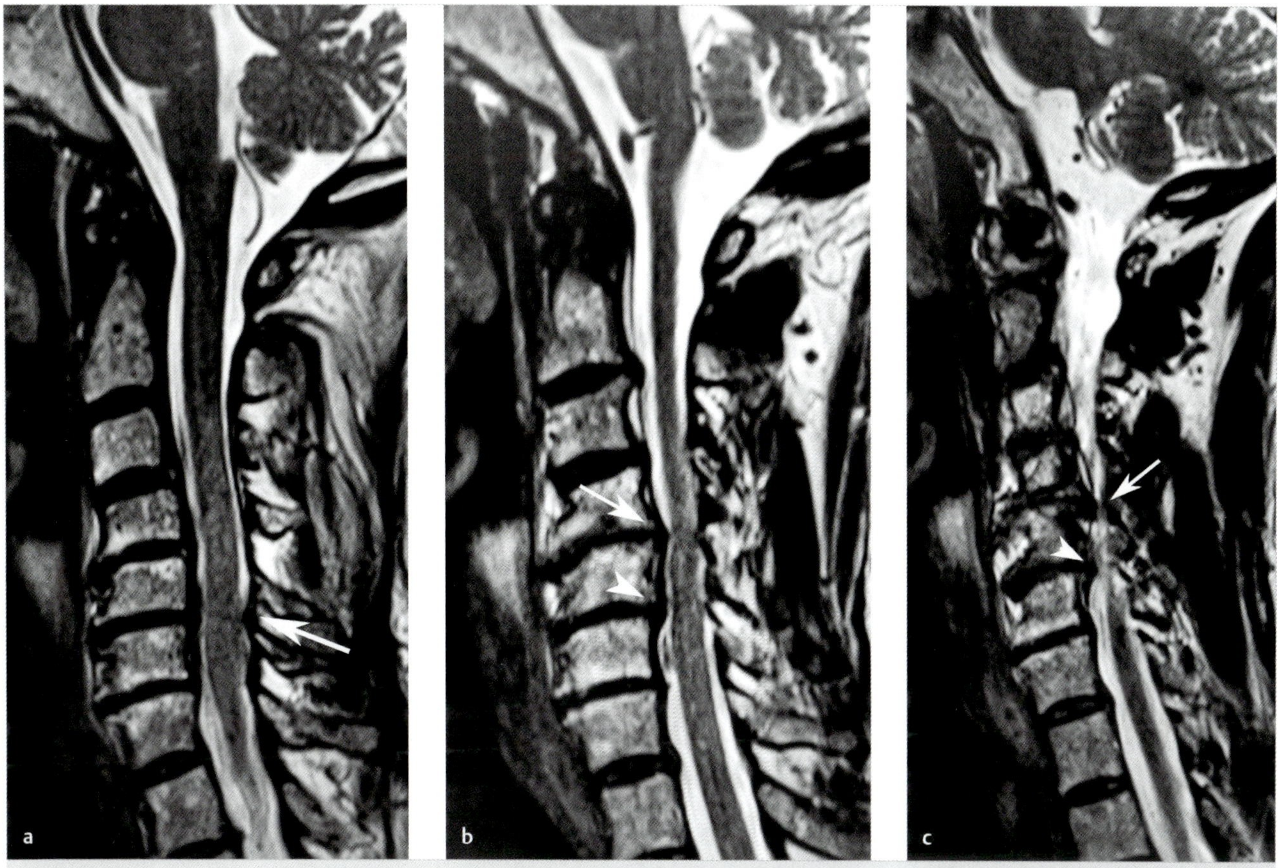

Fig. 15.26 Cervical stenosis. **(a)** A midline sagittal T2-weighted image shows multilevel degenerative disk disease with mild spondylolisthesis at C3–C4 and thickening of the posterior longitudinal ligament at multiple levels. There is focal thickening of the ligamentum flavum at the C5–C6 level (*arrow*). **(b)** A parasagittal T2-weighted image obtained several millimeters lateral to the midline shows effacement of the ventral cerebrospinal fluid (CSF) space and moderate stenosis at the C4–C5 level (*arrow*) caused by osteophyte formation and thickening of the posterior longitudinal ligament. Similar, but less severe, changes are seen at the C5–C6 level (*arrowhead*). **(c)** A parasagittal T2-weighted image obtained farther laterally in the plane of the neuroforamina shows severe foraminal stenosis at the C4–C5 level (*arrow*) and moderate foraminal stenosis at the C5–C6 level (*arrowhead*). (Reproduced with permission from, Zebala LP, Buchowski JM, Daftary AR, et al. The cervical spine. In: Khanna AJ, ed. MRI Essentials for the Spine Specialist. New York: Thieme; 2014:111–154.)

reported on the use of MRI to measure the space available for the cord as a technique for predicting recovery after cervical stabilization for patients with RA and atlantoaxial instability.[66,67] A cord space, or space available for the cord, of > 14 mm on MRI was associated with better clinical outcomes than was a space of < 10 mm, which was associated with a poor prognosis.[66,67] Flexion-extension MRI is particularly useful for evaluating patients with RA and those with instability at the OCJ and suboccipital cervical spine (► Fig. 15.28), especially because supine extension MRI does not account for the commonly occurring subluxations in such patients that are exaggerated with movement. Similar information can be obtained by combining the information obtained from a static (conventional) MRI study and flexion-extension cervical spine radiographs (► Fig. 15.9).

MRI can detect pannus formation in the cervical spine well before conventional radiographic signs become evident. In addition, involvement of the facet joints (inflammation, edema, and fusion) may be detected on MRI.[73] Patients with RA may also present with rheumatoid diskitis that appears as increased T2-weighted signal and decreased T1-weighted signal in the disk. The substantial differences between imaging and clinical features of RA in the spine have been documented and are well known.[74,75]

15.4 Infectious Conditions

The treatment of spinal infections continues to be a challenge despite advances in imaging, diagnostic testing, and antimicrobial therapy. A delay in diagnosis is common because spinal infections often have an early indolent course and early symptoms may be nonspecific (e.g., neck pain, muscle spasm), leading to a misdiagnosis of more common spinal ailments (e.g., muscle strain, degenerative disease). Spine infections may involve the vertebral body, posterior elements, intervertebral disks, epidural space, subdural space, subarachnoid space, or spinal cord.

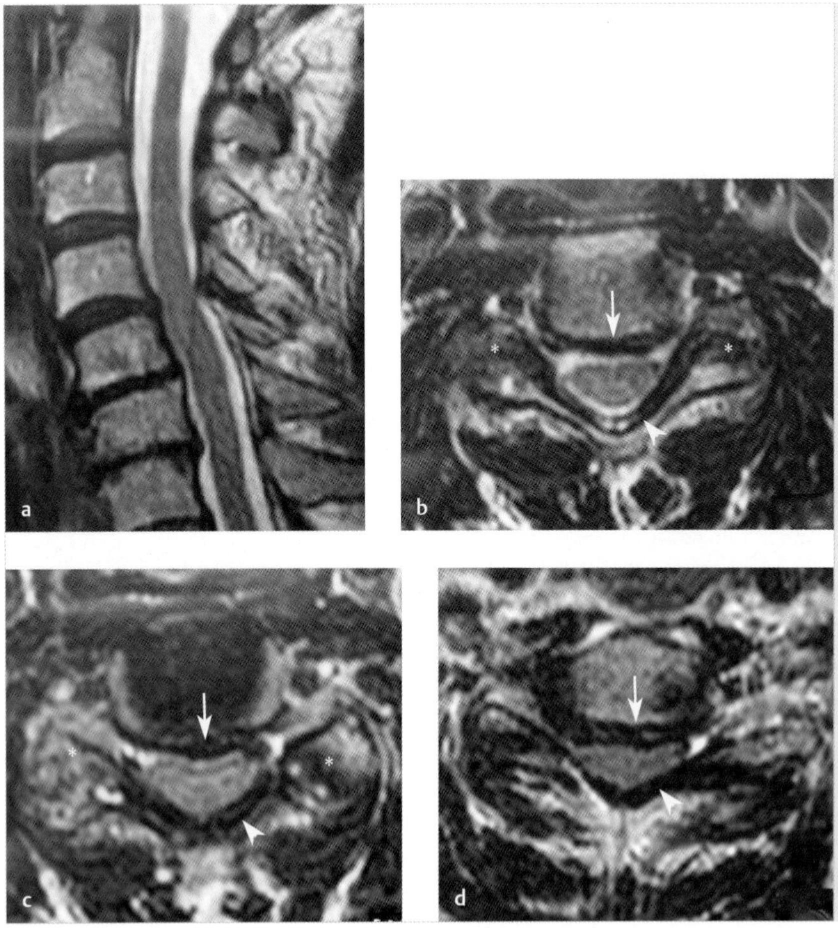

Fig. 15.27 Grading of cervical stenosis: mild to moderate-severe. **(a)** A sagittal T2-weighted image shows minimal spondylolisthesis at C4–C5 with moderate stenosis at this level. **(b)** An axial T2-weighted image at the C5–C6 level shows mild stenosis secondary to a central disk bulge (*arrow*), ligamentum flavum hypertrophy (*arrowhead*), and facet arthropathy (*asterisk*). **(c)** An axial T2-weighted image at the C4–C5 level shows moderate stenosis secondary to more substantial central disk bulge (*arrow*), ligamentum flavum hypertrophy (*arrowhead*), and facet arthropathy (*asterisk*). **(d)** An axial T2-weighted image (different patient) shows moderate-to-severe stenosis at the C5–C6 level as a result of even greater central disk bulge (*arrow*) and ligamentum flavum hypertrophy (*arrowhead*). (Reproduced with permission from, Zebala LP, Buchowski JM, Daftary AR, et al. The cervical spine. In: Khanna AJ, ed. MRI Essentials for the Spine Specialist. New York: Thieme; 2014:111–154.)

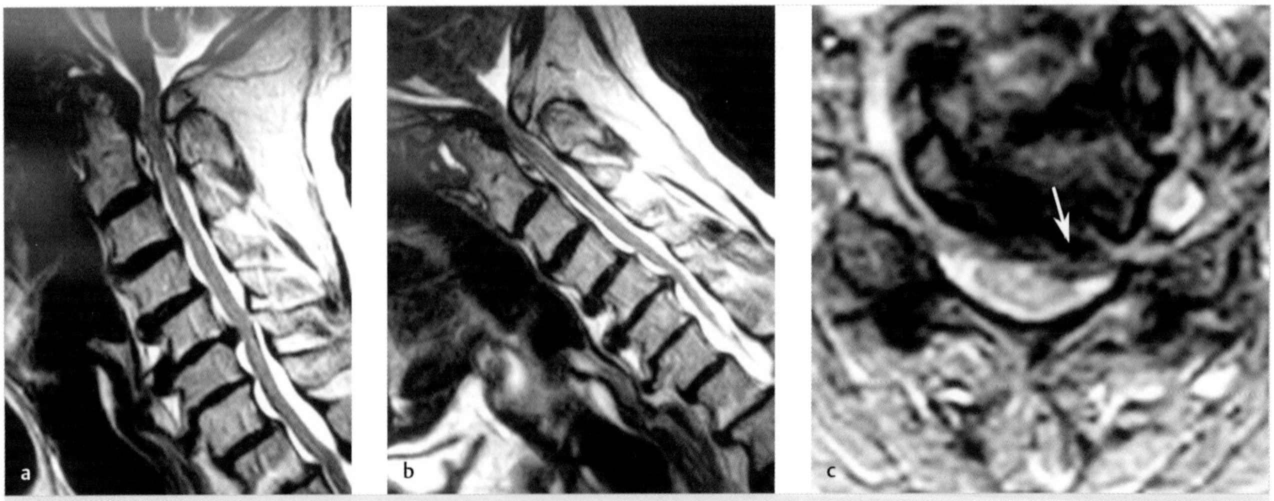

Fig. 15.28 Occipitocervical stenosis. **(a)** A sagittal T2-weighted image obtained with the patient in neutral position shows moderate stenosis at the occipitocervical junction (OCJ) and at the C5–C6 level. Multilevel degenerative disk disease is also seen. **(b)** A sagittal T2-weighted image in flexion shows exacerbation of the occipitocervical stenosis to severe. **(c)** An axial T2-weighted image at the C5–C6 level shows moderate stenosis at the C5–C6 level from degenerative changes and a left paracentral disk protrusion (*arrow*). (Reproduced with permission from, Zebala LP, Buchowski JM, Daftary AR, et al. The cervical spine. In: Khanna AJ, ed. MRI Essentials for the Spine Specialist. New York: Thieme; 2014:111–154.)

15.4.1 Cervical Vertebral Osteomyelitis and Diskitis

Infections of the cervical spine account for ~10% of spine infections and are less common than thoracic (~40%) or lumbar (~50%) spine infections.[76] Anatomic differences between the cervical and thoracolumbar spine (smaller canal diameter relative to the size of the spinal cord, intervertebral disks, and epidural space, and a vast venous plexus) may allow cervical spine infections to have a more aggressive and rapid progression that requires expedited treatment.[77] The clinical presentation of vertebral osteomyelitis and diskitis has variable signs and symptoms that do not vary with activity level, including fever (~50% of the time), weight loss, and neck or back pain. Neurologic symptoms vary according to the level of spinal involvement, spinal cord compression, spinal instability, or deformity.[20,21,76,77,78,79] Neurologic deficits secondary to spinal infection are more common in patients > 50 years old and in those with comorbidities such as diabetes, RA, and immunodeficiency.[20,76]

Bacterial inoculation of the spine may occur through hematogenous seeding, direct inoculation, or contiguous spread from local infection. *Staphylococcus aureus* is the most commonly cultured organism causing cervical osteomyelitis and diskitis.[76,77] It is found in 50 to 65% of culture-positive cases and accounts for > 80% of spinal infections in children.[80] Gram-negative infections (*Escherichia coli, Pseudomonas, Proteus*) may occur after genitourinary infections. Immunocompromised patients are susceptible to infections with atypical pathogens such as *Aspergillus, Candida, Nocardia asteroides,* and *Mycobacterium. Pseudomonas* infections may occur in intravenous drug abusers. Children with sickle cell disease may develop spine infections secondary to *Salmonella.*

Isolated diskitis is common in children because vascularity extends through the cartilaginous growth plate into the nucleus pulposus, allowing direct deposition of bacteria into the disk center. In adults, blood vessels reach only the annulus fibrosus, limiting bacterial deposition to the vertebral body metaphysis and end plate. In adult infections, intervertebral disk destruction may occur through bacterial proteolytic enzyme infiltration.

MRI is the imaging modality of choice for the diagnosis and evaluation of spinal infections and for monitoring the response to treatment.[77] High sensitivity (96%), specificity (93%), and accuracy (94%) have been reported for the MRI diagnosis of vertebral osteomyelitis.[61] MRI is more sensitive than conventional radiographs or CT and more specific than nuclear scintigraphy in identifying vertebral osteomyelitis.[77] Infectious spondylitis may present with findings such as low T1-weighted signal with or without high T2-weighted signal (high signal is often more evident on fat-suppressed T2-weighted or STIR images); increased T2-weighted signal within the intervertebral disk; contrast enhancement in the disk, subchondral marrow, and epidural space; erosion of end plates; epidural fluid collections; paraspinous soft-tissue abnormalities; and posterior element involvement (▶ Fig. 15.29).[20,77,79,81] Unfortunately, these imaging characteristics are the same as those of many spine abnormalities, including neoplastic disease. One can differentiate infection from other processes affecting the vertebral body bone marrow by noting that the epicenter of the former abnormality tends to be at the intervertebral disk. Conversely, neoplastic processes tend to have their epicenters within the vertebral body, and the edema tends not to cross the intervertebral disk. In addition, the vertebral end plate may have an irregular appearance because of infectious destruction, and disk height loss or collapse may occur with progressive infection. On gadolinium-enhanced images, disk enhancement is an essential factor for the diagnosis of diskitis, and enhancement of the vertebral subchondral bone may indicate a well-established and chronic infection.[20,77,79]

In comparison with other bacterial infections, *Mycobacterium tuberculosis* infection of the spine has some distinct differences:

- Intervertebral disks are damaged less or spared completely and may not show signal enhancement on T2-weighted images.[77]
- Tuberculous spondylodiskitis is a slow-growing process that is often associated with marked collapse of the vertebral bodies.
- Subligamentous spread of infection is often observed.
- Telescoping of one vertebral body disk into an adjacent level may be seen.

Gadolinium-enhanced MRI is essential for monitoring the efficacy of treatment of vertebral infection.[82] With appropriate treatment of the infection, a regression of the T2-weighted signal hyperintensity is observed.[79] Scar formation within the intervertebral disk is seen as a region of low signal intensity. A region of mottled signal intensity may also develop within the area of previous infection with associated contrast enhancement. Over time, osteophytic bridging may occur, followed by segmental fusion.[79] A lack of improvement on MRI and even deterioration of MRI features in the setting of clinical improvement do not necessarily indicate failure of treatment.[83,84]

In patients after surgery, evaluation for cervical spine infection may be complicated by the normal enhancement of the uninfected disk. MRI findings of infection in a patient after surgery include contrast enhancement of the subchondral bone and marrow adjacent to the infected disk.[77] Graft material and native vertebrae should not enhance within the first few days after spinal surgery. After several months, graft enhancement occurs, but it is often less intense and less uniform than that caused by infection. Bone graft usually has high signal intensity on T2-weighted images during the first postoperative year, and the signal decreases gradually as the bone graft is vascularized and fused.[77] An enhancing mass adjacent to the graft or a graft dislodgment is a sign of potential infection.[77]

15.4.2 Epidural Abscess

A spinal epidural abscess is a collection of purulent material outside the dura mater. An epidural abscess is usually associated with vertebral osteomyelitis, and direct extension from an adjacent infected vertebral body is the most common source for an epidural abscess.[77] Epidural abscesses are less common in the cervical spine than in the thoracic and lumbar spine and may be located anterior or posterior to the spinal cord.[77] Multiple spinal segments are usually involved (most commonly, C4–C7).[77]

Along with the increase in the number of patients with risk factors for spinal infections, the number of patients with

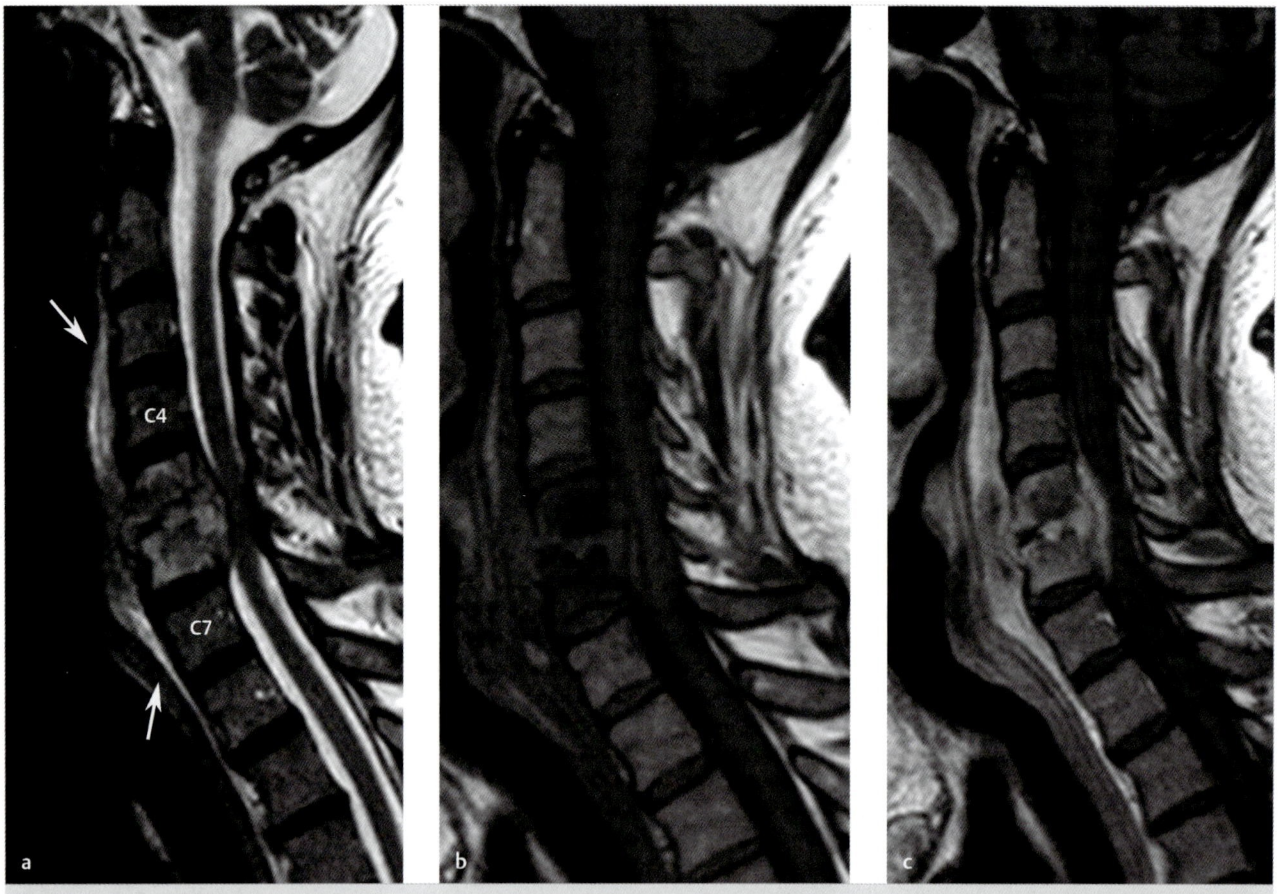

Fig. 15.29 Cervical spine diskitis and osteomyelitis. **(a)** A sagittal T2-weighted image shows obliteration of the C5–C6 disk space with associated edema in the C5–C6 vertebral bodies and an associated epidural component, which produces moderate spinal stenosis in a patient with infectious symptoms and findings. Note the prevertebral edema and soft-tissue fullness (between *arrows*). **(b)** Pregadolinium and **(c)** postgadolinium T1-weighted images show enhancement at the disk space, in the vertebral body's epidural component, and in the prevertebral space. (Reproduced with permission from, Zebala LP, Buchowski JM, Daftary AR, et al. The cervical spine. In: Khanna AJ, ed. MRI Essentials for the Spine Specialist. New York: Thieme; 2014:111–154.)

cervical epidural abscess is also increasing. The risk factors associated with vertebral osteomyelitis include the following:

- Age > 50 years.
- Alcoholism.
- Diabetes.
- Immunodeficiency (e.g., from medications, human immunodeficiency virus).
- Intravenous drug abuse.
- Male sex.
- Malignancy.
- Malnutrition.
- Obesity.
- Previous spinal procedure.
- Recent systemic illness.
- Tobacco use.
- Trauma.

These factors also increase the risk of developing an epidural abscess. The clinical presentation of an epidural abscess may be similar to that of vertebral osteomyelitis. Mass effect from the abscess compressing the spinal cord or nerve roots may present as radiculopathy, myelopathy, or paralysis.

As it is for vertebral osteomyelitis, MRI is the diagnostic study of choice for the evaluation of an epidural abscess.[20,77,79] Gadolinium-enhanced, fat-suppressed, T1-weighted images provide anatomic detail of the location and extension of the abscess and any associated vertebral infections.[77] T2-weighted and fat-suppressed T2-weighted images also show the boundaries of the epidural abscess and allow for the assessment of the degree of spinal cord compression. Gadolinium enhancement patterns vary from a thin, peripheral pattern, which may represent a collection of liquefied pus with a surrounding rim, to a homogeneous pattern seen with a phlegmon. The spinal cord may be evaluated for the level and amount of compression.

15.4.3 Intradural Infections

Intradural infections may be categorized as subdural abscess, leptomeningitis, or myelitis. A subdural abscess, which is clinically indistinguishable from an epidural abscess, is caused by direct extension from an epidural abscess, hematogenous spread, or iatrogenic contamination. Gadolinium-enhanced MRI shows the enhancing intradural-extramedullary abscess next to a compressed spinal cord. T2-weighted images show an associated signal intensity change within the spinal cord secondary to compression, ischemia, or myelitis.

Spinal leptomeningeal infections can be caused by many organisms, including *Neisseria meningitidis, Coccidioides immitis, Cryptococcus* sp., *Treponema pallidum,* and viral organisms. Gadolinium-enhanced MRI shows abnormal meningeal enhancement along the surface of the cord or nerve roots.[85] Meningeal enhancement can be seen incidentally over the brain, but meningeal enhancement of the spinal cord is abnormal.

Spinal cord infections and abscesses are uncommon and are associated with an increased mortality rate.[77,79] Hematogenous seeding of bacteria is the most common cause. Early cord infection shows increased T2-weighted signal and poorly defined enhancement with gadolinium.[77,79] Progressive infection may cause spinal cord cavitation, depicted as areas of low signal intensity on T1-weighted images and high signal intensity on T2-weighted images. In addition, the spinal cord may become edematous and enlarged from the infection, with MRI characteristics as described previously.

15.5 Other Pathologic Conditions

15.5.1 Tumors

Spine tumors are categorized by their anatomic location (see Chapter 21, Tumors of the Spine) as follows[78]:

- Extradural.
- Intradural-extramedullary.
- Intramedullary.

A reasonable differential diagnosis may be established by incorporating a clinical history, a physical examination, a basic understanding of possible tumor location, and the MRI examination findings.[78] A definitive diagnosis often requires a biopsy of the lesion.

MRI is an effective technique for imaging spine tumors because it accomplishes the following:

- Provides unparalleled soft-tissue detail.
- Allows evaluation of the neural elements.
- Shows important tissue characteristics of the tumor (e.g., vascularity, density, vascular perfusion, extent of marrow involvement).
- Allows assessment of the extent of spinal cord compression.

The entire spine needs to be evaluated because of possible skip lesions from intrathecal seeding, multiple primary sites, or a syrinx. The spinal cord can be screened with sagittal T1-weighted SE images and sagittal T2-weighted FSE images to obtain a myelogram-like examination of the spinal cord. Axial images may be helpful for specific areas of interest. Contrast enhancement improves the detection of most intramedullary and intradural-extramedullary tumors.[78] However, gadolinium enhancement may obscure the contrast between metastatic lesions and normal bone marrow if fat suppression is not applied.[86] Gradient-echo images usually are not helpful in imaging spinal cord tumors because of the limited ability to distinguish between soft tissue or tumor and CSF. For osseous tumors, gradient-echo imaging may show areas of calcification or hemorrhage within the tumor (see Chapter 21, Tumors of the Spine, for a more detailed discussion).[86]

15.5.2 Intrinsic Inflammatory Myelopathies

The most common cause of myelopathy is extrinsic compression. Although orthopaedic surgeons typically do not treat intrinsic inflammatory myelopathies, they should realize that they exist and can be differentiated from myelopathy secondary to extrinsic compression.[87] A basic understanding of these processes is important so that surgery is not considered for the treatment of a patient who presents with an intrinsic inflammatory myelopathy in the presence of incidentally noted or minimal stenosis. Briefly described in the following paragraphs are the most common inflammatory myelopathies affecting the cervical spinal cord and their appearance on MRI.[78]

Multiple Sclerosis

Approximately 60 to 75% of multiple sclerosis plaques outside the brain occur in the cervical spinal cord, and 90% of patients with cord plaques also have brain plaques.[88,89] Most plaques span two or fewer vertebral levels, occupy less than half the spinal cord diameter, and are located peripherally in the spinal cord.[89] MRI findings may include increased signal on T2-weighted sequences, decreased signal on T1-weighted images, patchy cord enhancement with gadolinium administration, and cord swelling or atrophy with larger plaques (▶ Fig. 15.30).[90]

Acute Transverse Myelopathy

Acute transverse myelitis is a monophasic, acute inflammatory condition of the entire spinal cord that produces motor, sensory, and sphincter impairment. There are multiple causes, including inflammatory processes, viral infections, vascular disorders, collagen vascular disease, postinfectious states, and idiopathic processes.[88] MRI findings vary, with T2-weighted pulse sequences showing areas of hyperintensity of various length and width often involving more than three or four spinal segments.[91] Enlargement of the spinal cord and gadolinium enhancement also vary.[92]

Subacute Necrotizing Myelopathy

Subacute necrotizing myelopathy is a rare, progressive myelopathy that usually occurs in elderly persons and often is attributed to spinal dural arteriovenous fistula, causing venous congestion, ischemia, and infarction of the spinal cord. Symptoms range from spastic to flaccid paraparesis, sensory abnormalities, and bowel and bladder dysfunction. MRI typically shows a long segment of fusiform cord swelling and edema with peripheral contrast enhancement.[88]

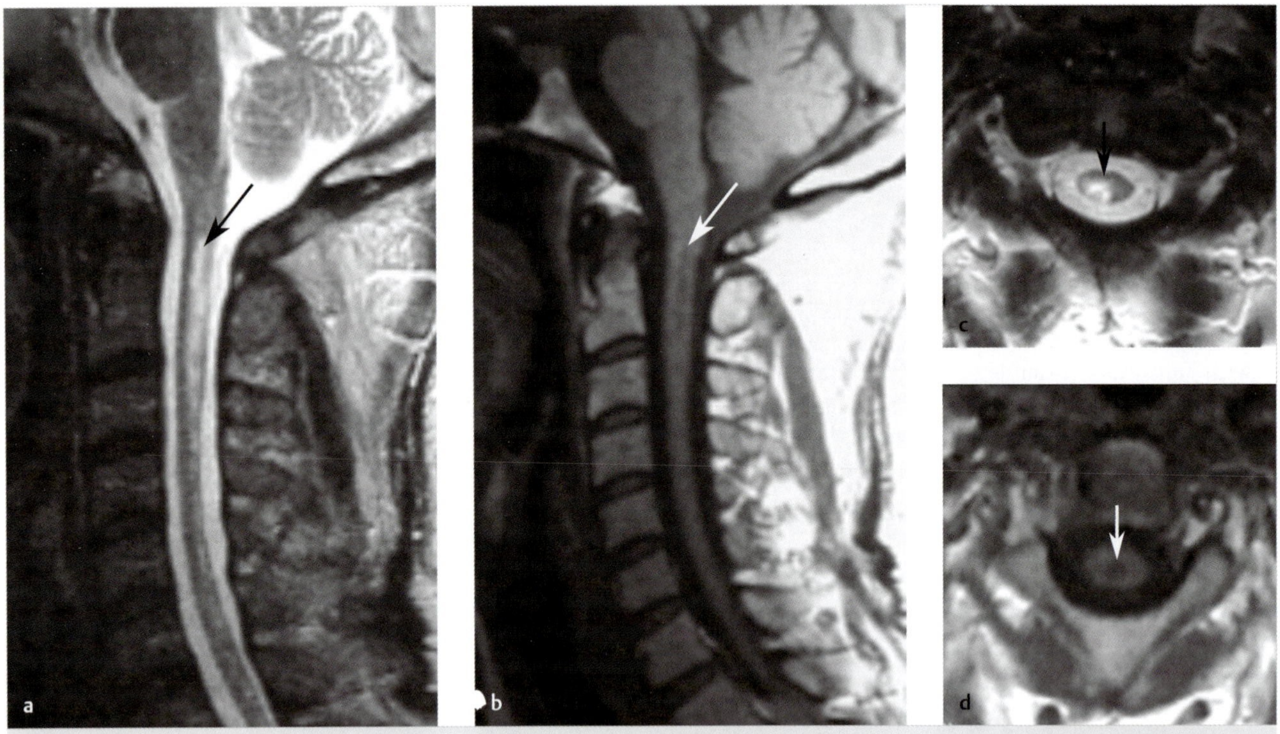

Fig. 15.30 Multiple sclerosis. **(a)** Sagittal T2-weighted, **(b)** sagittal T1-weighted, **(c)** axial T2-weighted, and **(d)** axial T1-weighted images show a focal region of increased **(a,c)** and decreased **(b,d)** signal within the spinal cord (*arrow* on each). In the appropriate clinical setting, these findings are compatible with multiple sclerosis; the diagnosis can be confirmed with lumbar puncture and cerebrospinal fluid (CSF) analysis. (Reproduced with permission from, Zebala LP, Buchowski JM, Daftary AR, et al. The cervical spine. In: Khanna AJ, ed. MRI Essentials for the Spine Specialist. New York: Thieme; 2014:111–154.)

Acquired Immune Deficiency Syndrome

Spinal cord disease in patients with acquired immune deficiency syndrome is common and includes human immunodeficiency virus myelitis and vacuolar myelopathy. Human immunodeficiency virus myelitis may be caused by direct human immunodeficiency virus infection, lymphoma, opportunistic infections, or metabolic and vascular disorders. Vacuolar myelopathy, a spongy degeneration primarily involving the posterior and lateral spinal columns causing progressive ataxia and paraparesis,[88] is the most common spinal cord disease associated with acquired immune deficiency syndrome.[93] T2-weighted MR images show cord atrophy and symmetric hyperintense focal lesions in the dorsal and lateral columns.[94] There is no cord swelling or gadolinium enhancement.

Viral Diseases

Viral infections of the spinal cord may be caused by multiple viruses affecting immunocompetent and immunocompromised patients. MRI characteristics of viral infection vary according to the causative organism and may include hyperintense areas on T2-weighted images; nerve root thickening, clumping, and enhancement; and diffuse atrophy.[88] Gadolinium enhancement varies by spinal cord area and characteristic, depending on which virus is causing the infection.

Bacterial, Parasitic, and Granulomatous Diseases

Clinical symptoms of myelitis, meningitis, and radiculitis can result from spinal cord invasion by bacterial, parasitic, or granulomatous infection. MRI findings vary and may include cord swelling, cord edema, rim-enhancing lesions, and nerve enhancement.[88]

Metabolic or Toxic Diseases

Subacute combined degeneration is a complication of vitamin B_{12} deficiency or nitrous oxide poisoning. The dorsal and lateral spinal columns show demyelination, axonal loss, and gliosis. MRI may show increased signal in the dorsal and lateral columns on T2-weighted images.[88] Radiation myelopathy is a progressive myelopathy typically seen in patients treated with radiation therapy for head or neck cancer. MRI may show cord swelling, edema, and contrast enhancement corresponding to cord necrosis, demyelination, and gliosis.[95]

15.5.3 Arthritides

Common arthritic conditions that affect the cervical spine and characteristic MRI findings are described in the following paragraphs. Imaging evaluation of these conditions often begins

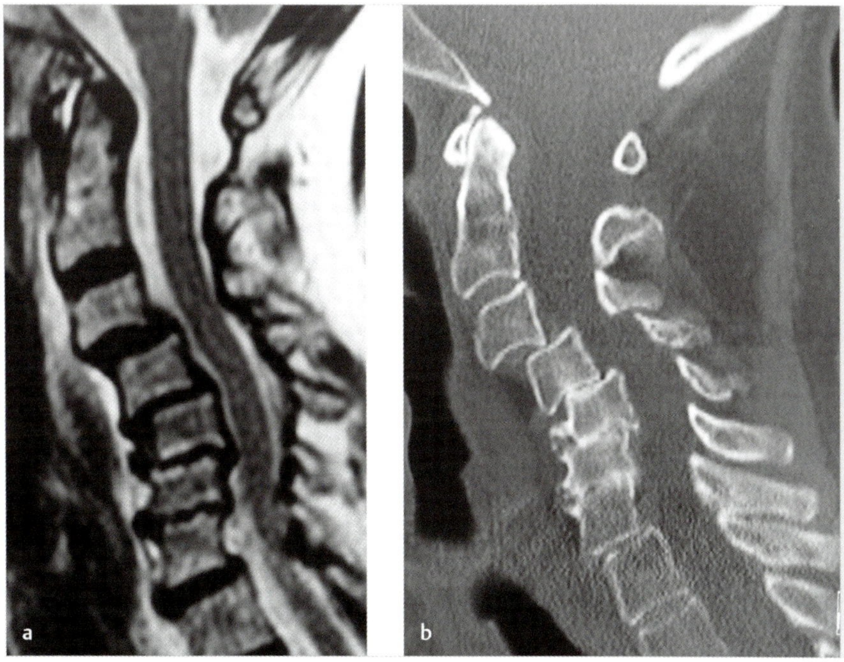

Fig. 15.31 Subaxial subluxation in rheumatoid arthritis (RA). (a) Sagittal T2-weighted and (b) sagittal reconstructed computed tomographic (CT) images show multilevel subaxial subluxation and degenerative disk disease. There is spondylolisthesis at C3–C4 and C4–C5 and retrolisthesis at C5–C6. Note the improved osseous detail provided by the CT image compared with the magnetic resonance (MR) image. (Reproduced with permission from, Zebala LP, Buchowski JM, Daftary AR, et al. The cervical spine. In: Khanna AJ, ed. MRI Essentials for the Spine Specialist. New York: Thieme; 2014:111–154.)

with conventional radiographs to assess the pattern and extent of osseous involvement. MRI is the preferred modality for the assessment of the spinal cord and neural elements.

Rheumatoid Arthritis

RA is the most common inflammatory arthropathy, and the cervical spine is the most common area of spinal involvement.[96] The destructive process is through an inflammatory synovitis, leading to bone, cartilage, ligament, and periarticular destruction. Clinical symptoms include pain, deformity, loss of mobility, paresthesias, myelopathy, radiculopathy, paralysis, and sudden death. MRI is useful for the evaluation of the craniocervical junction and for the assessment of atlantoaxial and subaxial subluxation, basilar invagination, and spinal cord compression (▸ Fig. 15.31).[96] In addition, MRI depicts the extent of periodontoid pannus formation, associated dens fractures, nodular fibrosis, and perivertebral erosions.[96] Patients with RA who are undergoing elective surgery for another musculoskeletal condition such as major joint replacement should be evaluated with cervical spine radiographs in flexion and extension views. If evidence of instability is noted on conventional radiographs, MRI should be considered to evaluate further, especially for atlantoaxial instability.

Juvenile Rheumatoid Arthritis

Juvenile RA is the most common connective tissue disorder in children and may present as one of three types: oligoarthritis (60%), polyarthritis (30%), or systemic disease (10%).[96] As it is for the adult form, MRI is excellent for identifying synovial hypertrophy, cartilage and bone destruction, and joint effusion in the juvenile form.[96]

Ankylosing Spondylitis

Ankylosing spondylitis, a seronegative spondyloarthropathy, is a chronic inflammatory arthropathy of unknown origin that affects ~1% of the general population[96] and predominantly involves the axial skeleton. Men are affected more often than women, and symptoms appear during late adolescence and early adulthood. The disease begins in the thoracolumbar and lumbosacral junctions and ascends to involve the thoracic and cervical spine.[96] MRI is useful for the evaluation of early development of ankylosing spondylitis,[97] acute fractures, advanced degenerative changes, vertebral body subluxations, epidural hematoma, cord compression, and deformity.[96] MRI findings often provide guidance for medical and surgical treatment.[98]

A common clinical scenario is one in which a patient with known or previously unknown ankylosing spondylitis presents with a complaint of neck pain after minor trauma. Conventional radiographs may show ankylosis of the cervical (or lumbar) spine but no evidence of fracture or displacement. Such patients may have an unrecognized nondisplaced fracture. MRI can be obtained to rule out the presence of a nondisplaced fracture through the ankylosed spine. Such fractures are best seen on fat-suppressed T2-weighted images.

Psoriatic Arthritis

Psoriatic arthritis may present before skin lesions. Axial skeleton radiographic findings are similar to those seen with RA.[96] MRI may show disk space narrowing and erosions of the apophyseal joints, vertebral end plates, and spinous processes. On MRI, the atlantoaxial damage in patients with psoriatic arthritis is indistinguishable from that of patients with RA.[96]

Amyloidosis

Amyloidosis is characterized by extracellular deposition of insoluble fibrillar proteins throughout the body.[96] In addition, amyloidosis displays primary, secondary, familial, and dialysis-associated patterns. The dialysis-associated form, β_2-microglobulin, has a particular affinity for the musculoskeletal system and mimics inflammatory arthritis in its destructive nature.[96] The classic triad of β_2-microglobulin deposition involves shoulder pain, carpal tunnel syndrome, and scapulohumeral arthritis. It is also associated with destructive spondyloarthropathy of the cervical spine.[99] Amyloid deposits are found in the intervertebral disks, ligaments, and synovial tissue; the deposits have affinity for the atlantoaxial region.[96,99] Amyloid arthritis findings may mimic those of degenerative change, infectious destruction, inflammatory arthritides, or tumor. MRI is useful for distinguishing amyloid deposition destruction from others in the differential diagnosis. Amyloid deposits exhibit low signal intensity on MRI sequences and have variable enhancement patterns on contrast-supplemented sequences.[96]

Gout

Gout, which is caused by an imbalance in uric acid metabolism, is characterized by polyarticular inflammation, soft-tissue tophi, gouty nephritis, and renal stones. The classic presentation is monoarticular inflammation involving the first metatarsophalangeal joint. Gouty involvement of the spine, especially cervical and lumbar regions, is rare and is seen in patients with long-standing peripheral articular manifestations.[96] MRI characteristics of gouty tophi include intermediate signal intensity on T1-weighted images, variable signal intensity on T2-weighted images, and variable contrast enhancement patterns.[100]

Calcium Pyrophosphate Dihydrate Deposition Disease

This common crystal-induced arthritis affects peripheral joints and occasionally the spine. Spinal involvement may include calcium deposition in the intervertebral disks or ligaments. Areas affected with calcium pyrophosphate dihydrate deposition appear as isointense or hypointense signal on T1-weighted images relative to brain tissue, mixed signal intensity on T2-weighted images, and marked peripheral enhancement with gadolinium.[96] Sometimes, calcification may surround the dens, producing a characteristic "crowned dens" sign.

15.6 Common Clinical Questions

1. Which MRI pulse sequence is the best for evaluating the integrity of the posterior ligamentous complex in patients with known or suspected cervical spine trauma?
   a) Axial T1-weighted images.
   b) Axial T2-weighted images.
   c) Sagittal T1-weighted images.
   d) Sagittal T2-weighted images.
   e) Sagittal STIR images.

2. What percentage of asymptomatic patients > 40 years old have evidence of degenerative disease on cervical spine MRI?
   a) 20%.
   b) 30%.
   c) 40%.
   d) 60%.
   e) 90%.

3. What diagnosis should be considered in a patient with clinical evidence of cervical radiculopathy and myelopathy and the single sagittal T2-weighted image shown in Figure 15.25b? What imaging study can be obtained to confirm this diagnosis?
   a) Multilevel disk protrusions; conventional radiographs.
   b) Multilevel disk herniations; conventional radiographs.
   c) Spinal tumor; MRI with and without gadolinium contrast enhancement.
   d) Ossification of the posterior longitudinal ligament; CT.
   e) Epidural abscess; MRI with and without gadolinium contrast enhancement.

4. What is the definition of absolute stenosis?
   a) AP canal diameter < 10 mm.
   b) AP canal diameter < 13 mm.
   c) Canal cross-sectional area < 100 mm^2.
   d) Torg ratio > 0.8.
   e) Torg ratio < 1.0.

5. What imaging study should be obtained to evaluate a patient with ankylosing spondylitis of the spine who presents with neck pain after a fall?
   a) Conventional radiographs only.
   b) Conventional radiographs and CT.
   c) Conventional radiographs and MRI.
   d) Single-photon emission CT scan.
   e) Three-phase bone scan.

References

[1] Henry M, Scarlata K, Riesenburger RI, et al. Utility of STIR MRI in pediatric cervical spine clearance after trauma. J Neurosurg Pediatr. 2013; 12(1): 30–36

[2] Lowery DW, Wald MM, Browne BJ, Tigges S, Hoffman JR, Mower WR, NEXUS Group. Epidemiology of cervical spine injury victims. Ann Emerg Med. 2001; 38(1):12–16

[3] Ackland HM, Cooper DJ, Malham GM, Stuckey SL. Magnetic resonance imaging for clearing the cervical spine in unconscious intensive care trauma patients. J Trauma. 2006; 60(3):668–673

[4] Carrino JA, Manton GL, Morrison WB, Vaccaro AR, Schweitzer ME, Flanders AE. Posterior longitudinal ligament status in cervical spine bilateral facet dislocations. Skeletal Radiol. 2006; 35(7):510–514

[5] Davis SJ, Teresi LM, Bradley WG, Jr, Ziemba MA, Bloze AE. Cervical spine hyperextension injuries: MR findings. Radiology. 1991; 180(1):245–251

[6] Flanders AE, Spettell CM, Tartaglino LM, Friedman DP, Herbison GJ. Forecasting motor recovery after cervical spinal cord injury: value of MR imaging. Radiology. 1996; 201(3):649–655

[7] Rizzolo SJ, Vaccaro AR, Cotler JM. Cervical spine trauma. Spine. 1994; 19 (20):2288–2298

[8] Silberstein M, Tress BM, Hennessy O. Delayed neurologic deterioration in the patient with spinal trauma: role of MR imaging. AJNR Am J Neuroradiol. 1992; 13(5):1373–1381

[9] Smith AS, Hurst GC, Duerk JL, Diaz PJ. MR of ballistic materials: imaging artifacts and potential hazards. AJNR Am J Neuroradiol. 1991; 12(3): 567–572

[10] Teitelbaum GP, Yee CA, Van Horn DD, Kim HS, Colletti PM. Metallic ballistic fragments: MR imaging safety and artifacts. Radiology. 1990; 175 (3):855–859

[11] Takhtani D, Melhem ER. MR imaging in cervical spine trauma. Magn Reson Imaging Clin N Am. 2000; 8(3):615–634

[12] Allen BL, Jr, Ferguson RL, Lehmann TR, O'Brien RP. A mechanistic classification of closed, indirect fractures and dislocations of the lower cervical spine. Spine. 1982; 7(1):1–27

[13] Khanna AJ, Kwon BK. Subaxial cervical spine injuries. In: Rao RD, Smuck M, eds. Orthopaedic knowledge update: spine 4. Rosemont, IL: American Academy of Orthopaedic Surgeons; 2012:221–233

[14] Bono CM, Schoenfeld A, Gupta G, et al. Reliability and reproducibility of subaxial cervical injury description system: a standardized nomenclature schema. Spine. 2011; 36(17):E1140–E1144

[15] Lin JL, Samuel S, Gray R, et al. Occult subaxial cervical disco-ligamentous injuries in computer tomography negative trauma patients. Eur Spine J. 2017; 26(4):1277–1283

[16] Vaccaro AR, Hulbert RJ, Patel AA, et al. Spine Trauma Study Group. The subaxial cervical spine injury classification system: a novel approach to recognize the importance of morphology, neurology, and integrity of the disco-ligamentous complex. Spine. 2007; 32(21):2365–2374

[17] Vaccaro AR, Madigan L, Schweitzer ME, Flanders AE, Hilibrand AS, Albert TJ. Magnetic resonance imaging analysis of soft tissue disruption after flexion-distraction injuries of the subaxial cervical spine. Spine. 2001; 26 (17):1866–1872

[18] Hart RA. Cervical facet dislocation: when is magnetic resonance imaging indicated? Spine. 2002; 27(1):116–117

[19] Lee JY, Nassr A, Eck JC, Vaccaro AR. Controversies in the treatment of cervical spine dislocations. Spine J. 2009; 9(5):418–423

[20] Boden SD, Lee RR, Herzog RJ. Magnetic resonance imaging of the spine. In: Frymoyer JW, ed. The adult spine: principles and practice. Philadelphia, PA: Lippincott-Raven; 1997:563–629

[21] Kaiser JA, Holland BA. Imaging of the cervical spine. Spine. 1998; 23(24): 2701–2712

[22] Mirvis SE. Use of MRI in acute spinal trauma. In: Uhlenbrock D, ed. MR imaging of the spine and spinal cord. New York: Thieme; 2004:437–465

[23] Kwon BK, Vaccaro AR, Grauer JN, Fisher CG, Dvorak MF. Subaxial cervical spine trauma. J Am Acad Orthop Surg. 2006; 14(2):78–89

[24] Li Q, Shen H, Li M. Magnetic resonance imaging signal changes of alar and transverse ligaments not correlated with whiplash-associated disorders: a meta-analysis of case-control studies. Eur Spine J. 2013; 22(1):14–20

[25] Ronnen HR, de Korte PJ, Brink PRG, van der Bijl HJ, Tonino AJ, Franke CL. Acute whiplash injury: is there a role for MR imaging? A prospective study of 100 patients. Radiology. 1996; 201(1):93–96

[26] Kwon BK, Hilibrand AS. Management of cervical fractures in patients with diffuse idiopathic skeletal hyperostosis. Curr Opin Orthop. 2003; 14(3): 187–192

[27] White ML. Cervical spine: MR imaging techniques and anatomy. Magn Reson Imaging Clin N Am. 2000; 8(3):453–470

[28] Quencer RM. The abnormal annulus fibrosus: can we infer the acuteness of an annular injury? AJNR Am J Neuroradiol. 2002; 23(7):1069

[29] Stadnik TW, Lee RR, Coen HL, Neirynck EC, Buisseret TS, Osteaux MJC. Annular tears and disk herniation: prevalence and contrast enhancement on MR images in the absence of low back pain or sciatica. Radiology. 1998; 206 (1):49–55

[30] Goldberg W, Mueller C, Panacek E, Tigges S, Hoffman JR, Mower WR, NEXUS Group. Distribution and patterns of blunt traumatic cervical spine injury. Ann Emerg Med. 2001; 38(1):17–21

[31] Adams VI. Neck injuries: I. Occipitoatlantal dislocation. A pathologic study of twelve traffic fatalities. J Forensic Sci. 1992; 37(2):556–564

[32] Adams VI. Neck injuries: III. Ligamentous injuries of the craniocervical articulation without occipito-atlantal or atlanto-axial facet dislocation. A pathologic study of 21 traffic fatalities. J Forensic Sci. 1993; 38(5):1097–1104

[33] Ahuja A, Glasauer FE, Alker GJ, Jr, Klein DM. Radiology in survivors of traumatic atlanto-occipital dislocation. Surg Neurol. 1994; 41(2):112–118

[34] Alker GJ, Jr, Oh YS, Leslie EV. High cervical spine and craniocervical junction injuries in fatal traffic accidents: a radiological study. Orthop Clin North Am. 1978; 9(4):1003–1010

[35] Goldberg AL, Baron B, Daffner RH. Atlantooccipital dislocation: MR demonstration of cord damage. J Comput Assist Tomogr. 1991; 15(1):174–175

[36] Bono CM, Vaccaro AR, Fehlings M, et al. Spine Trauma Study Group. Measurement techniques for upper cervical spine injuries: consensus statement of the Spine Trauma Study Group. Spine. 2007; 32(5):593–600

[37] Lee C, Woodring JH. Unstable Jefferson variant atlas fractures: an unrecognized cervical injury. AJNR Am J Neuroradiol. 1991; 12(6):1105–1110

[38] Spence KF, Jr, Decker S, Sell KW. Bursting atlantal fracture associated with rupture of the transverse ligament. J Bone Joint Surg Am. 1970; 52(3): 543–549

[39] Hadley MN, Walters BC, Grabb PA, et al. Management of vertebral artery injuries after nonpenetrating cervical trauma. Neurosurgery. 2002; 50(3) Suppl:S173–S178

[40] Even J, McCullough K, Braly B, et al. Clinical indications for arterial imaging in cervical trauma. Spine. 2012; 37(4):286–291

[41] Kathol MH. Cervical spine trauma. What is new? Radiol Clin North Am. 1997; 35(3):507–532

[42] Bowen BC, Pattany PM. Contrast-enhanced MR angiography of spinal vessels. Magn Reson Imaging Clin N Am. 2000; 8(3):597–614

[43] Bozzo A, Marcoux J, Radhakrishna M, Pelletier J, Goulet B. The role of magnetic resonance imaging in the management of acute spinal cord injury. J Neurotrauma. 2011; 28(8):1401–1411

[44] Eismont FJ, Arena MJ, Green BA. Extrusion of an intervertebral disc associated with traumatic subluxation or dislocation of cervical facets. Case report. J Bone Joint Surg Am. 1991; 73(10):1555–1560

[45] Robertson PA, Ryan MD. Neurological deterioration after reduction of cervical subluxation. Mechanical compression by disc tissue. J Bone Joint Surg Br. 1992; 74(2):224–227

[46] White AA, Southwick WO, Panjabi MM. Clinical instability in the lower cervical spine. A review of past and current concepts. Spine. 1976; 1(1): 15–27

[47] D'Alise MD, Benzel EC, Hart BL. Magnetic resonance imaging evaluation of the cervical spine in the comatose or obtunded trauma patient. J Neurosurg. 1999; 91(1) Suppl:54–59

[48] Stassen NA, Williams VA, Gestring ML, Cheng JD, Bankey PE. Magnetic resonance imaging in combination with helical computed tomography provides a safe and efficient method of cervical spine clearance in the obtunded trauma patient. J Trauma. 2006; 60(1):171–177

[49] Patel AA, Hurlbert RJ, Bono CM, Bessey JT, Yang N, Vaccaro AR. Classification and surgical decision making in acute subaxial cervical spine trauma. Spine. 2010; 35(21) Suppl:S228–S234

[50] Miyazaki M, Hymanson HJ, Morishita Y, et al. Kinematic analysis of the relationship between sagittal alignment and disc degeneration in the cervical spine. Spine. 2008; 33(23):E870–E876

[51] Miura J, Doita M, Miyata K, et al. Dynamic evaluation of the spinal cord in patients with cervical spondylotic myelopathy using a kinematic magnetic resonance imaging technique. J Spinal Disord Tech. 2009; 22(1):8–13

[52] Zhang L, Zeitoun D, Rangel A, Lazennec JY, Catonné Y, Pascal-Moussellard H. Preoperative evaluation of the cervical spondylotic myelopathy with flexion-extension magnetic resonance imaging: about a prospective study of fifty patients. Spine. 2011; 36(17):E1134–E1139

[53] Boden SD, McCowin PR, Davis DO, Dina TS, Mark AS, Wiesel S. Abnormal magnetic-resonance scans of the cervical spine in asymptomatic subjects. A prospective investigation. J Bone Joint Surg Am. 1990; 72(8): 1178–1184

[54] Boutin RD, Steinbach LS, Finnesey K. MR imaging of degenerative diseases in the cervical spine. Magn Reson Imaging Clin N Am. 2000; 8(3):471–490

[55] Uhlenbrock D. Degenerative disorders of the spine. In: Uhlenbrock D, ed. MR imaging of the spine and spinal cord. New York: Thieme; 2004:159–268

[56] Matsumoto M, Fujimura Y, Suzuki N, et al. MRI of cervical intervertebral discs in asymptomatic subjects. J Bone Joint Surg Br. 1998; 80(1):19–24

[57] Woods BI, Hilibrand AS. Cervical radiculopathy: epidemiology, etiology, diagnosis, and treatment. J Spinal Disord Tech. 2015; 28(5):E251–E259

[58] Boos N, Weissbach S, Rohrbach H, Weiler C, Spratt KF, Nerlich AG. Classification of age-related changes in lumbar intervertebral discs: 2002 Volvo Award in basic science. Spine. 2002; 27(23):2631–2644

[59] Mercer S, Bogduk N. The ligaments and annulus fibrosus of human adult cervical intervertebral discs. Spine. 1999; 24(7):619–626, discussion 627–628

[60] Fardon DF, Milette PC, Combined Task Forces of the North American Spine Society, American Society of Spine Radiology, and American Society of Neuroradiology. Nomenclature and classification of lumbar disc pathology. Recommendations of the Combined task Forces of the North American Spine Society, American Society of Spine Radiology, and American Society of Neuroradiology. Spine. 2001; 26(5):E93–E113

[61] Modic MT, Feiglin DH, Piraino DW, et al. Vertebral osteomyelitis: assessment using MR. Radiology. 1985; 157(1):157–166
[62] Modic MT, Steinberg PM, Ross JS, Masaryk TJ, Carter JR. Degenerative disk disease: assessment of changes in vertebral body marrow with MR imaging. Radiology. 1988; 166(1 Pt 1):193–199
[63] Matsunaga S, Sakou T. Ossification of the posterior longitudinal ligament of the cervical spine: etiology and natural history. Spine. 2012; 37(5): E309–E314
[64] Cowley P. Neuroimaging of spinal canal stenosis. Magn Reson Imaging Clin N Am. 2016; 24(3):523–539
[65] Pavlov H, Torg JS, Robie B, Jahre C. Cervical spinal stenosis: determination with vertebral body ratio method. Radiology. 1987; 164(3):771–775
[66] Boden SD. Rheumatoid arthritis of the cervical spine. Surgical decision making based on predictors of paralysis and recovery. Spine. 1994; 19(20): 2275–2280
[67] Boden SD, Dodge LD, Bohlman HH, Rechtine GR. Rheumatoid arthritis of the cervical spine. A long-term analysis with predictors of paralysis and recovery. J Bone Joint Surg Am. 1993; 75(9):1282–1297
[68] Smoker WRK. MR imaging of the craniovertebral junction. Magn Reson Imaging Clin N Am. 2000; 8(3):635–650
[69] Dreyer SJ, Boden SD. Natural history of rheumatoid arthritis of the cervical spine. Clin Orthop Relat Res. 1999(366):98–106
[70] Reiter MF, Boden SD. Inflammatory disorders of the cervical spine. Spine. 1998; 23(24):2755–2766
[71] Oda T, Fujiwara K, Yonenobu K, Azuma B, Ochi T. Natural course of cervical spine lesions in rheumatoid arthritis. Spine. 1995; 20(10):1128–1135
[72] Ross JS. Cervicomedullary and craniovertebral junctions. In: Modic MT, Masaryk TJ, Ross JS, eds. Magnetic resonance imaging of the spine. St. Louis, MO: Mosby-Year Book; 1994:191–215
[73] Joaquim AF, Ghizoni E, Tedeschi H, Appenzeller S, Riew KD. Radiological evaluation of cervical spine involvement in rheumatoid arthritis. Neurosurg Focus. 2015; 38(4):E4
[74] Bundschuh C, Modic MT, Kearney F, Morris R, Deal C. Rheumatoid arthritis of the cervical spine: surface-coil MR imaging. AJR Am J Roentgenol. 1988; 151(1):181–187
[75] Oostveen JCM, Roozeboom AR, van de Laar MAFJ, Heeres J, den Boer JA, Lindeboom SF. Functional turbo spin echo magnetic resonance imaging versus tomography for evaluating cervical spine involvement in rheumatoid arthritis. Spine. 1998; 23(11):1237–1244
[76] Tay BKB, Deckey J, Hu SS. Spinal infections. J Am Acad Orthop Surg. 2002; 10 (3):188–197
[77] Ruiz A, Post MJ, Sklar EM, Holz A. MR imaging of infections of the cervical spine. Magn Reson Imaging Clin N Am. 2000; 8(3):561–580
[78] Khanna AJ, Carbone JJ, Kebaish KM, et al. Magnetic resonance imaging of the cervical spine. Current techniques and spectrum of disease. J Bone Joint Surg Am. 2002; 84-A Suppl 2:70–80
[79] Uhlenbrock D, Henkes H, Weber W, Felber S, Kuehne D. Inflammatory disorders of the spine and spinal canal. In: Uhlenbrock D, ed. MR imaging of the spine and spinal cord. New York: Thieme; 2004:357–435
[80] Harris LF, Haws FP. Disc space infection. Ala Med. 1994; 63(7):12–14
[81] Renfrew DL. Infectious spondylitis. In: Renfrew DL, ed. Atlas of spine imaging. Philadelphia, PA: Saunders; 2003:259–280
[82] Bierry G, Jehl F, Prévost G, et al. Percutaneous inoculated rabbit model of intervertebral disc space infection: magnetic resonance imaging features with pathological correlation. Joint Bone Spine. 2008; 75(4):465–470
[83] Carragee EJ. The clinical use of magnetic resonance imaging in pyogenic vertebral osteomyelitis. Spine. 1997; 22(7):780–785
[84] Gillams AR, Chaddha B, Carter AP. MR appearances of the temporal evolution and resolution of infectious spondylitis. AJR Am J Roentgenol. 1996; 166(4):903–907
[85] Murphy KJ, Brunberg JA, Quint DJ, Kazanjian PH. Spinal cord infection: myelitis and abscess formation. AJNR Am J Neuroradiol. 1998; 19(2): 341–348
[86] Keogh C, Bergin D, Brennan D, Eustace S. MR imaging of bone tumors of the cervical spine. Magn Reson Imaging Clin N Am. 2000; 8(3):513–528
[87] DeSanto J, Ross JS. Spine infection/inflammation. Radiol Clin North Am. 2011; 49(1):105–127
[88] Finelli DA, Ross JS. MR imaging of intrinsic inflammatory myelopathies. Magn Reson Imaging Clin N Am. 2000; 8(3):541–560
[89] Tartaglino LM, Friedman DP, Flanders AE, Lublin FD, Knobler RL, Liem M. Multiple sclerosis in the spinal cord: MR appearance and correlation with clinical parameters. Radiology. 1995; 195(3):725–732
[90] Wiebe S, Lee DH, Karlik SJ, et al. Serial cranial and spinal cord magnetic resonance imaging in multiple sclerosis. Ann Neurol. 1992; 32(5):643–650
[91] Choi KH, Lee KS, Chung SO, et al. Idiopathic transverse myelitis: MR characteristics. AJNR Am J Neuroradiol. 1996; 17(6):1151–1160
[92] Pardatscher K, Fiore DL, Lavano A. MR imaging of transverse myelitis using Gd-DTPA. J Neuroradiol. 1992; 19(1):63–67
[93] Budka H. Neuropathology of myelitis, myelopathy, and spinal infections in AIDS. Neuroimaging Clin N Am. 1997; 7(3):639–650
[94] Chong J, Di Rocco A, Tagliati M, Danisi F, Simpson DM, Atlas SW. MR findings in AIDS-associated myelopathy. AJNR Am J Neuroradiol. 1999; 20 (8):1412–1416
[95] Wang PY, Shen WC, Jan JS. Serial MRI changes in radiation myelopathy. Neuroradiology. 1995; 37(5):374–377
[96] Janssen H, Weissman BN, Aliabadi P, Zamani AA. MR imaging of arthritides of the cervical spine. Magn Reson Imaging Clin N Am. 2000; 8(3):491–512
[97] Amrami KK. Imaging of the seronegative spondyloarthopathies. Radiol Clin North Am. 2012; 50(4):841–854
[98] Konca S, Keskin D, Cılız D, Bodur H, Sakman B. Spinal inflammation by magnetic resonance imaging in patients with ankylosing spondylitis: association with disease activity and outcome parameters. Rheumatol Int. 2012; 32(12):3765–3770
[99] Brzeski M, Fox JG, Boulton-Jones JM, Capell HA. Vertebral body collapse due to primary amyloidosis. J Rheumatol. 1990; 17(12):1701–1703
[100] Yu JS, Chung C, Recht M, Dailiana T, Jurdi R. MR imaging of tophaceous gout. AJR Am J Roentgenol. 1997; 168(2):523–527

Answers to Common Clinical Questions

1. Answer: e. Injury to posterior ligaments may be seen as areas of hyperintensity on T2-weighted images, especially fat-suppressed T2-weighted or STIR images. Sagittal STIR or fat-suppressed T2-weighted images are superior to T2-weighted images because they are more "fluid sensitive" and, thus, accentuate the edema seen with ligamentous injury.
2. Answer: d. Boden et al[53] reported that almost 60% of their asymptomatic patients > 40 years old had cervical spine degenerative disk disease on MRI. This fact is important in that the finding of degenerative changes, alone, on MRI is not an indication for surgical or other intervention. The patient should have clinical findings that correlate, are clinically significant, and/or are not amenable to or have not responded to nonoperative treatment.
3. Answer: d. Although it is difficult to make a diagnosis with a single image in a single plane from an MRI study, this image suggests the diagnosis of ossification of the posterior longitudinal ligament. The findings on MRI should be used to differentiate cervical disk disease and protrusions from ossification of the posterior longitudinal ligament. On most MR images showing cervical stenosis secondary to disk displacement, the abnormality and stenosis are based at the level of the disk, and stenosis is seen only behind the vertebral body in cases of disk extrusion and migration. Conversely, MRI of patients with ossification of the posterior longitudinal ligament shows stenosis at the level of the disk and also along the course of the posterior longitudinal ligament, which runs along the posterior aspect of the vertebral bodies. For patients with suspected ossification of the posterior longitudinal

ligament, CT imaging can be obtained to rule in or rule out this diagnosis, given that it provides optimal visualization of calcification and osseous detail.

4. Answer: a. There are several objective measures of cervical spinal stenosis. Relative stenosis is defined as an AP canal diameter of < 13 mm, and absolute stenosis is defined as an AP canal diameter of < 10 mm. The Torg or Pavlov ratio is calculated by dividing the AP canal diameter by the AP vertebral body diameter, with a ratio < 0.8 defined as stenotic. This ratio is often used to evaluate for congenital stenosis in athletes.
5. Answer: c. A common clinical scenario is one in which a patient with known or previously unknown ankylosing spondylitis presents with neck pain after minor trauma. Conventional radiographs may show ankylosis of the cervical (or lumbar) spine but no evidence of fracture or displacement. Such patients may have an unrecognized nondisplaced fracture. MRI can be obtained to rule out the presence of a nondisplaced fracture through the ankylosed spine. Such fractures are best seen on fat-suppressed T2-weighted images. CT imaging may not show a nondisplaced fracture. Single-photon emission CT imaging is best for the evaluation of isthmic spondylolisthesis. A three-phase bone scan may show increased radiotracer activity at the fracture site, but such activity may not be seen in the early postinjury time period, and the visibility of osseous detail and fracture pattern will be superior with MRI.

16 The Lumbar and Thoracic Spine

Gbolahan O. Okubadejo, Aditya R. Daftary, Jacob M. Buchowski, John A. Carrino, and A. Jay Khanna

Abstract

The typical MRI protocol of the lumbar spine for the evaluation of degenerative pathologies includes T2-weighted and T1-weighted images in both sagittal and axial planes. However, imaging protocols of the lumbar spine for specific indications can vary among institutions and should be modified when specific diagnoses such as infection, recurrent disk herniation, and tumor are being considered.

The initial evaluation of patients with known or suspected lumbar spine injury begins with conventional radiographs and/or CT imaging, which provides greater osseous detail and may reveal fractures or details that are not detected with conventional radiography. MRI provides soft-tissue visualization that is superior to that of conventional radiography or CT and is useful for the assessment of spinal cord injury, ligamentous injury, degree of spinal stenosis, and additional fracture evaluation.

MRI is the preferred initial advanced imaging modality for the evaluation of symptomatic lumbar spine degeneration and is highly sensitive and specific for the detection of degenerative changes. Despite this high sensitivity and specificity, it is important to understand that radiographic and MRI abnormalities do not always correlate with a symptomatic degenerative lesion.[134] Therefore, the spine specialist must correlate the findings on MRI with the patient's history and physical examination. Degenerative conditions that can be evaluated on lumbar spine MRI include disk displacement, disk degeneration, spinal stenosis, and spondylolisthesis. The nomenclature used for describing lumbar disk pathology should be consistent and applied uniformly, as shown in Chapter 15, The Cervical Spine.

Although the most common indication for MRI of the lumbar spine is the evaluation of degenerative conditions, this modality is also frequently and effectively used for the evaluation of patients with nondegenerative conditions such as trauma, infection, spinal tumors, various arthritides, and postoperative complications and findings.

Keywords: degenerative conditions, disks, end plates, imaging protocols, infectious conditions, thoracolumbar spine, trauma

16.1 Specialized Pulse Sequences and Imaging Protocols

As with the cervical spine and other regions in the musculoskeletal system, imaging protocols of the lumbar and thoracic spine for specific indications vary among institutions. However, the standard magnetic resonance imaging (MRI) of the lumbar and thoracic spine for degenerative pathologies usually includes the following pulse sequences:

- Sagittal T1-weighted spin-echo (SE).
- Sagittal T2-weighted fast spin-echo (FSE).
- Sagittal T2-weighted with fat suppression or sagittal short tau inversion recovery (STIR).
- Axial T1-weighted SE or axial gradient-echo.
- Axial T2-weighted FSE.

T1-weighted images are good for identifying anatomy and assessing the quantity of fat in neural foramina and the epidural spaces. They also help identify the presence of fracture lines. However, edema has low signal on T1-weighted images and may be difficult to identify. Signal on T1-weighted images increases in the presence of gadolinium contrast, so these images are used to assess for contrast enhancement. Contrast enhancement is particularly useful in differentiating recurrent disk pathology from scar tissue and in assessing infection, neoplasms, and vascular malformations. Contrast enhancement may be made more conspicuous by obtaining postgadolinium fat-suppressed images.

T2-weighted images are sensitive to edema, which is usually one of the early signs of pathology. Distinction between fat and fluid (edema) may be difficult on T2-weighted images. For this reason, fat suppression via a fat-suppressed T2-weighted or STIR image may be obtained to make edema more conspicuous. STIR images are preferred over fat-suppressed T2-weighted images for patients with spinal instrumentation because STIR images are less prone to magnetic susceptibility artifacts. T2-weighted and fat-suppressed T2-weighted or STIR images are extremely helpful in identifying ligamentous injury, subtle fractures, neoplasms, infection, and fluid collections, including joint effusions.

Highly T2-weighted images produce an "MR myelogram" that provides a nice perspective, which is similar to that of images obtained with conventional myelography and computed tomographic (CT) myelography. As with other myelographic images, these MR images can be used to evaluate for spinal stenosis. However, such images should always be interpreted in conjunction with other MR pulse sequences because they may be prone to artifacts that exaggerate or underestimate abnormalities, including the degree of stenosis.

By decreasing the degree to which protons are "flipped" during image acquisition (compared with T1-weighted and T2-weighted images, in which they are flipped by 90–180 degrees), gradient-echo images can be acquired much more quickly. Adjustments in the "flip angle," TR (repetition time), and TE (echo time) can create T1- and T2-weighting in these images. Gradient-echo images are very susceptible to magnetic susceptibility artifacts, which makes them useful for the detection of small areas of hemorrhage, such as those that occur with trauma and vascular malformations. Conversely, this susceptibility also causes gradient-echo images to overestimate canal and foraminal stenosis because of artifact from the adjacent bone. Advances in MRI techniques are decreasing the latter problem.[1] Because of the rapidity with which images are acquired, they can be obtained with higher resolution and even as a 3D volume, which makes isotropic voxels and reformations in multiple planes possible. As MR imaging protocols and imaging systems continue to evolve, image quality will likely improve and scan times will continue to decrease.[2,3,4]

16.2 Traumatic Conditions

Patients with suspected lumbar spine injuries should be evaluated initially with conventional radiographs. CT imaging offers greater osseous detail than do conventional radiographs and may reveal fractures or details that are not detected with radiography. MRI provides superior visualization of soft tissues compared with conventional radiographs or CT images and is useful for the assessment of ligamentous injury, degree of spinal stenosis, additional fracture evaluation, and associated findings such as epidural hematomas. Occult fractures not visible on conventional radiographs or CT images may be detected by the presence of vertebral body edema on MR images. Although MRI is extremely sensitive in identifying thoracolumbar spine fractures, their characteristics and the exact appearance of the osseous components can be challenging; CT may be a better choice for assessing these aspects of the fractures. MRI is indicated when neurologic deficit, vascular injury, or soft-tissue injury is suspected in the setting of trauma. It is also useful for the assessment of posttraumatic sequelae.

A systematic approach (see Chapter 3, A Systematic Approach to the Review of Spine MRI Studies) for the evaluation of lumbar spine MRI should be used to avoid missing pathologic conditions (see ▶ Table 16.1 for important lumbar spine structures to evaluate). In addition, it is essential that the MRI findings be interpreted in conjunction with other available imaging modalities, including conventional radiographs (with flexion and extension views if clinically indicated) and CT (see Chapter 4, Correlation of MRI with Other Imaging Studies).

Table 16.1 Evaluation of lumbar and thoracic spine trauma

Anatomy	Evaluation
Spinal column/ vertebral bodies	Alignment
	Vertebral body fracture
	Posterior element fracture
	Edema
	Degenerative change
Ligaments	Anterior longitudinal ligament
	Posterior longitudinal ligament
	Interspinous ligament
	Edema/rupture
Spinal cord	Edema
	Hemorrhage
	Compression
	Syrinx
Epidural space	Hematoma
	Disk herniation
	Osseous fragment

Source: Takhtani D, Melhem ER. MR imaging in cervical spine trauma. Magn Reson Imaging Clin N Am. 2000;8:615–634. Modified with permission.

16.2.1 Classification of Thoracolumbar Spine Trauma

Thoracolumbar spine trauma is a common and complex condition. There are many classification systems, all of which are based on a variety of factors such as mechanism of injury; morphology of fracture; involvement of columns; and presence, absence, or degree of neural compromise.[5,6,7,8] Like many classification systems, those for the evaluation of thoracolumbar spine trauma have not been universally accepted. This lack of acceptance may be the result of their complexity, lack of reproducibility, poor validity, or a combination thereof.

The Thoracolumbar Injury Classification and Severity Score recognizes the importance of the following three factors[9]:

- Fracture morphology (▶ Fig. 16.1).
- Integrity of the posterior ligamentous complex (stability or potential for neurologic compromise).
- Neurologic status of the patient.

Although a detailed review of this classification system is outside the scope of this chapter, these three components are used here to review and highlight the role of MRI in the evaluation of

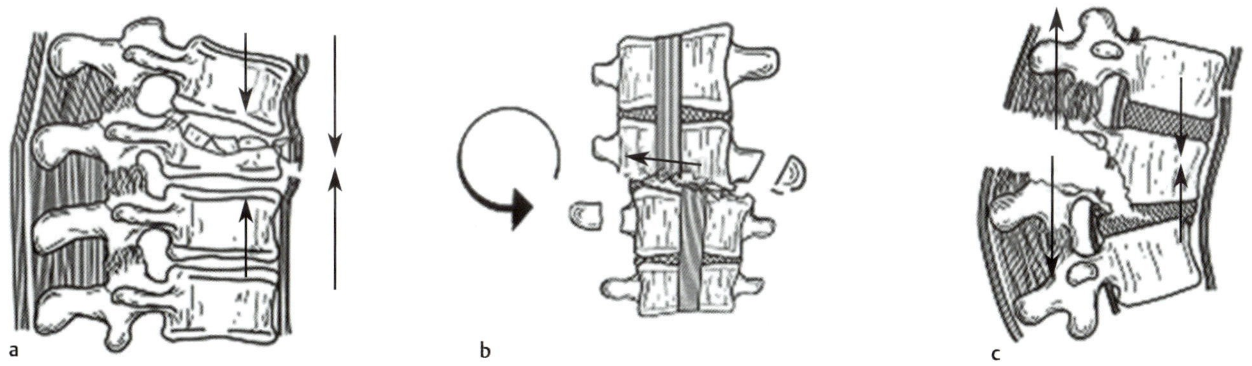

Fig. 16.1 Illustrations of the three major morphologic descriptors in the Thoracolumbar Injury Classification and Severity Score (compression, translation/rotation, and distraction). These descriptors are determined from a combination of conventional radiographs, computed tomographic (CT) images, and magnetic resonance imaging (MRI) sequences. **(a)** In compression, the vertebral body buckles under load to produce a compression or burst fracture. **(b)** In translation/rotation, the vertebral column is subjected to shear or torsional forces that cause the rostral part of the spinal column to translate or rotate with respect to the caudal part. **(c)** In distraction, the rostral spinal column becomes separated from the caudal segment because of distractive forces. Combinations of these morphologic patterns may occur. (Reproduced with permission from, Vaccaro AR, Lehman RA Jr, Hurlbert RJ, et al. A new classification of thoracolumbar injuries. The importance of injury morphology, the integrity of the posterior ligamentous complex, and neurologic status. Spine 2005;30:2325–2333.)

patients with thoracolumbar spine trauma. In addition, a systematic evaluation of these components and calculation of an injury severity score[9] can be used to guide the treatment of patients with thoracolumbar spine fractures.[10] The Thoracolumbar Injury Classification and Severity Score (▶ Table 16.2) provides prognostic information and has been found to be helpful in medical decision making.[10,11] Studies have shown that it has excellent reliability and validity.[12,13]

Table 16.2 Thoracolumbar Injury Classification and Severity Score

Injury characteristic	Qualifier	Points
Injury morphology		
Compression		1
	Burst	+ 1
Rotation/translation		3
Distraction		4
Neurologic status		
Intact		0
Nerve root		2
Spinal cord, conus medullaris	Incomplete	3
	Complete	2
Cauda equina		3
Posterior ligamentous complex integrity		
Intact		0
Suspected/indeterminate		2
Disrupted		3

Source: Patel AA, Vaccaro AR. Thoracolumbar spine trauma classification. J Am Acad Orthop Surg. 2010; 18(2):63–71.[10]
Note: +, one additional point given to the morphology.

16.2.2 Role of MRI in Thoracolumbar Spine Trauma

Evaluation of Fracture Morphology

The first element in the MRI evaluation of a thoracolumbar injury is the assessment of fracture morphology. The morphology description includes the type of fracture (e.g., compression, burst) and the position of various osseous fragments relative to their anatomic origin and to the spinal canal. As discussed above, for the assessment of the osseous components of a fracture, CT is superior to conventional radiography and MRI because of the excellent spatial resolution and osseous detail it provides (▶ Fig. 16.2). MRI may help provide additional information regarding the morphology of a fracture in a limited number of situations. For example, subtle fractures may be difficult to identify on CT or conventional radiographs, especially in patients with degenerative disk disease, where end-plate anatomy and vertebral morphology are affected by the degenerative changes. Furthermore, patients with osteoporosis or osteopenia may show less osseous reactive change, which typically enables the detection of subtle or subacute fractures on conventional radiographs. Fluid-sensitive pulse sequences such as fat-suppressed T2-weighted or short tau inversion recovery (STIR) images are excellent for identifying areas of subtle bone marrow edema and focusing attention on an area of potential osseous injury. This bone marrow edema often appears almost immediately after injury and can persist for several months or even a year thereafter.[14,15] It should be noted, however, that the differential considerations for bone marrow edema in a vertebral body are varied and include other entities such as tumors,

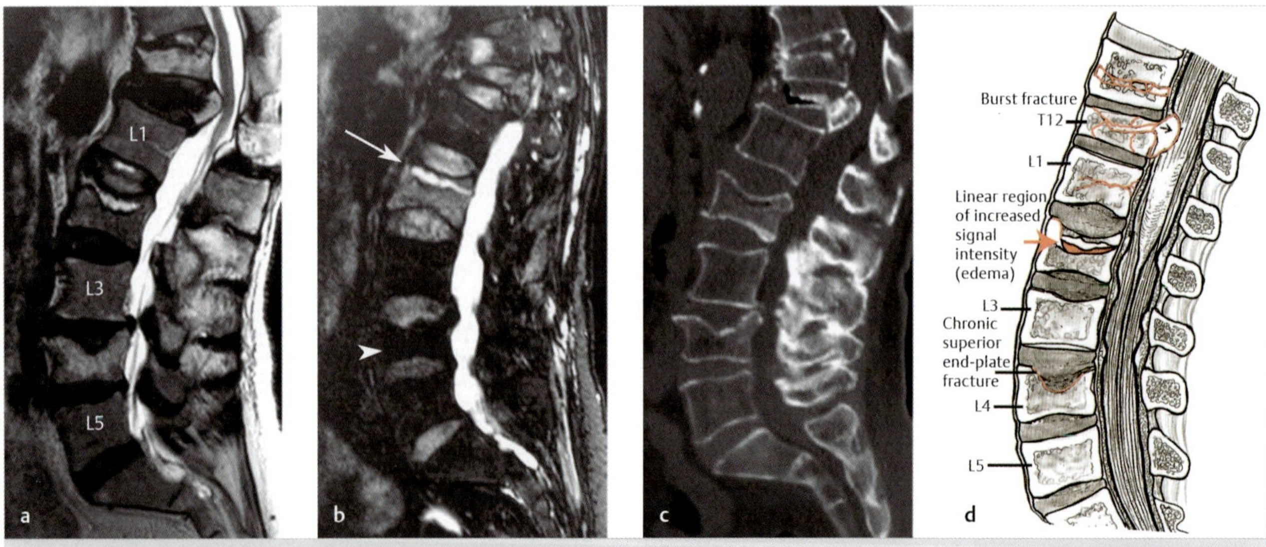

Fig. 16.2 Osteoporotic vertebral fractures. **(a)** A sagittal T2-weighted image shows multiple vertebral fractures, including vertebral compression fractures at L4, L2, and T11, and a burst fracture at T12. Note the bright T2-weighted signal fracture line at L2, characteristic of a benign osteoporotic fracture. **(b)** A sagittal short tau inversion recovery (STIR) image shows a linear region of increased signal intensity compatible with edema in the L2 vertebral body (*arrow*), which is compatible with an acute fracture. Note the diffuse edema in the vertebral body that could be mistaken for diffuse bone-marrow involvement by a neoplastic process. There is no increase in signal intensity in the L4 vertebral body (*arrowhead*), which is compatible with a chronic fracture. **(c)** A sagittal reconstructed computed tomographic (CT) image shows the osseous details of the fractures. The osseous margins are clearly defined, and the retropulsed posterior fragment characteristic of a benign osteoporotic fracture is evident at T12. **(d)** An illustration of the findings described in the preceding images. (Figure part **a, b, and c**: Reproduced with permission, from Okubadejo GO, Daftary A, Buchowski JM, et al. The lumbar and thoracic spine. In: Khanna AJ, ed. MRI for orthopaedic surgeons. New York: Thieme; 2010:269–315.) (Figure Part **d**: Reproduced with permission from, Okubadejo GO, Daftary A, Buchowski JM, et al. The lumbar and thoracic spine. In: Khanna AJ, ed. MRI essentials for the spine specialist. New York: Thieme; 2014:155–210.)

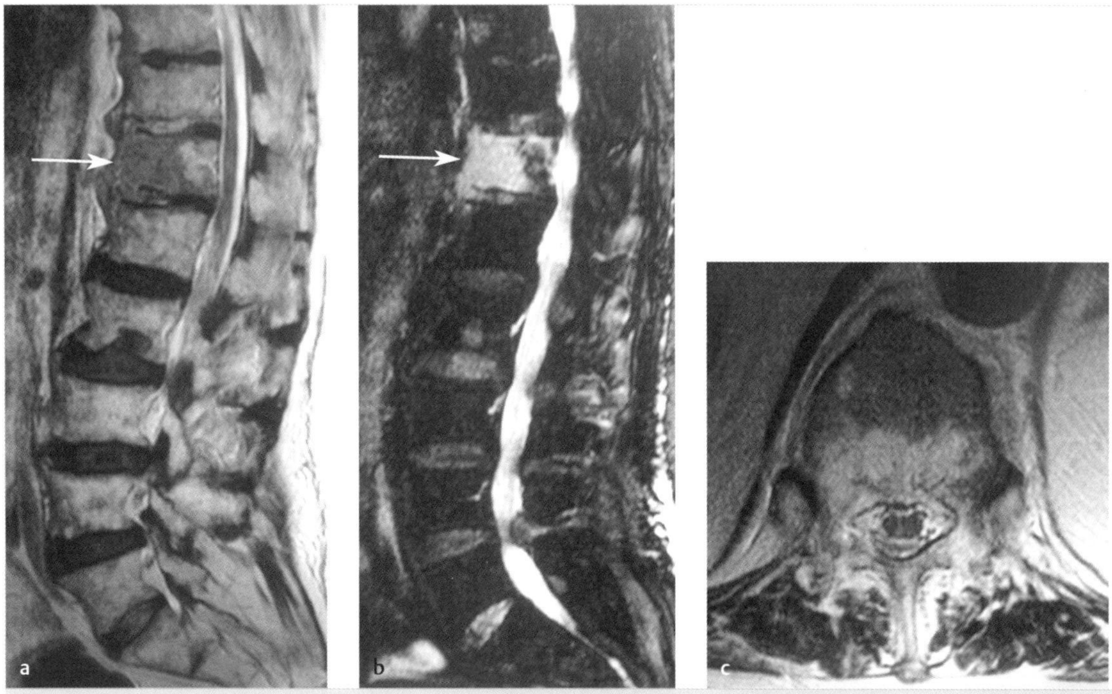

Fig. 16.3 Vertebral body metastasis in a patient with lung cancer. **(a)** A sagittal T2-weighted image shows heterogeneous bone-marrow signal intensity in multiple vertebral bodies (which can be seen with osteoporosis) but most prominently within the anterior half of the T12 vertebral body (*arrow*). Note that the anterior aspect of the vertebral body appears expanded because it is infiltrated with tumor. **(b)** A sagittal short tau inversion recovery (STIR) image shows markedly increased signal intensity in the same region (*arrow*). **(c)** An axial T2-weighted image shows heterogeneous signal intensity within the vertebral body. A percutaneous biopsy confirmed evidence of metastatic lung cancer. (Reproduced with permission from, Okubadejo GO, Daftary AR, Buchowski JM, et al. The lumbar and thoracic spine. In: Khanna AJ, ed. MRI for orthopaedic surgeons. New York: Thieme; 2010:269–315.)

end-plate degeneration, and infection. For this reason, correlation with other imaging findings, imaging techniques, and clinical information is important for making a definitive diagnosis.

For patients in whom vertebral compression fractures are associated with pain, vertebral augmentation procedures such as vertebroplasty or kyphoplasty may be considered as a treatment option. In a study of patients with chronic (1 year) vertebral compression fractures treated with vertebroplasty, Brown et al[15] found that clinical improvement was definitively correlated with the presence of preprocedural bone marrow edema. Therefore, it is essential that the MR images be reviewed for the absence, presence, and degree of bone marrow edema for each fracture (▶ Fig. 16.2).

Differentiating posttraumatic and osteoporotic fractures from neoplastic or pathologic fractures can be challenging (▶ Fig. 16.2, ▶ Fig. 16.3), especially in elderly patients. Neoplastic processes tend to fracture when most of the vertebral body is infiltrated with tumor (▶ Fig. 16.3). Key MRI features that suggest the presence of a malignant fracture include the following[16]:

- Convex posterior margin of the vertebral body (from tumor infiltration) (▶ Fig. 16.4).
- Abnormal signal in the posterior elements.
- Epidural mass and neural encasement by the same focal paraspinal mass.
- Presence of other osseous lesions.

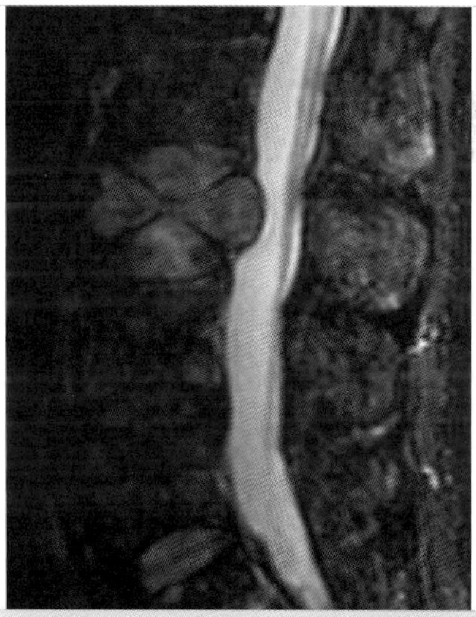

Fig. 16.4 A sagittal short tau inversion recovery (STIR) image shows a pathologic burst fracture of the L3 vertebral body in a patient with metastatic lung cancer. Note the diffusely increased signal within the vertebral body and the convex posterior margin of the vertebral body. (Reproduced with permission from, Okubadejo GO, Daftary AR, Buchowski JM, et al. The lumbar and thoracic spine. In: Khanna AJ, ed. MRI for orthopaedic surgeons. New York: Thieme; 2010:269–315.)

In the search for other lesions, care should be taken not to mistake additional osteoporotic vertebral fractures for metastatic lesions. A horizontal linear bright fracture line on T2-weighted images is considered the most reliable sign of a nonmalignant fracture (▶ Fig. 16.2). Other signs that decrease the likelihood of underlying tumor include a retropulsed fragment off the posterior aspect of the vertebral body, multiple fractures, and normal bone marrow signal.[16,17] Because contrast enhancement is often seen with acute benign fractures, it is no longer considered diagnostic for an underlying lesion or malignancy.[16,18]

Assessment of Stability

The term *spinal stability* refers to the ability of the spine to limit neurologic compromise under physiologic loads. Panjabi et al[19] have defined spinal stability as the degree of motion that prevents pain, neurologic deficit, and abnormal angulation. The definition can also be extended to include the ability of the spine to avoid the development of spinal deformity. Two key concepts in the MRI determination of spinal stability are the three-column concept and the assessment of the posterior ligamentous complex.

Three-Column Concept

More than 25 years ago, Denis[5] introduced the concept of the three-column spine and its clinical significance in the evaluation of spinal stability in patients with acute thoracolumbar injuries. Although the reliability and validity of the Denis system have been questioned,[13,20] it is still used frequently to help evaluate the degree of spinal instability. Spinal instability may be assessed based on the number of columns involved in an injury. The three columns are defined as follows (▶ Fig. 16.5):

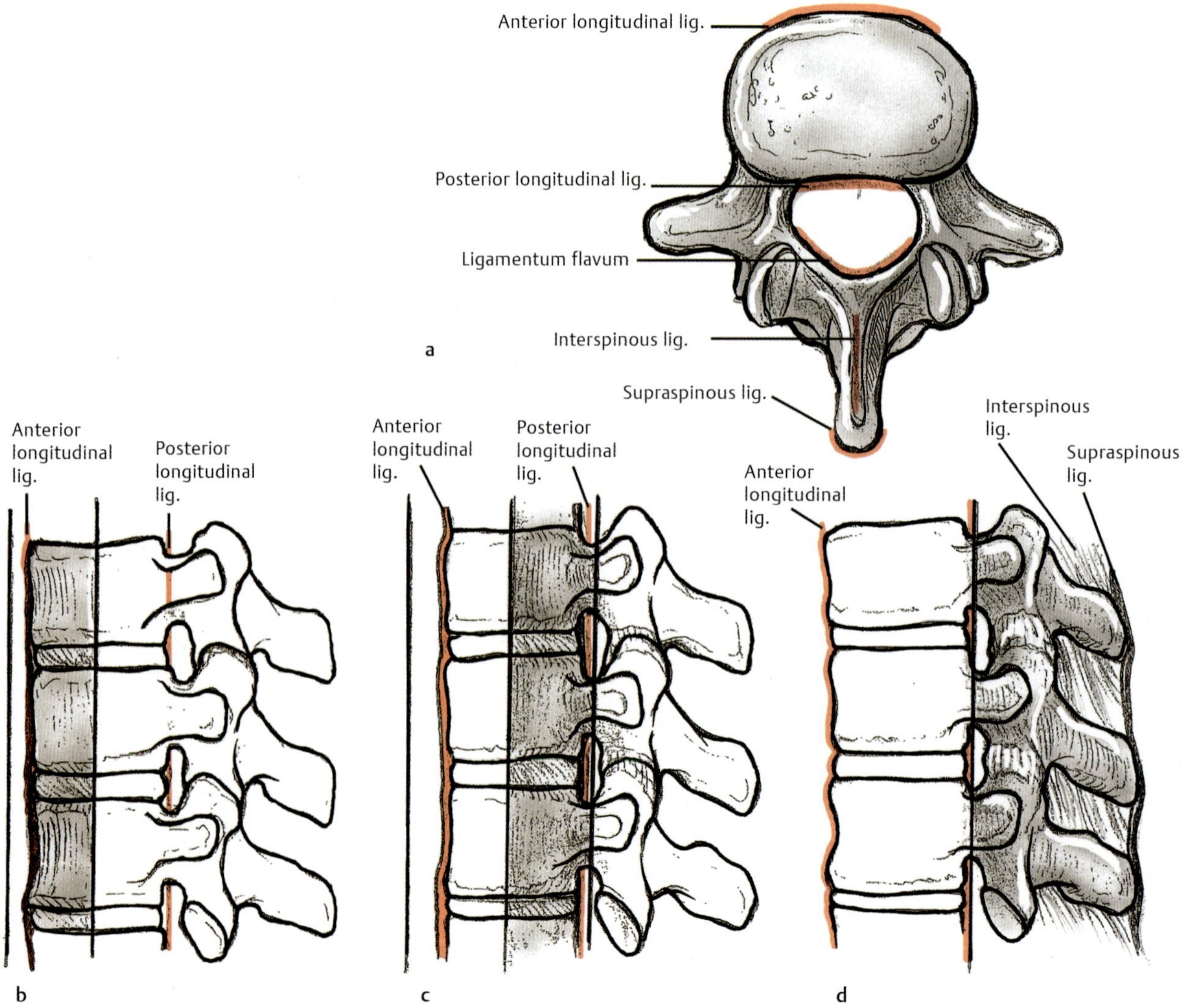

Fig. 16.5 Illustrations of the three columns of the spine as described by Denis.[5] **(a)** An axial view. The lateral views show the **(b)** anterior, **(c)** middle, and **(d)** posterior columns. (Reproduced with permission from, Okubadejo GO, Daftary A, Buchowski JM, et al. The lumbar and thoracic spine. In: Khanna AJ, ed. MRI essentials for the spine specialist. New York: Thieme; 2014:155–210.)

- *Anterior:* anterior longitudinal ligament and the anterior portion of the vertebral body and annulus.
- *Middle:* posterior vertebral body and annulus, and the posterior longitudinal ligament.
- *Posterior:* facet joints, posterior elements, and posterior ligaments (supraspinous and interspinous ligaments and ligamentum flavum).

If one column is involved, the spine is generally considered stable; with two-column involvement, the spine is variably stable, depending on the degree of involvement; and the involvement of all three columns leads to a highly unstable spine.

Posterior Ligamentous Complex

The posterior column and posterior ligamentous complex is an area of increasing concern in spinal stability (▶ Fig. 16.1c).[9,21,22,23] The components of the posterior ligamentous complex include the supraspinous ligament, interspinous ligament, ligamentum flavum, and the facet joint capsules.[9] The three ligaments that constitute the posterior ligamentous complex normally appear as dark and continuous bands on T1-weighted and T2-weighted images. When traumatized, they may show increased signal on fluid-sensitive pulse sequences (T2-weighted fat-suppressed and STIR) (▶ Fig. 16.6). Discontinuity of the dark signal of the fibers is also seen on MRI. It has been suggested that the MR images be reviewed with the intent of describing these ligaments as intact, indeterminate, or disrupted.[9]

Subtle fractures and dislocations of the facet joints and posterior elements are detected well on CT, but in some instances, the edema identified on MRI may be helpful in combination with close scrutiny of the CT images to identify subtle fractures. However, the true role of MRI in these instances is in identifying ligamentous injuries and hematomas; 28 to 47% of patients with thoracolumbar burst fractures are estimated to have disruption of the posterior ligamentous complex.[24]

Assessment of Neural Compromise

MRI plays its most vital role in the assessment of neural compromise and is excellent in its ability to determine the cause of compression. Neural compromise can be graded on MRI as mild, moderate, or severe (see the subsequent discussion of lumbar spinal stenosis). In addition to an evaluation of the degree of stenosis, the type of stenosis should also be described (central, lateral recess, or foraminal). In addition, one should note whether there is compression of specific neurologic structures such as the spinal cord or a specific nerve root. Common causes of neural compromise in patients after thoracolumbar spine trauma include the following:

- Burst fractures.
- Disk pathology.
- Epidural hematoma.
- Vertebral translation or dislocation.
- Penetrating trauma (▶ Fig. 16.7).

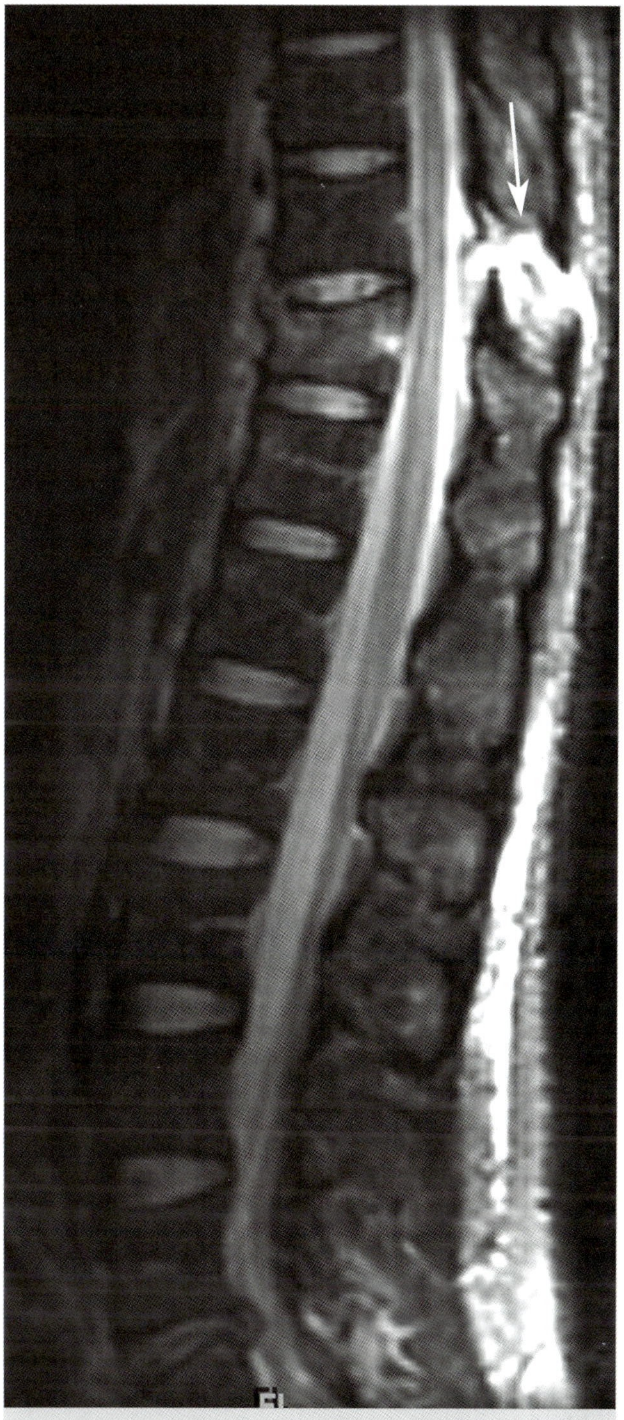

Fig. 16.6 A sagittal short tau inversion recovery (STIR) image shows a T11 flexion-distraction injury with compression fracture of T11 and an associated injury of the interspinous and supraspinous ligaments, as evidenced by increased signal intensity in the interspinous and supraspinous region between T10 and T11 (*arrow*). (Reproduced with permission from, Okubadejo GO, Daftary AR, Buchowski JM, et al. The lumbar and thoracic spine. In: Khanna AJ, ed. MRI for orthopaedic surgeons. New York: Thieme; 2010:269–315.)

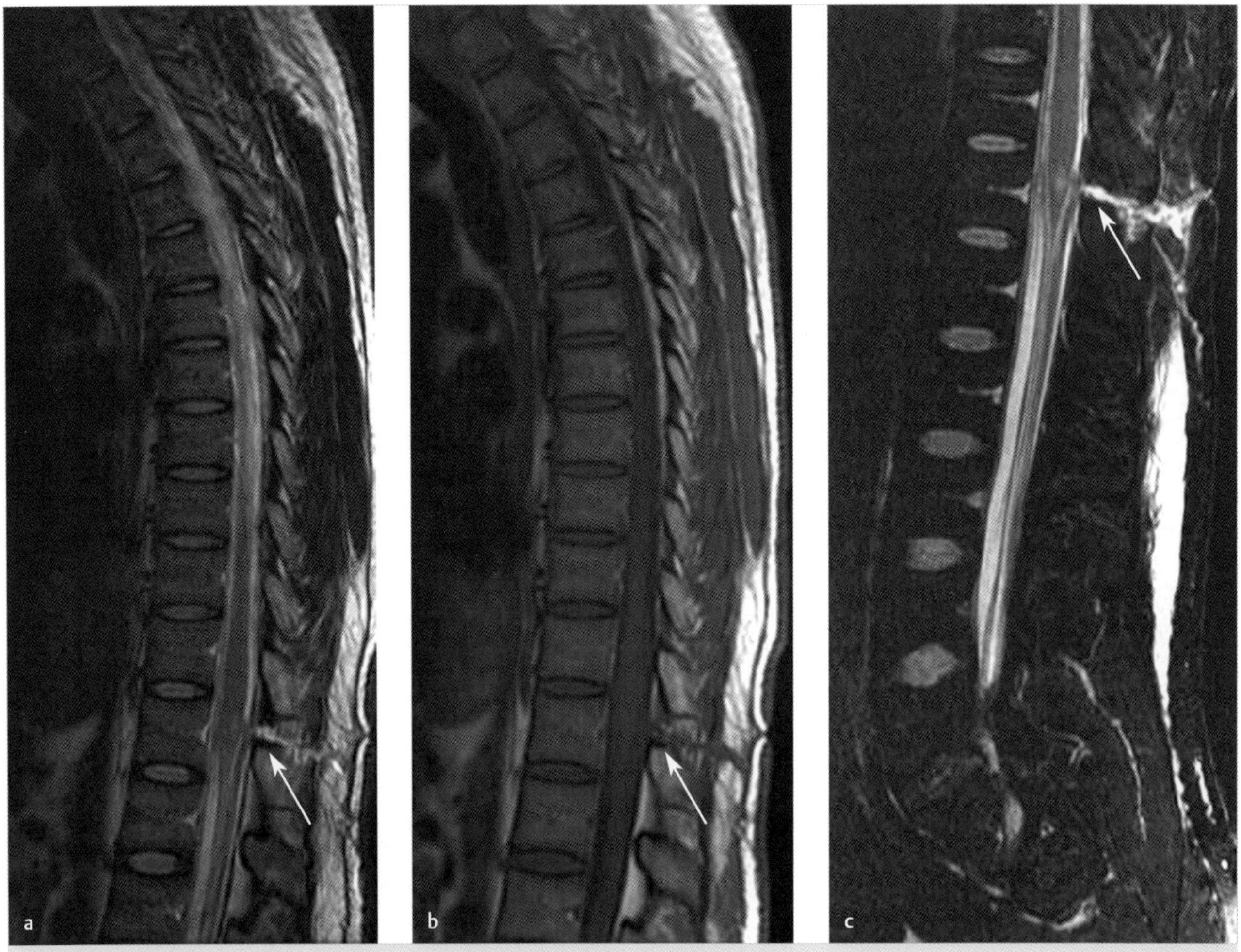

Fig. 16.7 Cord injury from a stab injury to the conus medullaris. **(a)** A sagittal T2-weighted image of the thoracic spine shows a linear track (*arrow*) from the skin to the conus medullaris with an associated region of increased signal within the conus medullaris, compatible with edema. **(b)** A sagittal T1-weighted image of the thoracic spine also shows the track (*arrow*) but does not show the edema within the conus medullaris. **(c)** A sagittal short tau inversion recovery (STIR) image of the lumbar spine accentuates the edema along the track (*arrow*) and also that within the conus medullaris. (Reproduced from Okubadejo GO, Daftary AR, Buchowski JM, et al. The lumbar and thoracic spine. In: Khanna AJ, ed. MRI for orthopaedic surgeons. New York: Thieme; 2010:269–315.)

Burst Fracture

Although CT is excellent for assessing the osseous component of a burst fracture, the associated neural compression and hematoma may be difficult to assess on CT, and MRI is far more accurate. It is important to differentiate a burst fracture (▶ Fig. 16.8) from a compression fracture (▶ Fig. 16.2). The former involves injury to the anterior and middle columns, whereas the latter involves injury to the anterior column only. The MR images should be evaluated carefully for the absence or presence and degree of stenosis, which can be secondary to the fracture alone or to preexisting degenerative changes, or to any combination thereof. Specifically, the sagittal T2-weighted images should be evaluated in the midline for the degree of posterior vertebral body wall encroachment on the spinal canal, CSF column, spinal cord, or cauda equina. Next, the parasagittal images should be evaluated for the same. Finally, the axial T2-weighted images can be reviewed to determine the location and degree of neural compromise in an orthogonal plane.

Disk Pathology

Traumatic compressive forces on the disk may lead to annular tears (also known as annular fissures), disk protrusions, extrusions, and sequestrations. Rupture of a few annular fibers leads to a small amount of fluid tracking from the nucleus pulposus to between the annular fibers, leading to a focus of high intensity on T2-weighted images. This finding of focal high intensity in the annulus is referred to as a *high-intensity zone* (▶ Fig. 16.9) and is suggestive of an annular tear. Although this finding may be seen in association with trauma, its level of importance is

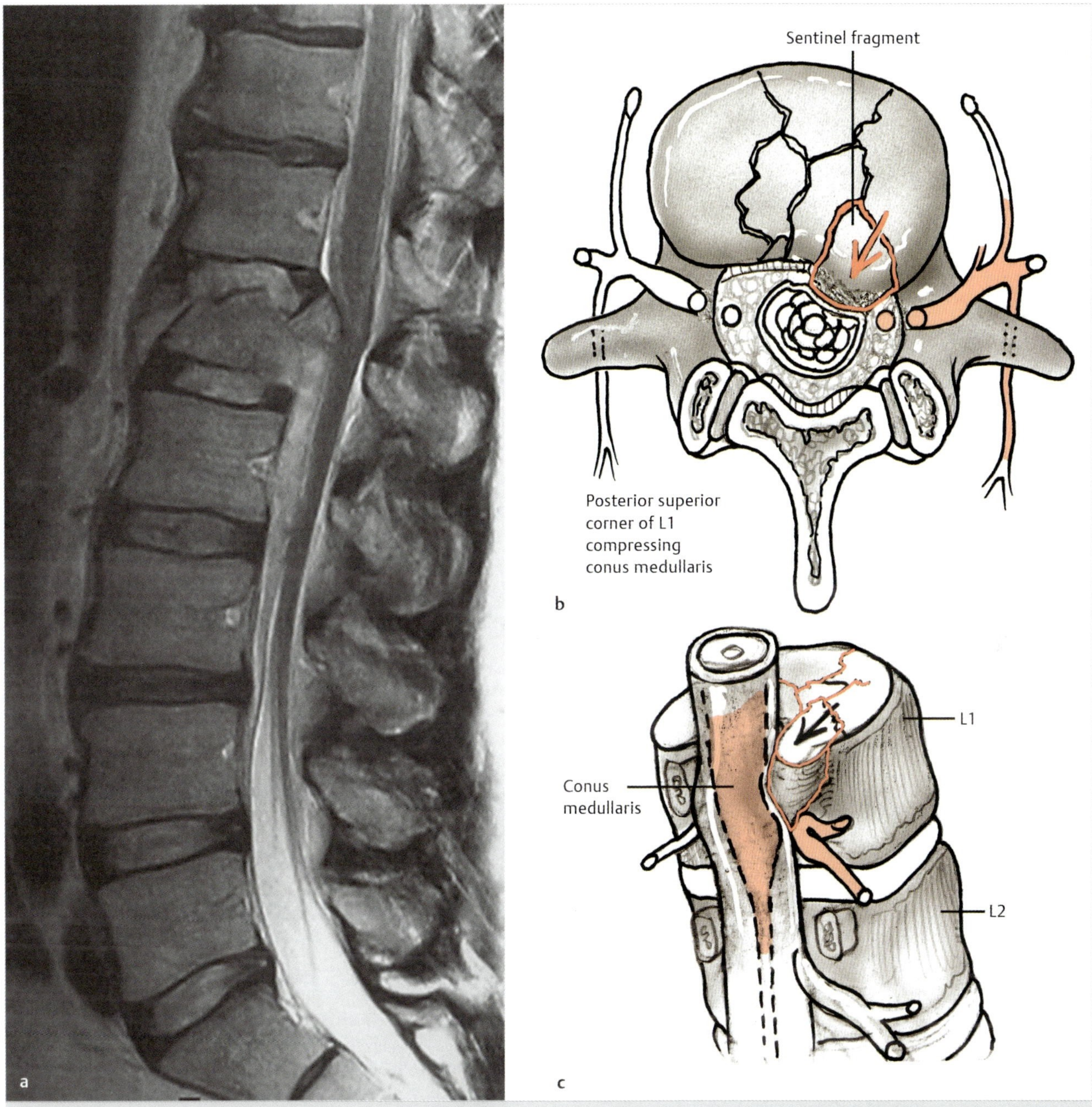

Fig. 16.8 **(a)** A sagittal T2-weighted image and illustrations in the **(b)** axial plane and **(c)** posterolateral perspective show an L1 burst fracture. Note that the posterior-superior margin of the vertebral body has displaced and rotated into the spinal canal. This displaced and rotated fragment *(arrow* on each) has been termed the *sentinel* or *culprit* fragment. (Figure part **a**: Reproduced with permission from, Okubadejo GO, Daftary AR, Buchowski JM, et al. The lumbar and thoracic spine. In: Khanna AJ, ed. MRI for orthopaedic surgeons. New York: Thieme; 2010:269–315.) (Figure part **b, c**: Reproduced with permission from, Okubadejo GO, Daftary A, Buchowski JM, et al. The lumbar and thoracic spine. In: Khanna AJ, ed. MRI essentials for the spine specialist. New York: Thieme; 2014:155–210.)

controversial because it is also seen as a natural process of disk degeneration and may or may not be associated with acute pain.[25,26,27] MRI is the modality of choice for assessing such abnormalities and associated areas for potential neurologic compromise (see the subsequent discussion of degenerative disk disease). The sagittal and axial T2-weighted images should be evaluated carefully for the presence of disk pathology such as protrusion, extrusions, and sequestrations. If present, the degree of neural compromise should be noted (see the subsequent sections).

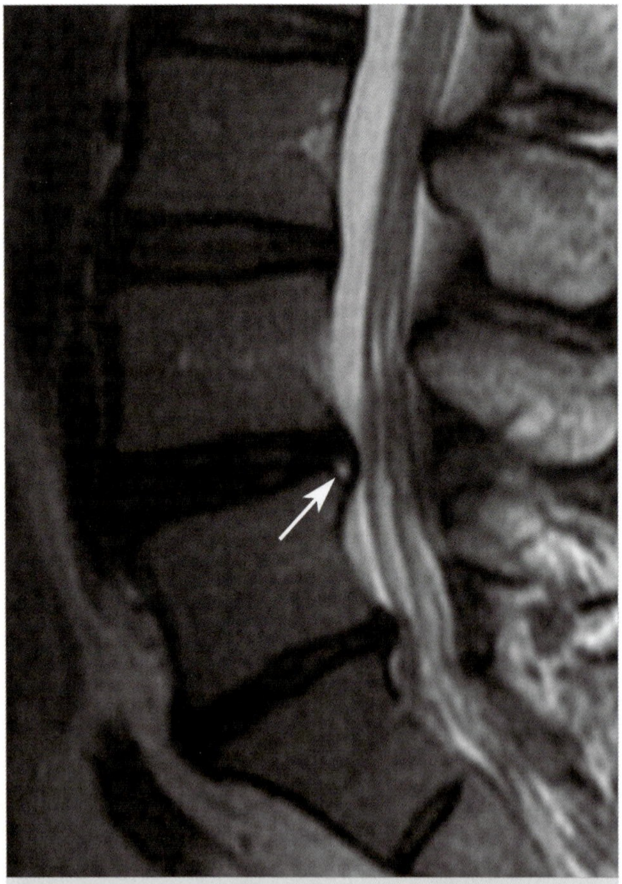

Fig. 16.9 A sagittal T2-weighted image shows a high-intensity zone at the posterior annulus of L4–L5 (*arrow*). Also noted is degenerative disk disease at L5–S1 with moderate loss of disk height. The L3–L4 disk is normal. (Reproduced with permission from, Okubadejo GO, Daftary AR, Buchowski JM, et al. The lumbar and thoracic spine. In: Khanna AJ, ed. MRI for orthopaedic surgeons. New York: Thieme; 2010:269–315.)

Epidural Hematoma

Hematomas may be seen occasionally in association with thoracolumbar spine trauma, and they can be difficult to differentiate from disk protrusions and extrusions. Hematomas often resolve spontaneously and may provide an explanation for patients who show a rapid and spontaneous resolution of apparent disk herniations.[28,29,30] Key differentiating features between a disk extrusion and a hematoma or fluid collection are the hematoma's larger size, different signal, obtuse margin along the posterior aspect of the vertebral body with maximum dimension at the midvertebral body level, and possible containment by the central septum (which attaches the posterior longitudinal ligament to the vertebral body).[31,32]

The signal pattern associated with epidural hemorrhage is related directly to the state of oxygenation of the blood that pools in the regions of interest adjacent to the cord. In the acute phase, T1-weighted images show signal that is isointense compared with that of the adjacent spinal cord, and T2-weighted images show heterogeneous areas of increased and decreased signal intensity. During the acute phase, deoxyhemoglobin is the main component of the hematoma. Deoxyhemoglobin appears isointense or slightly low in signal intensity compared with that of the normal spinal cord on T1-weighted images and as a hypointense signal on T2-weighted images. Within 2 to 4 days after injury, T1-weighted and T2-weighted images may show increased signal intensity.[24] By 8 to 10 days, the primary component of the hemorrhage is methemoglobin, which is hyperintense on T1-weighted images.[33]

Vertebral Translation or Dislocation

The posttraumatic translation of vertebral bodies may produce canal or foraminal narrowing with associated neural compression. Dislocation of the spine indicates an alteration of spinal alignment in all three planes and the displacement of one vertebral body relative to an adjacent one. Typical MRI signs of dislocations include the following:

- Altered facet joint anatomy with increased T2-weighted signal (or fluid) in the facet joints: the osseous anatomy is often better seen on CT, but edema and fluid on MRI help focus the search for a subtle injury.
- Disk herniation or pseudoherniation: with translation of one vertebral body in relation to the adjacent one, there may be uncovering of the disk, which gives the appearance of a herniation (pseudoherniation).
- Vertebral body translation: sagittal and coronal images are excellent for determining translation of vertebral bodies (▶ Fig. 16.10). Care should be taken when determining whether translations are the result of facet degeneration, osseous injury, facet joint displacement, or pars defects.

16.3 Nomenclature and Classification of Lumbar Disk Pathology

The nomenclature used for describing lumbar disk pathology should be consistent and applied uniformly. Fardon and Milette[34] have provided a comprehensive review of the nomenclature and classification of lumbar disk pathology. This nomenclature and classification scheme represents the recommendations of the combined task forces of the North American Spine Society, the American Society of Spine Radiology, and the American Society of Neuroradiology. Several other societies, including the American Academy of Orthopaedic Surgery, support the use of the nomenclature described here. Surgeons and radiologists involved in the care of patients with known or suspected lumbar disk pathology and the evaluation of their MR images should consider reviewing this publication[34] for additional details.

With this system, disk lesions are classified as follows:

- *Normal:* a young disk that is morphologically normal (no lesion).
- *Congenital/developmental variant:* disks that are congenitally abnormal or that have undergone changes in morphology secondary to abnormal growth of the spine.
- *Degenerative/traumatic lesion:* annular tear, degeneration, herniation.

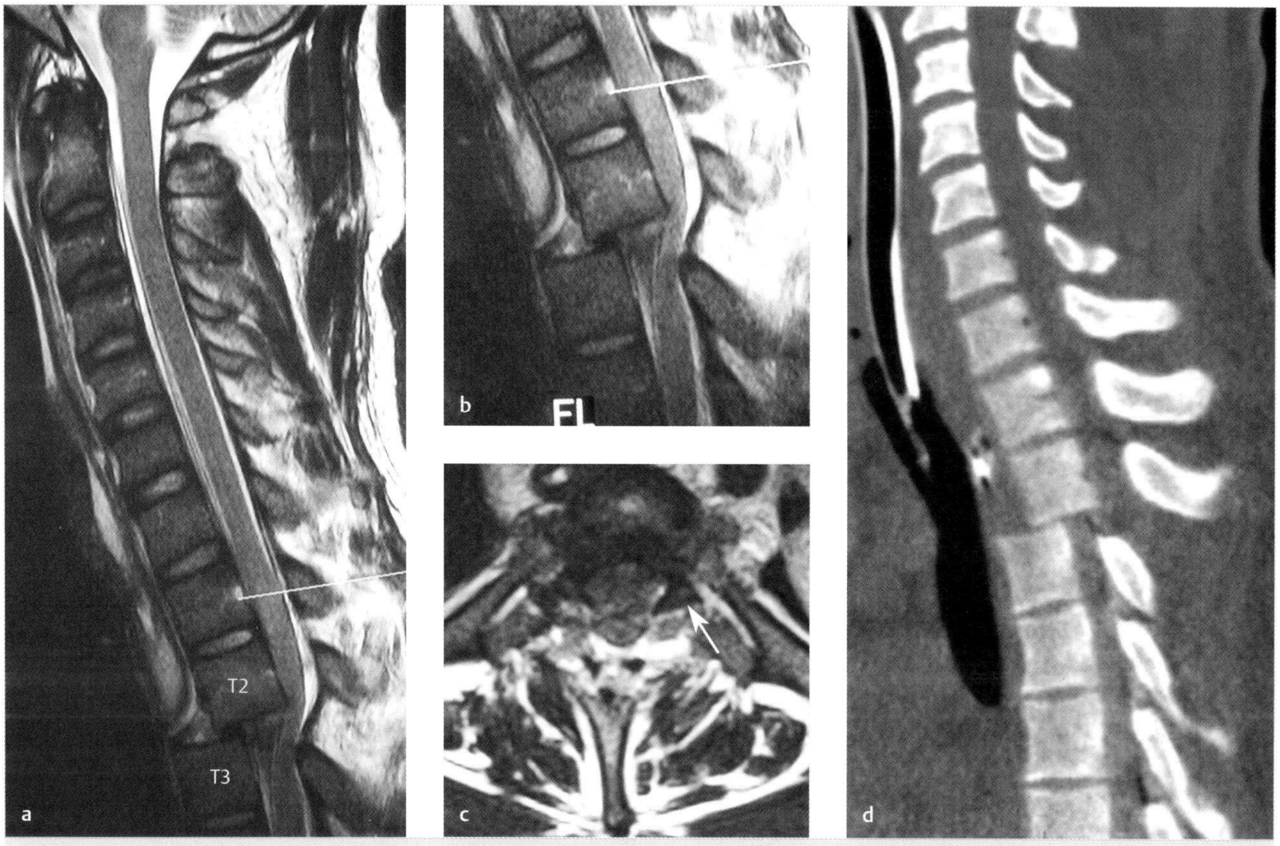

Fig. 16.10 T2–T3 dislocation. This **(a)** sagittal T2-weighted image and **(b)** enlarged image show anterior dislocation of T3 relative to T2 without fracture, with resultant severe cord compression, deformity, and acute signal change within the cord; the *line* on each points to the T1 vertebral body. **(c)** An axial T2-weighted image shows that the facets are "naked" or dissociated, a finding better seen on the left side (*arrow*). **(d)** A sagittal reconstructed computed tomographic (CT) image also shows the dislocation and confirms the absence of a fracture. (Reproduced with permission from, Okubadejo GO, Daftary AR, Buchowski JM, et al. The lumbar and thoracic spine. In: Khanna AJ, ed. MRI for orthopaedic surgeons. New York: Thieme; 2010:269–315.)

- *Inflammation/infection:* inflammatory spondylitis of subchondral end plate and bone marrow manifested as Modic type-1 MRI changes.[35,36,37,38]
- *Neoplasia:* all pathologic entities that may be primary or metastatic.
- *Morphologic variant of unknown importance.*

In the degenerative category, annular tears (also called annular fissures) are separations between annular fibers, avulsion of fibers from their vertebral body insertions, or other injuries of the fibers that involve one or multiple layers of the annular lamellae (▶ Fig. 16.11).

The degenerative process includes desiccation, fibrosis, narrowing of the disk space, diffuse bulging of the annulus beyond the disk space, extensive fissuring, mucinous degeneration of the annulus, defects and sclerosis of the end plates, and osteophytes at the vertebral apophyses. Degenerative changes can also be subcategorized as spondylosis deformans (changes in the disk associated with a normal aging process) or intervertebral osteochondrosis (consequences of a more clearly pathologic process) (▶ Fig. 16.12).

Herniation is defined as a localized displacement of disk contents beyond the borders of the intervertebral disk space (▶ Fig. 16.13a). The disk material may include nucleus, cartilage, fragmented apophyseal bone, annular tissue, or a combination of these. Most clinicians tend to describe disk pathology using the terms *bulge, herniation, extrusion,* and *sequestration.* Although the last two terms are often used correctly, there seems to be a high degree of interobserver variability in the use of the first two terms.

The currently accepted nomenclature is as follows: A herniation is considered "localized" if it involves < 50% of the disk circumference and "generalized" if it involves > 50%. A localized displacement is considered "focal" if < 25% of the disk circumference is involved (▶ Fig. 16.13b) and "broad-based" if the herniating disk content is between 25 and 50% (▶ Fig. 16.13c). Disk tissue noted circumferentially, between 50 and 100%, and beyond the edges of the ring apophyses is termed

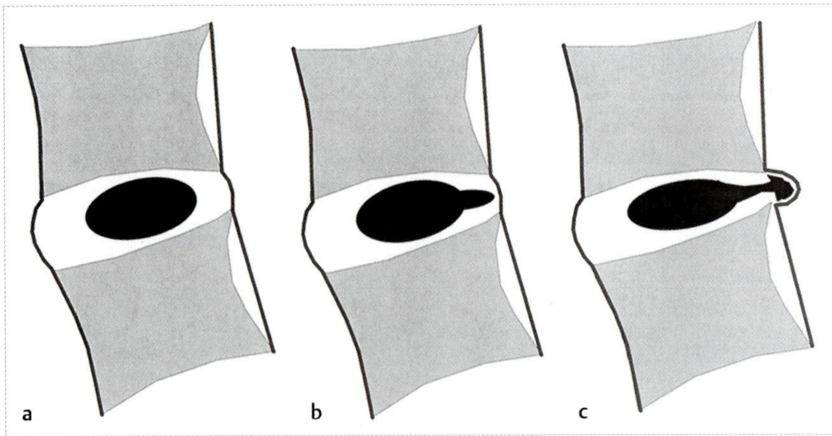

Fig. 16.11 Schematic sagittal illustrations show differentiating magnetic resonance imaging (MRI) features of disk pathology. **(a)** A normal disk. **(b)** An annular tear (radial tear, in this case). **(c)** A disk herniation. The term *tear* is used to refer to a localized radial, concentric, or horizontal disruption of the annulus without associated displacement of disk material beyond the limits of the intervertebral disk space. Nuclear material is shown in *black*, and the annulus (internal and external) corresponds to the white portion of the intervertebral space. (Reproduced from Milette PC. The proper terminology for reporting lumbar intervertebral disc disorders. Am J Neuroradiol 1997;18:1859–1866 with permission from Elsevier.)

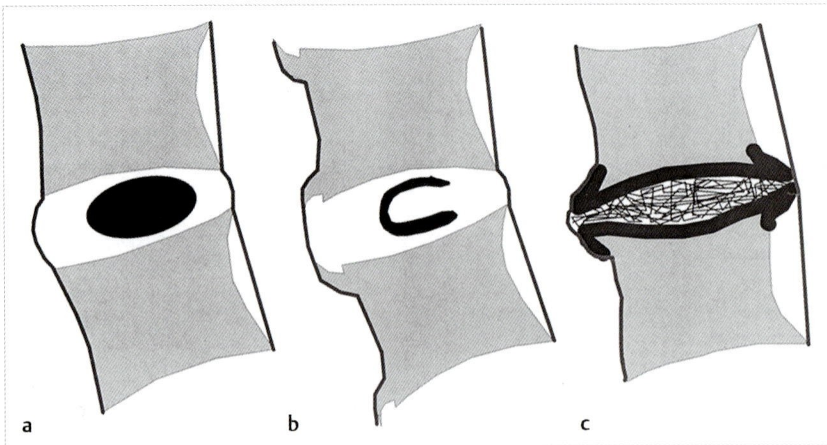

Fig. 16.12 Schematic sagittal illustrations show differentiating disk magnetic resonance imaging (MRI) characteristics. **(a)** Normal disk. **(b)** Spondylosis deformans. **(c)** Intervertebral osteochondrosis. Distinction among these three entities is usually possible on all imaging modalities, including conventional radiographs. (Reproduced from Milette PC. The proper terminology for reporting lumbar intervertebral disk disorders. Am J Neuroradiol 1997;18:1859–1866 with permission from Elsevier.)

bulging, which is not considered by some to be a form of herniation (▶ Fig. 16.13d). The terms *protrusion* (▶ Fig. 16.13e) and *extrusion* (▶ Fig. 16.13f) are also commonly used in the context of disk herniation. A protrusion is present if the greatest distance between the edges of the disk material beyond the disk space is less than the distance between the edges of the base in the same plane. The base is the cross-sectional area of disk material at the outer margin of the disk space of origin, where disk material displaced beyond the disk space is continuous with disk material within the disk space. An extrusion is present when any one distance between the edges of the disk material beyond the disk space is greater than the distance between the edges of the base (▶ Fig. 16.14) or when there is no continuity between the disk space and the disk fragment. Extrusion may be classified further as sequestered and migrated. Sequestration is noted if the displaced disk material is completely discontinuous with the parent disk. Migration consists of displacement of disk material away from the site of extrusion, regardless of whether or not there is sequestration (▶ Fig. 16.15).

Intravertebral herniation is a herniated disk in the craniocaudal direction through a defect in the vertebral body end plate. Herniations also can be described as contained or uncontained. Contained herniations are displacements of disk material that are retained by the outer annulus. Uncontained herniations are not retained by the outer annulus. Each abnormal presentation of disk pathology has specific features that can be detected with MRI (see the following section).

16.4 Degenerative Conditions

Along with cervical degenerative disorders, lumbar degenerative disk disease and associated stenosis are the most common indications for MRI of the spine. Most patients present with low back pain, lower extremity pain, or symptoms of neurogenic claudication. They usually have undergone at least 6 weeks of unsuccessful nonoperative management and often have been evaluated with conventional radiography. The purpose of MRI in this situation is most frequently to evaluate for the presence or absence of spinal stenosis, disk herniation, and degenerative disk disease.

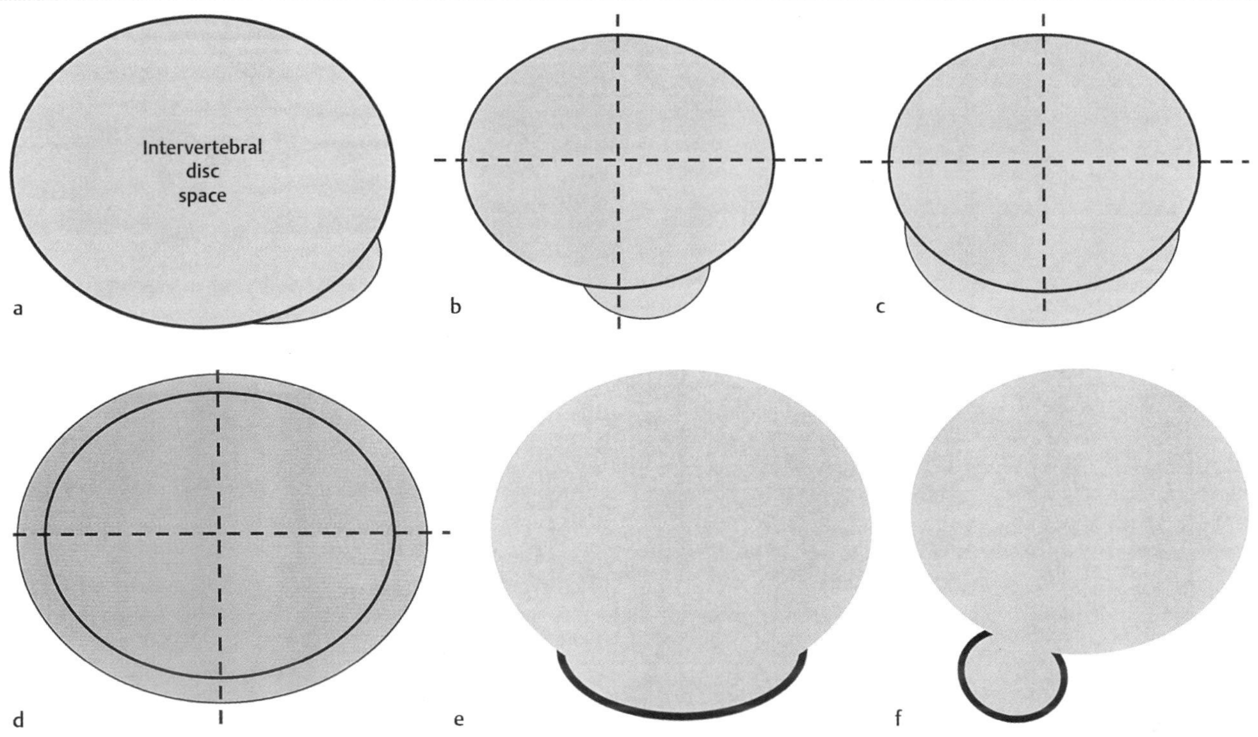

Fig. 16.13 Schematic drawings of disk herniation. In disk herniation, the interspace is defined, peripherally, by the edges of the vertebral ring apophyses, exclusive of osteophyte formations. **(a)** Localized extension of disk material beyond the intervertebral disk space, in a left posterior direction, which qualifies as a disk herniation. **(b)** By convention, a focal herniation involves < 25% (90 degrees) of the disk circumference. **(c)** By convention, a broad-based herniation involves between 25 and 50% (90–180 degrees) of the disk circumference. **(d)** Symmetrical presence (or apparent presence) of disk tissue "circumferentially" (50–100%) beyond the edges of the ring apophyses may be described as a "bulging disk" or "bulging appearance" and is not considered a form of herniation. *Bulging* is a descriptive term for the shape of the disk contour and not a diagnostic category. **(e)** Protrusion (see definition in text). **(f)** Extrusion (see definition in text). (Reproduced with permission from, Fardon DF, Milette PC. Nomenclature and classifi cation of lumbar disc pathology. Recommendations of the Combined Task Forces of the North American Spine Society, American Society of Spine Radiology, and American Society of Neuroradiology. Spine 2001;26:E93–E113.)

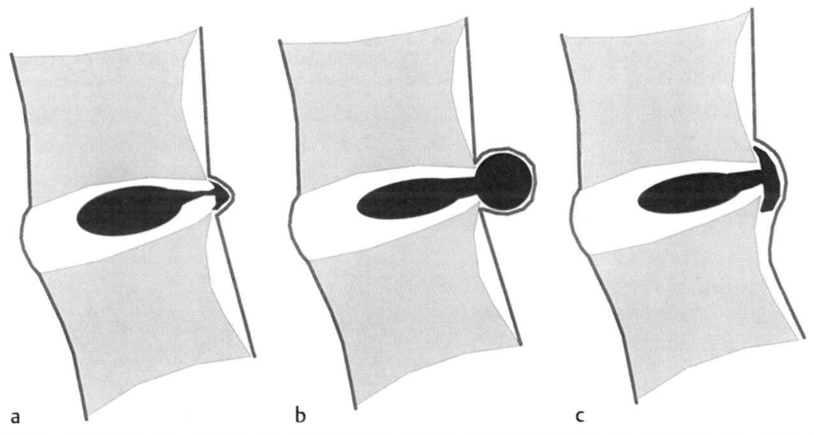

Fig. 16.14 Schematic drawings of protrusion and extrusion. When a large amount of disk material is displaced, distinction between **(a)** protrusion and **(b,c)** extrusion is usually possible only on sagittal magnetic resonance (MR) sections or sagittal computed tomographic (CT) reconstructions. **(c)** Although the shape of the displaced material is similar to that of a protrusion, the greatest craniocaudal diameter of the fragment is greater than the craniocaudal diameter of its base at the level of the parent disk, and the lesion therefore qualifies as an extrusion. In any situation, the distance between the edges of the base, which serves as reference for the definition of protrusion and extrusion, may differ from the distance between the edges of the aperture of the annulus, which cannot be assessed on CT images and is seldom appreciated on MR images. In the craniocaudal direction, the length of the base cannot exceed, by definition, the height of the intervertebral space. (Reproduced with permission from, Milette PC. Classification, diagnostic imaging, and imaging characterization of a lumbar herniated disc. Radiol Clin North Am 2000;38:1267–1292 with permission from Elsevier.)

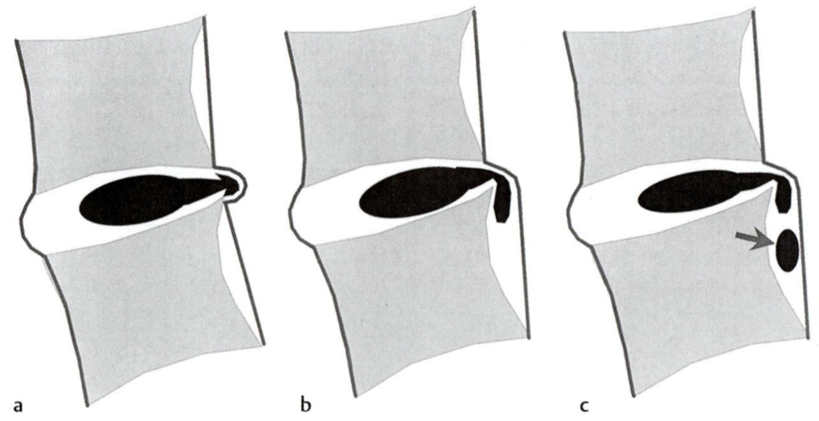

Fig. 16.15 Schematic drawings of various types of posterior central herniations. **(a)** A small subligamentous herniation (or protrusion) without substantial disk material migration. **(b)** A subligamentous herniation with downward migration of disk material under the posterior longitudinal ligament. **(c)** A subligamentous herniation with downward migration of disk material and sequestered fragment *(arrow)*. (Reproduced with permission from, Milette PC. Classification, diagnostic imaging, and imaging characterization of a lumbar herniated disc. Radiol Clin North Am 2000;38:1267–1292 with permission from Elsevier.)

Lumbar spine degeneration typically includes a constellation of changes such as degenerative disk disease, arthritic and hypertrophic changes involving the facet joints, and hypertrophy of the ligamentum flavum (see Chapter 15, The Cervical Spine, for a discussion of inflammatory arthropathies, including ankylosing spondylitis). It is important to note that patients exhibiting MRI changes may not necessarily be symptomatic.[39,40] A study of 33 asymptomatic, elite tennis players showed that 15% had normal MRI evaluations and 85% had abnormalities: 27% had pars lesions and 39% showed evidence of disk desiccation and bulging.[39] The high incidence of abnormal lumbar spine MRI studies was described by Boden et al[41] in 67 asymptomatic patients. A follow-up study of those 67 patients concluded that the MRI findings were not predictive of the development or duration of low back pain.[42]

16.4.1 Disks and End Plates

Degenerative Disk Disease

As noted above, Fardon and Milette[34] have suggested the use of the terms *normal, spondylosis deformans,* and *intervertebral osteochondrosis* to describe the degenerative lumbar disk (▶ Fig. 16.12). The changes seen on MRI correlate with the pathogenesis of degenerative disk disease, which results from the spectrum of changes that occur in the various parts of the vertebrodiscal complex.[43] The nucleus pulposus becomes increasingly hypointense on T2-weighted images because of desiccation. An alternative finding is the intervertebral disk vacuum phenomenon secondary to a collection of intradiscal nitrogen, which manifests as a linear area of signal void on T1-weighted and T2-weighted sequences. Gradient-echo sequences may show this particular finding even better than do T1-weighted and T2-weighted images.[44] Early signs of disk degeneration on MRI include infolding of the anterior annulus and a hypointense central region—often seen before any loss of disk signal intensity—which may be associated with reproduction of pain at diskography.[44] Advanced degeneration may present with a linear hyperintensity parallel to the end plate, which is thought to represent separation of the nucleus pulposus from the hyaline cartilage end plate.[44]

Pfirrmann et al[45] introduced a grading system for lumbar degenerative disk disease based on findings from sagittal T2-weighted MR images. This classification system describes five grades of progressively increasing degenerative disk disease. Its complexity may be the reason it is not commonly used by most clinicians. To summarize, the grading system describes the lumbar disk degenerative process as a continuum that progresses from a normal disk, to loss of the normal disk signal on T2-weighted images, to increasing loss of disk height, to degenerative end-plate changes and sclerosis.

Modic et al[36,37] described signal changes within the vertebral body bone marrow and end plate adjacent to degenerating disks. The first finding in the sequence of changes is fibrovascular ingrowth that results in diminished signal intensity on T1-weighted images and a corresponding increase in signal intensity on T2-weighted images (type 1) (▶ Fig. 16.16). The more chronic, type-2 changes involve a change from hematopoietic (red) to fatty (yellow) marrow, leading to relatively increased signal on T1-weighted images and slightly diminished signal intensity on T2-weighted images (▶ Fig. 16.17). Type-3 changes consist of decreased signal intensity on T1-weighted and T2-weighted sequences and are associated with subchondral sclerosis on radiographs (▶ Fig. 16.18).[35,44] Among the three types of degenerative end-plate changes, type-1 changes have been found to have the greatest correlation with the presence of discogenic back pain.[38,46,47,48]

In addition to an assessment of the type of lumbar degenerative disk disease using the methods just described, one should also describe the degree of lumbar disk degeneration by noting the amount of disk space height loss (▶ Fig. 16.19).

Annular Tears

Annular tears have a variable appearance on MRI, ranging from intermediate to high signal intensity on T2-weighted images. Studies have shown a correlation between high-signal-intensity annular

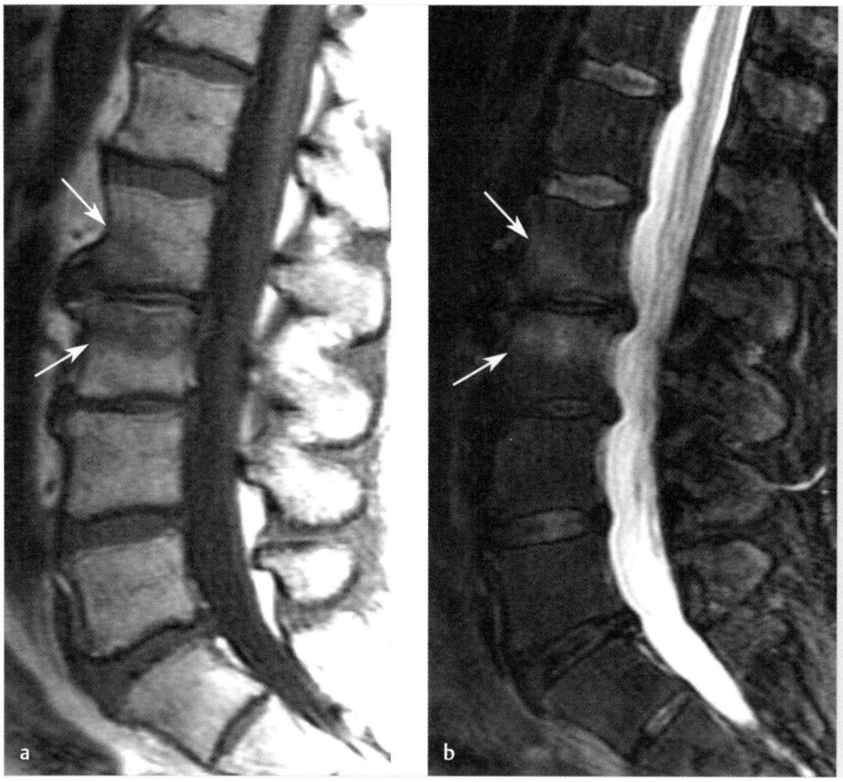

Fig. 16.16 Modic type-1 (fibrovascular) changes. Sagittal **(a)** T1-weighted and **(b)** fat-suppressed T2-weighted images show, at the L2–L3 level, the typical pattern (*arrow* on each) of decreased signal intensity on the T1-weighted image and increased signal on the T2-weighted image that is seen with Modic type-1 end-plate changes. (Reproduced with permission from, Okubadejo GO, Daftary AR, Buchowski JM, et al. The lumbar and thoracic spine. In: Khanna AJ, ed. MRI for orthopaedic surgeons. New York: Thieme; 2010:269–315.)

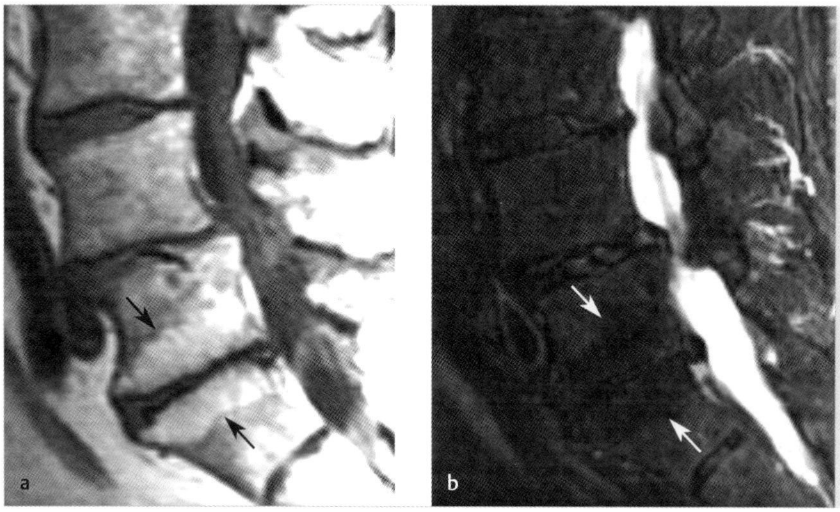

Fig. 16.17 Modic type-2 (fatty) changes. Sagittal **(a)** T1-weighted and **(b)** fat-suppressed T2-weighted images show, at the L5–S1 level, the typical pattern (*arrows* on each) of increased signal intensity on the T1-weighted image and decreased signal on the T2-weighted image that is seen with Modic type-2 end-plate changes. Note that degenerative changes and stenosis are also seen at other levels. (Reproduced with permission from, Okubadejo GO, Daftary AR, Buchowski JM, et al. The lumbar and thoracic spine. In: Khanna AJ, ed. MRI for orthopaedic surgeons. New York: Thieme; 2010:269–315.)

tears in the lumbar spine and painful concordant annular tears seen at provocative diskography.[49,50] Some investigators have suggested that the inflammation associated with these annular tears results in irritation of the adjacent nerve root, potentially leading to radiculopathy without overt mechanical nerve root compression.[50] T2-weighted sequences have been used to show the following three types of annular tears:

- Concentric.
- Radial.
- Transverse.

Concentric tears involve the entire extent of the annulus. Transverse tears occur at the periphery of the disk as a result of disruption of the Sharpey fibers. Radial tears extend from the nucleus through the annulus and may extend into the outer annulus, manifested on MRI as a high-intensity zone (▶ Fig. 16.9). The high-intensity zone is defined as a focal area of high signal intensity within the posterior annulus of the degenerating disk, separate from the nucleus. These high-intensity zones may also enhance after intravenous gadolinium administration.[44]

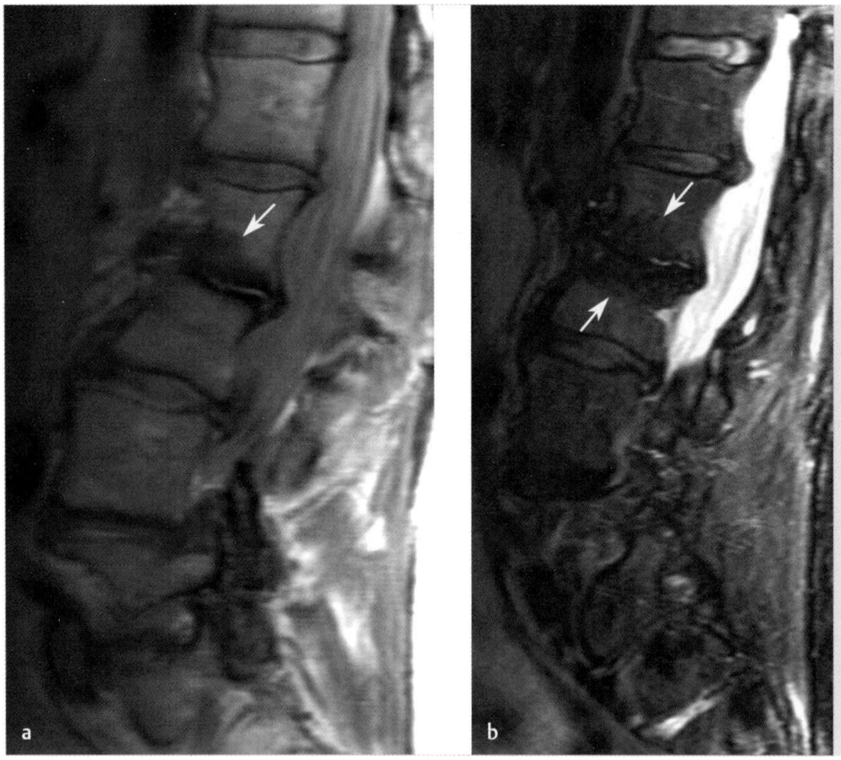

Fig. 16.18 Modic type-3 (sclerotic) changes. Sagittal **(a)** T1-weighted and **(b)** fat-suppressed T2-weighted images show, at the L2–L3 level, the typical pattern (*arrow[s]* on each) of decreased signal intensity that is seen with Modic type-3 end-plate changes. Note that degenerative changes are seen at other levels, and there is also evidence of lumbar scoliosis. (Reproduced with permission from, Okubadejo GO, Daftary AR, Buchowski JM, et al. The lumbar and thoracic spine. In: Khanna AJ, ed. MRI for orthopaedic surgeons. New York: Thieme; 2010:269–315.)

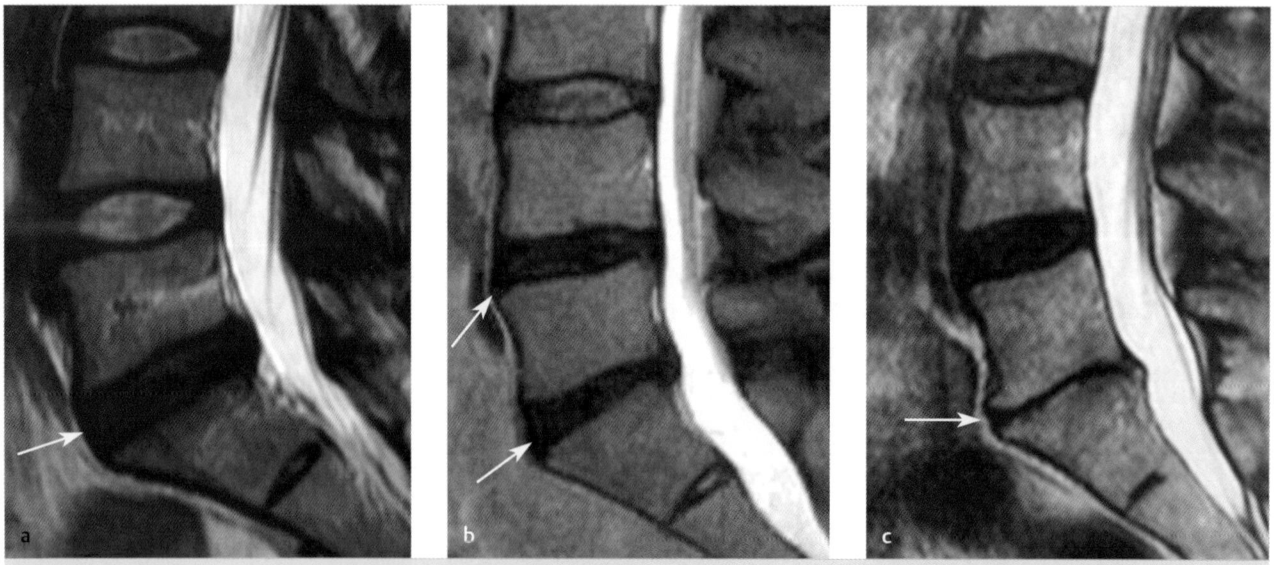

Fig. 16.19 Lumbar degenerative disk disease. The degree of disk T2-weighted signal and height loss should be evaluated and graded as **(a)** mild, **(b)** moderate, or **(c)** severe lumbar degenerative disk disease (*arrow[s]* on each). (Reproduced with permission from, Okubadejo GO, Daftary AR, Buchowski JM, et al. The lumbar and thoracic spine. In: Khanna AJ, ed. MRI for orthopaedic surgeons. New York: Thieme; 2010:269–315.)

Diskography can be used to further evaluate patients with annular tears. In addition to the morphologic information provided on fluoroscopic images and on postdiskography CT, the patient's pain response can be used to help predict whether an annular tear or other degenerative pathology is the cause of pain.[51,52] It is important to keep in mind, however, that the use of diskography in the diagnosis of discogenic low back pain continues to be debated and is not accepted at all centers.

Lumbar-Herniated Nucleus Pulposus

The terms used to describe the progressive states of herniated nucleus pulposus have been addressed previously (see section "Nomenclature and Classification of Lumbar Disk Pathology"). Shown here are the MRI appearances of each:

- Normal.
- Bulge (▶ Fig. 16.20).
- Protrusion (▶ Fig. 16.21).
- Extrusion (▶ Fig. 16.22).

The status of the annulus provides insight into the status of a herniated disk. A disk protrusion is a herniation with an intact annulus, confined by the posterior longitudinal ligament. Extrusions occur when the nuclear material breaches the outer annular fibers. If herniated disk material becomes detached from the parent disk, it is termed *sequestrated.* The sequestrated fragment can migrate superiorly, inferiorly, or occasionally, posterior to the thecal sac. Intradural disk herniation is very rare.[44]

It is often difficult to differentiate protrusion from extrusion. Several MRI signs may be used to aid this differentiation, including the following:

- If the AP diameter of the herniated disk is > 50% of the spinal canal diameter, then an extrusion is present in > 90% of cases.[44,53]
- Examination of the base of the disk shows that a protrusion usually has a broad base against the parent disk, which is broader than any other part of the hernia; an extrusion has a base that is narrower than the extruded material.
- Protrusions and extrusions can also be distinguished by their outlines. Protrusions are limited by the outer annular fibers and tend to have a smooth outline; in contrast, extrusions have a poorly defined outer margin.[44,54]

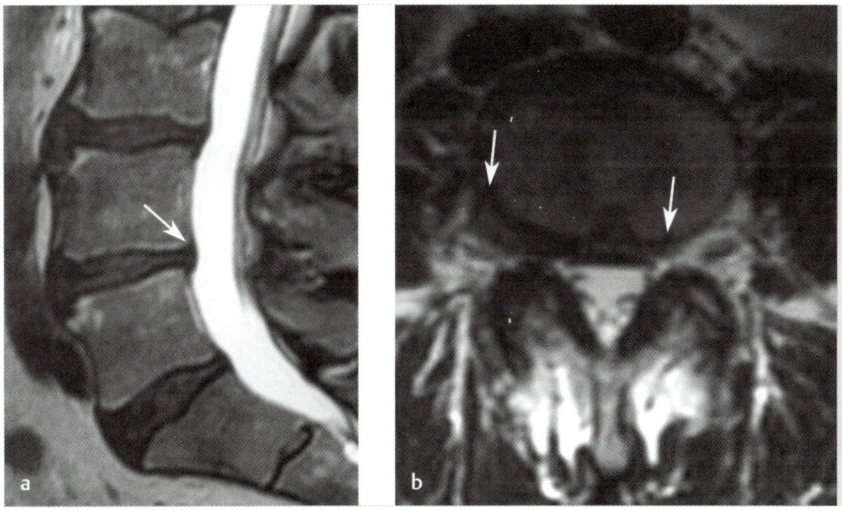

Fig. 16.20 Lumbar disk bulge. **(a)** Sagittal and **(b)** axial T2-weighted images show a right paracentral disk bulge that is asymmetric to the right, with extension into the right lateral recess and far laterally at the L4–L5 level (at *arrow* on **a** and between *arrows* on **b**). (Reproduced with permission from, Okubadejo GO, Daftary AR, Buchowski JM, et al. The lumbar and thoracic spine. In: Khanna AJ, ed. MRI for orthopaedic surgeons. New York: Thieme; 2010:269–315.)

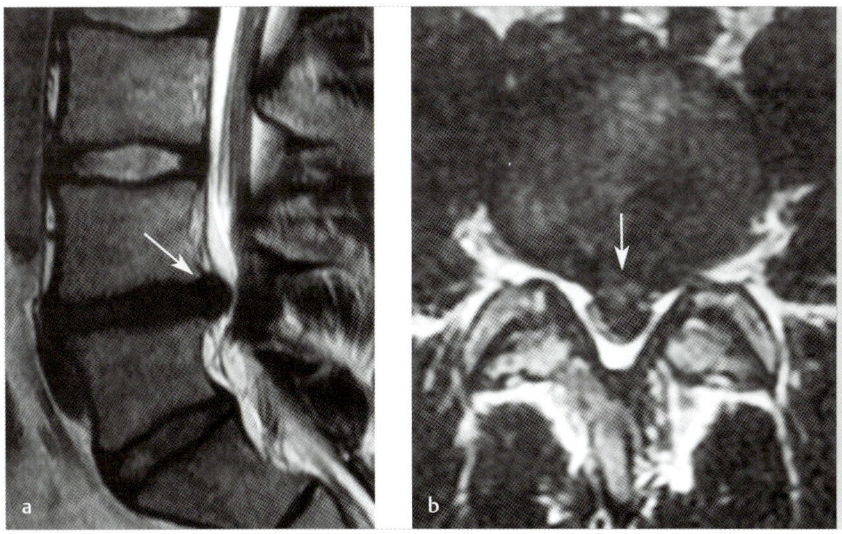

Fig. 16.21 Lumbar disk protrusion. **(a)** Sagittal and **(b)** axial T2-weighted images show a central disk protrusion at the L4–L5 level (*arrow* on each). (Reproduced with permission from, Okubadejo GO, Daftary AR, Buchowski JM, et al. The lumbar and thoracic spine. In: Khanna AJ, ed. MRI for orthopaedic surgeons. New York: Thieme; 2010:269–315.)

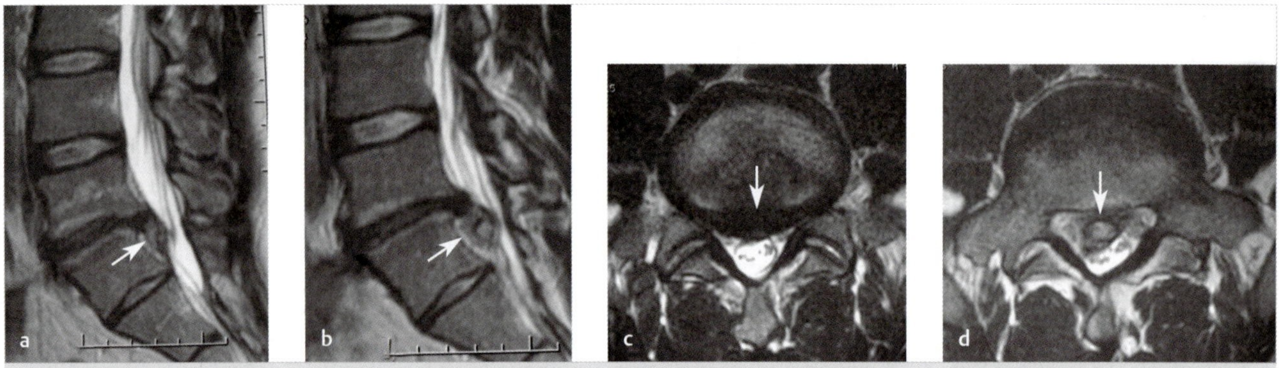

Fig. 16.22 Lumbar disk extrusion. (a) Midline sagittal and (b) parasagittal T2-weighted images show a large disk extrusion at the L4–L5 level and distal migration of the disk fragment (*arrow* on each) to behind the L5 vertebral body in a patient with transitional lumbosacral anatomy. Note the advanced degenerative disk disease at this level. (c) An axial T2-weighted image at the level of the L4–L5 disk shows what appears to be a central disk bulge (*arrow*). (d) However, an axial T2-weighted image at the L5 vertebral body level shows the disk extrusion (*arrow*). (Reproduced with permission from, Okubadejo GO, Daftary AR, Buchowski JM, et al. The lumbar and thoracic spine. In: Khanna AJ, ed. MRI for orthopaedic surgeons. New York: Thieme; 2010:269–315.)

When reviewing an MRI study that shows lumbar disk displacement, the clinician or radiologist should use the appropriate term to describe the morphology of the disk (bulge, protrusion, extrusion, sequestration) and should describe several key characteristics of the disk pathology, including the following (see ▶ Fig. 16.20, ▶ Fig. 16.21, ▶ Fig. 16.22 for examples of such descriptions):

- Level of the disk pathology.
- Precise location relative to the disk space.
- Size and degree of neural compression.

With regard to location of the disk pathology, the axial and sagittal T2-weighted images should be evaluated carefully to determine the location of the disk protrusion or other pathology. The following terms should be used to describe the location of the protrusion (primarily based on the appearance of the axial T2-weighted image) (▶ Fig. 16.23, ▶ Fig. 16.24):

- *Central* (▶ Fig. 16.25).
- *Posterolateral* or *lateral recess* (▶ Fig. 16.26).
- *Foraminal* (▶ Fig. 16.27).
- *Far lateral* (▶ Fig. 16.28).

Of all lumbar disk herniations, 90% are central or paracentral (5% are foraminal and 5% are far lateral).[55] It should be noted that a typical posterolateral disk protrusion compresses the traversing nerve root, whereas a far-lateral disk protrusion compresses the exiting nerve root. Thus, for example, a posterolateral disk protrusion at the L4–L5 level will likely produce L5 radiculopathy, whereas a far-lateral disk protrusion at the same level will likely produce L4 radiculopathy.

Another characteristic of the disk pathology that should be evaluated is its expected consistency at surgery. Specifically, the spine surgeon will benefit from knowing whether the disk can be expected to be "soft" or "hard." A soft disk protrusion consists primarily of nucleus pulposus, whereas hard disk pathology may consist of a chronic and desiccated disk protrusion or a posterior or posterolateral osteophyte (▶ Fig. 16.29). T2-weighted images occasionally show increased signal within the disk protrusion, a finding that often correlates with a soft disk at surgery.

Thoracic Disk Herniation

Thoracic disk herniations are rare, constituting only 1 to 2% of all disk herniations.[56] When they occur, they are seen most often in the lower thoracic spine, likely the result of the increased mobility and load in this region. They can also occur in association with Scheuermann disease. Sagittal T2-weighted images show thoracic disk herniations, and axial T2-weighted images allow additional characterization of the size, location, and morphology of the lesion (▶ Fig. 16.30).

Schmorl Nodes

Schmorl nodes represent herniations of the intervertebral disk through weak areas in the adjacent vertebral end plates and into the vertebral body.[57] They are found most commonly in the thoracic and lumbar spine and occur in ~10% of the population, with no dependency on age or sex.[58] Scheuermann kyphosis is one of several processes that is associated with Schmorl nodes and premature disk degeneration. Patients may be asymptomatic or have nonspecific pain that may not be related directly to the presence of the Schmorl node. When symptoms are the result of the Schmorl node(s), the patient may present with

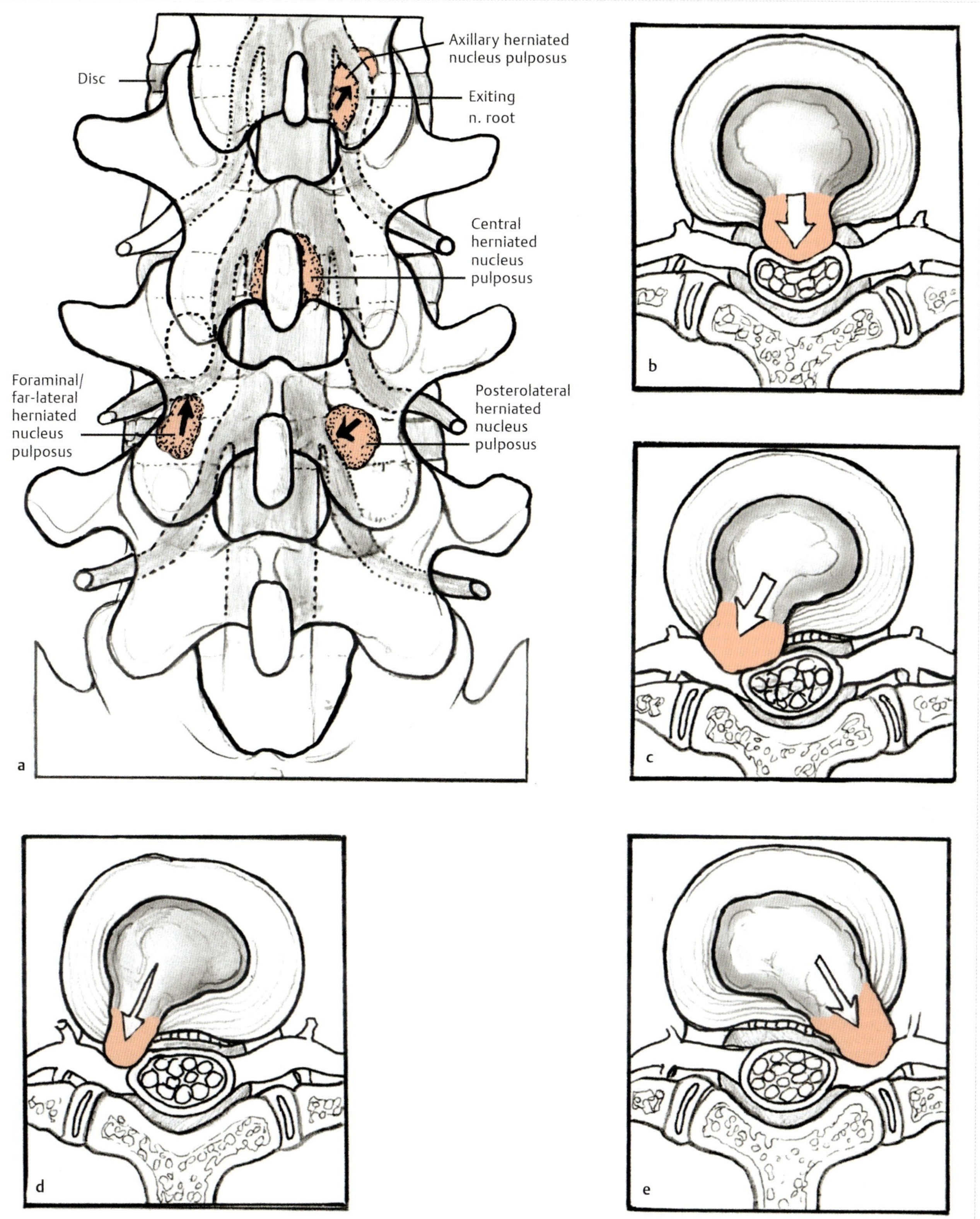

Fig. 16.23 Illustrations of types of herniated nucleus pulposus. **(a)** The posterior view shows their locations at the L2–L5 levels. The corresponding axial views show the **(b)** central, **(c)** posterolateral (paracentral), **(d)** lateral recess, and **(e)** far-lateral disk pathology. Each *arrow* indicates the direction of herniation. Abbreviation: n. root, nerve root. (Reproduced with permission from, Kerr SM, Patel DN, Vaccaro AR. Clinical features of herniated nucleus pulposus. In: Phillips FM, Lauryssen C, eds. The lumbar intervertebral disc. New York: Thieme, 2009:76–83.)

axial back pain. MRI provides the optimal detection of Schmorl nodes (▶ Fig. 16.30); they appear as extensions of disk material (with direct continuity with the disk) into the vertebral body, surrounded by a rim of low signal intensity secondary to reactive sclerosis.[44] Cases in which the Schmorl node is associated with increased T2-weighted signal in the adjacent bone marrow are more commonly associated with back pain and may represent an acute or subacute Schmorl node.[55,59]

16.4.2 Facets

Facet Arthropathy

Although it is now accepted that the facet joints may be a cause of pain in the degenerated spine, it is difficult to associate them with a particular clinical syndrome.[60,61,62] One of the earliest MRI findings of facet arthropathy is seen as fluid-like intra-articular signal intensity on sagittal or axial T2-weighted images (▶ Fig. 16.31). Observation of such fluid within the facet joints suggests the potential for dynamic instability on flexion-extension radiographs and, therefore, may affect the selection of surgical options for patients who demonstrate this finding.[63,64] Renfrew and Heithoff[31] described a practical and simple way to assess facet arthropathy:

- *Mild:* mild undulation of the margins with small (1–3 mm) osteophytes, minimal subchondral sclerosis, mild narrowing of articular cartilage, and < 25% increase in facet joint transverse dimension (▶ Fig. 16.32a).
- *Moderate:* more pronounced changes, osteophytes up to 3 to 5 mm, and 25 to 50% increase in facet transverse dimension (▶ Fig. 16.32b).
- *Severe:* additional progression of disease with near-complete loss of cartilage, osteophytes > 5 mm, and joint width > 50% of expected transverse dimension (▶ Fig. 16.32c).

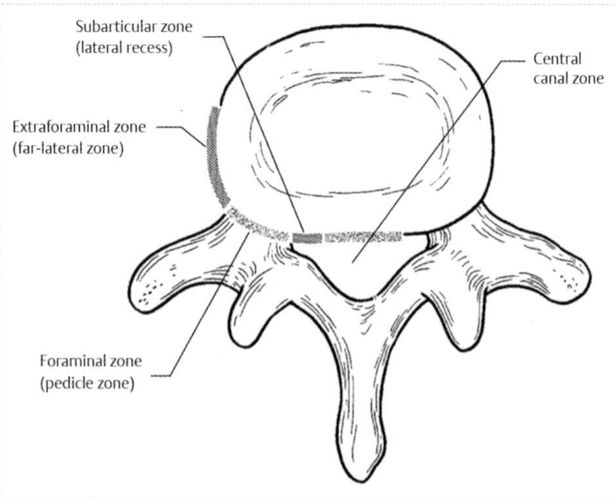

Fig. 16.24 Illustration shows the anatomic "zones" identified on axial images. (Reproduced with permission from, Wiltse LL, Berger PE, McCulloch JA. A system for reporting the size and location of lesions of the spine. Spine (Phila Pa 1976) 1997;22:1534–1537 with permission from Wolters Kluwer Health, Inc.)

Facet joint hypertrophy may cause canal, subarticular recess, or foraminal stenosis and neural compromise. Effusions may also be seen within facet joints, reflecting synovitis from osteoarthritis or a synovial proliferative process in inflammatory arthritis. Finally, asymmetric facet disease may predispose to degenerative disk disease and eventual scoliosis.[65,66,67]

Synovial Cyst

A synovial cyst, which originates most commonly from lumbar facet joints, may also cause neural compression and may appear on a sagittal T2-weighted image as a hyperintense cyst with a hypointense rim (▶ Fig. 16.33). T2-weighted MR images in the axial plane show the degree of lateral recess stenosis. Neural foramen stenosis may arise from a reduction in the height of the neural foramen because of degenerative narrowing of the intervertebral disk space, facet joint hypertrophy and osteophyte formation, or posterolateral encroachment from the disk in the form of bulges, protrusions, and extrusions. This compression is evaluated best on far-lateral parasagittal T1-weighted and T2-weighted images that show the neural

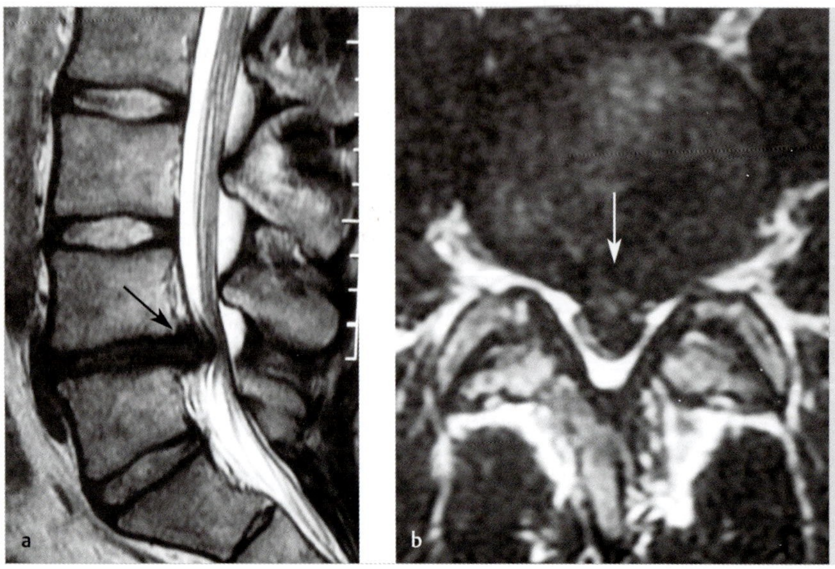

Fig. 16.25 Central disk protrusion. **(a)** Sagittal and **(b)** axial T2-weighted images show a central disk protrusion (*arrow* on each) at the L4–L5 level. (Reproduced with permission from, Okubadejo GO, Daftary AR, Buchowski JM, et al. The lumbar and thoracic spine. In: Khanna AJ, ed. MRI for orthopaedic surgeons. New York: Thieme; 2010:269–315.)

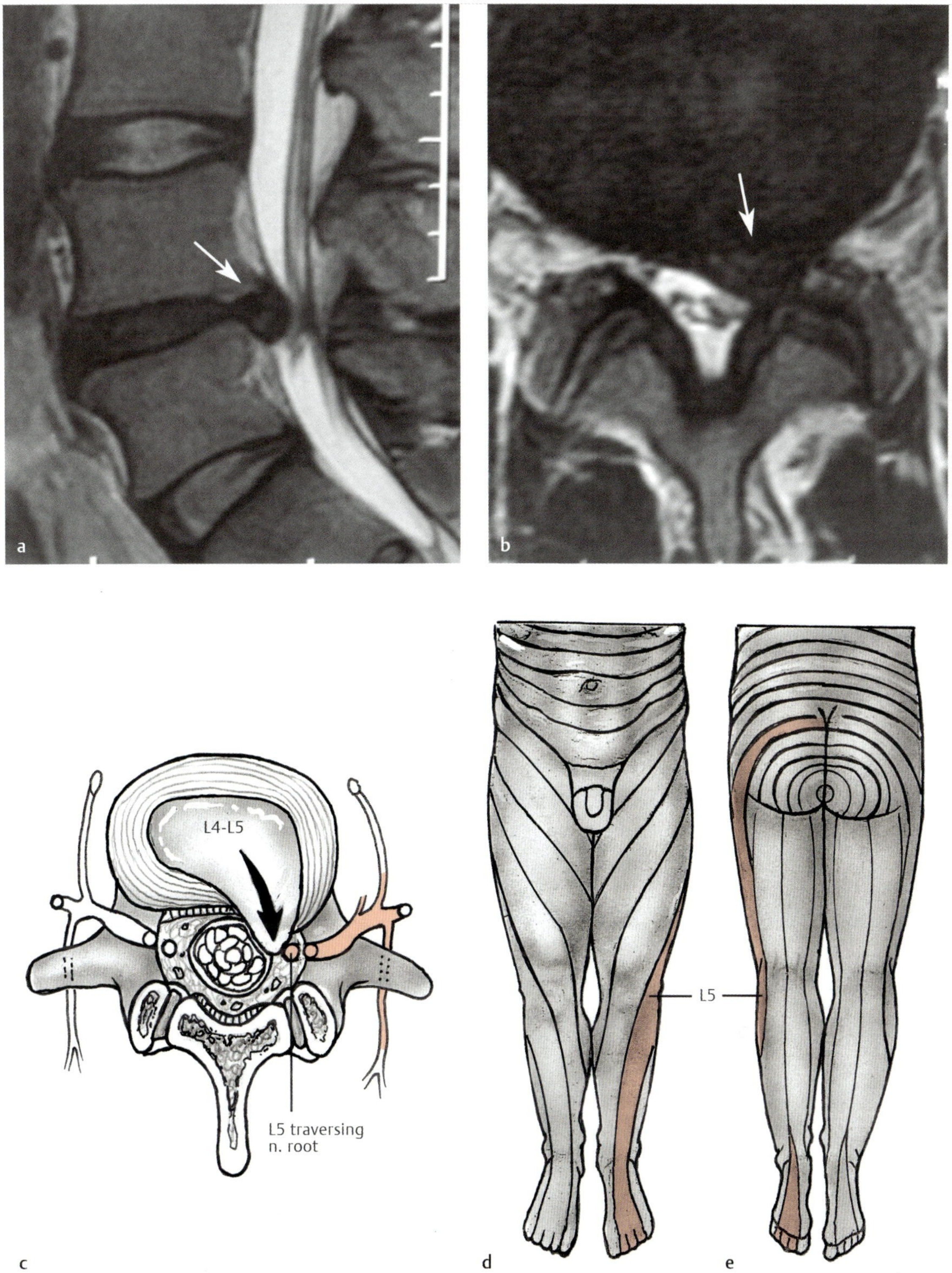

Fig. 16.26 Posterolateral disk protrusion. **(a)** Sagittal and **(b)** axial T2-weighted images and **(c)** an illustration show a left posterolateral disk protrusion (*arrow* on each) at the L4–L5 level that is in the subarticular zone and causes compression of the traversing L5 root. **(d)** Anterior and **(e)** posterior dermatomal maps show the distribution of pain or sensory deficit that may be seen in this patient. (Figure part **a** and **b**: Reproduced with permission from, Okubadejo GO, Daftary AR, Buchowski JM, et al. The lumbar and thoracic spine. In: Khanna AJ, ed. MRI for orthopaedic surgeons. New York: Thieme; 2010:269–315.) (Figure part **c**, **d**, and **e**: Reproduced with permission from, Okubadejo GO, Daftary A, Buchowski JM, et al. The lumbar and thoracic spine. In: Khanna AJ, ed. MRI essentials for the spine specialist. New York: Thieme; 2014:155–210.)

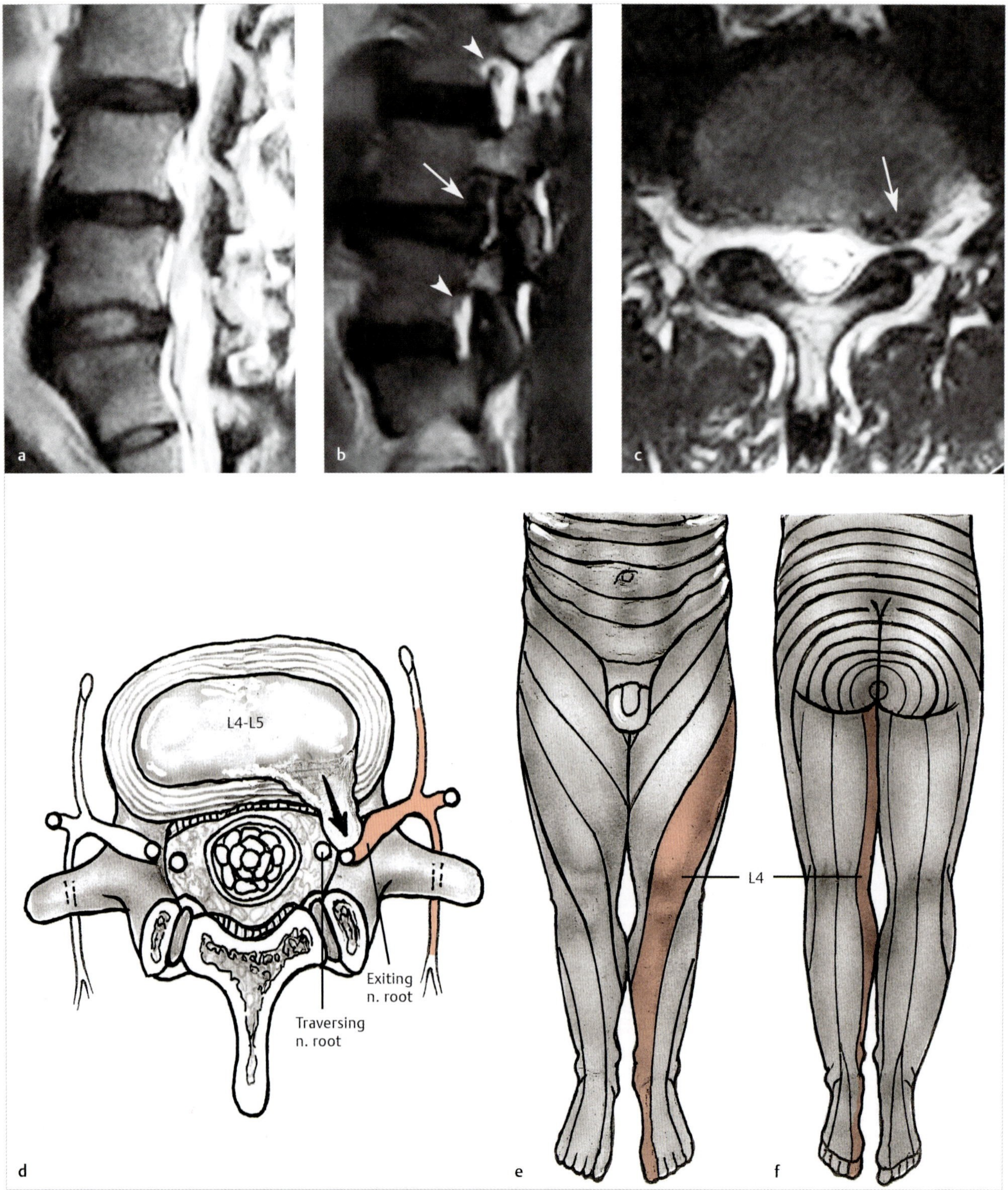

Fig. 16.27 Foraminal disk protrusion. **(a)** A sagittal T2-weighted image shows disk bulges at the L3–L4, L4–L5, and L5–S1 levels. **(b)** A parasagittal T2-weighted image at the level of the neural foramen shows disk material (*arrow*) within the left L4–L5 foramen, with resultant compression of the exiting L4 nerve root. Note the patency of the neural foramen at the L3–L4 and L5–S1 levels (*arrowheads*). **(c)** An axial T2-weighted image and **(d)** illustration at the L4–L5 level show a left-side disk protrusion (*arrow*) in the foraminal zone. **(e)** Anterior and **(f)** posterior dermatomal maps show the distribution of pain or sensory deficit that may be seen in this patient. (Figure part **a**, **b**, and **c**: Reproduced with permission from, Okubadejo GO, Daftary AR, Buchowski JM, et al. The lumbar and thoracic spine. In: Khanna AJ, ed. MRI for orthopaedic surgeons. New York: Thieme; 2010:269–315.) (Figure part **d**, **e**, and **f**: Reproduced with permission from, Okubadejo GO, Daftary A, Buchowski JM, et al. The lumbar and thoracic spine. In: Khanna AJ, ed. MRI essentials for the spine specialist. New York: Thieme; 2014:155–210.)

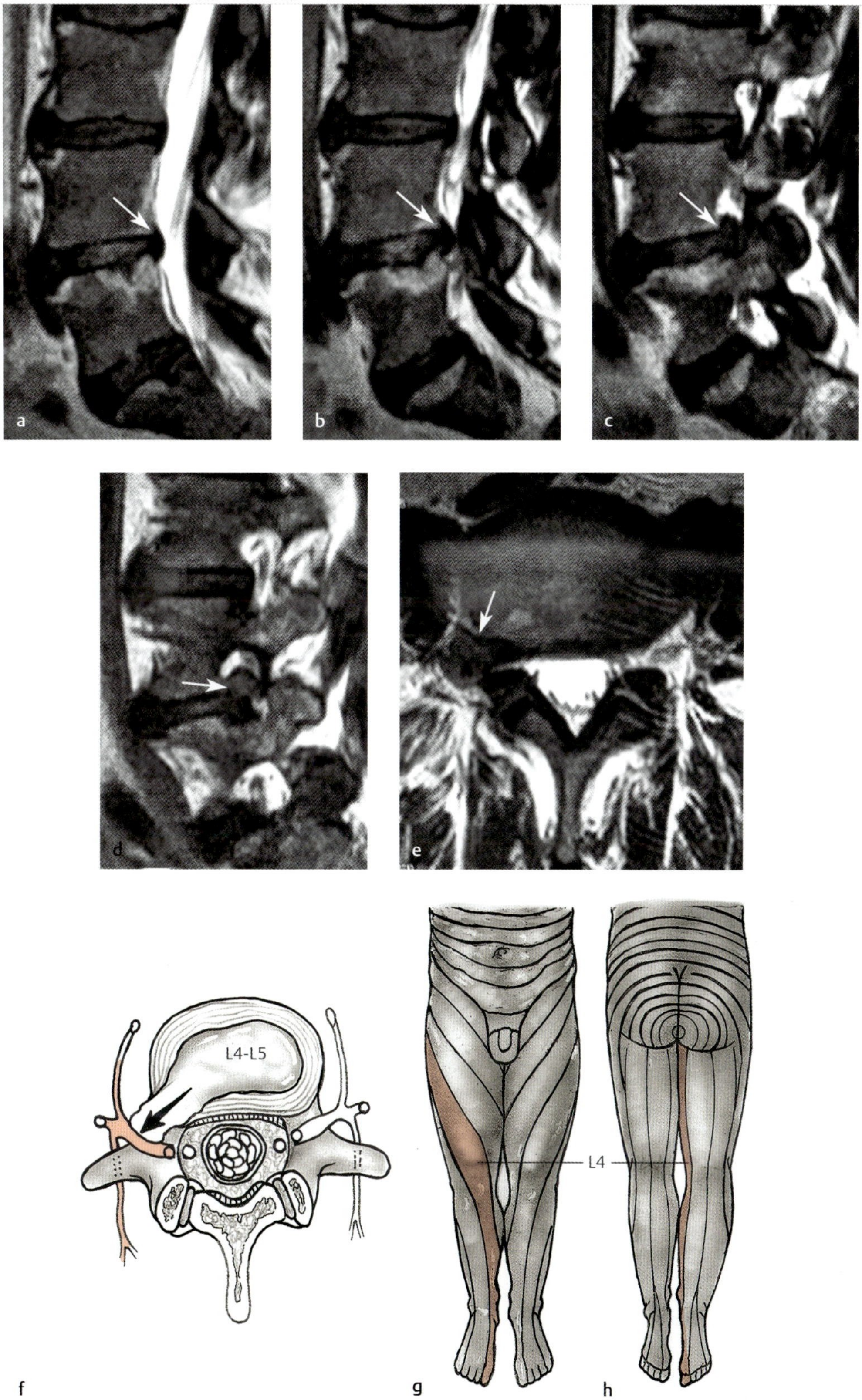

Fig. 16.28 Far-lateral disk protrusion. Sagittal T2-weighted images obtained in the **(a)** midline, **(b)** a few millimeters lateral to midline, **(c)** at the level of the pedicle, and **(d)** lateral to the pedicle and foramen show a right-side far-lateral disk herniation that is seen primarily on **d** (*arrow* on each) at the L4–L5 level. **(e)** The axial T2-weighted image (and **[f]** corresponding illustration) confirms that the disk protrusion is in the far-lateral zone (*arrow*) on the right side. **(g)** Anterior and **(h)** posterior dermatomal maps show the distribution of pain or sensory deficit that may be seen in this patient. (Figure part **a, b, c, d**, and **e**: Reproduced with permission from, Okubadejo GO, Daftary AR, Buchowski JM, et al. The lumbar and thoracic spine. In: Khanna AJ, ed. MRI for orthopaedic surgeons. New York: Thieme; 2010:269–315.) (Figure part **f, g**, and **h**: Reproduced with permission from, Okubadejo GO, Daftary A, Buchowski JM, et al. The lumbar and thoracic spine. In: Khanna AJ, ed. MRI essentials for the spine specialist. New York: Thieme; 2014:155–210.)

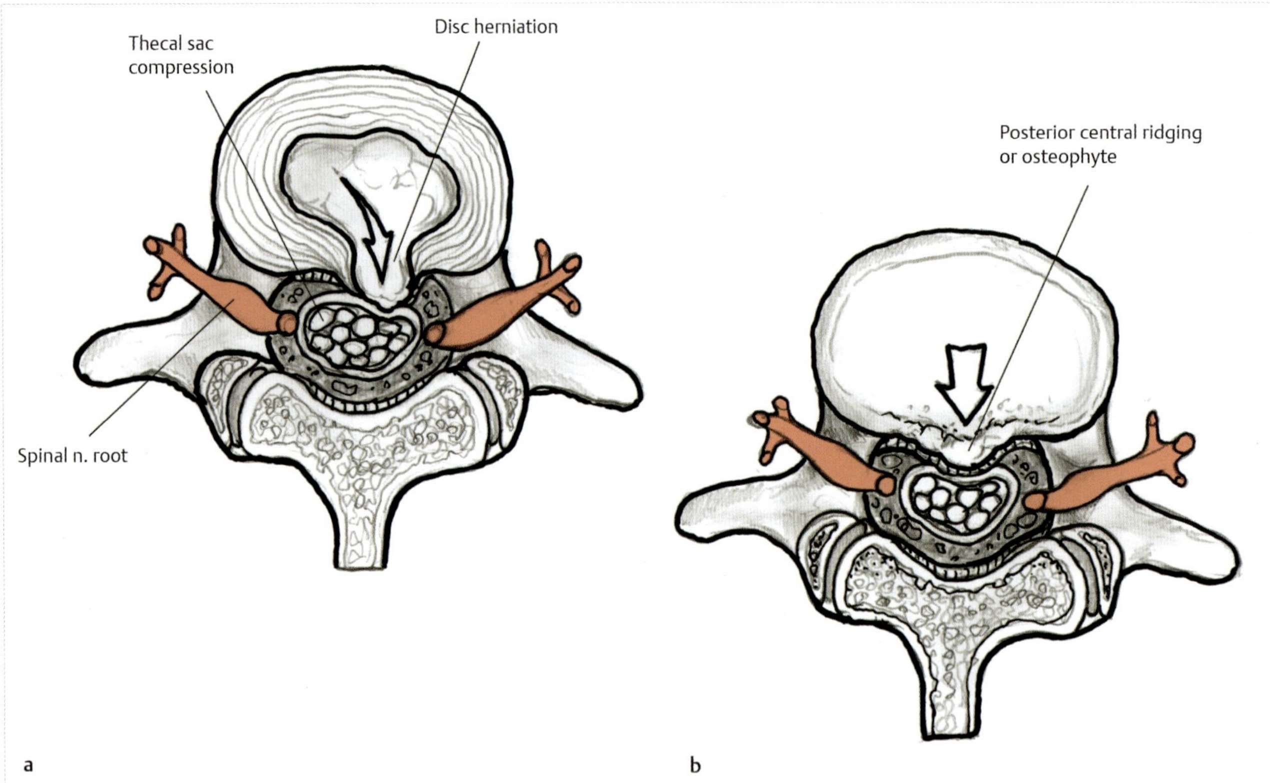

Fig. 16.29 Lumbar disk pathology. Illustrations show the difference between **(a)** soft and **(b)** hard disk pathology in the lumbar spine. The *arrow* on each indicates the direction of herniation. (Reproduced with permission from, Okubadejo GO, Daftary AR, Buchowski JM, et al. The lumbar and thoracic spine. In: Khanna AJ, ed. MRI for orthopaedic surgeons. New York: Thieme; 2010:269–315.)

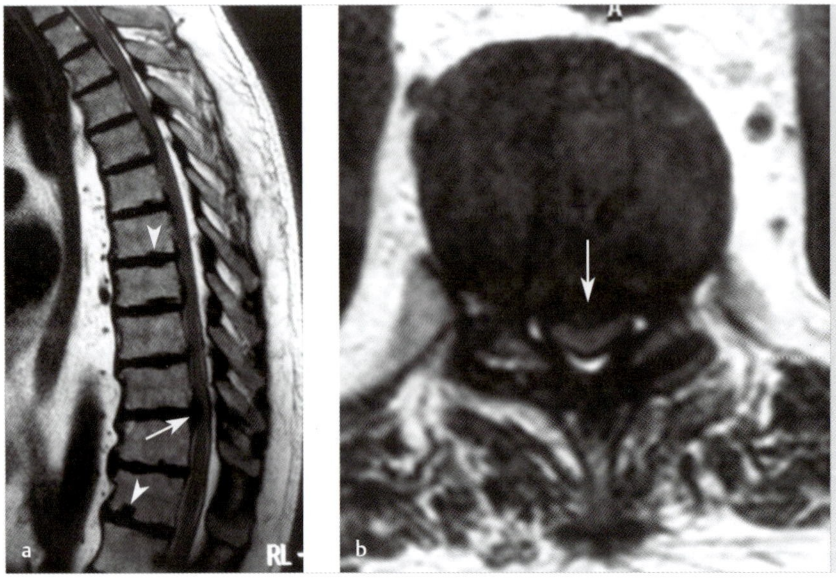

Fig. 16.30 Thoracic disk protrusion and stenosis. **(a)** Sagittal and **(b)** axial T2-weighted images show moderate-severe stenosis at the T10–T11 level secondary to a moderate-sized central disk protrusion (*arrow* on each) and underlying degenerative stenosis. Note the multilevel degenerative disk disease at other levels and the Schmorl nodes (**a**, *arrowheads*). (Reproduced with permission from, Okubadejo GO, Daftary AR, Buchowski JM, et al. The lumbar and thoracic spine. In: Khanna AJ, ed. MRI for orthopaedic surgeons. New York: Thieme; 2010:269–315.)

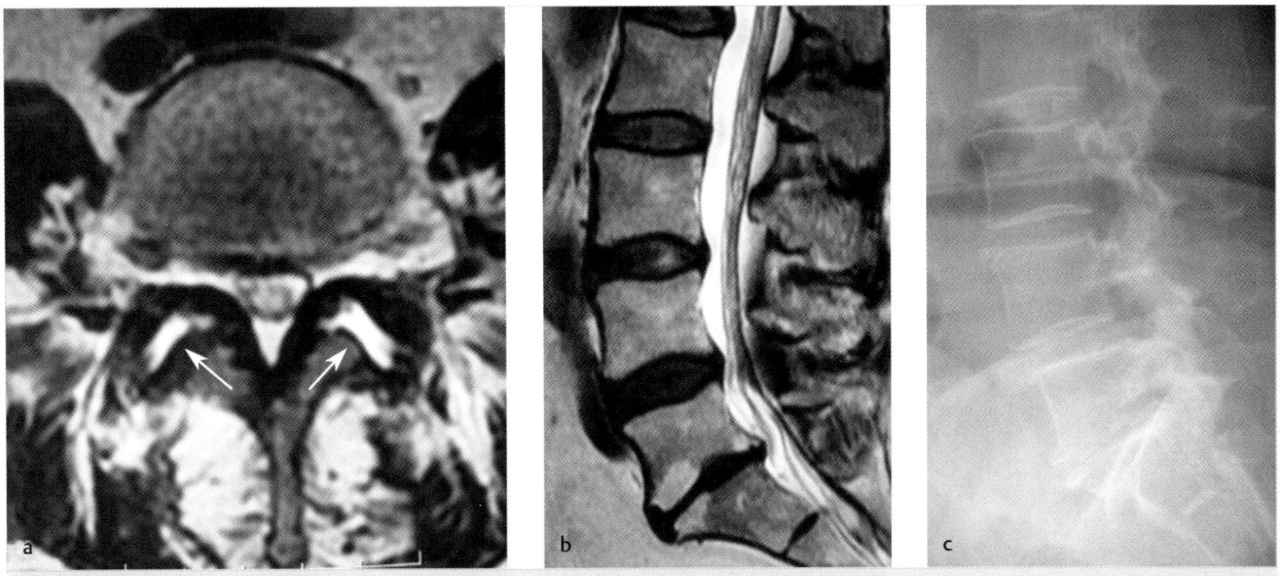

Fig. 16.31 Facet arthropathy and dynamic instability. **(a)** An axial T2-weighted image at the L4–L5 level shows bilateral facet arthropathy with fluid within and distending the L4–L5 facet joints (*arrows*). **(b)** A sagittal T2-weighted image (obtained with the patient in a supine position) shows evidence of stenosis at this level and suggests the possibility of a subtle L4–L5 spondylolisthesis. Advanced degenerative disk disease is also seen at the L5–S1 level. **(c)** A standing lateral radiograph shows an obvious Meyerding grade-1 spondylolisthesis at the L4–L5 level. This series of images shows that degenerative changes and excessive fluid within the facet joints may be associated with instability; given that magnetic resonance imaging (MRI) is performed with the patient in the supine position, the spondylolisthesis may not be seen on the sagittal magnetic resonance (MR) images. (Reproduced with permission from, Okubadejo GO, Daftary AR, Buchowski JM, et al. The lumbar and thoracic spine. In: Khanna AJ, ed. MRI for orthopaedic surgeons. New York: Thieme; 2010:269–315.)

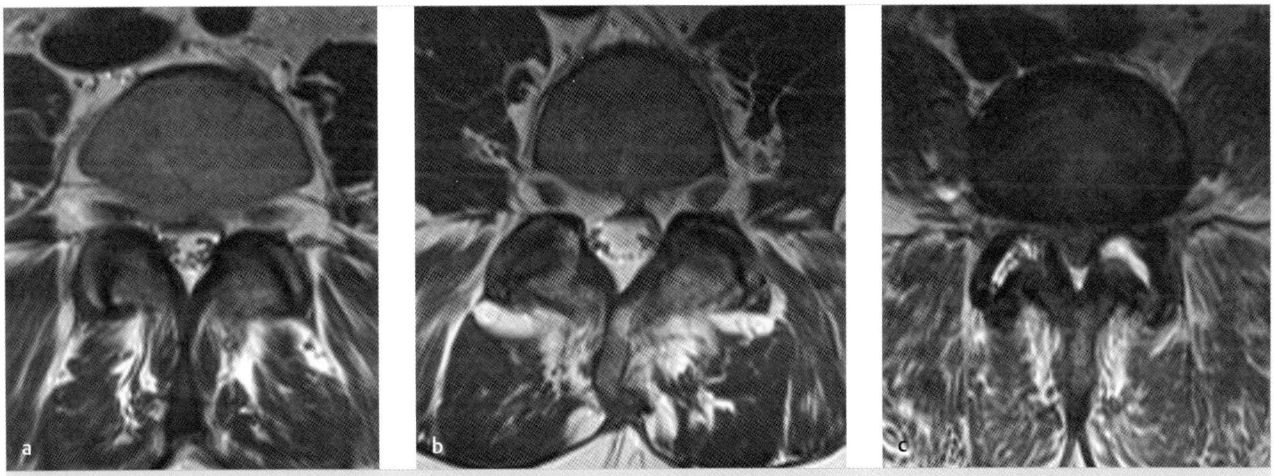

Fig. 16.32 Facet arthropathy. Axial T2-weighted images at the L4–L5 level in three patients show **(a)** mild, **(b)** moderate, and **(c)** severe facet arthropathy. (Reproduced with permission from, Okubadejo GO, Daftary AR, Buchowski JM, et al. The lumbar and thoracic spine. In: Khanna AJ, ed. MRI for orthopaedic surgeons. New York: Thieme; 2010:269–315.)

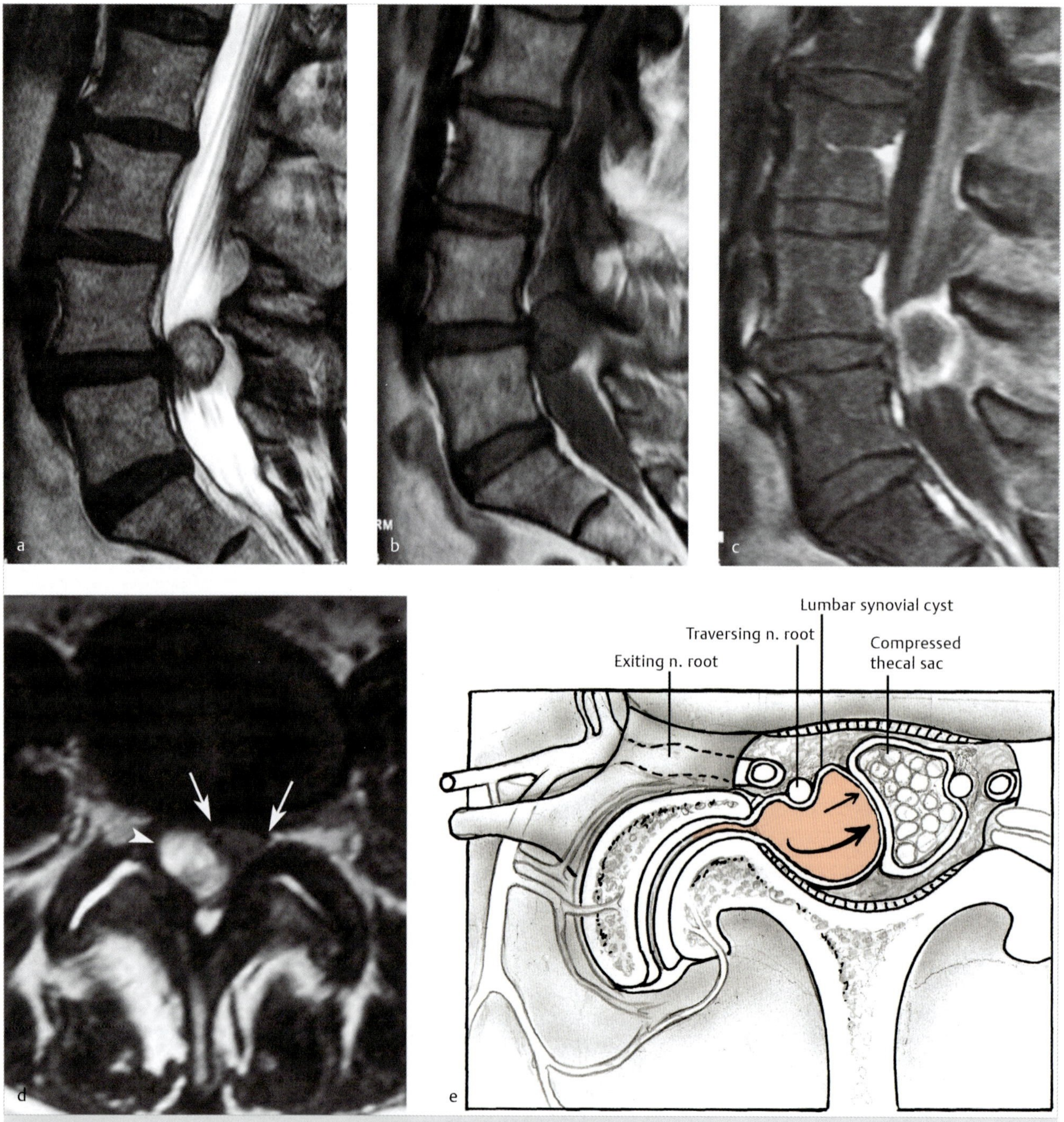

Fig. 16.33 Lumbar synovial cyst. Sagittal **(a)** T2-weighted, **(b)** T1-weighted, and **(c)** postgadolinium fat-suppressed T1-weighted Images show a large L4–L5 lesion compatible with a facet joint cyst when correlated with **(d)** the axial T2-weighted image. Note the intense peripheral enhancement of the lesion on **c**, the postgadolinium T1-weighted image. **(d)** The axial T2-weighted image shows that the cyst (*arrowhead*) likely originates from the right L4–L5 facet joint, and that the thecal sac (*between arrows*) is severely compressed and shifted toward the left. **(e)** An illustration in the axial plane shows the findings seen in the preceding images. (Figure part **a, b, c,** and **d**: Reproduced with permission from Okubadejo GO, Daftary AR, Buchowski JM, et al. The lumbar and thoracic spine. In: Khanna AJ, ed. MRI for orthopaedic surgeons. New York: Thieme; 2010:269–315.) (Figure part **e**: Reproduced with permission from Okubadejo GO, Daftary A, Buchowski JM, et al. The lumbar and thoracic spine. In: Khanna AJ, ed. MRI essentials for the spine specialist. New York: Thieme; 2014:155–210.)

foramina in cross-section.[68] On occasion, synovial cysts may contain air or may calcify, in which case they may not have the typical bright fluid signal on T2-weighted images and may appear gray or dark on all sequences.

16.4.3 Lumbar Spinal Stenosis

The term *spinal stenosis* describes the compression of the neural elements in the spinal canal, lateral recesses, or neural foramina. The evaluation of patients with known or suspected lumbar spinal stenosis is one of the primary indications for MRI of the lumbar spine.[69,70,71] Patients with lumbar stenosis typically present with combinations of radicular leg pain or weakness, neurogenic claudication, and low back pain. After nonoperative management fails for such patients and conventional radiographs have been obtained, MRI can be considered. The MR images should be evaluated to determine the degree (i.e., mild to severe), level (i.e., L1 to S1), and type (e.g., degenerative, congenital) of lumbar spinal stenosis.

The authors' suggested method for the assessment of lumbar spinal stenosis begins with a systematic evaluation of the midsagittal T2-weighted images. These images show the conus medullaris in the patient without scoliosis. The clinician or radiologist should carefully trace the posterior margin of the vertebral bodies and intervening disks to ensure that there is no effacement of the CSF space. Next, the dorsal margin of the thecal sac should be evaluated on these images to evaluate for focal hypertrophy of the ligamentum flavum. This procedure should be repeated on the parasagittal T2-weighted images in each direction (left and right from center) to evaluate for lateral recess and foraminal stenosis. After the sagittal T2-weighted images have been evaluated, the axial T2-weighted images are evaluated sequentially from the sacrum toward the upper lumbar spine. Specifically, CSF should be seen ventral to the cauda equina, which is often displaced posteriorly within the spinal canal, given that most studies are obtained with the patient in a supine position. The lateral recess and foraminal region should be evaluated bilaterally at each level to rule out stenosis secondary to disk, facet, or ligamentum flavum pathology.

Spinal stenosis may involve the neural foramina, lateral recesses, or central canal of the lumbosacral spine and is usually developmental or acquired in nature. Developmental spinal stenosis, which constitutes ~15% of all cases of spinal stenosis, is hereditary-idiopathic or associated with disorders of skeletal growth.[68] MRI of the hereditary form shows minor hypoplasia of the posterior osseous arch of the vertebrae, short pedicles, and narrowing of the cross-sectional area of the central spinal canal (▶ Fig. 16.34). Sagittal images may show progressive narrowing of the AP dimension of the spine in the caudal direction, indicating developmental spinal stenosis.

Acquired central spinal canal stenosis may arise from hypertrophic or degenerative changes of the intervertebral disks, facet joints, or ligamentum flavum (▶ Fig. 16.35). On MRI, central canal stenosis is characterized by compression of the thecal sac, best seen on sagittal and axial T2-weighted images. Fat-suppressed T2-weighted and STIR images provide a "myelographic effect," in which the CSF is seen as bright signal anterior and posterior to the neural elements on sagittal and axial images. Effacement, discontinuity, or displacement of this CSF space is seen in patients with focal and concentric spinal stenosis (▶ Fig. 16.36).

There are several objective measures of lumbar spinal stenosis.[72,73,74] Hamanishi et al[73] found that a cross-sectional area of < 100 mm^2 at more than two of three lumbar intervertebral levels was highly associated with the presence of intermittent neurogenic claudication. Speciale et al[74] evaluated observer variability in assessing lumbar spinal stenosis on MRI in relation to cross-sectional spinal canal area and found only a fair level of agreement among the observers; however, they found that the ability of the various readers to predict the degree of central stenosis was high.

Another method for evaluating the degree of lumbar spinal stenosis and its potential for contribution to clinical symptoms is the "sedimentation sign," a phenomenon named by

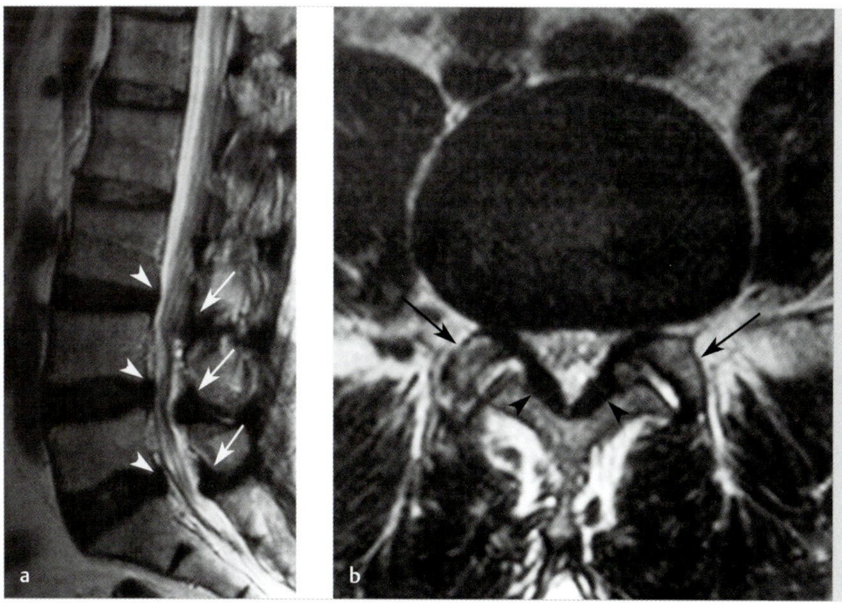

Fig. 16.34 Degenerative changes superimposed on congenital lumbar stenosis. **(a)** A sagittal T2-weighted image shows multilevel degenerative disk disease at L3–L4, L4–L5, and L5–S1, with evidence of stenosis from disk bulges at these levels (*arrowheads*), ligamentum flavum hypertrophy (*arrows*), and a generalized narrow appearance of the spinal canal relative to the anteroposterior (AP) diameter of the vertebral bodies. **(b)** An axial T2-weighted image at the L4–L5 level shows minimal to moderate stenosis secondary to underlying congenital stenosis with superimposed degenerative changes, including ligamentum flavum hypertrophy (*arrowheads*) and facet arthropathy (*arrows*). (Reproduced with permission from, Okubadejo GO, Daftary AR, Buchowski JM, et al. The lumbar and thoracic spine. In: Khanna AJ, ed. MRI for orthopaedic surgeons. New York: Thieme; 2010:269–315.)

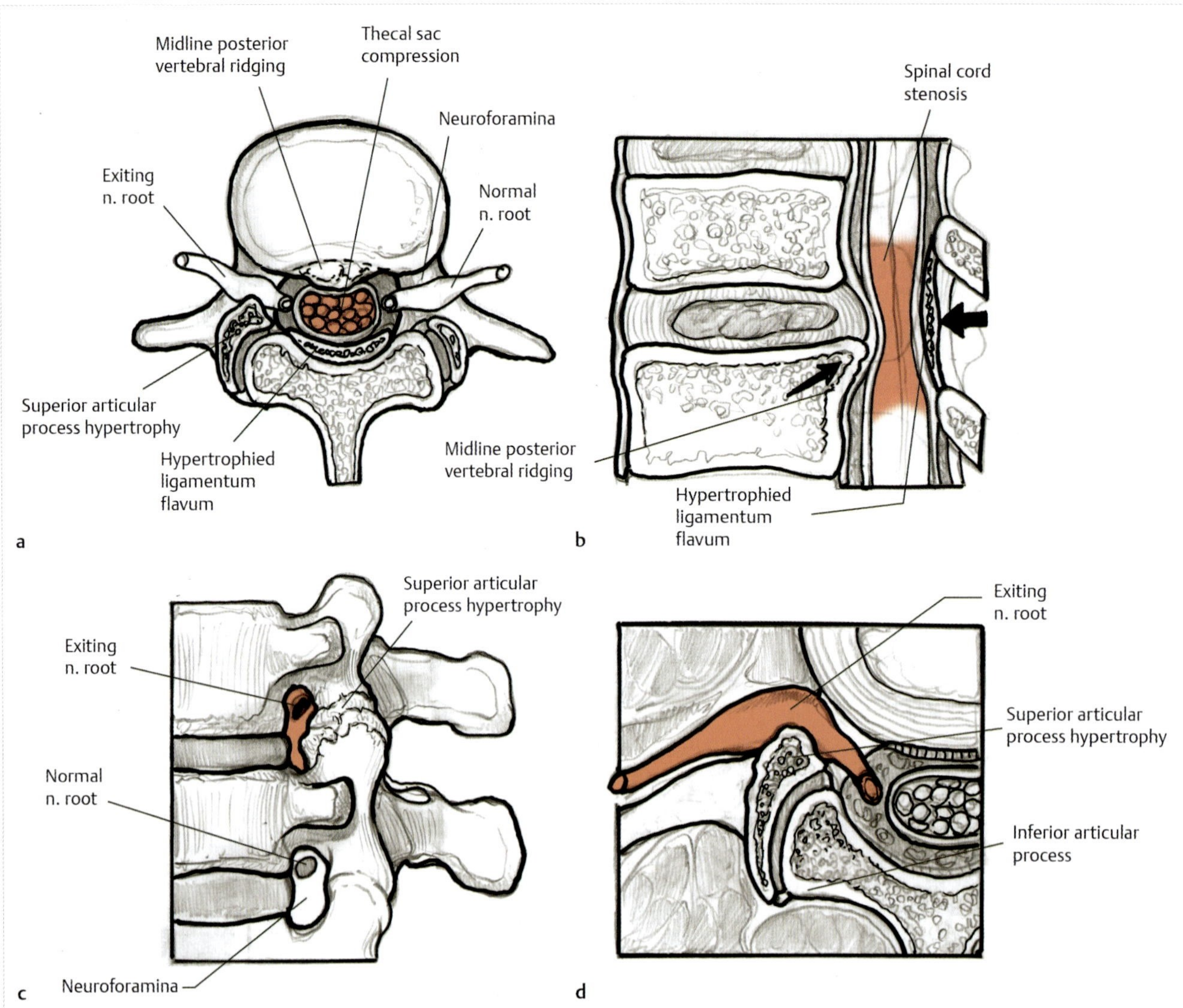

Fig. 16.35 Illustrations of the anatomic changes that lead to lumbar stenosis. **(a)** An axial view. **(b)** A midline sagittal view. **(c)** A parasagittal view at the level of the neural foramina. **(d)** A magnified axial view shows the left lateral recess and foramen. (Reproduced with permission from, Okubadejo GO, Daftary AR, Buchowski JM, et al. The lumbar and thoracic spine. In: Khanna AJ, ed. MRI for orthopaedic surgeons. New York: Thieme; 2010:269–315.)

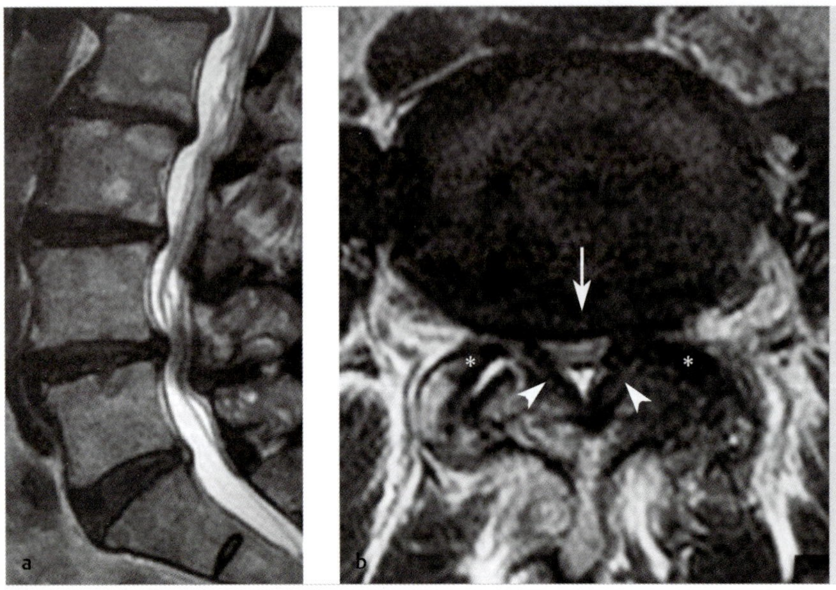

Fig. 16.36 Lumbar stenosis. **(a)** A sagittal T2-weighted image shows multilevel stenosis in the lumbar spine. **(b)** An axial T2-weighted image at the L4–L5 level shows moderate-severe stenosis secondary to contributions from a central disk bulge (*arrow*), ligamentum flavum hypertrophy (*arrowheads*), and facet arthropathy (*asterisks*). (Reproduced with permission from, Okubadejo GO, Daftary AR, Buchowski JM, et al. The lumbar and thoracic spine. In: Khanna AJ, ed. MRI for orthopaedic surgeons. New York: Thieme; 2010:269–315.)

Barz et al,[75] who also defined a positive sedimentation sign as an absence of sedimentation of nerve roots in patients with a diagnosis of lumbar spinal stenosis (▶ Fig. 16.37, ▶ Fig. 16.38). In patients without lumbar spinal stenosis, the lumbar nerve roots "sediment" to the dorsal part of the thecal sac (▶ Fig. 16.39). Conversely, in patients with symptomatic and morphologic central lumbar stenosis, such sedimentation is rarely seen.[75,76]

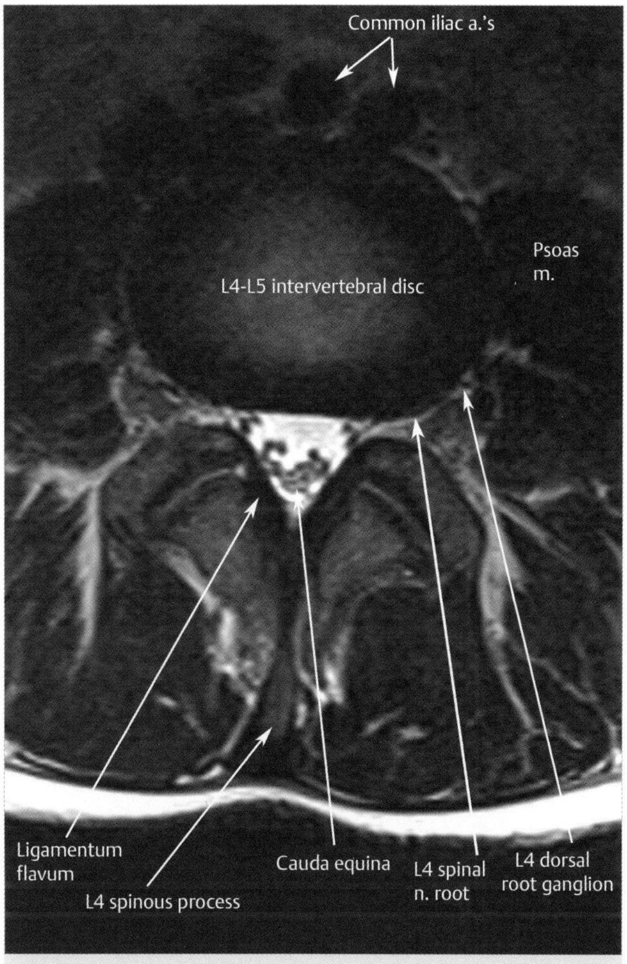

Fig. 16.37 An axial T2-weighted image of the lumbar spine at the L4–L5 level shows the cauda equina, L4 spinal nerve root, and L4 dorsal nerve root ganglion. Note the "sedimentation" of the nerve roots in the dorsal aspect of the thecal sac. (Reproduced with permission from, Okubadejo GO, Daftary AR, Buchowski JM, et al. The lumbar and thoracic spine. In: Khanna AJ, ed. MRI for orthopaedic surgeons. New York: Thieme; 2010:269–315.)

To show the clinical utility of the sedimentation sign and compare it with other, more traditional measures of lumbar stenosis, Fazal et al[77] reviewed the preoperative MRI studies of 71 consecutive patients who presented with lumbar spinal stenosis and underwent a lumbar decompressive procedure. They evaluated several radiographic parameters, including the sedimentation sign, and found that the sedimentation sign was noted to be positive in 120 of 134 (90%) operated levels. Based on this and other findings, those authors suggested that the sedimentation sign allows physicians to evaluate the degree of spinal stenosis objectively, and that the sign is most often present in patients who undergo lumbar decompressive surgery. They also found good correlation between the sedimentation sign and other radiographic parameters, including cross-sectional area, AP canal diameter, and degree of facet joint hypertrophy.[77]

Although the formal measurements of lumbar stenosis on MRI just described are well known, most clinicians and radiologists tend to grade the degree of spinal stenosis as mild, moderate, or severe. The authors use the following terms and definitions:

- *Mild:* stenosis in which the canal begins to assume a triangular shape, the thecal sac is not compressed, and there is minimal (< 2 mm) thickening of the ligamentum flavum. The AP canal diameter is > 75% of expected normal without nerve root crowding.
- *Moderate:* findings similar to those of mild stenosis but with compression and minimal flattening and deformity of the thecal sac. The AP canal diameter is between 50 and 75% of expected normal.
- *Severe:* advanced stenosis with very pronounced flattening and deformity of the thecal sac that is obvious on both sagittal and axial T2-weighted images. The ligamentum flavum is often thickened to > 4 mm. The AP canal diameter is < 50% of expected normal.

It should be noted that in some cases, canal narrowing can be downgraded if there is ample CSF surrounding the neural structures and upgraded if the surrounding CSF is scant. Similar terminology can be applied to grading stenosis in the subarticular recesses or foramina.

In addition to evaluating the degree of central and canal stenosis, the lateral recess, foraminal, and extraforaminal zones should also be assessed (▶ Fig. 16.24). Lateral recess and foraminal stenosis are most often the result of a combination of pathologies: facet arthropathy, ligamentum flavum hypertrophy, and disk bulge or protrusion. Specifically, hypertrophy of

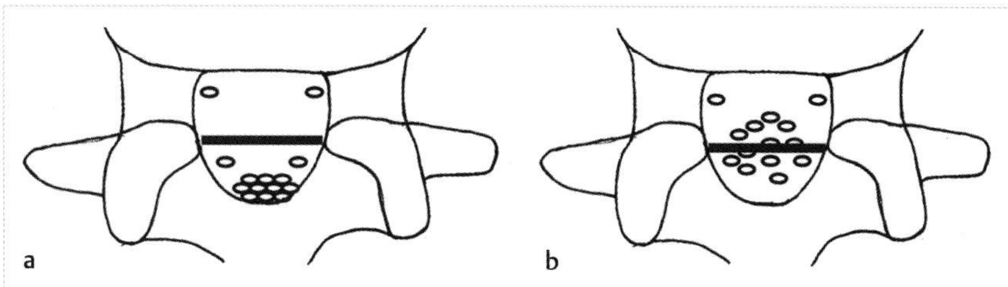

Fig. 16.38 An artist's sketch showing **(a)** negative and **(b)** positive sedimentation signs. (Reproduced with permission from Barz T, Melloh M, Staub LP, Lord SJ, Lange J, Roder CP, Theis JC, Merk HR. Nerve root sedimentation sign: evaluation of a new radiological sign in lumbar spinal stenosis. Spine (Phila Pa 1976) 2010;35(8):892–897. Reprinted by permission.)

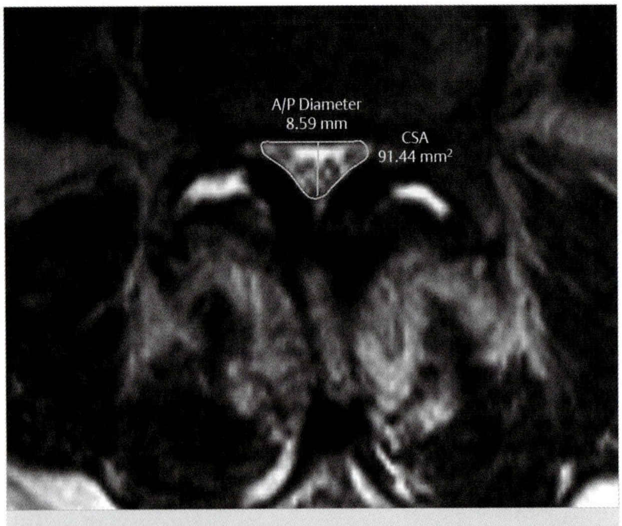

Fig. 16.39 An axial T2-weighted image of the lumbar spine shows the cross-sectional area and anteroposterior (AP) measurements and depicts a positive sedimentation sign. (Reproduced with permission from Fazal A, Yoo A, Bendo JA. Does the presence of the nerve root sedimentation sign on MRI correlate with the operative level in patients undergoing posterior lumbar decompression for lumbar stenosis? Spine J. 2013;13(8):837–842.)

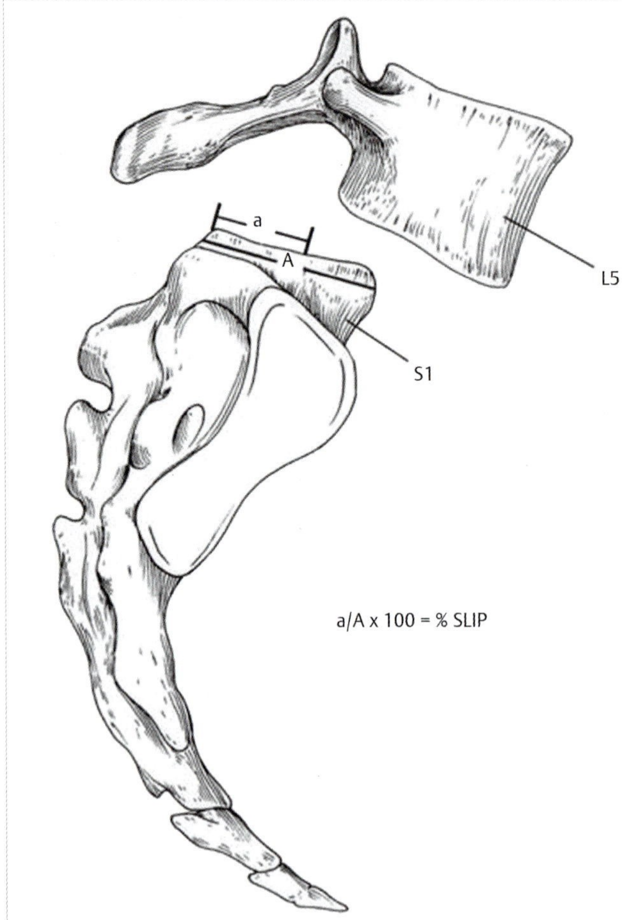

Fig. 16.40 An illustration of the Meyerding classification, which is used to quantify the degree of spondylolisthesis. Grade 1 is 0% to 25% slip, grade 2 is 26% to 50% slip, grade 3 is 51% to 75% slip, and grade 4 is 76% to 99% slip. *A* = width of the superior end plate of S1, *a* = distance between the posterior edge of the inferior end plate of L5 and the posterior edge of the superior end plate of S1. (Reproduced with permission from, Cavalier R, Herman MJ, Cheung EV, et al. Spondylolysis and spondylolisthesis in children and adolescents. I. Diagnosis, natural history, and nonsurgical management. J Am Acad Orthop Surg 2006;14:417–424. This reprinted illustration was modified with permission from Herman MJ, Pizzutillo PD, Cavalier R. Spondylolysis and spondylolisthesis in the child and adolescent athlete. Orthop Clin North Am 2003;34:461–467.)

the superior articular process from the caudal level often leads to the development of foraminal stenosis. In addition, degenerative disk disease with the associated loss of disk height and subsequent loss of foraminal height and volume can lead to the development or exacerbation of foraminal stenosis from other degenerative pathologies. Many clinicians and radiologists evaluate for the presence of foraminal stenosis in the axial plane. However, parasagittal images are also quite useful for confirming the presence of foraminal stenosis (▶ Fig. 16.27, ▶ Fig. 16.28). The normal foramen has an ovoid configuration on parasagittal images (see Chapter 13, Normal Spine MRI Anatomy), where the superior aspect of the foramen contains the exiting nerve root, and the inferior aspect of the foramen shows high signal intensity on both T1-weighted (from perineural fat) and T2-weighted (from CSF within the nerve root sleeve) images. On parasagittal images, patients with foraminal stenosis have progressive narrowing of the foramen, with resultant compression of the nerve root.

16.4.4 Cauda Equina Syndrome

Cauda equina syndrome is typically characterized by unilateral or bilateral sciatica, perianal or saddle anesthesia, bowel and bladder incontinence, and sensory and motor deficits in the lower extremities.[78] Often, it is caused by a space-occupying mass compressing against the cauda equina and/or conus medullaris. There can be numerous causes, including disk herniation, severe stenosis, trauma, tumor, or infection.[79,80]

MRI is the preferred imaging modality for the evaluation of the patient with suspected cauda equina syndrome. MRI allows visualization of space-occupying lesions within the spinal canal, as well as identification of compression of neural structures. Lumbar myelography with CT of the lumbar spine is indicated in patients who are unable to undergo MRI. Given that the treatment of cauda equina syndrome is urgent decompression, one of these imaging studies should be obtained without delay.

16.4.5 Spondylolisthesis

Spondylolisthesis is defined as anterior displacement of a vertebral body relative to the one caudal to it. Retrolisthesis is seen when the superior vertebral body is displaced posterior to the one caudal to it. Wiltse et al[81] classified lumbar spondylolisthesis on the basis of etiology: dysplastic, isthmic, degenerative, traumatic, iatrogenic, or pathologic. Meyerding[82] described the various degrees of forward slippage (from grade 1 to grade 4) based on a division of the superior surface of the lower vertebra into quarters (▶ Fig. 16.40). According to this system, a

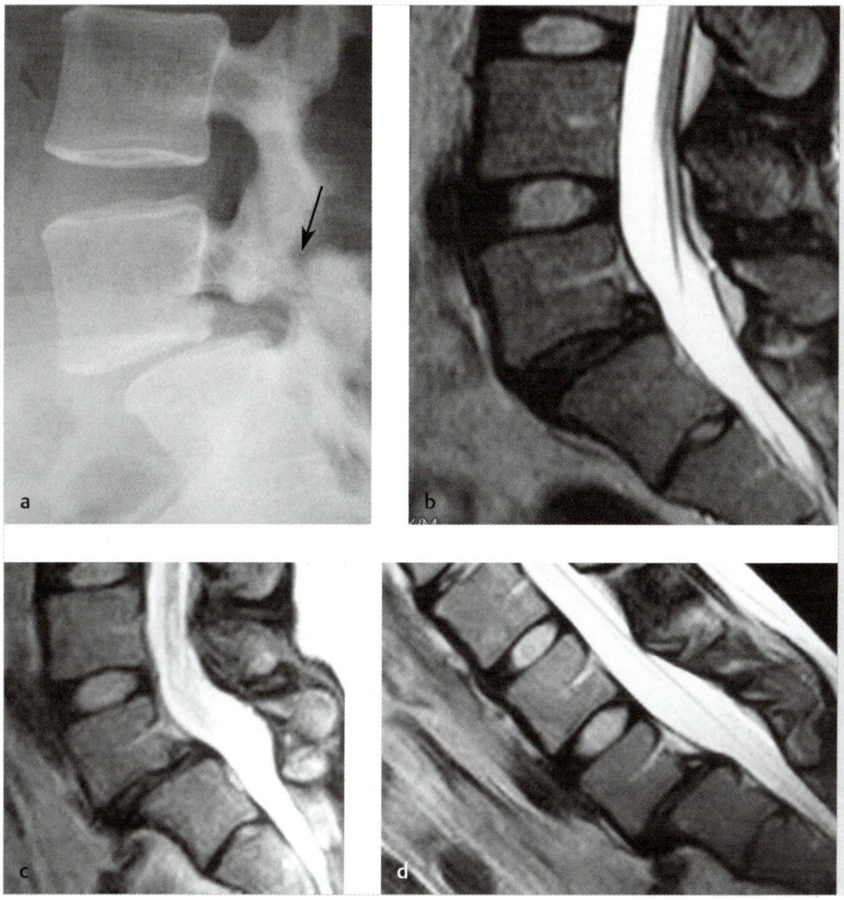

Fig. 16.41 Isthmic spondylolisthesis. **(a)** A lateral radiograph shows bilateral pars intra-articularis defects (*arrow*) at the L5–S1 level with Meyerding grade-2 spondylolisthesis. **(b)** A sagittal T2-weighted magnetic resonance (MR) image obtained via a closed system with the same patient in a supine position shows grade-1 spondylolisthesis. **(c)** A sagittal T2-weighted MR image obtained via an open magnetic resonance imaging (MRI) system with the patient in a standing position shows that the spondylolisthesis progresses to grade 2. **(d)** A sagittal T2-weighted image obtained via an open MRI system with the patient in a flexed position shows that the grade-2 spondylolisthesis progresses compared with images in the **(c)** neutral and **(b)** supine positions. (Reproduced with permission from, Okubadejo GO, Daftary AR, Buchowski JM, et al. The lumbar and thoracic spine. In: Khanna AJ, ed. MRI for orthopaedic surgeons. New York: Thieme; 2010:269–315.)

complete slip of L5 on S1 is termed *spondyloptosis*. Each manifestation of spondylolisthesis has specific associated MRI findings.

The system of Wiltse et al[81] details the features of spondylolisthesis as follows:

- *Dysplastic spondylolisthesis*: may present with degeneration and pseudobulging of the lumbosacral disk, with potential compression of the cauda equina between the neural arch of L4 and the superoposterior aspect of the sacrum (for a slip at L5). A parasagittal T1-weighted SE image may show severe compression of the exiting L5 nerve root.
- *Isthmic spondylolisthesis*: sagittal T2-weighted images often show obvious spondylolisthesis at the L5–S1 level (▶ Fig. 16.41). Parasagittal images at the level of the pedicle may show compression of the exiting L5 nerve root between the bulging L5–S1 disk and the undersurface of the L5 pedicle, along with reduction of foraminal height. The parasagittal images should also be scrutinized for the presence of a pars intra-articularis defect or reparative granulation tissue in that region; CT imaging may help confirm the presence of the pars defect.
- *Degenerative spondylolisthesis:* seen most commonly at the L4–L5 level. MRI can be used to evaluate narrowing of the central canal, lateral recesses, and neural foramina and compression of the cauda equina and exiting nerve roots. Facet joint cysts are not uncommon in the presence of degenerative spondylolisthesis. Sagittal and axial T2-weighted images delineate these entities clearly (▶ Fig. 16.42).
- *Traumatic spondylolisthesis:* MRI shows the associated soft-tissue injury, which may include rupture of the intervertebral disk and posterior ligamentous complex, as seen with bilateral facet dislocation (▶ Fig. 16.10).
- *Pathologic spondylolisthesis:* MRI shows very focal changes at the level of the pars intra-articularis depending on the specific pathology involved.
- *Iatrogenic spondylolisthesis:* may occur after laminectomy, facetectomy, and extensive resection of the facet joint and neural arch without fusion. MRI shows changes directly correlated to the specific areas altered during surgery.

Recently, the focus in spondylolisthesis has moved beyond the slippage of the vertebral bodies to include, among other issues, its etiologic factors and spinopelvic alignment. This change in focus has led to the development of more comprehensive classification systems that may be better at predicting progression of the disease, especially in younger individuals.[83,84,85]

16.4.6 Scoliosis

Scoliosis is a lateral curvature of the vertebral column in the coronal plane involving lateral and rotational vectors, and it may be associated with spinal cord or other neuronal abnormalities that are best visualized with MRI before operative intervention. The most common indication for MRI in patients with scoliosis is degenerative scoliosis. In this scenario, MRI is obtained to

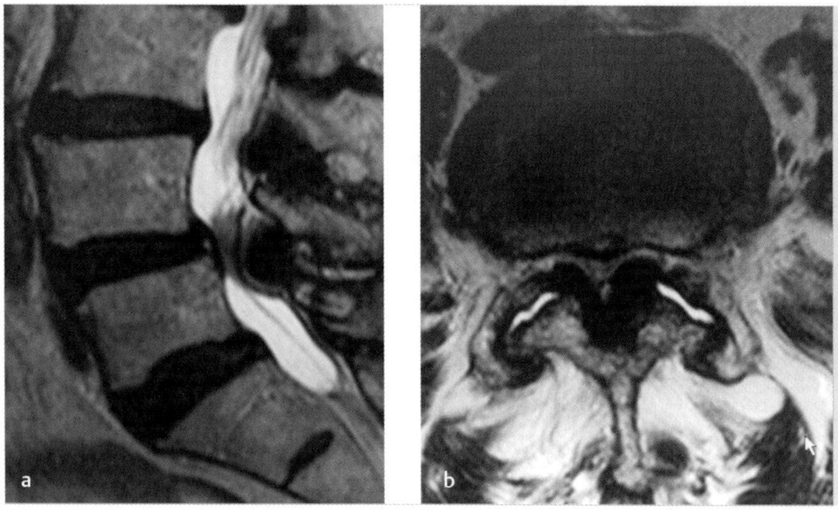

Fig. 16.42 Degenerative spondylolisthesis. (a) A sagittal T2-weighted image shows Meyerding grade-1 spondylolisthesis at the L4–L5 level with severe stenosis and evidence of a high-intensity zone at the posterior annulus of the L4–L5 disk. (b) An axial T2-weighted image shows severe stenosis from a central disk bulge, ligamentum flavum hypertrophy, and facet arthropathy. (Reproduced with permission from, Okubadejo GO, Daftary AR, Buchowski JM, et al. The lumbar and thoracic spine. In: Khanna AJ, ed. MRI for orthopaedic surgeons. New York: Thieme; 2010:269–315.)

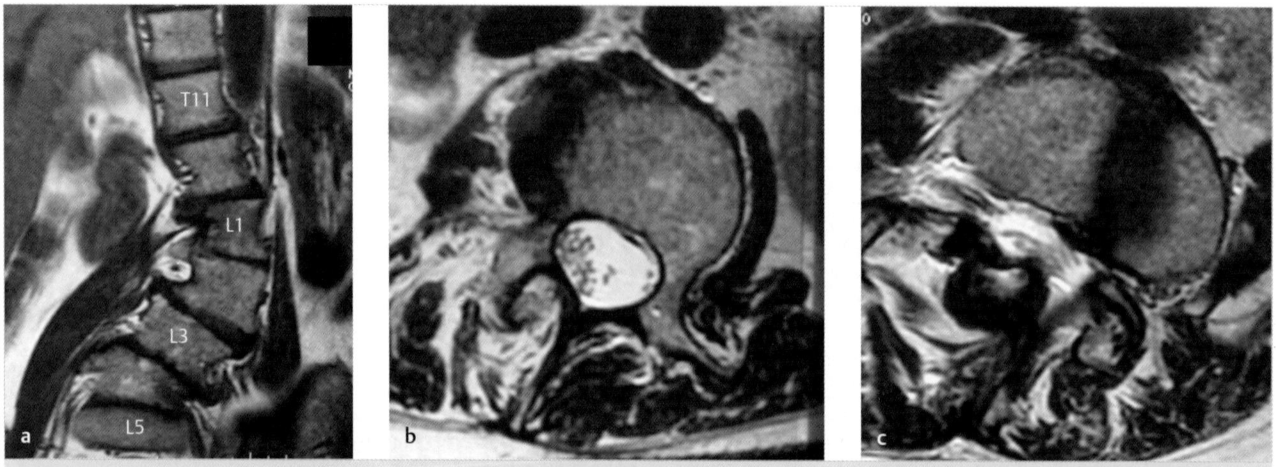

Fig. 16.43 Scoliosis. (a) A coronal T1-weighted image shows advanced thoracolumbar degenerative scoliosis that is primarily left convex with the apex of the curve at the L2 level. (b) An axial T2-weighted image at the L2 level shows rotation of the vertebral body but no substantial stenosis. (c) An axial T2-weighted image at the L3–L4 level shows rotation of the vertebral body level and moderate to severe stenosis secondary to degenerative changes. (Reproduced with permission from, Okubadejo GO, Daftary AR, Buchowski JM, et al. The lumbar and thoracic spine. In: Khanna AJ, ed. MRI for orthopaedic surgeons. New York: Thieme; 2010:269–315.)

evaluate for the presence, degree, and levels of stenosis. Because of the unique challenge of obtaining contiguous visualization of the spinal canal content in the scoliotic spine, specific protocols should be followed to obtain the best views. Redla et al[86] described the use of sagittal T1-weighted SE and T2-weighted FSE sequences, beginning from above the foramen magnum and including the brainstem down to the sacrum. However, for typical thoracolumbar scoliosis, MR images are obtained of the thoracic and lumbar spine only. When the curve is severe, sagittal sequences are obtained parallel to the two major portions of the curve and are planned from the coronal plane. Axial T1-weighted images are obtained through the apices of the curve, providing a second view of the cord. A coronal T1-weighted sequence also is obtained, especially to assess the vertebral bodies for congenital anomalies. In patients with degenerative stenosis, the sagittal and axial T2-weighted images should be evaluated in correlation with each other to determine the degree and type of stenosis at each level (▸ Fig. 16.43). This information helps determine the levels for decompression in a patient who is being considered for surgical intervention.

Aside from the evaluation of the patient with lumbar degenerative scoliosis and suspected stenosis, the indications for MRI in patients with scoliosis have been the subject of debate (see Chapter 17, MRI of the Pediatric Spine). Although some studies have shown that routine MRI is not indicated for patients with adolescent idiopathic scoliosis who have a typical right thoracic curve and who are neurologically intact,[87,88,89] others have found a high incidence of spinal cord abnormalities (18–26%) in patients with infantile and juvenile forms of scoliosis.[86,90] Those studies stressed the importance of MRI in children younger than 11 years. Spinal cord abnormality is suggested by several physical examination findings, including a left thoracic curve, absent abdominal reflexes, lower limb neurologic deficits, and cutaneous stigmata of occult spinal dysraphism.[86]

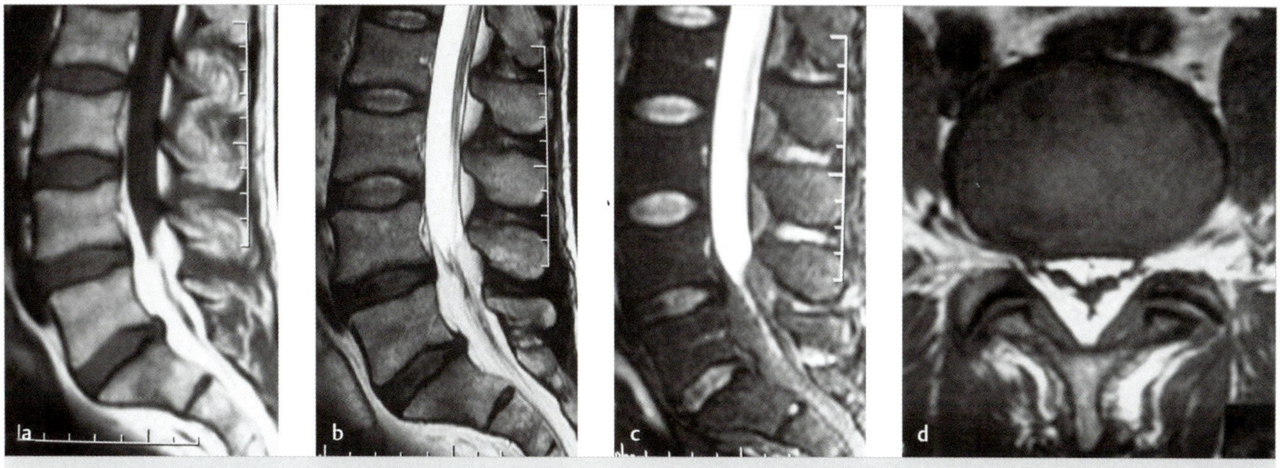

Fig. 16.44 Lumbar epidural lipomatosis. **(a)** Sagittal T1-weighted, **(b)** T2-weighted, and **(c)** short tau inversion recovery (STIR) images show advanced lumbar epidural lipomatosis extending from L4 to the sacrum with circumferential compression of the thecal sac. Note that the lipomatous tissue is most obvious on the T1-weighted image, blends in with the cerebrospinal fluid (CSF) on the T2-weighted image, and suppresses (becomes dark) on the STIR image. **(d)** An axial T1-weighted image at the L4–L5 level shows severe compression of the thecal sac by the extensive lumbar epidural lipomatosis. (Reproduced with permission from, Okubadejo GO, Daftary AR, Buchowski JM, et al. The lumbar and thoracic spine. In: Khanna AJ, ed. MRI for orthopaedic surgeons. New York: Thieme; 2010:269–315.)

MRI findings for abnormalities seen with scoliosis secondary to an underlying neurologic abnormality include the following:

- Tethered cord: thickened filum terminale and spinal lipoma, seen on sagittal T1-weighted SE and T2-weighted FSE images.
- Syringohydromyelia: dissection of CSF through the cord substance, best seen on T2-weighted images as increased signal within the cord, sometimes associated with sacculation.
- Diastematomyelia: a midline sagittal cleft of the spinal cord most commonly involving the lower thoracic and lumbar region, seen as two hemicords on MRI, with each having a single dorsal and ventral horn and a septum seen from the dorsal aspect of the vertebral body and extending into the cleft between the cords.
- Neurofibromatosis: a congenital condition that may show dural ectasia, pseudomeningocele, and neurofibromas on MRI.
- Pars defects: a common occurrence in patients with developmental scoliosis; may occur in up to 6.2% of patients with idiopathic scoliosis.[91]

16.4.7 Epidural Lipomatosis

Epidural lipomatosis is a condition in which there is excessive deposition of fat in the epidural space that, in turn, leads to spinal stenosis and neural compression. The syndrome is associated primarily with excessive glucocorticoid levels, which may be exogenous or endogenous but may also be spontaneous or idiopathic.[92,93,94] In the lumbar spine, epidural fat surrounding and compressing the thecal sac is the key finding. In the thoracic spine, the presence of > 6 mm of fat posterior to the cord is diagnostic. The characteristic feature of lumbar epidural lipomatosis is the presence of epidural tissue that follows the signal characteristics of subcutaneous fat on all pulse sequences, including fat-suppressed sequences (▶ Fig. 16.44). The primary differential consideration includes an intraspinal lipoma, which is typically focal and is often located in the anterior thoracic spine.[95] Other epidural abnormalities tend to have a low T1-weighted signal and can be excluded.

16.5 Infectious Conditions

16.5.1 Vertebral Osteomyelitis

Cases of vertebral osteomyelitis comprise between 2 and 4% of all skeletal infections.[96,97] MRI usually is the imaging modality of choice for the detection of this process, with a sensitivity of > 82% and a specificity of 53 to 94%.[98] Infection involving the vertebral body occurs through one of three primary routes[99]:

- Hematogenous (most common).
- Direct inoculation through surgery or penetrating trauma.
- Contiguous spread from an adjacent soft-tissue infection.

Hematogenous seeding occurs through nutrient arterioles of the vertebral bodies or by retrograde spread through the paravertebral venous plexus of Batson.[99,100,101] Infection then spreads from the vertebral body and marrow to the contiguous intervertebral disk and adjacent vertebral body, often sparing the central portion of the vertebral bodies.[99,100]

The MRI signal changes in patients with osteomyelitis include the following:

- Decreased signal intensity of the intervertebral disk and adjacent vertebral bodies, with a discernible margin between the two on T1-weighted images.
- Increased signal intensity of vertebral bodies adjacent to the involved disk on T2-weighted images.
- An abnormal configuration and increased signal intensity of the intervertebral disk with loss of the nuclear cleft on T2-weighted images (▶ Fig. 16.45).[97,102]

Gadolinium enhancement may be seen in adjacent vertebral bodies. However, gadolinium may also cause edematous mar-

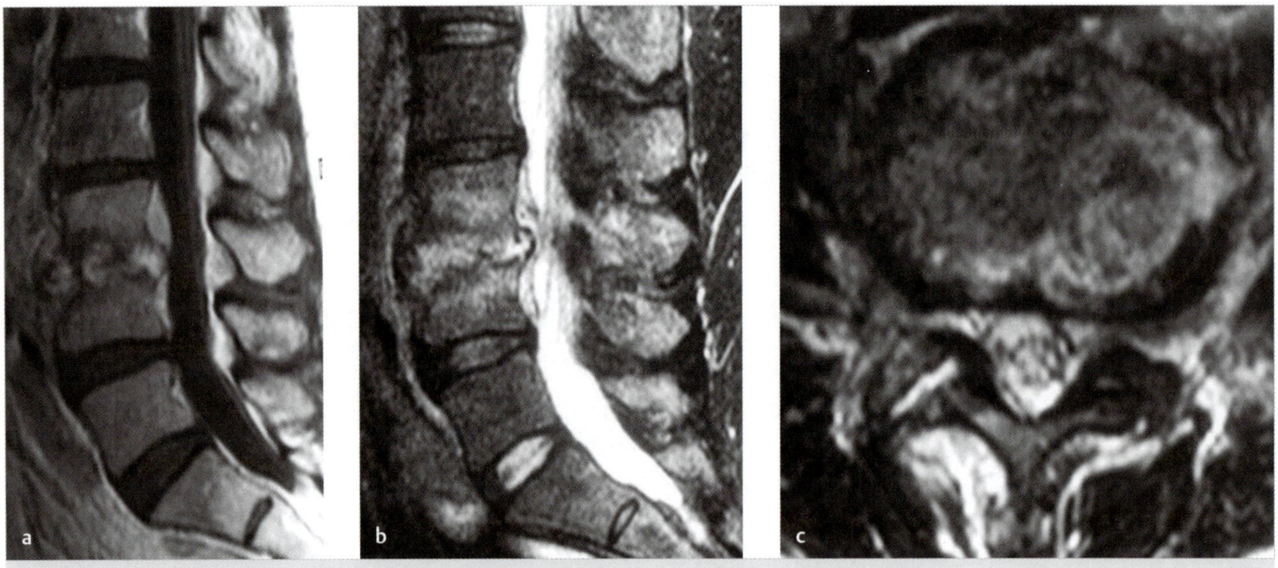

Fig. 16.45 Vertebral osteomyelitis and diskitis. **(a)** Sagittal postgadolinium T1-weighted and **(b)** short tau inversion recovery (STIR) images show enhancement and increased signal within the L3–L4 disk space and edema within the adjacent vertebral bodies in a patient with infectious symptoms and findings. **(c)** An axial T2-weighted image at the L3–L4 disk level also shows heterogeneous and increased signal within the disk space, compatible with diskitis. (Reproduced with permission from, Okubadejo GO, Daftary AR, Buchowski JM, et al. The lumbar and thoracic spine. In: Khanna AJ, ed. MRI for orthopaedic surgeons. New York: Thieme; 2010:269–315.)

row to blend in with the normal fatty marrow.[103] Combining fat-suppressed T1-weighted images with gadolinium contrast enhancement eliminates this problem.[102] STIR images may also be used for the MRI evaluation of osteomyelitis because they suppress the high signal intensity from fat and provide increased contrast.[104] STIR images are especially useful when combined with the anatomic detail from T1-weighted sequences.

The pattern of vertebral body involvement in vertebral osteomyelitis should be differentiated from that in patients with spinal tumors (see Chapter 21, Tumors of the Spine). Patients with vertebral osteomyelitis tend to have the epicenter of the pathologic change at the disk space, and those with tumors tend to have the epicenter at the vertebral body. In other words, infectious processes are based at and cross the disk space, whereas neoplastic processes typically are based in the vertebral body and do not cross the disk space.

16.5.2 Diskitis

Disk infection often causes edema, which leads to hyperintensity of the disk and the end plate on T2-weighted images; it also causes loss of definition of the vertebral end plates, inflammatory changes in the adjacent vertebral marrow, and gadolinium enhancement within the disk.[44,105,106] In addition, it is not uncommon to have an associated paraspinal inflammatory mass.

Spondylodiskitis, which essentially is diskitis with vertebral osteomyelitis, may be seen after lumbar disk surgery. It also may be seen after diskography or myelography.[107] Postoperative spondylodiskitis is believed to occur in 0.1 to 3% of patients.[107] Intraoperative contamination usually is the most common mechanism for infection. The most common infecting organisms are *Staphylococcus epidermidis* and *S. aureus*. MR images often show Modic type-1 changes at the level of the operated disk (vertebral end plate with decreased signal on T1-weighted images and increased signal intensity on T2-weighted images) and enhancement of the disk when contrast is used (▶ Fig. 16.46). No enhancing tissue should be seen outside the intervertebral space. Normal vertebral bone marrow has low signal intensity on T1-weighted images and high signal intensity on T2-weighted and contrast-enhanced images.[107] If a rim of soft tissue around the affected intervertebral space is noted to enhance, concern about septic spondylodiskitis arises, which can be ruled out with disk biopsy.

16.5.3 Epidural Abscess

An epidural abscess is a purulent epidural collection of material without involvement of the vertebral body or the disk space. Such collections usually are located anteriorly in the spinal canal and originate from the posterior aspect of the vertebral body and disk space. If the abscess originates from hematogenous sources, then it may be associated with a positive blood culture. MRI is very sensitive in the detection of these abscesses.[103] MRI is also useful in visualizing phlegmon and epidural abscesses, which usually are isointense or hypointense compared with the spinal cord on T1-weighted images, and which usually have high signal intensity on T2-weighted images (▶ Fig. 16.47).[104,107] The differentiation between epidural abscess and CSF may be difficult, necessitating gadolinium enhancement for better visualization. The high signal intensity of the enhancing mass can be distinguished easily from the lower signal intensity of the CSF and spine on T1-weighted images.[107] Sometimes, fat suppression is necessary to differentiate an abscess from epidural fat. Contrast enhancement also can aid in differentiating between epidural phlegmon and an abscess; dense homogeneous enhancement

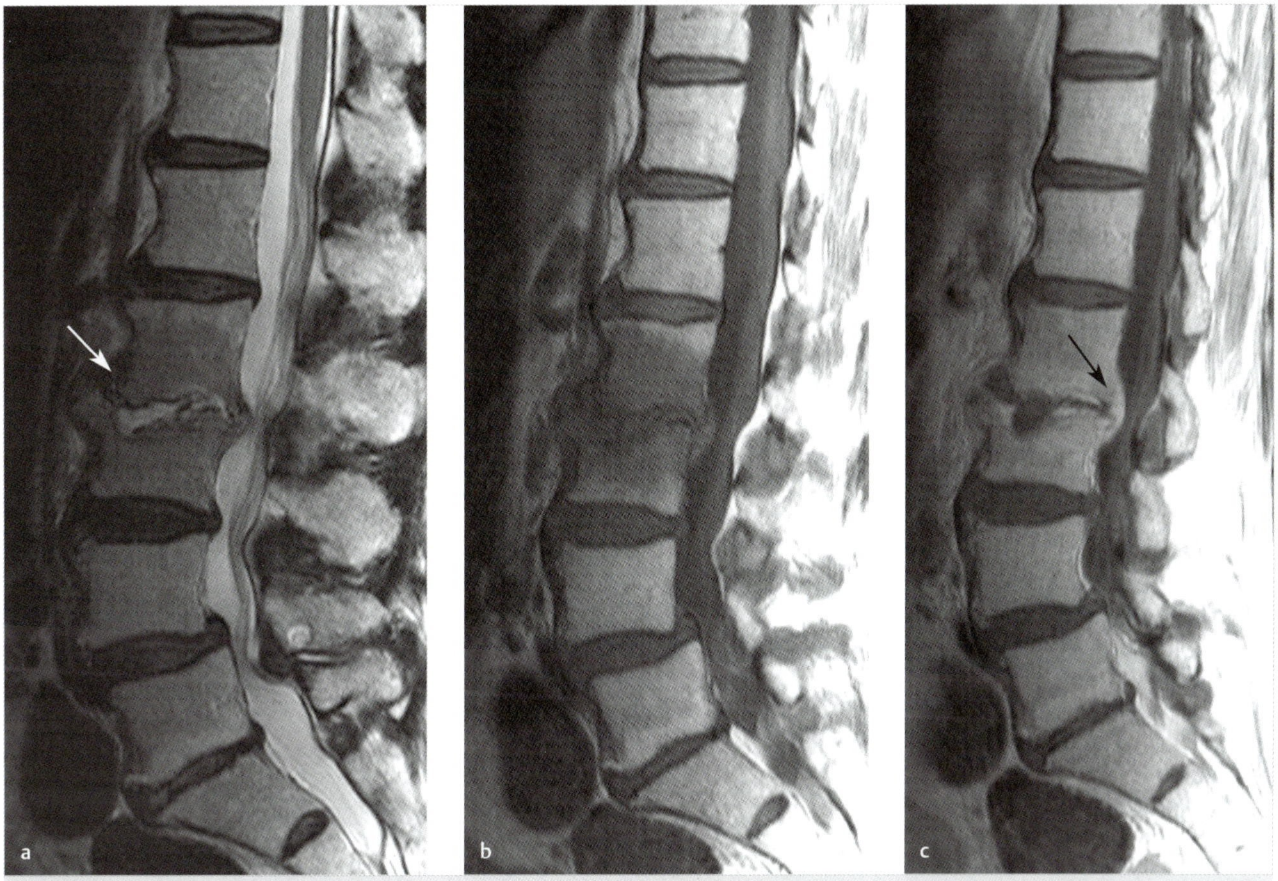

Fig. 16.46 Diskitis. Sagittal **(a)** T2-weighted, **(b)** T1-weighted, and **(c)** postgadolinium T1-weighted images show the typical findings of diskitis at the L2–L3 level (*arrows* on **a** and **c**). Note the increase in signal at the disk space on the T2-weighted image, the decrease in signal on the T1-weighted image, and the postgadolinium enhancement of the small epidural component (**c**, *arrow*). (Reproduced with permission from, Okubadejo GO, Daftary AR, Buchowski JM, et al. The lumbar and thoracic spine. In: Khanna AJ, ed. MRI for orthopaedic surgeons. New York: Thieme; 2010:269–315.)

of the mass suggests phlegmon, whereas peripheral or ring enhancement of the mass suggests an abscess. Paraspinal abscesses, also well visualized with MRI, usually have low signal intensity on T1-weighted images, and they are commonly associated with swelling of the psoas on T1-weighted images and increased signal on T2-weighted images. Gadolinium-enhanced images provide additional abscess delineation.

16.5.4 Tuberculosis

Tuberculosis has reappeared in the developed world because of the emergence of acquired immune deficiency syndrome; 5% of all cases of tuberculosis affect the musculoskeletal system.[108]

Tuberculosis usually results from hematogenous seeding. The rich vascular supply of the vertebral bodies makes the spine susceptible to infection. A vertebral body receives its blood supply inferiorly from the ascending branch of the posterior spinal artery and superiorly from the descending branch of this artery. These two arteries anastomose and create a network of vessels in the anterior epidural space. The network then leads to three or four arteries that enter the vertebral body through the nutrient foramen. Children are at increased risk for diskitis because they still have an arterial anastomosis between the vertebral end plate and the disk.[108] The intervertebral disk becomes less vascularized during adolescence. Arteries end within the vertebral bodies, which results in increased rates of infection within the bodies.[108]

Tuberculous osteomyelitis usually involves the ventral trabecular bone marrow adjacent to the intervertebral disk, and it spreads via the anterior longitudinal ligament to adjacent vertebral bodies. MR signs of tuberculosis infection are hypointense signal on T1-weighted images and hyperintense signal on T2-weighted images seen in the subchondral tissue. There also may be a hyperintense signal within the disk on T2-weighted images (▶ Fig. 16.48). As the disease progresses, it may lead to collapse of vertebral bodies, with an associated epidural abscess. Continuous destruction of the anterior cortices of single or contiguous vertebral bodies can lead to kyphotic deformity. Tuberculosis may also directly involve the spinal cord, a condition termed *tuberculosis myelitis*; it is usually seen in individuals < 30 years old. MRI with gadolinium is the best imaging modality for this phenomenon.[108]

It is not uncommon to see paraspinal involvement with abscess formation. In abscesses, gadolinium enhancement usually is seen only in the periphery, whereas granulation tissue enhances throughout. The observation of disk space sparing and enhancement of granulation tissue is highly suggestive of tuberculosis.[98]

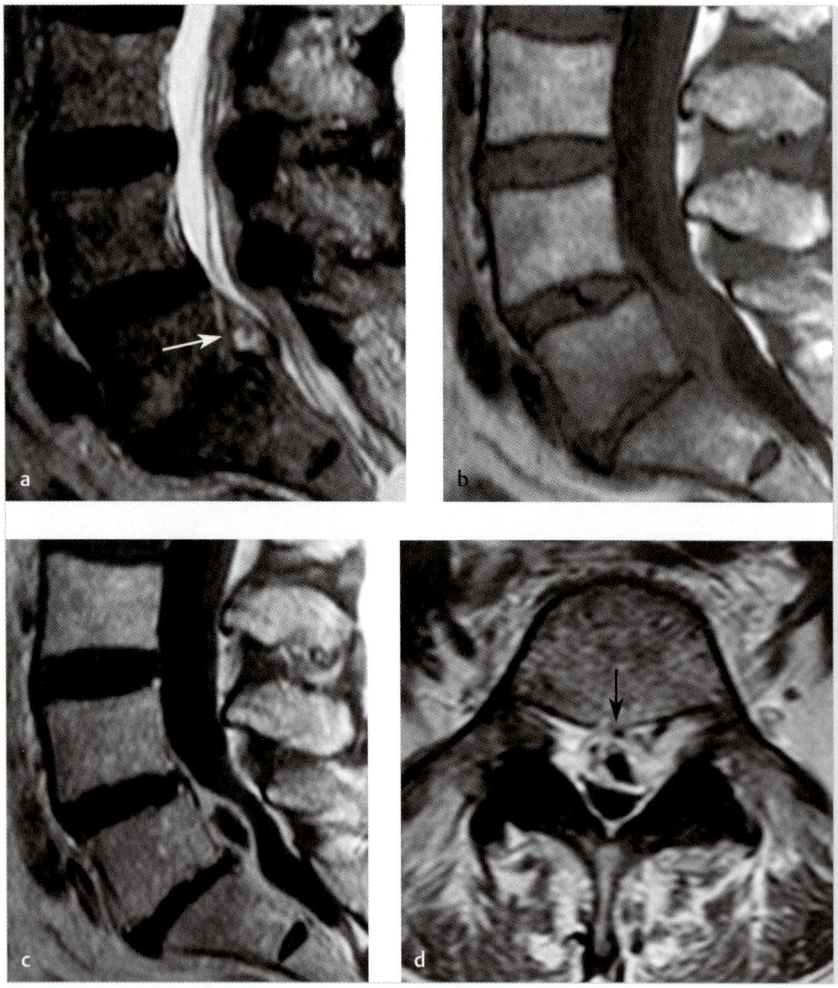

Fig. 16.47 Epidural abscess. (a) A sagittal T2-weighted image shows a ventral epidural collection (*arrow*) posterior to the L5 vertebral body in a patient with infectious symptoms and findings. (b) A sagittal T1-weighted image shows the same collection. (c) A sagittal postgadolinium T1-weighted image shows peripheral enhancement. (d) An axial postgadolinium T1-weighted image shows the ventral epidural collection (*arrow*), again with peripheral enhancement; the abscess is producing moderate to severe stenosis. (Reproduced with permission from, Okubadejo GO, Daftary AR, Buchowski JM, et al. The lumbar and thoracic spine. In: Khanna AJ, ed. MRI for orthopaedic surgeons. New York: Thieme; 2010:269–315.)

16.6 Postoperative MRI Findings

Previously, MRI had been considered to have limited use in evaluating the instrumented spine because of the resultant artifacts that were commonly seen. However, the introduction of titanium pedicle screws and specialized pulse sequences has improved the MRI visualization of the central spinal contents.[109,110,111,112,113,114] It is important to note that MRI may not always be the best imaging modality for the evaluation of the postoperative lumbar spine. Conventional radiographs are typically the starting point for the study of patients with instrumented lumbar fusion, given that they enable the evaluation of overall spinal alignment, position of instrumentation, and evidence of fusion. CT may be best for more precise determination of the presence or absence of fusion, infection, loosening, and postoperative fluid collections. The addition of myelography to CT imaging provides excellent determination of the presence and degree of spinal stenosis, or its absence.[115] MRI may be best for evaluating for the presence or absence of infection, postoperative fluid collection (such as hematoma or CSF), recurrent disk herniation, and residual or recurrent stenosis.[113]

Surgical procedures in the spine are typically performed with the following goals:

- Decompression of a stenotic spinal canal or neural foramen.
- Removal of herniated disk material.
- Stabilization and fusion of motion segments for existing instability (such as spondylolisthesis, scoliosis, or posttraumatic injury) or after iatrogenic instability (such as with facetectomy or multilevel laminectomies).
- Excision of tumor or infection.

According to the type of surgery performed and the clinical scenario, the spine surgeon and radiologist can use MRI (and other imaging modalities) to evaluate for various postsurgical findings.

16.6.1 After Decompression without Instrumentation/Fusion

Almost all decompressive procedures in the lumbar spine are performed via a posterior approach. These procedures include a midline laminectomy and bilateral foraminotomies, hemilaminotomy with foraminotomy, and hemilaminotomy with diskectomy. In most cases, careful review of the sagittal and axial images permits determination of the extent of bone removal during previous operations. Specifically, one should review the sagittal and axial T2-weighted images, follow the contour of the

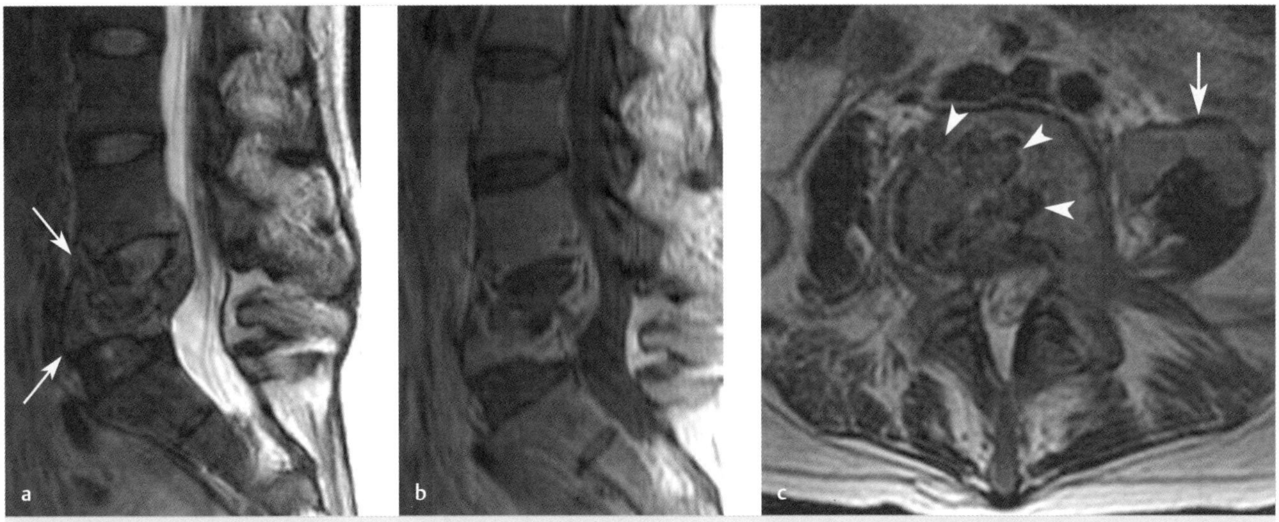

Fig. 16.48 Tuberculosis of the spine. Sagittal **(a)** T2-weighted and **(b)** T1-weighted images show destruction and partial collapse of the L5 vertebral body (between *arrows* on **a**) with relative preservation of the intervertebral disks. **(c)** An axial T2-weighted image at the L5 level shows signal change within the anterior aspect of the left psoas muscle (*arrow*), compatible with an abscess, and also heterogeneous signal within the vertebral body (*arrowheads*). (Reproduced with permission from, Okubadejo GO, Daftary AR, Buchowski JM, et al. The lumbar and thoracic spine. In: Khanna AJ, ed. MRI for orthopaedic surgeons. New York: Thieme; 2010:269–315.)

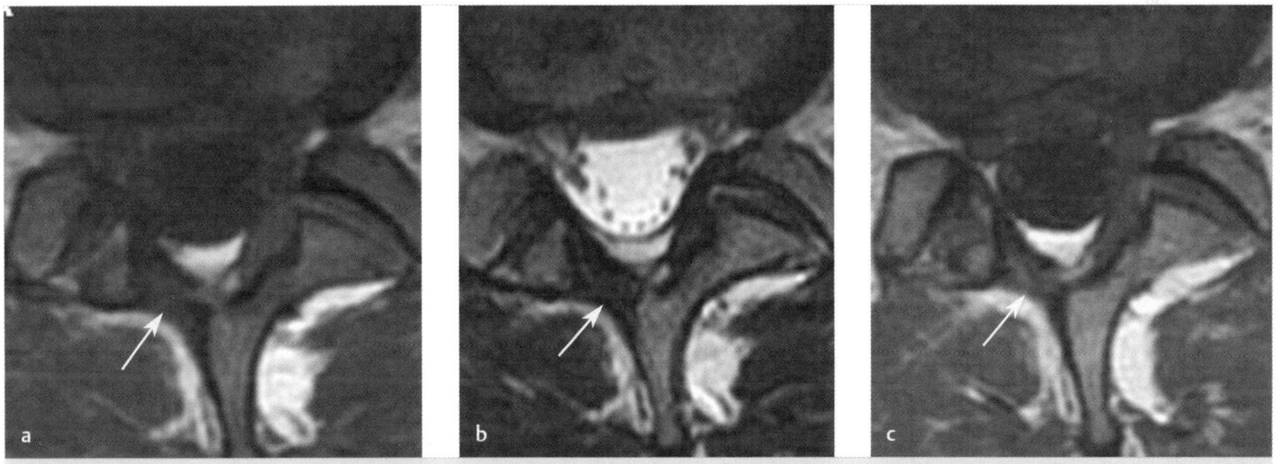

Fig. 16.49 Osseous defect after right L4–L5 hemilaminotomy. Axial **(a)** T1-weighted, **(b)** T2-weighted, and **(c)** postgadolinium T1-weighted images show partial removal of the right-side lamina, identifying the laminotomy site (*arrows* on each). (Reproduced with permission from, Thakkar RS, Malloy JP IV, Thakkar SC, Carrino JA, Khanna AJ. Imaging the postoperative spine. Radiol Clin North Am. 2012;50(4):731–747.)

thecal sac, and look for focal areas of posterior expansion of the thecal sac or for regions of compression of the thecal sac by scar tissue or recurrent/residual disk fragments. The axial T1-weighted images (which show more osseous detail than do T2-weighted images) should be carefully reviewed for areas of postsurgical absence of the osseous structures (▸ Fig. 16.49). If additional information may benefit the surgeon for preoperative planning, CT imaging may be considered.

After diskectomy, specific changes may be noted around the affected area, depending on the length of time between surgery and the imaging study. At the level of the disk, a high-signal-intensity band extending from the nucleus pulposus to the side of annular disruption may be seen on T2-weighted images up to 2 months after surgery. Annular enhancement may also be seen. There also may be a component of disk height loss, depending on the aggressiveness of the diskectomy. T1-weighted images show increased soft tissue within the anterior epidural space immediately after surgery; an epidural mass effect is observed in 80% of patients.[116] Anterior epidural soft-tissue edema with disruption of the posterior annular margin secondary to disk curettage can mimic the appearance of disk herniation. It can take from 2 to 6 months after surgery for a normal signal to return.[117,118] One should use caution when evaluating MRI studies during the first 6 weeks after surgery because there may be a large amount of tissue disruption and edema, producing a mass effect on the anterior thecal sac.

Nerve root enhancement secondary to breakdown of the blood–nerve barrier is another common finding during the immediate postoperative period. This enhancement decreases by 3 months after surgery and is virtually gone by 6 months.[116,119]

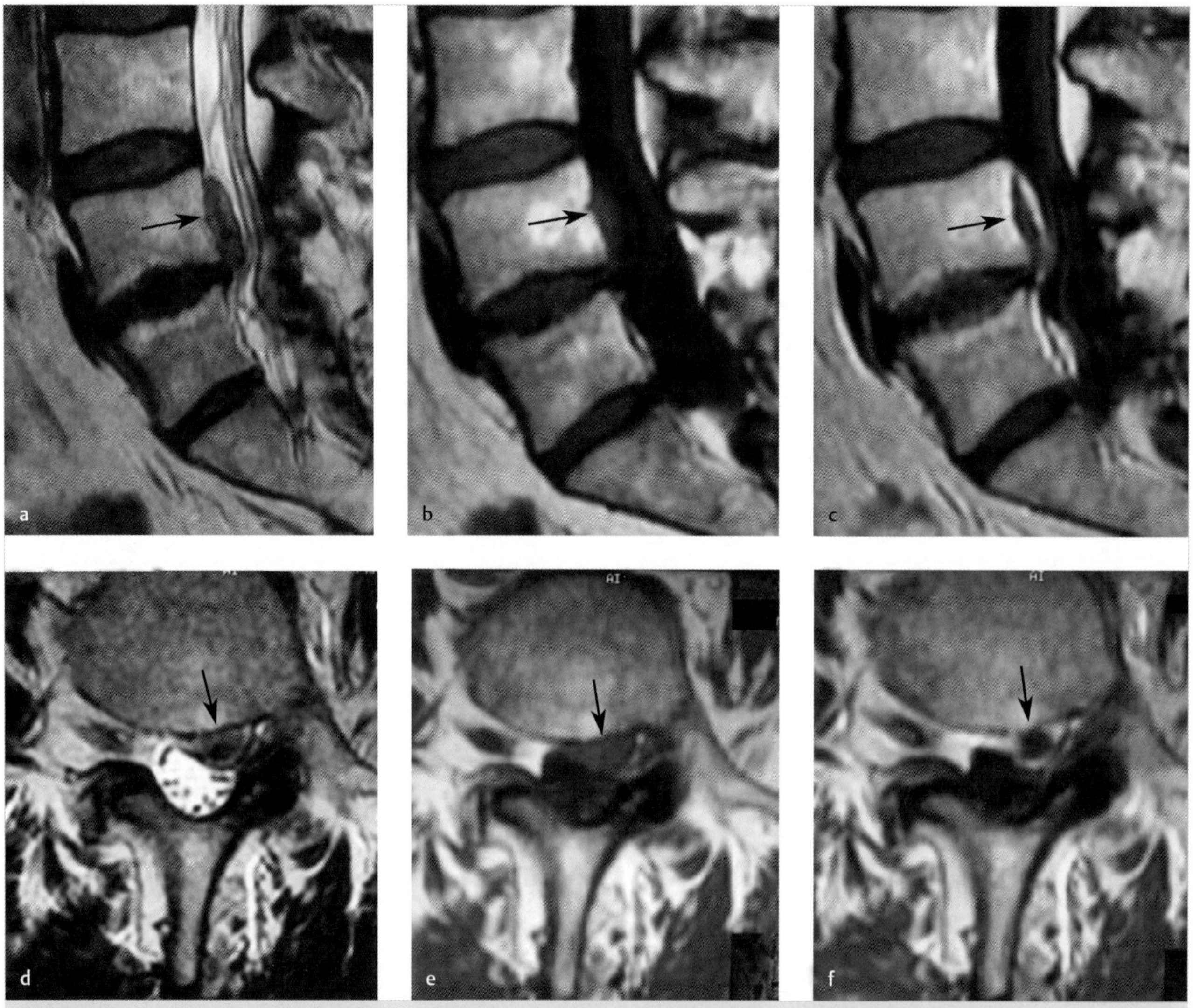

Fig. 16.50 Recurrent lumbar disk extrusion. Sagittal **(a)** T2-weighted, **(b)** T1-weighted, and **(c)** postgadolinium T1-weighted images in a patient with a history of L4–L5 diskectomy show a large disk extrusion *(arrow* on each) that has migrated proximally and is located behind the L4 vertebral body. Note that the disk is difficult to see on **b**, the T1-weighted image, and shows peripheral enhancement on **c**, the postgadolinium T1-weighted image. Axial **(d)** T2-weighted, **(e)** T1-weighted, and **(f)** postgadolinium T1-weighted images at the L4–L5 level show the left paracentral extradural lesion *(arrow* on each), which appears to be disk material on **d**, the T2-weighted image, and shows peripheral enhancement on **f**, the postgadolinium T1-weighted image, compared with **e**, the pregadolinium T1-weighted image. (Reproduced with permission from, Okubadejo GO, Daftary AR, Buchowski JM, et al. The lumbar and thoracic spine. In: Khanna AJ, ed. MRI for orthopaedic surgeons. New York: Thieme; 2010:269–315.)

Posterior soft-tissue changes continue to be seen up to 3 months after surgery. These changes include disruption and edema of the paraspinal muscles, with low signal intensity on T1-weighted images and high signal intensity on T2-weighted images. An enhancing subcutaneous track may be seen with gadolinium enhancement. After 6 months, all acute postoperative changes secondary to hemorrhage and edema usually have resolved.[116] The remaining scar tissue shows low to intermediate signal intensity on T1-weighted imaging and hypointensity on T2-weighted imaging.

Unfortunately, recurrent disk herniation is relatively common after surgery for a lumbar disk herniation. The reported incidence of recurrent disk herniation is 2 to 18%, and a large meta-analysis has indicated the rate is 7% in patients who undergo limited diskectomy and 3.5% in patients who undergo aggressive diskectomy.[120] Another recent series found the incidence of recurrent lumbar disk herniation to be 7%.[121] MRI can be used to differentiate recurrent disk herniation from scar tissue.[122,123,124,125,126] The importance of differentiating between recurrent disk herniation and scar tissue or epidural fibrosis lies in the fact that outcomes for revision surgery for recurrent disk herniation are substantially better than those for surgery in patients with only scar tissue and no recurrent disk herniation.[127,128,129,130,131] MRI in patients with recurrent disk herniation shows a focal extradural lesion, typically in the posterolateral or lateral recess region, that has peripheral enhancement with a central area of nonenhancement on postgadolinium T1-weighted images (▶ Fig. 16.50). Conversely, patients with epidural fibrosis show uniform enhancement of the epidural tissue.

16.6.2 After Instrumentation/Fusion

Stainless steel implants are considered superparamagnetic and produce the greatest degree of image degradation secondary to magnetic susceptibility artifacts.[131] Titanium and tantalum spinal implants, which are not superparamagnetic, produce less artifact than does stainless steel. Even with conventional T2-weighted and T1-weighted pulse sequences, the central canal can be visualized adequately in patients with titanium pedicle screws. These images can enable the detection of postoperative fluid collections (such as hematoma, seroma, pseudomeningocele, and abscess) and can even accurately show the degree of thecal sac compression from these fluid collections. In addition, the degree of adjacent-level stenosis at levels above and below an instrumented lumbar fusion can be seen well on sagittal and axial T2-weighted images (▶ Fig. 16.51).

The position of interbody fusion devices (such as those placed for transforaminal lumbar interbody fusion, posterior lumbar interbody fusion, and anterior lumbar interbody fusion) can also be assessed by MRI. These devices should be located within the confines of the interbody space, and the posterior aspect of the interbody device after a transforaminal or posterior lumbar interbody fusion procedure should be positioned within the posterior margin of the vertebral body. In cases of posterolateral graft extrusion into the spinal canal or neural foramen, patients often present with severe radicular pain and/or weakness. MR images show the contours of the interbody device compressing the thecal sac or nerve root and the associated inflammatory changes and epidural fibrosis (▶ Fig. 16.52).

16.6.3 Hematoma

Postoperative epidural hematoma typically develops within a few days after a posterior lumbar surgery that includes decompression, and it can occur after "small" decompressive procedures such as a microdiskectomy, as well as after larger procedures such as multilevel laminectomy (▶ Fig. 16.53) and posterior spinal fusion. Although CT is excellent for visualizing osseous detail and the precise location of spinal instrumentation relative to the spinal canal and neural foramen, MRI is superior for visualizing postoperative fluid collections (such as an epidural hematoma) and the size, location, and degree of compression of the thecal sac they produce.

16.6.4 Pseudomeningocele

A pseudomeningocele typically occurs in a patient who sustains a durotomy during an open surgical procedure or in a patient who undergoes resection of an intradural lesion. In both of these situations, there may be an incomplete closure of the dural opening, with resultant leakage of CSF into the operative site and posterior soft tissues. This collection of CSF is termed a *pseudomeningocele* because it is surrounded not by arachnoid and dura, but rather by a pseudomeninges of reactive fibrous tissue.[131] Pseudomeningoceles typically are well circumscribed, communicate with the subarachnoid space, and contain fluid that matches the signal characteristics of CSF, which is homogeneous and has low signal intensity on T1-weighted images and high signal intensity on T2-weighted images (▶ Fig. 16.54). Given that the pressure within a pseudomeningocele is often

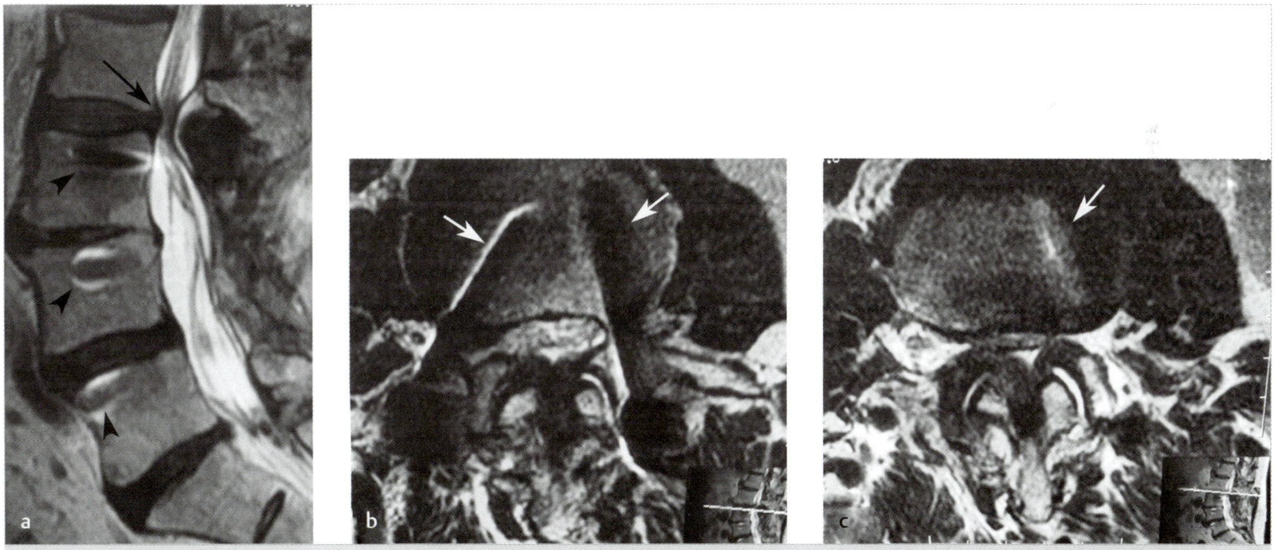

Fig. 16.51 Junctional lumbar stenosis above instrumented fusion. **(a)** A sagittal T2-weighted image shows junctional stenosis (*arrow*) at the L2–L3 level in a patient who has undergone L3–L5 laminectomy and instrumented fusion. Note the minimal artifact from the pedicle screws (*arrowheads*). **(b)** An axial T2-weighted image at the L3 pedicle screw level shows moderate to severe stenosis and also shows the pedicle screws (*arrows*). Note that the presence of the pedicle screws obscures the region of the lateral recess and foramen but does not prevent the evaluation of the status of the central canal. **(c)** An axial T2-weighted image at the L2–L3 level shows severe stenosis and only minimal residual artifact (*arrow*) from the pedicle screw below this level in the L3 vertebral body. Note the localizing sagittal image seen as an inset with each axial image **(b,c)**. (Reproduced with permission from Okubadejo GO, Daftary AR, Buchowski JM, et al. The lumbar and thoracic spine. In: Khanna AJ, ed. MRI for orthopaedic surgeons. New York: Thieme; 2010:269–315.)

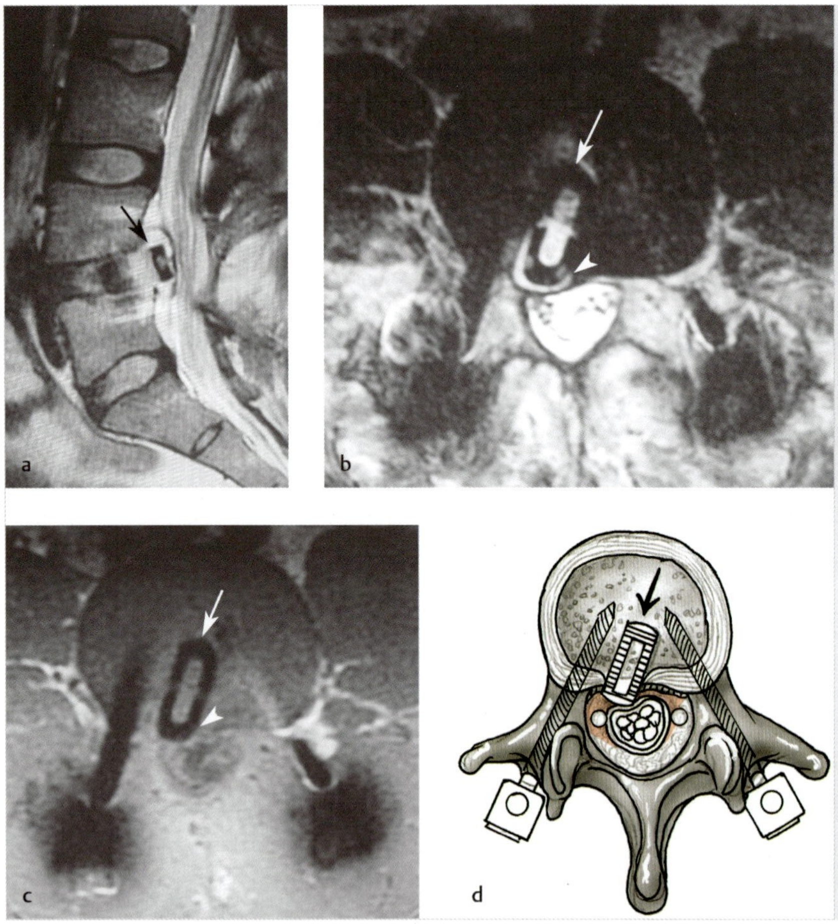

Fig. 16.52 Retropulsed interbody device. **(a)** A sagittal T2-weighted image shows retropulsion of an L4–L5 transforaminal interbody device (*arrow*) into the spinal canal. An axial **(b)** T2-weighted image, **(c)** T1-weighted image, and **(d)** illustration show that the interbody device (*arrow* on each) is retropulsed beyond the margin of the posterior vertebral body (*arrowhead* on **b** and **c**) and is producing right lateral recess stenosis. (Figure part **a**, **b**, and **c**: Reproduced with permission from Okubadejo GO, Daftary AR, Buchowski JM, et al. The lumbar and thoracic spine. In: Khanna AJ, ed. MRI for orthopaedic surgeons. New York: Thieme; 2010:269–315.) (Figure part **d**: Reproduced with permission from Okubadejo GO, Daftary A, Buchowski JM, et al. The lumbar and thoracic spine. In: Khanna AJ, ed. MRI essentials for the spine specialist. New York: Thieme; 2014:155–210.)

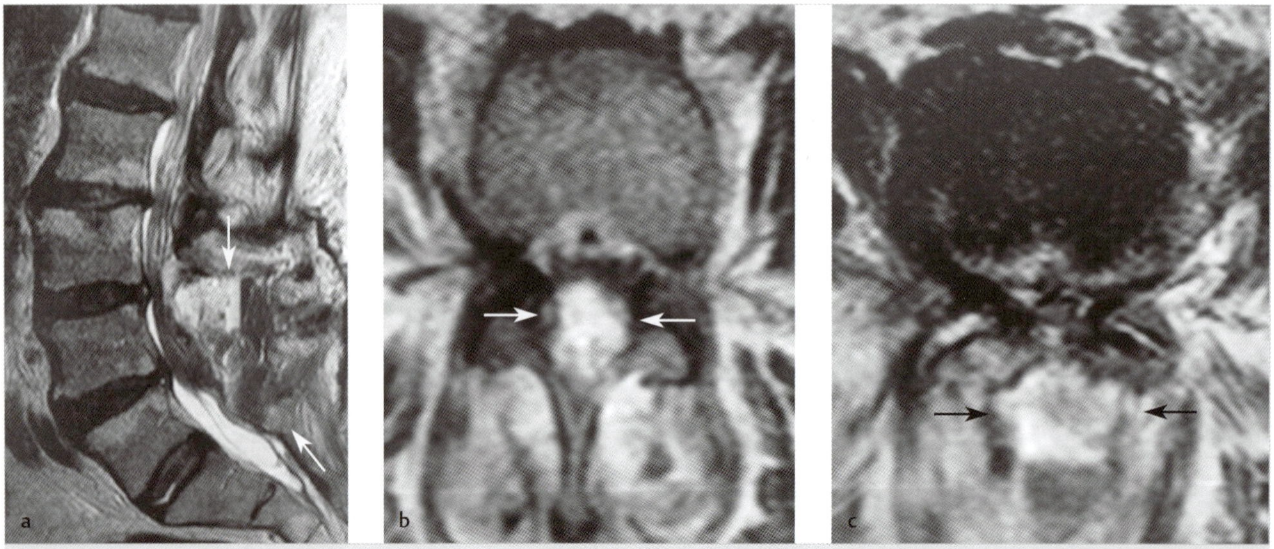

Fig. 16.53 Postoperative lumbar epidural hematoma. **(a)** A sagittal T2-weighted image shows a large and compressive fluid collection (between *arrows*) at the L3–L5 level in a patient after revision L4–L5 laminectomies. Axial T2-weighted images at the **(b)** L3–L4 and **(c)** L4–L5 levels show the hematoma (between *arrows* on each) and the associated compression of the thecal sac. (Reproduced with permission from, Okubadejo GO, Daftary AR, Buchowski JM, et al. The lumbar and thoracic spine. In: Khanna AJ, ed. MRI for orthopaedic surgeons. New York: Thieme; 2010:269–315.)

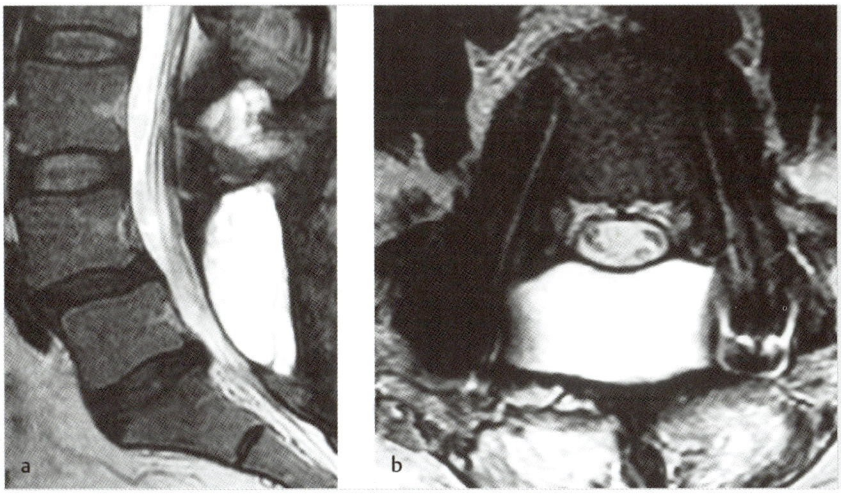

Fig. 16.54 Pseudomeningocele. **(a)** Sagittal and **(b)** axial T2-weighted images of a patient who sustained a durotomy during revision L4–S1 laminectomy and instrumented posterior fusion. The images show a well-circumscribed fluid collection that does not compress the thecal sac. Note that on **b**, the axial image at the L5 level, the central canal can be well visualized in the presence of pedicle screws. (Reproduced with permission from, Okubadejo GO, Daftary AR, Buchowski JM, et al. The lumbar and thoracic spine. In: Khanna AJ, ed. MRI for orthopaedic surgeons. New York: Thieme; 2010:269–315.)

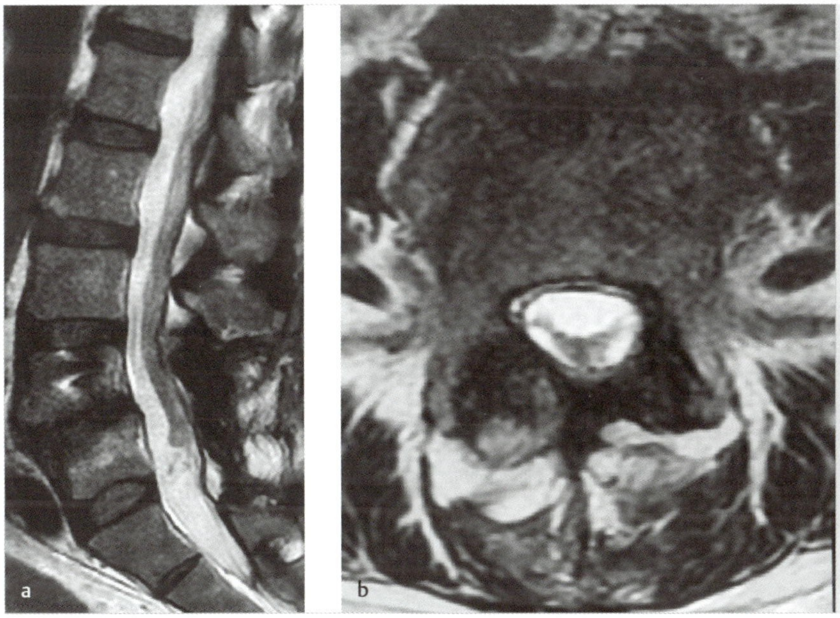

Fig. 16.55 Arachnoiditis. **(a)** Sagittal and **(b)** axial T2-weighted images of a patient after L4–L5 laminectomy and instrumented posterior fusion who had had several previous decompressive surgeries. Note the central adhesion of the nerve roots within the thecal sac into a central clump of soft-tissue signal (pseudocord) instead of their normal feathery appearance. **(b)** The axial image is at the L4–L5 level. (Reproduced with permission from, Okubadejo GO, Daftary AR, Buchowski JM, et al. The lumbar and thoracic spine. In: Khanna AJ, ed. MRI for orthopaedic surgeons. New York: Thieme; 2010:269–315.)

similar to that of the subarachnoid space, these collections often compress the thecal sac less than do postoperative epidural hematomas.[132]

16.6.5 Arachnoiditis

Signs of arachnoiditis include central adhesion of the nerve roots within the thecal sac into a central clump of soft-tissue signal (pseudocord) instead of their normal feathery appearance (► Fig. 16.55), peripheral adhesion of the nerve roots to the meninges (giving rise to an "empty" thecal sac sign), and an inflammatory mass that fills the thecal sac.[133] Various factors can lead to the development of arachnoiditis, including the trauma of the surgery itself, intradural blood after the repair of a durotomy, previous lumbar puncture, treated perioperative infection, and the previous use of myelographic contrast dye.[131]

16.7 Common Clinical Questions

1. Which of the following is *not* one of the criteria that the Thoracolumbar Injury Classification and Severity Score has recognized as being important in the evaluation of patients with thoracolumbar trauma?
   a) Fracture morphology.
   b) Integrity of the posterior ligamentous complex.
   c) Neurologic status of the patient.
   d) Integrity of the middle column.
   e) C and D.

2. What type of spondylolisthesis is shown in the images below?
   a) Degenerative.
   b) Isthmic.
   c) Iatrogenic.
   d) Pathologic.
   e) Traumatic.

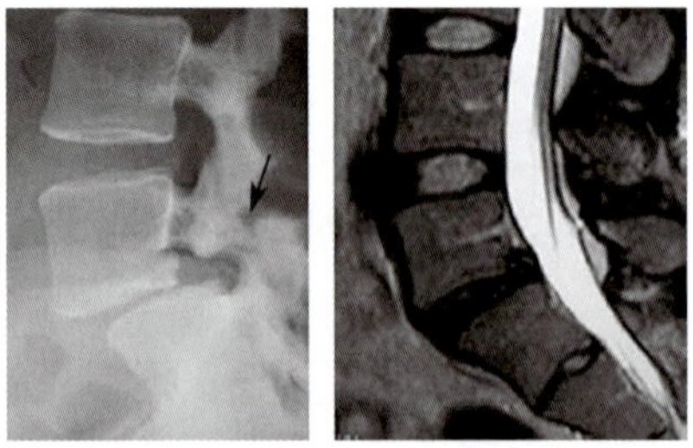

(Reproduced with permission from Okubadejo GO, Daftary A, Buchowski JM, et al. The lumbar and thoracic spine. In: Khanna AJ, ed. MRI essentials for the spine specialist. New York: Thieme; 2014:155–210.)

3. What type of disk pathology is seen in the images below?
   a) Bulge.
   b) Protrusion.
   c) Extrusion.
   d) Sequestration.
   e) Synovial cyst.

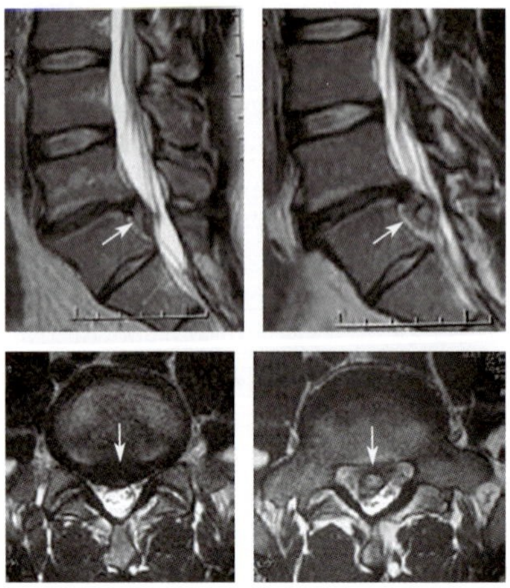

(Reproduced with permission from Okubadejo GO, Daftary A, Buchowski JM, et al. The lumbar and thoracic spine. In: Khanna AJ, ed. MRI essentials for the spine specialist. New York: Thieme; 2014:155–210.)

4. With what diagnosis are the images below most compatible?
   a) Spinal tumor.
   b) Tuberculosis.
   c) Vertebral compression fracture.
   d) Diskitis and osteomyelitis.
   e) These images are nondiagnostic, and a potential diagnosis cannot be suggested from this list without a biopsy.

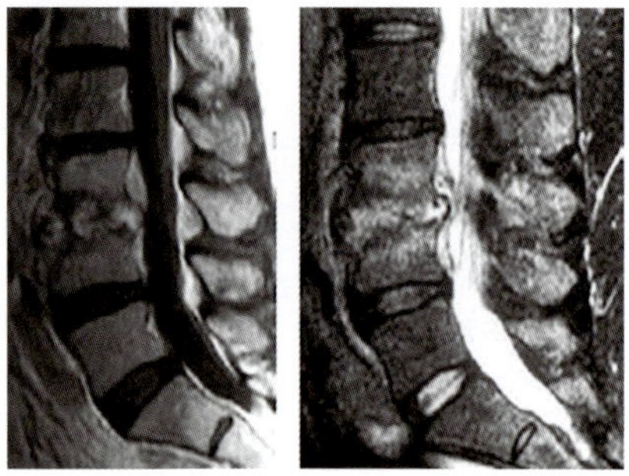

(Reproduced with permission from Okubadejo GO, Daftary A, Buchowski JM, et al. The lumbar and thoracic spine. In: Khanna AJ, ed. MRI essentials for the spine specialist. New York: Thieme; 2014:155–210.)

5. What is the most likely diagnosis shown in the images below in a patient who has recently undergone a posterior lumbar surgical procedure?
   a) Hematoma.
   b) Epidural abscess.
   c) Aneurysmal bone cyst.
   d) Pseudomeningocele.
   e) Myelomeningocele.

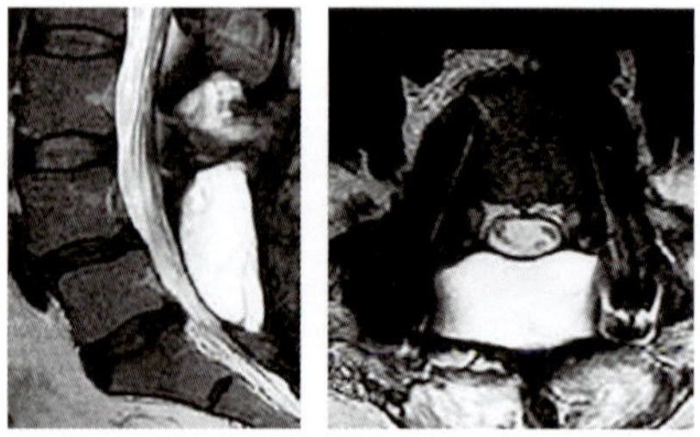

(Reproduced with permission from Okubadejo GO, Daftary A, Buchowski JM, et al. The lumbar and thoracic spine. In: Khanna AJ, ed. MRI essentials for the spine specialist. New York: Thieme; 2014:155–210.)

References

[1] Melhem ER, Benson ML, Beauchamp NJ, Lee RR. Cervical spondylosis: three-dimensional gradient-echo MR with magnetization transfer. AJNR Am J Neuroradiol. 1996; 17(4):705–711

[2] Longo MG, Fagundes J, Huang S, et al. Simultaneous multislice-based 5-minute lumbar spine MRI protocol: initial experience in a clinical setting. J Neuroimaging. 2017; 27(5):442–446

[3] Sayah A, Jay AK, Toaff JS, Makariou EV, Berkowitz F. Effectiveness of a rapid lumbar spine MRI protocol using 3D T2-weighted SPACE imaging versus a standard protocol for evaluation of degenerative changes of the lumbar spine. AJR Am J Roentgenol. 2016; 207(3):614–620

[4] Swami VG, Katlariwala M, Dhillon S, Jibri Z, Jaremko JL. Magnetic resonance imaging in patients with mechanical low back pain using a novel rapid-acquisition three-dimensional SPACE sequence at 1.5-T: a

pilot study comparing lumbar stenosis assessment with routine two-dimensional magnetic resonance sequences. Can Assoc Radiol J. 2016; 67 (4):368–378

[5] Denis F. The three column spine and its significance in the classification of acute thoracolumbar spinal injuries. Spine. 1983; 8(8):817–831

[6] Magerl F, Aebi M, Gertzbein SD, Harms J, Nazarian S. A comprehensive classification of thoracic and lumbar injuries. Eur Spine J. 1994; 3(4):184–201

[7] McCormack T, Karaikovic E, Gaines RW. The load sharing classification of spine fractures. Spine. 1994; 19(15):1741–1744

[8] Schroeder GD, Harrop JS, Vaccaro AR. Thoracolumbar trauma classification. Neurosurg Clin N Am. 2017; 28(1):23–29

[9] Vaccaro AR, Lehman RA, Jr, Hurlbert RJ, et al. A new classification of thoracolumbar injuries: the importance of injury morphology, the integrity of the posterior ligamentous complex, and neurologic status. Spine. 2005; 30(20):2325–2333

[10] Patel AA, Vaccaro AR. Thoracolumbar spine trauma classification. J Am Acad Orthop Surg. 2010; 18(2):63–71

[11] Joaquim AF, Fernandes YB, Cavalcante RAC, Fragoso RM, Honorato DC, Patel AA. Evaluation of the thoracolumbar injury classification system in thoracic and lumbar spinal trauma. Spine. 2011; 36(1):33–36

[12] Koh YD, Kim DJ, Koh YW. Reliability and validity of thoracolumbar injury classification and severity score (TLICS). Asian Spine J. 2010; 4(2):109–117

[13] Lewkonia P, Paolucci EO, Thomas K. Reliability of the thoracolumbar injury classification and severity score and comparison with the denis classification for injury to the thoracic and lumbar spine. Spine. 2012; 37 (26):2161–2167

[14] Blankenbaker DG, De Smet AA, Vanderby R, McCabe RP, Koplin SA. MRI of acute bone bruises: timing of the appearance of findings in a swine model. AJR Am J Roentgenol. 2008; 190(1):W1–W7

[15] Brown DB, Glaiberman CB, Gilula LA, Shimony JS. Correlation between preprocedural MRI findings and clinical outcomes in the treatment of chronic symptomatic vertebral compression fractures with percutaneous vertebroplasty. AJR Am J Roentgenol. 2005; 184(6):1951–1955

[16] Jung HS, Jee WH, McCauley TR, Ha KY, Choi KH. Discrimination of metastatic from acute osteoporotic compression spinal fractures with MR imaging. Radiographics. 2003; 23(1):179–187

[17] Kaplan PA, Orton DF, Asleson RJ. Osteoporosis with vertebral compression fractures, retropulsed fragments, and neurologic compromise. Radiology. 1987; 165(2):533–535

[18] Cuénod CA, Laredo JD, Chevret S, et al. Acute vertebral collapse due to osteoporosis or malignancy: appearance on unenhanced and gadolinium-enhanced MR images. Radiology. 1996; 199(2):541–549

[19] Panjabi MM, Thibodeau LL, Crisco JJ, III, White AA, III. What constitutes spinal instability? Clin Neurosurg. 1988; 34:313–339

[20] Wood KB, Khanna G, Vaccaro AR, Arnold PM, Harris MB, Mehbod AA. Assessment of two thoracolumbar fracture classification systems as used by multiple surgeons. J Bone Joint Surg Am. 2005; 87(7):1423–1429

[21] Bono CM, Vaccaro AR, Hurlbert RJ, et al. Validating a newly proposed classification system for thoracolumbar spine trauma: looking to the future of the thoracolumbar injury classification and severity score. J Orthop Trauma. 2006; 20(8):567–572

[22] Radcliff K, Su BW, Kepler CK, et al. Correlation of posterior ligamentous complex injury and neurological injury to loss of vertebral body height, kyphosis, and canal compromise. Spine. 2012; 37(13):1142–1150

[23] Rihn JA, Anderson DT, Harris E, et al. A review of the TLICS system: a novel, user-friendly thoracolumbar trauma classification system. Acta Orthop. 2008; 79(4):461–466

[24] Young PC, Petersilge CA. MR imaging of the traumatized lumbar spine. Magn Reson Imaging Clin N Am. 1999; 7(3):589–602

[25] Carrino JA, Lurie JD, Tosteson ANA, et al. Lumbar spine: reliability of MR imaging findings. Radiology. 2009; 250(1):161–170

[26] Mitra D, Cassar-Pullicino VN, McCall IW. Longitudinal study of high intensity zones on MR of lumbar intervertebral discs. Clin Radiol. 2004; 59 (11):1002–1008

[27] Peng B, Hou S, Wu W, Zhang C, Yang Y. The pathogenesis and clinical significance of a high-intensity zone (HIZ) of lumbar intervertebral disc on MR imaging in the patient with discogenic low back pain. Eur Spine J. 2006; 15(5):583–587

[28] Gundry CR, Heithoff KB. Epidural hematoma of the lumbar spine: 18 surgically confirmed cases. Radiology. 1993; 187(2):427–431

[29] Mochida K, Komori H, Okawa A, Muneta T, Haro H, Shinomiya K. Regression of cervical disc herniation observed on magnetic resonance images. Spine (Phila Pa 1976). 1998; 23(9):990–995, discussion 996–997

[30] Watanabe N, Ogura T, Kimori K, Hase H, Hirasawa Y. Epidural hematoma of the lumbar spine, simulating extruded lumbar disk herniation: clinical, discographic, and enhanced magnetic resonance imaging features. A case report. Spine. 1997; 22(1):105–109

[31] Renfrew DL, Heithoff KB. Degenerative disease. In: Renfrew DL, ed. Atlas of spine imaging. Philadelphia, PA: Saunders; 2003:11–128

[32] Schellinger D, Manz HJ, Vidic B, et al. Disk fragment migration. Radiology. 1990; 175(3):831–836

[33] Flanders AE, Tartaglino LM, Friedman DP, Aquilone LF. Magnetic resonance imaging in acute spinal injury. Semin Roentgenol. 1992; 27(4):271–298

[34] Fardon DF, Milette PC, Combined Task Forces of the North American Spine Society, American Society of Spine Radiology, and American Society of Neuroradiology. Nomenclature and classification of lumbar disc pathology. Recommendations of the Combined task Forces of the North American Spine Society, American Society of Spine Radiology, and American Society of Neuroradiology. Spine. 2001; 26(5):E93–E113

[35] Modic MT. Degenerative disc disease and back pain. Magn Reson Imaging Clin N Am. 1999; 7(3):481–491, viii

[36] Modic MT, Masaryk TJ, Ross JS, Carter JR. Imaging of degenerative disk disease. Radiology. 1988; 168(1):177–186

[37] Modic MT, Ross JS. Lumbar degenerative disk disease. Radiology. 2007; 245 (1):43–61

[38] Modic MT, Steinberg PM, Ross JS, Masaryk TJ, Carter JR. Degenerative disk disease: assessment of changes in vertebral body marrow with MR imaging. Radiology. 1988; 166(1 Pt 1):193–199

[39] Alyas F, Turner M, Connell D. MRI findings in the lumbar spines of asymptomatic, adolescent, elite tennis players. Br J Sports Med. 2007; 41 (11):836–841, discussion 841

[40] Wassenaar M, van Rijn RM, van Tulder MW, et al. Magnetic resonance imaging for diagnosing lumbar spinal pathology in adult patients with low back pain or sciatica: a diagnostic systematic review. Eur Spine J. 2012; 21(2):220–227

[41] Boden SD, Davis DO, Dina TS, Patronas NJ, Wiesel SW. Abnormal magnetic-resonance scans of the lumbar spine in asymptomatic subjects. A prospective investigation. J Bone Joint Surg Am. 1990; 72(3):403–408

[42] Borenstein DG, O'Mara JW, Jr, Boden SD, et al. The value of magnetic resonance imaging of the lumbar spine to predict low-back pain in asymptomatic subjects: a seven-year follow-up study. J Bone Joint Surg Am. 2001; 83(9):1306–1311

[43] Farshad-Amacker NA, Farshad M, Winklehner A, Andreisek G. MR imaging of degenerative disc disease. Eur J Radiol. 2015; 84(9):1768–1776

[44] Morgan S, Saifuddin A. MRI of the lumbar intervertebral disc. Clin Radiol. 1999; 54(11):703–723

[45] Pfirrmann CWA, Metzdorf A, Zanetti M, Hodler J, Boos N. Magnetic resonance classification of lumbar intervertebral disc degeneration. Spine. 2001; 26(17):1873–1878

[46] Thompson KJ, Dagher AP, Eckel TS, Clark M, Reinig JW. Modic changes on MR images as studied with provocative diskography: clinical relevance. A retrospective study of 2457 disks. Radiology. 2009; 250(3):849–855

[47] Toyone T, Takahashi K, Kitahara H, Yamagata M, Murakami M, Moriya H. Vertebral bone-marrow changes in degenerative lumbar disc disease. An MRI study of 74 patients with low back pain. J Bone Joint Surg Br. 1994; 76 (5):757–764

[48] Weishaupt D, Zanetti M, Hodler J, et al. Painful lumbar disk derangement: relevance of endplate abnormalities at MR imaging. Radiology. 2001; 218 (2):420–427

[49] Aprill C, Bogduk N. High-intensity zone: a diagnostic sign of painful lumbar disc on magnetic resonance imaging. Br J Radiol. 1992; 65(773):361–369

[50] Gundry CR, Fritts HM. Magnetic resonance imaging of the musculoskeletal system. Part 8. The spine, section 1. Clin Orthop Relat Res. 1997(338):275–287

[51] Stadnik TW, Lee RR, Coen HL, Neirynck EC, Buisseret TS, Osteaux MJC. Annular tears and disk herniation: prevalence and contrast enhancement on MR images in the absence of low back pain or sciatica. Radiology. 1998; 206 (1):49–55

[52] Yoshida H, Fujiwara A, Tamai K, Kobayashi N, Saiki K, Saotome K. Diagnosis of symptomatic disc by magnetic resonance imaging: T2-weighted and gadolinium-DTPA-enhanced T1-weighted magnetic resonance imaging. J Spinal Disord Tech. 2002; 15(3):193–198

[53] Herzog RJ. The radiologic assessment for a lumbar disc herniation. Spine. 1996; 21(24) Suppl:19S–38S
[54] Cassar-Pullicino VN. MRI of the ageing and herniating intervertebral disc. Eur J Radiol. 1998; 27(3):214–228
[55] Malfair D, Beall DP. Imaging the degenerative diseases of the lumbar spine. Magn Reson Imaging Clin N Am. 2007; 15(2):221–238, vi
[56] Dietze DD, Jr, Fessler RG. Thoracic disc herniations. Neurosurg Clin N Am. 1993; 4(1):75–90
[57] Peng B, Wu W, Hou S, Shang W, Wang X, Yang Y. The pathogenesis of Schmorl's nodes. J Bone Joint Surg Br. 2003; 85(6):879–882
[58] Hamanishi C, Kawabata T, Yosii T, Tanaka S. Schmorl's nodes on magnetic resonance imaging. Their incidence and clinical relevance. Spine. 1994; 19 (4):450–453
[59] Wagner AL, Murtagh FR, Arrington JA, Stallworth D. Relationship of Schmorl's nodes to vertebral body endplate fractures and acute endplate disk extrusions. AJNR Am J Neuroradiol. 2000; 21(2):276–281
[60] Jackson RP, Jacobs RR, Montesano PX. 1988 Volvo award in clinical sciences. Facet joint injection in low-back pain. A prospective statistical study. Spine. 1988; 13(9):966–971
[61] Revel M, Poiraudeau S, Auleley GR, et al. Capacity of the clinical picture to characterize low back pain relieved by facet joint anesthesia. Proposed criteria to identify patients with painful facet joints. Spine. 1998; 23(18): 1972–1976, discussion 1977
[62] Schwarzer AC, Aprill CN, Derby R, Fortin J, Kine G, Bogduk N. Clinical features of patients with pain stemming from the lumbar zygapophysial joints. Is the lumbar facet syndrome a clinical entity? Spine. 1994; 19(10):1132–1137
[63] Caterini R, Mancini F, Bisicchia S, Maglione P, Farsetti P. The correlation between exaggerated fluid in lumbar facet joints and degenerative spondylolisthesis: prospective study of 52 patients. J Orthop Traumatol. 2011; 12(2):87–91
[64] Cho BY, Murovic JA, Park J. Imaging correlation of the degree of degenerative L4–5 spondylolisthesis with the corresponding amount of facet fluid. J Neurosurg Spine. 2009; 11(5):614–619
[65] Boden SD, Riew KD, Yamaguchi K, Branch TP, Schellinger D, Wiesel SW. Orientation of the lumbar facet joints: association with degenerative disc disease. J Bone Joint Surg Am. 1996; 78(3):403–411
[66] Farfan HF, Sullivan JD. The relation of facet orientation to intervertebral disc failure. Can J Surg. 1967; 10(2):179–185
[67] Noren R, Trafimow J, Andersson GBJ, Huckman MS. The role of facet joint tropism and facet angle in disc degeneration. Spine. 1991; 16(5):530–532
[68] Jinkins JR. MR evaluation of stenosis involving the neural foramina, lateral recesses, and central canal of the lumbosacral spine. Magn Reson Imaging Clin N Am. 1999; 7(3):493–511, viii
[69] Alsaleh K, Ho D, Rosas-Arellano MP, Stewart TC, Gurr KR, Bailey CS. Radiographic assessment of degenerative lumbar spinal stenosis: is MRI superior to CT? Eur Spine J. 2017; 26(2):362–367
[70] de Schepper EIT, Overdevest GM, Suri P, et al. Diagnosis of lumbar spinal stenosis: an updated systematic review of the accuracy of diagnostic tests. Spine. 2013; 38(8):E469–E481
[71] Issack PS, Cunningham ME, Pumberger M, Hughes AP, Cammisa FP, Jr. Degenerative lumbar spinal stenosis: evaluation and management. J Am Acad Orthop Surg. 2012; 20(8):527–535
[72] Schroeder GD, Kurd MF, Vaccaro AR. Lumbar spinal stenosis: how is it classified? J Am Acad Orthop Surg. 2016; 24(12):843–852
[73] Hamanishi C, Matukura N, Fujita M, Tomihara M, Tanaka S. Cross-sectional area of the stenotic lumbar dural tube measured from the transverse views of magnetic resonance imaging. J Spinal Disord. 1994; 7(5):388–393
[74] Speciale AC, Pietrobon R, Urban CW, et al. Observer variability in assessing lumbar spinal stenosis severity on magnetic resonance imaging and its relation to cross-sectional spinal canal area. Spine. 2002; 27(10): 1082–1086
[75] Barz T, Melloh M, Staub LP, et al. Nerve root sedimentation sign: evaluation of a new radiological sign in lumbar spinal stenosis. Spine. 2010; 35(8):892–897
[76] Moses RA, Zhao W, Staub LP, Melloh M, Barz T, Lurie JD. Is the sedimentation sign associated with spinal stenosis surgical treatment effect in SPORT? Spine. 2015; 40(3):129–136
[77] Fazal A, Yoo A, Bendo JA. Does the presence of the nerve root sedimentation sign on MRI correlate with the operative level in patients undergoing posterior lumbar decompression for lumbar stenosis? Spine J. 2013; 13(8): 837–842
[78] Buchner M, Schiltenwolf M. Cauda equina syndrome caused by intervertebral lumbar disk prolapse: mid-term results of 22 patients and literature review. Orthopedics. 2002; 25(7):727–731
[79] Bagley CA, Gokaslan ZL. Cauda equina syndrome caused by primary and metastatic neoplasms. Neurosurg Focus. 2004; 16(6):11–18
[80] Harrop JS, Hunt GE, Jr, Vaccaro AR. Conus medullaris and cauda equina syndrome as a result of traumatic injuries: management principles. Neurosurg Focus. 2004; 16(6):19–23
[81] Wiltse LL, Newman PH, Macnab I. Classification of spondylolisis and spondylolisthesis. Clin Orthop Relat Res. 1976(117):23–29
[82] Meyerding HW. Spondylolisthesis; surgical fusion of lumbosacral portion of spinal column and interarticular facets; use of autogenous bone grafts for relief of disabling backache. J Int Coll Surg. 1956; 26(5 Part 1):566–591
[83] Hammerberg KW. New concepts on the pathogenesis and classification of spondylolisthesis. Spine. 2005; 30(6) Suppl:S4–S11
[84] Mac-Thiong JM, Labelle H. A proposal for a surgical classification of pediatric lumbosacral spondylolisthesis based on current literature. Eur Spine J. 2006; 15(10):1425–1435
[85] Mac-Thiong JM, Labelle H, Parent S, Hresko MT, Deviren V, Weidenbaum M, members of the Spinal Deformity Study Group. Reliability and development of a new classification of lumbosacral spondylolisthesis. Scoliosis. 2008; 3: 19
[86] Redla S, Sikdar T, Saifuddin A. Magnetic resonance imaging of scoliosis. Clin Radiol. 2001; 56(5):360–371
[87] O'Brien MF, Lenke LG, Bridwell KH, Blanke K, Baldus C. Preoperative spinal canal investigation in adolescent idiopathic scoliosis curves > or = 70 degrees. Spine. 1994; 19(14):1606–1610
[88] Slipman CW, Shin CH, Patel RK, et al. Etiologies of failed back surgery syndrome. Pain Med. 2002; 3(3):200–214, discussion 214–217
[89] Winter RB, Lonstein JE, Heithoff KB, Kirkham JA. Magnetic resonance imaging evaluation of the adolescent patient with idiopathic scoliosis before spinal instrumentation and fusion. A prospective, double-blinded study of 140 patients. Spine. 1997; 22(8):855–858
[90] Lewonowski K, King JD, Nelson MD. Routine use of magnetic resonance imaging in idiopathic scoliosis patients less than eleven years of age. Spine. 1992; 17(6) Suppl:S109–S116
[91] Fisk JR, Moe JH, Winter RB. Scoliosis, spondylolysis, and spondylolisthesis. Their relationship as reviewed in 539 patients. Spine. 1978; 3(3):234–245
[92] Al-Khawaja D, Seex K, Eslick GD. Spinal epidural lipomatosis: a brief review. J Clin Neurosci. 2008; 15(12):1323–1326
[93] Badami JP, Hinck VC. Symptomatic deposition of epidural fat in a morbidly obese woman. AJNR Am J Neuroradiol. 1982; 3(6):664–665
[94] Gero BT, Chynn KY. Symptomatic spinal epidural lipomatosis without exogenous steroid intake. Report of a case with magnetic resonance imaging. Neuroradiology. 1989; 31(2):190–192
[95] St. Amour TE, Hodges SE, Laakman RW, Tamas DE. Epidural lipomas, angiolipomas, and epidural lipomatosis. In: St. Amour TE, Hodges SC, Laakman RW, Tamas DE, eds. MRI of the spine. New York: Raven Press; 1994:501–507
[96] Jaramillo-de la Torre JJ, Bohinski RJ, Kuntz C, IV. Vertebral osteomyelitis. Neurosurg Clin N Am. 2006; 17(3):339–351, vii
[97] Modic MT, Feiglin DH, Piraino DW, et al. Vertebral osteomyelitis: assessment using MR. Radiology. 1985; 157(1):157–166
[98] Vaccaro AR, Betz RR, Zeidman SM, eds. Principles and practice of spine surgery. St. Louis, MO: Mosby; 2003
[99] Dagirmanjian A, Schils J, McHenry M, Modic MT. MR imaging of vertebral osteomyelitis revisited. AJR Am J Roentgenol. 1996; 167(6):1539–1543
[100] Ratcliffe JF. Anatomic basis for the pathogenesis and radiologic features of vertebral osteomyelitis and its differentiation from childhood discitis. A microarteriographic investigation. Acta Radiol Diagn (Stockh). 1985; 26(2): 137–143
[101] Batson OV. The vertebral vein system. Caldwell lecture, 1956. Am J Roentgenol Radium Ther Nucl Med. 1957; 78(2):195–212
[102] Dagirmanjian A, Schils J, McHenry MC. MR imaging of spinal infections. Magn Reson Imaging Clin N Am. 1999; 7(3):525–538
[103] Post MJD, Quencer RM, Montalvo BM, Katz BH, Eismont FJ, Green BA. Spinal infection: evaluation with MR imaging and intraoperative US. Radiology. 1988; 169(3):765–771
[104] Bertino RE, Porter BA, Stimac GK, Tepper SJ. Imaging spinal osteomyelitis and epidural abscess with short TI inversion recovery (STIR). AJNR Am J Neuroradiol. 1988; 9(3):563–564
[105] Brown R, Hussain M, McHugh K, Novelli V, Jones D. Discitis in young children. J Bone Joint Surg Br. 2001; 83(1):106–111
[106] Mahboubi S, Morris MC. Imaging of spinal infections in children. Radiol Clin North Am. 2001; 39(2):215–222

[107] Van Goethem JWM, Parizel PM, van den Hauwe L, Van de Kelft E, Verlooy J, De Schepper AMA. The value of MRI in the diagnosis of postoperative spondylodiscitis. Neuroradiology. 2000; 42(8):580–585
[108] Almeida A. Tuberculosis of the spine and spinal cord. Eur J Radiol. 2005; 55 (2):193–201
[109] Berquist TH. Imaging of the postoperative spine. Radiol Clin North Am. 2006; 44(3):407–418
[110] Gundry CR, Fritts HM. Magnetic resonance imaging of the musculoskeletal system. Part 8. The spine, section 2. Clin Orthop Relat Res. 1997(343):260–271
[111] Malik AS, Boyko O, Aktar N, Young WF. A comparative study of MR imaging profile of titanium pedicle screws. Acta Radiol. 2001; 42(3):291–293
[112] Rupp RE, Ebraheim NA, Wong FF. The value of magnetic resonance imaging of the postoperative spine with titanium implants. J Spinal Disord. 1996; 9 (4):342–346
[113] Thakkar RS, Malloy JP, IV, Thakkar SC, Carrino JA, Khanna AJ. Imaging the postoperative spine. Radiol Clin North Am. 2012; 50(4):731–747
[114] Viano AM, Gronemeyer SA, Haliloglu M, Hoffer FA. Improved MR imaging for patients with metallic implants. Magn Reson Imaging. 2000; 18(3): 287–295
[115] Zampolin R, Erdfarb A, Miller T. Imaging of lumbar spine fusion. Neuroimaging Clin N Am. 2014; 24(2):269–286
[116] Babar S, Saifuddin A. MRI of the post-discectomy lumbar spine. Clin Radiol. 2002; 57(11):969–981
[117] Annertz M, Jönsson B, Strömqvist B, Holtås S. Serial MRI in the early postoperative period after lumbar discectomy. Neuroradiology. 1995; 37(3): 177–182
[118] Ross JS. Magnetic resonance imaging of the postoperative spine. Semin Musculoskelet Radiol. 2000; 4(3):281–291
[119] Grand CM, Bank WO, Balériaux D, Matos C, Levivier M, Brotchi J. Gadolinium enhancement of vertebral endplates following lumbar disc surgery. Neuroradiology. 1993; 35(7):503–505
[120] McGirt MJ, Ambrossi GLG, Datoo G, et al. Recurrent disc herniation and long-term back pain after primary lumbar discectomy: review of outcomes reported for limited versus aggressive disc removal. Neurosurgery. 2009; 64 (2):338–344, discussion 344–345
[121] Kim MS, Park KW, Hwang C, et al. Recurrence rate of lumbar disc herniation after open discectomy in active young men. Spine. 2009; 34(1):24–29
[122] Bradley WG. Use of contrast in MR imaging of the lumbar spine. Magn Reson Imaging Clin N Am. 1999; 7(3):439–457, vii
[123] Bundschuh CV, Modic MT, Ross JS, Masaryk TJ, Bohlman H. Epidural fibrosis and recurrent disk herniation in the lumbar spine: MR imaging assessment. AJR Am J Roentgenol. 1988; 150(4):923–932
[124] Bundschuh CV, Stein L, Slusser JH, Schinco FP, Ladaga LE, Dillon JD. Distinguishing between scar and recurrent herniated disk in postoperative patients: value of contrast-enhanced CT and MR imaging. AJNR Am J Neuroradiol. 1990; 11(5):949–958
[125] Jinkins JR, Van Goethem JWM. The postsurgical lumbosacral spine. Magnetic resonance imaging evaluation following intervertebral disk surgery, surgical decompression, intervertebral bony fusion, and spinal instrumentation. Radiol Clin North Am. 2001; 39(1):1–29
[126] Sotiropoulos S, Chafetz NI, Lang P, et al. Differentiation between postoperative scar and recurrent disk herniation: prospective comparison of MR, CT, and contrast-enhanced CT. AJNR Am J Neuroradiol. 1989; 10(3): 639–643
[127] Bernard TN, Jr. Repeat lumbar spine surgery. Factors influencing outcome. Spine. 1993; 18(15):2196–2200
[128] Fandiño J, Botana C, Viladrich A, Gomez-Bueno J. Reoperation after lumbar disc surgery: results in 130 cases. Acta Neurochir (Wien). 1993; 122(1–2): 102–104
[129] Herron L. Recurrent lumbar disc herniation: results of repeat laminectomy and discectomy. J Spinal Disord. 1994; 7(2):161–166
[130] Jönsson B, Strömqvist B. Repeat decompression of lumbar nerve roots. A prospective two-year evaluation. J Bone Joint Surg Br. 1993; 75(6):894–897
[131] Van Goethem JWM, Parizel PM, Jinkins JR. Review article: MRI of the postoperative lumbar spine. Neuroradiology. 2002; 44(9):723–739
[132] Radcliff KE, Morrison W, Kepler C, et al. Distinguishing pseudomeningocele, epidural hematoma, and postoperative infection on postoperative MRI. J Spinal Disord Tech. 2013; 29(9):Epub ahead of print, Apr 3
[133] Gundry CR, Fritts HM. Magnetic resonance imaging of the musculoskeletal system: the spine. Clin Orthop Relat Res. 1998(346):262–278
[134] Burgstaller JM, Schüffler PJ, Buhmann JM, et al. LSOS Study Group. Is there an association between pain and magnetic resonance imaging parameters in patients with lumbar spinal stenosis? Spine. 2016; 41(17):E1053–E1062

Answers to Common Clinical Questions

1. Answer: d. The Thoracolumbar Injury Classification and Severity Score recognizes the importance of the following three factors when evaluating a patient with thoracolumbar trauma[9]: fracture morphology, integrity of the posterior ligamentous complex (stability or potential for neurologic compromise), and neurologic status of the patient.
2. Answer: b. The lateral radiograph shows bilateral pars interarticularis defects (*arrow*) at the L5–S1 level with Meyerding grade-1 spondylolisthesis, and the sagittal T2-weighted MR image shows the spondylolisthesis. The presence of the bilateral pars defects indicates that this is an isthmic spondylolisthesis, as described by Wiltse et al[81]; this type is most commonly seen at the L5–S1 level but can also be seen at other levels.
3. Answer: c. A disk herniation is defined as a localized displacement of disk contents beyond the borders of the intervertebral disk space. Most clinicians tend to describe disk pathology using the terms *bulge, protrusion, extrusion,* and *sequestration.* Although the last two terms are often used correctly, there seems to be a high degree of variability in the use of the first two terms. A protrusion is present if the greatest distance between the edges of the disk material beyond the disk space is less than the distance between the edges of the base in the same plane. The base is the cross-sectional area of disk material at the outer margin of the disk space of origin, where disk material displaced beyond the disk space is continuous with disk material within the disk space. An extrusion is present when any one distance between the edges of the disk material beyond the disk space is greater than the distance between the edges of the base or when there is no continuity between the disk space and the disk fragment. Extrusion may be classified further as sequestered and migrated. Sequestration is noted if the displaced disk material is completely discontinuous with the parent disk. Migration refers to displacement of disk material away from the site of extrusion, regardless of whether or not there is sequestration.
4. Answer: d. The pattern of vertebral body involvement in patients with vertebral osteomyelitis should be differentiated from that in patients with spinal tumors. Patients with vertebral osteomyelitis tend to have the epicenter of the pathologic change at the disk space, and those with tumors tend to have the epicenter at the vertebral body. The increased signal seen within the L3–L4 disk and adjacent vertebral bodies on the sagittal postgadolinium T1-weighted (**a**) and sagittal STIR (**b**) images has its epicenter at the disk space and is, therefore, most compatible with diskitis and vertebral osteomyelitis. A tumor would more likely "spare" the disk space, and tuberculous infection would likely do the same. The diagnosis of diskitis and osteomyelitis may be confirmed with a CT-guided biopsy, which would enable identification of the pathogen and selection of the appropriate antibiotic therapy. The increased signal with a vertebral compression fracture is seen in the vertebral body at the site of the fracture in patients with acute or subacute fractures, and the adjacent disk has normal signal.

5. Answer: d. These sagittal (**a**) and axial (**b**) T2-weighted images show a well-circumscribed fluid collection that does not compress the thecal sac in a patient who has undergone an L4–S1 laminectomy and instrumentation fusion procedure. A pseudomeningocele typically occurs in a patient who sustains a durotomy during an open surgical procedure or in a patient who undergoes resection of an intradural lesion. In both of these situations, there may be an incomplete closure of the dural opening, with resultant leakage of CSF into the operative site and posterior soft tissues. This collection of CSF is termed a *pseudomeningocele* because it is surrounded not by arachnoid and dura, but rather by a pseudomeninges of reactive fibrous tissue.[131] Pseudomeningoceles typically are well circumscribed, communicate with the subarachnoid space, and contain fluid that matches the signal characteristics of CSF, which is homogeneous and has low signal intensity on T1-weighted images and high signal intensity on T2-weighted images. Given that the pressure within a pseudomeningocele is usually similar to that of the subarachnoid space, these collections usually compress the thecal sac less than do postoperative epidural hematomas.[132]

17 MRI of the Pediatric Spine

A. Jay Khanna, Bruce A. Wasserman, and Paul D. Sponseller

Abstract

Magnetic resonance imaging (MRI) provides optimal imaging of the pediatric spine. Typical MR imaging protocols include sagittal and axial T2-weighted image. However, these imaging protocols, can vary across institutions and should be modified when specific diagnosis such as trauma, infection or tumor are being considered.

Appropriate interpretation of the pediatric spine MRI study is reliant upon noting and appreciating the differences between the normal anatomy of the adult spine and that of the pediatric spine at different stages of development.

As with adults, evaluation of the pediatric spine MRI study is best when the physician is familiar with a differential diagnosis and considerations including trauma, infections, neoplasm and the different types of spinal dysraphism.

Although MRI is an excellent imaging modality for the pediatric spine, it is important to correlate MRI findings with those from conventional radiographs, CT, and other types of imaging studies when indicated.

Keywords: pediatric spine, dysraphism, scoliosis, kyphosis, dysplasia

17.1 Specialized Pulse Sequences and Imaging Protocols

Standard pulse sequences for spinal imaging include spin-echo (SE) T1-weighted and fast spin-echo (FSE) T2-weighted images. The FSE technique enables the acquisition of T2-weighted images without prolonged imaging times. T1-weighted images enable the evaluation of anatomic detail, including that of the osseous structures and soft tissues. T2-weighted images are primarily used to evaluate the spinal cord and enhance lesion conspicuity. Because cerebrospinal fluid (CSF) is bright on T2-weighted images and the spinal cord retains its intermediate signal, the T2-weighted images maximize the CSF to neural tissue contrast and therefore enable optimal delineation of the spinal cord and nerve roots. T2-weighted images are very sensitive to pathologic changes in tissue, including any processes in which cells and the extracellular matrix have increased water content. This pathologic change is usually shown as an increase in signal intensity on T2-weighted images, which increases the conspicuity of most pathologic processes affecting the spine.

Open magnetic resonance imaging (MRI) systems are becoming more frequently used, especially for pediatric imaging. Although these systems often have significantly lower field strengths than closed magnets and thus usually produce studies of inferior overall quality, the open environment provides young patients with access to their parents and makes the experience less intimidating for patients with claustrophobia. Open systems are also helpful for procedures that might benefit from MRI guidance. When possible, however, the authors recommend that MR imaging be performed using closed 1.5-T or 3-T MRI systems.

17.2 Pediatric Sedation Protocols

Formal sedation is often required for the successful MRI evaluation of the pediatric patient, and multiple studies and reviews have evaluated and recommended specific sedation protocols.[1] The American Academy of Pediatrics has published guidelines for the elective sedation of pediatric patients,[2] but compliance with these guidelines is not mandatory. The American Academy of Pediatrics has stated that careful medical screening and patient selection by knowledgeable medical personnel are needed to exclude patients at high risk for life-threatening hypoxia.[3] Also, monitoring using their guidelines is necessary for the early detection and management of life-threatening hypoxia.[4] The American Academy of Pediatrics recommends that, before an examination in which sedation is to be used, children up to 3 years old should ingest nothing by mouth for 4 hours, and children 3 to 6 years old should ingest nothing by mouth for 6 hours.[3]

Although multiple protocols exist for the specific administration of various medications for pediatric sedation and although practices vary among institutions, a few agents are essential for most sedation protocols. Oral chloral hydrate is recommended for children < 18 months old. However, the use of oral chloral hydrate is controversial because of its variable absorption, paradoxical effects, and nonstandardized dosing regimen. Older or larger children usually receive intravenous pentobarbital, with or without fentanyl. Although some studies have reported the successful administration of sedation by trained nurses,[1,6] patients who may benefit from the expertise of an anesthesiologist include those with substantial comorbidities, such as the following:

- Cardiopulmonary disease.
- Skeletal dysplasias.
- Neuromuscular disease.
- Abnormal airway anatomy.

An important consideration after sedation for pediatric MRI is the need for strict adherence to established discharge criteria, including the following[5]:

- Return to baseline vital signs.
- Level of consciousness close to baseline.
- Ability to maintain a patent airway.

Because of the potential risks associated with anesthesia and sedation in the young patient, there is a trend toward referring pediatric patients who require sedation to hospitals with pediatric anesthesiologists. Alternate techniques include sleep deprivation and rapid, segmental scanning; the latter permits the acquisition of high-quality images without the use of sedation. The surgeon referring pediatric patients for MR images of the spine should be familiar with the sedation protocols and level of expertise at the selected facilities. It is important to note that sedation protocols vary greatly from institution to institution and that no protocol is 100% safe, which emphasizes the need for monitoring, careful patient selection, and evaluation. The authors advise consultation with the pediatric anesthesiologists at the referring physician's institution when sedating patients for MRI studies.

17.3 Normal Pediatric MRI Anatomy

To better understand and predict the MRI appearance of pathologic processes involving the spine, one should have a basic understanding of the normal MRI anatomy.[7,8] Because most orthopaedic surgeons are more familiar with the normal anatomy of the adolescent (▶ Fig. 17.1) and adult spines than with that of the pediatric spine, the salient points of the former two are presented first as a framework for understanding and differentiating the pediatric spine (for a full discussion of the adult spine anatomy, see Chapter 2, Normal MRI Anatomy of the Musculoskeletal System).

17.3.1 Adolescents and Adults

The lumbar spine is the most frequently imaged region in both children and adults. The lumbar spinal canal transitions from a round appearance in its proximal portion to a more triangular one distally. The lumbar facet joints are covered with 2 to 4 mm of hyaline cartilage. This cartilage can be nicely visualized on FSE pulse sequences and with gradient-echo pulse sequences. The epidural space and ligaments should also be carefully evaluated. The epidural fat is seen as high signal intensity on T1-weighted images; the ligamentum flavum shows minimally higher T1-weighted signal than the other ligaments. The conus medullaris, usually located at the L1–L2 level, is best seen as a regional enlargement of the spinal cord on the sagittal images. The filum terminale extends from the conus medullaris to the distal thecal sac. The traversing nerve roots pass distally from the conus medullaris and extend anteriorly and laterally. These nerve roots exit laterally underneath the pedicle and into the neural foramen. The intervertebral disk, consisting of the cartilaginous end plates, annulus fibrosus, and the nucleus pulposus, normally shows increased T2 signal in its central portion. It is important to note that CSF pulsations often create artifacts that degrade the image in the lumbar spine; those artifacts must not be mistaken for a pathologic process.

Evaluation of the cervical spine begins with the vertebral bodies. A mild lordosis is noted on sagittal images. On axial images, the spinal canal is triangular, with the base located anteriorly. It is important to note the normal variant dark band at the base of the dens that represents a remnant of the subdental synchondrosis; it should not be mistaken for a fracture. In adults, the facet joints are small and triangular, whereas in children they are relatively larger and flat. The spinal cord is elliptical in cross-section in the cervical spine. It is important to recognize that there is a difference in signal between the normal gray and white matter of the spinal cord. This signal heterogeneity should not be

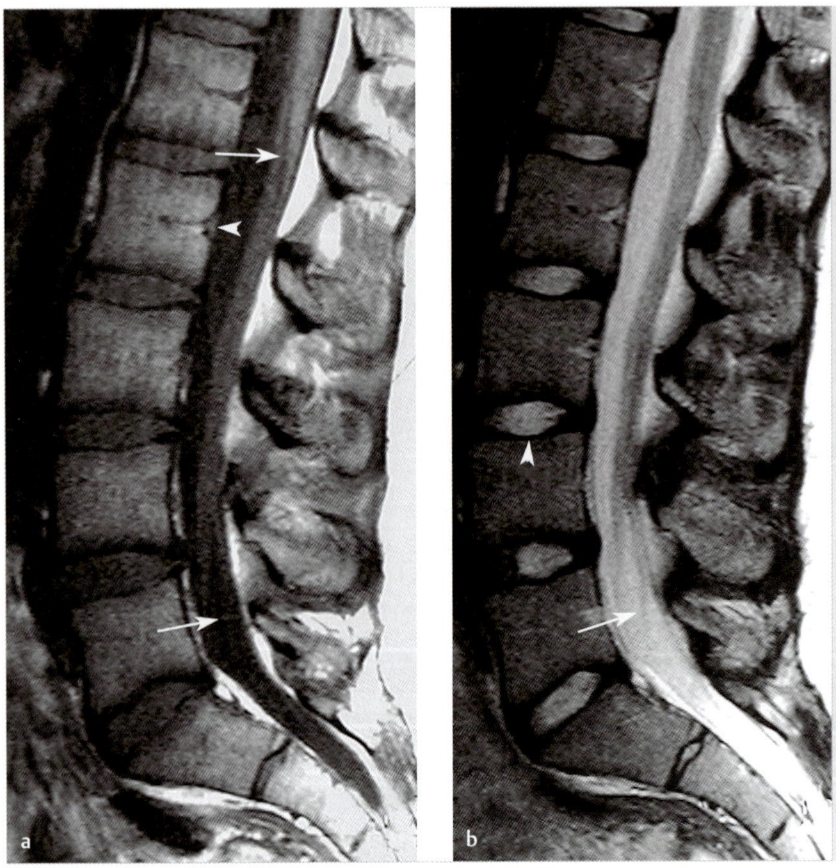

Fig. 17.1 Normal lumbar spine in a 16-year-old girl. **(a)** A sagittal T1-weighted image shows dark cerebrospinal fluid (CSF) (*arrow with small head*), the conus medullaris terminating at the L1–L2 level (*arrow with large head*), and the basivertebral channel (*arrowhead*). Note the normal rectangular appearance of the vertebral bodies and the lumbar lordosis. **(b)** A sagittal T2-weighted image shows bright CSF (*arrow*) and a bright nucleus pulposus (*arrowhead*). (Reproduced with permission from, Khanna AJ, Wasserman BA, Sponseller PD. The Pediatric Spine. In: Khanna AJ, ed. MRI for orthopaedic surgeons. New York: Thieme; 2010:338–349.)

mistaken for intramedullary pathology. The intervertebral disks are similar in appearance to, but smaller than, those seen at the thoracic and lumbar levels. An important anatomic feature of the cervical spine is the prominent epidural venous plexus, which is not present in the thoracic or lumbar spine.

The thoracic vertebral bodies are relatively constant in size, and the spinal canal is relatively round. Abundant epidural fat is present posteriorly, but there is less anteriorly than in the lumbosacral region. The cord is more round than in the cervical or lumbar regions, and the cord segment lies between two and three levels above the corresponding vertebral body. The intervertebral disks are thinner than the disks in the lumbar spine. The appearance of the CSF is more variable in the thoracic spine than that in the lumbar region because of more prominent CSF pulsations, but it is most commonly seen as a region of low signal dorsal to the spinal cord on T1-weighted images. This artifact is often most severe at the apex of curves, including the thoracic kyphosis. Techniques are available for minimizing this artifact, including gating to the pulse or cardiac cycle.

17.3.2 Children

Differences between the Pediatric and Adult Spine

Understanding the normal adult and adolescent spine leads to appreciation of the dynamic development of the pediatric spine. The MRI appearance of the growing spine is quite complex. Multiple substantial changes occur in the vertebral ossification center and the intervertebral disks that markedly alter the overall appearance of the spine, especially between infancy and 2 years of age.[9] In general, the vertebral ossification centers are incompletely ossified early in childhood, and the disks are thicker and have higher water content than those in the adult. The spinal canal and neural foramina are larger, and there is less curvature. In addition, the overall signal intensity of the vertebral bodies is lower than that of the adult spine on T1-weighted images because of the abundance of red (hematopoietic) marrow relative to yellow (fat) marrow in the pediatric, adolescent, and young adult spine.

By understanding the MRI appearance of this development process, the clinician is better equipped to differentiate normal from pathologic states. Sze et al[9] have characterized the MRI evolution of the pediatric spine between infancy and 2 years of age, and Goske et al[7] have described this dynamic process through the age of 10 years (see details later).

Full-Term Infant

In the newborn, the overall size of the vertebral body is small relative to the spinal canal, and the spinal cord ends at approximately the L2 level. The lumbar spine does not show the usual lordosis and is straight. The vertebral bodies show markedly low signal intensity on T1-weighted images, with a thin central hyperintense band that likely represents the basivertebral plexus. The spongy bone of the ossification center is ellipsoidal rather than rectangular and is often mistaken for a disk. The intervertebral disk is relatively narrow and often contains a thin, bright central band on T2-weighted images that represents the notochordal remnants.

Age: 3 Months

At 3 months, the osseous component of the vertebral body has increased and the amount of hyaline cartilage has decreased, with a resultant rectangular appearance to the vertebral bodies. The ossification centers begin to increase in signal intensity, starting at the end plates and progressing centrally. The neural foramina have not substantially changed at this age, remaining relatively large and ovoid in shape.

Age: 2 Years

At 2 years, the spine has begun to show its normal curvature, most likely because of the effects of weightbearing (▶ Fig. 17.2). The ossified portion of the vertebral body increases substantially in size and begins to assume its adult appearance, with near-complete ossification of the pedicles and the articular processes. The disk space and nucleus pulposus become longer and thinner. The cartilaginous end plate has decreased in size and is often difficult to identify. The neural foramen also begins to take its adult appearance as its inferior portion narrows.

Age: 10 Years

At 10 years, the spinal curvature resembles that of an adult (▶ Fig. 17.3). The ossification of the vertebral bodies and posterior elements is nearly complete, with a resultant decrease in the spinal canal diameter. The vertebral bodies also develop concave superior and inferior contours. The nucleus pulposus becomes smaller at this age and spans approximately half of the disk space in the sagittal plane. The neural foramina continue to narrow inferiorly.

17.3.3 Conus Medullaris

The spinal cord extends to the inferior aspect of the osseous spinal column in early fetal life.[7] Because of the more rapid longitudinal growth of the vertebral bodies relative to the spinal cord, the conus medullaris is repositioned in the upper lumbar spine by birth. It is important to note the location of the conus medullaris on every pediatric spine MRI study (▶ Fig. 17.1, ▶ Fig. 17.2). A conus level below the L2–L3 interspace in children > 5 years old is abnormal and indicates possible tethering.[10,11] Saifuddin et al[12] reviewed the MRI findings of 504 normal adult spines and found that the average conus position was the lower third of LI (range, middle third of T12 to the upper third of L3).

17.4 Pathologic Processes Involving the Pediatric Spine

17.4.1 Infection

Infectious processes involving the pediatric spine include osteomyelitis, diskitis, epidural abscess, and paraspinal abscess.[1,13,14,15] In general, the MRI signal characteristics of infection include a region of low T1 signal intensity and high T2 signal intensity in bone and soft tissue.

MRI is more sensitive than conventional radiographs or computed tomography (CT) and is more specific than nuclear

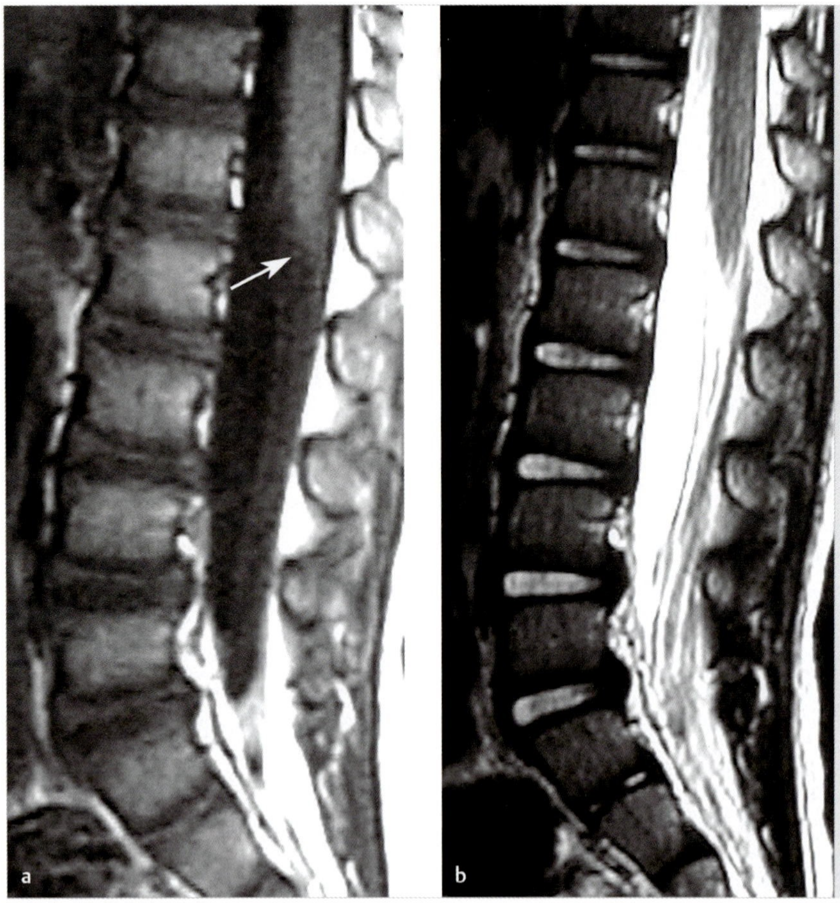

Fig. 17.2 Normal lumbar spine in a 2-year-old boy. **(a)** A sagittal T1-weighted image shows rectangular vertebral bodies and a wide, thin intervertebral disk. Note that the conus medullaris terminates at the L1–L2 level (*arrow*). **(b)** A sagittal T2-weighted image shows increased disk signal compared with that seen on the T1-weighted image. (Reproduced with permission from, Khanna AJ, Wasserman BA, Sponseller PD. The Pediatric Spine. In: Khanna AJ, ed. MRI for orthopaedic surgeons. New York: Thieme; 2010:338–349.)

scintigraphy in identifying vertebral osteomyelitis.[16,17] MRI provides the optimal means of imaging osteomyelitis (▶ Fig. 17.4). Marrow edema can be detected on short tau inversion recovery (STIR) images, and enhancement of the disk and adjacent vertebral bodies on postgadolinium, fat-suppressed T1-weighted images helps to confirm the diagnosis. The specificity of MRI for infection is higher in children than in adults because one of the primary confounding findings, degenerative arthritis, can be removed from the differential diagnosis. A key concept in both children and adults is differentiating osteomyelitis from neoplastic disease. An important characteristic that may help make this differentiation is the fact that infectious processes are more likely to cross intervertebral disks than are neoplastic conditions (▶ Fig. 17.5).

Diskitis, seen as a disruption of the normally well-defined disk-vertebral borders on T1-weighted images and as an increase in signal of the disk on T2-weighted images,[1] may obliterate the horizontal cleft within the intervertebral disk normally seen on T2-weighted images (▶ Fig. 17.6). The abnormal signal seen in infectious diskitis is classically associated with surrounding soft-tissue inflammation and reactive end-plate changes. Compared with adult patients, pediatric patients are more likely to develop primary diskitis because of increased blood supply to the disk. Adults are more likely to develop infectious diskitis after surgery or from contiguous spread from primary end-plate osteomyelitis.

Epidural abscesses are rare, but when they do develop, it is usually after surgery or vertebral osteomyelitis. The diagnosis of epidural abscesses can be made in the patient who has a collection in the epidural space and a clinical history that supports infection.[13] Gadolinium-enhanced T1-weighted images often show a peripheral rim of enhancement that represents the abscess wall.

17.4.2 Trauma

An important role of MRI is to evaluate for the presence of neural injury in the pediatric patient who has sustained substantial trauma to the spine and who has an abnormal neurologic examination or is unresponsive. The initial evaluation is performed with conventional radiographs, which are often normal. MRI evaluation may then be performed to evaluate for osseous, ligamentous, intervertebral disk, cord, and nerve root injury.[18] Although CT enables better evaluation of osseous detail and displaced fractures, MRI enables improved evaluation of nondisplaced fractures because of its ability to detect marrow signal abnormalities (▶ Fig. 17.6). MRI is also useful in its ability to help determine the age of the fracture and to evaluate for posttraumatic myelopathy. MRI, however, is not the optimal method for evaluating spondylolysis. CT offers increased spatial resolution and the ability to define accurately the osseous defect, whereas radionuclide imaging can show increased radiotracer activity in the region of the defect.

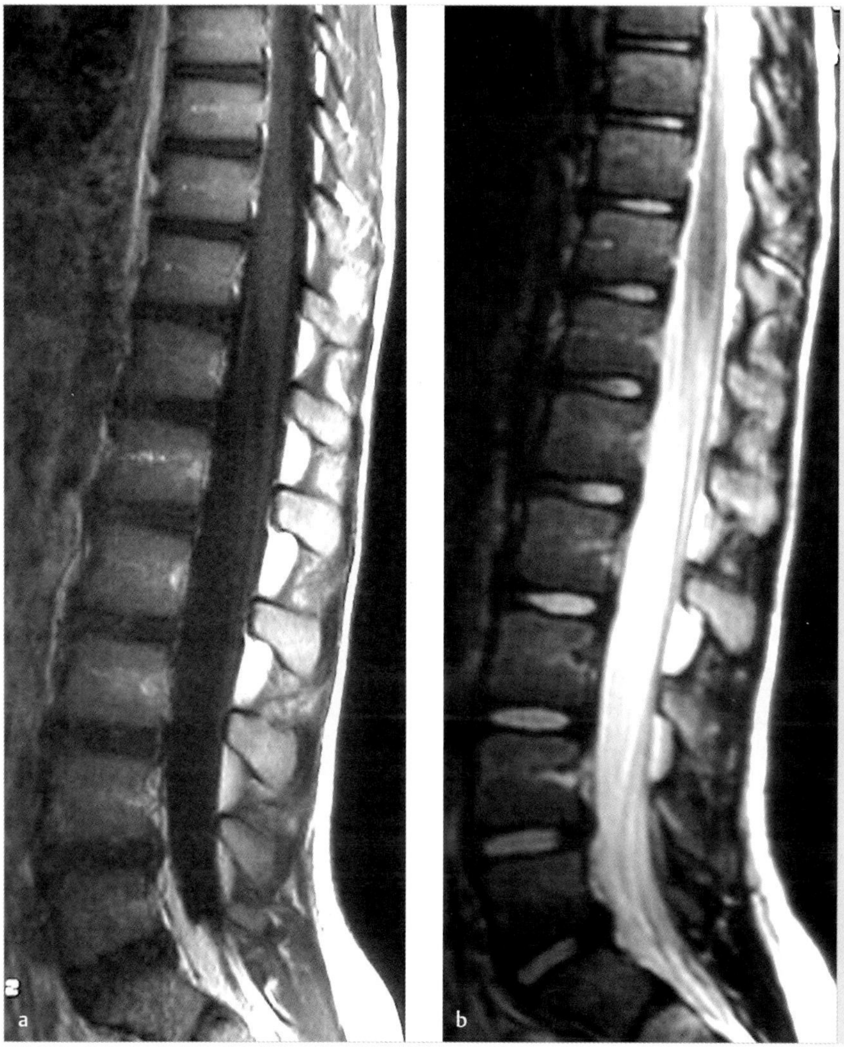

Fig. 17.3 This 10-year-old girl has a normal lumbar spine with normal lordosis. **(a)** A sagittal T1-weighted image. **(b)** A sagittal T2-weighted image. Note that the posterior elements are well formed, with a resultant decrease in the canal diameter. (Reproduced with permission from, Khanna AJ, Wasserman BA, Sponseller PD. The Pediatric Spine. In: Khanna AJ, ed. MRI for orthopaedic surgeons. New York: Thieme; 2010:338–349.)

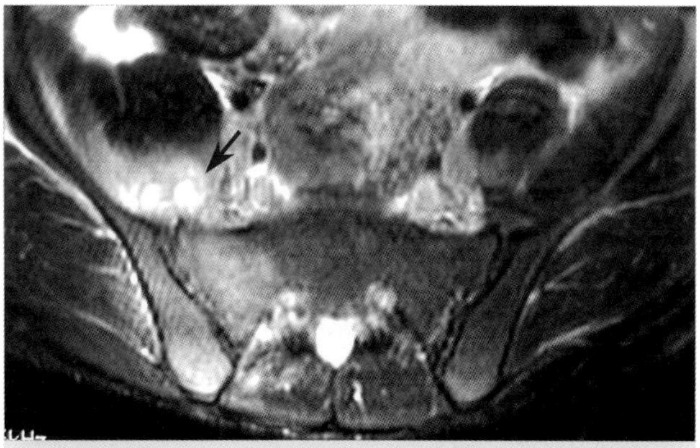

Fig. 17.4 This axial T2-weighted image in a 15-year-old boy with infectious symptoms and complaints of low back pain shows increased T2-weighted signal in the region of the right sacroiliac joint and an associated soft-tissue component at the anterior aspect of the joint (*arrow*), compatible with a sacroiliac joint infection. (Reproduced with permission from, Khanna AJ, Wasserman BA, Sponseller PD. The Pediatric Spine. In: Khanna AJ, ed. MRI for orthopaedic surgeons. New York: Thieme; 2010:338–349.)

With regard to acute disk herniation in the pediatric age group, it is important to note that this herniation represents more of a fracture with a hinge-like displacement of fibrocartilage and displacement of the entire disk and vertebral end plate than extrusion of a disk fragment, as is seen in the adult population.[19] Such avulsion fractures are often occult on conventional radiographs and are better detected with CT and MRI.[19] Axial MR images show the fracture fragment as an area of low signal intensity protruding into the spinal canal, and the sagittal images show a low-signal-intensity region in the shape of a Y or 7 on all pulse sequences.[19]

Spinal cord injury without radiographic abnormality (SCIWORA) is an established entity seen after pediatric spine trauma.[20,21] The characteristic hypermobility and ligamentous laxity of the pediatric osseous cervical and thoracic spine predispose children to a spinal cord injury without radiographic abnormality-type injury.[20] The elasticity of the osseous pediatric spine as well as the relatively large size of the head enable deformation of the musculoskeletal structures beyond physiologic limits, which results in cord trauma followed by spontaneous reduction of the spine.[20]

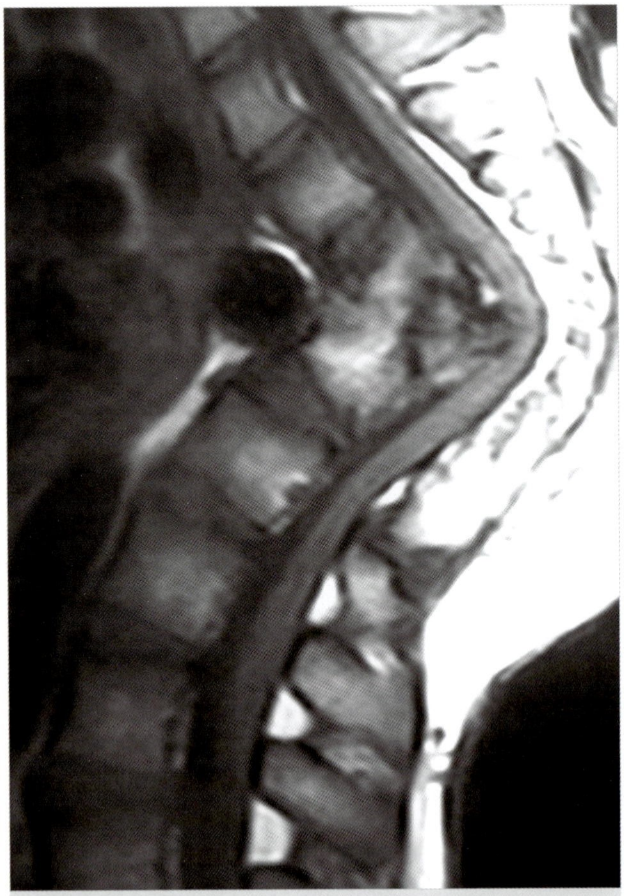

Fig. 17.5 In this 16-year-old girl with a history of tuberculosis, a sagittal T1-weighted image shows destruction of three consecutive midthoracic vertebral bodies with associated kyphosis and gibbus deformity, compatible with tuberculous osteomyelitis. (Reproduced with permission from, Khanna AJ, Wasserman BA, Sponseller PD. The Pediatric Spine. In: Khanna AJ, ed. MRI for orthopaedic surgeons. New York: Thieme; 2010:338–349.)

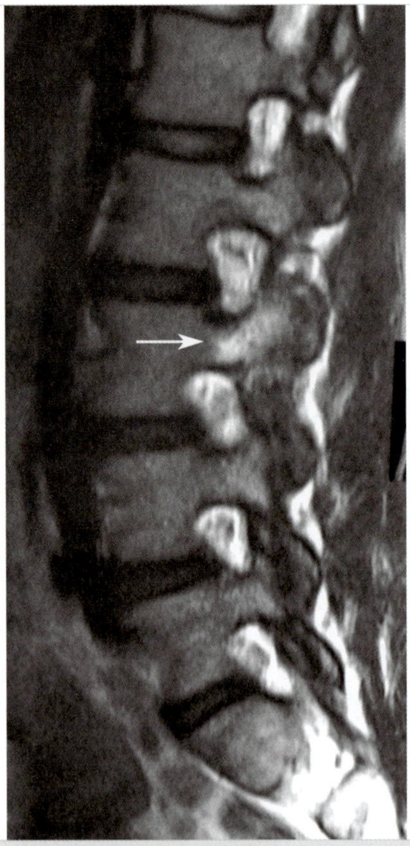

Fig. 17.6 In this 12-year-old boy with persistent low back pain and normal radiographs, a parasagittal T2-weighted image shows an area of increased signal (*arrow*) within the region of the pars intra-articularis, compatible with edema from an acute or subacute nondisplaced pars intra-articularis fracture. (Reproduced with permission from, Khanna AJ, Wasserman BA, Sponseller PD. The Pediatric Spine. In: Khanna AJ, ed. MRI for orthopaedic surgeons. New York: Thieme; 2010:338–349.)

As with other types of spinal cord injuries, the most important predictor of outcome is the severity of neurologic injury. A patient with a complete neurologic deficit after spinal cord injury without radiographic abnormality has a poor prognosis for recovery of neurologic function. The role of MRI in spinal cord injury without radiographic abnormality syndrome is to define the degree of neural injury, rule out occult fractures and subluxation that may require surgical intervention, and evaluate for the presence of ligamentous injury.[22,23] The T2-weighted and STIR images should show increased signal in the cord or vertebral body.[24] The increased T2 signal in the cord is compatible with edema and can range from a partial, reversible contusion to complete transection of the cord.

17.5 Imaging of Spinal Dysraphism

Spinal dysraphism is a general term used to describe a wide range of anomalies resulting from incomplete fusion of the midline mesenchyme, bone, and neural elements. The osseous abnormalities consist of defects within the neural arch with partial or complete absence of the spinous processes, laminae, or other components of the posterior elements. MRI has been shown to be the best modality for the evaluation of spinal dysraphism.[25,26,27,28]

To better understand the MRI of spinal dysraphism, it is important to have a basic knowledge of its various types. A classification system has been proposed that permits the systematic evaluation of a patient with a suspected spinal dysraphism (▶ Table 17.1).[26] By using this clinical classification system, the differential diagnosis can be rapidly narrowed to one of three categories: spinal dysraphism with a non-skin-covered back mass, spinal dysraphism with a skin-covered back mass, and spinal dysraphism with no back mass. The final diagnosis can then be selected from the identified category based on the lesion's MRI characteristics.

Myelomeningoceles represent a common type of spina bifida, the most common form of spinal dysraphism (▶ Fig. 17.7). It most often presents as a non-skin-covered back mass in the lumbosacral region, although it can also be seen at higher levels. This mass may or may not be covered by leptomeninges containing a variable amount of neural tissue. The sac herniates through a defect in the posterior elements of the spine. The spinal cord usually contains a dorsal cleft, is splayed open, and is often tethered within the sac.[26] Progressive scoliosis is seen in 66% of patients; Arnold-Chiari type-II malformation, in 90 to 99%; diastematomyelia, in 30 to 40%; and syringohydromyelia, in 40 to 80%.[29] Scarring can occur at the surgical site after sac closure, and it is important to monitor these patients for the signs and symptoms of the tethered cord syndrome.

Table 17.1 Classification of spinal dysraphism

Category	Types
Spinal dysraphism with a non-skin-covered back mass	Myelomeningocele
	Myelocele
Spinal dysraphism with a skin-covered back mass	Lipomeningocele
	Myelocystocele
	Simple posterior meningocele
Spinal dysraphism without a back mass	Diastematomyelia
	Dorsal dermal sinus
	Intradural lipoma
	Tight filum terminale
	Anterior sacral meningocele
	Lateral thoracic meningocele
	Hydromyelia
	Split notochord syndrome
	Caudal regression syndrome

Source: (Modified with permission fro, Byrd et al 1996.26 Modified with permission from, Byrd SE, Darling CF, McLone DG, Tomita T. MR imaging of the pediatric spine. Magn Reson Imaging Clin N Am. 1996; 4(4):797–833).[26]

Of the entities presenting with a skin-covered back mass in the presence of spinal dysraphism, lipomeningocele is the most common. The lipomeningocele consists of lipomatous tissue that is continuous with the subcutaneous tissue of the back and also insinuates through the dysraphic defect and dura and into the spinal canal. The spinal cord often contains a dorsal defect at the level of the lipomatous tissue and may be tethered at this level. The essential MRI feature of this lesion is that the lipomatous tissue matches the signal characteristics of subcutaneous fat on all pulse sequences, including fat-suppressed pulse sequences.

Occult spinal dysraphism presents without a back mass and includes many entities (▶ Fig. 17.1). Diastematomyelia is characterized by a sagittal splitting of the spinal cord, conus medullaris, or filum terminale into two segments, often in the thoracic or lumbar spine. The dural tube and arachnoid are undivided in approximately half of the patients; in such patients, clinical findings are rare, and surgery is not indicated. In the other half, the dural tube and arachnoid are completely or partially split at the level of the spinal cord cleft, which results in tethering of the cord and subsequent clinical symptoms. Coronal T1-weighted and T2-weighted images best define the

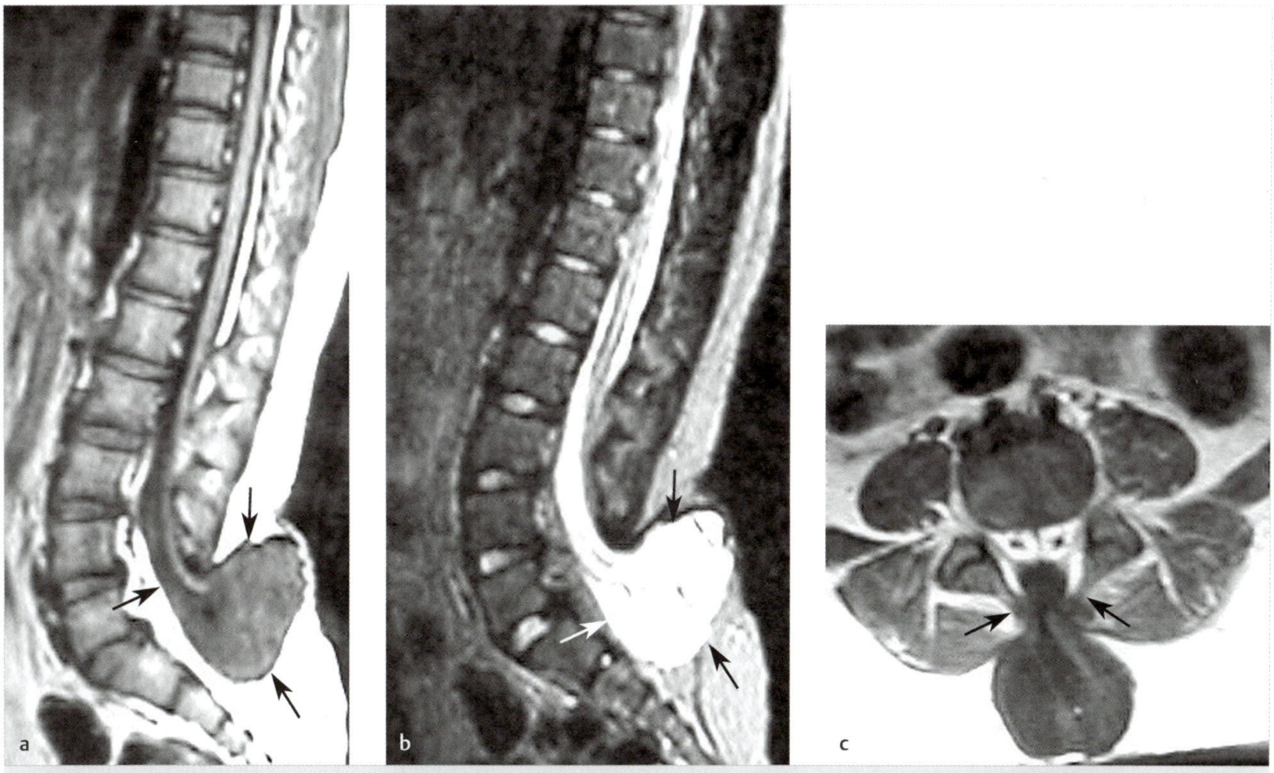

Fig. 17.7 A 6-year-old girl with a myelomeningocele. **(a)** A sagittal T1-weighted image shows a low back mass contiguous with the contents of the spinal canal (*arrows*). **(b)** A sagittal T2-weighted image shows that the mass is filled with high-signal-intensity fluid, compatible with cerebrospinal fluid (CSF) (*arrows*). **(c)** An axial T1-weighted image confirms the communication of the mass with the spinal canal through a defect in the posterior elements (*arrows*). (Reproduced with permission from, Khanna AJ, Wasserman BA, Sponseller PD. The Pediatric Spine. In: Khanna AJ, ed. MRI for orthopaedic surgeons. New York: Thieme; 2010:338–349.)

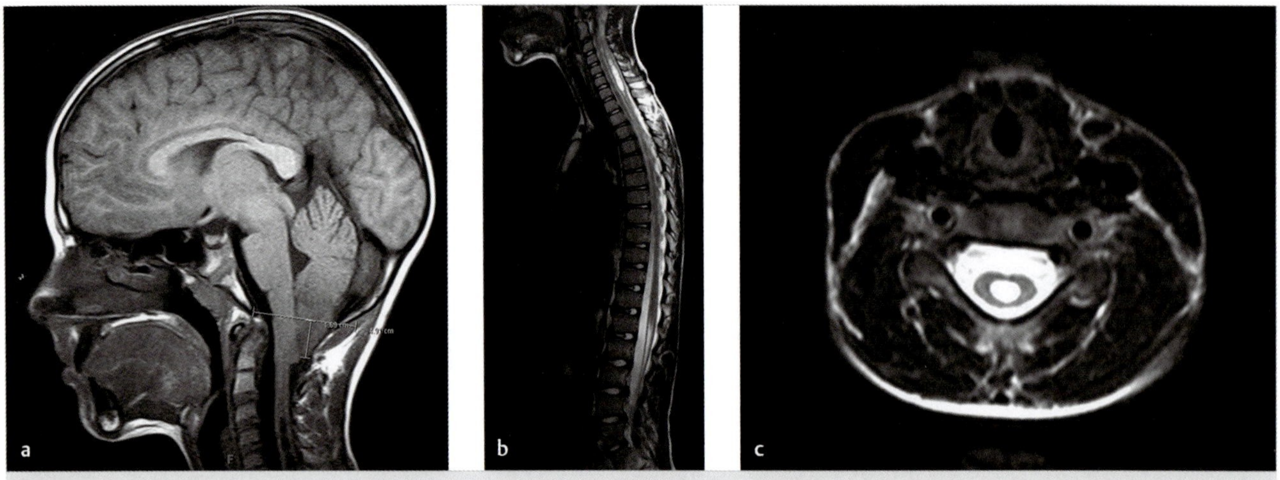

Fig. 17.8 A 9-year-old boy with a large syrinx of the cervical spine. **(a)** A sagittal T1-weighted image of the brain and upper cervical spine showing an Arnold Chiari type-I malformation and a syrinx of the upper cervical spine (*lines* showing 4.91 cm of cerebellar tonsil ectopia below the level of the foramen magnum). **(b)** A sagittal T2-weighted image of the entire spine showing a large syrinx extending from C4–C7. **(c)** An axial T2-weighted image at the C6 level confirms that the syrinx is located in the center of the spinal cord. (Reproduced with permission from, Khanna AJ, Wasserman BA, Sponseller PD. The Pediatric Spine. In: Khanna AJ, ed. MRI Essentials for the Spine Specialist. New York: Thieme; 2014:237–250.)

sagittal split in the cord; the findings should be confirmed on axial images. The osseous spur or fibrous band that occurs between each hemicord appears dark on T1-weighted and T2-weighted images and can be better visualized on CT.

Another important entity often seen in patients with spinal dysraphism is syringohydromyelia, or syrinx (▶ Fig. 17.8). A syrinx is a longitudinal cavity within the spinal cord that may or may not communicate with the central canal. Multiple theories exist to explain the etiology of a syrinx, including developmental and trauma-, inflammation-, ischemia-, and pressure-related causes. Sagittal MR images show a linear, low T1 signal intensity and high T2 signal intensity within the parenchyma of the spinal cord. Identification of a syrinx is sometimes an indication for contrast administration to exclude an underlying enhancing lesion.

17.5.1 Chiari Malformations

Chiari malformations are frequently seen in patients with spinal dysraphism. Chiari type-I malformations consist of cerebellar tonsillar ectopia, in which the cerebellar tonsils extend below the level of the foramen magnum.[30] The commonly quoted measurement for the degree of herniation of the tonsils below the foramen magnum is 5 mm. Mikulis et al[31] reported a variation by age in the upper limit of normal: 6 mm in the first decade of life, 5 mm in the second and third decades, and 3 mm by the ninth decade. In Chiari type-I malformations, the brainstem is spared, and the fourth ventricle remains in its normal location. Chiari type-I malformations are associated with syringohydromyelia,[32] craniovertebral junction anomalies, and basilar invagination. Chiari type-II malformations are more advanced and consist of downward displacement of the brainstem and inferior cerebellum into the cervical spinal canal, with a decrease in the size of the posterior fossa.

17.5.2 Tethered Cord Syndrome

The tethered cord syndrome, an important problem, is seen in a substantial number of patients with spinal dysraphism, especially those who have undergone surgical closure of the defect.[33,34] During fetal life, the spinal cord extends to the sacrococcygeal level. Because of the more rapid growth of the vertebral column after birth, the cord ascends to the L1–L2 level in the newborn. During the formation of a spinal dysraphic defect such as myelomeningocele, the open neural elements often attach to the peripheral ectoderm, resulting in spinal cord tethering. After surgical closure of the sac, there is a tendency for the spinal cord to become adherent at the repair site. As the child grows, this adherence may result in tethering of the cord and prevention of cephalad cord migration, with eventual symptoms. Thus, tethered cord should be ruled out as the potential cause of any deterioration in neurologic function in patients with spinal dysraphic and related conditions, including the following:

- Myelomeningoceles.
- Myeloceles.
- Lipomeningoceles.
- Diastematomyelia.

MRI has been proposed as the initial, and possibly the only, imaging modality for a patient with a suspected tethered spinal cord.[11] The sagittal images should be evaluated to determine the level of the conus medullaris (▶ Fig. 17.9). A conus level below the L2–L3 interspace in children > 5 years old is abnormal and an indication of possible tethering.[10,11] In addition, the tethered cord is often displaced posteriorly in the spinal canal. Other findings include lipoma or scar tissue within the epidural space and increased thickness of the filum terminale.[11]

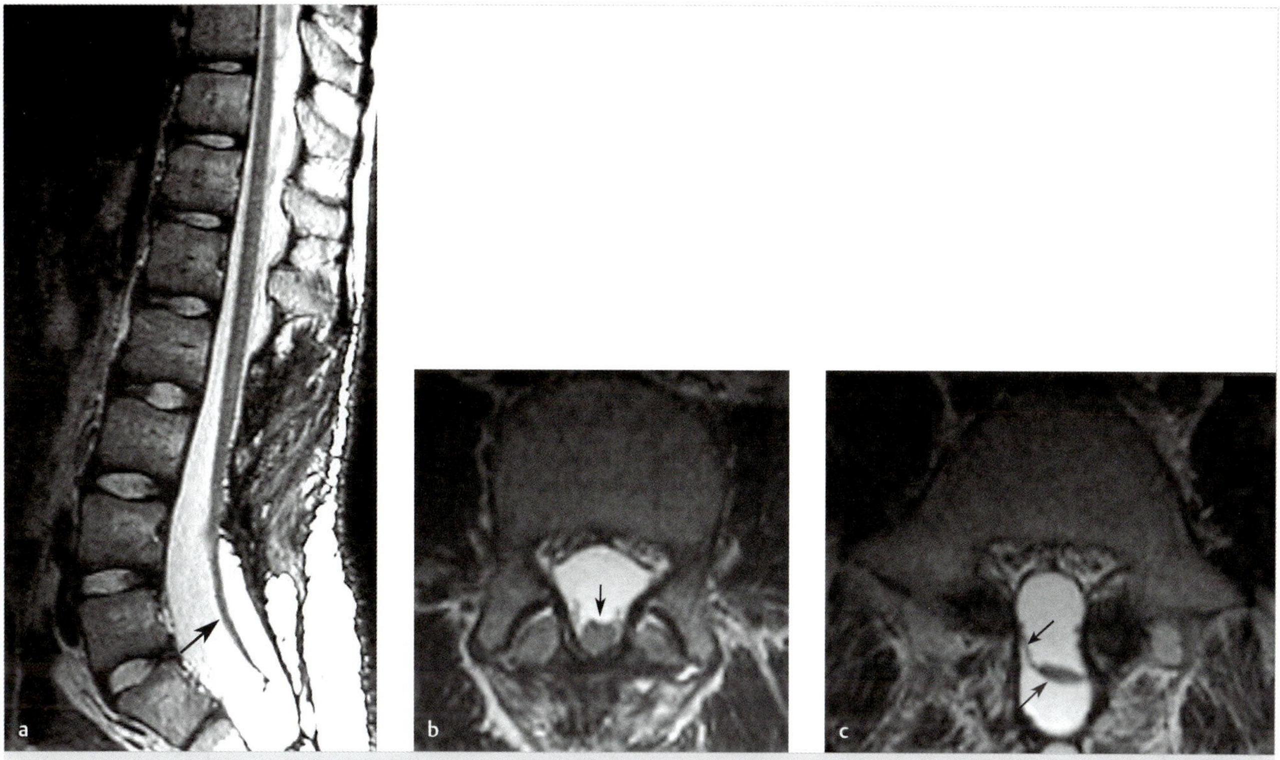

Fig. 17.9 This 14-year-old boy had a history of lipomeningocele. After surgical resection, he developed bowel and bladder dysfunction and new lower extremity paresthesias. **(a)** A sagittal T2-weighted image shows the cord to extend to approximately the L4 level and the filum terminale to extend to the S1 level (*arrow*), compatible with a tethered cord syndrome. **(b)** An axial T2-weighted image at the L4 level shows the cord to be located posteriorly within the thecal sac (*arrow*). **(c)** An axial T2-weighted image at the L5 level shows the placode (*arrow with a small head*) with a right-side nerve root coursing anteriorly and laterally (*arrow with a large head*). (Reproduced with permission from, Khanna AJ, Wasserman BA, Sponseller PD. The Pediatric Spine. In: Khanna AJ, ed. MRI for orthopaedic surgeons. New York: Thieme; 2010:338–349.)

It is important to note that although MRI can determine if a spinal cord is anatomically tethered, these findings should be correlated with the patient's symptoms and serial physical examinations before surgical release is considered.

17.6 Controversies with MRI of the Pediatric Spine

As with any diagnostic test, there remain several areas for which the use of MRI of the pediatric spine is controversial, including the specific indications for the following:

- Imaging of scoliosis.
- Imaging of tethered cord syndrome.
- Imaging in the presence of spinal instrumentation.

17.6.1 Scoliosis

Idiopathic scoliosis most often presents with a right-side lower thoracic curve. The purpose of MRI in the imaging of scoliosis is to detect intraspinal pathology, which is most frequently associated with left lower thoracic curves, an abnormal neurologic examination, and a young age at presentation.[35,36,37,38,39,40] Do et al[36] concluded that MRI is not indicated before spinal arthrodesis in a patient with an adolescent idiopathic scoliosis curve pattern and normal physical and neurologic examinations.

One particular area of controversy is the pediatric patient with back pain in the presence of scoliosis. In the authors' experience, young patients with typical idiopathic scoliosis often complain of intermittent and vague back pain at some point during their clinical course. In a retrospective study of 2,442 patients, Ramirez et al[2] found that a left thoracic curve or an abnormal neurologic examination was most predictive of an underlying pathologic condition. They found a significant association between back pain and an age of > 15 years, skeletal maturity, postmenarchal status, and a history of injury. Their conclusion was that it is unnecessary to perform extensive diagnostic studies on every patient with scoliosis and back pain. Based on clinical experience and a review of the literature, the current authors recommend obtaining an MRI in patients with scoliosis with a left lower thoracic curve, abnormal neurologic findings, infantile scoliosis, or juvenile scoliosis. Because coronal images are especially useful in evaluating patients with scoliosis, they should be a part of the routine imaging protocol.

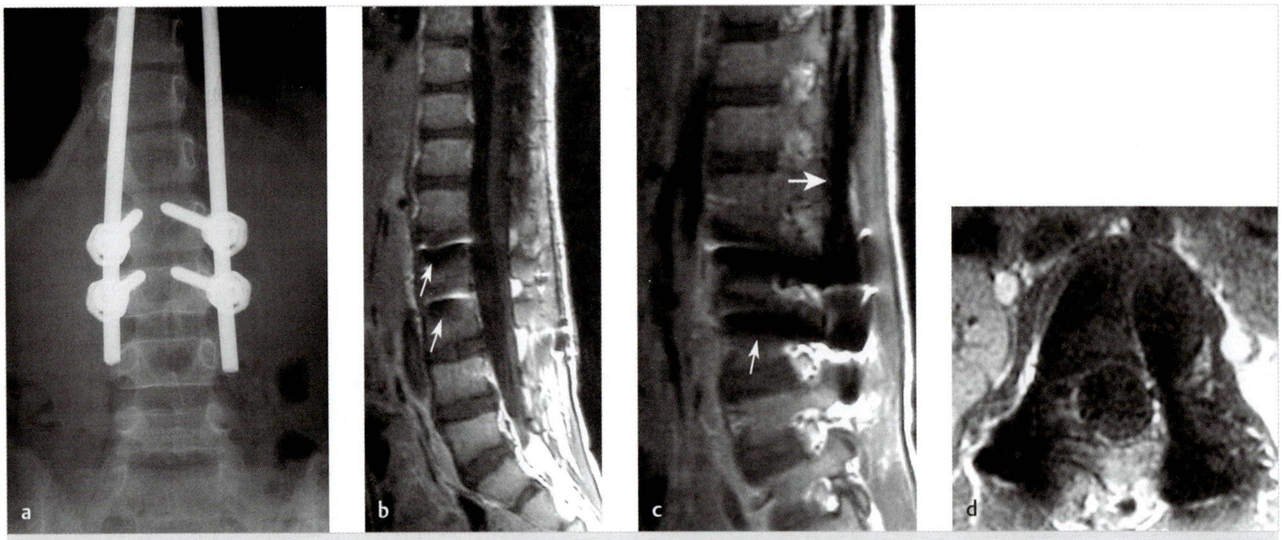

Fig. 17.10 A 6-year-old boy with a history of high-grade astrocytoma underwent resection, multilevel laminectomy, and posterior spinal arthrodesis from T4–L3 with titanium pedicle screws, hooks, and rods. **(a)** An anteroposterior (AP) radiograph 6 weeks after surgery. **(b)** A midline sagittal postgadolinium T1-weighted image enables visualization of the canal contents with only minimal artifact from the pedicle screws (*arrows*). **(c)** A parasagittal postgadolinium T1-weighted image shows a rod (*arrow with a large head*) and a pedicle screw (*arrow with a small head*), neither of which substantially degrades the image. **(d)** An axial postgadolinium T1-weighted image also shows the pedicle screws and a patent spinal canal. (Reproduced with permission from, Khanna AJ, Wasserman BA, Sponseller PD. The Pediatric Spine. In: Khanna AJ, ed. MRI for orthopaedic surgeons. New York: Thieme; 2010:338–349.)

17.6.2 Evaluation of the Tethered Cord Syndrome

As mentioned previously, the imaging of the tethered cord syndrome remains controversial. A dilemma arises when the MRI findings of tethered cord syndrome are noted and a decision with regard to nonoperative versus operative treatment has to be made. It is important to remember that although anatomic tethering of the cord can be easily identified by MRI, the determining factor for surgical intervention is the clinical history and examination, preferably obtained on a serial basis.

17.6.3 Imaging in the Presence of Implants

MRI of the spine in the presence of instrumentation is generally safe but limited because image artifacts produced by implants vary in degree based on the type of metal used and the pulse sequence used. Titanium produces less image degradation from artifact because it is less ferromagnetic than stainless steel.[41,42] However, with appropriate imaging techniques, clinically useful information can be safely obtained in the presence of both types of implants.[43] Specialized pulse sequences can help reduce the degree of tissue-obscuring artifact produced by spinal hardware and improve image quality compared with conventional T1-weighted SE pulse sequences.[44] For example, the metal-artifact-reduction pulse sequence has been shown to substantially reduce the amount of tissue-obscuring artifact produced by spinal hardware.[44] The current authors use MRI to evaluate pediatric spines with stainless steel or titanium implants (▶ Fig. 17.10), but the fact that the latter produces substantially less artifact affects the implant choice for a patient who may require follow-up MRI evaluation.

17.7 Common Clinical Questions

1. Pediatric patients with which of the following diagnoses may benefit from the expertise of an anesthesiologist when undergoing MRI examination of the spine?
   a) Cardiopulmonary disease.
   b) Skeletal dysplasias.
   c) Neuromuscular disease.
   d) Abnormal airway anatomy.
   e) All of the above.

2. At what age does the spine begin to show its normal curvature (i.e., lumbar lordosis)?
   a) At birth.
   b) 3 months.
   c) 2 years.
   d) 10 years.
   e) 16 years.

3. What is the typical location of the conus medullaris on a sagittal T2-weighted image of the lumbar spine in a patient who is ≥ 5 years old?
   a) T11.
   b) L1–L2.
   c) L3.
   d) L3–L4.
   e) The lumbosacral junction (L5–S1).

4. What is the most common type of spinal dysraphism?
   a) Diastematomyelia.
   b) Lipomeningocele.
   c) Myelocele.
   d) Caudal regression syndrome.
   e) Myelomeningocele.

5. Which of the following is NOT an indication for MR imaging of the spine in a pediatric patient with scoliosis?
   a) Low back pain.
   b) Left lower thoracic curve.
   c) Abnormal neurologic findings.
   d) Infantile scoliosis.
   e) Juvenile scoliosis.

References

[1] du Lac P, Panuel M, Devred P, Bollini G, Padovani J. MRI of disc space infection in infants and children. Report of 12 cases. Pediatr Radiol. 1990; 20(3):175–178

[2] Ramirez N, Johnston CE, II, Browne RH. The prevalence of back pain in children who have idiopathic scoliosis. J Bone Joint Surg Am. 1997; 79(3): 364–368

[3] American Academy of Pediatrics Committee on Drugs. American Academy of Pediatrics Committee on Drugs: Guidelines for monitoring and management of pediatric patients during and after sedation for diagnostic and therapeutic procedures. Pediatrics. 1992; 89(6 Pt 1):1110–1115

[4] Vade A, Sukhani R, Dolenga M, Habisohn-Schuck C. Chloral hydrate sedation of children undergoing CT and MR imaging: safety as judged by American Academy of Pediatrics guidelines. AJR Am J Roentgenol. 1995; 165(4):905–909

[5] Malviya S, Voepel-Lewis T, Prochaska G, Tait AR. Prolonged recovery and delayed side effects of sedation for diagnostic imaging studies in children. Pediatrics. 2000; 105(3):E42

[6] Khanna AJ, Wasserman BA, Sponseller PD. Magnetic resonance imaging of the pediatric spine. J Am Acad Orthop Surg. 2003; 11(4):248–259

[7] Goske MJ, Modic MT, Yu S. Pediatric spine: normal anatomy and spinal dysraphism. In: Modic MT, Masaryk TJ, Ross JS, eds. Magnetic resonance imaging of the spine. St. Louis, MO: Mosby-Year Book; 1994:352–387

[8] Rossi A, Martinetti C, Morana G, Severino M, Tortora D. Diagnostic approach to pediatric spine disorders. Magn Reson Imaging Clin N Am. 2016; 24(3): 621–644

[9] Sze G, Baierl P, Bravo S. Evolution of the infant spinal column: evaluation with MR imaging. Radiology. 1991; 181(3):819–827

[10] Barson AJ. The vertebral level of termination of the spinal cord during normal and abnormal development. J Anat. 1970; 106(Pt 3):489–497

[11] Moufarrij NA, Palmer JM, Hahn JF, Weinstein MA. Correlation between magnetic resonance imaging and surgical findings in the tethered spinal cord. Neurosurgery. 1989; 25(3):341–346

[12] Saifuddin A, Burnett SJD, White J. The variation of position of the conus medullaris in an adult population. A magnetic resonance imaging study. Spine. 1998; 23(13):1452–1456

[13] Auletta JJ, John CC. Spinal epidural abscesses in children: a 15-year experience and review of the literature. Clin Infect Dis. 2001; 32(1):9–16

[14] Modic MT, Feiglin DH, Piraino DW, et al. Vertebral osteomyelitis: assessment using MR. Radiology. 1985; 157(1):157–166

[15] Rossi A. Pediatric spinal infection and inflammation. Neuroimaging Clin N Am. 2015; 25(2):173–191

[16] Fernandez M, Carrol CL, Baker CJ. Discitis and vertebral osteomyelitis in children: an 18-year review. Pediatrics. 2000; 105(6):1299–1304

[17] Miller GM, Forbes GS, Onofrio BM. Magnetic resonance imaging of the spine. Mayo Clin Proc. 1989; 64(8):986–1004

[18] Huisman TA, Wagner MW, Bosemani T, Tekes A, Poretti A. Pediatric spinal trauma. J Neuroimaging. 2015; 25(3):337–353

[19] Banerian KG, Wang AM, Samberg LC, Kerr HH, Wesolowski DP. Association of vertebral end plate fracture with pediatric lumbar intervertebral disk herniation: value of CT and MR imaging. Radiology. 1990; 177(3):763–765

[20] Kriss VM, Kriss TC. SCIWORA (spinal cord injury without radiographic abnormality) in infants and children. Clin Pediatr (Phila). 1996; 35(3):119–124

[21] Pang D, Pollack IF. Spinal cord injury without radiographic abnormality in children: the SCIWORA syndrome. J Trauma. 1989; 29(5):654–664

[22] Boese CK, Oppermann J, Siewe J, Eysel P, Scheyerer MJ, Lechler P. Spinal cord injury without radiologic abnormality in children: a systematic review and meta-analysis. J Trauma Acute Care Surg. 2015; 78(4):874–882

[23] Farrell CA, Hannon M, Lee LK. Pediatric spinal cord injury without radiographic abnormality in the era of advanced imaging. Curr Opin Pediatr. 2017; 29(3):286–290

[24] Henry M, Scarlata K, Riesenburger RI, et al. Utility of STIR MRI in pediatric cervical spine clearance after trauma. J Neurosurg Pediatr. 2013; 12(1):30–36

[25] Altman NR, Altman DH. MR imaging of spinal dysraphism. AJNR Am J Neuroradiol. 1987; 8(3):533–538

[26] Byrd SE, Darling CF, McLone DG, Tomita T. MR imaging of the pediatric spine. Magn Reson Imaging Clin N Am. 1996; 4(4):797–833

[27] Huisman TAGM, Rossi A, Tortori-Donati P. MR imaging of neonatal spinal dysraphia: what to consider? Magn Reson Imaging Clin N Am. 2012; 20(1): 45–61

[28] O'Neill BR, Gallegos D, Herron A, et al. Use of magnetic resonance imaging to detect occult spinal dysraphism in infants. J Neurosurg Pediatr. 2017; 19(2): 217–226

[29] Modic MT, Yu S. Normal anatomy. In: Modic MT, Masaryk TJ, Ross JS, eds. Magnetic resonance imaging of the spine. St. Louis, MO: Mosby-Year Book; 1994:37–79

[30] Poretti A, Ashmawy R, Garzon-Muvdi T, Jallo GI, Huisman TA, Raybaud C. Chiari type 1 deformity in children: pathogenetic, clinical, neuroimaging, and management aspects. Neuropediatrics. 2016; 47(5):293–307

[31] Mikulis DJ, Diaz O, Egglin TK, Sanchez R. Variance of the position of the cerebellar tonsils with age: preliminary report. Radiology. 1992; 183(3):725–728

[32] Strahle J, Muraszko KM, Kapurch J, Bapuraj JR, Garton HJL, Maher CO. Chiari malformation Type I and syrinx in children undergoing magnetic resonance imaging. J Neurosurg Pediatr. 2011; 8(2):205–213

[33] Hall WA, Albright AL, Brunberg JA. Diagnosis of tethered cords by magnetic resonance imaging. Surg Neurol. 1988; 30(1):60–64

[34] Heinz ER, Rosenbaum AE, Scarff TB, Reigel DH, Drayer BP. Tethered spinal cord following meningomyelocele repair. Radiology. 1979; 131(1):153–160

[35] Diab M, Landman Z, Lubicky J, Dormans J, Erickson M, Richards BS, members of the Spinal Deformity Study Group. Use and outcome of MRI in the surgical treatment of adolescent idiopathic scoliosis. Spine. 2011; 36 (8):667–671

[36] Do T, Fras C, Burke S, Widmann RF, Rawlins B, Boachie-Adjei O. Clinical value of routine preoperative magnetic resonance imaging in adolescent idiopathic scoliosis. A prospective study of three hundred and twenty-seven patients. J Bone Joint Surg Am. 2001; 83(4):577–579

[37] Evans SC, Edgar MA, Hall-Craggs MA, Powell MP, Taylor BA, Noordeen HH. MRI of "idiopathic" juvenile scoliosis. A prospective study. J Bone Joint Surg Br. 1996; 78(2):314–317

[38] Gupta P, Lenke LG, Bridwell KH. Incidence of neural axis abnormalities in infantile and juvenile patients with spinal deformity. Is a magnetic resonance image screening necessary? Spine. 1998; 23(2):206–210

[39] Mejia EA, Hennrikus WL, Schwend RM, Emans JB. A prospective evaluation of idiopathic left thoracic scoliosis with magnetic resonance imaging. J Pediatr Orthop. 1996; 16(3):354–358

[40] Schwend RM, Hennrikus W, Hall JE, Emans JB. Childhood scoliosis: clinical indications for magnetic resonance imaging. J Bone Joint Surg Am. 1995; 77 (1):46–53

[41] Rudisch A, Kremser C, Peer S, Kathrein A, Judmaier W, Daniaux H. Metallic artifacts in magnetic resonance imaging of patients with spinal fusion. A comparison of implant materials and imaging sequences. Spine. 1998; 23(6): 692–699

[42] Rupp R, Ebraheim NA, Savolaine ER, Jackson WT. Magnetic resonance imaging evaluation of the spine with metal implants. General safety and superior imaging with titanium. Spine. 1993; 18(3):379–385

[43] Lyons CJ, Betz RR, Mesgarzadeh M, Revesz G, Bonakdarpour A, Clancy M. The effect of magnetic resonance imaging on metal spine implants. Spine. 1989; 14(7):670–672

[44] Chang SD, Lee MJ, Munk PL, Janzen DL, MacKay A, Xiang QS. MRI of spinal hardware: comparison of conventional T1-weighted sequence with a new metal artifact reduction sequence. Skeletal Radiol. 2001; 30(4):213–218

Answers to Common Clinical Questions

1. Answer: e. Although several studies have reported the successful administration of sedation by trained nurses, pediatric patients with each of the diagnoses listed here may benefit from the expertise of an anesthesiologist when undergoing an MRI examination of the spine.
2. Answer: c. The spine has usually begun to show its normal curvature (i.e., lumbar lordosis) by 2 years of age, most likely because of the effects of weightbearing.
3. Answer: b. A conus level below the L2–L3 interspace in children > 5 years old is abnormal and indicates possible tethering. A review of the MRI findings of 504 normal adult spines found that the average conus position was the lower third of LI (range, middle third of T12 to the upper third of L3).[12]
4. Answer: e. Myelomeningocele is the most common form of spinal dysraphism. It most often presents as a non-skin-covered back mass in the lumbosacral region, although it can also be seen at higher levels. This mass may or may not be covered by leptomeninges containing a variable amount of neural tissue. The sac herniates through a defect in the posterior elements of the spine.
5. Answer: a. One particular area of controversy for obtaining MRI is the pediatric patient with back pain in the presence of scoliosis. In the current authors' experience, young patients with typical idiopathic scoliosis often complain of intermittent and vague back pain at some point during their clinical course, and at least one large study has found that MRI is not indicated before spinal arthrodesis in a patient with an adolescent idiopathic scoliosis curve pattern and a normal physical and neurologic examination.

18 MRI of the Peripheral Nervous System

Shivani Ahlawat and Laura M. Fayad

Abstract

MRI is an ideal modality for assessment of peripheral nerves because of its inherent contrast resolution and ability to visualize direct and indirect signs of nerve pathology. MRI of the peripheral nervous system is a reliable and noninvasive tool for evaluation of normal nerves, abnormal nerves, and the regional skeletal muscles and has been shown to have good surgical correlation. It can provide important guidance in the treatment of patients with peripheral nerve disorders. MR indications for the evaluation of peripheral nerves continue to evolve with the emergence of advanced techniques and new applications.

Keywords: lower extremity, magnetic resonance imaging, nerve abnormalities, nerve anatomy, peripheral nerve disorder, upper extremity

Peripheral neuropathy can be a major cause of pain and functional impairment. Although the diagnosis of peripheral neuropathy is primarily based on a combination of clinical examination and electrophysiological testing, magnetic resonance imaging (MRI) is being used increasingly, especially in challenging cases.[1] Operative management of peripheral nerve disorders is also increasing, with estimates approaching 100,000 peripheral nerve surgeries annually.[2] Most cases of peripheral neuropathy presenting to orthopaedic surgeons comprise entrapment neuropathies in the upper and lower extremities related to mechanical causes such as entrapment in a fibrous or fibro-osseous tunnel (e.g., carpal or cubital tunnel syndrome) or to a dynamic cause related to limb positioning (e.g., snapping triceps syndrome). Occasionally, space-occupying lesions intrinsic or extrinsic to the affected nerve such as an anomalous muscle or adjacent scar, neoplasm, or osteophyte can lead to nerve irritation or mass effect with deviation of the course of a peripheral nerve (▶ Fig. 18.1). In patients with a clinically confounding presentation, MRI can visualize directly the primary signs of peripheral nerve pathology such as abnormal signal intensity, caliber, course, continuity, and presence or absence of a neoplasm, in addition to secondary signs that include skeletal muscle denervation. Of note, high-resolution MRI of the peripheral nervous system can affect the diagnostic determinations and therapeutic recommendations made by peripheral nerve surgeons.[3] This chapter describes MRI techniques used in the evaluation of peripheral nerve disorders, followed by a discussion of the normal and abnormal appearance on MRI of peripheral nerves in the upper and lower extremities.

18.1 Technical Considerations

High-resolution MRI of the peripheral nerves is possible because of various recent technical innovations, including higher field strengths (e.g., 3 T rather than 1.5 T); 3D isotropic, volumetric sequences that enable multiplanar reformations in any plane; improved fat-suppression methods; and improved coil design. Typically, a smaller field of view enabling higher resolution is preferred; however, in some cases, inclusion of more proximal or, rarely, distal anatomic regions is necessary. For example, in a challenging case of suprascapular neuropathy, a larger field of view that includes the brachial plexus and the affected shoulder may be needed to evaluate the brachial plexus for a potential underlying plexopathy while simultaneously assessing the shoulder joint for a possible spinoglenoid or suprascapular notch paralabral cyst. A combination of 2D and 3D anatomic and fluid-sensitive sequences are used in various planes to optimize a protocol to answer the clinical question and evaluate the anatomic region of interest. Non–fat-suppressed, routine anatomic sequences such as T1-weighted imaging are produced with high resolution using higher field strength, thin slice selection with minimal or no interslice gap, and smaller field of view. Fluid-sensitive sequences, generated by nulling the fat signal, are used to assess abnormal or elevated peripheral nerve signal because of increased endoneurial fluid. The short tau inversion recovery (STIR) sequence generates excellent fat suppression. Chemical frequency selective fat suppression also can be used but may produce heterogeneous fat suppression, particularly in the periphery of the field of view.

In addition to the routine 2D sequences in at least two planes of imaging, high-resolution anatomic and fluid-sensitive 3D sequences can be performed. These 3D sequences are performed with isotropic voxel resolution and enable

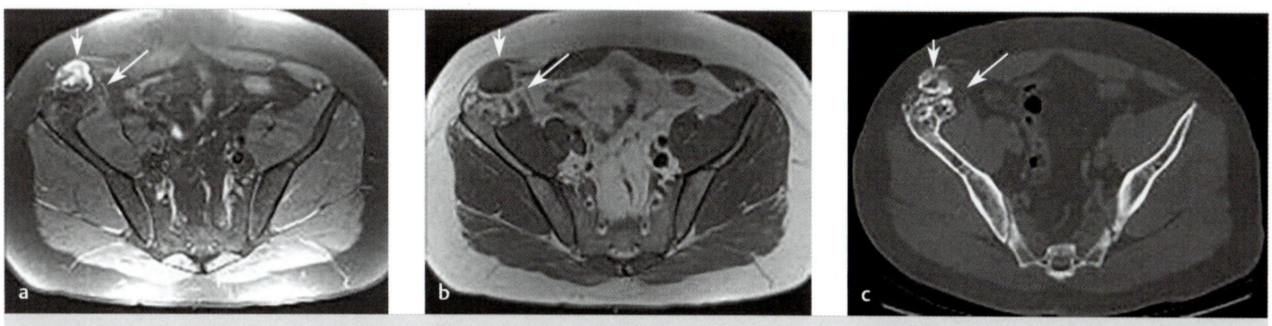

Fig. 18.1 **(a)** Axial T1-weighted and **(b)** fat-suppressed T2-weighted images show a large exophytic mass emanating from the right anterior superior iliac spine (*short arrows*), deviating the right lateral femoral cutaneous nerve (*long arrows*). The skeletal lesion is contiguous with the adjacent iliac bone cortex and medullary cavity, better seen on the **(c)** computed tomography (CT) image, which shows the features of an osteochondroma.

multiplanar reconstructions to visualize a peripheral nerve along its longitudinal course. Such 3D sequences can be performed with or without fat suppression; however, a high-quality 3D sequence requires a formidable time commitment by the patient, which may not be feasible, especially in patients with severe pain. Experimental sequences such as diffusion-weighted imaging and diffusion tensor imaging are emerging techniques being used for evaluation of peripheral nerve neoplasms, entrapment, and trauma.[4,5,6,7,8,9,10] These techniques can be challenging to implement and interpret because of air–tissue interfaces and the nonlinear course of the peripheral nerves and are, therefore, not routinely used. Diffusion-weighted imaging can be optimized to suppress vascular signal such that nerve-selective, 3D sequences are generated.[11,12] It is important to note that as the diffusion gradient is added to 3D MR sequences, the signal-to-noise ratio is reduced and the image quality can be degraded. Disadvantages of diffusion-weighted nerve-selective 3D MRI include susceptibility to local field heterogeneity, sensitivity to motion artifacts, and the potential failure of fat suppression.[11,12]

Contrast material is not administered routinely for the evaluation of peripheral nerves. A normal peripheral nerve should not enhance because of a preserved peripheral nerve–blood barrier. An abnormal nerve (e.g., secondary to trauma or the presence of a neoplasm) may enhance after contrast administration. Although there are few data regarding the added value of intravenous contrast material in the evaluation of peripheral nerve disorders, contrast may be useful for certain clinical indications, including neoplasms or previous peripheral nerve surgery.

18.2 Nerve Anatomy

Knowledge of the microscopic peripheral nerve architecture is necessary to understand the normal and abnormal MR appearance. A normal peripheral nerve consists of an axon, the basic functional unit of the nerve. Each axon is surrounded by the endoneurium, and multiple axons bundled together form a nerve fascicle. The perineurium surrounds each fascicle, and multiple fascicles are encased within an epineurium. ▶ Table 18.1 contrasts the MR appearance of normal and abnormal peripheral nerves (▶ Fig. 18.2, ▶ Fig. 18.3). The MR appearance of secondary findings of peripheral neuropathy, including various stages of skeletal muscle denervation, is also included (▶ Fig. 18.4).

18.3 Nerve Abnormalities

Peripheral nerves can be affected by many abnormalities that can be broadly categorized as focal and systemic conditions. Focal conditions include entrapment syndromes at fibrous or

Table 18.1 MR appearance of normal and abnormal peripheral nerves

MR sequences	Type	Normal nerve	Abnormal nerve	
			Primary findings	Secondary findings
Anatomic	T1	Smooth, round, or ovoid structure similar or smaller in caliber to adjacent vessels; isointense signal intensity to adjacent muscle; a rim of hyperintense fat signal	Deviated course; abnormal caliber; effacement of perineural fat; nerve discontinuity; presence of neurogenic neoplasm	Mass effect (e.g., because of adjacent osteophyte, mass lesion); skeletal muscle denervation (loss of muscle bulk and fatty replacement)
Fluid-sensitive	Fat-suppressed T2, STIR	Isointense to minimally hyperintense relative to skeletal muscle	Abnormal peripheral nerve signal; architectural distortion; presence of neurogenic neoplasm	Skeletal muscle denervation (edema-like signal)

Abbreviations: MR, magnetic resonance; STIR, short tau inversion recovery.

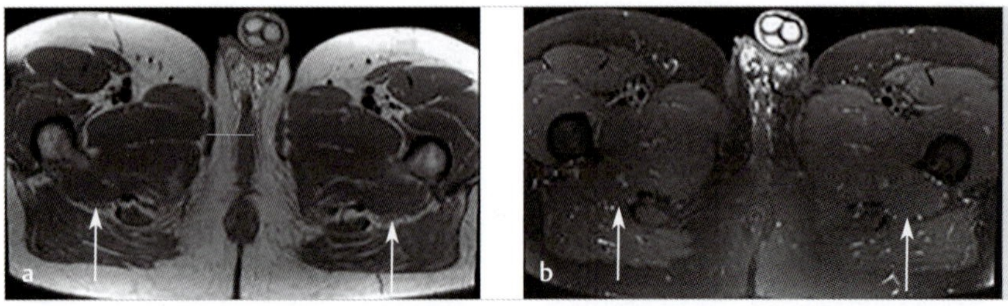

Fig. 18.2 Normal bilateral sciatic nerves (*arrows*) in the proximal thigh just distal to the ischial tuberosities on **(a)** axial T1-weighted and **(b)** fat-suppressed T2-weighted images. Note isointense signal intensity relative to the skeletal muscles on anatomic and fluid-sensitive sequences. There is no deviation of course, and the fat surrounding the sciatic nerves is preserved.

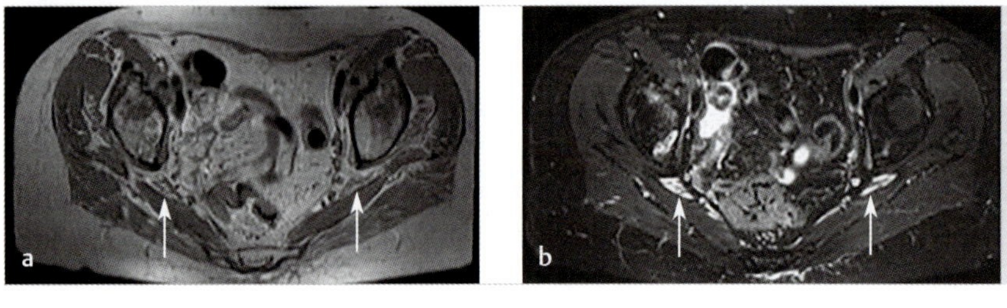

Fig. 18.3 Abnormal bilateral sciatic nerves (*arrows*) at the level of the sciatic foramen in a patient with previous radiation therapy on **(a)** axial intermediate-weighted and **(b)** fat-suppressed T2-weighted sequences. Note the enlarged caliber and elevated signal on fluid-sensitive sequences. The surrounding fat planes and usual nerve architecture or "fascicular pattern" are preserved.

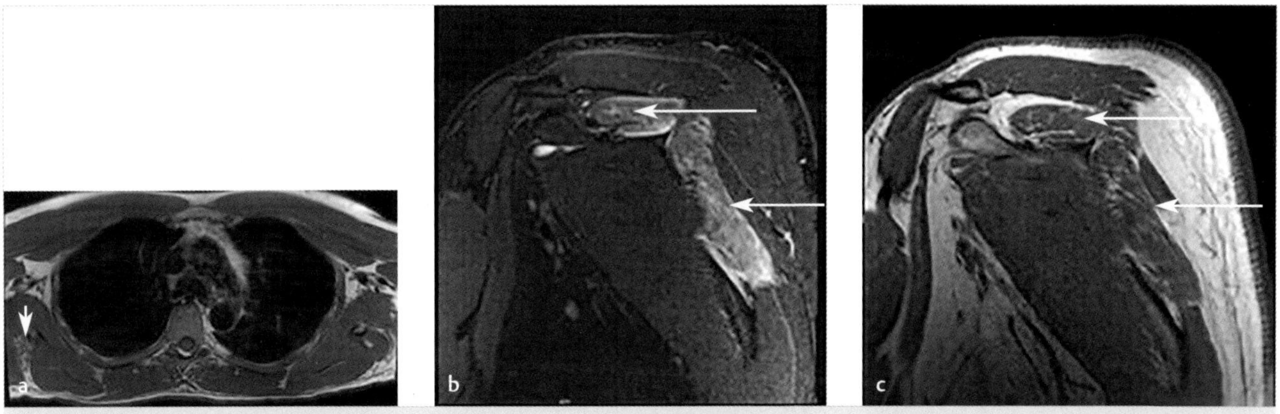

Fig. 18.4 Skeletal muscles provide important clues regarding chronic denervation. **(a)** Axial T1-weighted image through the upper chest shows asymmetric right teres minor atrophy (*arrow*), indicating chronic denervation in the axillary nerve distribution. A lesion at the level of the quadrilateral space should be sought in such a case. **(b)** Sagittal fluid-sensitive and **(c)** anatomic sequences show edema-like signal, disproportionate fatty replacement, and loss of muscle bulk (*arrows*) indicating acute-on-chronic (or ongoing) denervation in the supraspinatus and infraspinatus muscles. Involvement of both muscles suggests abnormality in the suprascapular nerve proximal to the suprascapular notch.

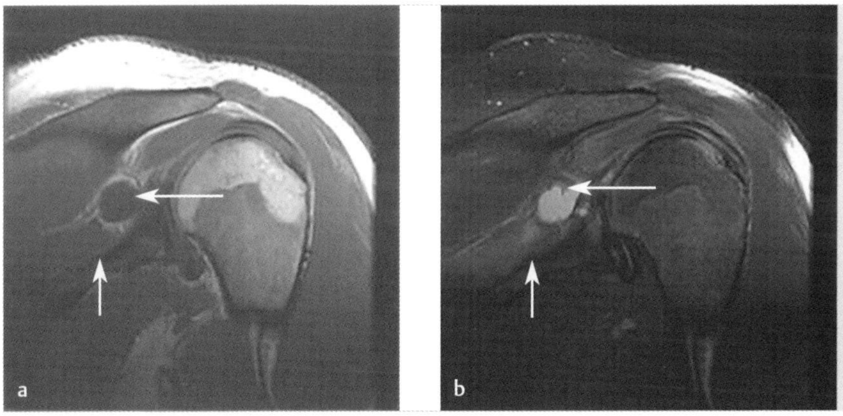

Fig. 18.5 **(a)** Coronal oblique anatomic and **(b)** fluid-sensitive sequences through the posterior left shoulder show a paralabral cyst in the spinoglenoid notch (*long arrows*) with isolated acute denervation myopathy in the infraspinatus muscle (*short arrows*). Note the absence of substantial loss of muscle bulk and fatty replacement, both features suggesting chronicity.

fibro-osseous tunnels, nerve injury related to penetrating or blunt trauma, neoplasms, and traction-related neuropathy caused by repetitive trauma (▶ Fig. 18.5). Systemic or multifocal diseases include hereditary disorders such as Charcot-Marie-Tooth disease, infections or inflammatory conditions like Parsonage-Turner syndrome or chronic demyelinating polyneuropathy, and neurocutaneous syndromes, including neurofibromatosis type 1, type 2, and schwannomatosis. Other systemic or diffuse neuropathic processes such as vasculitis and metabolic conditions (diabetes mellitus or vitamin deficiency) can also lead to multifocal neuropathy. A thorough history and physical examination combined with electrodiagnostic studies such as electromyography and nerve conduction velocity studies is the method by which patients with peripheral neuropathy have been traditionally evaluated. MRI is an emerging modality to assess patients with peripheral neuropathy, particularly in atypical or challenging cases of localized disease and occasionally multifocal or diffuse disease, and is part of the standard of care at specialized peripheral nerve centers. An important and specific advantage of MRI is that skeletal muscle denervation can be detected before signs of denervation are detectable by electromyography.

The most common indications for MRI of the peripheral nervous system are nerve entrapment, injury, and evaluation of a mass. Peripheral nerve entrapment can be caused by increased pressure within a fibrous or fibro-osseous tunnel because of variant anatomy or a space-occupying lesion. The purpose of MRI in the assessment of potential entrapment neuropathy is to confirm the clinical suspicion and to identify factors contributing to entrapment. Most entrapment sites such as in carpal tunnel syndrome do not require imaging to confirm the diagnosis but MRI can be helpful in the assessment of atypical cases and can detect variant anatomy. For example, in carpal tunnel syndrome, a persistent median artery, bifid or trifid median nerve, anomalous muscle, flexor tenosynovitis, or a mass such as a schwannoma may be identified by MRI (▶ Fig. 18.6). ▶ Table 18.2 and ▶ Table 18.3 list the larger peripheral nerves of the upper and lower extremities with their common entrapment sites and associated sensorimotor innervations. Discussion of each of the peripheral nerves is beyond the scope of this chapter; therefore, only the most common upper and lower extremity entrapment sites are reviewed.

The most common entrapment in the upper extremity is of the median nerve at the level of the carpal tunnel, then the ulnar nerve at the cubital tunnel. Qualitative anatomic fluid-sensitive sequences, in addition to more advanced imaging with quantitative T2-mapping, diffusion-weighted imaging, and

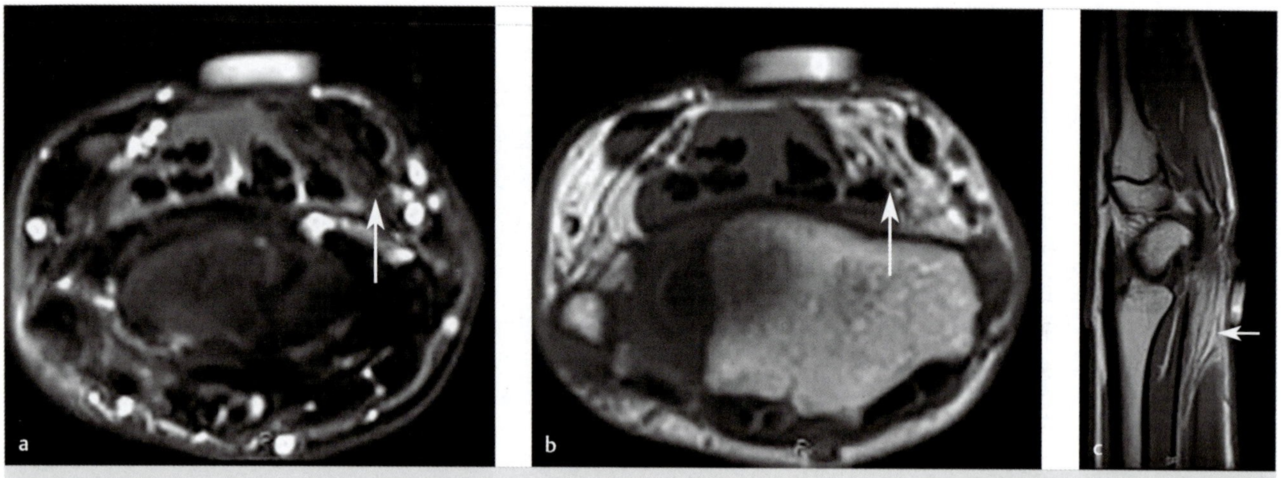

Fig. 18.6 (a) Axial fluid-sensitive and (b) anatomic images just proximal to the carpal tunnel show enlargement of the median nerve with presence of fat signal within the nerve (*arrows*). This finding is seen more clearly on the (c) sagittal non-fat-suppressed image, confirming the diagnosis of median nerve fibrolipomatous hamartoma.

Table 18.2 Common upper extremity entrapment syndromes: motor and sensory innervations of the upper extremity nerves and associated clinical presentation of neuropathy

Nerve	Innervation	Common entrapment site	Clinical presentation
Axillary	Sensory: skin over the lateral upper arm; motor: teres minor and deltoid	Quadrilateral space	Loss of arm abduction, weak flexion, extension, and rotation of the shoulder joint
Median	Sensory: lateral palm (not fingers) via the palmar cutaneous branch and radial 3.5 fingers via the common and proper digital branches; motor: forearm—anterior compartment of the forearm (except ulnar half of the flexor digitorum profundus and flexor digitorum quadratus; hand—recurrent branch to the thenar eminence (opponens pollicis, abductor pollicis brevis and superficial part of flexor pollicis brevis); first and second lumbricals of the hand	Pronator teres syndrome, anterior interosseous syndrome, carpal tunnel syndrome	Weakness in flexion of radial half of the fingers and thumb, loss of abduction and opposition of thumb; ape hand deformity with hyperextended index finger and thumb, and an adducted thumb; benediction sign—inability to flex thumb, index, and long finger when trying to make a fist; loss of sensation in lateral 3.5 fingers, including their nail beds and the thenar region
Posterior interosseous	Motor: extensor digitorum, extensor digiti minimi, extensor carpi ulnaris, abductor pollicis longus, extensor pollicis longus and brevis, extensor indicis	Arcade of Frohse	Isolated motor syndrome with finger drop and radial wrist deviation on extension
Radial	Sensory: arm and forearm skin (posteriorly and laterally), dorsal hand skin (including first web space); motor: muscular branches—triceps brachii (medial and lateral heads), anconeus, brachioradialis, extensor carpi radialis longus; deep branch—extensor carpi radialis brevis, supinator	Axilla: Saturday night palsy, mid-arm, proximal forearm, distal forearm: Wartenberg syndrome (entrapment deep to brachioradialis tendinous insertion)	Loss of forearm extension and supination; wrist drop because of lack of finger and hand extension
Suprascapular	Sensory: acromioclavicular and glenohumeral joints; motor: supraspinatus muscle and infraspinatus muscle (through the spinoglenoid notch)	Suprascapular notch, spinoglenoid notch	Decreased abduction and external rotation of the humerus and wasting of the supraspinatus and infraspinatus muscles
Ulnar	Sensory: small finger and the medial half of the ring finger, and the corresponding part of the palm; motor: flexor carpi ulnaris, flexor digitorum profundus, lumbrical muscles, opponens digiti minimi, flexor digiti minimi, abductor digiti minimi, interossei, adductor pollicis	Cubital tunnel, Guyon canal	Paresthesias at the ring and small finger and intrinsic hand weakness

diffusion tensor imaging have been reported in the evaluation of idiopathic carpal tunnel syndrome.[13,14,15,16] Primary MRI features associated with the clinical diagnosis of carpal tunnel syndrome are a smaller cross-sectional diameter of the nerve in the carpal tunnel compared with the diameter of the nerve proximal to the tunnel, bowing of the flexor retinaculum at the level of the hamate, and hyperintensity of the nerve proximal and distal to the site of compression.[17] Secondary signs of carpal

Table 18.3 Common lower extremity entrapment syndromes: motor and sensory innervations of the lower extremity nerves and associated clinical presentation of neuropathy

Nerve	Innervation	Common entrapment site	Clinical presentation
Common peroneal	All sensory and motor functions of superficial and deep peroneal nerves	Fibular head	Weak foot extension and foot eversion, leading to foot drop; paresthesia along the lateral lower leg and dorsal foot
Deep peroneal	Sensory: ankle joint (critical for ankle stability), the sinus tarsi, and the tarsal and metatarsophalangeal joints of the middle three digits; motor: anterior tibialis, extensor hallucis longus, extensor digitorum longus, and peroneus tertius muscles; the extensor digitorum brevis muscle	Fibular head	Weak foot extension
Femoral	Sensory: distal medial thigh, anteromedial knee joint, and medial leg and foot; motor: Iliacus and psoas in the pelvis; anterior division—pectineus and sartorius; posterior division—quadriceps	Inguinal ligament	Quadriceps muscle weakness; mild pain near the inguinal ligament; numbness in the medial leg and calf
Inferior calcaneal	Motor: abductor digiti minimi, lateral one-half of the quadratus plantae, flexor digitorum brevis, calcaneal periosteum, long plantar ligament, and adjacent vessels	First site: between the deep fascia of the abductor hallucis muscle and the medial plantar margin of the quadratus plantae; second site: more distally as the nerve passes along the anterior aspect of the medial calcaneal tuberosity	Chronic heel pain that may be mistaken clinically for plantar fasciitis
Intermetatarsal	Sensory: adjacent toes	Second and third intermetatarsal spaces	Pain on weightbearing; paresthesias affecting contiguous halves of two toes
Lateral femoral cutaneous	Sensory: anterolateral thigh; motor: none	Anterior superior iliac spine	Paresthesia or numbness to anterolateral thigh
Lateral plantar	Sensory: lateral sole of the midfoot and forefoot and the lateral one and one-half toes; motor: remaining muscles of the foot	Tarsal tunnel	Sensory abnormalities involving the lateral one-third of the plantar aspect of the foot
Medial plantar	Sensory: medial two-thirds of the plantar surface of the foot; motor: flexor digitorum brevis, abductor hallucis, flexor hallucis brevis, and first lumbrical	Tarsal tunnel	Sensory abnormalities involving the medial two-thirds of the foot
Posterior tibial	All sensory and motor functions of medial and lateral plantar nerves	Tarsal tunnel	Paresthesias along the plantar aspect of the foot and toes that worsen with activity and positive Tinel sign at the tarsal tunnel
Proper digital	Sensory: the skin on the medial side of the great toe; motor: flexor hallucis brevis	Plantar medial to hallux metatarsal head	Paresthesias along the medial and plantar aspects of the great toe metatarsal shaft and the great toe metatarsophalangeal joint
Proximal tibial	Motor: deep and superficial posterior compartment muscles, including the plantaris, popliteus, gastrocnemius, soleus, posterior tibial, flexor digitorum longus, and flexor hallucis longus	Soleal sling	Weakness of the plantar flexors and invertors of the foot; sensory loss in the heel and occasionally along the distribution of the sural nerve
Sciatic	Sensory: all sensation below the knee; motor: knee flexion by innervation of the posterior thigh muscles and all functions below the knee	Sciatic foramen	Weak foot extension and foot eversion leading to foot drop; paresthesia and anesthesia along the lateral lower leg and dorsal foot
Superficial peroneal	Sensory: distal two-thirds of the lateral leg and from the dorsum of the foot; motor: peroneus longus and brevis muscles	Fibular head	Weak foot eversion; numbness and tingling along the lateral aspect of the lower leg and the dorsum of the foot
Sural	Sensory: lateral aspect of the ankle and foot up to the base of the fifth toe	Not applicable	Pain and paresthesias along the lateral foot

tunnel syndrome are thenar muscle denervation edema and/or atrophy and fatty replacement. Similarly, cubital tunnel syndrome is a common entrapment neuropathy in the upper extremity (▶ Fig. 18.7). It can be seen in various clinical scenarios, including overhead throwing athletes (e.g., baseball pitchers), and is related to valgus stress and resultant ulnar nerve stretch injury. MRI enables the detection of primary signs of neuropathy, including an increased nerve size and signal intensity on fluid-sensitive sequences.[18] Of note, increased signal on fluid-sensitive sequences alone is not a reliable sign of peripheral neuropathy, particularly in the cubital tunnel because increased signal can be present in as many as 60% of healthy subjects.[19] Hence, additional signs of neuropathy must be sought, which include abnormal size, deviation of the course of the usual nerve, and muscle denervation (▶ Fig. 18.8).

The most common entrapment neuropathy in the lower extremity is the common peroneal nerve at the fibular head. Common peroneal nerve injury occurs most commonly at the level of the fibular neck and includes compression- and traction-type injuries. Causes of extrinsic compression or mass effect include prolonged knee crossing, tight casts, tibiofibular joint ganglions, neoplasms, aneurysms, traumatic episodes that result in proximal tibiofibular joint dislocation, and compartment syndrome. Causes of traction-related injury include repetitive ankle inversion and pronation (e.g., cycling, running), generalized multiligamentous laxity, and genu varum.[20] MRI

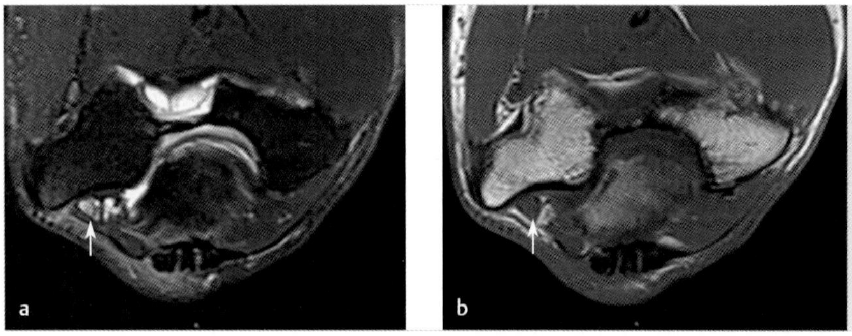

Fig. 18.7 **(a)** Axial fluid-sensitive and **(b)** anatomic images through the cubital tunnel show an enlarged ulnar nerve (*arrows*) with elevated fluid signal in a patient with ulnar neuropathy. Note the normal position of the ulnar nerve posterior to the medial humeral epicondyle.

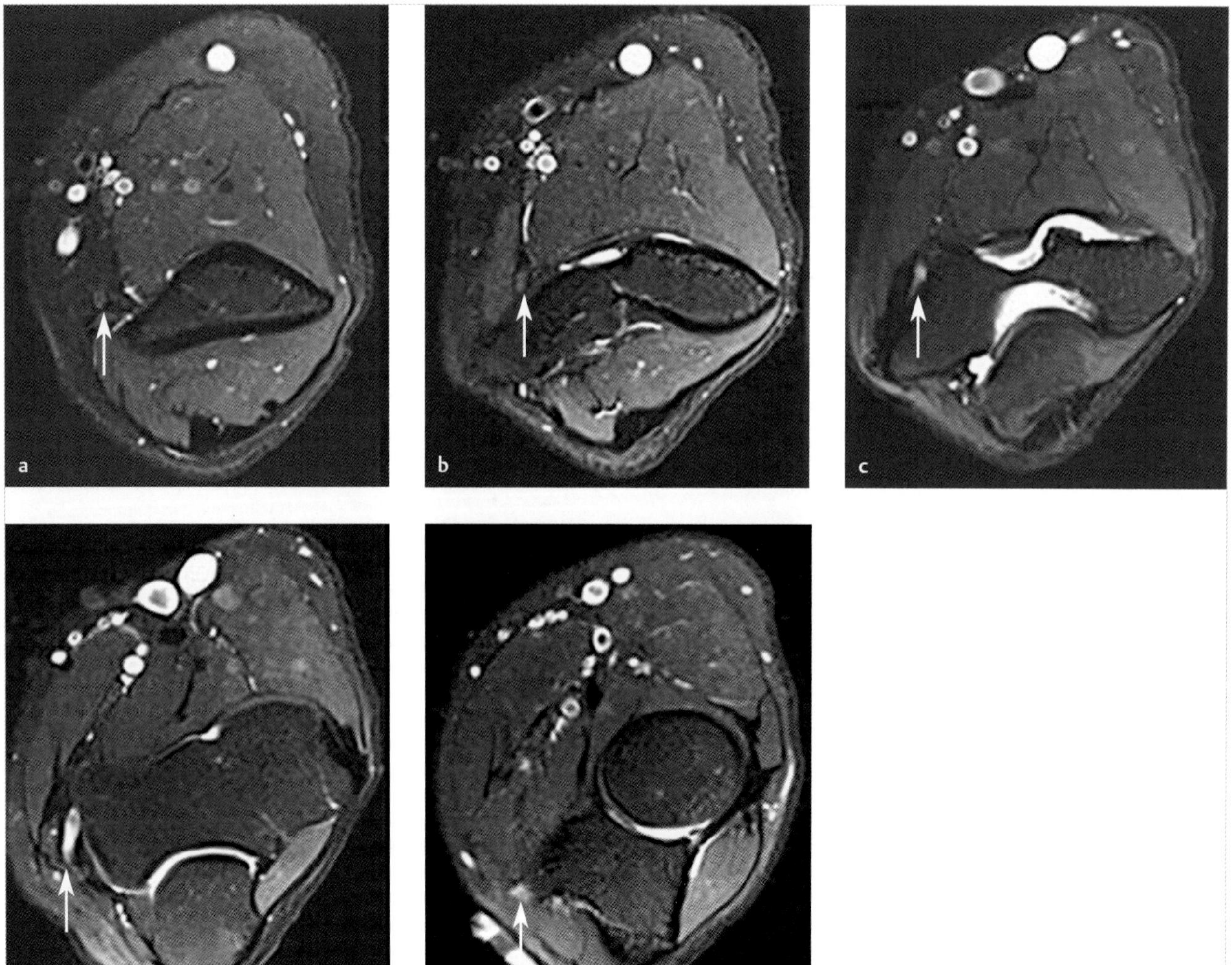

Fig. 18.8 **(a–e)** Sequential axial fluid-sensitive sequences extending proximal, through, and distal to the cubital tunnel show an abnormal position of the ulnar nerve anterior to the medial epicondyle because of previous submuscular transposition (*arrows*). The nerve is located deep to the flexor Pronator mass and is increased in signal intensity and enlarged in caliber with distorted internal architecture because of postsurgical entrapment.

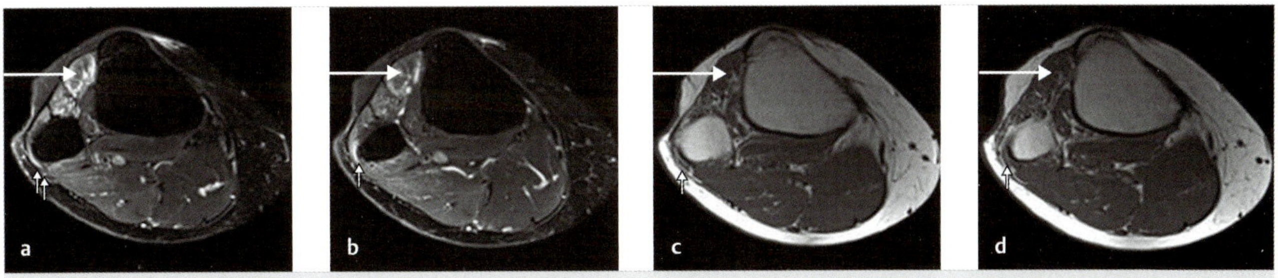

Fig. 18.9 **(a,b)** Sequential axial fluid-sensitive and **(c,d)** anatomic images through the fibular head show an abnormal common peroneal nerve (*short arrows*) with increased signal on fluid-sensitive sequences. The common peroneal nerve is thickened without discontinuity. There is also denervation myopathy in the anterolateral calf musculature (*long arrows*).

can show elevated common peroneal nerve signal intensity at the fibular fibro-osseous tunnel, as well as potential intrinsic or extrinsic lesions (▶ Fig. 18.9).

18.4 Accuracy and Effect of MRI of the Peripheral Nerves

Peripheral nerve surgery is becoming more common; therefore, the need for preoperative evaluation of peripheral nerves is greater. High-resolution MRI is performed more frequently and for an increasing number of indications. Unlike electrodiagnostic testing, MRI is noninvasive and may be more suitable for young patients and people with bleeding diatheses. In a recent systematic review on the accuracy of MRI in distinguishing normal from abnormal peripheral nerves, the pooled sensitivity and specificity of elevated signal on fluid-sensitive sequences were 77% (95% CI, 73–81%) and 67% (63–71%), respectively. The pooled sensitivity and specificity of nerve caliber enlargement were 63% (95% CI, 57–88%) and 84% (80–88%), respectively.[21] The pooled sensitivity and specificity for nerve flattening were 31% (95% CI, 24–37%) and 94% (87–94%),[21] respectively, making nerve flattening one of the most specific signs. It is important to note that most studies of MRI and peripheral neuropathy use convenience samples with retrospective analyses, and some include only patients suspected of peripheral nerve disease, rather than conducting robust prospective analyses. Hence, MRI remains an emerging modality in this area rather than an established technique. A recent publication of a prospective cohort study of patients with peripheral neuropathy showed the role of MRI on diagnostic and therapeutic decisions made by peripheral nerve surgeons.[3] The study emphasized that MRI can localize the affected peripheral nerve segments, improve diagnostic confidence, and narrow the differential diagnosis.[3] In addition, for patients with peripheral neuropathy, MRI can have a therapeutic effect, changing the indication, acuity, approach, and anticipated operative time for a surgical procedure.[3]

18.5 Common Clinical Questions

1. Which of the following technical parameters is used to generate high-resolution MRI for evaluation of peripheral nerves?
   a) Lower field strength.
   b) Thick slice selection.
   c) Larger field of view.
   d) No interslice gap.

2. The endoneurium encases each:
   a) Axon.
   b) Fascicle.
   c) Epineurium.
   d) Perineurium.

3. All of the following are focal peripheral nerve disorders, except:
   a) Entrapment syndromes at fibrous or fibro-osseous tunnels.
   b) Nerve injury related to penetrating or blunt trauma.
   c) Traction-related neuropathy caused by repetitive trauma.
   d) Charcot-Marie-Tooth disease.

4. The most common entrapment in the upper extremity is of the:
   a) Ulnar nerve at the cubital tunnel.
   b) Median nerve at the level of the carpal tunnel.
   c) Axillary nerve in the quadrilateral space.
   d) Suprascapular nerve in the spinoglenoid notch.

5. The most specific primary MRI feature of peripheral neuropathy is:
   a) Elevated signal on fluid-sensitive sequences.
   b) Nerve caliber enlargement.
   c) Nerve flattening.
   d) Skeletal muscle denervation.

References

[1] Filler AG, Maravilla KR, Tsuruda JS. MR neurography and muscle MR imaging for image diagnosis of disorders affecting the peripheral nerves and musculature. Neurol Clin. 2004; 22(3):643–682, vi–vii

[2] Siemionow M, Brzezicki G. Chapter 8: Current techniques and concepts in peripheral nerve repair. Int Rev Neurobiol. 2009; 87:141–172

[3] Chhabra A, Belzberg AJ, Rosson GD, et al. Impact of high resolution 3 tesla MR neurography (MRN) on diagnostic thinking and therapeutic patient management. Eur Radiol. 2016; 26(5):1235–1244

[4] Andreou A, Sohaib A, Collins DJ, et al. Diffusion-weighted MR neurography for the assessment of brachial plexopathy in oncological practice. Cancer Imaging. 2015; 15:6

[5] Boyer RB, Kelm ND, Riley DC, et al. 4.7-T diffusion tensor imaging of acute traumatic peripheral nerve injury. Neurosurg Focus. 2015; 39(3):E9

[6] Breckwoldt MO, Stock C, Xia A, et al. Diffusion tensor imaging adds diagnostic accuracy in magnetic resonance neurography. Invest Radiol. 2015; 50(8): 498–504

[7] Breitenseher JB, Kranz G, Hold A, et al. MR neurography of ulnar nerve entrapment at the cubital tunnel: a diffusion tensor imaging study. Eur Radiol. 2015; 25(7):1911–1918

[8] Markvardsen LH, Vaeggemose M, Ringgaard S, Andersen H. Diffusion tensor imaging can be used to detect lesions in peripheral nerves in patients with chronic inflammatory demyelinating polyneuropathy treated with subcutaneous immunoglobulin. Neuroradiology. 2016; 58(8):745–752

[9] Mürtz P, Kaschner M, Lakghomi A, et al. Diffusion-weighted MR neurography of the brachial and lumbosacral plexus: 3.0T versus 1.5T imaging. Eur J Radiol. 2015; 84(4):696–702

[10] Simon NG, Lagopoulos J, Gallagher T, Kliot M, Kiernan MC. Peripheral nerve diffusion tensor imaging is reliable and reproducible. J Magn Reson Imaging. 2016; 43(4):962–969

[11] Chhabra A, Soldatos T, Subhawong TK, et al. The application of three-dimensional diffusion-weighted PSIF technique in peripheral nerve imaging of the distal extremities. J Magn Reson Imaging. 2011; 34(4):962–967

[12] Chhabra A, Subhawong TK, Bizzell C, Flammang A, Soldatos T. 3T MR neurography using three-dimensional diffusion-weighted PSIF: technical issues and advantages. Skeletal Radiol. 2011; 40(10):1355–1360

[13] Barcelo C, Faruch M, Lapègue F, Bayol MA, Sans N. 3-T MRI with diffusion tensor imaging and tractography of the median nerve. Eur Radiol. 2013; 23 (11):3124–3130

[14] Cha JG, Han JK, Im SB, Kang SJ. Median nerve T2 assessment in the wrist joints: preliminary study in patients with carpal tunnel syndrome and healthy volunteers. J Magn Reson Imaging. 2014; 40(4):789–795

[15] Lindberg PG, Feydy A, Le Viet D, Maier MA, Drapé JL. Diffusion tensor imaging of the median nerve in recurrent carpal tunnel syndrome - initial experience. Eur Radiol. 2013; 23(11):3115–3123

[16] Naraghi A, da Gama Lobo L, Menezes R, et al. Diffusion tensor imaging of the median nerve before and after carpal tunnel release in patients with carpal tunnel syndrome: feasibility study. Skeletal Radiol. 2013; 42(10):1403–1412

[17] Monagle K, Dai G, Chu A, Burnham RS, Snyder RE. Quantitative MR imaging of carpal tunnel syndrome. AJR Am J Roentgenol. 1999; 172(6):1581–1586

[18] Bäumer P, Dombert T, Staub F, et al. Ulnar neuropathy at the elbow: MR neurography: nerve T2 signal increase and caliber. Radiology. 2011; 260(1): 199–206

[19] Husarik DB, Saupe N, Pfirrmann CW, Jost B, Hodler J, Zanetti M. Elbow nerves: MR findings in 60 asymptomatic subjects-normal anatomy, variants, and pitfalls. Radiology. 2009; 252(1):148–156

[20] Peck E, Finnoff JT, Smith J. Neuropathies in runners. Clin Sports Med. 2010; 29(3):437–457

[21] Kwee RM, Chhabra A, Wang KC, Marker DR, Carrino JA. Accuracy of MRI in diagnosing peripheral nerve disease: a systematic review of the literature. AJR Am J Roentgenol. 2014; 203(6):1303–1309

Answers to Common Clinical Questions

1. Answer: d. No interslice gap. High-resolution MRI can be performed using higher field strength, thin-slice selection with minimal or no interslice gap, and smaller field of view.
2. Answer: a. Axon. A normal peripheral nerve consists of an axon, the basic functional unit of the nerve. Each axon is surrounded by the endoneurium, and multiple axons bundled together form a nerve fascicle.
3. Answer: d. Charcot-Marie-Tooth disease. Peripheral nerves can be affected by many abnormalities that can be broadly categorized as focal and systemic conditions. Focal conditions include entrapment syndromes at fibrous or fibro-osseous tunnels, nerve injury related to penetrating or blunt trauma, neoplasms, and traction-related neuropathy caused by repetitive trauma. Systemic or multifocal diseases include hereditary disorders such as Charcot-Marie-Tooth disease, infections or inflammatory conditions like Parsonage-Turner syndrome or chronic demyelinating polyneuropathy, and neurocutaneous syndromes, including neurofibromatosis type 1, type 2, and schwannomatosis.
4. Answer: b. Median nerve at the level of the carpal tunnel. The most common entrapment in the upper extremity is of the median nerve at the level of the carpal tunnel, then the ulnar nerve at the cubital tunnel.
5. Answer: c. Nerve flattening. Unlike electrodiagnostic testing, MRI is noninvasive and may be more suitable for young patients and people with bleeding diatheses. In a recent systematic review on the accuracy of MRI in distinguishing normal from abnormal peripheral nerves, the pooled sensitivity and specificity of elevated signal on fluid-sensitive sequences were 77% (95% CI, 73–81%) and 67% (63–71%), respectively. The pooled sensitivity and specificity of nerve caliber enlargement were 63% (95% CI, 57–88%) and 84% (80–88%), respectively.[21] The pooled sensitivity and specificity for nerve flattening were 31% (95% CI, 24–37%) and 94% (87–94%),[21] respectively, making nerve flattening one of the most specific signs.

Part V

Tumors

V

19 Soft-Tissue Tumors

Carol D. Morris, Adam S. Levin, Raj M. Amin, and Laura M. Fayad

Abstract:
Magnetic resonance imaging (MRI) is the imaging modality of choice for evaluating soft-tissue masses. The aim of this chapter is to provide an overview of the MRI features of benign and malignant soft-tissue tumors. Lipomas are the most common of the benign soft-tissue neoplasms, and are characterized by homogeneous signal that is isointense to subcutaneous fat. Additional benign soft-tissue tumors with characteristic MRI appearances include ganglion cysts, hemangiomas, neurofibromas, schwannomas, tenosynovial giant cell tumor, and reactive lesions. MRI is also essential in the evaluation of malignant soft-tissue tumors, including sarcomas, lymphomas, and metastatic carcinoma. By the end of this chapter, the reader will be familiar with the characteristic findings and considerations when interpreting MRI for each of these neoplasms.

Keywords: MRI, tumor, neoplasm, soft tissue, benign, malignant, lipoma, sarcoma

19.1 Introduction

The cause of most benign and soft-tissue tumors is largely unknown. Benign soft-tissue masses outnumber malignant soft-tissue masses by at least 100 to 1. It is estimated that approximately 12,000 new cases of soft-tissue sarcoma are diagnosed in the United States annually. Clinically, benign and malignant tumors present with similar painless soft-tissue fullness. On imaging, benign soft-tissue masses tend to be superficial in location and < 5 cm in size, whereas soft-tissue sarcomas tend to occur deep in the fascia and are often larger. Treatment of soft-tissue masses depends on multiple factors. Many benign tumors can be followed clinically, whereas others may require excision for symptomatic reasons. Tumors that are not clearly benign on clinical examination and imaging warrant biopsy. Malignant tumors typically require referral to an Orthopaedic or surgical oncologist. Soft-tissue sarcomas are best treated in a multidisciplinary fashion through a combination of surgery, radiation, and/or chemotherapy.

Magnetic resonance imaging (MRI) is the imaging modality of choice for evaluating soft-tissue masses because of its excellent contrast resolution. Various MRI sequences are available for evaluating soft-tissue masses, and the most obvious application for MRI is to define the extent of the mass before resection. However, MRI is also useful for characterizing soft-tissue lesions as benign or malignant, identifying histologic characteristics (e.g., lipomatous content, myxoid content), determining treatment response, and detecting tumor recurrence.

Conventional MRI with T1-weighted images, fluid-sensitive sequences (fat-suppressed T2-weighted or short tau inversion recovery [STIR]), and static postcontrast imaging is the mainstay for evaluating soft-tissue tumors. Soft-tissue mass character and anatomic location are well displayed with T1-weighted imaging. Fluid-sensitive imaging shows potentially aggressive features of a mass such as perilesional edema and heterogeneity. After contrast administration, the degree of vascularity and cellularity of a mass can be assessed by how much enhancement occurs. More recent techniques refine the resolution of postcontrast imaging such that small areas of enhancement can be identified with high resolution.[1,2] Emerging techniques that provide functional information for the assessment of soft-tissue tumors include dynamic contrast enhancement and quantitative diffusion-weighted imaging, both of which can be integrated into a routine clinical examination[3,4] and are becoming more widely used (▶ Fig. 19.1). In addition to using these sequences to characterize soft-tissue masses for malignancy,

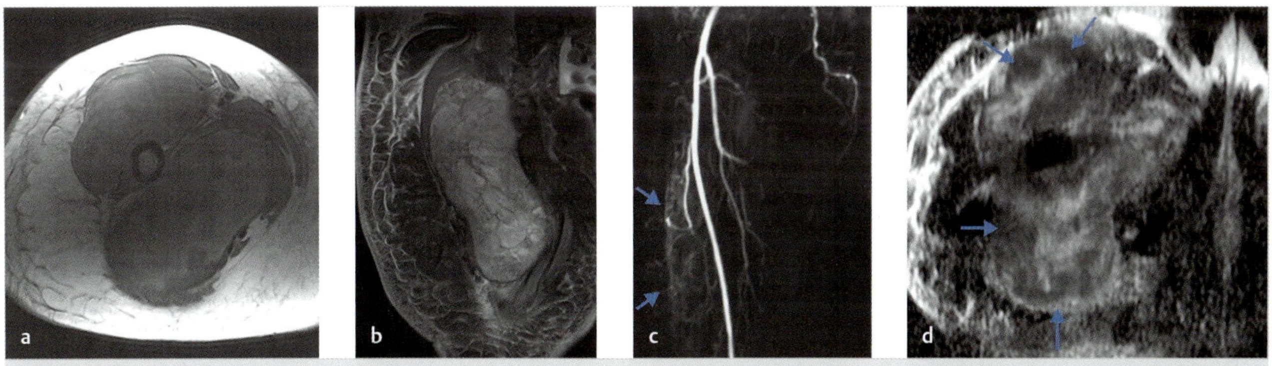

Fig. 19.1 High-grade sarcoma following neoadjuvant treatment. Axial T1W **(a)** and sagittal fat-suppressed T2W imaging **(b)** show a large heterogeneous mass. Tumor extent is well-delineated on these conventional anatomic sequences. However, in addition, coronal DCE-MR imaging **(c)** shows early arterial enhancement (*arrows*) within areas of viable tumor and axial ADC map from diffusion-weighted imaging **(d)** shows low ADC regions (*arrows*) again corresponding to viable treatment. DCE-MRI and DWI are sequences that provide information regarding vascularity and cellularity important to understanding tumor biology and treatment response.

these sequences can help assess treatment response after neoadjuvant therapy.[5,6] MR spectroscopy is a means of metabolic imaging with MRI and is still under investigation.[7,8]

For the common soft-tissue entities discussed below, the conventional MRI features of these lesions will be reviewed. The appearance of these lesions on more advanced sequences (including functional imaging and MR spectroscopy) is beyond the scope of this chapter.

19.2 Benign Tumors

19.2.1 Lipoma (▶ Fig. 19.2)

Lipomas are the most commonly diagnosed soft-tissue neoplasm, accounting for 30 to 50% of all mesenchymal lesions.[1,3,7,9] Most of them arise between the fourth and seventh decades of life. On examination, patients present with a painless, soft, mobile soft-tissue mass.[3,5,7,9] Most lipomas are superficial and < 5 cm in size and most commonly occur on the trunk, shoulder, upper arm, and neck.[3,5,7,9] Occasionally, because of their ubiquitous distribution, they present as painful, deep masses secondary to compression of neurovascular structures or viscera.[3] If conspicuous and asymptomatic, nonoperative treatment is preferred. Excision is reserved for severe disfigurement or symptoms.

Lipomas characteristically appear on MRI as masses with homogeneous signal isointense to subcutaneous fat on all pulse sequences.[9] Superficial lesions are typically well-circumscribed, whereas deeper lesions are typically more infiltrative.[10] On T1- and T2-weighted images without fat suppression, lipomas have homogeneous high signal intensity, indicative of lipid content. On fluid-sensitive sequences (fat-suppressed T2-weighted or STIR), they have low signal intensity with the lipid signal suppressed, and a few thin internal septations (without nodularity) may be present. Postcontrast T1-weighted images should show no enhancement or may show mild enhancement of thin, curvilinear septa.[11]

19.2.2 Ganglion Cyst (▶ Fig. 19.3)

Ganglion cyst is the most common mass of the hand and wrist. It typically presents in women between the fifth and sixth decades of life.[12,13] Although no cause has been determined, 10% of cases are associated with a traumatic event.[13] On physical examination, these cysts are small, translucent masses presenting on the extensor surface of the distal upper extremity near the dorsal band of the scapholunate ligament.[14] Although most are asymptomatic, some may cause mild pain, tenderness, and decreased range of motion.[15] Elsewhere in the body, they are known to occur around any joint but do not typically maintain communication with the capsule.[14,15] Treatment primarily involves observation and aspiration. The latter method has not been proven effective because lesions commonly recur. Adjunct therapies, including sclerosing agents, hyaluronidase, splinting, and steroid injections, have not shown evidence of benefit.[15] Surgical excision is indicated in symptomatic cases when nonoperative treatment has failed.[15]

Ganglion cysts appear on MRI as well-defined, round or oval masses of fluid signal intensity, which are uni- or multiloculated and may contain a few thin septations. They are located near joints or tendons. A track extending to the joint may be identified, and, if chronic, remodeling of the adjacent bone may also be present.[16] On T1-weighted images, ganglia are isointense to slightly hyperintense to muscle and hypointense to neighboring fat.[17] On T2-weighted images, they appear as high-signal-intensity lesions with internal low-signal-intensity lines, which represent thin septations, resulting in a compartmentalized appearance.[17,18] In addition to fluid, the high signal intensity may be because of high protein content in the ganglion.[17] Postcontrast T1-weighted images show enhancement of the thin fibrous wall and thin septations but do not show internal or nodular enhancement.[16,19,20]

19.2.3 Hemangioma (▶ Fig. 19.4)

The term soft-tissue "hemangioma" is often used by clinicians to encompass vascular malformations and congenital hemangiomas, and the MRI appearance has hence been described as a well-defined, lobulated soft-tissue mass or an infiltrative lesion.[12] However, true hemangiomas are considered tumors of infancy that typically involute (or may become noninvoluting congenital hemangiomas), whereas vascular malformations are congenital lesions that do not regress. This category of soft-tissue mass conservatively represents approximately 7% of benign soft-tissue masses.[21,22] Although most are found in infants,

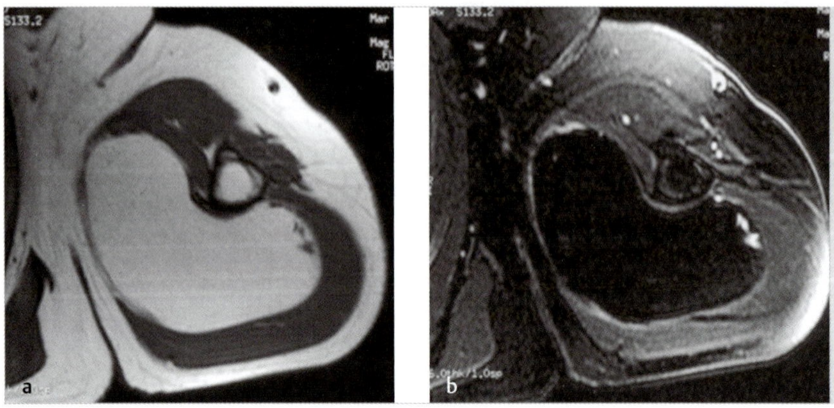

Fig. 19.2 Lipoma. Axial T1W image (a) shows a large soft tissue mass of homogeneous signal intensity similar to subcutaneous fat. On fat suppressed T2W imaging (b), the signal within the mass suppresses.

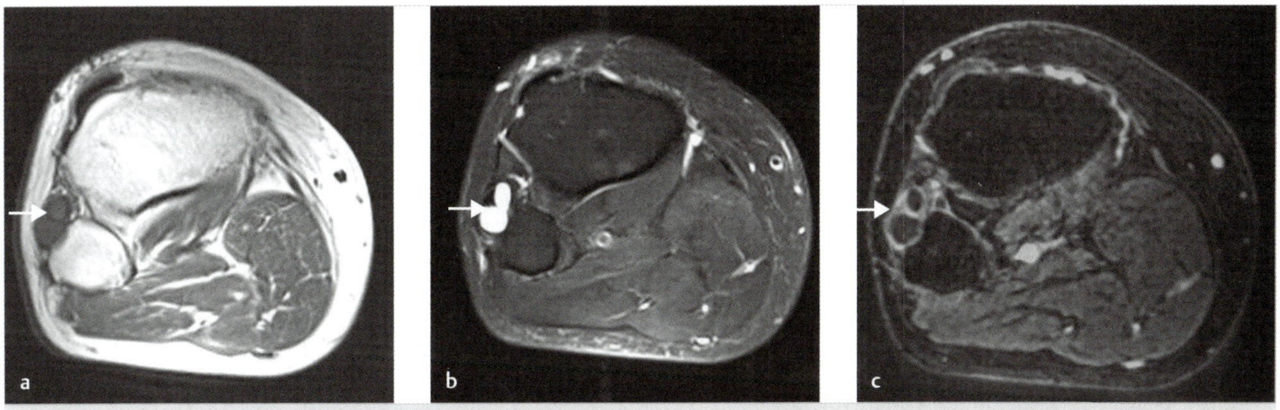

Fig. 19.3 Ganglion. Axial T1W image (a) shows lobular lesion in the soft tissues near the tibiofibular joint. Axial fat suppressed T2W (b) shows fluid signal intensity of the lesion. Axial postcontrast fat-suppressed T1W image (c) shows only peripheral enhancement and no central enhancement of the lesion, indicating it is a ganglion.

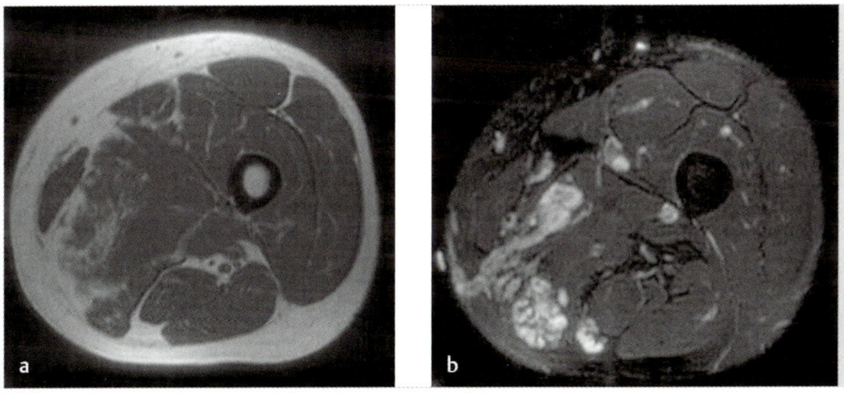

Fig. 19.4 Vascular malformation. Axial T1W image (a) shows a multifocal lesion infiltrating the muscles and subcutaneous tissues, relatively isointense to muscle and interspersed with lipid signal. Axial T2W image (b) shows the lesion extent to better advantage with fluid signal intensity. Note the infiltrative appearance with lack of mass effect and the cross-sectional architecture showing analogous to a "bunch of grapes."

hemangiomas may develop in adults often before the third decade of life.[22,23] Clinical presentation depends largely on location and depth of involvement. When they are confined to the cutaneous and subcutaneous tissues, hemangiomas tend to be painless. Cutaneous lesions are nodular and are intensely red, whereas subcutaneous lesions are more globus, soft masses with overlying blue epidermal discoloration.[23,24] Deeper-seated lesions often present as chronic thigh or calf pain.[22] Observation is the preferred treatment because of their spontaneous resolution. Intervention is reserved for painful lesions and consists of laser, sclerotherapy, or surgical excision.[23] Depending on the histological subtype, soft-tissue hemangiomas recur at a rate of 9 to 28%.[24]

On T1-weighted images, both types of vascular lesions typically appear as intermediate signal relative to skeletal muscle and may contain foci of high signal, which represent adipose tissue or slow-flow blood.[25,26,27,28] On T2-weighted images, high-signal-intensity areas in a lobular or multilobulated configuration (similar to a bunch of grapes) represent stagnant blood within vascular spaces.[27] Low-signal-intensity foci on T1- or T2-weighted images may represent high-flow blood (a signal void), thrombosed vessels, phleboliths, or dense fatty tissue.[21,27,29] On postcontrast T1-weighted images, these vascular lesions show prominent enhancement of areas corresponding to high signal intensity on T2-weighted images. Dilated feeding and draining vessels may also be visualized on postcontrast T1-weighted images and can be further assessed by MR angiography.[21,27] If phleboliths are present, they will show blooming artifact on gradient echo images.[28]

19.2.4 Neurofibroma (▶ Fig. 19.5)

Neurofibromas represent a heterogeneous mixture of nonneoplastic cells occurring sporadically and in association with neurofibromatosis type 1.[30,31,32] Onset is between the second and third decades of life; a suspect mass occurring before adolescence is highly unlikely to be a neurofibroma.[33] Physical examination, prognosis, and treatment of the patient with a neurofibroma is highly dependent on histological subtype. Spontaneous lesions are almost always nodular superficial neurofibromas restricted to the dermis and subcutaneous tissue.[34] Neurofibromas intimately associated with the fascicles of deep or superficial nerves, called plexiform neurofibromas, are almost always in the setting of neurofibromatosis type 1.[34] About 10% of the latter type of neurofibroma may undergo malignant degeneration to malignant peripheral nerve sheath tumors.[34] The workup and treatment of neurofibromas require a multimodal approach. Surgical excision is reserved for painful or disfiguring cutaneous neurofibromas. Typically, surgery is avoided in patients with neurofibromatosis type 1 because of the large number of tumors, unless the neurofibromas threaten

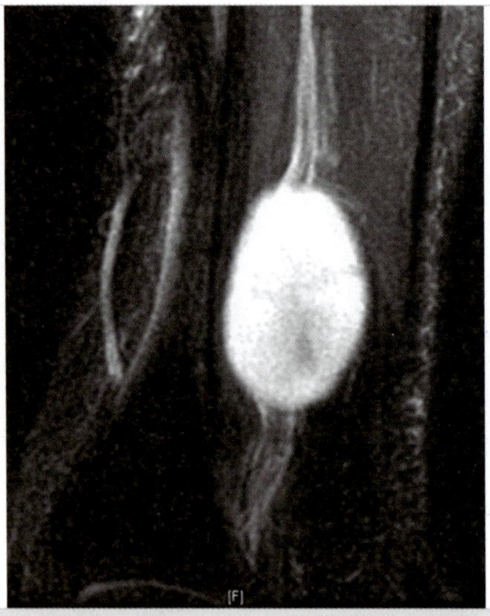

Fig. 19.5 Neurofibroma. Sagittal fluid-sensitive sequence shows an ovoid mass of fairly homogeneous hyperintensity with an internal area of low signal (the "target sign"). The mass is continuous with adjacent nerve.

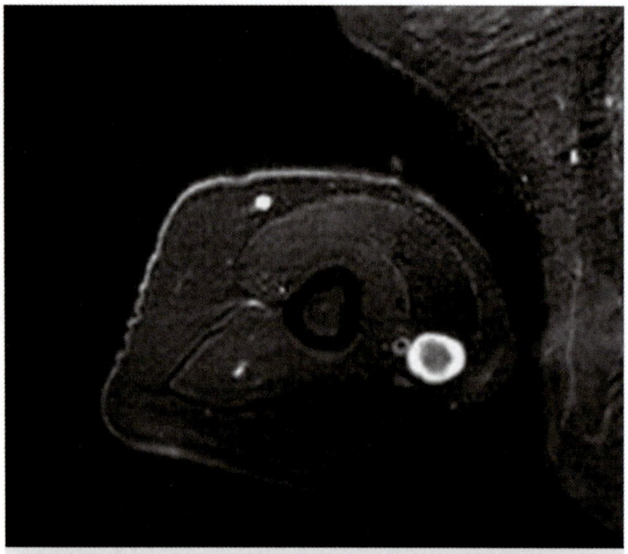

Fig. 19.6 Schwannoma. Similar to ▸ Fig. 19.5 (neurofibroma), a soft tissue mass is identified on this fat-suppressed image, with a clear "target sign." Features of neurofibromas and schwannomas overlap.

organ function.[35] Whereas neurofibromatosis type 1–related fibromas are likely to recur, isolated neurofibromas are very unlikely to recur after surgical excision.[35,36]

Neurofibromas can be localized, diffuse, or plexiform in morphology.[37] Localized neurofibromas appear as a well-defined, fusiform mass arising centrally within a nerve.[38,39] These lesions are typically iso- to hypointense relative to muscle on T1-weighted images,[37] and there is often a peripheral rim of high signal intensity, which represents a rim of normal fat that is preserved and displaced as the tumor enlarges ("split-fat sign").[19,38] Another feature of neurofibromas on T1-weighted images is vertically oriented high-intensity soft tissue extending from the ends of the mass. This finding is called the "string sign" and represents the normal nerve as it continues through the nerve sheath tumor.[19] On T2-weighted images, neurofibromas appear hyperintense and can have low signal centrally and higher signal peripherally. This finding is characteristic of neurofibromas and is called the "target sign."[19,37,38,40,41] The central low signal represents dense fibrocollagenous tissue, and the peripheral high signal represents myxomatous tissue with a high water content.[37] On postcontrast T1-weighted images, neurofibromas typically show enhancement of the central region greater than peripheral regions.[38]

Diffuse neurofibromas present as a poorly defined infiltrative mass extending along connective tissue septa, which appears as a predominantly low-signal reticulated branching pattern with honeycomb appearance on T2-weighted images. This finding results from the high collagen composition of the tumor.[37] Plexiform neurofibromas have a rope-like or "bag-of-worms" appearance because of nodular thickening and expansion of long nerves and their branches.[37,42]

Distinguishing neurofibromas from malignant peripheral nerve sheath tumors, especially in patients with neurofibromatosis type 1, can be challenging. Diffusion-weighted imaging and MR spectroscopy have been used successfully for the characterization of peripheral nerve sheath tumors.[43,44] On diffusion-weighted imaging, malignant peripheral nerve tumors show a greater degree of restricted diffusion than benign neurofibromas; thus, diffusion-weighted imaging is helpful when deciding whether a lesion has the potential for malignancy and requires biopsy.

19.2.5 Schwannoma (▸ Fig. 19.6)

Schwannomas are a histologically homogeneous entity representing approximately 5% of soft-tissue tumors.[35,45] These lesions occur sporadically between the second and fifth decades of life and are found most commonly in the head, neck, and flexor surfaces of the appendicular skeleton.[35,46] Multiple schwannomas are associated with defects in the neurofibromin 2 gene.[46] Clinically, these are indolent and painless lesions, usually < 5 cm in size.[35,45,47] When superficial, some schwannomas exhibit Tinel's sign.[45] Deep lesions often present with waxing and waning symptoms of pain and neurodeficits.[35] Treatment is aided by the well-encapsulated and extraneural nature of schwannomas.[45,48] The eccentric displacement of non-neoplastic tissue allows for preservation of the affected nerve function after resection.[45,47,48] These lesions are unlikely to recur after complete surgical excision.[46]

Schwannomas appear as fusiform masses eccentrically positioned in relation to the parent nerve, rather than centrally positioned as is the case with neurofibromas.[39] These lesions share similar MRI characteristics with neurofibromas. Schwannomas also show the split-fat sign, target sign, fascicular sign, and contrast enhancement. However, reportedly, the target sign is more commonly seen in neurofibromas, whereas the fascicular sign is more commonly seen in schwannomas.[38] Schwannomas can have homogeneous or heterogeneous enhancement as well as areas of necrosis that can mimic malignancy, especially in so-called "ancient schwannomas."[49]

Distinguishing schwannomas from malignancy can be challenging. Again, the techniques of diffusion-weighted imaging and MR spectroscopy have been used to characterize peripheral nerve sheath tumors but are not as widely used as conventional MRI.[43,44]

19.2.6 Tenosynovial Giant Cell Tumor/ Pigmented Villonodular Synovitis (▶ Fig. 19.7)

Soft-tissue giant cell tumors are benign lesions presenting in women twice as often as men, typically beginning in the third to fourth decades of life.[35,50] They are subdivided into diffuse-type and localized tumors.[35,50] After ganglion cysts, tenosynovial giant cell tumors are the most common tumors of the hand.[50] Typically, the localized form is a solitary, indolent, subcutaneous nodule with epidermal involvement reserved for the most distal fingertip lesions.[35,51] In contrast, the diffuse type is locally aggressive, often invading soft tissue and nearby osseous cortex. Clinically, the diffuse type presents as a periarticular, firm mass around the knee or hip.[52] Asymptomatic lesions are best treated nonoperatively, whereas symptomatic lesions may benefit from surgery or newer targeted therapies.[53]

Pigmented villonodular synovitis and tenosynovial giant cell tumors share similar MRI features because of their similar histological composition. Pigmented villonodular synovitis characteristically appears as diffuse intra-articular involvement of a villous mass with hemosiderin deposition.[54] On T1-weighted images, pigmented villonodular synovitis regions show low signal intensity, which is isointense to muscle.[55,56] On fluid-sensitive images, synovial fluid appears as high signal intensity, whereas hemosiderin-laden nodular thickening and villous projections of the synovium appear as intermediate or absent signal.[55,56] On postcontrast T1-weighted images, pigmented villonodular synovitis has homogeneous enhancement.[55] On gradient-echo sequences, decreased signal intensity, often more prominent in the periphery (blooming artifact), reflects the hemosiderin deposits.[25,55]

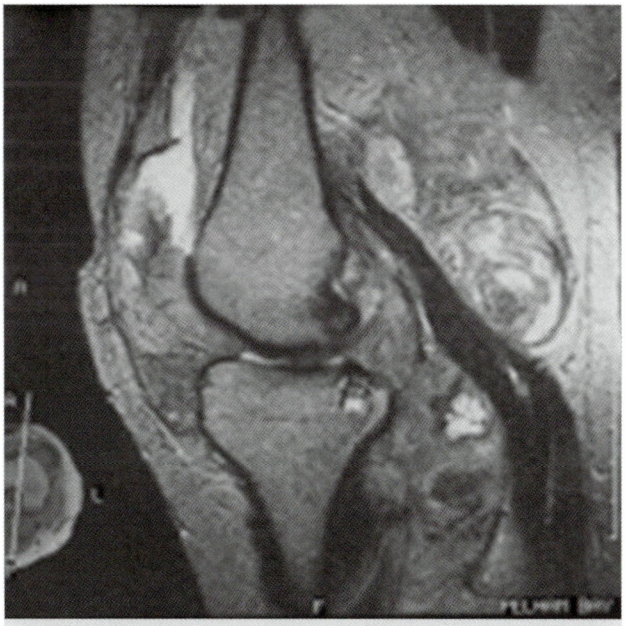

Fig. 19.7 Pigmented vilonodular synovitis (PVNS). Sagittal T2W image shows a large joint effusion with low signal intensity masses, typical of PVNS.

Tenosynovial giant cell tumor of the tendon sheath appears as an extra-articular focal mass adjacent to or surrounding a tendon sheath rather than within the joint.[19,54,57] This lesion is hypointense to isointense to muscle on T1- and T2-weighted images. This characteristic MRI feature is the result of hemosiderin and collagen within the lesion.[19,57,58] Postcontrast T1-weighted images show avid enhancement because of abundant proliferative capillaries and inflammatory cell infiltrates in the collagenous stroma.[57,58]

19.2.7 Reactive Lesions

Reactive lesions are the most common soft-tissue pathology seen in clinical practice. Often a thorough patient history and physical examination are sufficient for diagnosis; however, clinicians must be wary of the many similarities between these benign masses and rarer malignant sarcomas.

Hematoma (▶ Fig. 19.8)

Hematomas are often seen in the setting of blunt trauma; less frequently, they are described as spontaneous occurrences in the truncal musculature of patients with underlying hematologic conditions or in those who are on anticoagulation therapy.[52,59,60,61] There is considerable overlap in the clinical presentation of hematomas and soft-tissue tumors. Clinical follow-up is key to ensure timely resolution of the hematoma. Masses that do not regress as expected warrant further evaluation.

The MRI appearance of soft-tissue hematomas is age-dependent and reflects the respective hemoglobin degradation product that predominates as the hematoma evolves. Generally, hyperacute blood (a few hours old) shows intermediate signal intensity on T1-weighted images and high signal intensity on T2-weighted images, which represents the high water content of oxyhemoglobin.[25,62] Acute hematomas (1–2 days old) shows intermediate signal intensity on T1-weighted images and low signal intensity on T2-weighted images, which represents intracellular deoxyhemoglobin.[25,62] Early subacute hematomas (2–7 days old) show high signal intensity on T1-weighted images, which is first observed as a peripheral rim. The latter finding is because of formation of intracellular methemoglobin, which has a similar structure to gadolinium. Early subacute hematomas show low signal intensity on T2-weighted images.[25,62] Late subacute hematomas (7–28 days old) have high signal intensity on T1- and T2-weighted images, which represents extracellular methemoglobin. Acute and subacute hematomas may be surrounded by high signal intensity in the surrounding muscle, representing diffuse edema. Chronic hematomas (> 28 days old) have low signal intensity on T1- and T2-weighted images, especially around the periphery, which represents hemosiderin deposition and fibrosis.[25,62] However, hematomas are often heterogeneous and may cause repeat bleeding.[19]

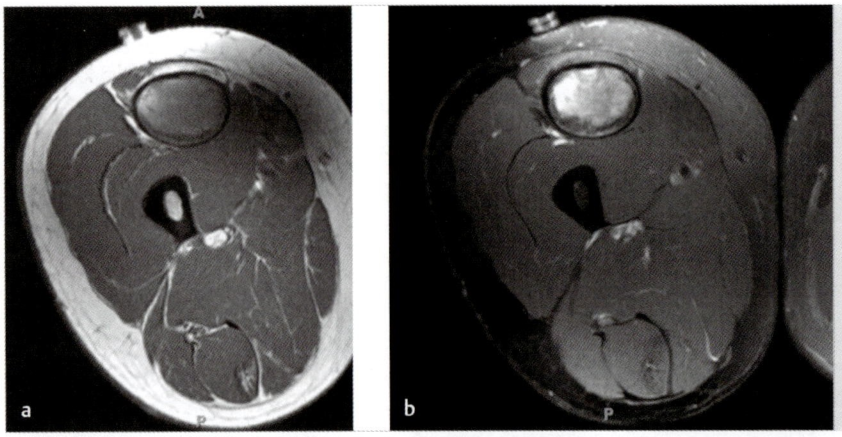

Fig. 19.8 Hematoma. Axial T1W **(a)** and fat-suppressed T2W **(b)** images show a soft tissue mass of increased T1 and T2 signal with surrounding hemosiderin rim, characteristic of a hematoma. (Reproduced with permission from, Fayad LM, Wang X, Salibi N, Barker PB, Jacobs MA, Machado AJ, Weber KL, Bluemke DA. A feasibility study of quantitative molecular characterization of musculoskeletal lesions by proton MR spectroscopy at 3 T. AJR Am J Roentgenol. 2010 Jul;195(1):W69-75)

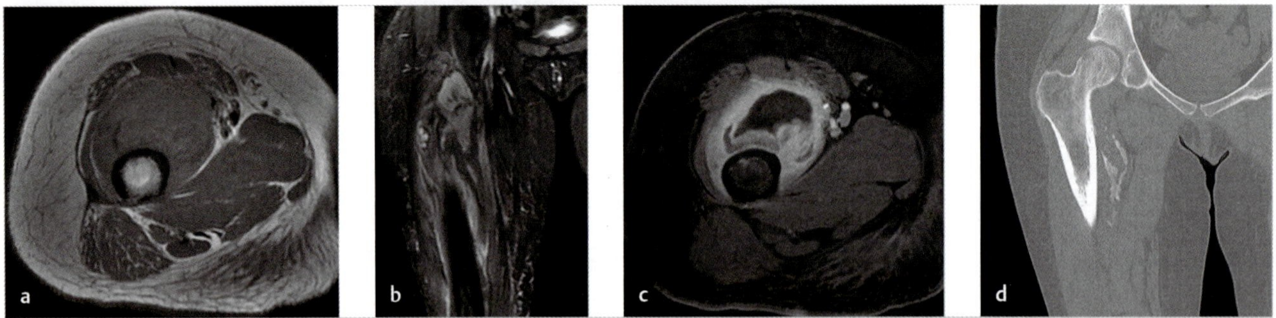

Fig. 19.9 Myositis Ossificans. Axial T1W **(a)**, coronal STIR **(b)** and axial fat-suppressed T1W **(c)** images show a mass with marked surrounding edema, with heterogeneous signal and peripheral enhancement, features of early myositis ossificans. Eight weeks later, CT **(d)** shows zonal pattern of ossification that is characteristic of this entity.

Myositis Ossificans (▶ Fig. 19.9)

Myositis ossificans is a reactive osseous lesion of soft tissue. Although often seen in young patients as a complication of a soft-tissue hematoma, it may occur in patients of any age with a nidus for ossification. Symptoms consist of continued pain at the site of previous trauma, gradual firmness of the associated mass, persistent discoloration of the overlying skin, and decreased flexibility of the affected muscle group.[63] Radiographs show soft-tissue ossification 3 to 6 weeks after the inciting trauma.[64] Treatment consists of observation, symptomatic therapy, and nonsteroidal anti-inflammatory medications. Most symptoms self-resolve within 3 to 6 months.[63] Surgical resection is reserved for lesions causing severe mobility deficits, and recurrence is uncommon after local excision.

The appearance of myositis ossificans depends on the age of the lesion. Early lesions (< 8 weeks old) are ill-defined and isointense to muscle on T1-weighted images and may only be associated with mass effect.[65] They have heterogeneous (predominantly high) signal intensity centrally on T2-weighted images[66] because of proliferating fibroblasts and myofibroblasts.[65] Curvilinear, irregular low-signal-intensity foci on T2-weighted images represent mineralization.[65] Perilesional edema is diffuse.[19,66,67] In addition, early on, postcontrast T1-weighted images show diffuse enhancement with fine neovascularization because of hypervascularity.[65,68]

In the subacute stage (approximately 8 weeks old), on T1-weighted images, the center is isointense and the border of the lesion has low signal intensity, representing a rim of ossification.[66] T2-weighted images show high signal intensity centrally, a rim of low signal intensity, and persistent perilesional edema.

Late lesions (> 8 weeks old) are well defined with high signal intensity and a rim of low signal intensity on T1- and T2-weighted images.[65] Progressive ossification of the lesion occurs in the periphery.[65] At this stage, surrounding edema has resolved and there is no enhancement because of avascularity.[65,68]

Abscess (▶ Fig. 19.10)

Soft-tissue abscesses represent 2% of all emergency department visits per year.[69,70,71] Although soft-tissue abscesses can occur in any patient, risk factors are diabetes, history of intravenous drug use, human immunodeficiency virus, and recent surgery.[71] Patients present with enlarging, warm, and erythematous lesions. Pain and exquisite tenderness are expected, with cellulitis being a common comorbid condition. Often, clinical examination is sufficient for diagnosis. Adjunct imaging modalities include radiography, CT, and sonography, which help physicians decide between bedside versus formal operative irrigation and debridement. Patients with surrounding cellulitis or with signs of systemic or osseus infection warrant antibiotic therapy in addition to debridement.

Soft-tissue abscesses appear as low-signal-intensity lesions on T1-weighted images and as high-intensity lesions with surrounding high-signal-intensity edema on T2-weighted images. The internal signal can be homogeneous or heterogeneous depending on the relative composition of proteinaceous debris,

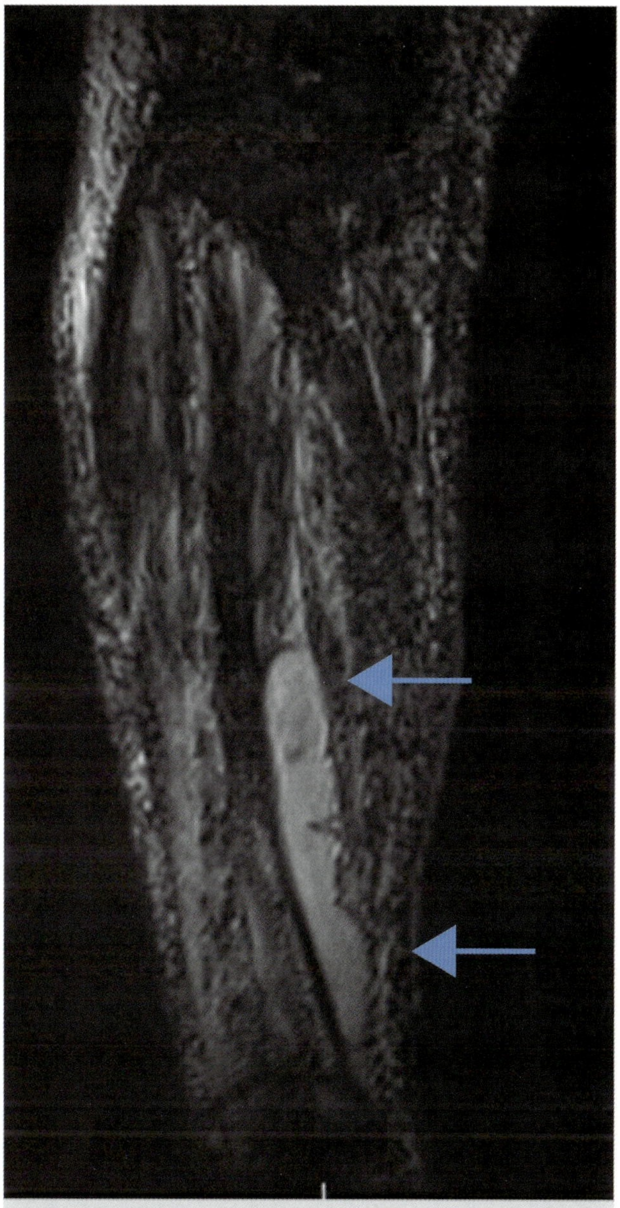

Fig. 19.10 Abscess. Coronal STIR shows elongated fluid collection in the calf with surrounding cellulitis.

necrosis, hemorrhage, or intralesional gas, especially on T2-weighted images.[72,73,74] On T1- and T2-weighted images, a surrounding low-signal-intensity rim represents the capsule and regions of signal absence indicate gas.[74] Postcontrast T1-weighted images show avid rim enhancement of the cellular and inflammatory components, which appear thick and irregular in the acute phase and thin and regular with chronicity.[75] The central necrotic components of the abscess do not enhance.[25,73]

Benign Adenopathy

The differential diagnosis for adenopathy is broad and includes benign and malignant disorders, as well as systemic disease.[76,77] Acute, in contrast to chronic, lymphadenopathy presents with tender, warm, and sometimes erythematous nodes.[77] These characteristics, when localized, are typically secondary to infection in the dependent draining region.[76] Nodal size also provides guidance as to the cause. Pathologic nodes are typically > 1 cm in the upper half of the body and 2 cm in the lower half.[76] Any node of > 3 cm is worrisome.[76]

Benign lymph nodes appear markedly hypointense to fat on T1-weighted images, moderately hypointense on proton density–weighted images, and hyperintense on T2-weighted images.[78] Reactively, enlarged lymph nodes appear elongated and oval or with a curvilinear appearance of the cortex if a fatty hilum is seen. In comparison, malignant lymph nodes are round.[78] Benign lymph nodes enhance uniformly on postcontrast T1-weighted images, without rim enhancement and central low intensity suggesting central necrosis.[78] On dynamic contrast-enhanced MRI, benign lymphadenopathy shows gradual increase in enhancement without a peak, whereas malignant lymph nodes show peak enhancement 60 to 80 seconds after contrast administration.[79] On ultrasmall superparamagnetic iron oxide–enhanced MRI, benign lymph nodes will have low signal intensity on T2- and T2*-weighted images because of susceptibility effect and T2 shortening that occurs as a result of phagocytosis of the particles by macrophages within the lymph node. In contrast, malignant lymph nodes lack normal structure and macrophage content and therefore appear unchanged on T2-weighted images because of lack of particle uptake.[80]

19.3 Malignant Tumors

19.3.1 Soft-Tissue Sarcoma

Soft-tissue sarcomas are malignant neoplasms of mesenchymal origin that can arise in any part of the body with connective tissue. Although soft-tissue sarcomas are of great concern to clinicians, they are outnumbered by their benign counterparts by 100-fold, they represent < 1% of cancer diagnosis annually, and they account for only 2% of cancer-related deaths. Approximately 50% of soft-tissue sarcomas occur in the extremities, with most arising in the lower extremity. On clinical examination, soft-tissue sarcomas present as enlarging, painless, firm, fixed masses. Any mass of > 5 cm and deep to the fascia should raise concern for a soft-tissue sarcoma. MRI is the imaging modality of choice for evaluation of a suspected soft-tissue sarcoma. Staging and biopsy are necessary to guide treatment. Patients with a suspected or biopsy-proven sarcoma are best treated in specialty centers with multimodality capability, including surgery, radiation, and chemotherapy.

Liposarcoma (▶ Fig. 19.11)

Liposarcoma is the most common subtype of soft-tissue sarcoma, accounting for 15 to 25% of all sarcomas.[81] They typically arise as a slowly enlarging mass in the sixth to eighth decades of life. Several subtypes exist, of which well-differentiated liposarcoma is the most common. As with all soft-tissue sarcomas, treatment depends on grade, location, and extent of disease.

The MR appearance of liposarcomas varies according to subtype. In general, MR features suggestive of liposarcoma in comparison to lipomas include prominent thick or nodular septa, large dimension, and neurovascular involvement.[7,25,82]

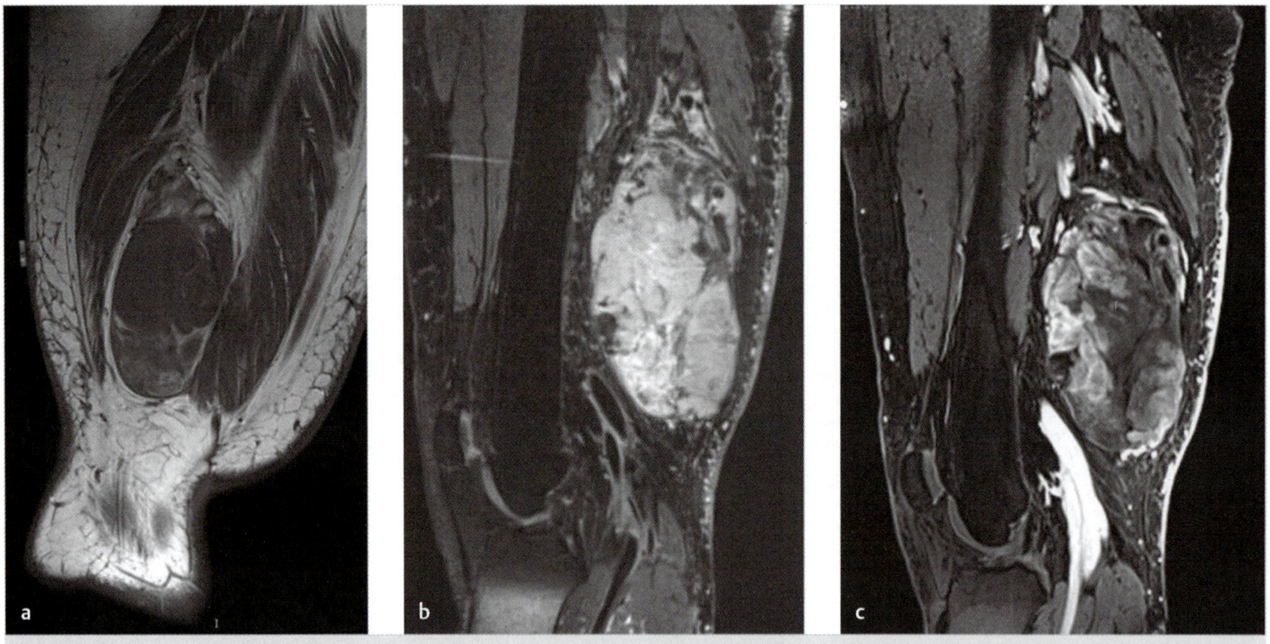

Fig. 19.11 Myxoid liposarcoma. Coronal T1W **(a)**, and fat-suppressed sagittal T2W **(b)** and sagittal post-contrast T1W **(c)** images show a large mass with internal lipid signal (denoted by high T1 signal areas), myxoid areas (denoted by high T2 signal) and enhancement following contrast administration.

Well-differentiated liposarcomas (similar to atypical lipomatous tumors of the extremities) appear as well-circumscribed masses that show fat signal intensity on T1- and T2-weighted images and contain internal septa, which appear as low internal signals on T1-weighted images and high internal signals on T2-weighted images.[83,84] On postcontrast T1-weighted images, well-differentiated liposarcomas show no or minimal enhancement, except for the nonlipomatous thick, nodular septa, which show avid enhancement.[7,82,83]

Myxoid liposarcomas typically appear as well-circumscribed, lobulated lesions, which are hypointense or isointense to muscle on T1-weighted images and have high signal intensity (close to water signal) on T2-weighted images. The latter finding corresponds to the high myxoid matrix composition and dearth of mature fat.[84] These tumors characteristically show homogeneous internal signal because of the myxoid matrix.[83,84] Low-signal-intensity septations represent fibrous tissue bands.[83] They may have a thick, low-signal-intensity rim, which represents a pseudocapsule.[83] Pleomorphic liposarcomas have a variable appearance, with heterogeneous internal signal. Depending on the degree of pleomorphism, these tumors have varying degrees of hemorrhage and necrosis, altering their appearance on MRI. Myxoid and pleomorphic liposarcomas show avid enhancement on postcontrast T1-weighted images, which correlates to the amount of vascularity and cellularity.[83]

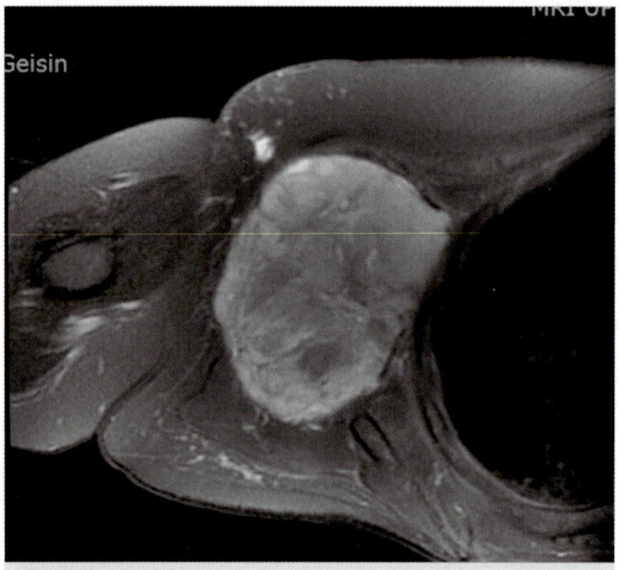

Fig. 19.12 MFH. Axial fat-suppressed T2W image shows a large heterogeneous mass. Features are nonspecific, although suspicious for malignancy.

Undifferentiated Pleomorphic Sarcoma (► Fig. 19.12)

Undifferentiated pleomorphic sarcoma, previously called malignant fibrous histiocytoma, arises in the sixth and seventh decades of life. Its name implies a lack of a known cellular differentiation pathway. Advanced pathology techniques have allowed reclassification of tumors previously referred to as malignant fibrous histiocytoma with more exact terminology.

Malignant fibrous histiocytoma typically appears as a well-defined, large (approximately 10 cm on average) lesion, most commonly located in the thigh.[85] On T1-weighted images, malignant fibrous histiocytoma has intermediate signal intensity, slightly higher than muscle. The signal may be homogeneous or heterogeneous on T1-weighted images, depending on the amount of hemorrhage or necrosis.[86,87] On T2-weighted images, malignant fibrous histiocytoma often has heterogeneous signal intensity because of hemorrhage, necrosis, or fibrous bands.[85,86] Postcontrast T1-weighted images show enhancement of the solid non-necrotic components.[87] If calcifications are present, they appear as low-signal-intensity foci on T1- and T2-weighted images.[86]

Synovial Sarcoma

Although synovial sarcomas occur in para-articular regions, there is no evidence to suggest a relationship with the joint capsule or lineage consistent with synovial cells.[88] Synovial sarcoma occurs at a mean age of 34 years, with > 40% arising before the third decade of life. Anatomically, 60% occur around the large joints of the lower extremity within associated tendons and bursae. The t(x;18) translocation is diagnostic of synovial sarcoma.[88]

Synovial sarcomas can appear as well-defined lobulated lesions or, occasionally, as poorly defined lesions. They are located close to a joint and may show involvement of the adjacent bone but do not originate in the joint.[89] Neurovascular encasement may be present if the origin is a nearby intramuscular site, resulting in a split-fat sign (rim of fat surrounding the tumor).[90] On T1-weighted images, synovial sarcomas are typically of intermediate signal.[91] Foci of high signal intensity on T1-weighted images and corresponding low signal intensity on T2-weighted images represent areas of hemorrhage.[25,89,91] On T2-weighted images, the signal intensity is heterogeneous, including hyperintense, hypointense, and isointense compared with fat; this finding has been referred to as a triple-signal pattern.[89,91] The hyperintense signal likely represents hemorrhage or necrosis; the intermediate signal likely represents solid cellular components; and the hypointense signal likely represents calcifications or fibrotic collagenous components.[90] Synovial sarcomas have also been described as having a "bowl of grapes" appearance, which refers to its multilobulated contour with areas of hemorrhage and fluid levels.[90] Postcontrast T1-weighted images show avid enhancement or enhancement of solid nodular foci, whereas necrotic and cystic areas remain unenhanced.[92]

Myxofibrosarcoma (▶ Fig. 19.13)

A unique characteristic of myxofibrosarcoma is its subcutaneous location.[93,94,95] The lack of natural boundaries in the subcutaneous tissue allows for extension of the tumor along the fascia. As a result, obtaining negative margins is a surgical challenge. These tumors are associated with higher rates of local recurrence compared with other soft-tissue sarcomas.

Myxofibrosarcomas can present as diffuse, infiltrative, spreading mass-like areas along fascial planes or as focal, well-demarcated lesions.[96] These tumors show central low signal intensity on T1-weighted images and high signal intensity on T2-weighted images because of their myxoid component.[96] If acute hemorrhage is present within the tumor, it appears as high signal intensity on T1-weighted images and can settle into a fluid–fluid layer with time.[87] Postcontrast T1-weighted images show nodular and peripheral enhancement of the solid, nonmyxomatous components. If more vascular and cellular elements are present, enhancement of the lesion appears more homogeneous.[87] A characteristic feature of myxofibrosarcomas is tapered fascial enhancement extending from the lesion, called the tail sign,

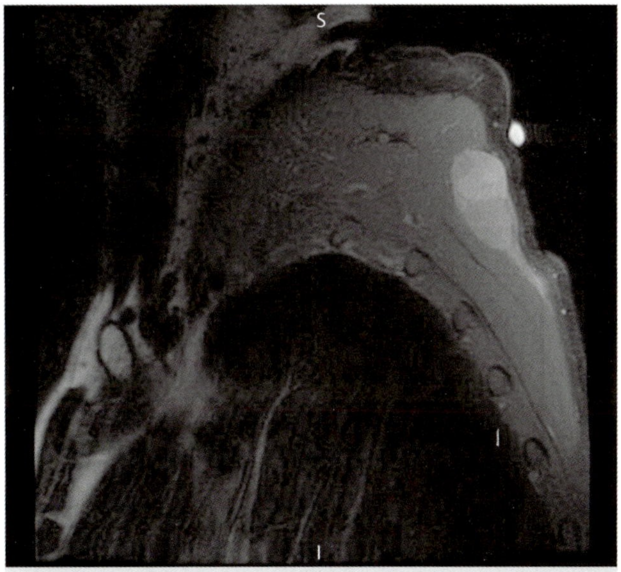

Fig. 19.13 Myxofibrosarcoma. Sagittal T2W image shows a mass with fascial extension, characteristic of this entity.

although this lesion can also be present in undifferentiated sarcomas.[95] T2-weighted images appear heterogeneous if hemorrhage and necrosis are present,[87] and perilesional edema can be present.[96]

19.3.2 Lymphoma

Lymphoma is a clonal proliferation of lymphocytes at various degrees of differentiation. The most common type of lymphoma is non-Hodgkin's B-cell lymphoma. Patients may present with a broad spectrum of symptoms depending on disease burden, from palpable adenopathy to night sweats and weight loss. Occasionally, an extra-nodal soft-tissue mass may be present.[97] Treatment typically combines radiation and chemotherapy depending on staging. Survival is related to rate of disease dissemination rather than histologic stage.

Soft-tissue lymphomas appear as superficial, lobular lesions or as deeper, infiltrative lesions.[98] The involved muscles are enlarged and typically involve multiple muscle compartments while preserving the intramuscular fat planes.[99,100] They characteristically extend along neurovascular bundles and through subcutaneous tissue.[25,98,99,101] On T1-weighted images, lymphomas show variable signal intensity but are predominantly isointense to muscle.[99,101] However, with the application of fat suppression to T1-weighted images, lymphomas may show high signal intensity relative to muscle.[25] On fluid-sensitive images, they appear as intermediate-signal-intensity lesions.[25,101] After contrast administration, there is diffuse enhancement within the tumor, which can be homogeneous or heterogeneous.[25,98,100] Thick, irregular enhancement of surrounding fascicles can also be seen.[99]

19.3.3 Metastatic Carcinoma (▶ Fig. 19.14)

Metastatic carcinoma of the soft tissue is rare compared with that of the bone.[102] When metastatic lesions are found, pulmonary

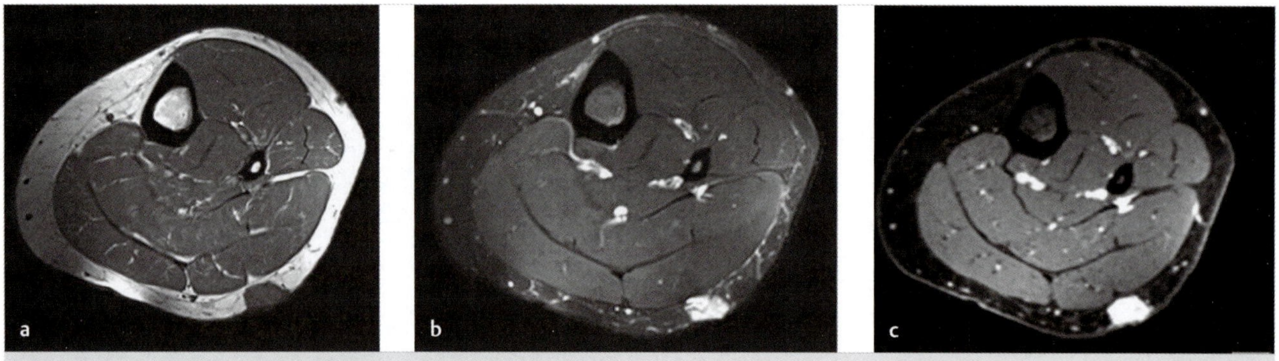

Fig. 19.14 Metastatic disease. Axial T1W **(a)**, T2 W **(b)** and fat-suppressed post-contrast T1W **(c)** images shows a soft tissue mass in the subcutaneous tissues of the calf. This has nonspecific features, but enhancement following contrast confirms this is a solid tumor rather than cyst, and metastatic disease was diagnosed by biopsy.

adenocarcinoma and squamous cell carcinoma, renal cancer, and colorectal cancer are the primary culprits, in decreasing order.[102,103] Masses may be singular or multifocal.[102] Treatment is primarily nonoperative. Overall survival is poor in patients with soft-tissue metastatic carcinoma.[102,104]

Soft-tissue metastases typically have nonspecific MRI findings. On T1-weighted images, they are hypointense to fat and isointense to muscle. On T2-weighted images, they typically show high signal intensity compared with muscle and may have perilesional edema.[105] The appearance of metastases is related to their hypercellularity and high nuclear–cytoplasmic ratio, and with hemorrhage or necrosis, the lesions may become heterogeneous.[25] Postcontrast T1-weighted images show enhancement of these lesions,[105] sometimes with extensive peritumoral enhancement and sometimes with central nonenhancing necrosis.[106]

19.4 Summary

Imaging of soft tissue tumors relies heavily on MRI as modality of choice. A variety of soft tissue tumors have characteristic MRI appearances that are worth familiarizing. Malignant soft tissue tumors require appropriate imaging for clinical decision making.

References

[1] Weiss SW. Lipomatous tumors. Monogr Pathol. 1996; 38:207–239

[2] Ahlawat S, Morris CD, Fayad LM. Three-dimensional volumetric MRI with isotropic resolution: improved speed of acquisition, spatial resolution and assessment of lesion conspicuity in patients with recurrent soft tissue sarcoma. Skeletal Radiol. 2016; 45(5):645–652

[3] Fletcher CDM, Unni KK, Mertens F, eds. Pathology & Genetics: Tumours of Soft Tissue and Bone. Lyon: IARC Press; 2002

[4] Del Grande F, Ahlawat S, Subhawong T, Fayad LM. Characterization of indeterminate soft tissue masses referred for biopsy: What is the added value of contrast imaging at 3.0 tesla? J Magn Reson Imaging. 2017; 45(2): 390–400

[5] Rydholm A, Berg NO. Size, site and clinical incidence of lipoma. Factors in the differential diagnosis of lipoma and sarcoma. Acta Orthop Scand. 1983; 54(6):929–934

[6] Soldatos T, Ahlawat S, Montgomery E, Chalian M, Jacobs MA, Fayad LM. Multiparametric assessment of treatment response in high-grade soft-tissue sarcomas with anatomic and functional MR imaging sequences. Radiology. 2016; 278(3):831–840

[7] Kransdorf MJ, Bancroft LW, Peterson JJ, Murphey MD, Foster WC, Temple HT. Imaging of fatty tumors: distinction of lipoma and well-differentiated liposarcoma. Radiology. 2002; 224(1):99–104

[8] Fayad LM, Jacobs MA, Wang X, Carrino JA, Bluemke DA. Musculoskeletal tumors: how to use anatomic, functional, and metabolic MR techniques. Radiology. 2012; 265(2):340–356

[9] Murphey MD, Carroll JF, Flemming DJ, Pope TL, Gannon FH, Kransdorf MJ. From the archives of the AFIP: benign musculoskeletal lipomatous lesions. Radiographics. 2004; 24(5):1433–1466

[10] Matsumoto K, Hukuda S, Ishizawa M, Chano T, Okabe H. MRI findings in intramuscular lipomas. Skeletal Radiol. 1999; 28(3):145–152

[11] Hosono M, Kobayashi H, Fujimoto R, et al. Septum-like structures in lipoma and liposarcoma: MR imaging and pathologic correlation. Skeletal Radiol. 1997; 26(3):150–154

[12] Rozbruch SR, Chang V, Bohne WH, Deland JT. Ganglion cysts of the lower extremity: an analysis of 54 cases and review of the literature. Orthopedics. 1998; 21(2):141–148

[13] Teh J, Whiteley G. MRI of soft tissue masses of the hand and wrist. Br J Radiol. 2007; 80(949):47–63

[14] Thornburg LE. Ganglions of the hand and wrist. J Am Acad Orthop Surg. 1999; 7(4):231–238

[15] Gude W, Morelli V. Ganglion cysts of the wrist: pathophysiology, clinical picture, and management. Curr Rev Musculoskelet Med. 2008; 1(3–4):205–211

[16] Kim JY, Jung SA, Sung MS, Park YH, Kang YK. Extra-articular soft tissue ganglion cyst around the knee: focus on the associated findings. Eur Radiol. 2004; 14(1):106–111

[17] Feldman F, Singson RD, Staron RB. Magnetic resonance imaging of para-articular and ectopic ganglia. Skeletal Radiol. 1989; 18(5):353–358

[18] Kransdorf MJ, Murphey MD. MR imaging of musculoskeletal tumors of the hand and wrist. Magn Reson Imaging Clin N Am. 1995; 3(2):327–344

[19] Helms CA, Major NM, Anderson MW, Kaplan P, Dussault R. Musculoskeletal MRI. Philadelphia: Saunders; 2009

[20] Wu JS, Hochman MG. Soft-tissue tumors and tumorlike lesions: a systematic imaging approach. Radiology. 2009; 253(2):297–316

[21] Teo EL, Strouse PJ, Hernandez RJ. MR imaging differentiation of soft-tissue hemangiomas from malignant soft-tissue masses. AJR Am J Roentgenol. 2000; 174(6):1623–1628

[22] Wierzbicki JM, Henderson JH, Scarborough MT, Bush CH, Reith JD, Clugston JR. Intramuscular hemangiomas. Sports Health. 2013; 5(5):448–454

[23] Richter GT, Friedman AB. Hemangiomas and vascular malformations: current theory and management. Int J Pediatr. 2012; 2012:645678

[24] Greenspan A, McGahan JP, Vogelsang P, Szabo RM. Imaging strategies in the evaluation of soft-tissue hemangiomas of the extremities: correlation of the findings of plain radiography, angiography, CT, MRI, and ultrasonography in 12 histologically proven cases. Skeletal Radiol. 1992; 21(1):11–18

[25] De Schepper AM, Vanhoenacker F, Gielen J, Parizel PM, eds. Imaging of Soft Tissue Tumors. Berlin: Springer; 2005

[26] Fayad LM, Hazirolan T, Bluemke D, Mitchell S. Vascular malformations in the extremities: emphasis on MR imaging features that guide treatment options. Skeletal Radiol. 2006; 35(3):127–137

[27] Suh JS, Hwang G, Hahn SB. Soft tissue hemangiomas: MR manifestations in 23 patients. Skeletal Radiol. 1994; 23(8):621–625

[28] Walker EA, Song AJ, Murphey MD. Magnetic resonance imaging of soft-tissue masses. Semin Roentgenol. 2010; 45(4):277–297

[29] Cohen EK, Kressel HY, Perosio T, et al. MR imaging of soft-tissue hemangiomas: correlation with pathologic findings. AJR Am J Roentgenol. 1988; 150(5):1079–1081

[30] Blakley P, Louis DN, Short MP, MacCollin M. A clinical study of patients with multiple isolated neurofibromas. J Med Genet. 2001; 38(7):485–488

[31] Rodriguez FJ, Folpe AL, Giannini C, Perry A. Pathology of peripheral nerve sheath tumors: diagnostic overview and update on selected diagnostic problems. Acta Neuropathol. 2012; 123(3):295–319

[32] Williams VC, Lucas J, Babcock MA, Gutmann DH, Korf B, Maria BL. Neurofibromatosis type 1 revisited. Pediatrics. 2009; 123(1):124–133

[33] Friedman JM. Neurofibromatosis 1. 1998 Oct 2 [updated 2025 Apr 3]. In: Adam MP, Feldman J, Mirzaa GM, Pagon RA, Wallace SE, Amemiya A, editors. GeneReviews® [Internet]. Seattle (WA): University of Washington, Seattle; 1993–2025

[34] Mautner VF, Asuagbor FA, Dombi E, et al. Assessment of benign tumor burden by whole-body MRI in patients with neurofibromatosis 1. Neuro-oncol. 2008; 10(4):593–598

[35] Goldblum JR, Folpe AL, Weiss SW. Benign tumors of peripheral nerves. In: Enzinger and Weiss's Soft Tissue Tumors. Philadelphia: Saunders; 2014:784–854

[36] Evans HL. Sporadic superficial diffuse neurofibromas with repeated local recurrence over many years and a tendency toward malignant change: a report of 3 cases. Am J Surg Pathol. 2013; 37(7):987–994

[37] Murphey MD, Smith WS, Smith SE, Kransdorf MJ, Temple HT. From the archives of the AFIP. Imaging of musculoskeletal neurogenic tumors: radiologic-pathologic correlation. Radiographics. 1999; 19(5):1253–1280

[38] Jee WH, Oh SN, McCauley T, et al. Extraaxial neurofibromas versus neurilemmomas: discrimination with MRI. AJR Am J Roentgenol. 2004; 183(3): 629–633

[39] Lin J, Martel W. Cross-sectional imaging of peripheral nerve sheath tumors: characteristic signs on CT, MR imaging, and sonography. AJR Am J Roentgenol. 2001; 176(1):75–82

[40] Suh JS, Abenoza P, Galloway HR, Everson LI, Griffiths HJ. Peripheral (extracranial) nerve tumors: correlation of MR imaging and histologic findings. Radiology. 1992; 183(2):341–346

[41] Vilanova JC, Woertler K, Narváez JA, et al. Soft-tissue tumors update: MR imaging features according to the WHO classification. Eur Radiol. 2007; 17 (1):125–138

[42] Sullivan TP, Seeger LL, Doberneck SA, Eckardt JJ. Case report 828: plexiform neurofibroma of the tibial nerve invading the medial and lateral gastrocnemius muscles and plantaris muscle. Skeletal Radiol. 1994; 23(2): 149–152

[43] Demehri S, Belzberg A, Blakeley J, Fayad LM. Conventional and functional MR imaging of peripheral nerve sheath tumors: initial experience. AJNR Am J Neuroradiol. 2014; 35(8):1615–1620

[44] Fayad LM, Wang X, Blakeley JO, et al. Characterization of peripheral nerve sheath tumors with 3T proton MR spectroscopy. AJNR Am J Neuroradiol. 2014; 35(5):1035–1041

[45] Beaman FD, Kransdorf MJ, Menke DM. Schwannoma: radiologic-pathologic correlation. Radiographics. 2004; 24(5):1477–1481

[46] Kurtkaya-Yapicier O, Scheithauer B, Woodruff JM. The pathobiologic spectrum of Schwannomas. Histol Histopathol. 2003; 18(3):925–934

[47] Walker EA, Fenton ME, Salesky JS, Murphey MD. Magnetic resonance imaging of benign soft tissue neoplasms in adults. Radiol Clin North Am. 2011; 49(6):1197–1217, vi

[48] Wippold FJ, II, Lubner M, Perrin RJ, Lämmle M, Perry A. Neuropathology for the neuroradiologist: Antoni A and Antoni B tissue patterns. AJNR Am J Neuroradiol. 2007; 28(9):1633–1638

[49] Lee YS, Kim JO, Park SE. Ancient schwannoma of the thigh mimicking a malignant tumour: a report of two cases, with emphasis on MRI findings. Br J Radiol. 2010; 83(991):e154–e157

[50] Lucas DR. Tenosynovial giant cell tumor: case report and review. Arch Pathol Lab Med. 2012; 136(8):901–906

[51] Briët JP, Becker SJ, Oosterhoff TCh, Ring D. Giant cell tumor of tendon sheath. Arch Bone Jt Surg. 2015; 3(1):19–21

[52] Horvai AE, Link T. Tenosynovial giant cell tumor, diffuse type. In: Bone and Soft Tissue Pathology. Philadelphia: Saunders; 2012:62–63

[53] Dercle L, Chisin R, Ammari S, et al. Nonsurgical giant cell tumour of the tendon sheath or of the diffuse type: are MRI or 18F-FDG PET/CT able to provide an accurate prediction of long-term outcome? Eur J Nucl Med Mol Imaging. 2015; 42(3):397–408

[54] Jelinek JS, Kransdorf MJ, Shmookler BM, Aboulafia AA, Malawer MM. Giant cell tumor of the tendon sheath: MR findings in nine cases. AJR Am J Roentgenol. 1994; 162(4):919–922

[55] Llauger J, Palmer J, Rosón N, Cremades R, Bagué S. Pigmented villonodular synovitis and giant cell tumors of the tendon sheath: radiologic and pathologic features. AJR Am J Roentgenol. 1999; 172(4):1087–1091

[56] Spritzer CE, Dalinka MK, Kressel HY. Magnetic resonance imaging of pigmented villonodular synovitis: a report of two cases. Skeletal Radiol. 1987; 16(4):316–319

[57] De Beuckeleer L, De Schepper A, De Belder F, et al. Magnetic resonance imaging of localized giant cell tumour of the tendon sheath (MRI of localized GCTTS). Eur Radiol. 1997; 7(2):198–201

[58] Demouy EH, Kaneko K, Bear HM, Rodriguez RP. Giant cell tumor of the plantar tendon sheath: role of MR imaging in diagnosis. Case report. Clin Imaging. 1993; 17(2):153–155

[59] Baoge L, Van Den Steen E, Rimbaut S, et al. Treatment of skeletal muscle injury: a review. ISRN Orthop. 2012; 2012:689012

[60] Conforti M. The treatment of muscle hematomas. In: Bisciotti N, Eirale C, eds. Muscle Injuries in Sport Medicine. Croatia: InTech; 2013:203–220

[61] Dohan A, Darnige L, Sapoval M, Pellerin O. Spontaneous soft tissue hematomas. Diagn Interv Imaging. 2015; 96(7–8):789–796

[62] Bush CH. The magnetic resonance imaging of musculoskeletal hemorrhage. Skeletal Radiol. 2000; 29(1):1–9

[63] Safran MR, Zachazewski J, Stone DA. Myositis ossificans. In: Instructions for Sports Medicine Patients. Philadelphia: Saunders; 2012:667–668

[64] Lau J, Hartin CW, Jr, Ozgediz DE. Myositis ossificans requires multiple diagnostic modalities. J Pediatr Surg. 2012; 47(9):1763–1766

[65] Kransdorf MJ, Meis JM, Jelinek JS. Myositis ossificans: MR appearance with radiologic-pathologic correlation. AJR Am J Roentgenol. 1991; 157(6):1243–1248

[66] De Smet AA, Norris MA, Fisher DR. Magnetic resonance imaging of myositis ossificans: analysis of seven cases. Skeletal Radiol. 1992; 21(8):503–507

[67] Kransdorf MJ, Meis JM. From the archives of the AFIP. Extraskeletal osseous and cartilaginous tumors of the extremities. Radiographics. 1993; 13(4): 853–884

[68] Yaghmai I. Myositis ossificans: diagnostic value of arteriography. AJR Am J Roentgenol. 1977; 128(5):811–816

[69] Gaspari R. US guided versus blindI&D for treatment of soft tissue abscesses in the ED. Accessed February 21, 2017 at: https://clinicaltrials.gov/ct2/show/study/NCT02264392

[70] Heilpern KL. Skin and soft tissue abscesses: the case for culturing abscess fluid. Ann Emerg Med. 2007; 50(1):64–66

[71] Nalmas S, Bishburg E, Shah M, Chan T. Skin and soft tissue abscess: 1 year's experience. J Cutan Med Surg. 2009; 13(5):257–261

[72] Beaman FD, Kransdorf MJ, Andrews TR, Murphey MD, Arcara LK, Keeling JH. Superficial soft-tissue masses: analysis, diagnosis, and differential considerations. Radiographics. 2007; 27(2):509–523

[73] Hopkins KL, Li KC, Bergman G. Gadolinium-DTPA-enhanced magnetic resonance imaging of musculoskeletal infectious processes. Skeletal Radiol. 1995; 24(5):325–330

[74] Wall SD, Fisher MR, Amparo EG, Hricak H, Higgins CB. Magnetic resonance imaging in the evaluation of abscesses. AJR Am J Roentgenol. 1985; 144(6): 1217–1221

[75] Lalam RK, Cassar-Pullicino VN, Tins BJ. Magnetic resonance imaging of appendicular musculoskeletal infection. Top Magn Reson Imaging. 2007; 18 (3):177–191

[76] Armitage JO, Bierman PJ. Approach to the patient with lymphadenopathy and splenomegaly. In: Goldman L, Schafer AI, eds. Goldman-Cecil Medicine. Philadelphia: Saunders; 2016:1138–1142.e1132

[77] Tower RL, Camitta BM. Lymphadenopathy. In: Kliegman RM, Stanton BF, St Geme JW, Schor NF, eds. Nelson Textbook of Pediatrics. Philadelphia: Elsevier; 2016:2413–2415.e2412

[78] Taupitz M, Beyersdorff D. Intra-abdominal Lymph nodes. In: Hamm B, Krestin GP, Laniado M, Nicolas V, Taupitz M, eds. MR Imaging of the Abdomen and Pelvis. Stuttgart: Thieme; 2009:331–340

[79] Laissy JP, Gay-Depassier P, Soyer P, et al. Enlarged mediastinal lymph nodes in bronchogenic carcinoma: assessment with dynamic contrast-enhanced MR imaging. Work in progress. Radiology. 1994; 191(1):263–267

[80] Harisinghani MG, Saini S, Weissleder R, et al. MR lymphangiography using ultrasmall superparamagnetic iron oxide in patients with primary

abdominal and pelvic malignancies: radiographic-pathologic correlation. AJR Am J Roentgenol. 1999; 172(5):1347–1351

[81] Goldblum JR, Folpe AL, Weiss SW. Liposarcoma. In: Enzinger and Weiss's Soft Tissue Tumors. Philadelphia: Saunders; 2014:484–523

[82] Jaovisidha S, Suvikapakornkul Y, Woratanarat P, Subhadrabandhu T, Nartthanarung A, Siriwongpairat P. MR imaging of fat-containing tumours: the distinction between lipoma and liposarcoma. Singapore Med J. 2010; 51(5): 418–423

[83] Arkun R, Memis A, Akalin T, Ustun EE, Sabah D, Kandiloglu G. Liposarcoma of soft tissue: MRI findings with pathologic correlation. Skeletal Radiol. 1997; 26(3):167–172

[84] Jelinek JS, Kransdorf MJ, Shmookler BM, Aboulafia AJ, Malawer MM. Liposarcoma of the extremities: MR and CT findings in the histologic subtypes. Radiology. 1993; 186(2):455–459

[85] Miller TT, Hermann G, Abdelwahab IF, Klein MJ, Kenan S, Lewis MM. MRI of malignant fibrous histiocytoma of soft tissue: analysis of 13 cases with pathologic correlation. Skeletal Radiol. 1994; 23(4):271–275

[86] Mahajan H, Kim EE, Wallace S, Abello R, Benjamin R, Evans HL. Magnetic resonance imaging of malignant fibrous histiocytoma. Magn Reson Imaging. 1989; 7(3):283–288

[87] Murphey MD, Gross TM, Rosenthal HG. From the archives of the AFIP. Musculoskeletal malignant fibrous histiocytoma: radiologic-pathologic correlation. Radiographics. 1994; 14(4):807–826, quiz 827–828

[88] Thway K, Fisher C. Synovial sarcoma: defining features and diagnostic evolution. Ann Diagn Pathol. 2014; 18(6):369–380

[89] Jones BC, Sundaram M, Kransdorf MJ. Synovial sarcoma: MR imaging findings in 34 patients. AJR Am J Roentgenol. 1993; 161(4):827–830

[90] Murphey MD, Gibson MS, Jennings BT, Crespo-Rodríguez AM, Fanburg-Smith J, Gajewski DA. From the archives of the AFIP: imaging of synovial sarcoma with radiologic-pathologic correlation. Radiographics. 2006; 26(5): 1543–1565

[91] Mahajan H, Lorigan JG, Shirkhoda A. Synovial sarcoma: MR imaging. Magn Reson Imaging. 1989; 7(2):211–216

[92] Walker EA, Salesky JS, Fenton ME, Murphey MD. Magnetic resonance imaging of malignant soft tissue neoplasms in the adult. Radiol Clin North Am. 2011; 49(6):1219–1234, vi

[93] Horvai AE, Link T. Myxofibrosarcoma. In: Bone and Soft Tissue Pathology. Philadelphia: Saunders; 2012:279–280

[94] Li W, Li D, Zhu X, Lu S, He C, Yang Q. Low-grade myxofibrosarcoma following a metal implantation in femur: a case report. Diagn Pathol. 2014; 9:6

[95] Yoo HJ, Hong SH, Kang Y, et al. MR imaging of myxofibrosarcoma and undifferentiated sarcoma with emphasis on tail sign; diagnostic and prognostic value. Eur Radiol. 2014; 24(8):1749–1757

[96] Kaya M, Wada T, Nagoya S, et al. MRI and histological evaluation of the infiltrative growth pattern of myxofibrosarcoma. Skeletal Radiol. 2008; 37 (12):1085–1090

[97] Carroll G, Breidahl W, Robbins P. Musculoskeletal lymphoma: MRI of bone or soft tissue presentations. J Med Imaging Radiat Oncol. 2013; 57 (6):663–673

[98] Suresh S, Saifuddin A, O'Donnell P. Lymphoma presenting as a musculoskeletal soft tissue mass: MRI findings in 24 cases. Eur Radiol. 2008; 18(11):2628–2634

[99] Chun CW, Jee WH, Park HJ, et al. MRI features of skeletal muscle lymphoma. AJR Am J Roentgenol. 2010; 195(6):1355–1360

[100] Hosono M, Kobayashi H, Kotoura Y, Tsuboyama T, Tsutsui K, Konishi J. Involvement of muscle by malignant lymphoma: MR and CT appearances. J Comput Assist Tomogr. 1995; 19(3):455–459

[101] Lee VS, Martinez S, Coleman RE. Primary muscle lymphoma: clinical and imaging findings. Radiology. 1997; 203(1):237–244

[102] Molina-Garrido MJ, Guillén-Ponce C. Muscle metastasis of carcinoma. Clin Transl Oncol. 2011; 13(2):98–101

[103] Rosai J. Soft tissues. In: Rosai & Ackerman's Surgical Pathology. Philadelphia: Elsevier; 2011:2105–2232

[104] Perisano C, Spinelli MS, Graci C, et al. Soft tissue metastases in lung cancer: a review of the literature. Eur Rev Med Pharmacol Sci. 2012; 16 (14):1908–1914

[105] Sudo A, Ogihara Y, Shiokawa Y, Fujinami S, Sekiguchi S. Intramuscular metastasis of carcinoma. Clin Orthop Relat Res. 1993(296):213–217

[106] Tuoheti Y, Okada K, Osanai T, et al. Skeletal muscle metastases of carcinoma: a clinicopathological study of 12 cases. Jpn J Clin Oncol. 2004; 34(4):210–214

20 Bone Tumors

Keith T. Aziz, Jonathan A. Forsberg, Edward F. McCarthy, Laura M. Fayad, Carol D. Morris, and Adam S. Levin

Abstract

MRI offers several advantages to plain radiographs in the evaluation of bone tumors. The aim of this chapter was to provide an overview of the features of benign and malignant bone tumors when evaluated with MRI. Although the clinical presentation of bone tumors is typically nonspecific, MRI allows for narrowing the differential diagnoses based on characteristic findings that we have outlined in this chapter. Examples of benign bone tumors covered in this chapter include osteoid osteoma, osteoblastoma, chondroblastoma, periosteal chondroma, enchondroma, osteochondroma, giant cell tumor, aneurysmal bone cyst, unicameral bone cyst, nonossifying fibroma and fibrous dysplasia. Malignant bone tumors that are covered include osteosarcoma, Ewing sarcoma and chondrosarcoma. By the end of this chapter, the reader will be familiar with the characteristic findings and considerations when interpreting MRI for each of these benign and malignant bone tumors.

Keywords: benign tumor, extremity, malignant tumor, osseous tumor, tumor characterization

20.1 Introduction

Osseous tumors and tumor-like lesions are often found incidentally on radiographs, and clinical presentation is frequently nonspecific, with features that may indicate any of several abnormal processes and injuries. A detailed history is valuable when attempting to differentiate benign conditions from aggressive tumor-like lesions, malignancies, or osseous neoplasms. A history of pain that awakens the patient during sleep or pain unrelieved by rest should prompt concern about a potential neoplasm or malignancy. Patient age and anatomic location of the lesion should be considered when a tumor or tumor-like lesion is noted because these factors can be highly associated with certain pathologies.

Radiographs and advanced cross-sectional imaging are key components of a thorough assessment, and familiarity with the imaging appearance of neoplastic processes is critical in appropriately managing patients. Magnetic resonance imaging (MRI) is used increasingly as an assessment tool in orthopaedic practice because its availability, cost, and diagnostic accuracy have improved. In the presence of bone tumors, MRI is used primarily for staging and preoperative planning. It offers a number of advantages versus conventional radiographs when assessing a lesion, particularly for establishing the extent of the lesion and determining its internal characteristics. These advantages include earlier visualization of bone loss and periosteal reaction, superior visualization of intramedullary involvement and soft-tissue invasion, and optimal assessment of intra-articular involvement, if any. Assessing tumor response to neoadjuvant therapy, detecting posttreatment recurrence, and improving tumor characterization require advanced imaging techniques that are beyond the scope of this chapter.[1]

Although these advantages emphasize the importance of MRI in musculoskeletal medicine, it must be emphasized that diagnosis typically cannot be based on MRI findings alone. A diagnosis should be made on the basis of appropriate imaging, discussion with a musculoskeletal radiologist and pathologist, patient history, and physical examination. This section focuses on the MRI characteristics of osseous lesions in the extremities.

20.2 Benign Tumors

20.2.1 Osteoid Osteoma

Osteoid osteomas are relatively common, painful benign skeletal neoplasms, classically presenting with pain that is worse at night and that frequently awakens the patient from sleep.[2,3,4,5] This lesion represents ~2 to 3% of all skeletal lesions.[6,7,8,9] It is most frequently observed in male patients between the ages of 10 and 20 years. The lesion most often occurs in lower extremity long bones; however, it can be seen in nearly any location, including the spine.[9,10,11,12] The underlying lesion is referred to as a nidus, which is radiolucent, often with a thick rim of dense reactive bone.[9,13]

Classically, a patient presents with progressively worsening pain that is relieved with nonsteroidal anti-inflammatory drugs.[9,14,15,16] The nidus has been shown to produce prostaglandins, which often irritate adjacent tissues.[17,18] The inflammation caused by the nidus may be so profound that it may cause scoliosis or growth plate disturbances in skeletally immature patients.[19,20,21]

Although osteoid osteoma can often be identified on plain radiographs, in certain cases, cross-sectional imaging is required for definitive diagnosis. Typically, computed tomography (CT) is optimal for identifying a small nidus; however, some diagnostic features can be identified by MRI, as well.

Optimally, the nidus would be identified as a small focus that has variable signal intensity on T1- and T2-weighted images.[22,23,24] However, in some cases the nidus is not definitively identified but the extensive surrounding inflammatory reaction is. Tissue surrounding the lesion has increased signal on T2-weighted images, presumably because of inflammation and edema.[22,23,24] Gadolinium causes enhancement of the lesion that can be better identified when combined with fat-suppression techniques.[25] When an osteoid osteoma is suspected, T1-weighted imaging with gadolinium can provide superior results, showing the nidus of the osteoid osteoma 82% of the time on the arterial phase, and with conspicuity equal to that of thin-segment CT.[24]

Although augmentation of MRI with contrast and targeted sequencing can improve the accuracy of MRI for diagnosing osteoid osteoma, the increased cellular infiltrate, edema, and vascularity around the nidus frequently prevent accurate diagnosis with MRI compared with other modalities.[26,27] MRI is not the ideal imaging modality for all lesions. In the case of osteoid osteoma, in which the lesion is often small and consists of an osseous abnormality, the excellent spatial resolution and osseous detail provided by CT make it a better choice than MRI when conventional radiography is insufficient for diagnosis. Treating osteoid osteoma may consist of long-term nonsteroidal anti-inflammatory drugs or aspirin, RF ablation, or surgical excision (▶ Fig. 20.1).[9,14,15,16,28]

20.2.2 Osteoblastoma

Osteoblastomas account for ~4% of benign primary skeletal tumors and cause many symptoms that are similar to those of osteoid osteoma, notably local pain, swelling, and tenderness that is worse at night.[29] Osteoblastomas present most frequently in the second through third decades of life and affect men twice as frequently as women.[30,31,32] The lesion is commonly located in the ankle, femur, proximal humerus, or spine.[29] Although osteoblastomas are histologically similar to osteoid osteomas, they may have distinct clinical and radiologic progression. Unlike osteoid osteomas, osteoblastomas are typically larger and can show progressive growth.[33,34]

Osteoblastomas are well visualized on plain radiographs but can have a variable presentation on imaging, especially because ~25% of lesions have a more aggressive radiographic appearance.[35,36] Osteoblastomas can have an analogous appearance to a large osteoid osteoma, can be primarily lytic, or can have a similar appearance to osteosarcoma. Most osteoblastomas are hypointense to isointense compared with muscle on T1-weighted images.[35,37] The presentation on T2-weighted imaging is varied and may be hypointense, isointense, or hyperintense, depending on the mineralized matrix and internal composition.[37,38] Osteoblastomas are highly vascular and enhance avidly after contrast administration.[37,38] Cross-sectional imaging often shows paravertebral atrophy, which may be a cause of scoliosis (similar to osteoid osteomas).[39] Treating osteoblastoma typically consists of curettage with local adjuvant treatment, though more destructive lesions may benefit from en bloc resection (▶ Fig. 20.2).[29,37]

20.2.3 Chondroblastoma

Chondroblastoma is a rare cartilaginous primary bone tumor that accounts for < 1% of all primary bone tumors.[40] Patients frequently present with pain and occasionally stiffness or joint effusion because the tumor often localizes to the epiphysis or apophysis.[40,41,42] Nearly 70% of chondroblastomas present in the second decade of life.[43,44] Chondroblastomas are two to three times as common in men as in women.[43] Anatomically, femur, humerus, and tibia are most commonly affected, with lesions originating in the epiphysis with extension into the metaphysis in up to 50% of cases.[41,43,45]

Plain radiographs typically show a well-circumscribed lytic epiphyseal lesion, often with a sclerotic rim and occasionally

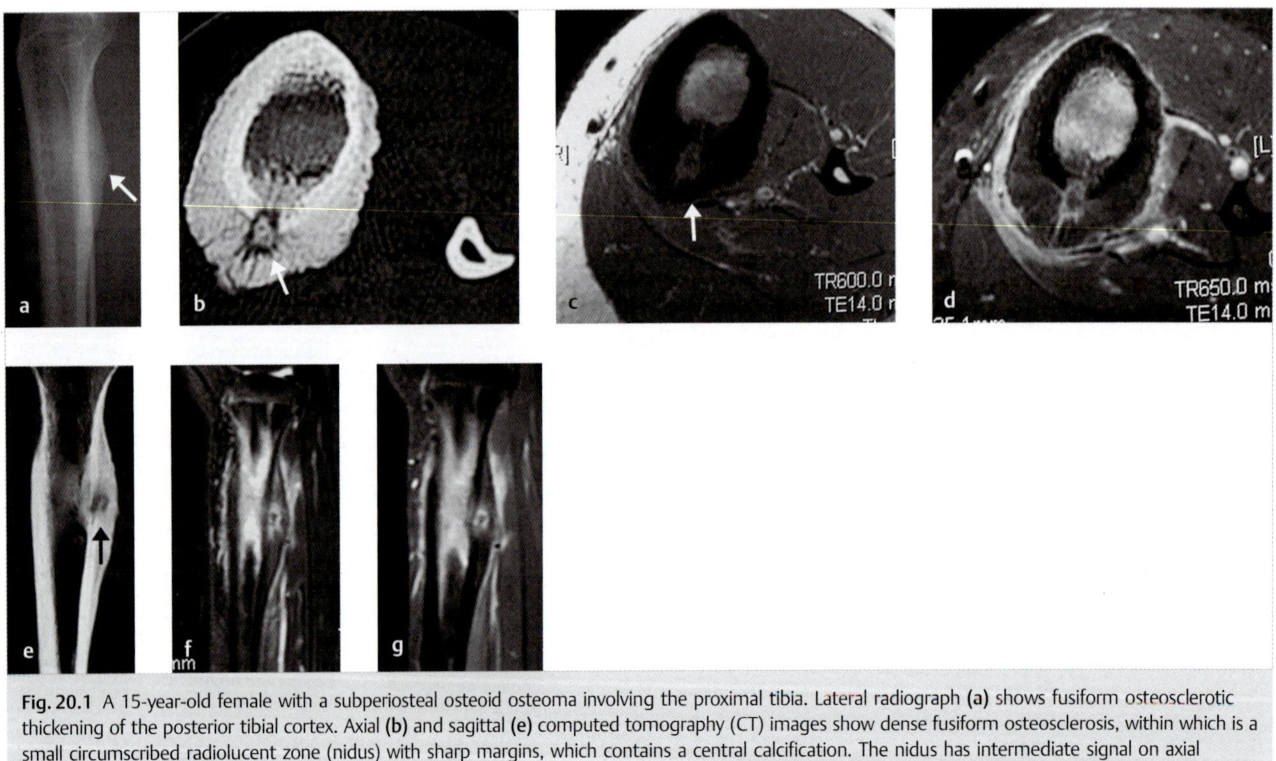

Fig. 20.1 A 15-year-old female with a subperiosteal osteoid osteoma involving the proximal tibia. Lateral radiograph **(a)** shows fusiform osteosclerotic thickening of the posterior tibial cortex. Axial **(b)** and sagittal **(e)** computed tomography (CT) images show dense fusiform osteosclerosis, within which is a small circumscribed radiolucent zone (nidus) with sharp margins, which contains a central calcification. The nidus has intermediate signal on axial T1-weighted imaging (T1WI) **(c)**, and high signal on sagittal fat-suppressed (FS) T2-weighted imaging (T2WI) **(f)**. The small central calcification in the nidus has low signal on T1WI and FS T2WI. The thickened cortex adjacent to the nidus has low and slightly high signal on FS T2WI, and is associated with periosteal reaction with high signal. The nidus shows gadolinium (Gd)-contrast enhancement on axial **(d)** and sagittal **(g)** FS T1WI. Prominent Gd-contrast enhancement is seen at the periosteal reaction, and mild diffuse enhancement is seen in the cortical thickening adjacent to the enhancing nidus. Poorly defined zones of high signal on FS T2WI and corresponding Gd-contrast enhancement on FS T1WI are also seen in the marrow adjacent to the lesion. (Figure part **a**, **b**, **c**, and **d**: Reproduced with permission from, Meyers S. MRI findings. In: Meyers S, ed. MRI of Bone and Soft Tissue Tumors and Tumorlike Lesions. 1st Edition. Thieme; 2007.) (Figure part **e**, **f**, and **g**: Reproduced with permission from, Meyers S. Lesions associated with thickening of bone cortex. In: Meyers S, ed. MRI of Bone and Soft Tissue Tumors and Tumor like Lesions. 1st Edition. Stuttgart: Georg Thieme Verlag KG; 2007.)

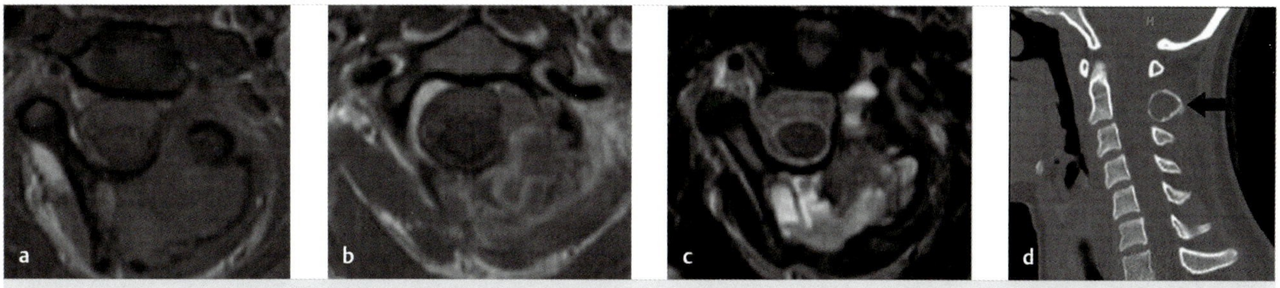

Fig. 20.2 Left-side cervical osteoblastoma. Axial (a) precontrast and (b) postcontrast T1-weighted images showing a lesion similar to (but larger than) the osteoid osteoma shown in Fig. 21.5. The lesion shows heterogeneous contrast enhancement with infiltration into the epidural space. (c) An axial T2-weighted image also shows the lesion. (d) A sagittal computed tomography (CT) reconstruction highlights the osseous destruction and expansion associated with the osteoblastoma in the spinous process (*arrow*). (Reproduced with permission from, Extradural Tumors. In: Khanna A, ed. MRI Essentials for the Spine Specialist. 1st Edition. Thieme; 2014.)

with periosteal reaction.[46,47] On MRI, the lesion is typically isointense to muscle on T1-weighted images.[47] On T2-weighted images, the lesion is fairly heterogeneous, with some features suggesting chondroid matrix.[45,47,48] The periphery of the tumor shows hypointensity and is often associated with prominent marrow edema and surrounding soft-tissue reaction.[43,45,48] A fluid–fluid level within the tumor is seen in ~20% of cases, although it may occur in up to 50% of chondroblastomas in the foot[49] and is often associated with secondary aneurysmal bone cyst (ABC) formation. Although chondroblastomas are benign, occasionally they develop benign lung metastases.[50] Chondroblastomas are treated by bone grafting, curettage, or local adjuvant, although 7 to 13% may recur after intralesional treatment (▶ Fig. 20.3).[45,51]

20.2.4 Periosteal Chondroma

Periosteal chondroma is a rare cartilage tumor that arises within the periosteum and accounts for ~1 to 2% of all cartilaginous tumors.[52,53,54,55] Periosteal chondromas often present initially with localized swelling, followed by mild to moderate pain.[55,56] The lesion presents most commonly in patients < 30 years of age, with the greatest frequency during the first and second decades of life.[55,56] The most common locations are the small bones of the hands and feet, although periosteal chondroma may occur in the long bones such as the proximal humerus and proximal tibia.[52,53,54,55,56] Periosteal chondromas are often present at the metaphysis or at the insertion site of a tendon or ligament. Despite their rarity, periosteal chondromas have a fairly distinct radiographic appearance, which helps facilitate their diagnosis.

On plain radiographs, there is a juxtacortical lesion that causes scalloping of the adjacent cortex, with lobules of calcified cartilage in approximately half of all lesions.[52,54] On T1-weighted images, the lesion is hypointense to isointense compared with muscle and shows a sharp demarcation compared with the underlying cortex.[52,55,57] A well-defined, smooth scalloping of the cortex is evident. On T2-weighted and short tau inversion recovery (STIR) images, the lesion will appear hyperintense with an intact periosteum.[52,55,57] If enhancement occurs with gadolinium, it commonly occurs at the periphery where the vascular supply for the lesion is located (▶ Fig. 20.4).[52,55,57]

20.2.5 Enchondroma

Enchondromas are fairly common benign tumors that comprise lobules of hyaline cartilage.[16,58] The lesion is often centrally located in the metaphyseal or metadiaphyseal region.[9,16,58] This is one of the most common lesions of the short tubular bones of the hands and feet, with some reports suggesting that up to half of all enchondromas present in the hand.[9,34,58] Enchondromas are commonly discovered incidentally while evaluating other processes. Although typically asymptomatic, these lesions may present with an abnormal fracture. Enchondromas may present at any age, though they are thought to develop during embryogenesis or early childhood.

On conventional radiographs, the lesion appears lucent, often with the characteristic ring and arc or stippled calcifications that are characteristic of cartilage lesions.[34,59] However, this lesion can appear without these findings if the cartilaginous components of the lesion have not yet calcified. Advanced cross-sectional imaging has been advocated as a noninvasive way to assess the malignant potential of cartilaginous lesions.[60] On T1-weighted MRI, the lesion is typically isointense to skeletal muscle. Less frequently, an area of high signal may be seen, representing intermixed intramedullary fat on a non–fat-suppressed image.[61,62,63] On T2-weighted images, there is high signal intensity in a pattern similar to that of articular cartilage, likely because of the ratio of water content to mucopolysaccharide in the hyaline cartilage.[61,62] With mineralization, there will be signal voids within the enchondroma. These lesions also enhance with gadolinium in a lobular pattern.[60,62,63] When diagnosed with a high degree of certainty, there is no need to biopsy an asymptomatic enchondroma because the lesion can be serially monitored.

It is important to attempt to differentiate between enchondroma and low-grade chondrosarcoma or atypical chondroid neoplasm because the distinction can be subtle. The main clinical symptom that favors a chondrosarcoma is pain, and there are several MRI features that suggest chondrosarcoma,

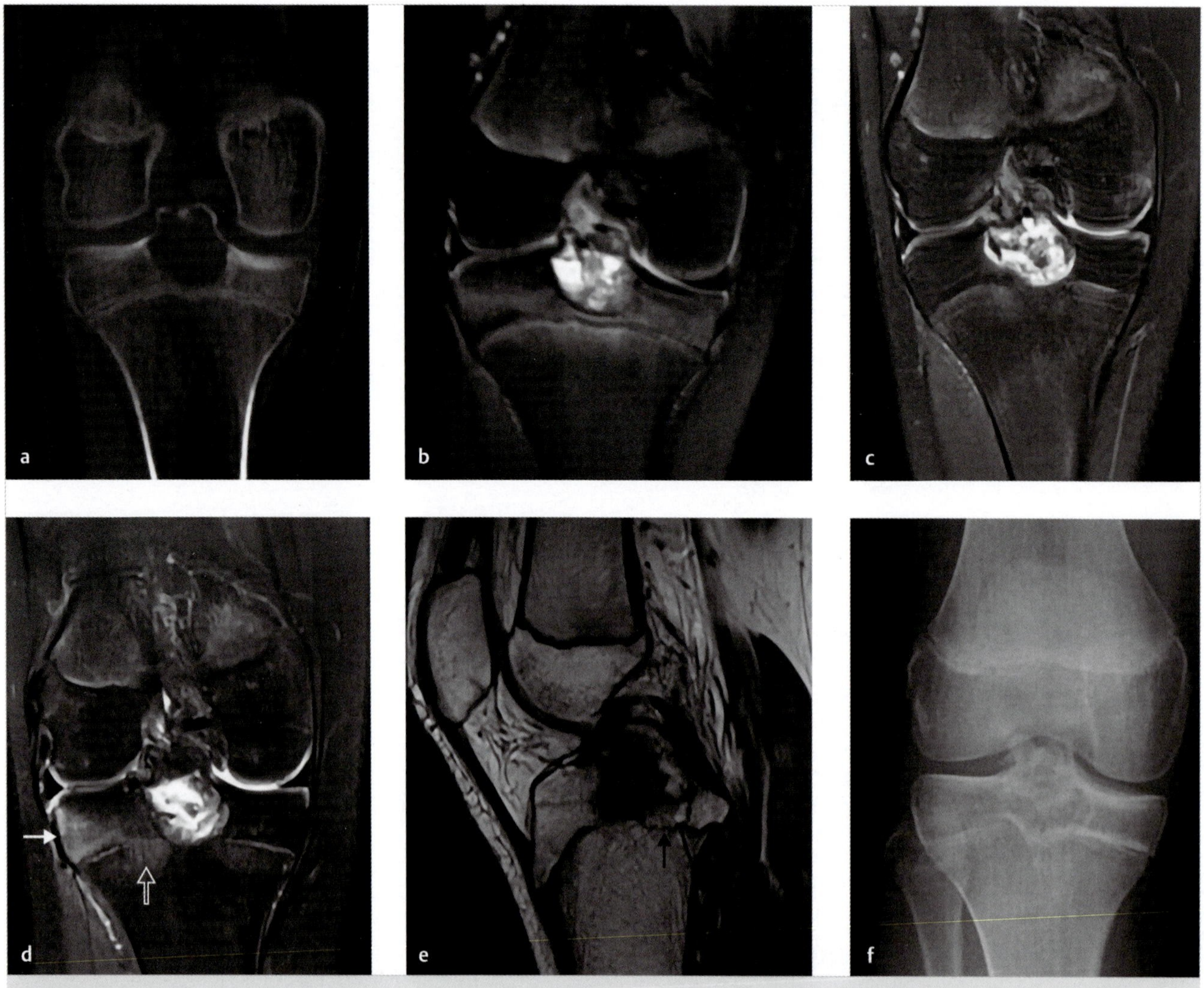

Fig. 20.3 (a) Coronal computed tomography reformatted image of a 13-year-old patient with a proximal tibial epiphyseal chondroblastoma. **(b)** Coronal short tau inversion recovery image showing the lesion and surrounding edema in the proximal tibial epiphysis, secondary to the tumor. **(c)** Coronal proton-density fat-suppressed (PDFS) image at 6 months following radiofrequency ablation of the lesion showing that the lesion has not yet filled in with fatty marrow; however, the perilesional edema has resolved, suggesting the lesion was successfully ablated. **(d)** Coronal PDFS image at 18 months following ablation. There is now stress-related edema at the lateral aspect of the proximal tibia (solid arrow) and bridging marrow/partial fusion across the physis (open arrow), better shown on the sagittal T1 image **(e**, arrow) and the radiograph **(f)**. Premature closure of the physis is a complication of radiofrequency ablation secondary to thermal injury. (Reproduced with permission from, Winn N, Lalam R. Imaging of the knee and surrounding structures following tumor surgery. Seminars in Musculoskeletal Radiology. Thieme Medical Publishers. 2018; 22(4):481–505.)

including cortical destruction, endosteal scalloping, periosteal reaction, and soft-tissue extension.[60] Studies have suggested that a lesion size larger than 5 cm, lesional filling of > 90% of the medullary diameter, growth of the lesion over time, and pain caused by the lesion suggest chondrosarcoma.[59,60]

It is important to be aware of rare, nonhereditary syndromes characterized by multiple osteochondromas, which include Ollier disease and Maffucci syndrome.[64,65,66] Enchondromas in these syndromes may be in a few or several bones.[64,65,66] Patients with either syndrome are at risk for malignancy.[64,65,66] Grossly, there are often growth disturbances because of disruption of the epiphyseal plate, and patients with Maffucci syndrome also have characteristic soft-tissue hemangiomas that may be noted as phleboliths on conventional radiographs (▶ Fig. 20.5).

20.2.6 Osteochondroma

Osteochondromas are the most common benign skeletal tumor and may account for as many as 32% of benign skeletal lesions.[9] Osteochondromas are believed to be derived from a portion of the physis that grows diagonally or perpendicularly to the surface of the bone, away from the joint. In some patients, these may be caused by an abnormal focus of metaplastic cartilage from congenital deficiency, radiation, or trauma.[9,34,67,68] One

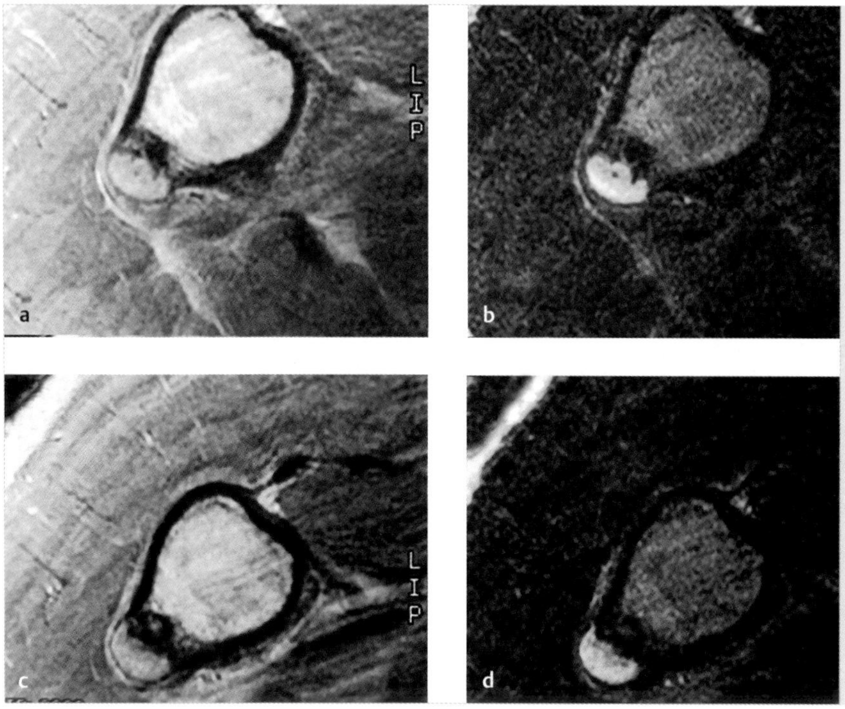

Fig. 20.4 A 28-year-old man with a sessile-type juxtacortical/periosteal chondroma involving the metadiaphyseal region of the humerus. The lesion has heterogeneous predominantly high signal as well as zones of intermediate and low signal on sagittal **(a, c)** fat-suppressed (FS) T2-weighted imaging (T2WI) and axial **(b)** T2WI. The lesion has intermediate signal on axial **(b)** proton density–weighted imaging (PDWI). Periosteal thickening at the base of the lesion is seen as irregular zones of low signal at the outer cortical margin. The lesion shows irregular zones of gadolinium (Gd)-contrast enhancement on sagittal **(d)** T1-weighted imaging (T1WI) and sagittal FS T1WI. (Reproduced with permission from, Meyers S. MRI findings. In: Meyers S, ed. MRI of Bone and Soft Tissue Tumors and Tumorlike Lesions. 1st Edition. Stuttgart: Thieme; 2007.)

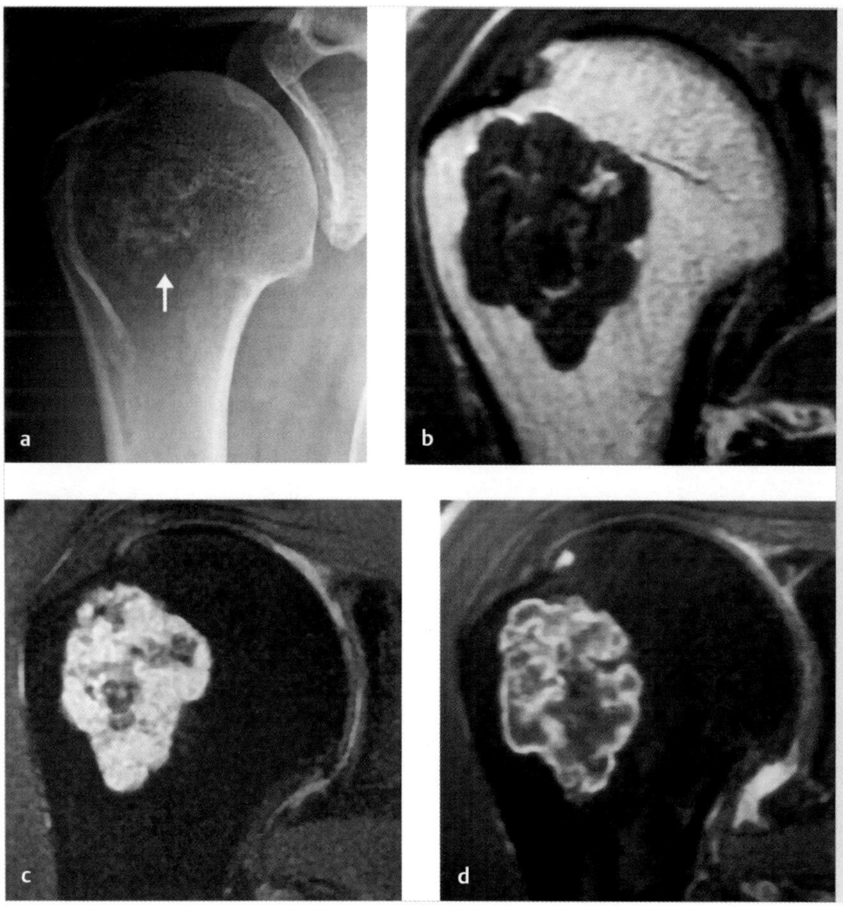

Fig. 20.5 A 46-year-old man with an enchondroma in the metadiaphyseal portion of the proximal humerus, which has chondroid mineralization (*arrow*) on anteroposterior radiograph **(a)**. The lesion has predominantly intermediate signal on coronal proton density–weighted imaging **(b)** and high signal on fat-suppressed (FS) T2-weighted imaging **(c)** as well as zones of low signal corresponding to mineralized chondroid matrix. The lesion shows peripheral lobular contrast enhancement on coronal FS T1-weighted imaging **(d)**. (Reproduced with permission from, Solitary Intramedullary Metadiaphyseal Lesions. In: Hollenberg G, Weinberg E, Meyers S, eds. Differential Diagnosis in Musculoskeletal MRI. 1st Edition. Thieme; 2015.)

study has described the prevalence of osteochondromas in the general population to be as high as 2%.[69] The lesion is most frequently diagnosed during the first four decades of life, with those patients with multiple hereditary exostosis (MHE) commonly presenting early in childhood.[34]

Osteochondromas are characterized by their morphology and are described as sessile or pedunculated. The lesion arises from the surface bone, with the medullary canal and the cortex of the bone being contiguous with the stalk of the lesion. The surface of the osteochondroma is covered in a cartilaginous cap, which is thought to consist of physeal cartilage. This cartilage cap is the site of growth and typically diminishes after skeletal maturity.[34] Although the lesion is commonly asymptomatic, patients may report pain with range of motion (mechanical irritation), or they may have bursae formation, decreased range of motion, fracture, or neurologic or vascular sequelae from direct compression by the lesion.[34,69,70] Rarely, the lesion can undergo malignant degeneration.

Plain radiographs are often diagnostic of osteochondromas and show a lesion with cortical and medullary components that are continuous with the host bone cortex and medullary cavity. The appearance of the cartilage cap of the osteochondroma can vary from imperceptible to a characteristic thick cartilaginous mineralization with ring and arc calcifications. MRI is frequently not indicated in initial diagnosis but can be used to diagnose complications and to rule out malignancy in a symptomatic lesion. T1-weighted MRI shows the tumor's relationship with the affected bone's medullary canal and cortex, confirming the smooth cortical and medullary continuity with the rest of the bone. T2-weighted images show high signal intensity in the cartilage cap, secondary to the high water content. The perichondrium can be appreciated as a thin peripheral zone on T2-weighted images.[71] There may be areas of signal dropout on T2 imaging because of calcifications within the cartilage cap. MRI allows precise measurement of the cartilage cap, and a cartilage cap exceeding 2 cm in adults suggests malignant transformation.[71,72] The measurements of the cartilage thickness in children are variable and do not appear to be related to malignancy.

MHE is a hereditary condition in which patients present with several osteochondromas located diffusely throughout the body.[73] MHE is caused by an autosomal-dominant inactivating mutation in the *EXT1*, *EXT2*, or *EXT3* gene.[74,75] Clinically, these patients present with a number of osteochondromas and often have growth disturbances and malalignment of the affected limbs.[74,75] Because of the multiple osteochondromas, it is more likely for these patients to have symptomatic lesions than patients with solitary osteochondromas, and patients with MHE are at increased risk of developing malignant transformation (▶ Fig. 20.6).[74]

20.2.7 Giant Cell Tumor (GCT)

GCT of the bone is a locally aggressive benign bone tumor that represents ~5% of all primary bone neoplasms.[76] It is most frequently observed in young adults, with a predilection for patients between 20 and 40 years of age.[77,78] GCTs are typically found in the epiphysis and can include the epiphyseal-metaphyseal region.[77,78] GCTs most frequently occur around the knee but may occur in any long bone.[77,78] The lesion causes lytic destruction of the affected bone.[77,78] Because of the destructive nature of the lesion, abnormal fracture or subchondral collapse may be a component of the presentation in anywhere from 11 to 37% of patients.[79,80] Although clinically benign, GCTs have a decreased rate of "benign" lung metastases and an increased rate of local recurrence, with the likelihood of developing a lung metastasis increasing with each recurrence.[81]

Conventional radiographs typically show a poorly marginated lytic lesion with a well-defined nonsclerotic rim. Internal matrix is not typically seen, and associated periosteal reaction is uncommon, though some reactive bone formation may be seen on imaging or pathology. Although the diagnosis may be suspected on plain radiographs, the multiplanar

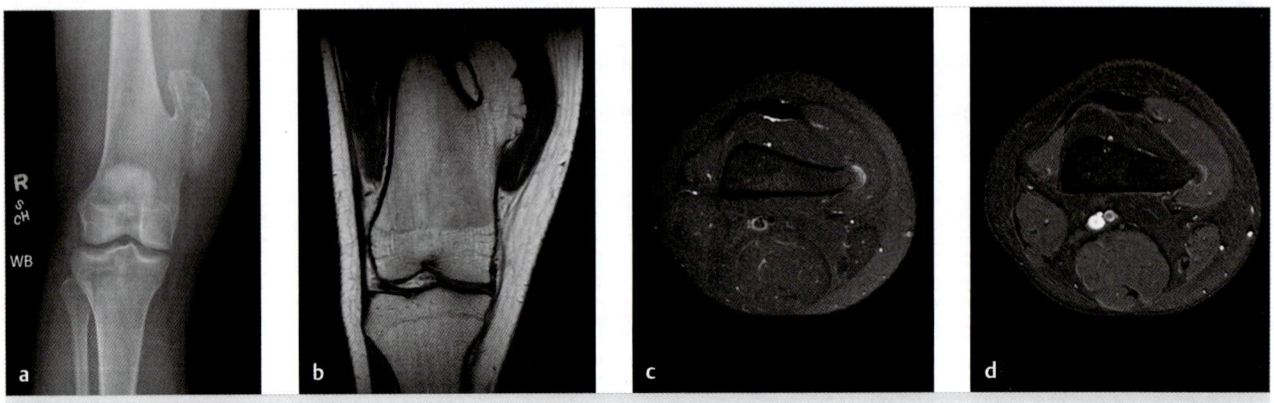

Fig. 20.6 Osteochondromas are typically noted in the metaphysis, and point away from the joint, as seen in this anteroposterior (AP) radiograph of the knee **(a)**. **(b)** Coronal T1 sequences demonstrating complete cortical and medullary continuity with the underlying bone. Axial fat-saturated T2 images **(c)** demonstrating a small cartilage cap, and fat-saturated post-gadolinium images **(d)** showing minimal peripheral enhancement of the cartilage cap.

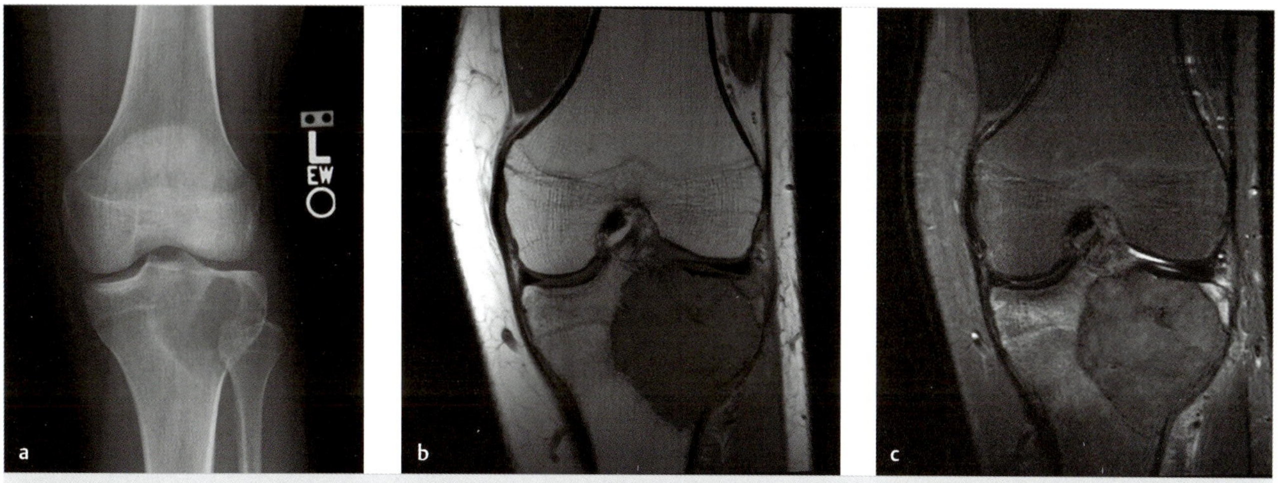

Fig. 20.7 Anteroposterior (AP) radiograph **(a)** demonstrating a lytic lesion involving the epiphysis of the proximal tibia in giant cell tumor of bone. Coronal T1 **(b)** sequences are isointense to muscle, though may be hypointense in some patients. **(c)** On fluid-sensitive sequences like this coronal short tau inversion recovery (STIR) image, giant cell tumors may be hyperintense, though this can have variable appearances due to hemosiderin deposition in some tumors. Some may have secondary aneurysmal bone cyst formation, not evident on these images.

images provided by MRI can be useful for evaluating the extent of the lesion and for detailing the aggressive features and soft-tissue involvement. The MRI signal characteristics of GCT are somewhat inconsistent because ~60% of all GCTs appear dark on all pulse sequences because of hemosiderin deposition.[82,83] Secondary ABC formation may occur, as well.[84] The remaining 40% of GCTs appear isointense to skeletal muscle on T1-weighted images and hyperintense on T2-weighted images.[82,83,85] T1- and T2-weighted images show the aggressive nature of the lesion with typical perilesional edema and can detail any soft-tissue extension that is usually contained by a reactive osseous rim.[83,86] GCTs are typically managed with curettage and bone grafting or cement, though more aggressive tumors can be treated with wide excision. The recurrence rate of GCTs can be reduced to ~10 to 29% using local adjuvants such as argon beam coagulation, exothermic reaction of standard bone cement, high-speed bur after curettage, hydrogen peroxide, liquid nitrogen, or phenol (▶ Fig. 20.7).[87]

20.2.8 ABC

Aneurysmal bone cyst (ABCs) are destructive, benign, cystic expansile lesions that account for ~9% of primary bone lesions.[34] ABCs may occur at any age, but most lesions occur in patients < 20 years old.[88,89] ABCs presenting in older patients are often secondary to other neoplastic processes because a preexisting lesion is observed in ~30% of ABCs overall.[90,91] Anatomically, ABCs most frequently occur around the knee in the distal femur or proximal tibia, followed by the posterior spinal elements, but they can occur in any bone.[34,90,91] These lesions may extend across an open physis but rarely show contiguous involvement of adjacent bones.[92] ABCs can be seen secondary to GCT of bone,[84,93,94] chondroblastoma, nonossifying fibroma (NOF), osteoblastoma, as well as other bone lesions.[84,93,94]

On conventional radiographs, ABCs have a variable appearance but frequently show an eccentric, expansile, lytic lesion with a blown-out osseous cortex.[84,93,94] MRI shows a well-defined lesion with a rim of low signal intensity, typically with internal septations and multiple fluid–fluid levels.[95,96] On T1-weighted images, there is increased signal in the dependent and nondependent fluid believed to be secondary to methemoglobin.[97,98] On T2-weighted imaging, there are fluid–fluid levels of low and high signal related to blood products; and occasionally, perilesional edema is present. After contrast administration, enhancement will be seen in the fibrous tissue of the internal septations but without internal enhancement to suggest a solid neoplasm.[96,97,98] However, secondary ABCs will, in part, display the imaging characteristics of the antecedent lesion with associated cyst formation.

It is important to distinguish a primary ABC from telangiectatic osteosarcoma.[49,99,100] Telangiectatic osteosarcoma shows nodularity in its septations along the rim, which correspond to nests of tumor cells. Similarly, an associated soft-tissue mass occurs in telangiectatic osteosarcoma in 89% of cases.[49,99,100] One of the best ways to distinguish between these lesions is to identify a solid-enhancing component or necrotic tissue associated with hemorrhagic tissue.[100,101]

A variant of ABC has been described, in which the lesion lacks the cystic cavities typically seen, known as a solid ABC.[102] Previous research has shown that 5 to 7.5% of primary ABCs are solid.[102,103] These often have imaging and abnormal features that overlap with GCT of bone, making the diagnosis somewhat challenging (▶ Fig. 20.8).

20.2.9 Unicameral Bone Cyst (UBC)

UBCs are commonly encountered benign cystic lesions, representing ~3% of all bone lesions.[104,105] UBCs most frequently occur within the first two decades of life, with 75 to 85% of UBCs occurring in patients < 25 years of age.[16,104,105] The most common locations include the proximal humerus and proximal femur.[105,106] Some believe that UBCs occur as a result of temporary cessation of medullary bone formation by the

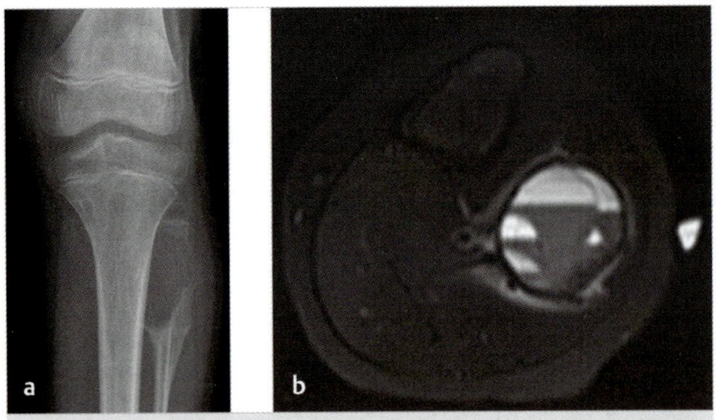

Fig. 20.8 Frontal radiograph of the knee **(a)** showing a lucent expansile lesion in the proximal fibula. Corresponding axial, fat-saturated, T2-weighted magnetic resonance (MR) image of the lesion **(b)** showing multiple fluid–fluid levels. (Reproduced with permission from, Case 19. In: Bindra J, Boutin R, eds. Top 3 Differentials in Musculoskeletal Imaging: A Case Review. 1st Edition. Thieme; 2020.)

epiphyseal plate, which allows for the development of a single-chambered cyst filled with serous fluid.[16] The anatomic location within the bone is typically metaphyseal, although UBCs have been observed in the diaphysis,[16,106] likely after longitudinal growth of the physis away from the lesion. UBCs are most often found in men, with reported ratios as high as 3:1.[104,105] Clinically, most patients with UBCs are asymptomatic unless there is a completed or impending abnormal fracture.[16,104,105]

Conventional radiographs are frequently sufficient to diagnose a UBC, especially when considering patient age, sex, anatomic location, and presentation. However, advanced cross-sectional imaging may be obtained on occasion. On MRI, UBCs show characteristics that are consistent with fluid-filled lesions. On T1-weighted sequences, UBCs show a uniform low signal intensity because of the serous fluid component in the lesion.[106] On fluid-sensitive images, UBCs show high signal consistent with a fluid cavity, although low-signal areas with the fluid–fluid levels can be dark because of the presence of blood products.[106] In addition, the cystic cavity in UBCs will often have multiple incomplete septations within a large cavity. Postgadolinium imaging can typically help confirm the cystic nature of the lesion because the cyst wall will enhance around the periphery of the lesion without internal enhancement.

20.2.10 NOF

NOF is a common benign lesion localized to the metaphysis of children and is believed to be present in 30 to 40% of skeletally immature children.[107,108] This lesion occurs in the metaphysis of long bones, most commonly the femur and tibia.[107] Commonly, the lesions ossify, become sclerotic, and ultimately heal. Fibrous cortical defects describe a similar process localized to the cortex, and the terms fibrous cortical defect, fibroxanthoma, metaphyseal fibrous defect, and NOF are often used interchangeably. In the absence of abnormal fracture or stress fracture, there are often no associated symptoms, and most lesions are discovered incidentally.

On conventional radiographs, NOFs have a characteristic appearance, showing an eccentric, well-defined lytic lesion with a well-defined sclerotic rim.[16] MRI findings can vary and depend on the amount of fibrous tissue relative to other tissue within the lesion, including collagen, hemorrhagic tissue, and osseous trabeculae. Most commonly, the lesion shows low signal intensity on T1-weighted MRI.[109,110] On T2-weighted MRI, NOFs are hypointense to muscle with septations.[109,110] MRI characteristics often reflect the presence of collagen, fibrous tissue, and hemosiderin within the lesion.[109,110] On occasion, NOFs show secondary ABC formation with fluid–fluid levels. Given the variable presentation of NOFs on MRI, it is helpful to compare and correlate findings with conventional radiographs. Unless these lesions cause an abnormal fracture, they typically need no therapy, and often casting is sufficient for treating an abnormal fracture (▶ Fig. 20.9).[111,112]

20.2.11 Fibrous Dysplasia

Fibrous dysplasia is a relatively common developmental disorder that accounts for ~5 to 7% of all benign bone lesions[34] As opposed to being a neoplastic process, this disorder is characterized by failure to form normal lamellar bone.[113] Fibrous dysplasia is characterized by the extent of osseous involvement and can affect one bone (monostotic fibrous dysplasia) or multiple bones (polyostotic fibrous dysplasia).[34,113,114] Monostotic fibrous dysplasia represents ~75% of cases, and patients typically present within the first or second decade of life.[113,115,116] Patients can present at any age, though lesions from fibrous dysplasia, are thought to represent developmental anomalies.[113,115,116] The presenting symptoms are most commonly pain and abnormal fracture.[113]

Conventional radiographs are often diagnostic, showing intramedullary lesions having a "ground-glass" appearance.[16] Affected bones may have a remodeled contour with gross deformity and narrowing of the cortex,[16] occasionally with surrounding sclerosis. Although plain radiographs are typically diagnostic, lesions are occasionally evaluated with cross-sectional imaging. On T1-weighted images, the lesion has low signal intensity and is isointense to skeletal muscle.[117,118,119] There is some variable signal intensity on T2-weighted radiographs, with data suggesting that 79% of all lesions were hypointense and 21% were hyperintense compared with muscle.[117,119] After contrast administration, there is enhancement within the lesion, distinguishing it from a cyst. Because of the variability in presentation on MRI, correlation with conventional radiography is important for diagnosis.[117,119]

Approximately one in five patients presents with polyostotic disease, and these cases are occasionally associated with café-au-lait spots, McCune-Albright syndrome, and other endocrinopathies such as precocious puberty.[34,113] The underlying cause of fibrous dysplasia is a mutation in a gene involved in the G-protein family of receptors (▶ Fig. 20.10).[34,113]

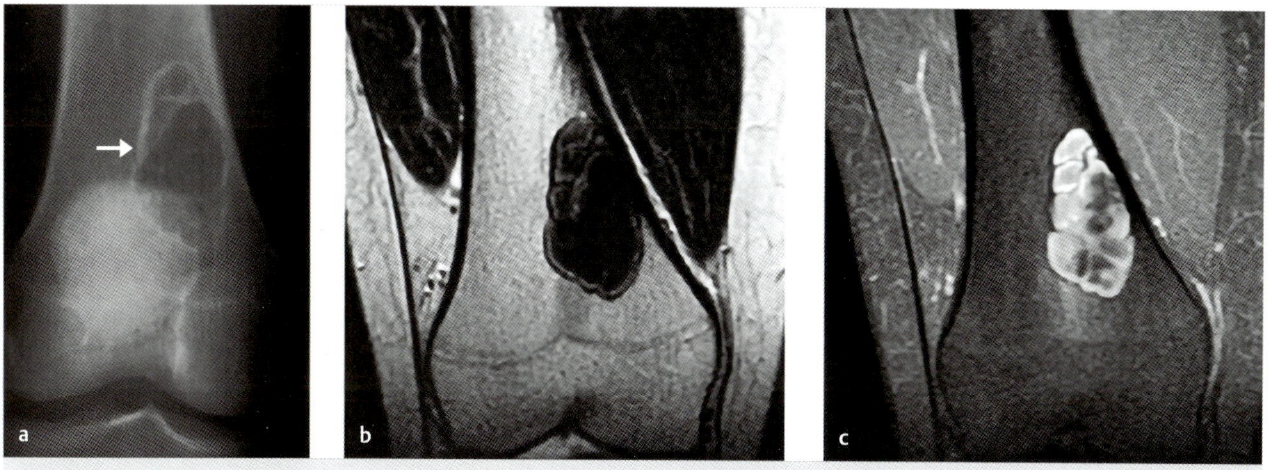

Fig. 20.9 Nonossifying fibroma in the distal femur of a 17 years old. The radiolucent lesion (*arrow*) has a thin sclerotic border on anteroposterior radiograph **(a)** and has heterogeneous mostly low signal on coronal T2-weighted imaging **(b)**. The lesion shows heterogeneous gadolinium-contrast enhancement on coronal fat-suppressed T1-weighted imaging **(c)**. (Reproduced with permission from, 10.5 Solitary Intramedullary Lesions with Well-Circumscribed Margins. In: Hollenberg G, Weinberg E, Meyers S, eds. Differential Diagnosis in Musculoskeletal MRI. 1st Edition. Thieme; 2015.)

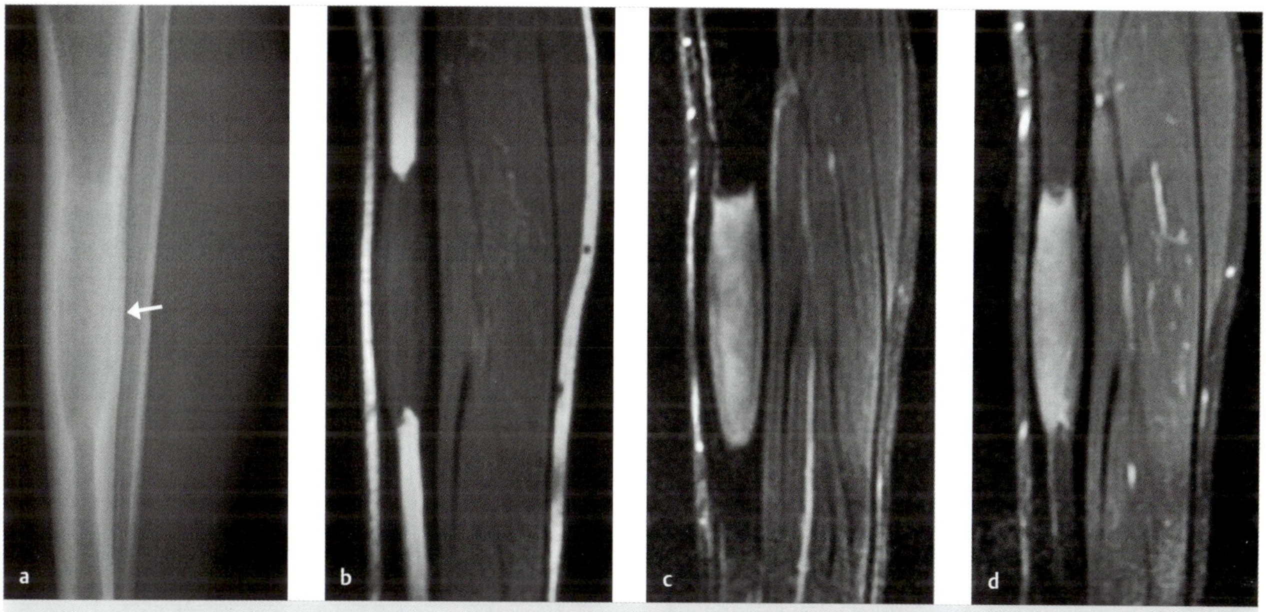

Fig. 20.10 A 19-year-old man with fibrous dysplasia involving the diaphysis of the tibia. The lesion (*arrow*) has increased attenuation with a ground-glass radiographic appearance and is associated with slight expansion and thinning of adjacent cortical margins **(a)**. The lesion has low-intermediate signal on sagittal T1-weighted imaging (T1WI) **(b)**, slightly high signal on sagittal, fat-suppressed (FS) T2-weighted imaging **(c)**, and shows gadolinium (Gd)-contrast enhancement on sagittal FS T1WI **(d)**. (Reproduced with permission from, Solitary Intramedullary Diaphyseal Lesions. In: Hollenberg G, Weinberg E, Meyers S, eds. Differential Diagnosis in Musculoskeletal MRI. 1st Edition. Thieme; 2015.)

20.3 Malignant Tumors

20.3.1 Osteosarcoma

Osteosarcoma is the most common primary malignant tumor of bone in children, and represents 20% of all primary malignant bone tumors,[120] second only to multiple myeloma.[121,122] Osteosarcoma most frequently occurs in adolescents and young adults, although there is a bimodal distribution with an additional incidence peak during late adulthood.[123] Osteosarcomas are a heterogeneous group of malignancies and vary in histologic and radiographic presentation.[16,123] In addition, the patterns of growth and aggressiveness of each lesion depend on the grade, histologic subtype, and location.[16] Variants of osteosarcoma include conventional high-grade intramedullary osteosarcoma, high-grade surface osteosarcoma, parosteal osteosarcoma, periosteal osteosarcoma, small cell osteosarcoma, telangiectatic osteosarcoma, and well-differentiated intramedullary osteosarcoma.[16]

Clinically, patients often present with nonspecific symptoms of pain and swelling, and the most common anatomic location of osteosarcomas is around the knee in the distal femur or proximal tibia.[16] The variety in growth patterns of osteosarcoma mirrors the variety in osteosarcoma subtypes, but they share their formation of osteoid by sarcoma cells. This can often be appreciated as disorganized or mottled radiodensity on conventional radiographs, though unmineralized osteoid may not show calcification at presentation.[16,124] A Codman's triangle of periosteal elevation is often seen on imaging, though this is a nonspecific finding. Although radiographs are often suspicious for the diagnosis, cross-sectional imaging provides exceptionally valuable information regarding anatomic involvement for surgical planning and matrix formation and can highlight the presence of skip metastasis when planning resection. In addition, MRI may be used to predict the histologic response to chemotherapy.[125]

Osteosarcomas often show replacement of metaphyseal bone marrow, cortical destruction, and extension into the surrounding soft tissue.[126,127] These masses often show low signal and appear isointense to muscle on T1-weighted images.[126,127] On T2-weighted and STIR sequences, osteosarcoma has high signal intensity and is often heterogeneous in signal appearance[126,127] though may have some signal dropout if mineralization occurs. T1-weighted images are frequently preferred in assessing the presence of skip metastases, as well as the anatomic involvement for surgical planning.

Periosteal osteosarcomas typically show cortical thickening, scalloping, and extension into the soft tissue.[128] This anatomic subtype most commonly shows a chondroblastic phenotype, which may be evident on MRI, with high signal intensity on T2-weighted images.[128]

Parosteal osteosarcomas appear to arise on the cortex surface, almost as if stuck onto the outside of the bone.[128] These typically are low grade and osteoblastic, which is reflected by an often densely sclerotic appearance with low signal on T1-weighted images and often low signal on T2-weighted images, as well.

Telangiectatic osteosarcomas often show multiple septations and fluid–fluid levels similar to ABCs,[129] though an underlying solid component is seen. Characteristic features that help distinguish ABC from telangiectatic osteosarcoma include the growth of nests of tumor cells along the septations in telangiectatic osteosarcoma, which appear on MRI as nodules along the rim septations.[49] Also, associated enhancing solid components and soft-tissue mass extension occur with telangiectatic osteosarcoma in 89% of cases, which do not typically occur with ABCs.[49,126,130] MRI has proven to be useful in determining prognosis of patients with osteosarcoma because the tumor response to chemotherapy can be assessed efficiently before acquiring tissue for histologic analysis (▶ Fig. 20.11).[126]

20.3.2 Ewing Sarcoma

Ewing sarcoma is another malignancy that constitutes ~10% of all primary bone tumors.[131,132] Ewing sarcoma has a peak incidence in adolescence and is the second most common malignant bone tumor in children.[132] There is an increased incidence in men, and the disease is rarely observed in nonwhite patients.[133,134] There is extensive heterogeneity in anatomic location and presentation, but the femur and pelvis are the most common locations.[16] Clinically, Ewing sarcoma presents as a painful, rapidly growing mass with symptoms often present for > 6 months.[132,135,136,137] Because of the highly aggressive nature, it is not uncommon for patients to present with metastases and systemic symptoms of fatigue, fever, and weight loss, which can be seen in other small, round, blue cell tumors.[132]

Conventional radiographs frequently show an aggressive and permeative pattern of lytic destruction with a wide zone of transition.[137] The lesion is often localized to the diaphysis, with an accompanying soft-tissue mass that is best evaluated with cross-sectional imaging.[137] On MRI, the lesion shows marrow replacement and cortical erosion, with bone destruction best visualized on T1-weighted images.[118,137] On T2-weighted and STIR images, there is evidence of increased signal and surrounding edema.[118,137,138] There is often much heterogeneity in the signal characteristics of Ewing sarcoma, which becomes more impressive as the size of the lesion increases.[137] Heterogeneity is often because of necrosis or internal hemorrhage, which often occurs in Ewing sarcoma because of its aggressiveness and rapid growth (▶ Fig. 20.12).[137]

20.3.3 Chondrosarcoma

Chondrosarcoma is the third most common primary bone malignancy, followed by myeloma and osteosarcoma.[139] Approximately 3.5% of all biopsied bone tumors are chondrosarcomas, and it is most frequently observed in the fourth and fifth decades of life.[140,141] Chondrosarcomas are categorized as surface or intramedullary lesions and may arise primarily or secondary to preexisting benign lesions such as osteochondromas or enchondromas.[16] Chondrosarcomas are most frequently observed around the distal femur, proximal tibia, pelvis, and proximal humerus.[16] There are several anatomic subtypes, which include central chondrosarcoma, periosteal chondrosarcoma, and surface chondrosarcoma. Histologic variants include clear cell chondrosarcoma, dedifferentiated chondrosarcoma, and mesenchymal chondrosarcoma. Most chondrosarcomas are central intramedullary chondrosarcoma,[142,143] which shares similar imaging characteristics to many of the aforementioned subtypes. Plain radiographs often show the characteristic rings and arcs of cartilage calcification with accompanying cortical destruction and soft-tissue extension. Cross-sectional imaging is used for evaluating the extent of anatomic involvement in these tumors.

On T1-weighted MRI, chondrosarcomas present as marrow-replacing lesions and have low to intermediate signal intensity.[139,144] On T2-weighted imaging, chondrosarcomas show high signal intensity secondary to the high water content of the unmineralized component of the lesion.[139,144] Dynamic MRI is a technique in which gadolinium is administered and serial MRIs of a given region are obtained to visualize the enhancement pattern. This method may help to differentiate a low-grade chondrosarcoma from an enchondroma.[145] The postgadolinium enhancement curve of a chondrosarcoma shows rapid enhancement and perfusion, whereas less active lesions such as endochondromas show more delayed enhancement (▶ Fig. 20.13).[145]

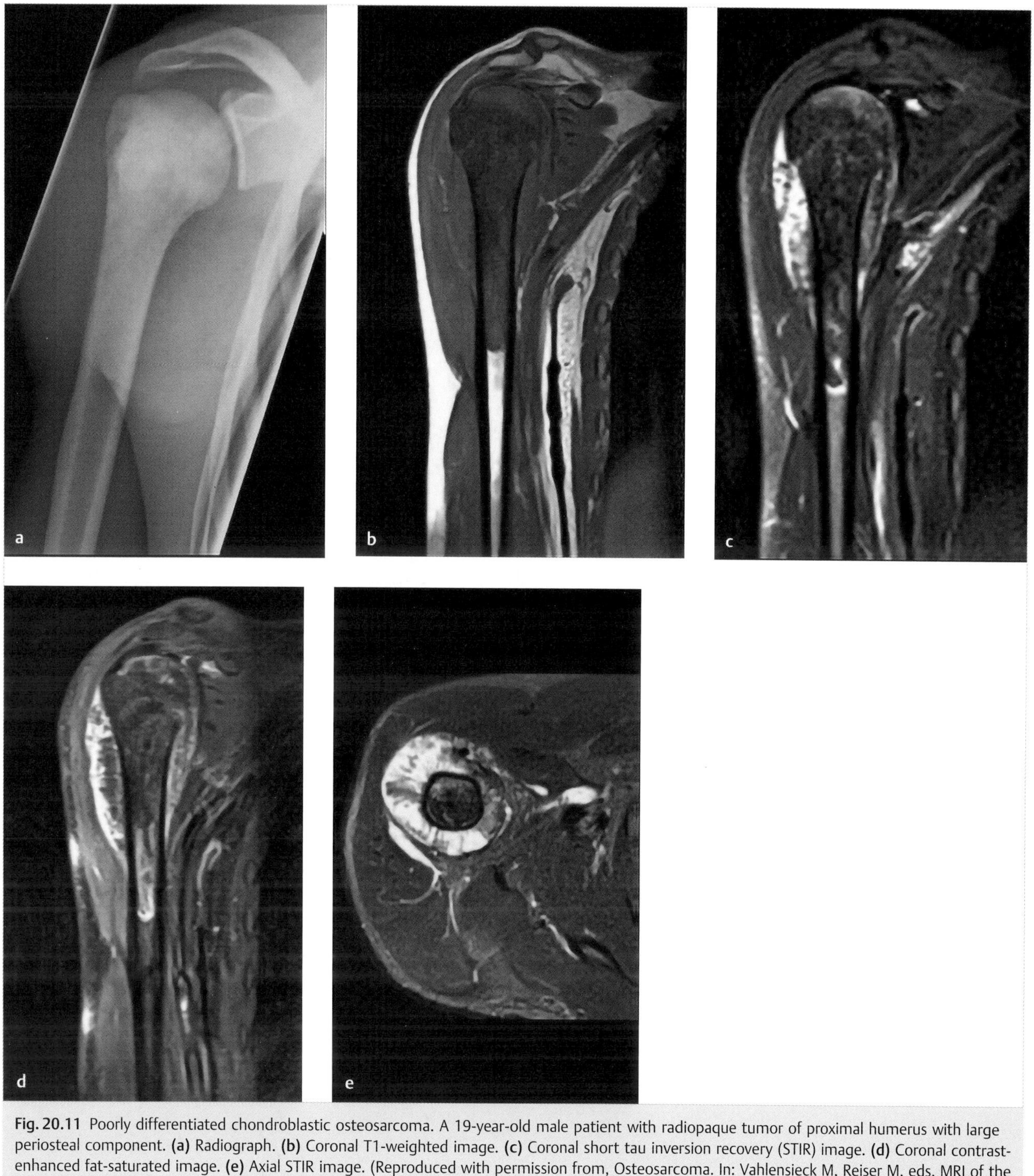

Fig. 20.11 Poorly differentiated chondroblastic osteosarcoma. A 19-year-old male patient with radiopaque tumor of proximal humerus with large periosteal component. **(a)** Radiograph. **(b)** Coronal T1-weighted image. **(c)** Coronal short tau inversion recovery (STIR) image. **(d)** Coronal contrast-enhanced fat-saturated image. **(e)** Axial STIR image. (Reproduced with permission from, Osteosarcoma. In: Vahlensieck M, Reiser M, eds. MRI of the Musculoskeletal System. 2nd Edition. Thieme; 2017.)

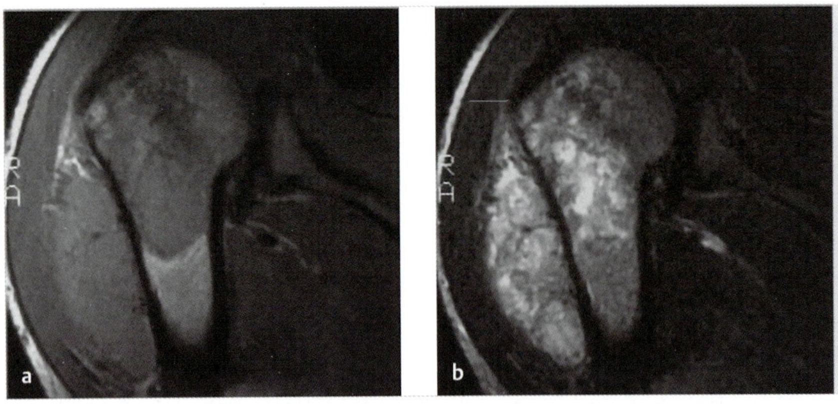

Fig. 20.12 Ewing sarcoma. A heterogeneous lesion involving the proximal humerus and extending into the lateral soft tissue is seen. The tumor depicts intermediate signal intensity on **(a)** proton density-weighted imaging (PDWI, coronal) and high signal intensity on **(b)** T2WI (coronal). (Reproduced with permission from, Localized Bone and Bone Marrow Disease. In: Burgener F, Meyers S, Tan R, et al, eds. Differential Diagnosis in Magnetic Resonance Imaging. 1st Edition. Thieme; 2002.)

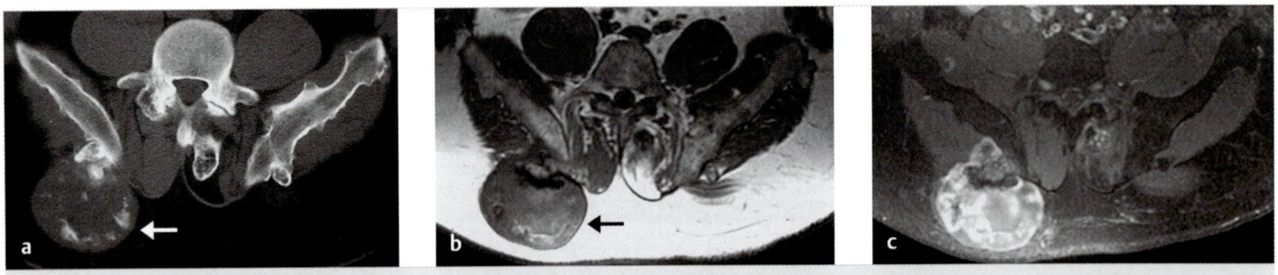

Fig. 20.13 A 30-year-old man who has multiple hereditary exostoses and a secondary low-grade chondrosarcoma arising from an osteochondroma at the posterior right iliac bone. Axial computed tomography (CT) image **(a)** showing multiple protrusions of cortical and medullary bone relative to the cortical bone of the pelvis representing benign osteochondromas, as well as a chondrosarcoma at the dorsal right iliac bone (*arrow*). The chondrosarcoma contains soft tissue attenuation and foci of chondroid mineralization associated with adjacent bone destruction. The chondrosarcoma has mostly intermediate signal on axial proton density-weighted imaging (PDWI) **(b)** as well as small foci with low and high signal. The tumor shows prominent heterogeneous gadolinium (Gd)-contrast enhancement on axial fat-suppressed (FS) T1-weighted imaging (T1WI) **(c)**. (Reproduced with permission from, Meyers S. Prognosis and treatment. In: Meyers S, ed. MRI of Bone and Soft Tissue Tumors and Tumorlike Lesions. 1st Edition. Stuttgart: Thieme; 2007.)

20.4 Common Clinical Questions

1. Which of the following most typically represents clinical features of osteoid osteoma?
   a) Pain worse at night in a young patient.
   b) Leg claudication in an older patient with walking.
   c) Painless swelling of the limb.
   d) Multiple pulmonary emboli.

2. All of the following MRI features suggest chondrosarcoma instead of enchondroma, EXCEPT:
   a) Cortical destruction.
   b) Endosteal scalloping.
   c) Periosteal reaction.
   d) Soft tissue extension.
   e) Sub 1 cm well circumscribed cartilage lesion centrally located in metaphysesal region.

3. All of the following are common primary bone malignancies, EXCEPT:
   a) Alveolar rhabdomyosarcoma.
   b) Chondrosarcoma.
   c) Myeloma.
   d) Osteosarcoma.

4. Aneursymal bone cysts have which of the following imaging characteristics:
   a) Destructive, cystic, expansile lesions with fluid-fluid levels.
   b) Sclerotic cortical defects in metaphysis.
   c) Poorly marginated lytic lesions with well defined non sclerotic rim.
   d) Mushroom like expansile cartilage lesion with well defined stalk.

5. Which of the following represent clinical imaging features of giant cell tumors:
   a) Destructive, cystic, expansile lesions with fluid fluid levels.
   b) Sclerotic cortical defects in metaphysis.
   c) On radiograph, poorly marginated lytic lesions with well defined non sclerotic rim.
   d) Mushroom like expansile cartilage lesion with well defined stalk.

References

[1] Fayad LM, Jacobs MA, Wang X, Carrino JA, Bluemke DA. Musculoskeletal tumors: how to use anatomic, functional, and metabolic MR techniques. Radiology. 2012; 265(2):340–356

[2] Pettine KA, Klassen RA. Osteoid-osteoma and osteoblastoma of the spine. J Bone Joint Surg Am. 1986; 68(3):354–361
[3] Sherman MS. Osteoid osteoma; review of the literature and report of 30 cases. J Bone Joint Surg Am. 1947; 29(4):918–930
[4] Sim FH, Dahlin CD, Beabout JW. Osteoid-osteoma: diagnostic problems. J Bone Joint Surg Am. 1975; 57(2):154–159
[5] Swee RG, McLeod RA, Beabout JW. Osteoid osteoma. Detection, diagnosis, and localization. Radiology. 1979; 130(1):117–123
[6] Chuang SY, Wang SJ, Au MK, Huang GS. Osteoid osteoma in the talar neck: a report of two cases. Foot Ankle Int. 1998; 19(1):44–47
[7] Greenspan A. Benign bone-forming lesions: osteoma, osteoid osteoma, and osteoblastoma. Clinical, imaging, pathologic, and differential considerations. Skeletal Radiol. 1993; 22(7):485–500
[8] Klein MH, Shankman S. Osteoid osteoma: radiologic and pathologic correlation. Skeletal Radiol. 1992; 21(1):23–31
[9] Unni KK. Dahlin's bone tumors: general aspects and data on 11,087 cases. Philadelphia, PA: Lippincott-Raven Publishers; 1996
[10] Goldman AB, Schneider R, Pavlov H. Osteoid osteomas of the femoral neck: report of four cases evaluated with isotopic bone scanning, CT, and MR imaging. Radiology. 1993; 186(1):227–232
[11] Kaweblum M, Lehman WB, Bash J, Strongwater A, Grant AD. Osteoid osteoma under the age of five years. The difficulty of diagnosis. Clin Orthop Relat Res. 1993(296):218–224
[12] Resnick D, Kyriakos M, Greenway GD. Tumor like diseases of bone: imaging and pathology of specific lesions. In: Diagnosis of bone and joint disorders. Philadelphia, PA: WB Saunders; 1995:3648–3697
[13] Edeiken J, DePalma AF, Hodes PJ. Osteoid osteoma. (Roentgenographic emphasis). Clin Orthop Relat Res. 1966; 49(49):201–206
[14] Healey JH, Ghelman B. Osteoid osteoma and osteoblastoma. Current concepts and recent advances. Clin Orthop Relat Res. 1986(204):76–85
[15] Kattapuram SV, Kushner DC, Phillips WC, Rosenthal DI. Osteoid osteoma: an unusual cause of articular pain. Radiology. 1983; 147(2):383–387
[16] McCarthy EF, Frassica FJ. Pathology of bone and joint disorders: with clinical and radiographic correlation. Philadelphia, PA: WB Saunders; 1998
[17] Makley JT, Dunn MJ. Prostaglandin synthesis by osteoid osteoma. Lancet. 1982; 2(8288):42
[18] Mungo DV, Zhang X, O'Keefe RJ, Rosier RN, Puzas JE, Schwarz EM. COX-1 and COX-2 expression in osteoid osteomas. J Orthop Res. 2002; 20(1):159–162
[19] Keim HA, Reina EG. Osteoid-osteoma as a cause of scoliosis. J Bone Joint Surg Am. 1975; 57(2):159–163
[20] Norman A, Dorfman HD. Osteoid-osteoma inducing pronounced overgrowth and deformity of bone. Clin Orthop Relat Res. 1975(110):233–238
[21] Uehara M, Takahashi J, Kuraishi S, et al. Osteoid osteoma presenting as thoracic scoliosis. Spine J. 2015; 15(12):e77–e81
[22] Glass RB, Poznanski AK, Fisher MR, Shkolnik A, Dias L. MR imaging of osteoid osteoma. J Comput Assist Tomogr. 1986; 10(6):1065–1067
[23] Houang B, Grenier N, Gréselle JF, et al. Osteoid osteoma of the cervical spine. Misleading MR features about a case involving the uncinate process. Neuroradiology. 1990; 31(6):549–551
[24] Liu PT, Chivers FS, Roberts CC, Schultz CJ, Beauchamp CP. Imaging of osteoid osteoma with dynamic gadolinium-enhanced MR imaging. Radiology. 2003; 227(3):691–700
[25] Gaeta M, Minutoli F, Pandolfo I, Vinci S, D'Andrea L, Blandino A. Magnetic resonance imaging findings of osteoid osteoma of the proximal femur. Eur Radiol. 2004; 14(9):1582–1589
[26] Davies M, Cassar-Pullicino VN, Davies AM, McCall IW, Tyrrell PN. The diagnostic accuracy of MR imaging in osteoid osteoma. Skeletal Radiol. 2002; 31(10):559–569
[27] Hosalkar HS, Garg S, Moroz L, Pollack A, Dormans JP. The diagnostic accuracy of MRI versus CT imaging for osteoid osteoma in children. Clin Orthop Relat Res. 2005(433):171–177
[28] Rosenthal DI, Hornicek FJ, Wolfe MW, Jennings LC, Gebhardt MC, Mankin HJ. Percutaneous radiofrequency coagulation of osteoid osteoma compared with operative treatment. J Bone Joint Surg Am. 1998; 80(6):815–821
[29] Papagelopoulos PJ, Galanis EC, Sim FH, Unni KK. Clinicopathologic features, diagnosis, and treatment of osteoblastoma. Orthopedics. 1999; 22(2):244–247, quiz 248–249
[30] Nakatani T, Yamamoto T, Akisue T, et al. Periosteal osteoblastoma of the distal femur. Skeletal Radiol. 2004; 33(2):107–111
[31] Nomikos GC, Murphey MD, Kransdorf MJ, Bancroft LW, Peterson JJ. Primary bone tumors of the lower extremities. Radiol Clin North Am. 2002; 40(5):971–990
[32] Temple HT, Mizel MS, Murphey MD, Sweet DE. Osteoblastoma of the foot and ankle. Foot Ankle Int. 1998; 19(10):698–704
[33] Atesok KI, Alman BA, Schemitsch EH, Peyser A, Mankin H. Osteoid osteoma and osteoblastoma. J Am Acad Orthop Surg. 2011; 19(11):678–689
[34] Hakim DN, Pelly T, Kulendran M, Caris JA. Benign tumours of the bone: a review. J Bone Oncol. 2015; 4(2):37–41
[35] Kroon HM, Schurmans J. Osteoblastoma: clinical and radiologic findings in 98 new cases. Radiology. 1990; 175(3):783–790
[36] Lucas DR, Unni KK, McLeod RA, O'Connor MI, Sim FH. Osteoblastoma: clinicopathologic study of 306 cases. Hum Pathol. 1994; 25(2):117–134
[37] Pelargos PE, Nagasawa DT, Ung N, et al. Clinical characteristics and diagnostic imaging of cranial osteoblastoma. J Clin Neurosci. 2015; 22(3):445–449
[38] Pettersson H, Gillespy T, III, Hamlin DJ, et al. Primary musculoskeletal tumors: examination with MR imaging compared with conventional modalities. Radiology. 1987; 164(1):237–241
[39] Saifuddin A, Sherazi Z, Shaikh MI, Natali C, Ransford AO, Pringle JA. Spinal osteoblastoma: relationship between paravertebral muscle abnormalities and scoliosis. Skeletal Radiol. 1996; 25(6):531–535
[40] Qasem SA, DeYoung BR. Cartilage-forming tumors. Semin Diagn Pathol. 2014; 31(1):10–20
[41] Miller TT. Bone tumors and tumorlike conditions: analysis with conventional radiography. Radiology. 2008; 246(3):662–674
[42] Romeo S, Hogendoorn PC, Dei Tos AP. Benign cartilaginous tumors of bone: from morphology to somatic and germ-line genetics. Adv Anat Pathol. 2009; 16(5):307–315
[43] Brower AC, Moser RP, Gilkey FW, Kransdorf MJ. Chondroblastoma. In: Cartilaginous tumors of the skeleton Mosby-Year Book, St Louis. St. Louis, MO: Mosby-Year Book; 1990:74–113
[44] Jaffe HL, Lichtenstein L. Benign chondroblastoma of bone: a reinterpretation of the so-called calcifying or chondromatous giant cell tumor. Am J Pathol. 1942; 18(6):969–991
[45] Lin PP, Thenappan A, Deavers MT, Lewis VO, Yasko AW. Treatment and prognosis of chondroblastoma. Clin Orthop Relat Res. 2005; 438(438):103–109
[46] Brower AC, Moser RP, Kransdorf MJ. The frequency and diagnostic significance of periostitis in chondroblastoma. AJR Am J Roentgenol. 1990; 154(2):309–314
[47] Weatherall PT, Maale GE, Mendelsohn DB, Sherry CS, Erdman WE, Pascoe HR. Chondroblastoma: classic and confusing appearance at MR imaging. Radiology. 1994; 190(2):467–474
[48] Oxtoby JW, Davies AM. MRI characteristics of chondroblastoma. Clin Radiol. 1996; 51(1):22–26
[49] Keenan S, Bui-Mansfield LT. Musculoskeletal lesions with fluid-fluid level: a pictorial essay. J Comput Assist Tomogr. 2006; 30(3):517–524
[50] Roberts PF, Taylor JG. Multifocal benign chondroblastomas: report of a case. Hum Pathol. 1980; 11(3):296–298
[51] Suneja R, Grimer RJ, Belthur M, et al. Chondroblastoma of bone: long-term results and functional outcome after intralesional curettage. J Bone Joint Surg Br. 2005; 87(7):974–978
[52] Brien EW, Mirra JM, Luck JV, Jr. Benign and malignant cartilage tumors of bone and joint: their anatomic and theoretical basis with an emphasis on radiology, pathology and clinical biology. II. Juxtacortical cartilage tumors. Skeletal Radiol. 1999; 28(1):1–20
[53] Nojima T, Unni KK, McLeod RA, Pritchard DJ. Periosteal chondroma and periosteal chondrosarcoma. Am J Surg Pathol. 1985; 9(9):666–677
[54] Robinson P, White LM, Sundaram M, et al. Periosteal chondroid tumors: radiologic evaluation with pathologic correlation. AJR Am J Roentgenol. 2001; 177(5):1183–1188
[55] Zheng K, Yu X, Xu S, Xu M. Periosteal chondroma of the femur: a case report and review of the literature. Oncol Lett. 2015; 9(4):1637–1640
[56] Boriani S, Bacchini P, Bertoni F, Campanacci M. Periosteal chondroma. A review of twenty cases. J Bone Joint Surg Am. 1983; 65(2):205–212
[57] Woertler K, Blasius S, Brinkschmidt C, Hillmann A, Link TM, Heindel W. Periosteal chondroma: MR characteristics. J Comput Assist Tomogr. 2001; 25 (3):425–430
[58] Milgram JW. The origins of osteochondromas and enchondromas. A histopathologic study. Clin Orthop Relat Res. 1983(174):264–284
[59] Marco RA, Gitelis S, Brebach GT, Healey JH. Cartilage tumors: evaluation and treatment. J Am Acad Orthop Surg. 2000; 8(5):292–304
[60] Murphey MD, Flemming DJ, Boyea SR, Bojescul JA, Sweet DE, Temple HT. Enchondroma versus chondrosarcoma in the appendicular skeleton: differentiating features. Radiographics. 1998; 18(5):1213–1237, quiz 1244–1245

[61] Aoki J, Sone S, Fujioka F, et al. MR of enchondroma and chondrosarcoma: rings and arcs of Gd-DTPA enhancement. J Comput Assist Tomogr. 1991; 15 (6):1011–1016
[62] Cohen EK, Kressel HY, Frank TS, et al. Hyaline cartilage-origin bone and soft-tissue neoplasms: MR appearance and histologic correlation. Radiology. 1988; 167(2):477–481
[63] Woertler K. Benign bone tumors and tumor-like lesions: value of cross-sectional imaging. Eur Radiol. 2003; 13(8):1820–1835
[64] Lewis RJ, Ketcham AS. Maffucci's syndrome: functional and neoplastic significance. Case report and review of the literature. J Bone Joint Surg Am. 1973; 55(7):1465–1479
[65] Liu J, Hudkins PG, Swee RG, Unni KK. Bone sarcomas associated with Ollier's disease. Cancer. 1987; 59(7):1376–1385
[66] Schwartz HS, Zimmerman NB, Simon MA, Wroble RR, Millar EA, Bonfiglio M. The malignant potential of enchondromatosis. J Bone Joint Surg Am. 1987; 69(2):269–274
[67] D'Ambrosia R, Ferguson AB, Jr. The formation of osteochondroma by epiphyseal cartilage transplantation. Clin Orthop Relat Res. 1968; 61(61): 103–115
[68] Libshitz HI, Cohen MA. Radiation-induced osteochondromas. Radiology. 1982; 142(3):643–647
[69] Antonio ZP, Alejandro RM, Luis MRJ, José GR. Femur ostochondroma and secondary pseudoaneurysm of the popliteal artery. Arch Orthop Trauma Surg. 2006; 126(2):127–130
[70] Murphey MD, Jelinek JS, Temple HT, Flemming DJ, Gannon FH. Imaging of periosteal osteosarcoma: radiologic-pathologic comparison. Radiology. 2004; 233(1):129–138
[71] Lee JK, Yao L, Wirth CR. MR imaging of solitary osteochondromas: report of eight cases. AJR Am J Roentgenol. 1987; 149(3):557–560
[72] Hudson TM, Springfield DS, Spanier SS, Enneking WF, Hamlin DJ. Benign exostoses and exostotic chondrosarcomas: evaluation of cartilage thickness by CT. Radiology. 1984; 152(3):595–599
[73] Schmale GA, Conrad EU, III, Raskind WH. The natural history of hereditary multiple exostoses. J Bone Joint Surg Am. 1994; 76(7):986–992
[74] Kivioja A, Ervasti H, Kinnunen J, Kaitila I, Wolf M, Böhling T. Chondrosarcoma in a family with multiple hereditary exostoses. J Bone Joint Surg Br. 2000; 82(2):261–266
[75] Wuyts W, Van Hul W, De Boulle K, et al. Mutations in the EXT1 and EXT2 genes in hereditary multiple exostoses. Am J Hum Genet. 1998; 62(2):346–354
[76] Manaster BJ, Doyle AJ. Giant cell tumors of bone. Radiol Clin North Am. 1993; 31(2):299–323
[77] Chakarun CJ, Forrester DM, Gottsegen CJ, Patel DB, White EA, Matcuk GR, Jr. Giant cell tumor of bone: review, mimics, and new developments in treatment. Radiographics. 2013; 33(1):197–211
[78] Turcotte RE. Giant cell tumor of bone. Orthop Clin North Am. 2006; 37(1): 35–51
[79] Murphey MD, Nomikos GC, Flemming DJ, Gannon FH, Temple HT, Kransdorf MJ. From the archives of AFIP. Imaging of giant cell tumor and giant cell reparative granuloma of bone: radiologic-pathologic correlation. Radiographics. 2001; 21(5):1283–1309
[80] van der Heijden L, Dijkstra PD, Campanacci DA, Gibbons CL, van de Sande MA. Giant cell tumor with pathologic fracture: should we curette or resect? Clin Orthop Relat Res. 2013; 471(3):820–829
[81] Szendröi M. Giant-cell tumour of bone. J Bone Joint Surg Br. 2004; 86(1):5–12
[82] Aoki J, Tanikawa H, Ishii K, et al. MR findings indicative of hemosiderin in giant-cell tumor of bone: frequency, cause, and diagnostic significance. AJR Am J Roentgenol. 1996; 166(1):145–148
[83] James SLJ, Davies AM. Giant-cell tumours of bone of the hand and wrist: a review of imaging findings and differential diagnoses. Eur Radiol. 2005; 15 (9):1855–1866
[84] Biesecker JL, Marcove RC, Huvos AG, Miké V. Aneurysmal bone cysts. A clinicopathologic study of 66 cases. Cancer. 1970; 26(3):615–625
[85] Herman SD, Mesgarzadeh M, Bonakdarpour A, Dalinka MK. The role of magnetic resonance imaging in giant cell tumor of bone. Skeletal Radiol. 1987; 16(8):635–643
[86] Vidyadhara S, Rao SK. Techniques in the management of juxta-articular aggressive and recurrent giant cell tumors around the knee. Eur J Surg Oncol. 2007; 33(2):243–251
[87] Becker WT, Dohle J, Bernd L, et al. Arbeitsgemeinschaft Knochentumoren. Local recurrence of giant cell tumor of bone after intralesional treatment with and without adjuvant therapy. J Bone Joint Surg Am. 2008; 90(5): 1060–1067
[88] Koskinen EV, Visuri TI, Holmström T, Roukkula MA. Aneurysmal bone cyst: evaluation of resection and of curettage in 20 cases. Clin Orthop Relat Res. 1976(118):136–146
[89] Vergel De Dios AM, Bond JR, Shives TC, McLeod RA, Unni KK. Aneurysmal bone cyst. A clinicopathologic study of 238 cases. Cancer. 1992; 69(12):2921–2931
[90] Kransdorf MJ, Sweet DE. Aneurysmal bone cyst: concept, controversy, clinical presentation, and imaging. AJR Am J Roentgenol. 1995; 164(3):573–580
[91] Rapp TB, Ward JP, Alaia MJ. Aneurysmal bone cyst. J Am Acad Orthop Surg. 2012; 20(4):233–241
[92] Adamsbaum C, Kalifa G, Seringe R, Dubousset J. Direct Ethibloc injection in benign bone cysts: preliminary report on four patients. Skeletal Radiol. 1993; 22(5):317–320
[93] Bonakdarpour A, Levy WM, Aegerter E. Primary and secondary aneurysmal bone cyst: a radiological study of 75 cases. Radiology. 1978; 126(1):75–83
[94] Levy WM, Miller AS, Bonakdarpour A, Aegerter E. Aneurysmal bone cyst secondary to other osseous lesions. Report of 57 cases. Am J Clin Pathol. 1975; 63(1):1–8
[95] Beltran J, Simon DC, Levy M, Herman L, Weis L, Mueller CF. Aneurysmal bone cysts: MR imaging at 1.5 T. Radiology. 1986; 158(3):689–690
[96] Munk PL, Helms CA, Holt RG, Johnston J, Steinbach L, Neumann C. MR imaging of aneurysmal bone cysts. AJR Am J Roentgenol. 1989; 153(1):99–101
[97] Cory DA, Fritsch SA, Cohen MD, et al. Aneurysmal bone cysts: imaging findings and embolotherapy. AJR Am J Roentgenol. 1989; 153(2):369–373
[98] Revel MP, Vanel D, Sigal R, et al. Aneurysmal bone cysts of the jaws: CT and MR findings. J Comput Assist Tomogr. 1992; 16(1):84–86
[99] Hoffer FA. Primary skeletal neoplasms: osteosarcoma and ewing sarcoma. Top Magn Reson Imaging. 2002; 13(4):231–239
[100] Murphey MD, wan Jaovisidha S, Temple HT, Gannon FH, Jelinek JS, Malawer MM. Telangiectatic osteosarcoma: radiologic-pathologic comparison. Radiology. 2003; 229(2):545–553
[101] Murphey MD, Robbin MR, McRae GA, Flemming DJ, Temple HT, Kransdorf MJ. The many faces of osteosarcoma. Radiographics. 1997; 17(5):1205–1231
[102] Sanerkin NG, Mott MG, Roylance J. An unusual intraosseous lesion with fibroblastic, osteoclastic, osteoblastic, aneurysmal and fibromyxoid elements. "Solid" variant of aneurysmal bone cyst. Cancer. 1983; 51(12): 2278–2286
[103] Bertoni F, Bacchini P, Capanna R, et al. Solid variant of aneurysmal bone cyst. Cancer. 1993; 71(3):729–734
[104] Kadhim M, Sethi S, Thacker MM. Unicameral bone cysts in the humerus: treatment outcomes. J Pediatr Orthop. 2016; 36(4):392–399
[105] Weinman J, Servaes S, Anupindi SA. Treated unicameral bone cysts. Clin Radiol. 2013; 68(6):636–642
[106] Pretell-Mazzini J, Murphy RF, Kushare I, Dormans JP. Unicameral bone cysts: general characteristics and management controversies. J Am Acad Orthop Surg. 2014; 22(5):295–303
[107] Betsy M, Kupersmith LM, Springfield DS. Metaphyseal fibrous defects. J Am Acad Orthop Surg. 2004; 12(2):89–95
[108] Caffey J. On fibrous defects in cortical walls of growing tubular bones: their radiologic appearance, structure, prevalence, natural course, and diagnostic significance. Adv Pediatr. 1955; 7:13–51
[109] Jee WH, Choe BY, Kang HS, et al. Nonossifying fibroma: characteristics at MR imaging with pathologic correlation. Radiology. 1998; 209(1):197–202
[110] Kransdorf MJ, Utz JA, Gilkey FW, Berrey BH. MR appearance of fibroxanthoma. J Comput Assist Tomogr. 1988; 12(4):612–615
[111] Arata MA, Peterson HA, Dahlin DC. Pathological fractures through non-ossifying fibromas. Review of the Mayo Clinic experience. J Bone Joint Surg Am. 1981; 63(6):980–988
[112] Drennan DB, Maylahn DJ, Fahey JJ. Fractures through large non-ossifying fibromas. Clin Orthop Relat Res. 1974(103):82–88
[113] Riddle ND, Bui MM. Fibrous dysplasia. Arch Pathol Lab Med. 2013; 137(1): 134–138
[114] Feller L, Wood NH, Khammissa RA, Lemmer J, Raubenheimer EJ. The nature of fibrous dysplasia. Head Face Med. 2009; 5:22
[115] Mirra JM, Gold RH. Fibrous dysplasia. In: Mirra JM, Piero P, Gold RH, eds. Bone tumors. Philadelphia, PA: Lea and Febiger; 1989:191–226
[116] Wilner D. Radiology of bone tumors and allied disorders. Philadelphia, PA: WB Saunders; 1982
[117] Jee WH, Choi KH, Choe BY, Park JM, Shinn KS. Fibrous dysplasia: MR imaging characteristics with radiopathologic correlation. AJR Am J Roentgenol. 1996; 167(6):1523–1527

[118] Miller SL, Hoffer FA. Malignant and benign bone tumors. Radiol Clin North Am. 2001; 39(4):673–699
[119] Utz JA, Kransdorf MJ, Jelinek JS, Moser RP, Jr, Berrey BH. MR appearance of fibrous dysplasia. J Comput Assist Tomogr. 1989; 13(5):845–851
[120] Salunke AA, Chen Y, Tan JH, Chen X, Khin LW, Puhaindran ME. Does a pathological fracture affect the prognosis in patients with osteosarcoma of the extremities?: a systematic review and meta-analysis. Bone Joint J. 2014; 96-B(10):1396–1403
[121] Brenner W, Bohuslavizki KH, Eary JF. PET imaging of osteosarcoma. J Nucl Med. 2003; 44(6):930–942
[122] Ottaviani G, Jaffe N. The epidemiology of osteosarcoma. Cancer Treat Res. 2009; 152:3–13
[123] Mirabello L, Troisi RJ, Savage SA. Osteosarcoma incidence and survival rates from 1973 to 2004: data from the Surveillance, Epidemiology, and End Results Program. Cancer. 2009; 115(7):1531–1543
[124] Suresh S, Saifuddin A. Radiological appearances of appendicular osteosarcoma: a comprehensive pictorial review. Clin Radiol. 2007; 62(4):314–323
[125] Jeon DG, Song WS, Cho WH, Kong CB, Cho SH. Proximal tumor location and fluid-fluid levels on MRI predict resistance to chemotherapy in stage IIB osteosarcoma. Clin Orthop Relat Res. 2014; 472(6):1911–1920
[126] Baunin C, Schmidt G, Baumstarck K, et al. Value of diffusion-weighted images in differentiating mid-course responders to chemotherapy for osteosarcoma compared to the histological response: preliminary results. Skeletal Radiol. 2012; 41(9):1141–1149
[127] Schima W, Amann G, Stiglbauer R, et al. Preoperative staging of osteosarcoma: efficacy of MR imaging in detecting joint involvement. AJR Am J Roentgenol. 1994; 163(5):1171–1175
[128] Murphey MD, Choi JJ, Kransdorf MJ, Flemming DJ, Gannon FH. Imaging of osteochondroma: variants and complications with radiologic-pathologic correlation. Radiographics. 2000; 20(5):1407–1434
[129] Tsai JC, Dalinka MK, Fallon MD, Zlatkin MB, Kressel HY. Fluid-fluid level: a nonspecific finding in tumors of bone and soft tissue. Radiology. 1990; 175 (3):779–782
[130] Saifuddin A. The accuracy of imaging in the local staging of appendicular osteosarcoma. Skeletal Radiol. 2002; 31(4):191–201
[131] Larsson SE, Lorentzon R. The geographic variation of the incidence of malignant primary bone tumors in Sweden. J Bone Joint Surg Am. 1974; 56(3):592–600
[132] Lawlor ER, Sorensen PH. Twenty years on: what do we really know about Ewing sarcoma and what is the path forward? Crit Rev Oncog. 2015; 20 (3–4):155–171
[133] Herzog CE. Overview of sarcomas in the adolescent and young adult population. J Pediatr Hematol Oncol. 2005; 27(4):215–218
[134] Lim SM, Yoo CJ, Han JW, et al. Incidence and survival of pediatric soft tissue sarcomas: comparison between adults and children. Cancer Res Treat. 2015; 47(1):9–17
[135] Hasegawa SL, Davison JM, Rutten A, Fletcher JA, Fletcher CD. Primary cutaneous Ewing's sarcoma: immunophenotypic and molecular cytogenetic evaluation of five cases. Am J Surg Pathol. 1998; 22(3):310–318
[136] Machado I, Llombart B, Calabuig-Fariñas S, Llombart-Bosch A. Superficial Ewing's sarcoma family of tumors: a clinicopathological study with differential diagnoses. J Cutan Pathol. 2011; 38(8):636–643
[137] Murphey MD, Senchak LT, Mambalam PK, Logie CI, Klassen-Fischer MK, Kransdorf MJ. From the radiologic pathology archives: Ewing sarcoma family of tumors: radiologic-pathologic correlation. Radiographics. 2013; 33 (3):803–831
[138] Grier HE. The Ewing family of tumors. Ewing's sarcoma and primitive neuroectodermal tumors. Pediatr Clin North Am. 1997; 44(4):991–1004
[139] Douis H, Saifuddin A. The imaging of cartilaginous bone tumours. II. Chondrosarcoma. Skeletal Radiol. 2013; 42(5):611–626
[140] Giuffrida AY, Burgueno JE, Koniaris LG, Gutierrez JC, Duncan R, Scully SP. Chondrosarcoma in the United States (1973 to 2003): an analysis of 2890 cases from the SEER database. J Bone Joint Surg Am. 2009; 91(5): 1063–1072
[141] Herget GW, Uhl M, Opitz OG, Adler CP, Südkamp NP, Knöller S. The many faces of chondrosarcoma of bone, own cases and review of the literature with an emphasis on radiology, pathology and treatment. Acta Chir Orthop Traumatol Cech. 2011; 78(6):501–509
[142] Arora RS, Alston RD, Eden TO, Geraci M, Birch JM. The contrasting age-incidence patterns of bone tumours in teenagers and young adults: implications for aetiology. Int J Cancer. 2012; 131(7):1678–1685
[143] Terek RM. Recent advances in the basic science of chondrosarcoma. Orthop Clin North Am. 2006; 37(1):9–14
[144] Parlier-Cuau C, Bousson V, Ogilvie CM, Lackman RD, Laredo JD. When should we biopsy a solitary central cartilaginous tumor of long bones? Literature review and management proposal. Eur J Radiol. 2011; 77(1): 6–12
[145] De Coninck T, Jans L, Sys G, et al. Dynamic contrast-enhanced MR imaging for differentiation between enchondroma and chondrosarcoma. Eur Radiol. 2013; 23(11):3140–3152

Answers to Common Clinical Questions

1. Answer: a. Pain worse at night in young patient.
2. Answer: e. Sub 1 cm well circumscribed cartilage lesion centrally located in metaphysesal region.
3. Answer: a. Alveolar rhabdomyosarcoma.
4. Answer: a. Destructive, cystic, expansile lesions with fluid fluid levels.
5. Answer: c. On radiograph, poorly marginated lytic lesions with well defined, non sclerotic rim.

21 Tumors of the Spine

Daniel M. Sciubba, Patricia L. Zadnik, Bruce A. Wasserman, and Ziya L. Gokaslan

Abstract

Spinal tumors are extradural, intradural-extramedullary, or intramedullary, and most are metastatic tumors. Diagnosis involves identifying the compartment location, generating a preimaging differential diagnosis, incorporating patient information to narrow the differential diagnosis, and using various imaging modalities.

Magnetic resonance imaging (MRI) is the preferred modality for spinal tumors. However, MRI should be complemented by conventional radiography and/or computed tomography. The MRI protocol for suspected spine tumors includes T1- and T2-weighted images and gadolinium-enhanced images in the axial and sagittal planes.

Extradural primary benign tumors have characteristic MRI and patient characteristics that differentiate them from malignant tumors. They include hemangioma, osteoid osteoma, giant cell tumor, osteochondroma, aneurysmal bone cyst, and eosinophilic granuloma. Extradural primary malignant tumors include multiple myeloma, solitary bone plasmacytoma, chordoma, and sarcomas.

Intradural-extramedullary lesions arise from within the dura. MRI typically displays a widened ipsilateral subarachnoid space in which the cord and roots are displaced away from the mass. Nerve-sheath tumors and meningiomas account for > 80% of such masses.

Intramedullary tumors grow from the spinal cord itself and account for 20% of intraspinal neoplasms in adults and 30 to 35% of intraspinal neoplasms in children. Nearly 90% of these tumors are gliomas. Less common lesions include hemangioblastomas and metastases. On MRI, classic intramedullary lesions show a diffuse, multisegmental, smoothly enlarged cord or filum terminale mass with gradual surrounding subarachnoid effacement. Many lesions are associated with syringomyelia or cyst-like cavities within the cord, extending within the central canal of the cord or eccentric to the canal in a longitudinal orientation.

Keywords: benign tumors, computed tomography, conventional radiography, lesions, magnetic resonance imaging, metastatic tumors, spine tumors

21.1 Introduction

Spine tumors are traditionally classified by anatomic location into the following three compartments[1,2,3,4]: extradural, intradural-extramedullary, and intramedullary. The extradural compartment consists of all structures outside the dura, including the osseous structures, the paravertebral region and paraspinal musculature, and the epidural space. Although orthopaedic surgeons most commonly treat tumors of the extradural compartment, they must have an understanding of the other two compartments to provide comprehensive patient care and to communicate effectively with neurosurgical colleagues.

Spine tumors are also classified by origin as primary or metastatic. Although many primary lesions occur in the spinal cord, nerve roots, dura, and osseous spine, most lesions within the spine are metastatic tumors.[5,6,7] Such lesions occur mostly in the extradural compartment, especially in the osseous structures. As systemic therapies for metastatic disease have improved and the life expectancy of such patients has increased, the incidence of metastatic spread to the spine has also increased.

Up to 40% of patients with cancer develop visceral or osseous metastases, and the spinal column is the most common site of osseous metastases.[7,8,9,10,11] Prostate, lung, and breast cancer account for most of such lesions.[3,6] Metastases can occur in any compartment of the spinal column but the vertebral body is the site most commonly affected (approximately 85% of occurrences)[1,12] followed by the paravertebral region, epidural space, and intradural compartment. Although any segment of the spine can be affected, such lesions typically occur in the thoracic spine (approximate rate, 70%) followed by the lumbar spine (20%) and the cervical spine and sacrum (10%).[1,12]

Epidemiologic data suggest that most patients with suspected spine tumors eventually are shown to have metastatic (rather than primary) disease in the vertebral body (rather than in other locations), and that metastatic and primary lesions (benign and malignant) can occur within any segment and compartment of the spine and in men or women of almost any age. Although most lesions have particular identifying characteristics, it is imperative that, to efficiently and effectively diagnose a spine tumor, the orthopaedic surgeon take the following steps when reviewing imaging[10]:

1. The compartment location of the lesion in the spinal column (extradural, intradural-extramedullary, or intramedullary) must be identified. Such localization may narrow the differential diagnosis.
2. The clinician generates a preimaging differential diagnosis according to patient demographic and clinical characteristics such as age, sex, medical history, and neurologic signs and symptoms (▶ Table 21.1). Such a meticulous evaluation not only guides the type and location of such imaging but also provides insight as to the true underlying pathology. In this way, imaging serves to corroborate or refute, rather than merely suggest, the previously hypothesized differential diagnosis.
3. The patient's demographic information and clinical presentation are used to narrow the differential diagnosis. For example, tumors that present in children often are extremely rare in adults and vice versa. In addition, for patients with a history of cancer, neck pain or back pain should be assumed to be a symptomatic spinal metastasis until proven otherwise.
4. Various imaging modalities (conventional radiography, computed tomography [CT], or magnetic resonance imaging [MRI]) can be used to determine a working diagnosis. Although these steps often lead to the correct diagnosis, the working diagnosis based on current imaging techniques is not always accurate. Therefore, image-guided or open biopsy often has a role in obtaining a definitive diagnosis before the initiation of a treatment plan (i.e., surgery, radiation therapy, chemotherapy).

Table 21.1 Differential diagnosis of spine lesion by anatomic compartment

Compartment	Malignant	Benign	Nontumorous growths
Extradural	Chordoma	Aneurysmal bone cyst	
	Ewing sarcoma	Eosinophilic granuloma	
	Leukemia; chondrosarcoma	Giant cell tumor	
	Lymphoma	Hemangioma	
	Metastases	Osteoblastoma	
	Myeloma	Osteochondroma	
	Osteosarcoma	Osteoid osteoma	
Intradural extramedullary	Malignant nerve sheath	Hemangiopericytoma	Arachnoid cyst
	Metastases	Meningioma	Dermoid
	Tumors	Nerve-sheath tumors	Epidermoid
		Neurofibroma	Lipoma
		Paraganglioma	
		Schwannoma	
Intramedullary	Astrocytoma	Astrocytoma	
	Metastases	Hemangioblastoma	
		Ependymoma	

MRI is the preferred imaging modality for evaluating most disorders of the spine, including spine tumors.[13,14,15,16] MRI is more sensitive than conventional radiography, CT, or bone scanning in detecting primary malignant bone tumors and metastatic lesions in the spine[17,18] because MRI provides superior resolution of soft-tissue structures such as the intervertebral disks, spinal cord, nerve roots, meninges, and paraspinal musculature. In addition, MRI provides clarity at the bone–soft-tissue interface, yielding precise anatomic detail of osseous compression or invasion of neural and paraspinal structures.

Despite this excellent anatomic and soft-tissue depiction, MRI is limited in its detection of calcifications and small osseous fragments and is subject to metal-induced artifact when used in the instrumented spine (usually with stainless steel or titanium), which may prevent accurate assessment of neural compression and necessitate a fluoroscopic or CT myelogram for optimal evaluation. CT also provides superior osseous detail and permits resolution of calcification in areas within or around soft-tissue structures. Therefore, the ideal method of evaluating a patient with a suspected or known spinal mass involves a combination of conventional radiography and/or CT imaging with MRI.

This chapter describes image interpretation techniques that permit identification of the compartment and the MRI appearance of the most common tumors in each location, facilitating the systematic and efficient creation of a differential diagnosis (▶ Table 21.1) for any spine tumor evaluated with MRI.

21.2 Specialized Pulse Sequences and Imaging Protocols

MRI protocols vary widely among institutions and in relation to the spinal region involved. Despite such variation, the MRI protocol for any patient suspected of having a spine tumor should include T1-weighted and T2-weighted images and gadolinium-enhanced studies in the axial and sagittal planes.[2,19,20,21] Gadolinium enhancement often provides improved anatomic detail of spinal tumors and may supply signature clues to the underlying pathology.[19] Because of the high signal intensity of fat within an adult's marrow on T1-weighted images, fat-suppression techniques are useful in evaluating osseous lesions that enhance with contrast.[2] Similarly, enhancing lesions in the epidural space are better seen with fat suppression, particularly in the lumbar spine in which the epidural space is composed primarily of fat. Gradient-echo sequences are not as useful for assessing spine tumors unless hemorrhage is suspected. Conversely, diffusion-weighted imaging, which often shows restricted diffusion in a vertebral body with a tumor, may be helpful in distinguishing benign from pathologic compression fractures.[13,22] Consultation with a neuroradiologist is advisable for the selection of the ideal imaging protocol.

21.3 Extradural Tumors

Extradural masses typically arise from the osseous spine, intervertebral disks, and adjacent soft tissues. With MRI, the hallmark of such lesions is focal displacement of the thecal sac away from the mass, with an obliterated subarachnoid space and compressed spinal cord (▶ Fig. 21.1). The dura often appears to be draped over the mass. The most common malignant extradural masses are metastases (▶ Fig. 21.2), followed by primary malignant tumors of the spine.[12] The most common benign extradural masses are degenerative and traumatic lesions such as disk herniations, osteophytes, and fractures, followed by primary benign tumors of the spine.[12] This chapter discusses extradural neoplastic lesions of the spine, both malignant and benign.

21.3.1 Metastatic Disease

The spinal column is the most common site of osseous metastases, and the most common extradural malignant spine tumors in adults are metastatic lesions.[12] Autopsy studies show vertebral metastases in up to 40% of patients with systemic cancer, with 5% of adults presenting with epidural spinal cord compression.[6,9,11,23]

Most spine metastases in adults arise from lung, breast, or prostate cancer, followed less frequently by lymphoma, melanoma, renal cancer, sarcoma, and multiple myeloma.[5,6] Approximately 5% of children with solid malignant tumors develop spinal metastases with cord compression.[24] In children, spinal metastases are typically caused by Ewing sarcoma or neuroblastoma, followed by osteogenic sarcoma, rhabdomyosarcoma, Hodgkin disease, soft-tissue sarcoma, and germ-cell tumors.[24]

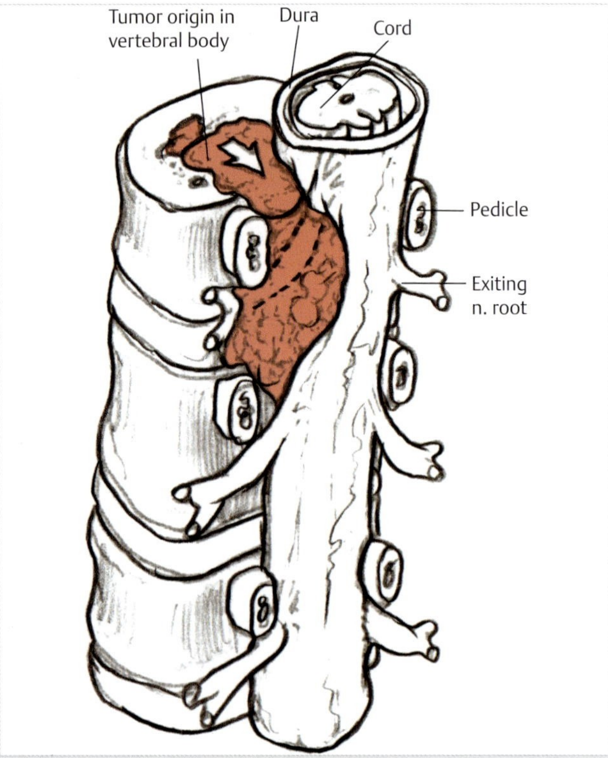

Fig. 21.1 Illustration of posterior oblique view depicting the characteristics of an extradural mass. The spinal cord and dura are displaced. The depicted mass extends from the vertebral body (*arrow*) into the extradural space. (Reproduced with permission from, Sciubba DM, Zadnik PL, Wasserman BA, Gokaslan ZL. Tumors of the Spine. In: Khanna AJ, ed. MRI Essentials for the Spine Specialist. New York: Thieme; 2014:211–236.)

In adults, the initial site of metastatic tumor growth in the spine typically is the posterior vertebral body, followed by the epidural space and pedicle.[25] Conversely, metastatic tumors in children invade the spinal canal via the neural foramina, causing circumferential cord compression.[5] Spinal metastases in adults can occur at any level but they usually involve the lower thoracic and lumbar spine because of the higher proportion of red bone marrow in those locations.[17,25]

MRI is the method of choice for imaging metastatic spine disease because of its unparalleled ability to delineate epidural and paraspinous soft-tissue involvement. Imaging patterns of such lesions can show focal lytic, focal blastic/sclerotic, diffuse homogeneous, and diffuse inhomogeneous lesions.[12,18,26] The most common pattern is multifocal lytic lesions, which are hypointense on T1-weighted images and hypointense to hyperintense on T2-weighted images (▶ Fig. 21.3). Sclerotic lesions tend to be hypointense on T1- and T2-weighted images. Diffuse homogeneous and inhomogeneous lesions are hypointense on T1-weighted images and hyperintense on T2-weighted images; however, the signal pattern can be variable and depends on the degree of fatty marrow. Contrast enhancement of such lesions is extremely variable, as well.

MRI also may be useful for distinguishing benign osteoporotic fractures from pathologic tumor-related fractures.[13,22,27,28] Benign fractures typically have marrow signal intensity identical to that of neighboring normal vertebral bodies. Pathologic fractures are more hypointense on T1-weighted images and more hyperintense on T2-weighted images than normal vertebral bodies.[27] In addition, diffusion-weighted images, combined with apparent diffusion coefficient mapping, often show more extensive restricted diffusion with pathologic fractures than with osteoporotic fractures.[2] The identification of epidural or paraspinal soft-tissue involvement is also helpful in confirming a pathologic cause.

MRI may be used to further identify the vascularity of spinal metastatic tumors. Gradient-echo images are helpful to identify

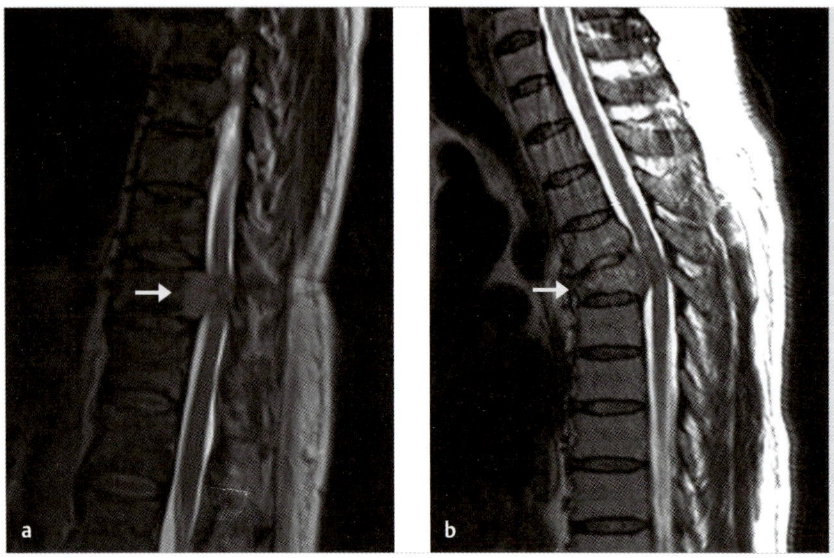

Fig. 21.2 Sagittal T2-weighted images of extradural metastatic lesions show compression and distortion of the underlying dura and spinal cord in two patients. **(a)** Prostate metastasis (*arrow*) to the thoracic spine with epidural extension. **(b)** Non-small-cell lung cancer metastasis to the upper thoracic spine with epidural extension. Loss of vertebral body height is noted (*arrow*). (Reproduced with permission from, Sciubba DM, Zadnik PL, Wasserman BA, Gokaslan ZL. Tumors of the Spine. In: Khanna AJ, ed. MRI Essentials for the Spine Specialist. New York: Thieme; 2014:211–236.)

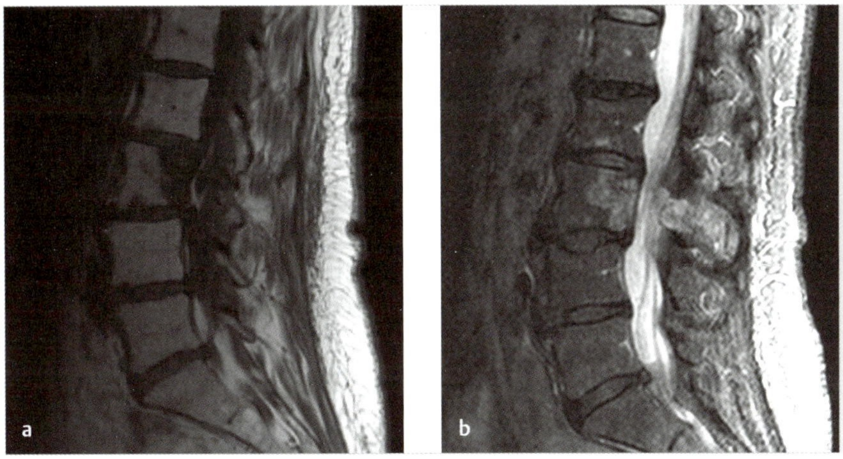

Fig. 21.3 Lumbar spine metastasis from breast carcinoma. **(a)** A sagittal T1-weighted image shows a hypointense lesion occupying the L3 vertebral body. **(b)** The disease extent is more evident on this sagittal fat-suppressed T2-weighted image. (Reproduced with permission from, Sciubba DM, Zadnik PL, Wasserman BA, Gokaslan ZL. Tumors of the Spine. In: Khanna AJ, ed. MRI Essentials for the Spine Specialist. New York: Thieme; 2014:211–236.)

blood products; postcontrast T1-weighted sequences may help to identify vascular-flow voids; and T2-weighted fast spin-echo sequences further highlight vascular lesions. Spinal magnetic resonance angiography may be used to visualize venous and arterial anatomy in greater detail. Spinal magnetic resonance angiography can be performed with or without contrast because vascular-flow voids can be reconstructed into three-dimensional images using postprocessing algorithms to generate maximum-intensity projection images. Maximum-intensity projections can create a three-dimensional image of large intradural vessels, and these data may be useful to identify target vessels for formal spinal angiography and embolization. Preoperative embolization of vascular lesions can reduce intraoperative bleeding and reduce surgical time.

21.3.2 Primary Benign Tumors

Benign primary tumors of the extradural compartment of the spine have characteristic MRI findings and patient demographic characteristics that help differentiate them from malignant lesions.

Vertebral Hemangioma

Vertebral hemangioma is the most common spinal axis tumor.[28,29] This benign vascular tumor of the vertebral body, often discovered incidentally on imaging, can be associated with vertebral body collapse and epidural extension with spinal cord compression. On rare occasions, it may exhibit aggressive growth.[30,31] MRI sequences of the typical (fatty) hemangioma show lesions that are hyperintense on T1- and T2-weighted images with robust contrast enhancement (▶ Fig. 21.4).[32] Vertebral hemangiomas are one of the very few spinal tumors that show increased signal intensity on T1- and T2-weighted images. Occasionally, such lesions are more vascular and may appear isointense or hypointense on T1-weighted images, making them difficult to distinguish from metastases. Although CT images show the typical "polka dot" appearance on axial images and the typical "corduroy" or "jailhouse striation" pattern on sagittal images as a result of the thickened trabeculae, MRI is the best modality for characterizing the epidural extent and cord compromise of aggressive lesions. Although such lesions primarily involve the vertebral body, 10 to 15% have concomitant involvement of the posterior elements.[29] Multiple lesions are seen in 25 to 30% of patients.[33]

Osteoid Osteoma

This benign, osteoid-producing tumor is usually < 1.5 cm in size and often surrounded by a ring of sclerotic bone. Almost all of these lesions involve the neural arch, and most occur within the lumbar spine, followed by the cervical, thoracic, or sacral regions. Bone scintigraphy and CT are more helpful than MRI for detecting and characterizing these lesions. The nidus is hypointense or isointense on T1-weighted images and varies from hypointense to hyperintense on T2-weighted images, often with surrounding hyperintensity that likely is related to a local inflammatory response (▶ Fig. 21.5).[34,35,36] The rapid enhancement pattern, typically located within the nidus, is best seen on dynamic sequences (e.g., serial postcontrast images). The surrounding reactive zone enhances more slowly with such imaging. Of note, up to 70% of patients may present with scoliosis related to muscle spasm, with concavity on the side of the tumor.[37] Patients often report severe night pain.[38]

Osteoblastoma

Osteoblastomas, also known as giant osteoid osteomas, are similar histologically to osteoid osteomas but are differentiated largely by size (> 1.5 cm). Patient symptoms also can help to distinguish these lesions. Osteoblastomas cause dull pain as opposed to the intense night pain caused by osteoid osteomas.[39,40,41] Occasionally, osteoblastomas possess atypical features and behave aggressively.[41] Like osteoid osteomas, these lesions originate in the neural arch but exhibit greater mass expansion.[12] Thus, they may be centered in the pedicle, lamina, transverse or spinous process, articular pillar, or pars interarticularis with extension into the vertebral body. The lesion is hypointense or isointense on T1-weighted images and isointense or hyperintense on T2-weighted images, with

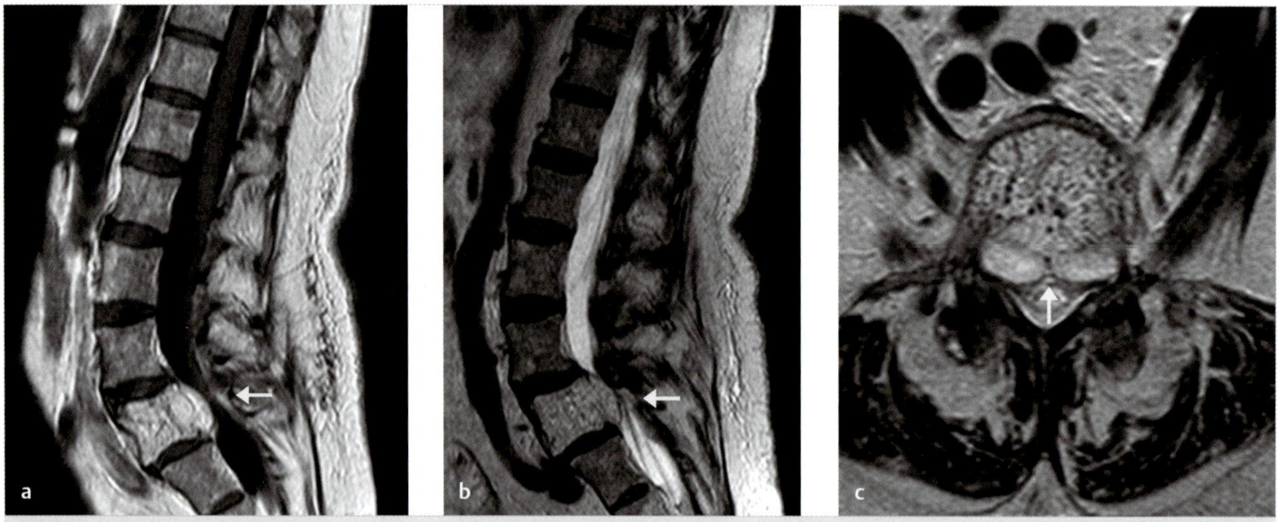

Fig. 21.4 Lumbar vertebral hemangioma. This asymptomatic lesion is centered in the vertebral body and appears hyperintense on **(a)** T1-weighted postcontrast and **(b)** T2-weighted sagittal images (*arrow on each*). **(c)** On axial T2-weighted imaging, the classic "polka dot" appearance of the vertebral body is noted, with infiltration into the anterior epidural space divided by a cleavage plane formed by the midline septum (*arrow*). This spinal hemangioma is somewhat atypical in that there is involvement of the posterior wall and extension into the spinal canal. Most hemangiomas remain confined to the vertebral body. (Reproduced with permission from, Sciubba DM, Zadnik PL, Wasserman BA, Gokaslan ZL. Tumors of the Spine. In: Khanna AJ, ed. MRI Essentials for the Spine Specialist. New York: Thieme; 2014:211–236.)

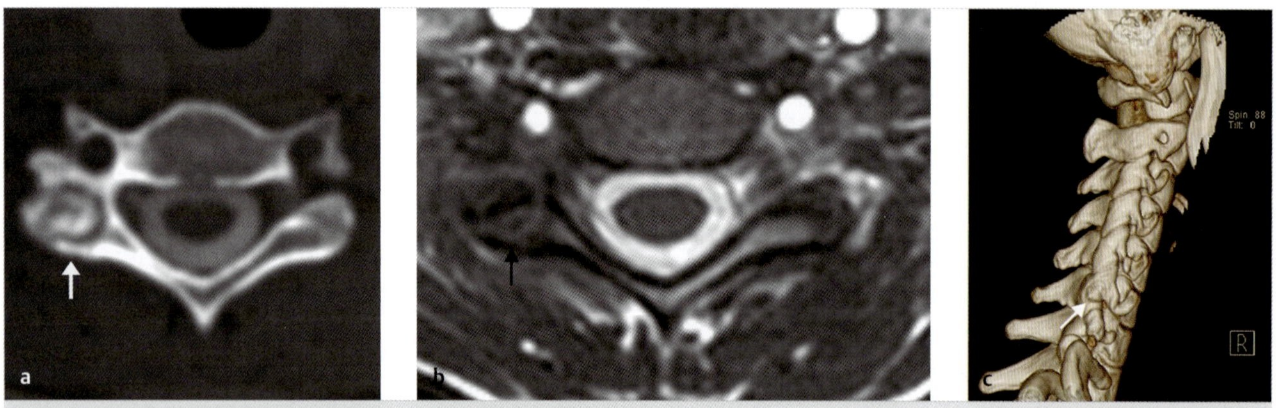

Fig. 21.5 Right-side cervical osteoid osteoma. **(a)** An axial computed tomography myelogram shows the characteristic hyperdense center with sclerotic rim (*arrow*). **(b)** An axial T2-weighted image shows a hypointense center (*arrow*) corresponding to sclerotic bone, surrounded by a region of high signal intensity corresponding to reactive edema. **(c)** On three-dimensional computed tomography reconstruction, the osseous outgrowth corresponding to the osteoma (*arrow*) is seen. (Reproduced with permission from, Sciubba DM, Zadnik PL, Wasserman BA, Gokaslan ZL. Tumors of the Spine. In: Khanna AJ, ed. MRI Essentials for the Spine Specialist. New York: Thieme; 2014:211–236.)

extensive peritumoral edema (flare phenomenon). Fluid–fluid levels are often present within the lesion (▶ Fig. 21.6). Contrast enhancement is variable.[40]

Giant Cell Tumor

Giant cell tumors are locally aggressive, lytic tumors in the vertebral body and sacrum and are named for the osteoclast-like giant cells that are present on histology.[28,37] Hemorrhage is common secondary to the hypervascular stroma of these lesions. MRI shows expansile lesions with hypointense to isointense signal on T1-weighted images and isointense to hyperintense signal on T2-weighted images (▶ Fig. 21.7). Contrast enhancement is often heterogeneous, commonly surrounding areas of necrosis, blood, and/or cystic cavities with fluid–fluid levels.[42] Such lesions can undergo sarcomatous transformation (10% of cases) to become malignant giant cell tumors.[37] Therefore, patients with these tumors must be monitored with MRI or CT because of the risk of recurrence. It is important to note that the differential diagnosis of midline tumors in the sacrum includes giant cell tumor, chordoma, aneurysmal bone cyst, plasmacytoma, and metastases in adults and sacrococcygeal teratoma in children.[43]

Osteochondroma

Osteochondroma, also known as osteocartilaginous exostosis, consists of cartilage-covered osseous protuberances with a

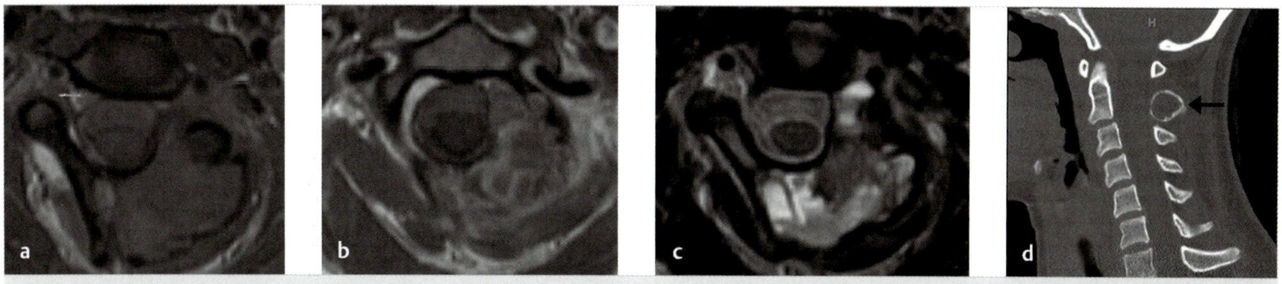

Fig. 21.6 Left-side cervical osteoblastoma. Axial **(a)** precontrast and **(b)** postcontrast T1-weighted images show a lesion similar to but larger than the osteoid osteoma shown in **Fig.** 21.5. The lesion shows heterogeneous contrast enhancement with infiltration into the epidural space. **(c)** An axial T2-weighted image also shows the lesion. **(d)** A sagittal computed tomography reconstruction highlights the osseous destruction and expansion associated with the osteoblastoma in the spinous process (*arrow*). (Reproduced with permission from, Sciubba DM, Zadnik PL, Wasserman BA, Gokaslan ZL. Tumors of the Spine. In: Khanna AJ, ed. MRI Essentials for the Spine Specialist. New York: Thieme; 2014:211–236.)

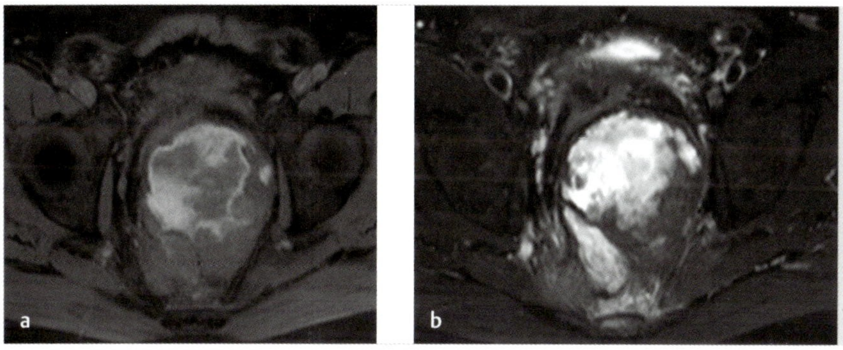

Fig. 21.7 Sacral giant cell tumor. This expansile lesion shows heterogeneous enhancement on **(a)** a coronal postcontrast T1-weighted image and high signal intensity on **(b)** an axial fat-suppressed T2-weighted image. (Reproduced with permission from, Sciubba DM, Zadnik PL, Wasserman BA, Gokaslan ZL. Tumors of the Spine. In: Khanna AJ, ed. MRI Essentials for the Spine Specialist. New York: Thieme; 2014:211–236.)

medullary cavity that is contiguous with the parent bone.[44,45] These lesions grossly appear to be cauliflower- or mushroom-shaped with cartilaginous caps. Only 5% of these growths occur within the spine (compared with 85% in long-bone metaphyses) but when they do, they are located mostly in the cervical spine, particularly at C2.[43] These lesions most commonly arise from the spinous and transverse processes but they also may arise from the vertebral body. On T1- and T2-weighted images, they appear as central hyperintense lesions surrounded by hypointense calcified cortex.[46] The cartilaginous cap is hypointense to isointense on T1-weighted images and isointense to hyperintense on T2-weighted images and exhibits peripheral enhancement of cartilage.[45] MRI is the preferred imaging modality for measuring the cartilaginous cap and determining the status of regional neural and musculoskeletal tissue. Thickening of the cap (> 1 cm) should raise concern for malignant transformation to chondrosarcoma. CT may be used for evaluating the osseous structure of the lesion, confirming the contiguity of the medullary cavity with the parent bone, and evaluating for fractures.

Aneurysmal Bone Cyst

These lesions are expansile benign neoplasms containing thin-walled cavities filled with blood and blood products that occur most commonly in patients < 20 years old. A substantial proportion of aneurysmal bone cysts are associated with preexisting osseous lesions such as an osteoblastoma, giant cell tumor, chondroblastoma, nonossifying fibroma, or fibrous dysplasia.[37,47,48,49,50,51] They arise in the neural arch but most extend into the vertebral body. The classic presentation is a balloon-like expansile remodeling of bone, leaving a thinned "eggshell" cortex. On T1- and T2-weighted images, the lesions appear as lobulated neural-arch masses, commonly with extension into the vertebral body, epidural space, and adjacent vertebral bodies and ribs.[47] Intratumoral cysts contain fluid–fluid levels secondary to blood breakdown products (▶ Fig. 21.8); however, visualization of these levels often requires the patient to be motionless for several minutes before imaging. Contrast enhancement may be present at the periphery of the tumor and in the septations. Vertebral body collapse may occur secondary to the extensive vertebral body destruction associated with such lesions.

Eosinophilic Granuloma

This lytic lesion of the vertebral body classically presents with a single collapsed vertebral body (vertebra plana) in patients < 10 years old (▶ Fig. 21.9) and consists of a benign proliferation of Langerhans cell histiocytes. The lesions are hyperintense on T2-weighted images but present with variable intensity on T1-weighted images. Contrast enhancement is robust.[12,52]

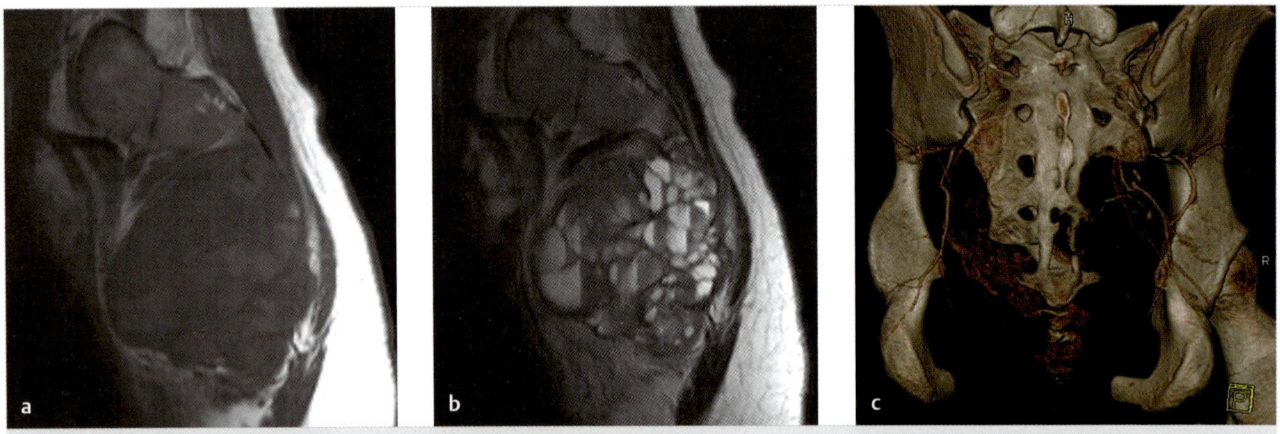

Fig. 21.8 Aneurysmal bone cyst. Sagittal **(a)** T1-weighted and **(b)** T2-weighted images of the sacrum show a large T1-hypointense tumor with multiple cysts containing fluid–fluid levels indicative of blood breakdown products. **(c)** A three-dimensional computed tomography reconstruction shows a posterior coronal view of osseous destruction of the sacrum secondary to tumor growth. (Reproduced with permission from, Sciubba DM, Zadnik PL, Wasserman BA, Gokaslan ZL. Tumors of the Spine. In: Khanna AJ, ed. MRI Essentials for the Spine Specialist. New York: Thieme; 2014:211–236.)

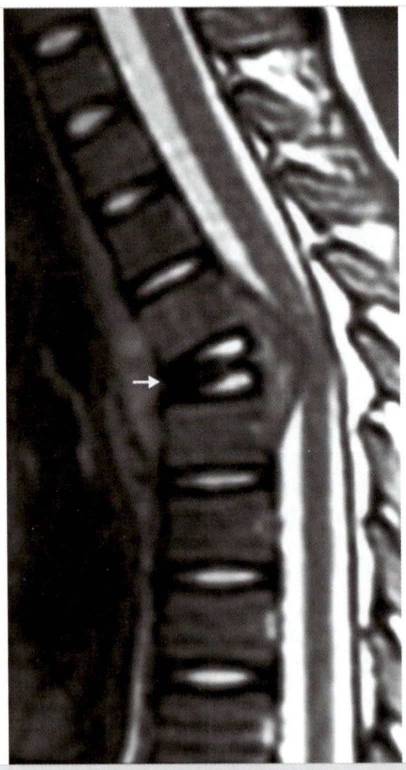

Fig. 21.9 A sagittal T2-weighted image of an eosinophilic granuloma shows the typical finding of a vertebra plana (*arrow*). In this case, there is also an epidural mass that displaces the spinal cord. Note the associated kyphotic deformity. (Reproduced with permission from, Sciubba DM, Zadnik PL, Wasserman BA, Gokaslan ZL. Tumors of the Spine. In: Khanna AJ, ed. MRI Essentials for the Spine Specialist. New York: Thieme; 2014:211–236.)

21.3.3 Primary Malignant Tumors

Multiple Myeloma

Multiple myeloma is the multifocal, metastatic, and systemic presentation of a solitary bone plasmacytoma.[53] Like solitary bone plasmacytomas, focal lesions appear in the vertebral bodies with low to intermediate signal intensity on T1-weighted images compared with normal bone marrow, and they appear hyperintense on T2-weighted images. Postgadolinium enhancement is often present (▶ Fig. 21.10). Multiple myeloma also is shown on MRI by diffuse marrow involvement at multiple spinal levels.[54] Compared with other metastatic lesions, which usually have early pedicle involvement, multiple myeloma usually involves the pedicle late in the course of disease.[43]

Solitary Bone Plasmacytoma

Solitary plasmacytoma presents as a mass of monoclonal plasma cells from bone or soft tissue and may precede multiple myeloma by several years.[55] Clinical differentiation from multiple myeloma requires a biopsy-proven solitary lesion, the absence of other such lesions in the skeleton, and the absence of anemia, hypercalcemia, and renal involvement suggesting systemic myeloma.[56,57,58] Such lesions are lytic, destructive, and often accompanied by compression fractures associated with soft-tissue masses and fractures that may lead to severe collapse (vertebra plana). T1-weighted images show a solitary lesion centered in the vertebral body that is hypointense or isointense compared with muscle and can show curvilinear low-signal areas and/or cortical infolding caused by end-plate fractures. In most cases, the posterior elements are involved, and neural compression is varied. T2-weighted images show heterogeneous signal within the lesion with focal hyperintensities. Mild to moderate diffuse contrast enhancement is common, and peripheral (rim) contrast enhancement is rare.[59] Scanning of the entire skeleton is mandatory to identify a secondary lesion, which occurs in the spine in one-third of patients.[43,60]

Chordoma

These malignant tumors arising from notochord remnants typically present in one of two histologic patterns. The more common type, known as a typical chordoma, is composed of lobules and sheets of physaliphorous cells, which contain intracytoplasmic

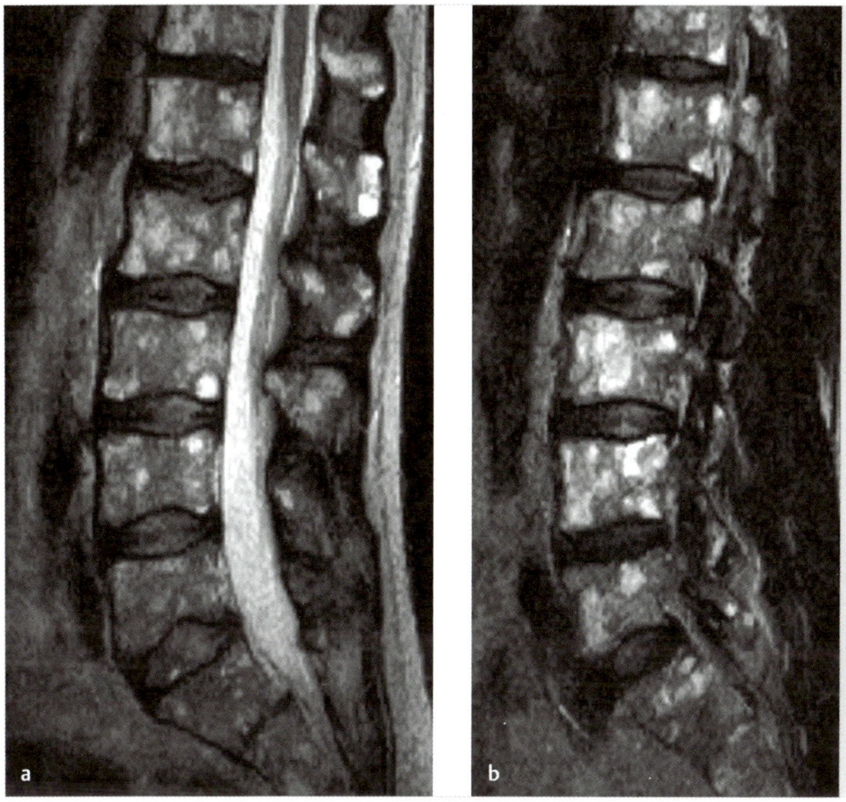

Fig. 21.10 Multiple myeloma. **(a)** Midsagittal and **(b)** parasagittal T2-weighted images of the lumbar spine show multiple, well-circumscribed, high-signal-intensity lesions throughout the lumbar spine. The diagnosis of multiple myeloma can be confirmed by correlation with computed tomography imaging and also with urine and serum-protein electrophoresis. (Reproduced with permission from, Sciubba DM, Zadnik PL, Wasserman BA, Gokaslan ZL. Tumors of the Spine. In: Khanna AJ, ed. MRI Essentials for the Spine Specialist. New York: Thieme; 2014:211–236.)

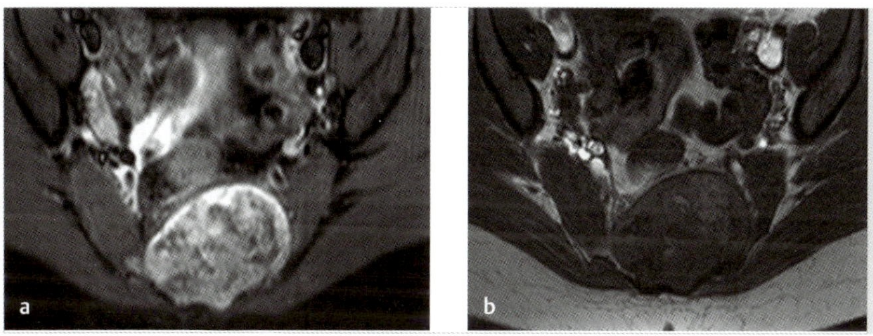

Fig. 21.11 This **(a)** axial fat-suppressed T2-weighted image of a sacral chordoma shows a hyperintense lesion that has extended into the pelvis and left gluteal muscles. **(b)** The lesion appears mostly hypointense with focal regions of hyperintensity, likely representing hemorrhage or mucinous material on an axial T1-weighted image. (Reproduced with permission from, Sciubba DM, Zadnik PL, Wasserman BA, Gokaslan ZL. Tumors of the Spine. In: Khanna AJ, ed. MRI Essentials for the Spine Specialist. New York: Thieme; 2014:211–236.)

vacuoles and abundant mucin.[61] The less common type contains cartilaginous foci and is termed chondroid chordoma.[12,61] Chordomas present as lytic, destructive lesions arising in the midline of the spinal column at any location from clivus to coccyx but they are found more commonly at the sacrococcygeal (50%) and sphenooccipital (clival) (35%) areas and less commonly in the cervical, thoracic, and lumbar vertebral bodies (15%).[43] For lesions within the vertebral bodies, a cervical location (particularly at C2) is most common, followed by lumbar and thoracic areas. Chordomas often are several centimeters in size at discovery, usually involve two or more adjacent vertebrae, and involve the intervertebral disks, surrounding paravertebral soft tissues, and spinal canal. On T1-weighted images, the lesions are hypointense or isointense to bone marrow. On T2-weighted images, lesions are hyperintense compared with intervertebral disks and cerebrospinal fluid secondary to the high intratumoral mucin content and are septated by low-signal fibrous bands (▶ Fig. 21.11). Short-tau inversion recovery or fat-suppressed T2-weighted images can help in defining borders with neighboring soft tissues. Contrast-enhanced images range from contrast blush to robust enhancement.[62,63]

Sarcomas

Chondrosarcoma

These malignant, lytic tumors of chondrocytes are characterized by the formation of cartilaginous matrix. They can occur as primary tumors or as malignant degeneration of osteochondromas and enchondromas, can cause cortical disruption, and can extend into surrounding soft tissues.[64,65] Chondrosarcomas can occur wherever cartilage exists,[66] and approximately 5% occur in the spine.[43] T2-weighted images show high signal intensity in areas of hyaline cartilage and low signal intensity in areas of mineralized matrix. T1-weighted images are helpful in delineating soft-tissue invasion. Contrast-enhanced images show strong enhancement of the septa with "ring and arc" patterns that

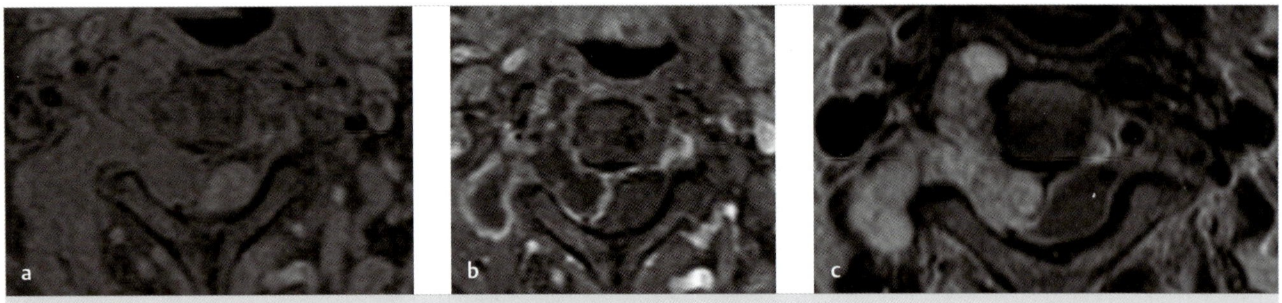

Fig. 21.12 These axial **(a)** precontrast and **(b)** postcontrast T1-weighted images show an exophytic, cauliflower-shaped lesion, found to be a chondrosarcoma, arising from the lateral mass of C2. **(c)** The lesion shows the "ring and arc" pattern on an axial T2-weighted image. (Reproduced with permission from, Sciubba DM, Zadnik PL, Wasserman BA, Gokaslan ZL. Tumors of the Spine. In: Khanna AJ, ed. MRI Essentials for the Spine Specialist. New York: Thieme; 2014:211–236.)

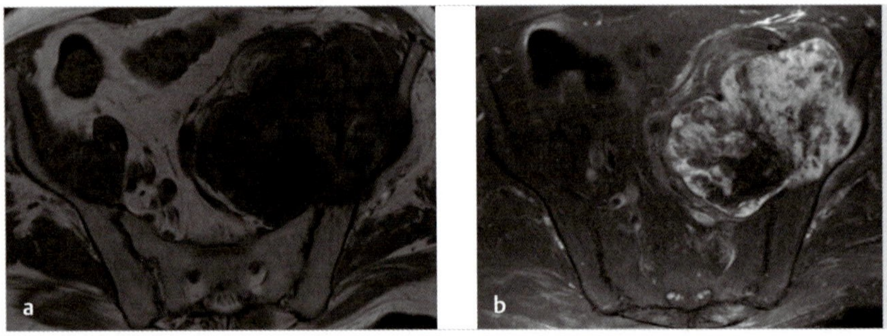

Fig. 21.13 Osteosarcoma. **(a)** An axial T1-weighted image of a left-side osteosarcoma of the sacrum and ilium. **(b)** The lesion is hyperintense on an axial postgadolinium, fat-suppressed T1-weighted image with a central hypointense, cystic/necrotic area. (Reproduced with permission from, Sciubba DM, Zadnik PL, Wasserman BA, Gokaslan ZL. Tumors of the Spine. In: Khanna AJ, ed. MRI Essentials for the Spine Specialist. New York: Thieme; 2014:211–236.)

delineate areas of hyaline cartilage, cystic mucoid tissue, and necrosis, none of which enhances with contrast (▶ Fig. 21.12).[67]

Osteosarcoma/Osteogenic Sarcoma

Of all primary osteogenic sarcomas, 4% occur in the spine and sacrum, primarily in the posterior spinal elements.[68] These malignant, lytic tumors of osteoblasts are characterized by the formation of immature, woven osteoid and can occur as primary tumors or as malignant degeneration in individuals with Paget disease, irradiated bone, or bone infarcts. These tumors present primarily in the vertebral bodies, commonly with extension into the posterior elements and typically have focal areas of low signal on all pulse sequences, secondary to matrix mineralization (▶ Fig. 21.13).[69] In the telangiectatic form, T2-weighted images may show fluid–fluid levels.

Ewing Sarcoma

The spine is a rare site for Ewing sarcoma. When it does occur, it usually represents a metastatic tumor from another site of origin.[70] Usually centered in the vertebral body or sacrum, Ewing sarcoma often causes a "moth-eaten" or permeative type of bone destruction rather than extensive bone loss.[71] Fifty percent of these lesions have an extraosseous, noncalcified soft-tissue mass.[68,72] On T1-weighted images, these lesions are hypointense to isointense compared with surrounding bone marrow, and the cortex usually is preserved despite extraosseous tumor spread. On T2-weighted images, lesions are hyperintense. MRI is the ideal imaging modality for delineating extension of soft-tissue mass. Because Ewing sarcoma is histologically a small, round-cell tumor, it can be radiographically identical to primitive neuroectodermal tumors, Langerhans cell histiocytosis, lymphoma, leukemia, myeloma, and metastatic neuroblastoma. Ewing sarcoma may also have imaging characteristics similar to those of osteomyelitis. In addition, patients with Ewing sarcoma may present with vertebral body collapse, similarly to patients with Langerhans cell histiocytosis.[73]

21.3.4 Other Tumors

Neuroblastic Tumors

These embryonal tumors, which are derived from neural crest cells, exist as a spectrum ranging from the most benign ganglioneuromas, to intermediate-differentiated ganglioneuroblastomas, to the most malignant neuroblastomas. These tumors present almost exclusively in patients < 10 years old and almost exclusively as abdominal or thoracic paraspinal masses with intraspinal extension.[12] The lesions are typically large and extend through a widened neural foramen, creating dumbbell-shaped morphologies and compressing the spinal cord (▶ Fig. 21.14). The lesions are hypointense to isointense on T1-weighted images and hypointense to hyperintense on T2-weighted images. Although classically they present as paraspinal masses, they may appear as metastatic lesions within vertebral bodies. Contrast enhancement varies but often surrounds areas of internal hemorrhage or necrosis.[74,75]

Angiolipoma

These benign lesions of adipose and vascular elements present in the spine primarily as epidural masses. They rarely present in an intramedullary location.[76] Because the lesions

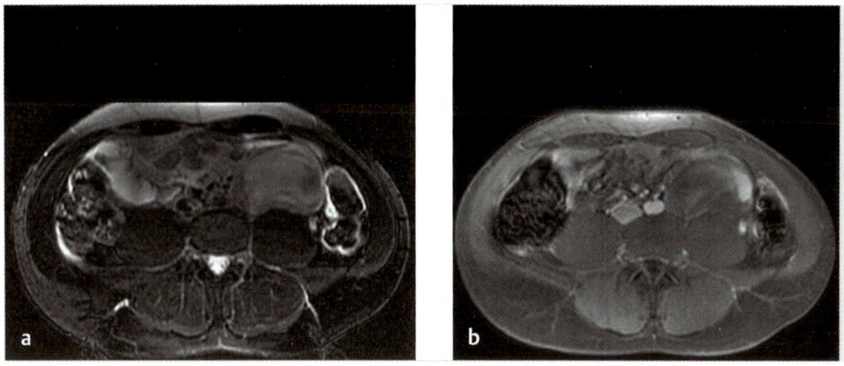

Fig. 21.14 Left-side paraspinal ganglioneuroma. **(a)** An axial T2-weighted fat-suppressed image shows a lesion adjacent to the vertebral body and anterior to the psoas muscle. The lesion is hyperintense compared with muscle. **(b)** An axial postgadolinium T1-weighted image shows the lesion to be isointense compared with muscle, with sparse intralesional and peripheral enhancement.(Reproduced with permission from, Sciubba DM, Zadnik PL, Wasserman BA, Gokaslan ZL. Tumors of the Spine. In: Khanna AJ, ed. MRI Essentials for the Spine Specialist. New York: Thieme; 2014:211–236.)

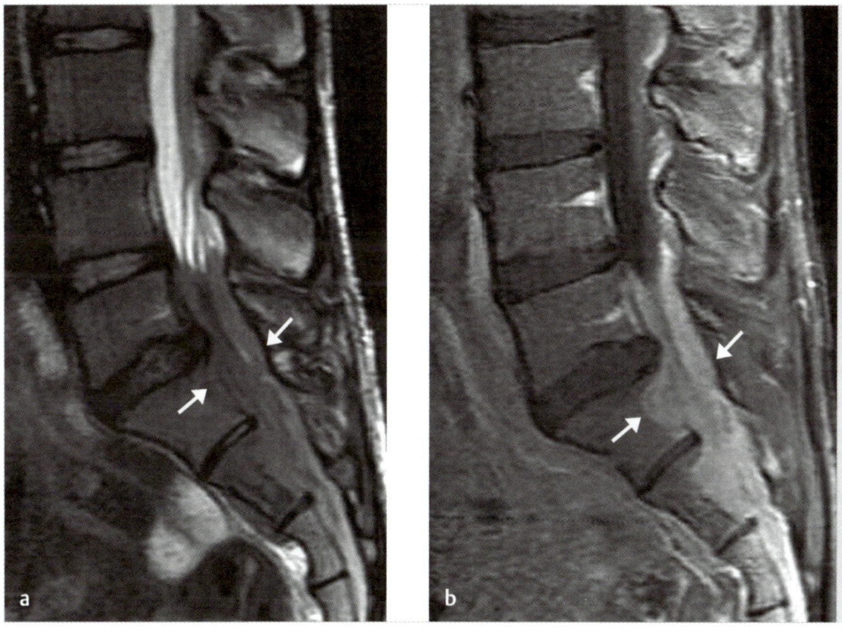

Fig. 21.15 Epidural B-cell lymphoma surrounding and compressing the caudal thecal sac in the lumbosacral spine. **(a)** On a sagittal T2-weighted image, the lesion is isointense compared with the nerve roots and fills the spinal canal, expanding the canal at S1 (*arrows*). **(b)** On a sagittal postgadolinium T1-weighted image, the lesion (*arrows*) shows robust enhancement. (Reproduced with permission from, Sciubba DM, Zadnik PL, Wasserman BA, Gokaslan ZL. Tumors of the Spine. In: Khanna AJ, ed. MRI Essentials for the Spine Specialist. New York: Thieme; 2014:211–236.)

are composed of fat and vascular tissues, MRI shows heterogeneous signal intensity. On T1-weighted images, most lesions are hyperintense with isointense to hypointense areas around prominent vascular components. The lesion may appear heterogeneous on T2-weighted images but it has high signal intensity. Therefore, fat-suppressed T1-weighted images with contrast are most useful for defining this lesion and often show heterogeneous enhancement. Interestingly, these lesions do not show vascular-flow voids. These lesions may destroy adjacent bone in the anterior epidural space, although only rarely in the posterior epidural space.[77]

Lymphoma

Lymphoreticular neoplasms present with variable imaging manifestations within the spine.[78,79] The following locations of the spine may be affected: epidural space (most common), osseous structures, lymphomatous meninges (within the subarachnoid space), or intramedullary (least common).[43] Lymphomas of the spine are usually metastatic lesions, not primary lesions arising in the spine.[80] Only 3 to 4% of all malignant bone tumors are primary osseous lymphomas. In the spine, non-Hodgkin lymphoma is far more common than Hodgkin disease, and > 80% of such lesions are of B-cell origin.[81]

MRI is ideal for defining the spinal compartment within which the tumor resides. Epidural lesions are isointense on T1-weighted images and variable but often isointense or hyperintense compared with the spinal cord on T2-weighted images (▶ Fig. 21.15). Osseous lesions are hypointense compared with normal marrow on T1-weighted images and isointense to hyperintense on T2-weighted images. Leptomeningitis lymphomas result in thickening of the nerve roots, occasionally with focal nodules, which are isointense compared with the spinal cord on T1- and T2-weighted images. Intramedullary masses show cord thickening that is isointense compared with the spinal cord on T1-weighted images and hyperintense with surrounding edema on T2-weighted images. Contrast-enhanced images show diffuse uniform enhancement regardless of the location, with a diagnostic accuracy of 99%.[43]

21.4 Intradural-Extramedullary Tumors

These lesions arise within the dura but not from within the spinal cord. Classic MRI findings include a widened ipsilateral subarachnoid space in which the cord and roots are displaced away from the mass (▶ Fig. 21.16). Nerve-sheath tumors

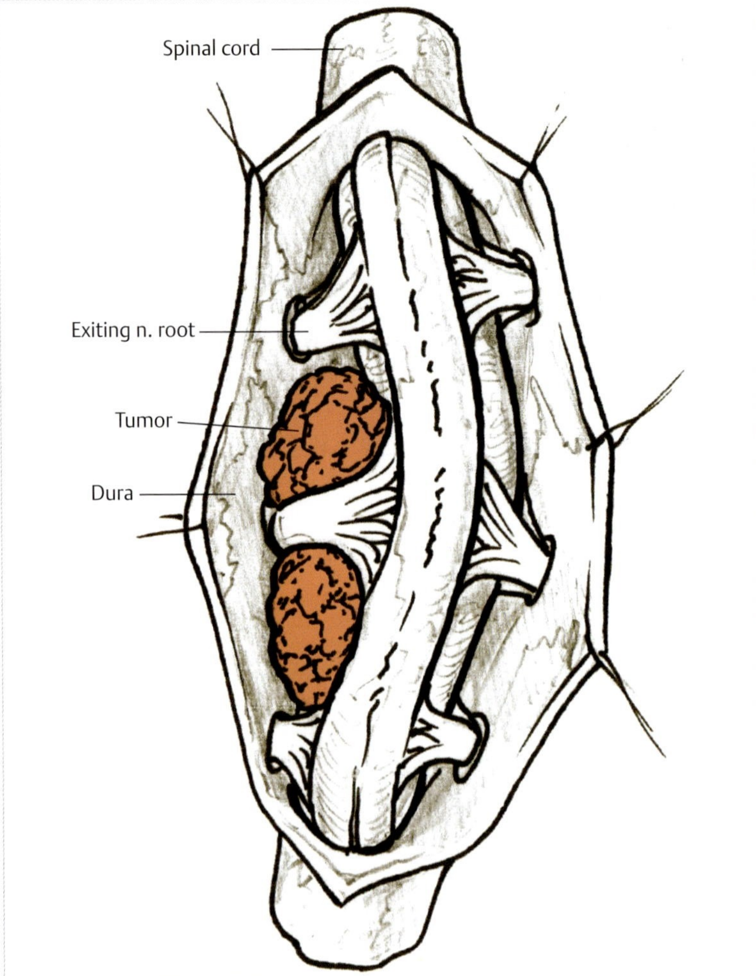

Fig. 21.16 Illustration of the dorsal view depicts the imaging characteristics of an intradural-extramedullary mass. (Reproduced with permission from, Sciubba DM, Zadnik PL, Wasserman BA, Gokaslan ZL. Tumors of the Spine. In: Khanna AJ, ed. MRI Essentials for the Spine Specialist. New York: Thieme; 2014:211–236.)

(schwannomas and neurofibromas) and meningiomas account for > 80% of such masses.[82]

21.4.1 Meningioma

Most of these tumors are slow growing, benign (> 95%), and based on the dura mater.[83] CT imaging may provide added detail because these tumors can calcify; however, MRI is still the ideal imaging modality.[83] Classically, the lesions are isointense compared with the spinal cord on T1-weighted images and isointense to hyperintense on T2-weighted images (▶ Fig. 21.17). Focal areas of hypointensity occur in the presence of calcifications or flow voids. Contrast-enhanced T1-weighted images show prominent enhancement, sometimes with a broad-based dural attachment (dural "tails"). Most lesions are solitary and occur most commonly in the thoracic spine (80%), followed by the cervical spine (16%) and lumbar spine (4%).[84,85] Compared with nerve-sheath tumors, which are usually anterolateral, meningiomas are usually located dorsal to the cord.[84,85]

21.4.2 Schwannoma

These benign neoplasms of the peripheral nerve sheaths are the most common intradural-extramedullary masses and appear as well-circumscribed lesions that may be intradural-extramedullary (75%), completely extradural-paraspinal (15%), or intradural and extradural (dumbbell-shaped).[12] T1-weighted images often show an isointense to hypointense lesion relative to the spinal cord that may be associated with adjacent osseous erosion such as widening of the neural foramen or vertebral scalloping.[86,87] In contrast to meningiomas, most schwannomas are hyperintense on T2-weighted images. Postgadolinium T1-weighted images show enhancement that may be homogeneous, heterogeneous, or rim enhancing around cystic areas (▶ Fig. 21.18). Hemorrhage and cystic degeneration are more common with schwannomas than with neurofibromas. Solitary lesions are usually sporadic but when these lesions occur at multiple concurrent sites, the diagnosis of type-2 neurofibromatosis should be considered.

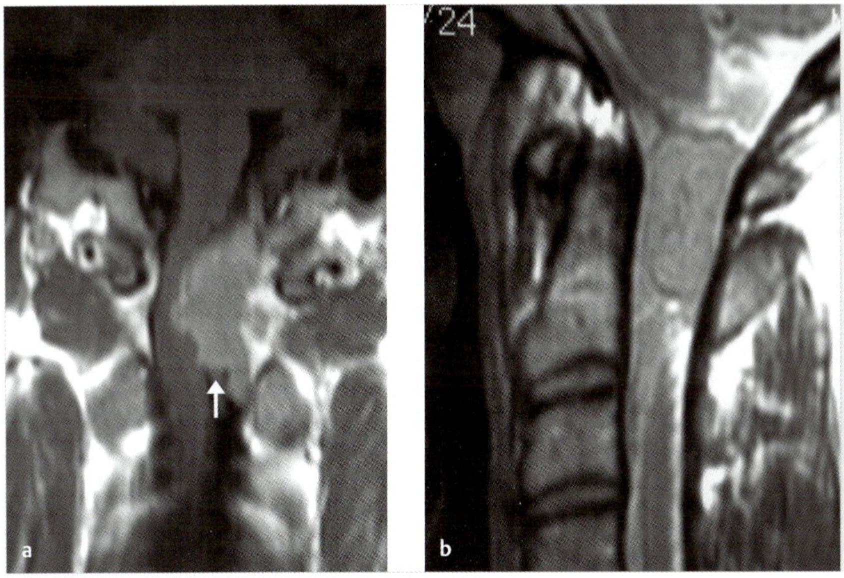

Fig. 21.17 Cervical meningioma. (a) A coronal postgadolinium T1-weighted image shows a widely dural-based lesion (*arrow*) that enhances and is hyperintense compared with the spinal cord. (b) On a sagittal T2-weighted image, the lesion is slightly hyperintense compared with the spinal cord, showing cord displacement and widening of the ipsilateral cerebrospinal fluid space, characteristic of intradural-extramedullary lesions. (Reproduced with permission from, Sciubba DM, Zadnik PL, Wasserman BA, Gokaslan ZL. Tumors of the Spine. In: Khanna AJ, ed. MRI Essentials for the Spine Specialist. New York: Thieme; 2014:211–236.)

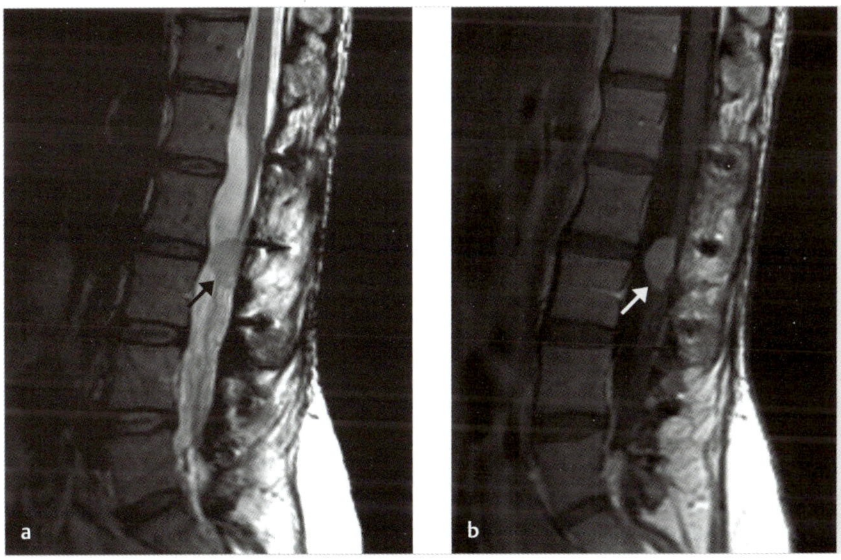

Fig. 21.18 Sagittal images of a schwannoma in the lumbar spine. (a) The lesion (*arrow on each*) is slightly hyperintense compared with the cord on a T2-weighted image and (b) shows strong homogeneous contrast enhancement with gadolinium on a T1-weighted image. (Reproduced with permission from, Sciubba DM, Zadnik PL, Wasserman BA, Gokaslan ZL. Tumors of the Spine. In: Khanna AJ, ed. MRI Essentials for the Spine Specialist. New York: Thieme; 2014:211–236.)

21.4.3 Neurofibroma

These benign neoplasms of the peripheral nerve sheaths can present as focal, diffuse, or plexiform lesions. They can undergo transformation to malignant tumors. Neurofibromas have MRI characteristics (▸ Fig. 21.19) similar to those of schwannomas but they often occur as multiple lesions in a patient with the stigmata of familial neurofibromatosis[88]:

- Vertebral anomalies.
- Meningoceles.
- Dural ectasia.
- Intramedullary astrocytomas.
- Short-segment thoracic scoliosis or kyphosis.
- Axillary or inguinal freckling.
- Café-au-lait spots.
- Optic glioma.
- Lisch nodules (hamartomas of the iris) of type-1 neurofibromatosis.

Therefore, if lesions that look like a schwannoma or neurofibroma on imaging occur in an individual with characteristics of type-1 neurofibromatosis, the lesions are likely to be neurofibromas, not schwannomas.[89] Even when isolated, these lesions are usually associated with type-1 neurofibromatosis. Unlike schwannomas, neurofibromas on T2-weighted images often have a peripheral area of high signal intensity surrounding a central area of low to intermediate signal intensity known as a target sign. Also unlike schwannomas, neurofibromas typically lack a cystic component.

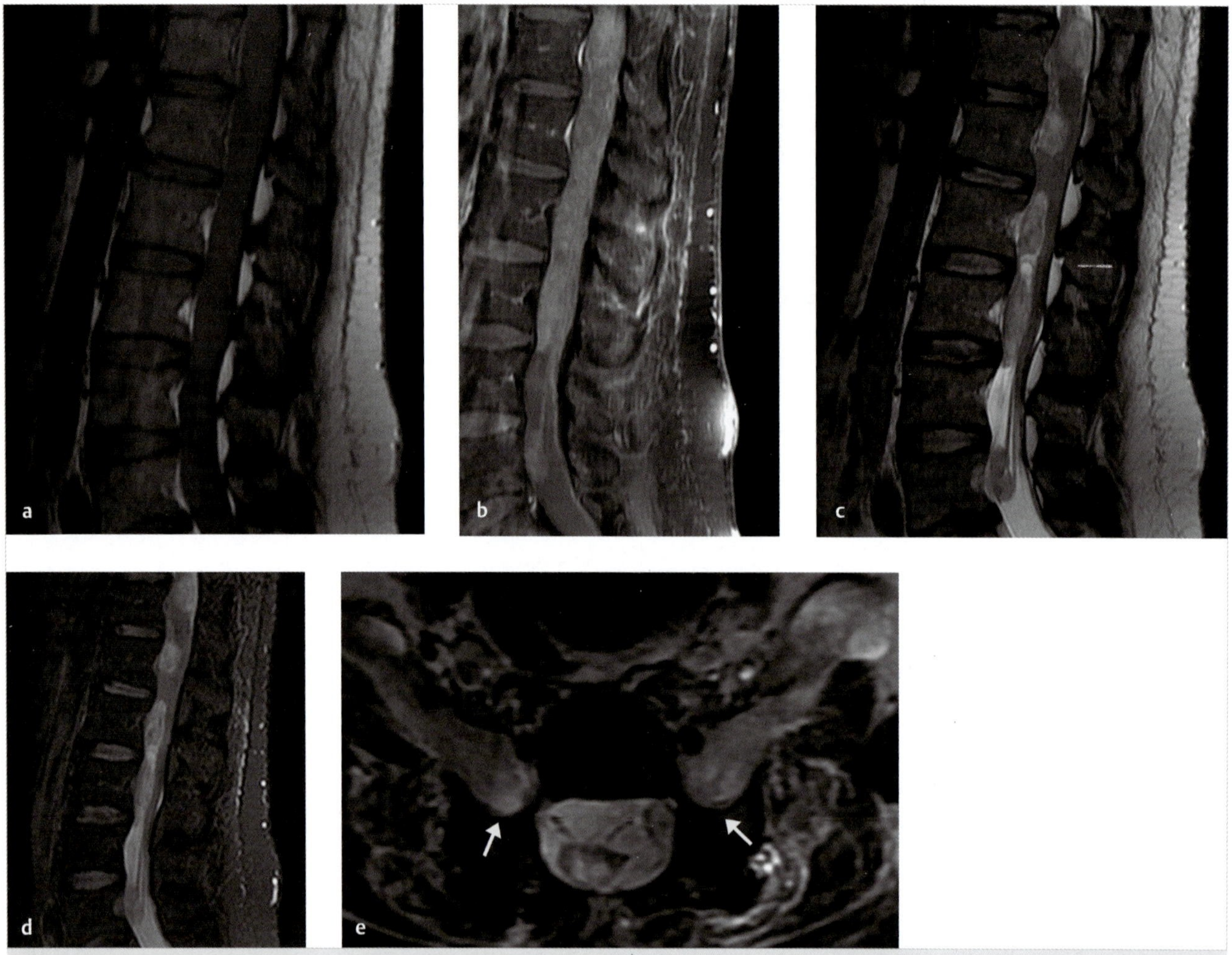

Fig. 21.19 Multiple thoracolumbar neurofibromas. Sagittal T1-weighted images show isointense lesions **(a)** precontrast that **(b)** enhance postcontrast. Sagittal **(c)** T2-weighted and **(d)** fat-suppressed T2-weighted images show hyperintense lesions. **(e)** Axial T2-weighted image shows foraminal widening by bilateral neurofibromas (*arrows*). (Reproduced with permission from, Sciubba DM, Zadnik PL, Wasserman BA, Gokaslan ZL. Tumors of the Spine. In: Khanna AJ, ed. MRI Essentials for the Spine Specialist. New York: Thieme; 2014:211–236.)

21.4.4 Malignant Peripheral Nerve-Sheath Tumor

These malignant spindle-cell sarcomas of neural origin involve the spinal roots, neural plexuses, peripheral nerves, and end organs and are divided into malignant schwannomas and neurofibrosarcomas. Approximately 50 to 60% are associated with type-1 neurofibromatosis. They most commonly present as large (> 5 cm), infiltrative, hemorrhagic soft-tissue masses.[83] MRI is the preferred imaging modality. The lesions are hyperintense compared with surrounding fat on T2-weighted images and on short-tau inversion recovery images and isointense compared with muscle on T1-weighted images (▶ Fig. 21.20). T1-weighted images with contrast show marked enhancement. Infiltration into surrounding soft tissue may lead to indistinct margins. Hemorrhage and necrosis within the mass may be seen, resulting in heterogeneous signal. Intradural-extramedullary masses often show a dumbbell configuration with widening of the intervertebral foramina and erosion of the pedicles. Because of this characteristic, these lesions may be difficult to distinguish from benign spinal schwannomas. Therefore, a malignant peripheral nerve-sheath tumor should be suspected in the presence of sudden growth in a preexisting schwannoma or neurofibroma.

21.4.5 Hemangiopericytoma

Although radiographically very similar to meningiomas, these dural-based lesions are hypervascular, more locally aggressive, and more prone to metastasis. They often erode and replace adjacent bone and exhibit large soft-tissue components. MRI shows multilobular masses hypointense on T1-weighted images and hyperintense on T2-weighted images.[89,90] T1-weighted images with contrast and fat suppression show robust, homogeneous enhancement. Malignant meningiomas may look similar to hemangiopericytomas but meningiomas often possess finger-like processes rather than the lobules of hemangiopericytomas.

21.5 Intramedullary Tumors

These lesions of the spinal cord itself account for 5 to 10% of all central nervous system tumors, 20% of intraspinal neoplasms in

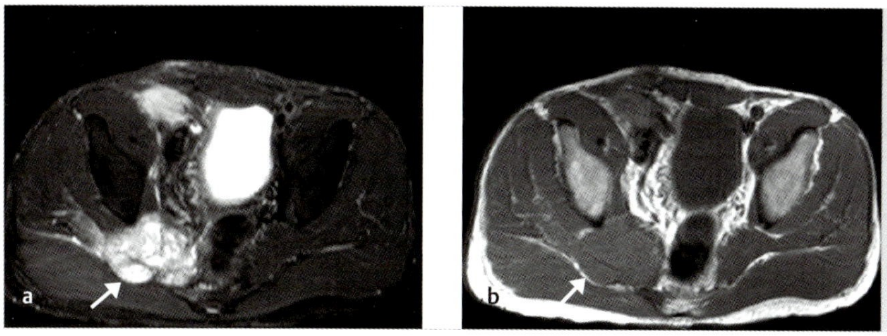

Fig. 21.20 Right-side sacral malignant peripheral nerve-sheath tumor. Compared with muscle, the lesion (*arrow on each*) is **(a)** hyperintense on an axial fat-suppressed T2-weighted image and **(b)** isointense on an axial T1-weighted image. (Reproduced with permission from, Sciubba DM, Zadnik PL, Wasserman BA, Gokaslan ZL. Tumors of the Spine. In: Khanna AJ, ed. MRI Essentials for the Spine Specialist. New York: Thieme; 2014:211–236.)

adults, and 30 to 35% of intraspinal neoplasms in children.[43] More than 90% of these lesions are gliomas.[91] Of spinal cord gliomas, > 95% are ependymomas and low-grade astrocytomas, with ependymomas being more common (60%) than astrocytomas (30%).[43,92,93,94] In children, however, astrocytomas are more common.[95] The remaining lesions include hemangioblastomas and metastases but these lesions are very rare.[96]

MRI is the diagnostic modality of choice for evaluating possible spinal cord tumors and myelopathy. Classic MRI findings show a diffuse, multisegmental, smoothly enlarged cord or filum terminale mass with gradual surrounding subarachnoid effacement. Many lesions are associated with syringomyelia or cyst-like cavities within the cord, extending within the central canal of the cord or eccentric to the canal in a longitudinal orientation (▶ Fig. 21.21).

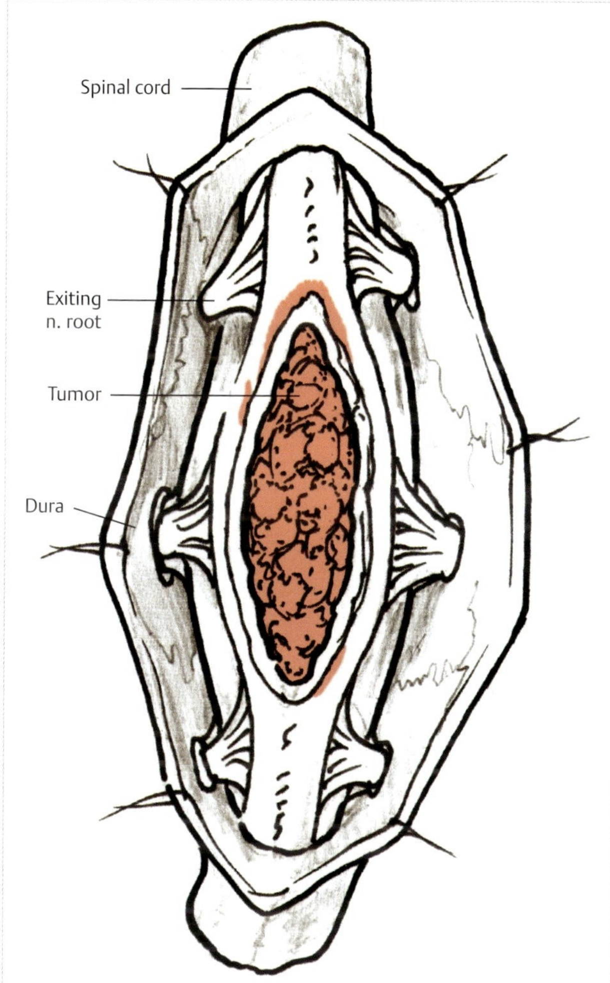

Fig. 21.21 Illustration of the dorsal view depicts the characteristics of an intramedullary mass. The mass diffusely enlarges the cord over multiple spinal segments. (Reproduced with permission from, Sciubba DM, Zadnik PL, Wasserman BA, Gokaslan ZL. Tumors of the Spine. In: Khanna AJ, ed. MRI Essentials for the Spine Specialist. New York: Thieme; 2014:211–236.)

21.5.1 Ependymoma and Low-Grade Astrocytoma

Ependymomas and low-grade astrocytomas appear nearly identical on MRI.[20,97] Widening of the cord secondary to infiltration and syringomyelia are most obvious on T2-weighted images, in which the hyperintense cerebrospinal fluid signal is contrasted against the less intense cord signal. In addition, such lesions typically possess high signal intensity on T2-weighted images. T1-weighted images usually show lesions that are isointense or hypointense relative to the surrounding spinal cord (▶ Fig. 21.22).[20,97]

Mixed-signal lesions are seen if hemorrhage (more typical of ependymomas), tumor necrosis, or cyst formation has occurred. With the administration of contrast, intramedullary tumors typically show robust enhancement, often in a nodular, peripheral, or heterogeneous pattern. Such lesions usually are located in the cervical and/or thoracic spinal cord.[98] Ependymomas more commonly have a "cap sign," referring to a focal hypointensity on T2-weighted images that appears in areas of hemosiderin at the cranial or caudal margin of the tumor. A helpful tool for learning to identify intramedullary spinal cord tumors, most specifically ependymomas, is recalling the five Cs:

- Central within the cord.
- Cervical in location.
- Contrast-enhancing.
- Associated with cysts.
- Cap sign.

Unlike cellular or mixed ependymomas, which typically occur in the cervical spine, myxopapillary ependymomas typically occur in the conus medullaris and filum terminale.[99,100,101] Because these lesions typically are slow growing, vertebral body scalloping is common, with a large conus lesion that fills the entire lumbosacral thecal sac. The neural foramina also may be enlarged. Interestingly, although these lesions grow from ependymal cells of the conus and filum, making them intramedullary in origin, they most commonly appear like intradural-extramedullary masses because there is no widening of the cord at the level of the cauda equina. Therefore, cerebrospinal fluid signal on T2-weighted images creates a meniscus-like sign around the lesion (▶ Fig. 21.23).

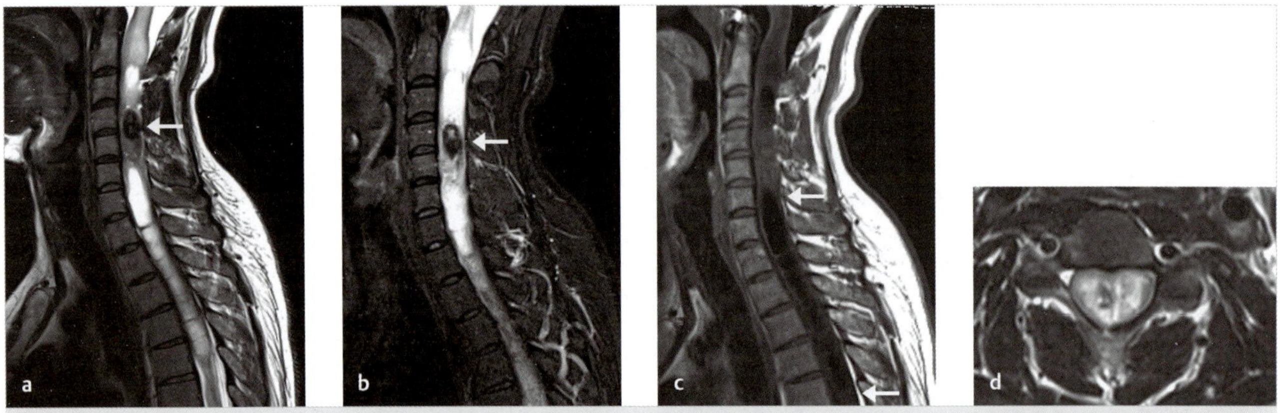

Fig. 21.22 Cervical ependymoma. Sagittal **(a)** T2-weighted and **(b)** short tau inversion recovery images show a large cervical ependymoma centered at C4–C5 but with abnormal cord signal extending from C2 to C7. Note the hypointense hemosiderin "cap" (*arrows on each*). **(c)** A sagittal T1-weighted image shows that the tumor is located at C4–C5 and that the abnormal cord-signal change extending below the lesion is secondary to the formation of a septated syrinx (*between arrows*). A syrinx also extends cranially from the lesion. **(d)** An axial T2-weighted image shows that the lesion is located within the spinal cord, which is seen as a thin sliver of low-signal intensity surrounding the lesion. (Reproduced with permission from, Sciubba DM, Zadnik PL, Wasserman BA, Gokaslan ZL. Tumors of the Spine. In: Khanna AJ, ed. MRI Essentials for the Spine Specialist. New York: Thieme; 2014:211–236.)

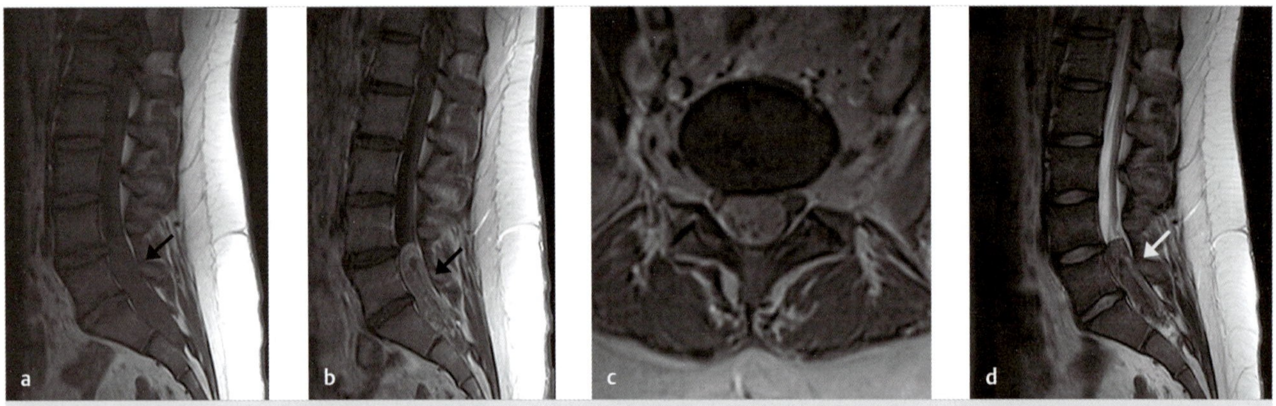

Fig. 21.23 Myxopapillary ependymoma of the lumbar region. **(a)** A sagittal T1-weighted precontrast image shows a hypointense lesion (*arrow*). **(b)** Sagittal and **(c)** axial T1-weighted postcontrast images show robust enhancement of the lesion (*arrow on* ***b***). **(d)** A sagittal T2-weighted image shows the lesion (*arrow*) is heterogeneously hypointense. Although derived from the filum, ependymomas in this segment of the spine reside in the intradural-extramedullary compartment. (Reproduced with permission from, Sciubba DM, Zadnik PL, Wasserman BA, Gokaslan ZL. Tumors of the Spine. In: Khanna AJ, ed. MRI Essentials for the Spine Specialist. New York: Thieme; 2014:211–236.)

Paragangliomas are rare tumors that most commonly present in the cauda equina where they often are indistinguishable from myxopapillary ependymomas.[81] On MRI, these lesions are typically seen as well-defined areas of intense enhancement after contrast administration. Because of their high degree of vascularity, paragangliomas often show prominent foci of high-velocity signal loss ("flow voids"), corresponding to enlarged feeding arteries and/or draining veins.

21.5.2 Hemangioblastoma

Hemangioblastomas typically appear as highly vascular nodules within the subpial compartment. Thus, they lie closer to the surface of the cord than do ependymomas and astrocytomas.[102] They are associated with extensive cyst formation that diffusely enlarges the cord in up to 70% of patients.[103] Because of the highly vascular nature of such lesions, robust homogeneous contrast enhancement within the tumor nodule is the rule, and MRI almost always shows prominent flow voids (▶ Fig. 21.24). Multiple lesions can occur in the presence of von Hippel–Lindau syndrome, with rare extensive involvement of the leptomeninges, referred to as leptomeningeal hemangioblastomatosis.[104] When a spinal hemangioblastoma is suspected on MRI, it is advisable to image the entire central nervous system to exclude multiple lesions.

21.5.3 Intramedullary Metastases

Intramedullary metastases are rare, representing only 4 to 8.5% of all central nervous system metastases.[43] Most spinal cord metastases are localized to the pia mater, in which they appear as a thin rim of enhancement along the cord surface on post-contrast T1-weighted images. In addition, edema disproportionate to a focal, small cord lesion suggests metastasis, even if isolated.[105] Primary malignancies accounting for such lesions are most commonly lung and breast carcinomas, lymphoma, leukemia, or melanoma.[19,106] In 20% of patients, intramedullary metastasis is the first presentation of cancer for the patient.[43]

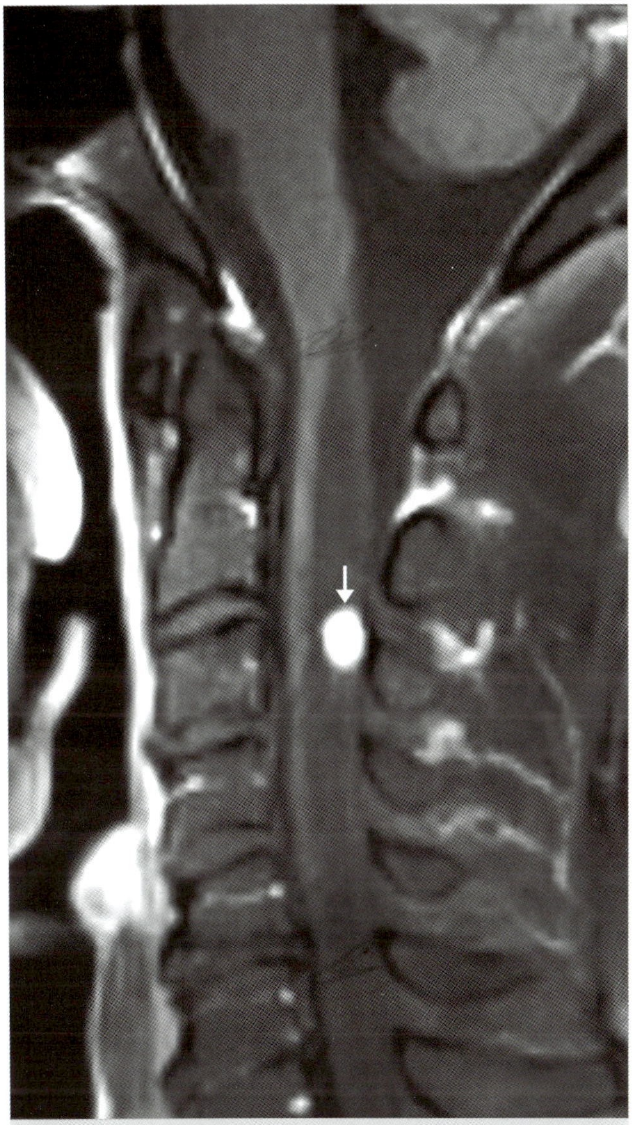

Fig. 21.24 A sagittal postgadolinium fat-suppressed T1-weighted image of a cervical hemangioblastoma shows a small, eccentrically located, robustly enhancing tumor nodule (*arrow*) associated with a large cervicothoracic syrinx. (Reproduced with permission from, Sciubba DM, Zadnik PL, Wasserman BA, Gokaslan ZL. Tumors of the Spine. In: Khanna AJ, ed. MRI Essentials for the Spine Specialist. New York: Thieme; 2014:211–236.)

MRI with or without contrast can be helpful in distinguishing benign cysts or syrinxes from those associated with intramedullary tumors. Tumor cysts are smaller, more irregular, often eccentrically positioned within the cord, and almost always associated with an enhancing tumor, whereas benign cysts are rostral or caudal to the tumor, have smooth walls, cause symmetric cord expansion, and do not show contrast enhancement.[107]

Other lesions of the spinal cord that must be included in the differential diagnosis include autoimmune or inflammatory myelitis, cord ischemia or infarction, and arteriovenous malformations.[12]

21.6 Common Clinical Questions

1. All of the following features seen on a magnetic resonance image are associated with ependymoma, except:
   a) Central within the cord.
   b) Cervical in location.
   c) Osseous invasion.
   d) Contrast-enhancing.
   e) Associated with cysts.
   f) Cap sign.

2. True/False. Ependymomas and astrocytomas appear nearly identical on a magnetic resonance image. True or false?

3. A 19-year-old woman presents to your office with 2 months of worsening buttock pain and right-side leg weakness. Pelvic magnetic resonance imaging shows an expansile lesion with fluid–fluid levels. Her most likely diagnosis is:
   a) Chordoma.
   b) Giant cell tumor.
   c) Metastatic breast cancer.
   d) Osteochondroma.

4. True/False. Osteoid osteomas are larger than osteoblastomas. True or false?

5. Which of the following lesions is/are commonly identified in the neural arch?
   a) Hemangioma.
   b) Osteoid osteoma.
   c) Aneurysmal bone cyst.
   d) Eosinophilic granuloma.
   e) B and C.
   f) None of the above.

References

[1] Gebauer GP, Farjoodi P, Sciubba DM, et al. Magnetic resonance imaging of spine tumors: classification, differential diagnosis, and spectrum of disease. J Bone Joint Surg Am. 2008; 90 Suppl 4:146–162

[2] Khanna AJ, Shindle MK, Wasserman BA, et al. Use of magnetic resonance imaging in differentiating compartmental location of spinal tumors. Am J Orthop. 2005; 34(10):472–476

[3] Masaryk TJ. Neoplastic disease of the spine. Radiol Clin North Am. 1991; 29 (4):829–845

[4] Sevick RJ, Wallace CJ. MR imaging of neoplasms of the lumbar spine. Magn Reson Imaging Clin N Am. 1999; 7(3):539–553, ix

[5] Cappuccio M, Bandiera S, Babbi L, et al. Management of bone metastases. Eur Rev Med Pharmacol Sci. 2010; 14(4):407–414

[6] Perrin RG, Laxton AW. Metastatic spine disease: epidemiology, pathophysiology, and evaluation of patients. Neurosurg Clin N Am. 2004; 15 (4):365–373

[7] Sciubba DM, Petteys RJ, Dekutoski MB, et al. Diagnosis and management of metastatic spine disease. A review. J Neurosurg Spine. 2010; 13(1):94–108

[8] Constans JP, de Divitiis E, Donzelli R, Spaziante R, Meder JF, Haye C. Spinal metastases with neurological manifestations. Review of 600 cases. J Neurosurg. 1983; 59(1):111–118

[9] Eleraky M, Papanastassiou I, Vrionis FD. Management of metastatic spine disease. Curr Opin Support Palliat Care. 2010; 4(3):182–188

[10] Joyce D, O'Donoghue G, Kerin M. Metastatic breast disease: an all too common cause of back pain. BMJ Case Rep. 2010; 2010:Epub ahead of print, Jan 13

[11] Kamholtz R, Sze G. Current imaging in spinal metastatic disease. Semin Oncol. 1991; 18(2):158–169

[12] Osborn AG. Cysts, tumors, and tumorlike lesions of the spine and spinal cord. In: Osborn AG, ed. Diagnostic neuroradiology. St. Louis, MO: Mosby; 1994:876–918

[13] Pozzi G, Garcia Parra C, Stradiotti P, Tien TV, Luzzati A, Zerbi A. Diffusion-weighted MR imaging in differentiation between osteoporotic and neoplastic vertebral fractures. Eur Spine J. 2012; 21 Suppl 1:S123–S127

[14] Thawait SK, Marcus MA, Morrison WB, Klufas RA, Eng J, Carrino JA. Research synthesis: what is the diagnostic performance of magnetic resonance imaging to discriminate benign from malignant vertebral compression fractures? Systematic review and meta-analysis. Spine. 2012; 37(12):E736–E744

[15] Umutlu L, Forsting M, Ladd ME. Ultrahigh-field magnetic resonance imaging: the clinical potential for anatomy, pathogenesis, diagnosis and treatment planning in neck and spine disease. Neuroimaging Clin N Am. 2012; 22(2):363–371, xii

[16] Van Goethem JWM, van den Hauwe L, Ozsarlak O, De Schepper AMA, Parizel PM. Spinal tumors. Eur J Radiol. 2004; 50(2):159–176

[17] Algra PR, Bloem JL, Tissing H, Falke TH, Arndt JW, Verboom LJ. Detection of vertebral metastases: comparison between MR imaging and bone scintigraphy. Radiographics. 1991; 11(2):219–232

[18] Avrahami E, Tadmor R, Dally O, Hadar H. Early MR demonstration of spinal metastases in patients with normal radiographs and CT and radionuclide bone scans. J Comput Assist Tomogr. 1989; 13(4):598–602

[19] Chamberlain MC, Sandy AD, Press GA. Spinal cord tumors: gadolinium-DTPA-enhanced MR imaging. Neuroradiology. 1991; 33(6):469–474

[20] Sun B, Wang C, Wang J, Liu A. MRI features of intramedullary spinal cord ependymomas. J Neuroimaging. 2003; 13(4):346–351

[21] Switlyk MD, Hole KH, Skjeldal S, et al. MRI and neurological findings in patients with spinal metastases. Acta Radiol. 2012; 53(10):1164–1172

[22] Li KC, Poon PY. Sensitivity and specificity of MRI in detecting malignant spinal cord compression and in distinguishing malignant from benign compression fractures of vertebrae. Magn Reson Imaging. 1988; 6(5):547–556

[23] Tatsui H, Onomura T, Morishita S, Oketa M, Inoue T. Survival rates of patients with metastatic spinal cancer after scintigraphic detection of abnormal radioactive accumulation. Spine. 1996; 21(18):2143–2148

[24] Byrne TN. Spinal cord compression from epidural metastases. N Engl J Med. 1992; 327(9):614–619

[25] Algra PR, Heimans JJ, Valk J, Nauta JJ, Lachniet M, Van Kooten B. Do metastases in vertebrae begin in the body or the pedicles? Imaging study in 45 patients. AJR Am J Roentgenol. 1992; 158(6):1275–1279

[26] Wald JT. Imaging of spine neoplasm. Radiol Clin North Am. 2012; 50(4): 749–776

[27] Baker LL, Goodman SB, Perkash I, Lane B, Enzmann DR. Benign versus pathologic compression fractures of vertebral bodies: assessment with conventional spin-echo, chemical-shift, and STIR MR imaging. Radiology. 1990; 174(2):495–502

[28] Thakur NA, Daniels AH, Schiller J, et al. Benign tumors of the spine. J Am Acad Orthop Surg. 2012; 20(11):715–724

[29] Yochum TR, Lile RL, Schultz GD, Mick TJ, Brown CW. Acquired spinal stenosis secondary to an expanding thoracic vertebral hemangioma. Spine. 1993; 18 (2):299–305

[30] Bandiera S, Gasbarrini A, De Iure F, Cappuccio M, Picci P, Boriani S. Symptomatic vertebral hemangioma: the treatment of 23 cases and a review of the literature. Chir Organi Mov. 2002; 87(1):1–15

[31] Urrutia J, Postigo R, Larrondo R, Martin AS. Clinical and imaging findings in patients with aggressive spinal hemangioma requiring surgical treatment. J Clin Neurosci. 2011; 18(2):209–212

[32] Baudrez V, Galant C, Vande Berg BC. Benign vertebral hemangioma: MR-histological correlation. Skeletal Radiol. 2001; 30(8):442–446

[33] Djindjian M, Nguyen JP, Gaston A, Pavlovitch JM, Poirier J, Awad IA. Multiple vertebral hemangiomas with neurological signs. Case report. J Neurosurg. 1992; 76(6):1025–1028

[34] Gangi A, Alizadeh H, Wong L, Buy X, Dietemann JL, Roy C. Osteoid osteoma: percutaneous laser ablation and follow-up in 114 patients. Radiology. 2007; 242(1):293–301

[35] Harish S, Saifuddin A. Imaging features of spinal osteoid osteoma with emphasis on MRI findings. Eur Radiol. 2005; 15(12):2396–2403

[36] Liu PT, Chivers FS, Roberts CC, Schultz CJ, Beauchamp CP. Imaging of osteoid osteoma with dynamic gadolinium-enhanced MR imaging. Radiology. 2003; 227(3):691–700

[37] Luther N, Bilsky MH, Härtl R. Giant cell tumor of the spine. Neurosurg Clin N Am. 2008; 19(1):49–55

[38] Laurence N, Epelman M, Markowitz RI, Jaimes C, Jaramillo D, Chauvin NA. Osteoid osteomas: a pain in the night diagnosis. Pediatr Radiol. 2012; 42 (12):1490–1501, quiz 1540–1542

[39] Boriani S, Amendola L, Bandiera S, et al. Staging and treatment of osteoblastoma in the mobile spine: a review of 51 cases. Eur Spine J. 2012; 21(10):2003–2010

[40] Boriani S, Capanna R, Donati D, Levine A, Picci P, Savini R. Osteoblastoma of the spine. Clin Orthop Relat Res. 1992(278):37–45

[41] Harrop JS, Schmidt MH, Boriani S, Shaffrey CI. Aggressive "benign" primary spine neoplasms: osteoblastoma, aneurysmal bone cyst, and giant cell tumor. Spine. 2009; 34(22) Suppl:S39–S47

[42] Murphey MD, Nomikos GC, Flemming DJ, Gannon FH, Temple HT, Kransdorf MJ. From the archives of AFIP. Imaging of giant cell tumor and giant cell reparative granuloma of bone: radiologic-pathologic correlation. Radiographics. 2001; 21(5):1283–1309

[43] Ross JS. Chondrosarcoma. In: Ross JS, Brant-Zawadzki M, Moore KR, et al., eds. Diagnostic imaging: spine. Salt Lake City: Amirsys; 2004:IV-1–38-IV-31–41

[44] Lotfinia I, Vahedi P, Tubbs RS, Ghavame M, Meshkini A. Neurological manifestations, imaging characteristics, and surgical outcome of intraspinal osteochondroma. J Neurosurg Spine. 2010; 12(5):474–489

[45] Sharma MC, Arora R, Deol PS, Mahapatra AK, Mehta VS, Sarkar C. Osteochondroma of the spine: an enigmatic tumor of the spinal cord. A series of 10 cases. J Neurosurg Sci. 2002; 46(2):66–70, discussion 70

[46] Rodallec MH, Feydy A, Larousserie F, et al. Diagnostic imaging of solitary tumors of the spine: what to do and say. Radiographics. 2008; 28(4):1019–1041

[47] Boriani S, De Iure F, Campanacci L, et al. Aneurysmal bone cyst of the mobile spine: report on 41 cases. Spine. 2001; 26(1):27–35

[48] Cebula H, Boujan F, Beaujeux R, Boyer P, Froelich S. Giant cell tumor of the C2 colonized by an aneurismal bone cyst. Report of case. Neurochirurgie. 2012; 58(6):376–381

[49] Manaster BJ. Skeletal radiology. Chicago, IL: Year Book Medical Publishers; 1989

[50] Mankin HJ, Hornicek FJ, Ortiz-Cruz E, Villafuerte J, Gebhardt MC. Aneurysmal bone cyst: a review of 150 patients. J Clin Oncol. 2005; 23(27): 6756–6762

[51] Wu Z, Yang X, Xiao J, et al. Aneurysmal bone cyst secondary to giant cell tumor of the mobile spine: a report of 11 cases. Spine. 2011; 36(21):E1385–E1390

[52] Oguro K, Sakai H, Arai M, Igarashi T. Eosinophilic granuloma of bone: two case reports. Brain Dev. 2013; 35(4):372–375

[53] Bataille R, Harousseau JL. Multiple myeloma. N Engl J Med. 1997; 336(23): 1657–1664

[54] Moulopoulos LA, Dimopoulos MA, Alexanian R, Leeds NE, Libshitz HI. Multiple myeloma: MR patterns of response to treatment. Radiology. 1994; 193(2):441–446

[55] Holland J, Trenkner DA, Wasserman TH, Fineberg B. Plasmacytoma. Treatment results and conversion to myeloma. Cancer. 1992; 69(6):1513–1517

[56] Bolek TW, Marcus RB, Jr, Mendenhall NP. Solitary plasmacytoma of bone and soft tissue. Int J Radiat Oncol Biol Phys. 1996; 36(2):329–333

[57] He MX, Zhu MH, Zhang YM, Fu QG, Wu LL. [Solitary plasmacytoma of spine: a clinical, radiologic and pathologic study of 13 cases]. Zhonghua Bing Li Xue Za Zhi. 2009; 38(5):307–311

[58] Ota K, Tsuda T, Katayama N, et al. A therapeutic strategy for isolated plasmacytoma of bone. J Int Med Res. 2001; 29(4):366–373

[59] Shah BK, Saifuddin A, Price GJ. Magnetic resonance imaging of spinal plasmacytoma. Clin Radiol. 2000; 55(6):439–445

[60] Knobel D, Zouhair A, Tsang RW, et al. Rare Cancer Network. Prognostic factors in solitary plasmacytoma of the bone: a multicenter Rare Cancer Network study. BMC Cancer. 2006; 6:118

[61] Walcott BP, Nahed BV, Mohyeldin A, Coumans JV, Kahle KT, Ferreira MJ. Chordoma: current concepts, management, and future directions. Lancet Oncol. 2012; 13(2):e69–e76

[62] Boriani S, Weinstein JN, Biagini R. Primary bone tumors of the spine. Terminology and surgical staging. Spine. 1997; 22(9):1036–1044

[63] Soo MYS. Chordoma: review of clinicoradiological features and factors affecting survival. Australas Radiol. 2001; 45(4):427–434

[64] Hsieh PC, Xu R, Sciubba DM, et al. Long-term clinical outcomes following en bloc resections for sacral chordomas and chondrosarcomas: a series of twenty consecutive patients. Spine. 2009; 34(20):2233–2239
[65] Strike SA, McCarthy EF. Chondrosarcoma of the spine: a series of 16 cases and a review of the literature. Iowa Orthop J. 2011; 31:154–159
[66] Dorfman HD, Czerniak B. Bone tumors. St. Louis, MO: Mosby; 1998
[67] Aoki J, Sone S, Fujioka F, et al. MR of enchondroma and chondrosarcoma: rings and arcs of Gd-DTPA enhancement. J Comput Assist Tomogr. 1991; 15 (6):1011–1016
[68] Crim J. Osteosarcoma. In: Ross JS, Brant-Zawadzki M, Moore KR, et al., eds. Diagnostic imaging: spine. Salt Lake City: Amirsys; 2004:IV-1–42-IV-41–45
[69] Bramwell VHC. Osteosarcomas and other cancers of bone. Curr Opin Oncol. 2000; 12(4):330–336
[70] Dorwart RH, LaMasters DL, Watanabe TJ. Tumors. In: Newton T, Potts D, eds. Computed tomography of the spine and spinal cord. San Anselmo, CA: Clavadel Press; 1983:115–147
[71] Boriani S, Amendola L, Corghi A, et al. Ewing's sarcoma of the mobile spine. Eur Rev Med Pharmacol Sci. 2011; 15(7):831–839
[72] Crim J. Ewing sarcoma. In: Ross JS, Brant-Zawadzki M, Moore KR, et al., eds. Diagnostic imaging: spine. Salt Lake City: Amirsys; 2004:IV-1–50-IV-51–53
[73] Boyko OB, Cory DA, Cohen MD, Provisor A, Mirkin D, DeRosa GP. MR imaging of osteogenic and Ewing's sarcoma. AJR Am J Roentgenol. 1987; 148(2):317–322
[74] Lonergan GJ, Schwab CM, Suarez ES, Carlson CL. Neuroblastoma, ganglioneuroblastoma, and ganglioneuroma: radiologic-pathologic correlation. Radiographics. 2002; 22(4):911–934
[75] Sofka CM, Semelka RC, Kelekis NL, et al. Magnetic resonance imaging of neuroblastoma using current techniques. Magn Reson Imaging. 1999; 17(2): 193–198
[76] Guzey FK, Bas NS, Ozkan N, Karabulut C, Bas SC, Turgut H. Lumbar extradural infiltrating angiolipoma: a case report and review of 17 previously reported cases with infiltrating spinal angiolipomas. Spine J. 2007; 7(6):739–744
[77] Oge HK, Söylemezoglu F, Rousan N, Ozcan OE. Spinal angiolipoma: case report and review of literature. J Spinal Disord. 1999; 12(4):353–356
[78] De Fino C, Arena V, Hohaus S, Di Iorio R, Bozzoli V, Mirabella M. Intravascular large B-cell lymphoma presenting as slowly progressive paraparesis with normal MRI features. J Neurol Sci. 2012; 314(1–2):171–174
[79] Thornton E, Krajewski KM, O'Regan KN, Giardino AA, Jagannathan JP, Ramaiya N. Imaging features of primary and secondary malignant tumours of the sacrum. Br J Radiol. 2012; 85(1011):279–286
[80] Katzman GL. Lymphoma. In: Ross JS, Brant-Zawadzki M, Moore KR, et al., eds. Diagnostic imaging: spine. Salt Lake City: Amirsys; 2004:IV-1–54-IV-51–57
[81] Koeller KK, Rosenblum RS, Morrison AL. Neoplasms of the spinal cord and filum terminale: radiologic-pathologic correlation. Radiographics. 2000; 20 (6):1721–1749
[82] Li MH, Holtås S, Larsson EM. MR imaging of intradural extramedullary tumors. Acta Radiol. 1992; 33(3):207–212
[83] Burger PC, Shcheithauer BW, Vogel FS. Surgical pathology of the nervous system and its coverings. Philadelphia, PA: Churchill Livingstone; 2002
[84] Cohen-Gadol AA, Zikel OM, Koch CA, Scheithauer BW, Krauss WE. Spinal meningiomas in patients younger than 50 years of age: a 21-year experience. J Neurosurg. 2003; 98(3) Suppl:258–263
[85] Naderi S. Spinal meningiomas. Surg Neurol. 2000; 54(1):95
[86] Conti P, Pansini G, Mouchaty H, Capuano C, Conti R. Spinal neurinomas: retrospective analysis and long-term outcome of 179 consecutively operated cases and review of the literature. Surg Neurol. 2004; 61(1):34–43, discussion 44
[87] Murphey MD, Smith WS, Smith SE, Kransdorf MJ, Temple HT. From the archives of the AFIP. Imaging of musculoskeletal neurogenic tumors: radiologic-pathologic correlation. Radiographics. 1999; 19(5):1253–1280
[88] Uhlmann EJ, Plotkin SR. Neurofibromatoses. Adv Exp Med Biol. 2012; 724: 266–277
[89] Akhaddar A, Chakir N, Amarti A, et al. Thoracic epidural hemangiopericytoma. Case report. J Neurosurg Sci. 2002; 46(2):89–92, discussion 92
[90] Ackerman PD, Khaldi A, Shea JF. Intradural hemangiopericytoma of the thoracic spine: a case report. Spine J. 2011; 11(7):e9–e14
[91] Brant-Zawadzki M. Astrocytoma, spinal cord. In: Ross JS, Brant-Zawadzki M, Moore KR, et al., eds. Diagnostic imaging: spine. Salt Lake City: Amirsys; 2004:IV-1–102-IV-101–105
[92] Harrop JS, Ganju A, Groff M, Bilsky M. Primary intramedullary tumors of the spinal cord. Spine. 2009; 34(22) Suppl:S69–S77
[93] Houten JK, Cooper PR. Spinal cord astrocytomas: presentation, management and outcome. J Neurooncol. 2000; 47(3):219–224
[94] Parsa AT, Chi JH, Acosta FL, Jr, Ames CP, McCormick PC. Intramedullary spinal cord tumors: molecular insights and surgical innovation. Clin Neurosurg. 2005; 52:76–84
[95] Smith AB, Soderlund KA, Rushing EJ, Smirniotopolous JG. Radiologic-pathologic correlation of pediatric and adolescent spinal neoplasms: Part 1, Intramedullary spinal neoplasms. AJR Am J Roentgenol. 2012; 198(1):34–43
[96] Houten JK, Weiner HL. Pediatric intramedullary spinal cord tumors: special considerations. J Neurooncol. 2000; 47(3):225–230
[97] Lowe GM. Magnetic resonance imaging of intramedullary spinal cord tumors. J Neurooncol. 2000; 47(3):195–210
[98] McCormick PC, Torres R, Post KD, Stein BM. Intramedullary ependymoma of the spinal cord. J Neurosurg. 1990; 72(4):523–532
[99] Bagley CA, Kothbauer KF, Wilson S, Bookland MJ, Epstein FJ, Jallo GI. Resection of myxopapillary ependymomas in children. J Neurosurg. 2007; 106(4) Suppl Pediatrics:261–267
[100] Bagley CA, Wilson S, Kothbauer KF, Bookland MJ, Epstein F, Jallo GI. Long term outcomes following surgical resection of myxopapillary ependymomas. Neurosurg Rev. 2009; 32(3):321–334, discussion 334
[101] Sonneland PRL, Scheithauer BW, Onofrio BM. Myxopapillary ependymoma. A clinicopathologic and immunocytochemical study of 77 cases. Cancer. 1985; 56(4):883–893
[102] Pruksakorn P, Siwanuwatn R, Snabboon T. Spinal hemangioblastoma. Am J Med Sci. 2011; 342(3):240
[103] Murota T, Symon L. Surgical management of hemangioblastoma of the spinal cord: a report of 18 cases. Neurosurgery. 1989; 25(5):699–707, discussion 708
[104] Chu BC, Terae S, Hida K, Furukawa M, Abe S, Miyasaka K. MR findings in spinal hemangioblastoma: correlation with symptoms and with angiographic and surgical findings. AJNR Am J Neuroradiol. 2001; 22(1): 206–217
[105] Reddy P, Sathyanarayana S, Acharya R, Nanda A. Intramedullary spinal cord metastases: case report and review of literature. J La State Med Soc. 2003; 155(1):44–45
[106] Soga K, Irioka T, Yano T, Mizusawa H. Intramedullary spinal cord metastasis with a longitudinally extensive spinal cord lesion. Intern Med. 2011; 50(7): 795–796
[107] Brunberg JA, DiPietro MA, Venes JL, et al. Intramedullary lesions of the pediatric spinal cord: correlation of findings from MR imaging, intraoperative sonography, surgery, and histologic study. Radiology. 1991; 181(2):573–579

Answers to Common Clinical Questions

1. Answer: c. The magnetic resonance image features of ependymoma include a central location within the spinal cord, predilection for the cervical spine, postgadolinium contrast enhancement, association with cysts, and the cap sign, as described in this chapter.
2. Answer: True. Ependymomas and astrocytomas have nearly identical appearances on a magnetic resonance image. Therefore, they are typically differentiated by biopsy.
3. Answer: b. Of the options listed, giant cell tumor is the most compatible with the magnetic resonance image characteristics and age of the patient. Aneurysmal bone cyst would be another consideration but is not provided as an option in this question.
4. Answer: False. Osteoid osteomas are similar to but smaller than osteoblastomas. A size of 1.5 cm is typically used as the threshold to differentiate between these two diagnoses.
5. Answer: e. Osteoid osteomas and aneurysmal bone cysts are commonly identified in the neural arch (posterior elements). Aneurysmal bone cysts typically originate in the neural arch and extend into the vertebral body. Hemangiomas and eosinophilic granulomas are typically seen in the vertebral body.

Index

Note: Page numbers set **bold** or *italic* indicate headings or figures, respectively.

F

G

H

I

K

L

M

N

Z